Diabetes and Cardiovascular Disease

Second Edition

CONTEMPORARY CARDIOLOGY

CHRISTOPHER P. CANNON, MD
SERIES EDITOR

DIABETES AND CARDIOVASCULAR DISEASE

Second Edition

Edited by

MICHAEL T. JOHNSTONE, MD, CM, FRCP(C)

ARISTIDIS VEVES, MD, DSc

Beth Israel Deaconess Medical Center, Harvard Medical School, Boston, MA

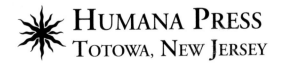

HUMANA PRESS
TOTOWA, NEW JERSEY

Production Editor: Melissa Caravella
Cover design by Patricia F. Cleary

Cover Illustration: From Fig. 2 in Chapter 22, "Peripheral Vascular Disease in Patients With Diabetes Mellitus," by Bernadette Aulivola, Allen D. Hamdan, and Frank W. LoGerfo.

For additional copies, pricing for bulk purchases, and/or information about other Humana titles, contact Humana at the above address or at any of the following numbers: Tel.: 973-256-1699; Fax: 973-256-8341; E-mail: orders@humanapr.com; or visit our Website: www.humanapress.com

This publication is printed on acid-free paper. ∞
ANSI Z39.48-1984 (American National Standards Institute) Permanence of Paper for Printed Library Materials.

Printed in the United States of America. 10 9 8 7 6 5 4 3 2 1

eISBN: 1-59259-908-7

Library of Congress Cataloging-in-Publication Data

Diabetes and cardiovascular disease / edited by Michael T. Johnstone and Aristidis Veves.-- 2nd ed.
    p. cm. -- (Contemporary cardiology)
  Includes bibliographical references and index.
  ISBN 1-58829-413-7 (alk. paper)
  1. Diabetic angiopathies. 2. Cardiovascular system--Diseases--Etiology.
I. Johnstone, Michael T. II. Veves, Aristidis. III. Series: Contemporary cardiology (Totowa, N.J. : unnumbered)
  RC700.D5D524 2005
  616.4'62--dc22

2005000629

DEDICATION

To my daughters, Jessica and Lauren, and my mother Rose
for their patience, love, inspiration, and support.
—MTJ

To my parents and my wife Maria.
—AV

PREFACE TO THE FIRST EDITION

The cause of diabetes mellitus is metabolic in origin. However, its major clinical manifestations, which result in most of the morbidity and mortality, are a result of its vascular pathology. In fact, the American Heart Association has recently stated that, "from the point of view of cardiovascular medicine, it may be appropriate to say, diabetes is a cardiovascular disease" (1). But diabetic vascular disease is not limited to just the macrovasculature. Diabetes mellitus also affects the microcirculation with devastating results, including nephropathy, neuropathy, and retinopathy. Diabetic nephropathy is the leading cause of end-stage renal disease in the United States, while diabetic retinopathy is the leading cause of new-onset blindness in working-age Americans.

The importance of this text on *Diabetes and Cardiovascular Disease* is evident by the magnitude of the population affected by diabetes mellitus. Over 10 million Americans have been diagnosed with diabetes mellitus, while another 5 million remain undiagnosed. The impact from a public health perspective is huge and increasing. As the population of the United States grows older, more sedentary, and obese, the risk of developing diabetes and its complications will increase.

Epidemiological studies have identified diabetes mellitus as a major independent risk factor for cardiovascular disease. Over 65% of patients with diabetes mellitus die from a cardiovascular cause. The prognosis of patients with diabetes mellitus who develop overt clinical cardiovascular disease is much worse than those cardiovascular patients free of diabetes mellitus.

The 24 chapters of *Diabetes and Cardiovascular Disease* focus on either clinical or basic aspects of diabetes and cardiovascular disease. Part I, Pathophysiology, reviews the mechanisms and risk factors for diabetic cardiovascular disease. Part II focuses on the heart in diabetes mellitus, including coronary artery disease and congestive heart failure. The peripheral vascular system is the subject of Part III, which addresses epidemiology, mechanisms, methods of assessment, and treatment of this macrovascular disease. Lastly, Part IV reviews the different microvascular effects in individuals with diabetes mellitus, including retinopathy, nephropathy, neuropathy, and microcirculation of the diabetic foot.

The aim of *Diabetes and Cardiovascular Disease* is to serve as a comprehensive review of both the basic and clinical aspects of diabetic vascular disease for the practicing clinician. The readership will include cardiologists, general internists, vascular specialists, family physicians, and medical students, along with other interested practitioners and allied health personnel. The text is also directed toward both clinical and basic research scientists, and emphasis has thus been given to both theoretical and practical points. Each chapter covers its topics in great detail and is accompanied by extensive references.

We are indebted to the many people who worked on this volume. In particular, we wish to thank those talented and dedicated physicians who contributed the many chapters in this text. We were fortunate to have the collaboration of a group of authors who were among the most prominent in their respective fields. We hope that our efforts will serve as a stimulus for further research in this increasingly important health concern.

We want to extend our deepest appreciation to Paul Dolgert and Craig Adams of Humana Press for guiding us through the preparation of this book. As well, we want to give a special thanks to Dr. Christopher Cannon, who saw the need for such a volume and gave us the opportunity to edit this text.

Michael T. Johnstone, MD
Aristides Veves, MD, DSc

REFERENCE

1. Grundy SM, Benjamin IJ, Burke GL, et al. AHA Scientific Statement-Diabetes and Cardiovascular Disease. Circulation 1999;100:1134-1146.

PREFACE

It has been only four years since the first edition of this very successful text, *Diabetes and Cardiovascular Disease*. During this time, interest in diabetes mellitus as a risk factor for cardiovascular disease has increased logarithmically, having been the subject of many studies now found in the cardiology literature as well as American Heart Association statements in *Circulation*. This higher level of attention is only a reflection of the increasing obesity and diabetes mellitus epidemic that continues to build in Western societies, and in particular, the United States.

With the substantial increase in information resulting from this research and the ever-increasing numbers of people afflicted by diabetes mellitus, the need for a text that summarizes the information obtained, diagnostic and therapeutic guidelines becomes increasingly important. We believe our second edition mirrors the increased attention focused on this disease process, which affects about 16 million people in the United States alone.

With this burgeoning interest in diabetic cardiovascular disease, it is challenging to keep up with all the important developments in the area. In an effort to do so, we have made significant changes to this second edition. All the chapters have been updated and new ones have been added. In particular, the chapters on hypertension and dyslipidemia, as well as heart failure, and coronary artery disease and diabetes mellitus have undergone extensive "makeovers."

We have reorganized the chapters, putting the basic science chapters in the first half of the text, with the clinical chapters now in the second half. We have moved the chapters on diabetes and dyslipidemia and hypertension to the clinical section of the text. The last chapter, "Diabetes Mellitus and Coronary Artery Disease," has not only been significantly redone, it is now at the end of the text in an effort to serve as a summary of the clinical macrovascular disease chapters.

In the basic section, we have added chapters on diabetes mellitus and PPARs by Dr. Plutzky, and PARP activation and the nitrosative state by Drs. Pacher and Szabó. The role of estrogens in diabetic vascular disease is discussed by Drs. Tsatsoulis and Economides, and finally the effect of adipocyte cytokines in the development of diabetes mellitus is discussed. On the clinical side, we have added chapters on interventional therapy in cardiac and peripheral vascular disease by Drs. Lorenz, Carrozza, and Garcia, as well as a chapter on cardiovascular surgery in diabetes by Drs. Khan, Voisine, and Sellke.

We again want to thank Craig Adams, Developmental Editor, and Paul Dolgert, the Editorial Director at Humana Press, as well as their office staff for their assistance in putting together this text. Also we want to give again a special thanks to Dr. Christopher Cannon whose vision it was to include such a text in the *Contemporary Cardiology* series.

Michael T. Johnstone, MD
Aristidis Veves, MD, DSc

CONTENTS

Part II. Clinical

Contributors

LLOYD PAUL AIELLO, MD, PhD, *Beetham Eye Institute, Joslin Diabetes Center, Harvard Medical School, Boston, MA*

ARESH J. ANWAR, MD, MRCP, *Division of Clinical Sciences, Warwick Medical School, University of Warwick and University Hospital of Coventry and Warwickshire, Coventry, UK*

BERNADETTE AULIVOLA, MD, *Division of Vascular Surgery, Department of Surgery, Beth Israel Deaconess Medical Center, Harvard Medical School, Boston, MA*

EDWARD J. BOYKO, MD, MPH, *Department of Medicine, University of Washington School of Medicine; Epidemiologic Research and Information Center, VA Puget Sound Health Care System, Seattle, WA*

JOSEPH P. CARROZZA, MD, *Department of Medicine, Beth Israel Deaconess Medical Center, Boston, MA*

JERRY CAVALLERANO, OD, PhD, *Joslin Diabetes Center, Harvard Medical School, Boston, MA*

DEBORAH CHYUN, RN, PhD, *Adult Advanced Practice Nursing Speciality, Yale University School of Nursing, New Haven, CT*

MYLAN C. COHEN, MD, MPH, *Maine Cardiology Associates, Maine Medical Center, Portland, ME; Department of Medicine, University of Vermont College of Medicine, Burlington, VT*

ALANNA COOLONG, MD, *Division of Cardiology, Maine Medical Center, Portland, ME*

S. J. CREELY, MD, *Division of Clinical Sciences, Warwick Medical School, University of Warwick and University Hospital of Coventry and Warwickshire, Coventry, UK*

PETER G. DANIAS, MD, PhD, *Department of Medicine, Beth Israel Deaconess Medical Center, Harvard Medical School, Boston, MA; Hygeia Hospital, Maroussi, Greece*

PANAYIOTIS ECONOMIDES, MD, *Research Division, Joslin Diabetes Center, Harvard Medical School, Boston, MA*

AMAL F. FARAG, MD, *Division of Endocrinology, New York Harbor Veterans Administration Center, Brooklyn, NY*

EDWARD P. FEENER, PhD, *Research Division, Joslin Diabetes Center, Harvard Medical School, Boston, MA*

LAWRENCE GARCIA, MD, *Department of Medicine, Beth Israel Deaconess Medical Center, Boston, MA*

DAVID GARDNER, MD, *Division of Endocrinology, University of Missouri, Columbia, MO*

ALINA GAVRILA, MD, *Division of Endocrinology and Metabolism, Department of Internal Medicine, Beth Israel Deaconess Medical Center, Boston, MA*

ELI GELFAND, MD, *Cardiovascular Division, Department of Medicine, Beth Israel Deaconess Medical Center, Boston, MA*

HENRY N. GINSBERG, MD, *College of Physicians and Surgeons of Columbia University, New York, NY*

ALLEN D. HAMDAN, MD, *Division of Vascular Surgery, Department of Surgery, Beth Israel Deaconess Medical Center, Harvard Medical School, Boston, MA*

ZHIHENG HE, MD, PhD, *Research Division, Joslin Diabetes Center, Department of Ophthalmology, Harvard Medical School, Boston, MA*

CHANTEL HILE, MD, *Department of Medicine, Beth Israel Deaconess Medical Center, Boston, MA*

MICHAEL T. JOHNSTONE, MD, CM, FRCP(C), *Cardiovascular Division, Department of Medicine, Beth Israel Deaconess Medical Center, Harvard Medical School, Boston, MA*

TANVEER A. KHAN, MD, *Division of Cardiothoracic Surgery, Beth Israel Deaconess Medical Center, Department of Medicine and Surgery, Harvard Medical School, Boston, MA*

LALITA KHAODHIAR, MD, *Joslin-Beth Israel Deaconess Foot Center, Beth Israel Deaconess Medical Center, Harvard Medical School, Boston, MA*

GEORGE L. KING, MD, *Research Division, Joslin Diabetes Center, Harvard Medical School, Boston, MA*

GEORGE P. KINZFOGL, MD, *Staff Cardiologist, Health Center of Metrowest, Framingham, MA*

SUDHESH KUMAR, MD, FRCP, *Division of Clinical Sciences, Warwick Medical School, University of Warwick and University Hospital of Coventry and Warwickshire, Coventry, UK*

FRANK W. LOGERFO, MD, *Division of Vascular Surgery, Department of Surgery, Beth Israel Deaconess Medical Center, Harvard Medical School, Boston, MA*

MARIA F. LOPES-VIRELLA, MD, PhD, *Division of Endocrinology, Diabetes and Medical Genetics, Department of Medicine, Medical University of South Carolina; Ralph H. Johnson Veterans Administration Medical Center, Charleston, SC*

DAVID P. LORENZ, MD, *Department of Medicine, Beth Israel Deaconess Medical Center, Harvard Medical School, Boston, MA*

RAYAZ A. MALIK, MB ChB, PhD, *Department of Medicine, Manchester Royal Infirmary, Manchester, UK*

CHRISTOS S. MANTZOROS, MD, *Division of Endocrinology and Metabolism, Department of Internal Medicine, Beth Israel Deaconess Medical Center, Boston, MA*

SAMY I. MCFARLANE, MD, MPH, *Department of Medicine, State University of New York Health Science Center at Brooklyn Kings, County Hospital Center, Brooklyn, NY*

KEIKO NARUSE, MD, PhD, *Research Division, Joslin Diabetes Center, Harvard Medical School, Boston, MA*

PÁL PACHER, MD, PhD, *Inotek Pharmaceuticals, Beverly, MA; Laboratory of Physiologic Studies, National Institute on Alcohol Abuse and Alcoholism, National Institutes of Health, Rockville, MD; Institute of Pharmacology and Pharmacotherapy, Semmelweis University, Budapest, Hungary*

WULF PALINSKI, MD, *Department of Medicine, University of California, San Diego, School of Medicine, San Diego, CA*

MELPOMENI PEPPA, MD, *Department of Geriatrics, Mount Sinai School of Medicine, New York, NY*

JORGE PLUTZKY, MD, *Cardiovascular Division, Brigham and Women's Hospital, Harvard Medical School, Boston, MA*

PETER D. REAVEN, MD, *Department of Medicine, Carl T. Hayden VA Medical Center, Phoenix, AZ*

BIJAN ROSHAN, MD, *Joslin Diabetes Center, Beth Israel Deaconess Medical Center, Harvard Medical School, Boston, MA*

RAYMOND R. RUSSELL, III, MD, PhD, *Department of Internal Medicine (Cardiovascular Medicine), Yale University School of Medicine, New Haven, CT*

ROLA SAOUAF, MD, *Department of Radiology, New York-Presbyterian Hospital, Columbia University College of Physicians and Surgeons, New York, NY*

DAVID J. SCHNEIDER, MD, *Department of Medicine, The University of Vermont College of Medicine, Burlington, VT*

FRANK W. SELLKE, MD, *Division of Cardiothoracic Surgery, Beth Israel Deaconess Medical Center, Harvard Medical School, Boston, MA*

SUKETU SHAH, MD, *Division of Endocrinology and Metabolism, Department of Internal Medicine, Beth Israel Deaconess Medical Center, Harvard Medical School, Boston, MA*

NICHOLAS L. SMITH, PhD, MPH, *Investigator, Cardiovascular Health Research Unit, University of Washington School of Medicine, Seattle, WA*

BURTON E. SOBEL, MD, *Department of Medicine, The University of Vermont College of Medicine, Burlington, VT*

RICHARD J. SOLOMON, MD, *Department of Medicine, The University of Vermont College of Medicine, Burlington, VT*

JAMES R. SOWERS, MD, FACP, *Department of Cardiovascular Medicine, University of Missouri, Columbia, MO*

HELMUT O. STEINBERG, MD, *Division of Endocrinology, Indiana University School of Medicine, Indianapolis, IN*

CSABA SZABÓ, MD, PhD, *Inotek Pharmaceuticals, Beverly, MA; Department of Human Physiology and Experimental Research, Semmelweis University, Budapest, Hungary*

ASHA THOMAS-GEEVARGHESE, MD, *Department of Medicine, College of Physicians and Surgeons of Columbia University, New York, NY; Medstar Research Institute, Washington, DC*

AGATHOCLES TSATSOULIS, MD, PhD, FRCP, *Division of Endocrinology, Department of Medicine, University of Ioannina Medical School, Ioannina, Greece*

CATHERINE TUCK, MD, *(Deceased) formerly Assistant Professor of Medicine, College of Physicians and Surgeons of Columbia University, New York, NY*

JAIME URIBARRI, MD, *Division of Nephrology, Mount Sinai School of Medicine, New York, NY*

DOUGLAS E. VAUGHAN, MD, *Division of Cardiovascular Medicine, Vanderbilt University Medical Center, Veterans Administration Medical Center, Nashville, TN*

ARISTIDIS VEVES, MD, DSc, *Joslin-Beth Israel Deaconess Foot Center, Beth Israel Deaconess Medical Center; Department of Surgery, Harvard Medical School, Boston, MA*

GABRIEL VIRELLA, MD, PhD, *Department of Microbiology and Immunology, Medical University of South Carolina, Charleston, SC*

HELEN VLASSARA, MD, *Department of Geriatrics, Mount Sinai School of Medicine, New York, NY*

PIERRE VOISINE, MD, *Division of Cardiothoracic Surgery, Beth Israel Deaconess Medical Center, Harvard Medical School, Boston, MA*

STEPHANIE G. WHEELER, MD, MPH, *Department of Medicine, University of Washington School of Medicine and VA Puget Sound Health Care System, Seattle, WA*

LAWRENCE H. YOUNG, MD, *Department of Internal Medicine (Cardiovascular Medicine), Yale University School of Medicine, New Haven, CT*

I

PATHOPHYSIOLOGY

1 Effects of Insulin on the Vascular System

Helmut O. Steinberg, MD

CONTENTS

INTRODUCTION

Over the last decade it has become clear that insulin, in addition to its actions on glucose, protein, and fatty acid metabolism also exhibits distinct effects on the vascular system. Importantly, elevated circulating insulin levels have been found to be an independent risk factor for cardiovascular disease (CVD). This observation raised the question regarding whether elevated insulin levels per se may cause macrovascular disease or whether the insulin levels are elevated to compensate for the insulin resistance seen in obesity, hypertension, and type 2 diabetes.

Because insulin resistance/hyperinsulinemia are associated with CVD, the question arises regarding whether insulin itself possesses direct vascular effects, which might accelerate atherosclerosis or cause hypertension. In fact, it has been shown over the last decade that insulin elicits a coordinated response at the level of the skeletal muscle vasculature, the heart, and the sympathetic nervous system (SNS). Insulin, in lean insulin-sensitive subjects, increases skeletal muscle and adipose tissue blood flow at physiological concentrations. Simultaneously, cardiac output and SNS activity increase. The majority of the increment in cardiac output is directed toward skeletal muscle suggesting that the blood-flow elevation as a result of insulin's vascular action may be instrumental in augmenting skeletal muscle glucose uptake. The role of the rise in sympathetic nervous system activity (SNSA) in response to insulin is less well understood. It has been proposed that the increase in SNS activity may counteract insulin's vasodilator effect to avoid a decrease in blood pressure levels. The insulin-induced change in SNS may also be important for blood-flow regulation in adipose tissue. Furthermore, insulin may also exert part of its cardiovascular effects indirectly via modulation of renal sodium and volume handling.

From: *Contemporary Cardiology: Diabetes and Cardiovascular Disease, Second Edition*
Edited by: M. T. Johnstone and A. Veves © Humana Press Inc., Totowa, NJ

It has been demonstrated that insulin's effect on skeletal muscle blood flow is mediated through the release of endothelium-derived nitric oxide (NO), the most potent endogenous vasodilator. Importantly, NO is not only a vasodilator but also exhibits a host of anti-atherosclerotic properties. In addition to its effect on NO release, insulin also modulates the response to other vasoactive hormones such as angiotensin II or norepinephrine (NE) at the level of the vascular endothelium and the vascular smooth muscle cell. Therefore, insulin's effect on the vasculature of normal subjects appears to have beneficial effects that may counteract blood pressure elevation and inhibit the atherosclerotic process.

Assessment of insulin's effect on the microcirculation in vivo has lagged behind the study of the macrocirculation mainly because of insufficient resolution of the current techniques. Nevertheless, data obtained with different techniques, such as tracer, positron emission tomography (PET) scanning, thermodilution, or most recently, pulsed ultrasound combined with microbubbles, suggest that hyperinsulinemia leads to the recruitment of capillaries in skeletal muscle. In fact most recently, contrast-enhanced ultrasonography directly demonstrated an increase in capillary density in response to hyperinsulinemia. Whether capillary recruitment augments insulin-mediated glucose uptake, and whether impaired insulin-mediated vasodilation contributes to decreased rates of insulin-mediated glucose uptake (insulin resistance) is still an open question. Further improvement of the methods to assess microvascular changes in response to insulin will help to better understand the effect of the insulin resistance on the microvasculature.

Insulin's vasodilator effect on skeletal muscle and adipose tissue vasculature is blunted in states of insulin resistance such as obesity, hypertension, and type 2 diabetes mellitus. Whether the cardiac response to insulin is affected in insulin resistance is unclear. Because impaired insulin-mediated vasodilation in obesity and type 2 diabetes suggested decreased production of NO, recent research has focused on vascular endothelial function in insulin-resistant states. There is now good evidence for impaired endothelial function and decreased NO production in obesity, hypertension, and type 2 diabetes. The mechanism(s) by which obesity and type 2 diabetes impair endothelial function are not fully elucidated but elevated free fatty acid (FFA) levels, increased endothelin-dependent vascular tone or increased levels of asymmetric dimethyl-arginine (ADMA) as observed in these insulin-resistant subjects may account, at least in part, for the vascular dysfunction.

The function of the vascular system is to allow the delivery of blood (oxygen and nutrients) to the tissues according to their unique metabolic needs. To accomplish this task for the ever-changing tissue requirements without compromising the blood supply of vital organs, the vascular system responds in a variety of ways. It responds at the local tissue level via the release of short-acting vasoactive hormones, which redirect blood flow from less active to more active tissue units. The vascular system reroutes blood flow from organs with (relatively) lesser needs to organ systems, which require higher rates of blood flow for example by activation of the SNS. Finally, if tissue requirements can not be met by the above mechanisms, cardiac output will increase to meet all requirements and to avoid dangerous reductions in blood pressure.

It is well established that insulin increases skeletal muscle glucose uptake and whole-body oxygen consumption. However, it was not until 1982 when it was first demonstrated in dogs (1) that insulin has direct effects on the vasculature. It took another decade to establish that insulin also exhibits vascular effects in humans. The following review will focus mainly on data obtained from human studies but data from animal or data from in vitro studies will be used when providing mechanistic insight into insulin's effects on the vasculature.

TECHNICAL CONSIDERATIONS

Before exploring insulin's vascular actions, several technical considerations should be made. In vivo studies of insulin's effect on the vascular system require, in most cases, systemic administration of glucose (euglycemic hyperinsulinemic clamp technique) to maintain stable glucose concentrations. Using the euglycemic hyperinsulinemic clamp technique *(2)* avoids hypoglycemia and the release of hormones such as epinephrine, NE, or cortisol, which can blunt the metabolic and vascular action of insulin. However, glucose metabolism will be increased by insulin administration and therefore, it may be difficult to dissociate insulin's vascular and metabolic effects. Furthermore, even small amounts of insulin may result in a decrease of systemic FFA levels or in an increase in SNSA, which may alter vascular responses to different stimuli.

The experimental conditions under which the data are obtained may influence the vascular response to insulin and other vasoactive substances. For example, the cardiovascular response in part may depend on whether the study is performed with the subject in the supine or upright sitting position *(3)*, whether the forearm or the leg are studied and so on. Finally, in regards to the assessment of skeletal muscle perfusion and blood pressure, the methods (strain gauge plethysmography vs thermodilution or PET scanning) have different sensitivities, which may explain part of the divergent observations in the literature. Similarly, results of vascular function studies may differ according to the methods. Interestingly, flowmediated vasodilation (FMD), the change in brachial artery diameter in response to ischemia, did not correlate with insulin sensitivity in a larger Canadian study.

PHYSIOLOGY

Insulin's Effects on Skeletal Muscle Blood Flow

Insulin increases skeletal muscle blood flow in lean insulin-sensitive subjects. This insulin effect is observed in the leg *(4,5)* and the forearm *(6)*. Insulin's vasodilator action occurs at physiological concentrations and in dose-dependent fashion (Fig. 1). Limb blood-flow rates nearly double at insulin levels in the high physiological range (~70–90 µU/mL). However, not all researchers have been able to observe the vasodilatory effects of insulin *(7)*, except after a prolonged infusion, or at very high (~3000 µU/mL) systemic insulin levels *(8)*. The reasons for these divergent findings are not clear but are likely a result of differences in sensitivity and reproducibility of the methods used to determine blood flow.

In lean, insulin-sensitive subjects, the onset of insulin-mediated increments in skeletal muscle blood flow occurs early during a euglycemic/hyperinsulinemic clamp with a half-life of approx 30 minutes, nearly identical to that of insulin's effect to increase glucose extraction *(9)*. A similar time course for insulin's vascular effect has also recently been described by Westerbacka and associates *(10)*, who studied the effect of euglycemic hyperinsulinemia on pulse wave reflection in the aorta. In this study, the authors measured the pressure difference (central aortic augmentation) between the early and late systolic pressure peaks using applanation tonometry. They found that pressure augmen-

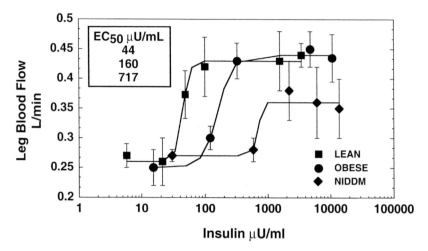

Fig. 1. Rates of leg blood flow in response to a wide range of steady-state insulin concentrations during euglycemic clamp studies in lean (●), obese (○) and obese type 2 diabetic (▲) subjects. The insert shows the insulin concentration required to achieve half-maximal increments in leg blood flow (EC50) in the different groups. (From ref. *11a*.)

tation and augmentation index decreased already after 30 minutes of hyperinsulinemia becoming statistically significant after 1 hour. Because wave-reflection is determined by compliance and vascular resistance, and because an early rise in skeletal muscle blood flow was not detected, which would indicate a fall in peripheral vascular resistance, the authors concluded that insulin at physiological concentrations (~60 μU/mL) affect the caliber or distensibility (compliance) of large arteries. Taken together, these studies provide evidence that insulin's effect on the vasculature occurs early in the course of hyperinsulinemia and parallels its effect on glucose metabolism.

Insulin does not only increase skeletal muscle blood flow at physiological concentrations but also augments the response to the endothelium-dependent vasodilator methacholine chloride. We have demonstrated *(11)* nearly a 50% augmentation of endothelium-dependent vasodilation at insulin levels of about 25 μU/mL. However, insulin did not change the leg blood-flow response to the endothelium-independent vasodilator sodium nitroprusside. In support of our observation, insulin, in the isolated rat aorta, did augment endothelium-dependent relaxation in response to the endothelium-dependent vasodilator acetylcholine but did not affect the response to sodium nitroprusside *(12)*. Taken together, these data indicate that insulin augments the production of but not the response to NO. In contrast to the above findings, euglycemic hyperinsulinemia was found to decrease FMD independent of insulin sensitivity or plasma lipid concentrations *(13)*. Because this *(13)* study did use a less well-defined model to estimate endothelial function *(14)* these results are difficult to interpret.

Because insulin augmented the endothelial response to methacholine chloride, we hypothesized that insulin causes skeletal muscle vasodilation via the release of NO. Using *NG*-monomethyl-L-arginine (L-NMMA), an inhibitor of NO synthase, we found that insulin's vasodilatory effects could be nearly completely annulled. The increment in leg blood flow was prevented by administration of L-NMMA into the femoral artery prior to initiating the systemic insulin infusion *(9)*. Moreover, leg blood flow, which nearly doubled in response to 4 hours of euglycemic hyperinsulinemia returned to baseline

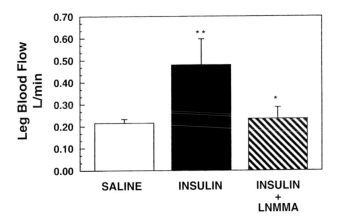

Fig. 2. Leg blood flow under basal conditions (saline), in response to 4 hours of euglycemic hyperinsulinemia alone (insulin) and with superimposed intrafemoral artery infusion of L-NMMA (insulin + L-NMMA). (From ref. *11a.*)

(Fig. 2) levels within 5 minutes of an infusion of L-NMMA into the femoral artery *(11)*. Our findings have been confirmed by others in humans *(15)* and in animals *(16)*. Thus, it is now well established that insulin increases skeletal muscle blood flow via release of endothelial-derived NO.

The notion that insulin acts via release of NO from endothelial cell is supported by the observation that insulin directly releases NO from human umbilical vein endothelial cells *(17)*. This insulin-mediated NO release occurred in a dose-dependent fashion and could be completely abolished by *N*(omega)-nitro-L-arginine methyl ester (L-NAME), an inhibitor of NO synthase.

Further investigation of the signaling pathway involved in insulin-mediated NO release revealed that genestein (an inhibitor of tyrosine kinase) nearly completely prevented the release of NO. Importantly, application of wortmannin, which inhibits phosphatidylinositol 3-kinase (PI3K), a signaling molecule required for insulin's effect to increase glucose uptake, caused about a 50% decrease in NO production. These in vitro results indicate that insulin induced release of NO is mediated through signaling pathways involving tyrosine kinase, PI3K, and Akt downstream from the insulin receptor *(18)*. Importantly, Akt has recently been shown to phosphorylate endothelial NO synthase (eNos), which results in increased activity of eNos *(19,20)*. Together, these findings suggest that insulin's metabolic and vascular actions share common signaling pathways. Thus, the similar time course of skeletal muscle vasodilation and glucose uptake in response to insulin's could be explained by a common signaling pathway. Moreover, impairment of a common signaling pathway in obesity, hypertension, or diabetes could lead to both blunting of insulin-mediated blood-flow increments and decreased rates of skeletal muscle glucose uptake. In this regard, it is important to note that mice deficient of eNOS were insulin resistant and mildly hypertensive *(21)*, but mice deficient of endothelial insulin receptors *(22)* exhibited normal glucose metabolism.

Insulin's Effects on the Heart

Our lab *(23)* investigated the effect of different insulin infusion rates on stroke volume in groups of lean normotensive volunteers (Fig. 3A). Hyperinsulinemia in the low physi-

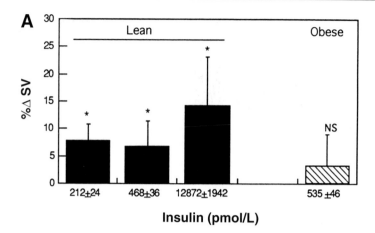

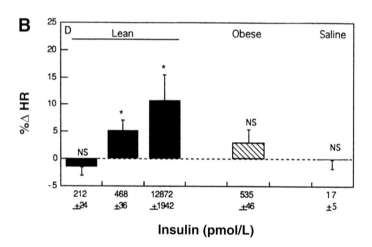

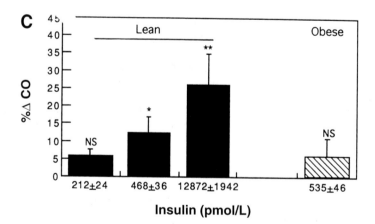

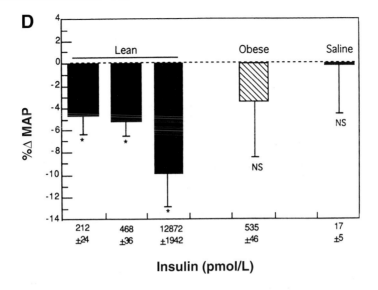

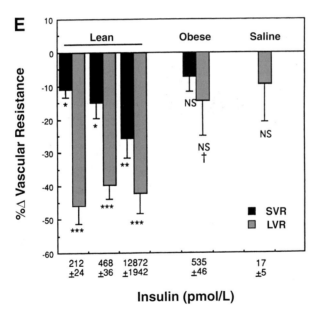

Fig. 3. Percent change (%Δ) from baseline in (**A**) stroke volume (SV), (**B**) heart rate (HR), (**C**) cardiac output (CO), (**D**) mean arterial blood pressure (MAP), and (**E**) total peripheral resistance (closed bar) and leg vascular resistance (hatched bar) during systemic hyperinsulinemic euglycemia and saline (control) infusion studies in lean and obese subjects. * $p < 0.05$, ** $p < 0.01$n and not significant (NS) vs baseline. (From ref. *11a*.)

ological range (35 ± 4 µU/mL) and in the high physiological range (78 ± 6 µU/mL) increased stroke volume by about 7%. A nearly 15% augmentation of stroke volume was observed with supraphysiological insulin concentrations (2145 ± 324 µU/mL). A similar effect of insulin on stroke volume was reported by ter Maaten and associates *(24),* who observed a nearly 13% rise at insulin levels of about 50 µU/mL. The increase in stroke volume could be a result of either a decrease in peripheral resistance (*see* Insulin's Effect on Blood Pressure and Vascular Resistance) or as a result of an increase in inotropy of the heart muscle. Experiments in the isolated beating heart or with heart muscle preparation indicate that insulin increases contractility of heart muscle. Taken together, these data indicate that insulin has a direct effect on the heart to increase cardiac stroke volume.

In addition to augmenting stroke volume, insulin increases heart rate. In our groups, heart rate did not change at low (~35 μU/mL) levels but increased by 5% and 10% at insulin concentrations of about 80 and about 2100 μU/mL, respectively (Fig. 3B). Thus, our data indicate that insulin increases heart rate in a dose-dependent fashion. Increments in heart rate in response to hyperinsulinemia were also found by others (5,6,25) but not by all (24). The reason for the discrepancy is not clear but differences in volume status or position during the study may explain in part the different observations. Whether the increase in heart rate is a direct insulin effect or whether it is mediated by activation of the SNS is not known.

As a result of the rise in heart rate and stroke volume in response to insulin, cardiac output increases. In our study groups, cardiac output increased by about 6%, 12%, and 26% in response to insulin concentrations of about 35, 80, and 2100 μU/mL (Fig. 3C). In support of our data, Ter Maaten and colleagues found about a 9% increase in cardiac output with insulin concentrations of about 50 μU/mL (24). Moreover, Fugman and associates' study replicated most of the above findings in a more recent study (26), demonstrating increased cardiac output in response to high physiological levels of insulin. These insulin effects are not only of academic interest but may have implications under conditions in which cardiac output needs to be augmented. For example, insulin's effect to increase cardiac output has been used to improve severe heart failure in patients undergoing cardiac surgery who were unresponsive to catecholamines and vasodilators (27).

Insulin's Effects on the Sympathetic/Parasympathetic Nervous System

Insulin has been shown to increase SNSA years before its vasodilator action was appreciated (28). Systemic insulin infusion causes a dose dependent rise in NE levels. In one study (6), NE levels in response to insulin increased from 199 ± 19 pg/mL under basal conditions to 258 ± 25 and 285 ± 95 pg/mL at insulin concentrations of 72 ± 8 and 144 ± 13 μU/mL, respectively. In the same study, skeletal muscle SNSA measured by microneurograpy exhibited an even more impressive rise in response to insulin. Microneurography allows to measure frequency and amplitude of electric activity directly at the level of sympathetic nerve fibers. Determined by microneurography, SNSA increased from baseline of about 380 U to about 600 and about 750 U in response to euglycemic hyperinsulinemia. Similar differences between the methods to assess changes in SNSA have been found by others (29), suggesting that plasma NE levels may underestimate the true effect of insulin to stimulate SNSA.

Interestingly, insulin modulates SNSA in a non-uniform manner. Van De Borne and colleagues (30) studied the effect of insulin on skeletal muscle SNSA with microneurography. The effect of hyperinsulinemia on cardiac SNSA and parasympathetic tone was assessed by power spectral analysis of the decrease in R-R interval. Power spectral analysis allows one to distinguish between low-frequency and high-frequency components of the changes in R-R intervals. The high frequency component is thought to reflect parasympathetic nervous system activity (PNSA; vagal tone) whereas the low-frequency component reflects SNSA. Additionally, systemic infusion of the β-blocker propranolol allows to distinguish the contribution of the PNS and the SNS on the R-R interval variability.

In response to hyperinsulinemia (84 ± 5 µU/mL), skeletal muscle SNSA increased more than twofold. In contrast, the SNSA effect on the reduction in R-R interval and variability in response to hyperinsulinemia was relatively small. This observation suggests that insulin's effect on the SNSA may be targeted specifically toward skeletal muscle the place of insulin's metabolic action. Interestingly, the increase in skeletal muscle SNSA may delay insulin's vasodilator action as proposed by Satori and associates (31).

The mechanism(s) for the increments in SNSA during hyperinsulinemia are not well understood. It may be mediated via the baroreceptor reflex to counteract insulin's vasodilator action, or may represent a direct insulin effect on the central nervous system. Moreover, coupling of insulin's effect on the SNS and its effect to increase glucose uptake/metabolism cannot be excluded. Although activation of the baroreceptor reflex in response to a decrease in blood pressure causes activation of the SNS, it can not explain all of the observed changes. First, time course of blood pressure decline and SNSA were different (6) and second, the increments in SNSA in response to insulin were nearly twice as those in response to blood pressure fall achieved by nitroglycerin infusion (32). In support of a direct role of insulin on SNSA at the level of the brain, injection of insulin directly into the third ventricle has been shown to increase SNSA in rats (33). This increase in SNSA activity could be abolished by generating a lesion in the surrounding the lateroventral portion of the third ventricle, a region implicated in the sympathetic neural control. Therefore, current evidence suggests a direct effect of insulin on the brain to increase SNSA, but other mechanisms cannot be excluded.

More recently it has been demonstrated that insulin also modulates PNSA. Unfortunately, no biochemical markers of PNSA exist that can be easily measured in vivo. As mentioned above, PNSA is studied by measuring the changes in R-R intervals using power spectral analysis. The PNSA (vagal component of heart rate control) is represented in the high frequency part of the spectrum.

In 1996, Bellavere and associates (34) reported a decrease in high-frequency variability of R-R intervals in response to hyperinsulinemia indicating that PNSA decreased. Similar results were obtained by Van De Borne and associates (30) in which euglycemic hyperinsulinemia decreased both R-R interval and the high-frequency variability of the R-R intervals. Moreover, this insulin-induced reduction of both R-R interval and high-frequency variability could not be suppressed by the β-blocker propranolol. These data indicate that the reduction in PNSA and not increments in SNS were likely responsible for the changes in R-R interval and variability. Furthermore, these data suggest that the effect of hyperinsulinemia on cardiac SNSA may be less than originally thought.

Taken together, the current data suggest that insulin's effect to stimulate SNSA may be mediated at least in part via a direct insulin effect on the brain. Furthermore, hyperinsulinemia appears to reduce parasympathetic tone at the level of the heart, which may contribute to the increments in heart rate.

Insulin's Effects on the Kidneys

The effect of euglycemic hyperinsulinemia on renal hemodynamics has not been studied by many groups. In one study (35), insulin at levels of about 100 µU/mL has been reported to increase renal plasma flow by 10% ± 5%. A similar rise in renal plasma flow has been reported in response to L-arginine-induced insulin secretion.

Insulin's effect on electrolyte handling is well established. Insulin has been found to cause antinatriuresis (36,37), antikaliuresis, and antiuricosuria in healthy volunteers. The antinatriuresis is achieved via a decrease in fractional sodium excretion. Fractional sodium excretion fell by 20% to 30% in response to euglycemic hyperinsulinemia with insulin levels of 50 to 60 µU/mL, well in the physiological range. Reductions in potassium and uric acid excretion in response to insulin were of similar magnitude (36). Based on animal studies (38), it was thought that insulin exerts the antinatriuretic effect at the level of the distal tubule in which the highest density of insulin receptors is found but it may be that the proximal tubule is the more likely site of insulin's antinatriuretic action in humans (39). The mechanism of the antikaliuretic and antiuricoretic effects of insulin are less well elucidated.

Insulin's Effect on Blood Pressure and Vascular Resistance

Insulin's effect on skeletal muscle vasculature, stroke volume, heart rate, cardiac output, SNS, and renal sodium handling can affect blood pressure. Blood pressure is determined by cardiac output and total peripheral resistance (TPR). In other words, blood pressure in response to insulin may increase, stay unchanged or decrease dependent on the changes in cardiac output and resistance. In lean, insulin-sensitive subjects, insulin causes a small but significant fall in blood pressure. In our study (23), hyperinsulinemia in the low (35 ± 4 µU/mL) and high (72 ± 6 µU/mL) physiological range caused about a 5% drop in mean arterial pressure (MAP), and supraphsyiological insulin concentrations 2100 ± 325 µU/mL were associated with about a 10% fall in MAP (Fig. 3D). However, although a drop in MAP has been reported by many groups, it has not been observed in all studies. MAP remained unchanged in a study reported by Scherrer (7) and even increased by nearly 7 mmHg in another study (24). The reasons for the different effect of euglycemic hyperinsulinemia on blood pressure are not clear.

The decrease in MAP in light of increased cardiac output indicates (29) a fall in TPR. In fact, TPR decreased in a dose-dependent fashion by 11.1 ± 2.2, 15.0 ± 4.7, and 26.0 ± 6.0% at insulin concentrations of 35 ± 4, 72 ± 6, and 2,100 ± 325 µU/mL, respectively (Fig. 3E). A similar decrease in TPR with comparable levels of hyperinsulinemia was also observed by Fugman and associates (26). Even more impressive than the fall in TPR was the drop in leg vascular resistance (LVR). LVR decreased by nearly 45% at an insulin concentration of 35 ± 4 µU/mL (Fig. 3E). Higher prevailing insulin levels did not result in further decrements in LVR. Similar decrements resistance have been observed by Anderson in the forearm (6,40) and by Vollenweider in the calf (29). However, in one study (24) in which both blood pressure and forearm blood flow increased, no changes in vascular resistance were detected.

Metabolic Implications of Insulin's Vascular Effects

Our lab has long championed the idea that insulin's vascular effects may contribute to the rate at which glucose is taken up by skeletal muscle, which represents the majority of insulin-sensitive tissues. In other words, insulin's vascular effects may determine, at least in part, insulin sensitivity and impairment of insulin's vascular effects may result in insulin resistance.

In support of this idea, we found that insulin's effect to increase skeletal muscle blood flow and cardiac output is positively and strongly associated with the rates of glucose uptake achieved in response to euglycemic hyperinsulinemia. In two studies (23,40) performed nearly 5 years apart, the correlation coefficient between leg blood-flow increments and whole-body glucose uptake were 0.63 and 0.56, indicating that blood flow

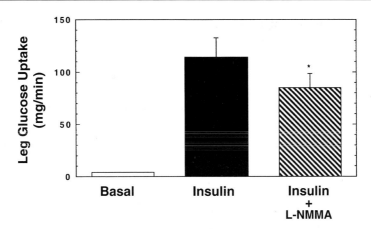

Fig. 4. Leg glucose uptake under basal conditions (basal), in response to 4 hours of euglycemic hyperinsulinemia alone (insulin) and with superimposed intrafemoral artery infusion of L-NMMA (insulin + L-NMMA). (From ref. *11a*.)

achieved during euglycemic hyperinsulinemia explains one-quarter to one-third of the variation in insulin sensitivity. Similarly, ter Maaten and associates *(24)* found that the correlation coefficent between percent increments in leg blood-flow and insulin-sensitivity index was 0.88, again suggesting that insulin's effect to augment blood flow contributes to rates of glucose uptake. Furthermore, cardiac output or changes in cardiac output in response euglycemic hyperinsulinemia also correlated significantly albeit not as strongly as leg blood flow with rates of whole-body glucose uptake *(23,24)*. Finally, the similar time courses *(9)* of insulin-mediated vasodilation and insulin-mediated glucose uptake suggest that metabolic and vascular actions of insulin might be coupled.

Taken together, these data suggest but do not prove that insulin's effects on metabolism and the vascular system are coupled. To test our hypothesis more rigidly, we assessed the effect of leg blood-flow changes on leg glucose uptake. In one set of studies *(41)*, we increased leg blood flow from 0.32 ± 0.12 L per minute during euglycemic hyperinsulinemia to 0.60 ± 0.12 L per minute ($p < 0.05$) by administering a intrafemoral artery infusion of the endothelium-dependent vasodilator methacholine chloride. As a result of the blood flow increments, leg glucose uptake increased from 87.6 ± 13.4 to 129.4 ± 21.8 mg per minute ($p < 0.05$). In a second set of studies *(42)*, we decreased leg blood flow during euglycemic hyperinsulinemia by nearly 50% via an intrafemoral artery infusion of the NO synthase inhibitor L-NMMA. The fall in leg blood flow induced by L-NMMA caused leg glucose uptake to decrease from 114 ± 18 to 85 ± 13 mg per minute ($p < 0.05$) representing about a 25% reduction of glucose uptake (Fig. 4), well in line with what had been predicted according to the experimentally defined correlation coefficients. In a third series of studies, we examined whether rates of skeletal muscle glucose uptake in response to changes in leg blood flow followed a noncapillary recruitment model as proposed by Renkin or whether changes in glucose uptake were dependent on capillary recruitment. The results of this study revealed that leg glucose uptake in response to pharmacological manipulation of blood flow were different than predicted by the Renkin model indicating that capillary recruitment is important for insulin's metabolic actions *(43)*. These findings are supported by studies by Bonadonna and associates *(44)* who looked at forearm glucose uptake using multiple tracer technique and Rattigan and associates *(45)* who measured glucose uptake in the isolated rat hindlimb. More recently, Coggins and associates *(46)*, using echo enhanced ultrasound provided more direct evidence for insulin's effect to recruit skeletal muscle capillaries in men. Together, these data provide strong evidence that insulin's vascular effects relate to its metabolic effects and that this metabolic effect is mediated by capillary recruitment.

The above discussed effects of insulin on the vascular system are also observed in response to meals. Depending on the amount of carbohydrate or fat ingested and the circulating insulin levels achieved, heart rate, stroke volume, skeletal muscle blood flow, and SNSA increase substantially, indicating that this coordinated cardiovascular response occurs under physiological conditions and may be necessary to maintain both metabolic and hemodynamic homeostasis. Postprandial hypotension, which is frequently observed in the elderly, may be a result of insufficient increments in heart rate and/or stroke volume to compensate for insulin's vasodilator effect.

Interactions Between Insulin and Norepinephrine and Angiotensin II

Because elevated insulin levels were associated with higher rates of hypertension, it was hypothesized that insulin might augment the action of vasoconstrictor hormones such as NE or angiotensin II. Indeed, earlier studies *(25,28)* reported that exogenous insulin enhanced the blood pressure response to NE. About a 20% and 40% reduction of the NE concentrations required to rise diastolic blood pressure by 20 mmHg was reported after 1 and 6 hours of euglycemic hyperinsulinemia. In contrast to this finding, we *(47)* observed that euglycemic hyperinsulinemia caused a right shift in the response to graded systemic infusions of NE. The reason(s) for the discrepant findings are not clear, but are likely a result of differences in study protocol and the method by which blood pressure was determined (intra-arterial vs cuff). Nevertheless, our data suggest that insulin attenuates vascular responsiveness to NE.

In support of this notion, Sakai and associates *(48)* reported that an intra-arterial infusion of insulin attenuated the vasoconstrictor response to NE by nearly 50%. Moreover, Lembo and coworkers also demonstrated that insulin-augmented β-adrenergic vasodilaton in response to isoproteronol and attenuated α-adrenergic vasoconstriction *(49)*. Furthermore, this insulin action was blocked by L-NMMA and inhibitor of NO synthase. These results indicate that insulin's modulatory effect on adrenergic response is mediated via the release of NO.

The effect of hyperinsulinemia on blood pressure the response to angiotensin II has been studied by a number of groups *(50–52)*. Insulin does not augment nor attenuate the blood pressure response to systemic angiotensin II infusion. However, Sakai and associates *(48)* demonstrated that insulin, when directly infused into a vessel, may modulate the vasoconstrictor response to angiotensin II. In their study, the direct intrabrachial artery infusion of insulin caused a more than 50% attenuation of the forearm blood-flow response to angiotensin II.

Insulin modulates the response to vasopressor hormones such as NE, vasopressin, and angiotensin II not only at the level of the vascular endothelium but also directly at the level of the vascular smooth muscle cell independent of the endothelium. Insulin attenuates agonist-evoked calcium transients *(53)* resulting in decreased vascular smooth muscle contractions. Whether this insulin effect at the level of the vascular smooth muscle can be explained by its effect on shared signaling pathways as described with angiotensin II *(54)* or by a different mechanism remains to be clarified. It is clear, however, that an imbalance between insulin's vasorelaxant effects and other vasoconstrictor hormones may result in the accelerated development of blood pressure elevation and macrovascular disease.

Interestingly, blood pressure elevation by systemic administration of NE *(47)* or angiotensin II *(51,55,56)* failed to decrease rates of insulin-mediated glucose uptake and induce insulin resistance. To the contrary and somewhat unexpectedly, the blood pressure elevation increased rates of insulin-mediated glucose uptake. The reason for this unexpected finding was most likely that limb blood flow increased, which allowed for the higher delivery rates of substrate, glucose, and insulin, and thus augment skeletal muscle glucose uptake.

Interactions Between Insulin and Adipocytokines

Adipose tissue has been shown to release a number of hormones that may interact with the vasculature. Leptin, a hormone secreted from the adipocyte, causes not only the release of NO from endothelial cells and but also augments insulin's effect to release NO *(57)*. Furthermore, adiponectin, another adipocyte-derived hormone, has been shown to cause the release of NO from endothelial cells *(58)*. Finally, interleukin-6, released from intra-abdominal fat cells may cause a decrease in endothelial NO production via increasing C-reactive protein *(59)* or via decreasing adiponectin secretion *(60)*.

PATHOPHYSIOLOGY: THE METABOLIC SYNDROME

The metabolic syndrome or syndrome X describes the clustering of a number of metabolic and hemodynamic abnormalities commonly seen in obesity and diabetes. More important, the metabolic syndrome is an independent risk factor for CVD. Syndrome X *(61,62)* is associated with resistance to insulin-mediated glucose uptake, glucose intolerance, hyperinsulinemia, increased very low-density lipoprotein triglyceride, decreased high-density lipoprotein cholesterol, increased plasminogen activator inhibitor-1, and hypertension. Because the classic risk factors can account for only about 50% of the increased rates of cardiovascular morbidity and mortality associated with obesity and type 2 diabetes *(63)*, other factors must play a role. One way to probe for potential candidates that might contribute to the higher rate of hypertension and the accelerated atherosclerotic process in insulin resistance is to evaluate the effect of obesity, hypertension, and type 2 diabetes on insulin's vascular effects.

The Metabolic Syndrome and Insulin's Effects on Skeletal Muscle Blood Flow

The effect of obesity, hypertension, and diabetes on insulin's vascular effects has been studied over the last years by a number of groups including our own. We *(64)* have demonstrated that obesity causes a left shift in the response to insulin's vasodilatory effect (Fig. 1). Importantly, the dose that achieves half maximal effect (ED) 50 for insulin's effect to increase skeletal muscle blood flow in the obese was nearly four times (~160 µU/mL) that of the lean (~45 µU/mL). Impaired insulin-mediated vasoadilation in the obese was confirmed by Vollenweider and associates *(65)*. They report about an 8% increment in calf blood flow in response to 2 hours of euglycemic hyperinsulinemia in obese subjects, which is in stark contrast to the 30% increment achieved in the lean subjects.

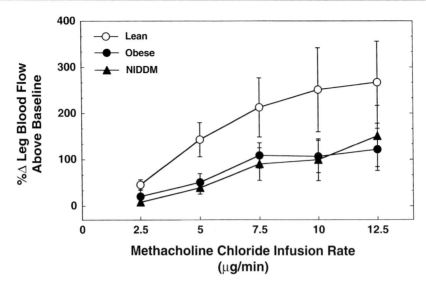

Fig. 5. Percent change (%Δ) from baseline in leg blood flow (LBF) in response to graded intrafemoral artery infusions of the endothelium dependent vasodilator methacholine chloride in groups of lean, obese, and obese type 2 diabetic subjects. (From ref. *11a*.)

Other evidence for impaired vascular action of insulin in obesity comes from a recent study by Westerbacka *(66)*. The authors studied the effect of obesity on insulin's ability to decrease arterial stiffness. In contrast to lean controls, arterial stiffness did not change in response to hyperinsulinemia with insulin levels of about 70 μU/mL, and decreased only slightly in response to insulin levels of about 160μU/mL.

Type 2 diabetes was associated with even more pronounced impairment of insulin-mediated vasodilation. In our study *(64)*, only supraphysiological hyperinsulinemia (~2000 μU/mL) achieved about a 33% rise in blood flow and the limitation in flow increments could not be overcome by higher insulin concentrations (Fig. 1).

Because insulin-mediated vasodilation, which depends on NO, is impaired in obesity and type 2 diabetes, we studied whether this impairment results from defective endothelial function or whether or defective NO activity. To this end, we generated dose–response curves for the leg blood-flow response to the endothelium-dependent vasodilator methacholine chloride and to the endothelium-independent vasodilator sodium nitroprusside. Leg blood-flow in response to methacholine increased threefold in the lean but only twofold in both obese and type 2 diabetics (Fig. 5). In contrast, the leg blood-flow response to sodium nitroprusside did not differ between lean, obese and type 2 diabetics. Resistance to leg blood-flow increments in response to the endothelium-dependent vasodilator bradykinin has also been recently reported in obesity *(67),* thus supporting our data that NO production is impaired.

In addition to obesity and type 2 diabetes, elevated blood pressure levels are associated with impaired insulin-mediated vasodilation *(68)*. Laine and associates *(67)* demonstrated that insulin-stimulated leg blood flow increased by 91% in the control subjects but only by 33% in the hypertensive subjects. This is important because hypertension has been shown by Forte and associates *(69)* to be associated with significantly decreased rates of NO production. Therefore, it is likely that in hypertension, impaired NO production is responsible for the blunted vasodilation in response to hyperinsulinemia.

Direct measurements of the effect of obesity and type 2 diabetes on NO production in skeletal muscle, however, have yielded conflicting data. In one preliminary study *(70)*, we measured insulin-induced changes in NO flux rates in subjects exhibiting a wide range of insulin sensitivity. NO flux was calculated by multiplying the concentration of nitrite and nitrate times leg blood-flow rates before and after 4 hours of euglycemic hyperinsulinemia. In this study, NO flux rates more than doubled in athletes who exhibited high insulin sensitivity but did not change in diabetics who were insulin resistant. However, Avogarro and associates *(71)*, who measured NO flux rates in the forearm in obese and type 2 diabetic subjects, were unable to detect a difference in NO flux between the two groups. The reason for the discrepant observations are not clear but further research will help to clarify this issue. More recently, measurements of whole-body NO production, using labeled l-arginine, the precursor of NO, revealed lower NO production rates in type 2 diabetics as compared to normal subjects *(72)*, which provides more direct evidence for impaired NO production in type 2 diabetes.

Taking the data together, basal whole-body NO production is decreased in hypertensive and in type 2 diabetic patients, and it is highly likely that obesity, hypertension, and type 2 diabetes exhibit impaired NO production in response to euglycemic hyperinsulinemia. Because NO is not only a potent vasodilator but also possesses a number of antiatherogenic properties, this defect in NO production could theoretically contribute to the increased rate of CVD in insulin-resistant states such as obesity, hypertension, or type 2 diabetes.

The mechanism(s) of impaired insulin-mediated vasodilation in obesity or type 2 diabetes are not known. One of the metabolic abnormalities consistently observed in insulin resistance is elevated FFA levels. Elevation of FFA levels also induces insulin resistance, which may be mediated, in part, via impairment of insulin-mediated vasodilation. Therefore, we studied the effect of FFA elevation on endothelial function in lean, insulin-sensitive subjects. The results of this study indicated that moderate two- or three-fold elevation of FFA levels sustained for 2 hours and achieved by systemic infusion of Intralipid plus heparin blunted the response to the endothelium-dependent vasodilator methacholine chloride (Fig. 6) but not to the endothelium-independent vasodilator sodium nitroprusside *(73)*. Similar results were reported by de Kreutzenberg and colleagues, who measured forearm vascular responses to before and after elevation of FFA *(74)*. Interestingly, the postischemic flow response was also impaired by FFA elevation *(75)*. Importantly, elevation of triglyceride levels alone in our studies did not cause endothelial dysfunction. This notion is supported by studies from patients with low lipoprotein lipase activity who exhibit normal endothelial function *(76)* despite markedly elevated triglyceride levels.

To further investigate the relation among elevated FFA levels, insulin sensitivity, and insulin-induced vasodilation, we investigated the time-course effect of FFA elevation on insulin-mediated increments in blood flow. Four to 8 but not 2 hours of FFA elevation reduced insulin-mediated vasodilation *(77)*. Furthermore, increments in NO flux in response to euglycemic hyperinsulinemia was nearly completely abrogated by superimposed FFA elevation. This effect on insulin-induced vasodilation was only observed when FFA elevation also caused insulin resistance. These data indicate that insulin-mediated vasodilation is coupled to insulin's effect on glucose uptake. In contrast, muscarinergic agonist-induced endothelium-dependent vasodilation appears to be regulated by other mechanisms as this signaling pathway can be disrupted by FFA elevations as short as 2 hours *(73)*. Indirect evidence for this proposed effect of FFA elevation on

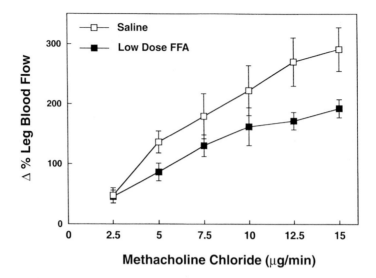

Fig. 6. Leg blood flow (LBF) increments (Δ%) in response to graded intrafemoral artery infusions of methacholine chloride during infusion of saline (open squares) or during 20% fat intralipid emulsion (closed squares) combined with heparin designed to increase systemic circulating free fatty acid levels two- or threefold. (From ref. *11a*.)

insulin-mediated vasodilation comes from muscle biopsy studies in response to hyperinsulinemic euglycemia with and without superimposed FFA elevation *(78)*. Dresner and colleagues *(78)* demonstrated that insulin resistance induced by FFA elevation was associated with decreased PI3K activity in skeletal muscle. Therefore, if insulin-signaling pathways are shared in endothelial cells and skeletal muscle, one may expect impaired insulin signaling in the endothelial cells in response to euglycemic hyperinsulinemia with superimposed FFA elevation.

Other evidence for the effect of elevated FFA levels to reduce endothelial NO production come from in vitro studies. Davda *(79)* and co-workers demonstrated a dose-dependent effect of oleic acid to impair NO release from cultured endothelial cells. Niu *(80)* and colleagues demonstrated that elevation of oleic acid attenuated the aortic strip relaxation in response to acetylcholine. Taken together, these findings from in vivo and in vitro studies strongly suggest a causal role of elevated FFA levels to impair endothelial function and decrease the rates of NO release.

Different mechanisms by which FFA may impair endothelial function could be via increased plasma levels of asymmetric dimethyl-L-arginine (ADMA) and/or via increased endothelin action. Lundman and associates *(81)* demonstrated that acute elevation of triglyceride (and likely elevated FFA) levels achieved by systemic infusion of a triglyceride emulsion was associated with elevation of ADMA levels and decreased flow-mediated vasodilation. Similarly, Fard and associates *(82)* showed that a high fat meal given to diabetic subjects resulted in increased plasma ADMA levels and impaired flow-mediated vasodilation.

Endothelin levels have been shown to increase in response to FFA elevation. Because elevated FFA levels are a hallmark of obesity and type 2 diabetes mellitus, Cardillo and associates *(83)* and Mather and associates *(84)* infused an inhibitor of endothelin, BQ 123 (specific inhibitor of the endothelin 1A receptor) directly into the brachial and femoral artery respectively. Both studies revealed more pronounced vasodilation in response to BQ123 in the obese and diabetic subjects, indicating an increased endothelin-dependent tone in the insulin-resistant subjects. Increased endothelin secretion in response to hyperinsulinemia may also contribute to the impaired vasodilation observed in insulin-resistant states (85).

The Metabolic Syndrome and Insulin's Effects on the Heart

Before discussing the effect of insulin on heart rate in insulin-resistant obese and diabetic subjects, two points should be made. First, basal heart rate and cardiac output (86) in obese and diabetic subjects is almost always increased as compared to lean subjects. Second, heart function in diabetes may be abnormal as a result of autonomic neuropathy. Thus, the data have to be interpreted with caution especially when comparing relative ($\Delta\%$) changes between insulin-sensitive and insulin-resistant groups.

The effect of insulin resistance on insulin-induced change in stroke volume has received little attention. Stroke volume did not change in our group of obese subjects (Fig. 3A) exposed to insulin concentrations of about 90 μU/mL. However, we may have failed to detect a small, less than 5% increase in stroke volume because of small group size. Muscelli and associates (87) however, report a near 10% rise in stroke volume at insulin concentrations of about 120 μU/mL. The reason for the different results is not clear. Groups were comparable in regards to body mass index or blood pressure. However, Muscelli and associates (87) used two-dimensional echocardiography whereas we used dye dilution technique to determine stroke volume. Thus, the discrepant results may be explained, at least in part, by different sensitivities of the methods by which cardiac output was determined.

We did not observe a change in heart rate in response to hyperinsulinemia about 90 μU/mL in our obese subjects (Fig. 3B). In contrast to our findings, Vollenweider and associates detected about a 10% increase in heart rate in obese subjects with insulin levels comparable to our study (~100 μU/mL). Heart rate was also found to rise in a dose-dependent fashion in response to hyperinsulinemia (88) in type 2 diabetics.

Because stroke volume and heart rate did not change in our obese group (Fig. 3C), cardiac output did not change either. However, other studies report a significant 15% increment in obesity (87). In type 2 diabetes, data on changes in cardiac output in response to hyperinsulinemia are not available. Nevertheless, because heart rate has been reported to increase in diabetics in response to hyperinsulinemia, it is reasonable to assume that cardiac output may increase as well. Taken together, the observations suggest that insulin's stimulatory effect on stroke volume, heart rate, and cardiac output may be intact in obese and type 2 diabetic subjects.

Insulin's action on the heart may extend well beyond modulation of hemodynamics. Cardiomyocytes possess insulin receptors which are important in postnatal development of the heart (89). It is not known whether impaired insulin receptor signaling in the cardiomyocyte plays a role in the increased incidence of left ventricular hypertrophy and congestive heart failure observed in obesity and diabetes.

The Metabolic Syndrome and Insulin's Effects on the Sympathetic/ Parasympathetic Nervous System

When assessing the SNSA by measuring NE no differences were detected between lean and obese subjects (29,90,91). Tack and colleagues used tritiated NE combined with forearm blood-flow measurements to assess the effect of hyperinsulinemia on SNSA in the forearm of lean type 2 diabetic and controls. The results of the study were that insulin increased arterial and venous NE concentrations in both groups. For example, 45 minutes of hyperinsulinemia caused arterial NE levels to increase by $63.8 \pm 14\%$ and $41.3 \pm 9.1\%$ in diabetic and control subjects respectively. In both groups, the rise in NE concentration was as a result of higher rates of total body and forearm NE spillover. The changes in NE concentration and spillover were comparable between the diabetic and controls. Unfortunately, no obese subjects were studied which would have allowed to distinguish the effects of diabetes (hyperglycemia) from those of obesity.

When measured by micro-neurography, basal skeletal muscle SNSA was found to be elevated more than twofold in obesity (90–92). In diabetes, no microneurography data are available. In response to euglycemic hyperinsulinemia, SNSA increased significantly (29). Although the relative rise in SNSA was blunted in the obese subjects, the absolute levels of SNSA achieved during hyperinsulinemia were comparable between lean and obese subjects. These data suggest that SNSA is nearly maximally stimulated in obese insulin-resistant subjects and that added hyperinsulinemia is unable to increase SNSA above levels achieved in lean controls.

Only two groups have thus far studied the effect of the metabolic syndrome on PNSA. Unfortunately, the data are somewhat contradictory. Muscelli and associates (93) report an increase in the low-frequency/high-frequency (LF/HF) ratio in response to euglycemic hyperinsulinemia in lean normal subjects but not in obese insulin-resistant subjects. The authors conclude that insulin alters cardiac control by enhancing sympathetic outflow and withdrawal parasympathetic tone. On the other hand, Laitinen and associates (94) demonstrate the opposite, an increase in the LF/HF in obese insulin-resistant subjects but not in the normal controls. Certainly, these opposite findings require clarification. Nevertheless, both studies suggest that the effect of hyperinsulinemia on PNSA is modulated by the presence of the metabolic syndrome.

The Metabolic Syndrome and Insulin's Effect on the Kidney

The effect of euglycemic hyperinsulinemia on renal hemodynamics in obesity has not been studied. In one study assessing the effect of euglycemic hyperinsulinemia on renal function in type 2 diabetes, no differences in estimated renal plasma flow were observed. Thus, the scarce data suggest that insulin's effect on renal blood flow is intact in obesity and type 2 diabetes.

Insulin's effect on electrolyte handling has been well studied in type 2 diabetes but data on obesity are not available. The antinatriuretic effect of insulin is well preserved in type 2 diabetes. Gans and associates (88) report a fall in fractional sodium excretion fell by $43 \pm 6\%$ and $57 \pm 9\%$ in response to euglycemic hyperinsulinemia with insulin levels of 64 ± 12 and 1113 ± 218 µU/mL, respectively. Because no control group was available in this study, it is not possible to determine whether the antinatriuretic response was normal or exaggerated in type 2 diabetes. Exaggerated antinatriuresis could lead to volume retention and contribute to the development of hypertension.

The Metabolic Syndrome and Insulin's Effect on Blood Pressure

Insulin's effect on the heart, the SNS, and the kidneys appear to be intact in subjects with the metabolic syndrome. This is in contrast to the impairment of insulin's effect to vasodilate skeletal muscle vasculature, which contributes to the decrease in peripheral vascular resistance during euglycemic hyperinsulinemia. Therefore, because the product of cardiac output and vascular resistance determine blood pressure, one might expect euglycemic hyperinsulinemia to result in blood pressure elevation. In our study, euglcycemic hyperinsulinemia did not alter blood pressure in the obese subjects (Fig. 3D). Other groups have reported that blood pressure in response to euglycemic hyperinsulinemia increased (29), decreased (95), or remained unchanged (96) in obese and diabetic subjects. Thus, the current data do not support the idea that hyperinsulinemia per se is causally related to the blood pressure elevation associated with the metabolic syndrome.

The Metabolic Syndrome and Interactions Between Insulin and Norepinephrine

Although there is great interest in the effect of the metabolic syndrome on the vascular responses to vasopressors such as NE or angiotensin II, few data are available in humans. We have demonstrated that the pressure response to systemic infusion of NE is augmented in obesity (47). At similar NE concentrations, the obese subjects exhibited a nearly 50% more pronounced blood pressure rise than the lean controls. Furthermore, insulin's effect to attenuate the pressure response to NE was abolished by obesity.

The effect of insulin resistance on the pressure response to angiotensin II was evaluated by Gaboury and associates (97) in normotensive and hypertensive subjects. In normotensive subjects, no relationship between insulin sensitivity and the blood pressure response to angiotensin II was detected. However, insulin sensitivity correlated inversely with the blood pressure response to angiotensin II in the hypertensive subjects.

Taken together, these data suggest that vascular responses to pressors may be increased in insulin resistance, which could contribute to the development of hypertension. The data also indicate that the relationship between insulin resistance and pressure responsiveness is not linear and may be modulated by additional factors that are poorly understood.

Interventions to Ameliorate the Effects of the Metabolic Syndrome on the Vascular System

If the increased rate of CVD associated with metabolic syndrome is partially mediated via the effects of insulin resistance on the vascular system, amelioration of insulin resistance should improve the abnormalities of the vascular system, which have been described above. In other words, maneuvers that improve insulin sensitivity should result in lower blood pressure, decreased heart rate, reduced SNSA, and improved endothelial function. Unfortunately, only a few studies have assessed the effect of improved insulin sensitivity on insulin-mediated vasodilation and endothelial function.

Weight loss is known to improve insulin sensitivity and to lower blood pressure (98). Weight loss also decreases heart rate and reduces the heightened SNSA (99,100). Although no studies have yet examined the effect of weight loss on endothelial function one would predict that endothelial function improves as well (101). However, it is unclear whether endothelial function would return to completely normal levels.

Troglitazone, a thiozolidenedione derivative, has been described to improve insulin sensitivity (102) and lower blood pressure in obese subjects. Furthermore, troglitazone decreased peripheral vascular resistance in diabetics (103), and pioglitazone decreased blood pressure in diabetic subjects (104). These data suggest that improvement of insulin sensitivity without changes in body fat content ameliorates cardiovascular abnormalities observed with the metabolic syndrome.

Our own findings *(105)* using 600 mg of troglitazone per day for 3 months in obese females suffering from polycystic ovary syndrome suggest a beneficial effect of troglitazone on both insulin-mediated vasodilation and the blood-flow responses to the endothelium-dependent vasodilator methacholine chloride. In contrast to our study, Tack and co-workers *(106)* found no effect of troglitazone (400 mg per day for 8 weeks) on insulin-induced blood-flow increments in obese insulin-resistant subjects despite a 20% improvement in insulin sensitivity. Thus, given the sparse and somewhat contradictory literature about the effect of increased insulin sensitivity on insulin-mediated increments in blood flow and endothelial function, further studies are required. Nevertheless, reduction of insulin resistance leading to improved endothelial and vascular system function may result in decreased cardiovascular morbidity and mortality in obese, hypertensive, and diabetic subjects.

CONCLUSION

Over the last 15 years, it has become established that insulin is a vascular hormone. Insulin's vascular actions extend beyond its effect to increase skeletal muscle blood flow and glucose uptake. Current data suggest that insulin modulates vascular tone, and vascular smooth muscle cell proliferation and migration via the release of NO and other yet unidentified mechanisms. Thus, insulin's effects on the vascular system may be important to prevent or delay the progression of CVD. The metabolic syndrome affects the vascular system at multiple levels. Resistance to the vascular actions of insulin may explain, at least in part, the abnormalities associated with the metabolic syndrome. The altered state of the vascular system in the metabolic syndrome may contribute to the higher rates of hypertension and macrovascular disease. Future research assessing the interaction between insulin's effect on the vasculature and newly discovered adipocytokines and other vasoactive hormones will better define the pathophysiological abnormalities underlying insulin-resistant states and help design therapies to improve endothelial function and reverse the accelerated atherosclerotic process.

ACKNOWLEDGMENTS

This work was supported by grants DK 42469, DK20542 (Dr. Baron), and MO1-RR750–19 (Dr. Steinberg) from the National Institutes of Health, and a Veterans Affairs Merit Review Award. Dr. Steinberg is recipient of the CAP award MO1-RR750–19 from the National Institutes of Health. The authors wish to thank Joyce Ballard for her expert and invaluable help in preparing the manuscript.

REFERENCES

1. Liang C-S, et al. Insulin infusion in conscious dogs. Effects on systemic and coronary hemodynamics, regional blood flows, and plasma catecholamines. J Clin Invest 1982;69:1321–1336.
2. DeFronzo RA, Tobin JD, Andres R. Glucose clamp technique: a method for quantifying insulin secretion and resistance. Am J Physiol 1979;237:E14–E23.
3. Ray CA, et al. Muscle sympathetic nerve responses to dynamic one leg exercise: effect of body posture. Am J Physiol 1993;264:H1–H7.
4. Laakso M, et al. Decreased effect of insulin to stimulate skeletal muscle blood flow in obese men. J Clin Invest 1990;85:1844–1852.
5. Scherrer U, et al. Suppression of insulin-induced sympathetic activation and vasodilation by dexamethasone in humans. Circulation 1993;88:388–394.

6. Anderson EA, et al. Hyperinsulinemia produces both sympathetic neural activation and vasodilation in normal humans. J Clin Invest 1991;87:2246–2252.
7. Scherrer U, Sartori C. Insulin as a vascular and sympathoexcitatory hormone: implications for blood pressure regulation, insulin sensitivity, and cardiovascular morbidity. Circulation 1997;96(11):4104–4113.
8. Utriainen T, et al. Methodological aspects, dose-response characteristics and causes of interindividual variation in insulin stimulation of limb blood flow in normal subjects. Diabetologia 1995;38:555–564.
9. Baron AD, et al. Effect of perfusion rate on the time course of insulin mediated skeletal muscle glucose uptake. Am J Physiol 1996;271:E1067–E1072.
10. Westerbacka J, et al. Diminished wave reflection in the aorta. A novel physiological action of insulin on large blood vessels. Hypertension 1999;33(5):1118–1122.
11. Steinberg HO, et al. Insulin-mediated skeletal muscle vasodilation is nitric oxide dependent. J Clin Invest 1994;94:1172–1179.
11a. Johnstone MT, Veves A. (Eds.) Diabetes and cardiovascular disease. Humana Press, Totowa, NJ: 2001.
12. Laight DW, et al. Pharmacological modulation of endothelial function by insulin in the rat aorta. J Pharm Pharmacol 1998;50(10):1117–1120.
13. Campia U, et al. Insulin Impairs Endothelium-Dependent Vasodilation Independent of Insulin Sensitivity or Lipid Profile. Am J Physiol Heart Circ Physiol 2004;286:H76–H82.
14. Bhagat K, Hingorani A, Vallance P. Flow associated or flow mediated dilatation? More than just semantics [editorial] [published erratum appears in Heart 1997 Oct;78(4):422]. Heart 1997;78(1):7–8.
15. Scherrer U, et al. Nitric oxide release accounts for insulin's vascular effects in humans. J Clin Invest, 1994;94:2511–2515.
16. Chen YL, Messina EJ. Dilation of isolated skeletal muscle arterioles by insulin is endothelium dependent and nitric oxide mediated. Am J Physiol 1996; 270:H2120–H2124.
17. Zeng G, Quon MJ. Insulin stimulated production of nitric oxide is inhibited by Wortmannin. Direct measurement in vascular endothelial cells. J Clin Invest 1996;98:894–898.
18. Zeng G, et al. Roles for insulin receptor, PI3-kinase, and Akt in insulin-signaling pathways related to production of nitric oxide in human vascular endothelial cells. Circulation 2000;101(13):1539–1545.
19. Dimmeler S, et al. Activation of nitric oxide synthase in endothelial cells by Akt- dependent phosphorylation. Nature 1999;399(6736):601–605.
20. Fulton D, et al. Regulation of endothelium-derived nitric oxide production by the protein kinase Akt. Nature 1999;399(6736):597–601.
21. Shankar RR, et al. Mice with gene disruption of both endothelial and neuronal nitric oxide synthase exhibit insulin resistance. Diabetes 2000;49(5):684–687.
22. Vincent D, et al. The role of endothelial insulin signaling in the regulation of vascular tone and insulin resistance. J Clin Invest 2003;111(9):1373–1380.
23. Baron AD Brechtel G. Insulin differentially regulates systemic and skeletal muscle vascular resistance. Am J Physiol (Endocrinol Metab 28), 1993;265:E61–E67.
24. ter Maaten JC, et al. Relationship between insulin's haemodynamic effects and insulin- mediated glucose uptake. Eur J Clin Invest 1998;28(4):279–284.
25. Gans ROB, et al. Exogenous insulin augments in healthy volunteers the cardiovascular reactivity to noradrenaline but not to angiotensin II. J of Clin Invest 1991;88:512–518.
26. Fugmann A, et al. Central and peripheral haemodynamic effects of hyperglycaemia, hyperinsulinaemia, hyperlipidaemia or a mixed meal. Clin Sci (Lond) 2003;105(6):715–721.
27. Kozlov IA, et al. [The use of ultra-high doses of insulin for the treatment of severe heart failure during cardiosurgical interventions]. Anesteziol Reanimatol 1992;3:22–27.
28. Rowe JW, et al. Effect of insulin and glucose infusions on sympathetic nervous system activity in normal man. Diabetes 1981;30(3):219–225.
29. Vollenweider P, et al. Impaired insulin-induced sympathetic neural activation and vasodilation in skeletal muscle in obese humans. J Clin Invest 1994;93:2365–2371.
30. Van De Borne P, et al. Hyperinsulinemia produces cardiac vagal withdrawal and nonuniform sympathetic activation in normal subjects. Am J Physiol 1999;276(1Pt 2):R178–R183.
31. Sartori C, Trueb L, Scherrer U. Insulin's direct vasodilator action in humans is masked by sympathetic vasoconstrictor tone. Diabetes 1996;45(Suppl 2):85A.
32. Rea RF, Hamdan M. Baroreflex control of muscle sympathetic nerve activity in borderline hypertension [see comments]. Circulation 1990;82(3):856–862.
33. Munzel MS, et al. Mechanisms of insulin action on sympathetic nerve activity. Clin Exp Hypertens 1995;17:39–50.

34. Bellavere F, et al. Acute effect of insulin on autonomic regulation of the cardiovascular system: a study by heart rate spectral analysis. Diabet Med 1996; 13:709–714.

35. Schmetterer L, et al. Renal and ocular hemodynamic effects of insulin. Diabetes 1997;46(11):1868–1874.

36. Muscelli E, et al. Effect of insulin on renal sodium and uric acid handling in essential hypertension. Am J Hypertens 1996;9(8):746–752.

37. Gans ROB, et al. Renal and cardiovascular effects of exogenous insulin in healthy volunteers. Clin Sci 1991;80:219–225.

38. DeFronzo RA, Goldberg M, Agus ZS. The effects of glucose and insulin on renal electrolyte transport. J Clin Invest 1976;58(1):83–90.

39. Trevisan R, et al. Role of insulin and atrial natriuretic peptide in sodium retention in insulin-treated IDDM patients during isotonic volume expansion. Diabetes 1990;39(3):289–298.

40. Anderson EA, et al. Insulin increases sympathetic nervous system activity but not blood pressure in borderline hypertensive humans. Hypertension 1992;19:621–627.

41. Baron AD, et al. Skeletal muscle blood flow independently modulates insulin-mediated glucose uptake. Am J Physiol 1994;266:E248–E253.

42. Baron AD, et al. Insulin-mediated skeletal muscle vasodilation contributes to both insulin sensitivity and responsiveness in lean humans. J ClinInvest 1995;96:786–792.

43. Baron AD, et al. Interaction between insulin sensitivity and muscle perfusion on glucose uptake in human skeletal muscle: evidence for capillary recruitment. Diabetes 2000;49(5):768–774.

44. Bonadonna R, et al. Role of tissue specific blood flow and tissue recruitment in insulin-mediated glucose uptake of human skeletal muscle. Circulation 1998;98:234–241.

45. Rattigan S, Clark MG, Barrett EJ. Hemodynamic actions of insulin in rat skeletal muscle. Evidence for capillary recruitment. Diabetes 1997;46:1381–1388.

46. Coggins M, et al. Physiologic hyperinsulinemia enhances human skeletal muscle perfusion by capillary recruitment. Diabetes 2001;50(12):2682–2690.

47. Baron AD, et al. Interactions between insulin and norepinephrine on blood pressure and insulin sensitivity. J Clin Invest 1994;93:2453–2462.

48. Sakai K, et al. Intra-arterial infusion of insulin attenuates vasoreactivity in human forearm. Hypertension 1993;22:67–73.

49. Lembo G, et al. Insulin modulation of an endothelial nitric oxide component present in the alpha-2 and beta adrenergic responses in human forearm. J Clin Invest 1997;100:2007–2014.

50. Gans RO, et al. Exogenous insulin augments in healthy volunteers the cardiovascular reactivity to noradrenaline but not to angiotensin II. J Clin Invest 1991; 88(2):512–518.

51. Buchanan TA, et al. Angiotensin II increases glucose utilization during acute hyperinsulinemia via a hemodynamic mechanism. J Clin Invest 1993;92:720–726.

52. Vierhapper H. Effect of exogenous insulin on blood pressure regulation in healthy and diabetic subjects. Hypertension 1985;7(6 Pt 2):II49–II53.

53. Touyz RM, Tolloczko B, Schiffrin EL. Insulin attenuates agonist-evoked calcium transients in vascular smooth muscle. Hypertension 1994;23(Suppl 1):I-25–I-28.

54. Folli F, et al. Angiotensin II inhibits insulin signaling in aortic smooth muscle cells at multiple levels. A potential role for serine phosphorylation in insulin/angiotensin II crosstalk. J Clin Invest 1997;100(9):2158–2169.

55. Morris AD, et al. Pressor and subpressor doses of angiotensin II increase insulin sensitivity in NIDDM. Dissociation of metabolic and blood pressure effects. Diabetes 1994;43(12):1445–1449.

56. Townsend RR, DiPette DJ. Pressor doses of angiotensin II increase insulin mediated glucose uptake in normotensive men. Am J Physiol 1993;265:E362–E366.

57. Vecchione C, et al. Cooperation between insulin and leptin in the modulation of vascular tone. Hypertension 2003;42(2):166–170.

58. Chen H, et al. Adiponectin stimulates production of nitric oxide in vascular endothelial cells. J Biol Chem 2003;278(45):45,021–45,026.

59. Verma S, et al. A self-fulfilling prophecy: C-reactive protein attenuates nitric oxide production and inhibits angiogenesis. Circulation 2002;106(8):913–919.

60. Fasshauer M, Paschke R. Regulation of adipocytokines and insulin resistance. Diabetologia 2003;46(12):1594–1603.

61. Reaven GM. Role of insulin resistance in human disease. Diabetes 1988;37: 1595–1607.

62. Reaven GM. Syndrome X: 6 years later. J Intern Med 1994;236(Suppl 736):13–22.

63. Pyorala K, Laakso M, Uusitupa M. Diabetes and atherosclerosis: an epidemiologic view. Diabetes Metab Rev 1987;3:463–524.

64. Laakso M, et al. Impaired insulin-mediated skeletal muscle blood flow in patients with NIDDM. Diabetes 1992;41:1076–1083.

65. Vollenweider L, et al. Insulin-induced sympathetic activation and vasodilation in skeletal muscle. Diabetes 1995;44:641–645.

66. Westerbacka J, et al. Marked resistance of the ability of insulin to decrease arterial stiffness characterizes human obesity. Diabetes 1999;48(4):821–827.

67. Laine H, et al. Insulin resistance of glucose uptake in skeletal muscle cannot be ameliorated by enhancing endothelium-dependent blood flow in obesity. J Clin Invest 1998;101:1156–1162.

68. Baron AD, et al. Skeletal muscle blood flow—a possible link between insulin resistance and blood pressure. Hypertension 1993;21:129–135.

69. Forte P, et al. Basal nitric oxide synthesis in essential hypertension. Lancet 1997;349(9055):837–842.

70. Steinberg HO, et al. Insulin mediated nitric oxide production is impaired in insulin resistance. Diabetes 1997;46(Suppl 1):24A.

71. Avogaro A, et al. Forearm nitric oxide balance, vascular relaxation, and glucose metabolism in NIDDM patients. Diabetes 1997;46:1040–1046.

72. Avogaro A, et al. L-arginine-nitric oxide kinetics in normal and type 2 diabetic subjects: a stable-labelled 15N arginine approach. Diabetes 2003;52(3):795–802.

73. Steinberg HO, et al. Elevated circulating free fatty acid levels impair endothelium-dependent vasodilation. J Clin Invest 1997;100:1230–1239.

74. de Kreutzenberg SV, et al. Plasma free fatty acids and endothelium dependent-vasodilation: effect of chain-length and cyclooxygenase inhibition. J Clin Endocrinol Metab 2000;85:793–798.

75. Lundman P, et al. Transient trigyleridemia decreases vascular reactivity in young, healthy mean without factors for coronary heart disease. Circulation 1997;96:3266–3268.

76. Chowienczyk PJ, et al. Preserved endothelial function in patients with severe hypertriglyceridemia and low functional lipoprotein lipase activity. J Am Coll Cardiol 1997;29(5):964–968.

77. Steinberg HO, et al. Free fatty acid elevation impairs insulin-mediated vasodilation and nitric oxide production. Diabetes 2000;49(7):1231–1238.

78. Dresner A, et al. Effects of free fatty acids on glucose transport and IRS-1-associated phosphatidylinositol 3-kinase activity. J Clin Invest 1999;103(2):253–259.

79. Davda RK, et al. Oleic acid inhibits endothelial nitric oxide synthase by a protein kinase C-independent mechanism. Hypertension 1995;26:764–770.

80. Niu XL, et al. Some similarities in vascular effects of oleic acid and oxidized low- density lipoproteins on rabbit aorta. J Mol Cell Cardiol 1995;27(1):531–539.

81. Lundman P, et al. Mild-to-moderate hypertriglyceridemia in young men is associated with endothelial dysfunction and increased plasma concentrations of asymmetric dimethylarginine. J Am Coll Cardiol 2001;38(1):111–116.

82. Fard A, et al. Acute elevations of plasma asymmetric dimethylarginine and impaired endothelial function in response to a high-fat meal in patients with type 2 diabetes. Arterioscler Thromb Vasc Biol 2000;20(9):2039–2044.

83. Cardillo C, et al. Enhanced vascular activity of endogenous endothelin-1 in obese hypertensive patients. Hypertension 2004;43(1):36–40.

84. Mather KJ, et al. ET-1A blockade improves endothelium-dependent vasodilation in insulin resistant obese and type 2 diabetic patients. Diabetes 2000;49(Suppl 1):585P.

85. Miller AW, et al. Enhanced endothelin activity prevents vasodilation to insulin in insulin resistance. Hypertension 2002;40(1):78–82.

86. Scaglione R, et al. Central obesity and hypertension: pathophysiologic role of renal haemodynamics and function. Int J Obes Relat Metab Disord 1995;19(6):403–409.

87. Muscelli E, et al. Autonomic and hemodynamic responses to insulin in lean and obese humans. J Clin Endocrinol Metab 1998;83(6):2084–2090.

88. Gans RO, Bilo HJ, Donker AJ. The renal response to exogenous insulin in non-insulin-dependent diabetes mellitus in relation to blood pressure and cardiovascular hormonal status. Nephrol Dial Transplant 1996;11(5):794–802.

89. Belke DD, et al. Insulin signaling coordinately regulates cardiac size, metabolism, and contractile protein isoform expression. J Clin Invest 2002;109(5):629–639.

90. Tack CJ, et al. Direct vasodilator effects of physiological hyperinsulin-aemia in human skeletal muscle. Eur J Clin Invest 1996;26:772–778.

91. Grassi G, et al. Sympathetic activation in obese normotensive subjects. Hypertension 1995;25:560–563.

92. Scherrer U, et al. Body fat and sympathetic nerve activity in healthy subjects. Circulation 1994;89:2634–2640.

93. Muscelli E, et al. Influence of duration of obesity on the insulin resistance of obese non- diabetic patients. Int J Obes Relat Metab Disord 1998;22(3):262–267.

94. Laitinen T, et al. Power spectral analysis of heart rate variability during hyperinsulinemia in nondiabetic offspring of type 2 diabetic patients: evidence for possible early autonomic dysfunction in insulin-resistant subjects. Diabetes 1999;48(6):1295–1299.

95. Gans ROB, et al. Acute hyperinsulinemia induces sodium retention and a blood pressure decline in diabetes mellitus. Hypertension 1992;20:199–209.

96. Tack CJ, et al. Effects of insulin on vascular tone and sympathetic nervous system in NIDDM. Diabetes 1996;45(1):15–22.

97. Gaboury CL, et al. Relation of pressor responsiveness to angiotensin II and insulin resistance in hypertension. J Clin Invest 1994;94:2295–2300.

98. Ikeda T, et al. Improvement of insulin sensitivity contributes to blood pressure reduction after weight loss in hypertensive subjects with obesity. Hypertension 1996;27(5):1180–1186.

99. Grassi G, et al. Body weight reduction, sympathetic nerve traffic, and arterial baroreflex in obese normotensive humans. Circulation 1998;97(20):2037–2042.

100. Esposito K, et al. Sympathovagal balance, nighttime blood pressure, and QT intervals in normotensive obese women. Obes Res 2003;11(5):653–659.

101. Nicoletti G, et al. Effect of a multidisciplinary program of weight reduction on endothelial functions in obese women. J Endocrinol Invest 2003;26(3):RC5–RC8.

102. Nolan JJ, et al. Improvement in glucose tolerance and insulin resistance in obese subjects treated with troglitazone. N Engl J Med 1994;331:1188–1193.

103. Ghazzi MN, et al. Cardiac and glycemic benefits of troglitazone treatment in NIDDM. The Troglitazone Study Group. Diabetes 1997;46(3):433–439.

104. Gerber P, et al. Effects of pioglitazone on metabolic control and blood pressure: a randomised study in patients with type 2 diabetes mellitus. Curr Med Res Opin 2003;19(6):532–539.

105. Paradisi G, et al. Troglitazone therapy improves endothelial function to near normal levels in women with polycystic ovary syndrome. J Clin Endocrinol Metab 2003;88(2):576–580.

106. Tack CJ, et al. Insulin-induced vasodilatation and endothelial function in obesity/insulin resistance. Effects of troglitazone. Diabetologia 1998;41(5):569–576.

2   Effects of Diabetes and Insulin Resistance on Endothelial Functions

Zhiheng He, MD, PhD, Keiko Naruse, MD, PhD, and George L. King, MD

Contents

INTRODUCTION

Cardiovascular complications have been the leading cause of mortality and morbidity in patients with diabetes and affect a variety of tissue and organs including retina, myocardium, nerves, skin, and kidney *(1–3)*. The incidence of coronary artery disease (CAD) in patients with diabetes or insulin-resistance syndrome is increased in subjects older than 30 years *(4,5)*. The Framingham study, which surveyed longitudinally more than 5000 patients with 18 years of follow-up indicated that major clinical manifestation of CAD were increased in diabetic patients, especially in women *(2)*. The risk of CAD increases with duration, reflecting the effect of the aging process, whereas in diabetic patients, both aging and duration of diabetes increased the risk of cardiac mortality: more than 50% of mortality in diabetic patients is related to cardiovascular disease (CVD). The incidence of cardiac or cerebrovascular disease is two to four times higher in diabetic patients than those of the general population *(6,7)*.

In patients with insulin-dependent diabetes mellitus (IDDM) who were followed for 20–40 years, the mortality as a result of CAD between the age of 30 and 55 years was 33%, whereas only 8% of the men and 4% of the women had died in nondiabetic population *(5)*. Unlike that of the general population, the risks of CAD in patients with IDDM are similar in men and women and increase at the same rate after age of 30. The incidence of CAD is also increased in noninsulin-dependent diabetes mellitus (NIDDM) and frequently occurs in families with CAD and NIDDM. Hyperinsulinemia and insulin resis-

From: *Contemporary Cardiology: Diabetes and Cardiovascular Disease, Second Edition*
Edited by: M. T. Johnstone and A. Veves © Humana Press Inc., Totowa, NJ

tance, which often precedes NIDDM, are risk factors for CAD. Several studies have shown that patients with NIDDM treated with insulin have a higher risk of CAD than those without insulin therapy, suggesting that severity of disease; loss of islet cell functions, or exogenous insulin treatment may also have an impact on CAD.

The influence of diabetes on CAD is synergistic with other factors, such as age, hypercholesterolemia, hypertension, and smoking. Additionally, diabetes itself is also an independent risk factor *(2,8–10)*. Although the increase in cardiovascular mortality probably has several causes, one of the specific factors pertaining to diabetes in the pathogenesis of diabetic vascular complications is hyperglycemia. This is well supported by both the Diabetes Control and Complication Trial (DCCT) and the United Kingdom Prospective Diabetes Study (UKPDS). The DCCT has clearly established that better glycemic control can prevent diabetic microangiopathy, such as retinopathy, nephropathy, and neuropathy, with improving trends observed in cardiovascular complications *(11)*. In the UKPDS *(3,12)*, more intensive glucose control was associated with a 12% reduction in the risk of pooled macrovascular and microvascular events. In a Japanese study, intensive insulin therapy in type 2 diabetic patients who were newly diagnosed, nonobese, and insulin sensitive (the Kumamoto trial) reduced the progression of retinopathy, nephropathy, and neuropathy, but too few events were seen to assess the impact of intensive glucose management on cardiovascular complications *(13)*. These results suggest that glycemic control with insulin can increase the survival of diabetic patients.

The second major risk factor specific for patients with diabetes or glucose intolerance is abnormalities of insulin actions in the vascular tissues. A substantial body of evidence exists for a relationship between insulin resistance and cardiovascular morbidity and mortality, suggesting an association among insulin sensitivity, hypertension, and endothelial function *(14–18)*. In this chapter, we first review the role of insulin resistance, hyperglycemia, and hypercholesterolemia in the vasculature and then describe cellular and functional abnormalities in endothelial cells.

Specific tissue responses or local factors are as important as systemic factors such as hyperglycemia in diabetes. The importance of tissue-specific responses or factors is demonstrated by differences in changes of vascular cells in the retina, renal glomeruli, and arteries (Table 1). In the retina, the number of endothelial cells appears to be increased, as exemplified by the formation of microaneurysms and neovascularization *(19)*. In contrast, endothelial cells in macrovessels are injured, as shown by pathological studies leading to the initiation of acceleration of the atherosclerotic process *(20,21)*.

INSULIN RESISTANCE

Hyperinsulinemia and insulin resistance have been shown to increase the risk of CVDs or atherosclerosis in diabetic states, and being a potential risk factor in the development of hypertension, not only in diabetic patients but also in the general population. The mechanism by which hyperinsulinemia or insulin resistance increases the risk of atherosclerosis is still unclear. Many theories have been suggested, including insulin-induced salt retention, directly enhancing proliferation of vascular smooth muscle cells (VSMCs) *(22,23)*, and indirectly regulating of endothelial cell homeostasis via the alteration of growth factors and cytokines in cells share extensive interaction with endothelial cells, such examples include fibroblasts, epithelial cells, VSMCs, and cardiomyocytes *(24–26)*.

We have characterized insulin receptors on the vascular cells and reported that they are identical to those in the nonvascular cells with respect to binding, structure, and tyrosine

Table 1
Alterations of Cell Numbers Observed in Various Vascular Tissues in Diabetes

	Retina	*Glomeruli*	*Macrovessels*
Endothelial cells	↑	↓	↓
Contractile cells	↓	↓	↑
Epithelial cells		↓	

phosphorylation activity *(23,27)*. The insulin receptor is a member of the tyrosine kinase family, and the activation of the receptor by insulin-binding results in autophosphorylation of receptor and activation of tyrosine kinase (Fig. 1). As in other cells, insulin receptors in vascular cells can activate at least two different signal transduction pathways; one is PI 3-kinase (PI3K) cascades and the other is Ras-mitogen-activated protein (MAP) kinase cascades. These signaling processes mediate the many actions of insulin in vascular cells, such as the regulation of cell growth, gene expression, protein synthesis, and glycogen incorporation. However, insulin receptors can mediate unusual functions in endothelial cells. We have demonstrated that endothelial cells can internalize insulin via a receptor-mediated process and transport the insulin across the endothelial cell without degradation *(28,29)*. In contrast, other types of endothelial cells, such as hepatocytes or adipocytes, will heavily degrade insulin when it is internalized. Another vascular-specific action of insulin is the activation or increased expression of nitric oxide (NO), resulting in localized vasodilation *(30–33)*. Mice null for insulin receptor specifically in endothelial cells (VENIRKO mice) were recently established *(34)*. Although only less than 5% of the insulin receptor mRNA expression was left in endothelial cells, these mice develop normally and did not show major differences in their vasculature as compared to their control litter mates except a mild reduction of gene expression for endothelial nitric oxide synthase (eNOS) and endothelin-1 in endothelial cells *(34)*. However, when challenged with hypoxia, VENIRKO mice developed more than 50% reduction in retinal neovascularization *(35)*. These results suggest that the alteration of insulin signaling might affect the expression of vascular regulators in endothelial cells and further affect vascular biology such as neovascularization.

Besides these actions, insulin has been reported to have many biological and physiological actions on vascular cells (Table 2). It is believed that hyperinsulinemia or insulin resistance can contribute to the acceleration of atherosclerosis by increasing the proliferation of aortic smooth muscle cells and the synthesis of extracellular matrix (ECM) proteins in the arterial wall (Fig. 2). However, the mitogenic actions of insulin on cells may not be significant in physiological conditions *(36)*, because insulin can only stimulate the growth of vascular cells at concentrations greater than 10 nmol/L. Only in severe insulin-resistant or hyperinsulinemic state can the plasma level of insulin may exert its growth-promoting actions in smooth muscle cells (SMCs) by enhancing the mitogenic action of more potent growth factors, such as platelet-derived growth factor and insulin-like growth factors *(37)*.

One of the best-characterized vascular effects of insulin is its vasodilatory action, which is mainly mediated by the production of NO *(31)*. Baron *(30)* reported that blood flow to the leg increased by two fold after 4 hours of hyperinsulinemia during a euglycemic-hyperinsulinemic clamp study. With superimposed infusion of *NG-*monomethyl-L-arginine (L-NMMA), an inhibitor of NO synthase, into the femoral artery,

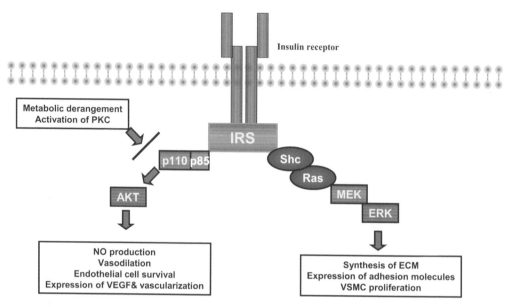

Fig. 1. Schematic diagram of the signaling pathways of insulin in vascular endothelial cells. Activation of either PI3K/Akt or Ras/MEK/MAP-kinase pathways can mediate most actions of insulin, with the former stimulating mainly anti-atherogenic effects, whereas the latter stimulating atherogenic actions. In diabetic or insulin-resistant states, metabolic derangements or activation of PKC has been suggested to selectively inhibit Insulin receptor-mediated activation of PI3K/Akt pathway, but spare the Ras/MEK/MAP pro-atherogenic arm of insulin's signaling cascade. This may in turn contribute to atherogenic lesion formation. IRS, insulin-receptor substrate; PI3K, phosphatidylinositol 3-kinase; MAPK, mitogen activated protein kinase.

Table 2
List of Effects of Insulin in Vascular Cells

Glucose incorporation into glycogen
Amino acid transport
Endothelin expression
eNOS expression and activation
VEGF expression in vascular smooth muscle cells
Tyrosine phosphorylation of various proteins
Exocytosis and receptor-mediated transcytosis
Basement matrix synthesis
Increased plasminogen activator inhibitor I
c-myc, c-fos expression
Protein synthesis
DNA synthesis
Cellular proliferation

the vasodilation was completely abrogated. It has also been reported that insulin-mediated vasodilation is impaired in states of insulin-resistant states (38). Consistent with this observation, obese nondiabetic subjects often have impaired endothelium-dependent vasodilation, especially relative to the patients with type 2 diabetes (32). These findings suggest that endothelial cell dysfunction may have genetic base and is involved in the risk

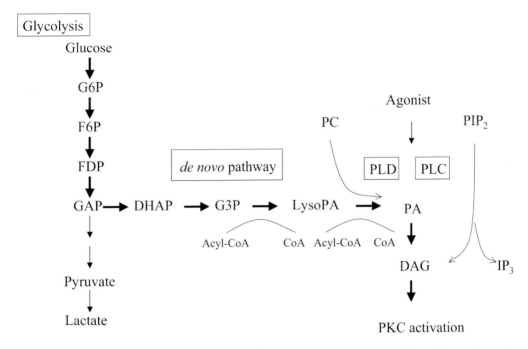

Fig. 2. Mechanism of DAG synthesis and PKC activation in diabetes mellitus. Hyperglycemia activates the de novo synthesis of DAG and leads to PKC activation. Acy-CoA, aceyl-coenzyme A; CoA, coenzyme A; DAG, diacylglycerol; DHAP, dihydroxyacetone phosphate; FDP, fructose 1,6-diphosphate; F6P, fructose 6 phosphate; GAP, glyceradehyde 3 phosphate; G3P, glycerol 3 phosphate; G6P, glucose 6 phosphate; IP3, inositol 1,4,5-triphosphate; LysoPA, lysophosphatidic acid; PA, phosphatidic acid; PC, phosphatidylcholine; PIP2, phosphatidylinositol 4,5-bisphosphate; PKC, protein kinase C; PLC, phospholipase C; PLD, phospholipase D.

of atherosclerosis in subjects with insulin resistance regardless whether they have diabetes *(32)*.

The effect of insulin on NO production in the endothelial cells may be biphasic, with rapid and delayed components. Relative to other stimulants of NO production, insulin is rather weak, with 10 to 100 times less maximum effects than acetylcholine. However, it is possible that the delayed-positive effect of insulin on eNOS expression has an important consequence in sustaining the level of eNOS expression, which will have a general effect on all the stimulators of NO production. The mechanism of insulin's effect on NO production appears to be mediated by the activation of PI3K pathway *(33)*. However, the acute effect appears to be an activation of eNOS, whereas the delayed effects are as a result of the upregulation of gene expression for eNOS.

Thus, in the vascular tissues, insulin has a variety of effects, which can be mediated by at least two signaling pathways involving PI3K and Ras-MAP kinase. At physiological concentrations, insulin mediates its effects through the activation of PI3K/Akt pathway, causing actions such as NO production. This effect can be interpreted as anti-atherogenic. In contrast, the effects mediated through Ras-MAP kinase pathway by insulin, for example, stimulation of ECM production; cell proliferation and migration, appears to be pro-atherogenic. The later effect requires the presence of high concentration of insulin that can be observed in insulin-resistant states. We have proposed that the increased risk of atherosclerosis in insulin-resistant states is caused by the loss of insulin's

Table 3
Proposed Mechanisms of the Adverse Effect of Hyperglycemis

Activation of the polyol pathway
Increases in the nonenzymatic glycation products
Activation of DAG-PKC cascade
Increases in oxidative stress
Enhanced flux via the hexosamine metabolism
Vascular inflammation
Altered expression and actions of growth factors and cytokines

action on PI3K/Akt pathway activation and the subsequent production of NO, whereas the activation of Ras-MAP kinase pathway remain intact. In support of this theory, we have documented that the activation of PI3K/Akt pathway and eNOS expression by insulin are significantly reduced in microvessels from insulin-resistant Zucker obese rats as compared to that of the healthy lean control rats, whereas the activation of Ras-MAP kinase pathway was not affected (33,39). These results have provided a molecular explanation for the clinical findings that both insulin deficiency (as in type 1 diabetic patients) and insulin-resistant states (as in patients with metabolic syndrome and type 2 diabetes) can lead to an acceleration of CVD.

HYPERGLYCEMIA

Hyperglycemia has been shown to be the main cause of microvascular complications in the DCCT (11) and UKPDS study (12). For cardiovascular complications, the contribution of hyperglycemia is probably also significant. Several biochemical mechanisms appear to explain the adverse effects of hyperglycemia on vascular cells (Table 3). This is not surprising because the metabolism of glucose and its metabolites can affect multiple cellular pathways. Glucose is transported into the vascular cells mostly by GLUT-1 transporters, which can be regulated by extracellular glucose concentration and other physiological stimulators, such as hypoxia (40). Once glucose is transported, it is metabolized to alter signal transduction pathways, such as the activation of diacylglycerol (DAG) and protein kinase C (PKC), or to increase flux through the mitochondria to change the redox potential (41–44). Lastly, another metabolic pathway (such as that of aldose reductase), which is normally inactive, can be used. In this review, we describe these theories and suggest that the common pathways for most of the adverse effects of hyperglycemia are mediated by alterations in signal transduction of such substances as DAG–PKC or other kinase and phosphatase.

Advance Glycation End-Products

Extended exposure of proteins to hyperglycemia can result in nonenzymatic reactions, in which the condensation of glucose with primary amines forms Schiff bases. These products can rearrange to form Amadori products and advanced glycation end-products (AGE). The glycation process occurs both intracellularly and extracellularly. It has been reported that the glycation modification target to intracellular signaling molecules and extracellular structure proteins alike, and furthermore, alter cellular functions. Multiple forms of proteins subjected to glycation have been identified with $N\epsilon$-(carboxymethyl)lysine (CML), pentosidine, and pyralline being the major form of AGEs presented in diabetic states.

A significant role for AGE in diabetic vascular complications is supported by their increased serum concentration in diabetic states *(45,46)*. Infusion of AGE into animals without diabetes reproduces some pathological abnormalities in vasculature similar to that in diabetes *(47)*. Furthermore, inhibition of AGE formation can partly prevent pathological changes in diabetic animals. Treatment of diabetic rats with aminoguanidine, an inhibitor of AGE formation and inducible nitric oxide synthase, can prevent the progression of both diabetic nephropathy *(48)* and retinopathy *(49)*, evidenced by the reduction of albuminuria; mesangial expansion; endothelial cell proliferation; pericyte loss; and even the formation of microaneurysms. Other inhibitors of protein glycation, such as OPB-9195 *(50)* or ALT-711 *(51)* have yielded similar results in animals with diabetes.

Recently, receptor for advanced glycation end-products (RAGE) has received substantial attention in its role in endothelial cell dysfunction in diabetes, especially in the development of atherosclerosis *(52)*. RAGE belongs to the immunoglobulin superfamily and has been reported to express in vascular cells including endothelial cells and SMCs *(53)*. Accumulation of RAGE has been reported in the vasculature in diabetic states *(46,47)*. Infusion of RAGE is associated with vascular hyperpermeability similar to that in diabetes and these changes can be neutralized in the presence of soluble RAGE (sRAGE) *(47)*, the extracellular domain of RAGE that disrupt AGE–RAGE interaction. Additionally, when mice deficient for apolipoprotein (apo)E (apoE–/–) were induced to have type 1-like diabetes by streptozotocin injection, they developed much more advanced atherosclerotic lesions in their aorta as compared to the apoE–/– mice without diabetes *(46)* and the progression of the atherosclerotic lesion can be reversed by intraperitoneal injection of sRAGE *(46)*. Although the molecular and cellular mechanisms underlying RAGE-induced vascular permeability change is still not fully understood, it is postulated that the induction of vascular oxidative stress *(54)*; activation of PKC and other intracellular signaling events *(55)*; and inflammation *(56)*.

These results provide supportive evidence suggesting an important role for AGE formation and RAGE activation in the development of diabetic vascular complications. The AGE–RAGE axis could therefore potentially be a target for clinical interventions. Indeed, aminoguanidine is currently being evaluated in a clinical trial for its effect on the progression of nephropathy in type 2 diabetes in 599 patients across United States and Canada *(57)*. However, majority of the results were obtained from animal studies and an affirmative role for AGE in the pathogenesis of diabetic vascular complications require further clinical evaluations.

Activation of the Polyol Pathway

Increased activity of the polyol pathway has been documented in culture studies using vascular cells exposed to diabetic level of D-glucose and in animals with diabetes *(58,59)*. In these studies, hyperglycemia has been shown to increase the activity of aldose reductase and enhances the reduction of glucose to sorbitol, then further oxidized to fructose by sorbitol dehydrogenase. Abnormality in the polyol pathway has been suggested to cause vascular damage in the following ways: (a) osmotic damage by the accumulation of sorbitol *(58)*; (b) induction of oxidative stress by increasing nicotinamide adenine dinucleotide phosphate (NADP)/NAD+ ratio and the activation of Na+/K+ adenosine triphosphate (ATP)ase *(59)*; and (c) reduction of NO in the vasculature by decreasing cellular NADPH, a cofactor used by aldose reductase to reduce glucose to sorbitol *(60)*. Multiple studies have shown that inhibition of aldose reductase, the key enzyme in the polyol pathway, could prevent the some pathological abnormalities in diabetic retinopathy, nephropathy, and neuropathy *(59)*. However, these results are not supported by data obtained from clinical trials using inhibitors of aldose reductase. A 3-year follow up of diabetic patients treated with Sorbinil (250 mg per day) failed to discern difference in retinopathy *(61)*, although another aldose reductase inhibitor Zenarestat has been shown to improve nerve conduction in diabetic peripheral polyneuropathy *(62)*. Based on the largely negative clinical data, a significant role for the activation of the polyol pathway in the pathogenesis of diabetic vascular complications has not been fully established.

Alteration in Oxidative Stress

Increases of oxidative stress by metabolic derangement has long been reported in diabetic states and proposed to cause vascular complications *(44,59,63,64)*. In diabetic states, induction of oxidative stress could be as a result of the increased production of superoxide anion via the induction of NADPH oxidase and mitochondrial pathway; decreases of superoxide clearance; lipid and protein modification; and the reduction of endogenous antioxidants such as ascorbic acid, vitamin E, and glutathione.

Several lines of evidence support a role of increased oxidative stress in the pathogenesis of diabetic vascular complications. Reactive oxygen species, an index of oxidative stress, has been reported to be increased and in diabetic patients with retinopathy *(65)* and other cardiovascular complications in the Framingham Heart Study *(66)* and correlate with the severity of these diseases. Furthermore, these results have been recapitulated in diabetic animals or even in vascular cells cultured in media containing high levels of D-glucose *(59,64)*.

Induction of oxidative stress has been suggested to induce vascular dysfunctions via multiple approaches including cellular DNA damage by activating the poly(ADP-ribose) polymerase *(67,68)*; reduction of NO bioavailability *(59)*, and the activation of other mechanisms known to induce vascular cell damage such as AGE formation, PKC activation, and induction of polyol pathway *(69)*. Additionally, evidence has shown that reactive oxygen species can cause severe disturbances in the regulation of coronary flow and cellular homeostasis, leading to the severe macrovascular lesions typically observed in diabetic patients after more than 10 years of disease *(70,71)*. Inhibition of reactive oxygen species also prevent the generation of AGE products and the activation of PKC in cultured endothelial cells *(69)*, suggesting that the auto-oxidative process plays an important role in the complex reaction cascade leading to AGE formation.

Several pathways in diabetic states, such as activation of PKC pathway, especially the β2 isoform *(72,73)*; AGE formation *(54)*, oxidized lipids *(64,66)*, and altered polyol activity *(59)* can lead to the activation of NADPH oxidase or flux through the mitochondrial respiratory chain *(69)* to generate reactive oxygen species that further increases tissue oxidative stress. On the other hand, oxidative stress can precedes formation of some AGE, such as pentosidine and CML, and activation of the DAG–PKC pathway *(74)*.

Although multiple studies using vascular cell in culture or diabetic animals have all supported that oxidative stress play an important role in vascular complications of diabetes. However, clinical studies have not yet provided conclusive results. The Heart Outcomes Prevention Evaluation Study (HOPE) has shown that treatment with vitamin E at a dose of 400 IU per day for a mean of 4.5 years has no apparent effect on cardiovascular outcomes in patients who had CVD or diabetes in addition to one other risk factor *(75)*. Similarly, the MICRO-HOPE study also yielded negative results showing

Table 4
Summary of DAG Levels and PKC Activities in Cultured Cells Exposed High Glucose
Condition and Tissues Isolated From Diabetic Animals

	Diacylglycerol	Protein kinase C
Cultured cells		
Retinal endothelial cells	↑	↑
Aortic endothelial cells	↑	↑
Aortic smooth muscle cells	↑	↑
Renal mesangial cells	↑	↑
Tissues		
Retina (diabetic rats and dogs)	↑	↑
Heart (diabetic rats)	↑	↑
Aorta (diabetic rats and dogs)	↑	↑
Renal glomeruli (diabetic rats)	↑	↑
Brain (diabetic rats)	→	→
Peripheral nerve (diabetic rats)	→	→

that 400 IU per day of vitamin E failed to show difference in cardiovascular outcomes and diabetic nephropathy (76). However, we have reported that oral vitamin E treatment at a dose as high as 1800 IU per day appears to be effective in normalizing retinal hemodynamic abnormalities and improving renal function in type 1 diabetic patients of short disease duration without inducing a significant changes in glycemic control (77). At this dose, vitamin E is capable of inhibiting PKC activity (74). These results suggest that high-dose vitamin E supplementation may reduce the risks of diabetic vascular complications by antioxidant-dependent and -independent pathways. These largely inconclusive clinical results have suggested that oxidative stress play a supporting rather than central role in the pathogenesis of diabetic vascular complications.

Activation of the DAG–PKC Pathway

One major advance in the understanding of diabetic vascular disease is the unraveling of changes in signal transduction pathways in diabetic states. One of the best-characterized signaling changes is the activation of DAG–PKC pathway. Such activation appears to be related to elevation of DAG, a physiological activator of PKC. Increases in total DAG contents have been demonstrated in a variety of tissues associated with diabetic vascular complications, including retina (78), aorta, heart (79), renal glomeruli (80), and nonvascular tissues as in the liver (81), but not in the brain and peripheral nerves of diabetic animals and patients (Table 4). Increasing glucose levels from 5 to 22 mol/L in the media elevated the cellular DAG contents in aortic endothelial cells and SMCs (79), retinal endothelial cells (78), and renal mesangial cells (82,83). The increase in DAG–PKC reaches maximum in 3–5 days after elevating glucose levels and remain chronically elevated for many years. In fact, we have already shown that euglycemic control by islet cell transplant after 3 weeks was not able to reverse the increases in DAG or PKC levels in the aorta of diabetic rats (79). These data suggest that the activation of DAG–PKC could be sustained chronically and is difficult to reverse, similar to pathways of diabetic complications.

DAG can be generated from multiple pathways. Agonist-induced formation of DAG depends mainly on hydrolysis of phosphatidylinositol by phospholipase C *(84)*. However, this mechanism is most likely minimally involved in diabetes, because inositol phosphate products were not found to be increased by hyperglycemia in aortic cells and glomerular mesangial cells *(85,86)*. When the fatty acids in DAG were analyzed *(87)*, DAG induced by high-glucose condition has predominantly palpitate- and oleic- acid–enriched composition, whereas DAG generated from hydrolysis of phosphatidylinositol has the composition of 1-stearoly-2-arachidonyl-*SN*-glycerol *(88)*. In labeling studies using [6–3H]- or [U-14C]- glucose, we have shown that elevated glucose increase the incorporation of glucose into the glycerol backbone of DAG in aortic endothelial cells (87), aortic SMCs *(89)*, and renal glomeruli *(90)*. These facts indicate that the increased DAG levels in high-glucose condition are mainly derived from the *de novo* pathway (Fig. 2).

It is also possible that DAG is produced through the metabolism of phosphatidylcholine as a result of the activation of phospholipase D *(91)*. One potential pathway for the increase in DAG is the result of glyco-oxidation inducing activation of the DAG pathway because oxidants such as H_2O_2 are known to activate DAG–PKC pathway (Fig. 3) *(92)*. We have reported that vitamin E, a well-studied antioxidant, has the additional interesting property of inhibiting the activation of DAG–PKC in vascular tissues and cultured vascular cells exposed to high glucose levels *(74)*. We have confirmed that vitamin E can inhibit PKC activation probably by decreasing DAG levels rather than inhibiting PKC, because the direct addition of vitamin E to purified PKC-α or -β isoforms in vitro has no inhibitory effect *(93)*.

PKC belongs to a family of serine-threonine kinases and plays a key role in intracellular signal transduction for hormones and cytokines. There are at least 11 isoforms of PKC and are classified as conventional PKCs (α, β1, β2, γ); novel PKCs (δ, ε, η, θ, μ); and atypical PKCs (ζ,λ) *(94,95)*. Multiple isoforms of PKC including α, β1, β2, δ, ε, and ζ are all expressed in endothelial cells *(79,96)*. Activation of PKC has been suggested to play key roles in the development of diabetic cardiovascular complications *(97)*.

The activation of PKC by hyperglycemia appears to be tissue-selective, because it has been noted in the retina, aorta, heart, and glomeruli but not in the brain and peripheral nerves in diabetic animals (Table 4). Among the various PKC isoforms, PKC-β and -δ appear to be preferentially activated in the aorta and heart of diabetic rats *(79)* and in cultured aortic SMCs exposed to high levels of glucose *(74)*. However, increases in multiple PKC isoforms were observed in some vascular tissues, such as PKC-α, -β2, and -ε in the retina and PKC-α, β1, and δ in the glomeruli in the glomeruli of diabetic rats *(98)*. Recently, we and others have shown that a number of in vivo abnormalities such as renal mesangial expansion, basement membrane thickening, blood flow, and monocyte activation in diabetic rats can be prevented or normalized using an orally effective specific inhibitor for PKC-β isoform LY333531 *(90)*. One of the early changes in the vasculature in diabetic states is the reduced bioavailability of endothelium-derived NO, which further aggravates endothelial dysfunctions. This process is apparently at least partly caused by the activation of PKC-β by hyperglycemia. Beckman and colleagues applied forearm hyperglycemic clamps on fourteen healthy subjects to mimic the effects and demonstrated that endothelium-dependent vasodilation in response to methacholine chloride is decreased in hyperglycemia as compared to that in euglycemic conditions *(99)*. The reduction of vasodilation can be normalized by oral treatment of PKC-β-selective inhibi-

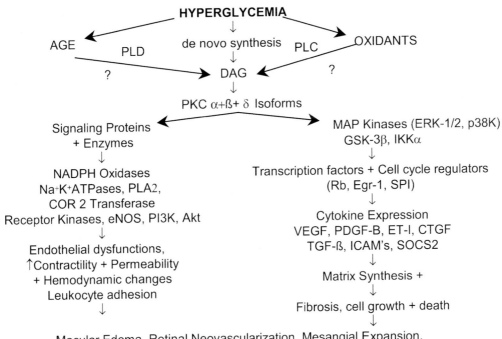

HYPERGLYCEMIA

AGE ← PLD — de novo synthesis — PLC → OXIDANTS

? → DAG ← ?

PKC α+ß+ δ Isoforms

Signaling Proteins + Enzymes ← → MAP Kinases (ERK-1/2, p38K) GSK-3β, IKKα

NADPH Oxidases Na+K+ATPases, PLA2, COR 2 Transferase Receptor Kinases, eNOS, PI3K, Akt

Transcription factors + Cell cycle regulators (Rb, Egr-1, SPI)

Endothelial dysfunctions, ↑Contractility + Permeability + Hemodynamic changes Leukocyte adhesion

Cytokine Expression VEGF, PDGF-B, ET-I, CTGF TGF-ß, ICAM's, SOCS2

Matrix Synthesis +

Fibrosis, cell growth + death

Macular Edema, Retinal Neovascularization, Mesangial Expansion, Proteinuria, Sensory Polyneuropathy + Cardiomyopathy

Fig. 3. Schematic diagram of pathways utilized by hyperglycemia to induce pathological changes in the vasculature. Hyperglycemia stimulates de novo synthesis of DAG that further activates multiple isoforms of PKC. Activation of the α, β, and δ isoforms have all been reported. This will in turn affect the activity of other intracellular signaling pathways such as the Ras/MEK/MAPK, p38 MAPK and PI3K/Akt pathways. Alteration of key enzymes determining cellular homeostasis, i.e., NADPH oxidase, Na+/K+-ATPase; eNOS, COR 2 transferase has also been documented. All these changes can have profound impact on the regulation of vascular cell biology including cell cycle progression, gene expression, endothelial cell dysfunctions and hemodynamic change that constitute the cellular basis of diabetic vascular complications. PLC; phospholipase D, PLC; Phospholipase C, eNOS; endothelial nitric oxide synthase, Rb, retinoblastoma; Egr-1, early growth response-1, GSK-3β; Glycogen synthase kinase-3β, IKKα; IκB kinaseα, VEGF; vascular endothelial growth factor, ANP; atrial natriuretic peptide; PDGF, platelet-derived growth factor; ET-1; endothelin-1, CTGF, connective tissue growth factor; TGF-β, transforming growth factor-β; ICAM, intercellular adhesion molecules; SOCS2, suppressor of cytokine signaling.

tor LY333531 (32 mg per day) *(99)*. These data support that the activation of PKC-β isoform is involved in the development of some aspects of diabetic vascular complications.

For a hyperglycemia-induced change to be credible as a causal factor of diabetic complications, it has to be shown to be chronically altered, to be difficult to reverse, to cause similar vascular changes when activated without diabetes, and to be able to prevent complications when it is inhibited. So far, we have presented evidence on the DAG–PKC activation that fulfills at least three of these criteria. Clinical studies using a PKC-β inhibitor are now in a phase II/III clinical trial to determine its usefulness in diabetic retinopathy *(100)* and neuropathy *(101)*.

DYSLIPIDEMIA

In more than half of all diabetic patients, especially those with type 2 diabetes and insulin resistance, decreases in high-density lipoprotein (HDL) cholesterol and hypertriglycemia have been reported *(102)*. Increases in low-density lipoprotein (LDL) cholesterol levels are also frequently observed in diabetic patients, but such increases are more frequently in those with poor glycemic control or in parallel with hypertriglycemia. Additionally, LDLs can be modified in diabetes, as in the formation of glycated or oxidized LDLs *(103,104)*, which have a decreased metabolism or are atherogenic.

Recent findings have shown that small, dense LDLs, and excess triglyceride-rich remnants, which are highly atherogenic, are increased in the insulin-resistant states *(105)*. Hyperinsulinemia and central obesity, which are commonly accompanied by insulin resistance and type 2 diabetes can lead to an overproduction of very low-density lipoproteins (VLDLs) *(106)*. VLDL particles contain a number of apolipoproteins and triglycerides. Increased free fatty acid and glucose levels can increase VLDL output from the liver, and elevated triglyceride levels can inhibit apoB degradation, resulting in increased secretion of VLDL. Lipoprotein lipase (LPL) activity in decreased in diabetic patients because insulin is a major regulator of LPL activity. Because LPL is necessary for the breakdown of chylomicrons and triglycerides and results in decreased clearance of VLDL, decreases in LPL activity are one of the causes for the increase in VLDLs. A decrease in LDL levels results in more glyceride-rich particles, fewer HDL particles, and much smaller, dense LDL particles in type 2 diabetic patients. Increased VLDL levels can accelerate the atherosclerotic process in several ways: VLDLs could be toxic for the metabolism and growth of endothelial cells *(107)*. Another possibility is that VLDLs from diabetic animals deposit more lipids in macrophages, which are precursors of foam cells in the arterial walls *(102)*.

HDLs, which are decreased in diabetic states, reduce the inhibitory effect of LDL on endothelium-mediated vasodilation *(108)*. Hypercholesterolemia increases the expression of endothelial adhesion molecules and platelets aggregability and adhesion *(109–112)*, and augmenting vasoconstriction.

Small, dense LDLs, which are known to be a potent risk factor for coronary heart disease, oxidize easily and are rapidly taken up by macrophages *(113)*, subsequently interacting with the endothelial cells, releasing vasoactive factors and becoming foam cells. Experimental and clinical data suggest that elevated serum levels of total and LDL cholesterol are associated with impaired endothelial functions *(114–116)*. Modified (mostly oxidized) LDLs impair endothelial function more than native LDLs at similar doses, based on in vitro vasodilator responses *(116,117)*. The levels of oxidized LDLs correlate better with impairment in endothelial function than cholesterol levels. Modified/oxidized LDL can affect gene expression (i.e., a decrease in eNOS expression and increase in endothelin-gene expression and production), which will promote vasoconstriction and hypertension.

Several studies have suggested that a key detrimental effect of hypercholesterolemia is to decrease NO availability *(113)*. Administration of the NO precursor L-arginine restores endothelial dysfunction induced by oxidized LDLs, suggesting an impairment in NO synthesis or decreased L-arginine availability *(115,116)*. In clinical studies, infusion of L-arginine can improve impaired endothelium-dependent vasodilation, including that as a result of hypercholesterolemia *(115,118)*.

CELLULAR AND FUNCTIONAL ALTERATIONS IN VASCULAR ENDOTHELIAL CELLS INDUCED BY DIABETIC STATE

Vascular Contractility and Blood Flow

Hemodynamic abnormalities such as blood flow and vascular contractility have been reported in many organs of diabetic animals or patients, including the kidney, retina, peripheral arteries, and microvessels of peripheral nerves. In the retina of diabetic patients and animals with a short duration and without clinical retinopathy, blood flow has been shown to be decreased *(119–123)*. One possible explanation for the decreased retinal blood flow in early stage of diabetes is as a result of an increase in vascular resistance at the microcirculatory level induced by PKC activation. We have reported that the decreased retinal blood flow can be mimicked by intravitreous injection of phorbol esters, which are PKC activators *(78)*. Furthermore, decreases in retinal blood flow in diabetic rats have been reported to be normalized by PKC inhibitors *(90)*. In addition to the retina, decreases in blood flow have also been reported in the peripheral nerves of diabetic animals by most investigators; these were normalized by PKC inhibitor, an aldose reductase inhibitor, and antioxidants respectively.

One of the possible mechanisms by which PKC activation could be causing vasoconstriction in the retina is by increased expression of endothelin-1 (ET-1). We have reported that the expression of ET-1, potent vasoconstrictor, is increased in the retina of diabetic rats and that intravitreous injection of endothelin-A receptor antagonist BQ123 prevented the decrease in retinal blood flow in diabetic rats *(124)*. The induction of ET-1 expression could also be normalized by LY333531, a PKC-β-selective inhibitor *(125)*. The decrease in blood flow to the retina could lead to local hypoxia, which is a potent inducer of vascular endothelial growth factor (VEGF); this factor can cause increases in permeability and microaneurysms, as observed in diabetic retina *(126,127)*.

Abnormalities in hemodynamic have been documented to precede diabetic nephropathy. Elevated renal glomerular filtration rate and modest increases in renal blood flow are characteristic finding in IDDM patients and experimental diabetic animals with poor glycemic control *(128–131)*. Diabetic glomerular filtration is likely to be the result of hyperglycemia-induced decreases in arteriolar resistance, especially at the level of afferent arteriole, resulting in an elevation of glomerular filtration pressure. This effect of hyperglycemia can be mimicked in vitro by incubating renal mesangial cells with elevated glucose levels that reduced cellular response to vasoconstriction. Several reports have suggested that the activation of PKC via the induction of prostaglandins may involve in this adverse effects of hyperglycemia *(132,133)*.

Changes in NO could also alter vascular contractility and blood flow. In the resistant vessels isolated from diabetic patients and animals, the relaxation phase after acetylcholine stimulation appears to be delayed *(134–137)*. These impaired vascular relaxation can be restored by PKC inhibitors and mimicked by phorbol ester in normal arteries *(137)*. The inhibition of PKC increased mRNA expression of eNOS in aortic endothelial cells *(138)*. We have observed reduced eNOS expression in microvasculature in Zucker fatty rats, which are the model of insulin resistance *(33)*.

Oral administration of effective specific inhibitor for PKCβ isoform LY333531 to diabetic rats for 2 weeks from the onset of the disease can normalize the retinal blood flow and glomerular filtration rate in parallel with inhibition of PKC activity *(90)*. Similarly, the renal albumin excretion rate can be improved after 8 weeks of such treatment. These data support the idea that the activation of PKCβ isoform is involved in the development of some aspects of diabetic vascular complications and endothelial dysfunctions.

Vascular Permeability and Neovascularization

Increased vascular permeability is another characteristic vascular abnormality in diabetic patients and animals, in which increased permeability can occur at as early as 4–6 weeks' duration of diabetes, suggesting endothelial cell dysfunctions *(139)*. Because the vascular barrier is formed by tight junctions between endothelial cells, the increase in permeability as a result of the abnormalities in the endothelial cells. The activation PKC can directly increase the permeability of albumin and other macromolecules through barriers formed by endothelial cells, probably by phosphorylating the cytoskeletal proteins forming the intercellular junctions *(140–142)*. Recently, PKC-β1 overexpression in human dermal microvascular endothelial cells has been reported to enhance phorbol ester-induced increase in permeability to albumin *(143)*. Thus, the actions of phorbol ester and hyperglycemia in endothelial-barrier functions are mediated in part through activation of PKC-β1 isoform.

PKC activation can also regulate vascular permeability and neovascularization via the expression of growth factors, such as VEGF/vascular permeability factor (VPF), which is increased in ocular fluids from diabetic patients and has been implicated in the neovascularization process of proliferative retinopathy *(144)*. We have reported that both the mitogenic and permeability-induced actions of VEGF/VPF are partly as a result of the activation of PKCβ via the tyrosine phosphorylation of phospholipase-δ *(145)*. The use of the PKCβ selective inhibitor LY333531 can decrease endothelial cell proliferation, angiogenesis, and permeability induced by VEGF *(145,146)*.

Na⁺-K⁺-ATPase

Na^+-K^+-ATPase, an integral component of the sodium pump, is involved in the maintenance of cellular integrity and functions such as contractility, growth and differentiation *(147)*. It is well established that Na^+/K^+-ATPase activity is generally decreased in the vascular and neuronal tissues of diabetic patients and experimental animals *(41,43,147–149)*. However, the mechanism by which hyperglycemia inhibits Na^+/K^+-ATPase activity have provided some conflicting results regarding the role of PKC. Phorbol esters have shown to prevent the inhibitory effect of hyperglycemia on Na^+/K^+ATPase, which suggest that PKC activity might be decreased in the diabetic condition.

However, we have reported that elevated glucose levels increased PKC and cytosolic phospholipase A2 (cPLA2) activities, resulting in increases of arachidonic acid release and prostaglandin E2 (PGE2) production and decrease in Na^+-K^+ ATPase activity *(150)*. Inhibitors of PKC or PLA2 prevented hyperglycemia-induced reduction in Na^+-K^+ ATPase activities in aortic smooth muscle cells and mesangial cells. The apparent paradoxical effects of phorbol ester and hyperglycemia in the enzymes of this cascade are probably as a result of the quantitative and qualitative differences of PKC stimulation induced by these stimuli. Phorbol ester, which is not a physiological activator, probably activated many PKC isoforms and increased PKC activity by 5–10 times, whereas hyperglycemia can only increase PKC activities by twofold, a physiologically relevant change that affected selective PKC isoforms. Thus, the results derived from the studies using phorbol esters are difficult to interpret with respect to their physiological significance.

Basement Membrane Thickening and Extracellular Matrix Expansion

Thickening of capillary basement membrane is one of the early structural abnormalities observed in almost all the tissues, including the vascular system in diabetes *(151)*. Because basement membrane can affect numerous cellular functions, such as in structure support, vascular permeability, cell adhesion, proliferation, differentiation, and gene expression, alterations in its components may cause vascular dysfunctions.

Histologically, increases in type IV and VI collagen, fibronectin and laminin and decreases in proteoglycans are observed in the mesangium of diabetic patients with nephropathy and probably in the vascular endothelium in general *(152,153)*. These effects can be replicated in mesangial cells incubated in increasing glucose levels that were prevented general PKC inhibitors *(154–156)*. Additionally, increased expression of transforming growth factor (TGF)-β has been implicated in the development of mesangial expansion and basement membrane thickening in diabetes. Because PKC activation can increase the production of ECM and TGF-β, it is not surprising that several reports have shown that PKC inhibitors can also prevent hyperglycemia- or diabetes-induced increases in ECM and TGF-β in mesangial cells or renal glomeruli *(98)*.

Thrombosis

The abnormalities in coagulation and platelet biology in type 2 diabetes patients are well documented *(157)*. The development of thrombosis within the vasculature depends on the balance between procoagulant and anti-thrombotic factors, which are shifted toward thrombosis in type 2 diabetes patients *(158)*. Plasminogen activator inhibitor(PAI-1) is produced by liver and endothelial cells and binds to the active site of both tissue plasminogen activator and urokinase plasminogen activator and neutralizes their activity *(159)*. Thus, increased expression of PAI-1 can lead to decreased fibrinolytic activity and predispose to thrombosis. Higher insulin concentration, similar to those seen in the plasma of diabetic patients, induced accumulation of PAI-1. It was also shown that using intact anesthetized rabbits with euglycemic-hyperinsulinemic or hyperproinsulinemic cramps, insulin or proinsulin could increase PAI-1 accumulation. Insulin alone dose not have a significant effect of PAI-I expression in normal subjects. However, elevated insulin levels with an environment of increased glucose and triglycerides, which is typical of type 2 diabetic patients, elicit an insulin-dependent increase in circulating PAI-1. The PAI-1 content in atherectomy specimens from type 2 diabetes patients also has been shown to increase in normal subject.

Abnormalities in renin–angiotensin system, which are seen in diabetic patients, are one of the inducer in PAI-1 accumulation. The contribution of the renin–angiotensin system to diabetic vascular complications has been attributed mainly to an increased responsiveness of vascular tissue to angiotensin II *(160)*. We observed that angiotensin II-induced PAI-1 and -2 expression in vascular endothelial and smooth muscle cells, which is partially dependent of PK C *(161)*. These data suggests that the therapy for decreasing insulin resistance and improvement of glycemic control can restore the fibrinolytic response.

CONCLUSION

It is likely that insulin resistance and hyperglycemia are responsible, directly or indirectly, for the abnormality of vascular endothelial functions in diabetic patients. New studies on the adverse effects of hyperglycemia have suggested that alterations in the signal transduction pathways induced by glycation products, oxidants, and redox potentials are important mechanisms in endothelial and vascular cell functions, because it may affect both antiatherogenic and atherogenic actions. Selective impairment of insulin-signaling through the PI 3K/Akt pathway causes the blunting of insulin's antiatherogenic actions. Hyperinsulinemia, when present concomitantly with insulin resistance, may enhance insulin's atherogenic actions. Agents that can improve insulin resistance in the endothelium and inhibit the adverse effects of hyperglycemia will ultimately prevent the microvascular and cardiovascular complications of diabetes.

REFERENCES

1. Krolewski AS, Warram JH, Rand LI, Kahn CR. Epidemiologic approach to the etiology of type I diabetes mellitus and its complications. N Engl J Med 1987;317:1390–1398.
2. Kannel WB, McGee DL. Diabetes and cardiovascular disease. The Framingham study. JAMA 1979;241:2035–2038.
3. Turner RC. The U.K. Prospective Diabetes Study. A review. Diabetes Care 1998;21 (Suppl 3):C35–C38.
4. Krolewski AS, Kosinski EJ, Warram JH, et al. Magnitude and determinants of coronary artery disease in juvenile-onset, insulin-dependent diabetes mellitus. Am J Cardiol 1987;59:750–755.
5. Knuiman MW, Welborn TA, McCann VJ, Stanton KG, Constable IJ. Prevalence of diabetic complications in relation to risk factors. Diabetes 1986;35:1332–1339.
6. Hanson RL, Imperatore G, Bennett PH, Knowler WC. Components of the "metabolic syndrome" and incidence of type 2 diabetes. Diabetes 2002;51:3120–3127.
7. Abbasi F, Brown BW Jr, Lamendola C, McLaughlin T, Reaven GM. Relationship between obesity, insulin resistance, and coronary heart disease risk. J Am Coll Cardiol 2002;40:937–943.
8. Steinberg D, Gotto AM Jr. Preventing coronary artery disease by lowering cholesterol levels: fifty years from bench to bedside. JAMA 1999;282:2043–2050.
9. Sosenko JM, Breslow JL, Miettinen OS, Gabbay KH. Hyperglycemia and plasma lipid levels: a prospective study of young insulin-dependent diabetic patients. N Engl J Med 1980;302:650–654.
10. Fuller JH, Shipley MJ, Rose G, Jarrett RJ, Keen H. Coronary-heart-disease risk and impaired glucose tolerance. The Whitehall study. Lancet 1980;1:1373–1376.
11. The DCCT Research Group. The effect of intensive treatment of diabetes on the development and progression of long-term complications in insulin-dependent diabetes mellitus. The Diabetes Control and Complications Trial Research Group. N Engl J Med 1993;329:977–986.
12. The UKPDS Group. Intensive blood-glucose control with sulphonylureas or insulin compared with conventional treatment and risk of complications in patients with type 2 diabetes (UKPDS 33). UK Prospective Diabetes Study (UKPDS) Group. Lancet 1998;352:837–853.
13. Ohkubo Y, Kishikawa H, Araki E, et al. Intensive insulin therapy prevents the progression of diabetic microvascular complications in Japanese patients with non-insulin-dependent diabetes mellitus: a randomized prospective 6-year study. Diabetes Res Clin Pract 1995;28:103–117.
14. Reaven GM. Banting lecture 1988. Role of insulin resistance in human disease. Diabetes 1988;37:1595–1607.
15. Despres JP, Lamarche B, Mauriege P, et al. Hyperinsulinemia as an independent risk factor for ischemic heart disease. N Engl J Med 1996;334:952–957.
16. Petrie JR, Ueda S, Webb DJ, Elliott HL, Connell JM. Endothelial nitric oxide production and insulin sensitivity. A physiological link with implications for pathogenesis of cardiovascular disease. Circulation 1996;93:1331–1333.
17. Natali A, Taddei S, Quinones Galvan A, et al. Insulin sensitivity, vascular reactivity, and clamp-induced vasodilatation in essential hypertension. Circulation 1997;96:849–855.
18. Stehouwer CD, Schaper NC. The pathogenesis of vascular complications of diabetes mellitus: one voice or many? Eur J Clin Invest 1996;26:535–543.
19. Frank RN. Diabetic retinopathy. N Engl J Med 2004;350:48–58.
20. Colwell JA, Lopes-Virella M, Halushka PV. Pathogenesis of atherosclerosis in diabetes mellitus. Diabetes Care 1981;4:121–133.
21. Beckman JA, Creager MA, Libby P. Diabetes and atherosclerosis: epidemiology, pathophysiology, and management. JAMA 2002;287:2570–2581.

22. Banskota NK, Taub R, Zellner K, Olsen P, King GL. Characterization of induction of protooncogene c-myc and cellular growth in human vascular smooth muscle cells by insulin and IGF-I. Diabetes 1989;38:123–129.
23. Banskota NK, Taub R, Zellner K, King GL. Insulin, insulin-like growth factor I and platelet-derived growth factor interact additively in the induction of the protooncogene c-myc and cellular proliferation in cultured bovine aortic smooth muscle cells. Mol Endocrinol 1989;3:1183–1190.
24. Miele C, Rochford JJ, Filippa N, Giorgetti-Peraldi S, Van Obberghen E. Insulin and insulin-like growth factor-I induce vascular endothelial growth factor mRNA expression via different signaling pathways. J Biol Chem 2000;275:21695–21702.
25. Jiang ZY, He Z, King BL, et al. Characterization of multiple signaling pathways of insulin in the regulation of vascular endothelial growth factor expression in vascular cells and angiogenesis. J Biol Chem 2003;278:31964–31971.
26. Poulaki V, Qin W, Joussen AM, et al. Acute intensive insulin therapy exacerbates diabetic blood-retinal barrier breakdown via hypoxia-inducible factor-1alpha and VEGF. J Clin Invest 2002;109:805–815.
27. King GL, Davidheiser S, Banskota NK, Oliver J, Inoguchi T. Insulin receptors and actions on vascular cells. In: Smith U, Bruun NE, Hedner T, Hokfelt B, (eds). Hypertension as an Insulin-Resistance Disorder. Genetic Factors and Cellular Mechanisms. Elsevier Science Publisher, Amsterdam, 1991, pp. 183–197.
28. King GL, Johnson SM. Receptor-mediated transport of insulin across endothelial cells. Science 1985;227:1583–1586.
29. Hachiya HL, Halban PA, King GL. Intracellular pathways of insulin transport across vascular endothelial cells. Am J Physiol 1988;255:C459–C464.
30. Baron AD. Insulin and the vasculature—old actors, new roles. J Investig Med 1996;44:406–412.
31. Scherrer U, Randin D, Vollenweider P, Vollenweider L, Nicod P. Nitric oxide release accounts for insulin's vascular effects in humans. J Clin Invest 1994;94:2511–2515.
32. Steinberg HO, Chaker H, Leaming R, Johnson A, Brechtel G, Baron AD. Obesity/insulin resistance is associated with endothelial dysfunction. Implications for the syndrome of insulin resistance. J Clin Invest 1996;97:2601–2610.
33. Kuboki K, Jiang ZY, Takahara N, et al. Regulation of endothelial constitutive nitric oxide synthase gene expression in endothelial cells and in vivo: a specific vascular action of insulin. Circulation 2000;101:676–681.
34. Vicent D, Ilany J, Kondo T, et al. The role of endothelial insulin signaling in the regulation of vascular tone and insulin resistance. J Clin Invest 2003;111:1373–1380.
35. Kondo T, Vicent D, Suzuma K, et al. Knockout of insulin and IGF-1 receptors on vascular endothelial cells protects against retinal neovascularization. J Clin Invest 2003;111:1835–1842.
36. King GL, Davidheiser S, Banskoto N, Oliver J, Inoguchi T. Insulin receptors and actions on vascular cells. In: Smith U, (ed). Nono Nordisk Foundation Symposium No. 5. Excepta Medica, Amsterdam, 1991, pp. 183–187.
37. Bornfeldt KE, Raines EW, Nakano T, Graves LM, Krebs EG, Ross R. Insulin-like growth factor-I and platelet-derived growth factor-BB induce directed migration of human arterial smooth muscle cells via signaling pathways that are distinct from those of proliferation. J Clin Invest 1994;93:1266–1274.
38. Balletshofer BM, Rittig K, Enderle MD, et al. Endothelial dysfunction is detectable in young normotensive first-degree relatives of subjects with type 2 diabetes in association with insulin resistance. Circulation 2000;101:1780–1784.
39. Jiang ZY, Lin YW, Clemont A, et al. Characterization of selective resistance to insulin signaling in the vasculature of obese Zucker (fa/fa) rats. J Clin Invest 1999;104:447–457.
40. Kaiser N, Sasson S, Feener EP, et al. Differential regulation of glucose transport and transporters by glucose in vascular endothelial and smooth muscle cells. Diabetes 1993;42:80–89.
41. Greene DA, Lattimer SA, Sima AA. Sorbitol, phosphoinositides, and sodium-potassium-ATPase in the pathogenesis of diabetic complications. N Engl J Med 1987;316:599–606.
42. Brownlee M. Advanced protein glycosylation in diabetes and aging. Annu Rev Med 1995;46:223–234.
43. King GL, Shiba T, Oliver J, Inoguchi T, Bursell SE. Cellular and molecular abnormalities in the vascular endothelium of diabetes mellitus. Annu Rev Med 1994;45:179–188.
44. Baynes JW. Role of oxidative stress in development of complications in diabetes. Diabetes 1991;40:405–412.
45. Berg TJ, Bangstad HJ, Torjesen PA, Osterby R, Bucala R, Hanssen KF. Advanced glycation end products in serum predict changes in the kidney morphology of patients with insulin-dependent diabetes mellitus. Metabolism 1997;46:661–665.

46. Park L, Raman KG, Lee KJ, et al. Suppression of accelerated diabetic atherosclerosis by the soluble receptor for advanced glycation endproducts. Nat Med 1998;4:1025–1031.

47. Wautier JL, Zoukourian C, Chappey O, et al. Receptor-mediated endothelial cell dysfunction in diabetic vasculopathy. Soluble receptor for advanced glycation end products blocks hyperpermeability in diabetic rats. J Clin Invest 1996;97:238–243.

48. Soulis-Liparota T, Cooper M. Papazoglou D, Clarke B, Jerums G. Retardation by aminoguanidine of development of albuminuria, mesangial expansion, and tissue fluorescence in streptozocin-induced diabetic rat. Diabetes 1991;40:1328–1334.

49. Hammes HP, Martin S, Federlin K, Geisen K, Brownlee M. Aminoguanidine treatment inhibits the development of experimental diabetic retinopathy. Proc Natl Acad Sci USA 1991;88:11555–11558.

50. Nakamura S, Makita Z, Ishikawa S, et al. Progression of nephropathy in spontaneous diabetic rats is prevented by OPB-9195, a novel inhibitor of advanced glycation. Diabetes 1997;46:895–899.

51. Wolffenbuttel BH, Boulanger CM, Crijns FR, et al. Breakers of advanced glycation end products restore large artery properties in experimental diabetes. Proc Natl Acad Sci USA 1998;95:4630–4634.

52. Schmidt AM, Stern D. Atherosclerosis and diabetes: the RAGE connection. Curr Atheroscler Rep 2000;2:430–436.

53. Brett J, Schmidt AM, Yan SD, et al. Survey of the distribution of a newly characterized receptor for advanced glycation end products in tissues. Am J Pathol 1993;143:1699–1712.

54. Wautier MP, Chappey O, Corda S, Stern DM, Schmidt AM, Wautier JL. Activation of NADPH oxidase by AGE links oxidant stress to altered gene expression via RAGE. Am J Physiol Endocrinol Metab 2001;280:E685–E694.

55. Yan SD, Schmidt AM, Anderson GM, et al. Enhanced cellular oxidant stress by the interaction of advanced glycation end products with their receptors/binding proteins. J Biol Chem 1994;269:9889–9897.

56. Hofmann MA, Drury S, Fu C, et al. RAGE mediates a novel proinflammatory axis: a central cell surface receptor for S100/calgranulin polypeptides. Cell 1999;97:889–901.

57. Freedman BI, Wuerth JP, Cartwright K, et al. Design and baseline characteristics for the aminoguanidine Clinical Trial in Overt Type 2 Diabetic Nephropathy (ACTION II). Control Clin Trials 1999;20:493–510.

58. Gabbay KH. Hyperglycemia, polyol metabolism, and complications of diabetes mellitus. Annu Rev Med 1975;26:521–536.

59. Brownlee M. Biochemistry and molecular cell biology of diabetic complications. Nature 2001;414:813–820.

60. Tesfamariam B. Free radicals in diabetic endothelial cell dysfunction. Free Radic Biol Med 1994;16:383–391.

61. Sorbinil Retinopathy Trial Research Group. A randomized trial of sorbinil, an aldose reductase inhibitor, in diabetic retinopathy. Sorbinil Retinopathy Trial Research Group. Arch Ophthalmol 1990;108:1234–1244.

62. Greene DA, Arezzo JC, Brown MB. Effect of aldose reductase inhibition on nerve conduction and morphometry in diabetic neuropathy. Zenarestat Study Group. Neurology 1999;53:580–591.

63. Giugliano D, Ceriello A, Paolisso G. Oxidative stress and diabetic vascular complications. Diabetes Care 1996;19:257–267.

64. Kuroki T, Isshiki K, King GL. Oxidative stress: the lead or supporting actor in the pathogenesis of diabetic complications. J Am Soc Nephrol 2003;14:S216–S220.

65. Augustin AJ, Dick HB, Koch F, Schmidt-Erfurth U. Correlation of blood-glucose control with oxidative metabolites in plasma and vitreous body of diabetic patients. Eur J Ophthalmol 2002;12:94–101.

66. Keaney JF Jr, Larson MG, Vasan RS, et al. Obesity and systemic oxidative stress: clinical correlates of oxidative stress in the Framingham Study. Arterioscler Thromb Vasc Biol 2003;23,434–439.

67. Dandona P, Thusu K, Cook S, et al. Oxidative damage to DNA in diabetes mellitus. Lancet 1996;347:444–445.

68. Garcia Soriano F, Virag L, Jagtap P, et al. Diabetic endothelial dysfunction: the role of poly(ADP-ribose) polymerase activation. Nat Med 2001;7:108–113.

69. Nishikawa T, Edelstein D, Du XL, et al. Normalizing mitochondrial superoxide production blocks three pathways of hyperglycaemic damage. Nature 2000;404,787–790.

70. Hamby RI, Zoneraich S, Sherman L. Diabetic cardiomyopathy. JAMA 1974;229:1749–1754.

71. Rosen P, Du X, Tschope D. Role of oxygen derived radicals for vascular dysfunction in the diabetic heart: prevention by alpha-tocopherol? Mol Cell Biochem 1998;188:103–111.

72. Inoguchi T, Li P, Umeda F, et al. High glucose level and free fatty acid stimulate reactive oxygen species production through protein kinase C—dependent activation of NAD(P)H oxidase in cultured vascular cells. Diabetes 2000;49:1939–1945.

73. Kitada M, Koya D, Sugimoto T, et al. Translocation of glomerular p47phox and p67phox by protein kinase C-beta activation is required for oxidative stress in diabetic nephropathy. Diabetes 2003;52:2603–2614.

74. Kunisaki M, Bursell SE, Umeda F, Nawata H, King GL. Normalization of diacylglycerol-protein kinase C activation by vitamin E in aorta of diabetic rats and cultured rat smooth muscle cells exposed to elevated glucose levels. Diabetes 1994;43:1372–1377.

75. Yusuf S, Dagenais G, Pogue J, Bosch J, Sleight P. Vitamin E supplementation and cardiovascular events in high-risk patients. The Heart Outcomes Prevention Evaluation Study Investigators. N Engl J Med 2000;342:154–160.

76. Lonn E, Yusuf S, Hoogwerf B, et al. Effects of vitamin E on cardiovascular and microvascular outcomes in high-risk patients with diabetes: results of the HOPE study and MICRO-HOPE substudy. Diabetes Care 2002;25:1919–1927.

77. Bursell SE, Clermont AC, Aiello LP, et al. High-dose vitamin E supplementation normalizes retinal blood flow and creatinine clearance in patients with type 1 diabetes. Diabetes Care 1999;22:1245–1251.

78. Shiba T, Inoguchi T, Sportsman JR, Heath WF, Bursell S, King GL. Correlation of diacylglycerol level and protein kinase C activity in rat retina to retinal circulation. Am J Physiol 1993;265:E783–E793.

79. Inoguchi T, Battan R, Handler E, Sportsman JR, Heath W, King GL. Preferential elevation of protein kinase C isoform beta II and diacylglycerol levels in the aorta and heart of diabetic rats: differential reversibility to glycemic control by islet cell transplantation. Proc Natl Acad Sci USA 1992;89:11059–11063.

80. Craven PA, DeRubertis FR. Protein kinase C is activated in glomeruli from streptozotocin diabetic rats. Possible mediation by glucose. J Clin Invest 1989;83:1667–1675.

81. Considine RV, Nyce MR, Allen LE, et al. Protein kinase C is increased in the liver of humans and rats with non-insulin-dependent diabetes mellitus: an alteration not due to hyperglycemia. J Clin Invest 1995;95:2938–2944.

82. Ayo SH, Radnik R, Garoni JA, Troyer DA, Kreisberg JI. High glucose increases diacylglycerol mass and activates protein kinase C in mesangial cell cultures. Am J Physiol 1991;261:F571–F577.

83. Studer RK, Craven PA, DeRubertis FR. Role for protein kinase C in the mediation of increased fibronectin accumulation by mesangial cells grown in high-glucose medium. Diabetes 1993;42:118–126.

84. Nishizuka Y. Intracellular signaling by hydrolysis of phospholipids and activation of protein kinase C. Science 1992;258:607–614.

85. King GL, Ishii H, Koya D. Diabetic vascular dysfunctions: a model of excessive activation of protein kinase C. Kidney International 1997;52:S77–S85.

86. Derubertis FR, Craven PA. Activation of protein kinase C in glomerular cells in diabetes. Mechanisms and potential links to the pathogenesis of diabetic glomerulopathy. Diabetes 1994;43:1–8.

87. Inoguchi T, Xia P, Kunisaki M, Higashi S, Feener EP, King GL. Insulin's effect on protein kinase C and diacylglycerol induced by diabetes and glucose in vascular tissues. Am J Physiol 1994;267:E369–E379.

88. Holub BJ, Kuksis A. Metabolism of molecular species of diacylglycerophospholipids. Adv Lipid Res 1978;16:1–125.

89. Xia P, Inoguchi T, Kern TS, Engerman RL, Oates PJ, King GL. Characterization of the mechanism for the chronic activation of diacylglycerol-protein kinase C pathway in diabetes and hypergalactosemia. Diabetes 1994;43:1122–1129.

90. Ishii H, Jirousek MR, Koya D, et al. Amelioration of vascular dysfunctions in diabetic rats by an oral PKC beta inhibitor. Science 1996;272:728–731.

91. Yasunari K, Kohno M, Kano H, Yokokawa K, Horio T, Yoshikawa J. Possible involvement of phospholipase D and protein kinase C in vascular growth induced by elevated glucose concentration. Hypertension 1996;28:159–168.

92. Taher MM, Garcia JG, Natarajan V. Hydroperoxide-induced diacylglycerol formation and protein kinase C activation in vascular endothelial cells. Arch Biochem Biophys 1993;303:260–266.

93. Kunisaki M, Bursell SE, Clermont AC, et al. Vitamin E prevents diabetes-induced abnormal retinal blood flow via the diacylglycerol-protein kinase C pathway. Am J Physiol 1995;269:E239–E246.

94. Mellor H, Parker PJ. The extended protein kinase C superfamily. Biochem J 1998;332(Pt 2):281–292.

95. Way KJ, Chou E, King GL. Identification of PKC-isoform-specific biological actions using pharmacological approaches. Trends Pharmacol Sci 2000;21:181–187.

96. Park JY, Takahara N, Gabriele A, et al. Induction of endothelin-1 expression by glucose: an effect of protein kinase C activation. Diabetes 2000;49:1239–1248.

97. Way KJ, Katai N, King GL. Protein kinase C and the development of diabetic vascular complications. Diabet Med 2001;18:945–959.

98. Koya D, Jirousek MR, Lin YW, Ishii H, Kuboki K, King GL. Characterization of protein kinase C beta isoform activation on the gene expression of transforming growth factor-beta, extracellular matrix components, and prostanoids in the glomeruli of diabetic rats. J Clin Invest 1997;100:115–126.

99. Beckman JA, Goldfine AB, Gordon MB, Garrett LA, Creager MA. Inhibition of protein kinase Cbeta prevents impaired endothelium- dependent vasodilation caused by hyperglycemia in humans. Circ Res 2002;90:107–111.

100. Aiello LP. The potential role of PKC beta in diabetic retinopathy and macular edema. Surv Ophthalmol 2002;47(Suppl 2):S263–S269.

101. Bastyr III E, Price K, Skljarevski V, Lledo A, Vignati L. Ruboxistaurin (RBX) mesylate treatment in patients with diabetic peripheral neuropathy (DPN) improves clinical global impression (CGI) and correlates with change in patient symptoms and signs. Diabetes 2003;52:A191.

102. Ledet T, Neubauer B, Christensen NJ, Lundbaek K. Diabetic cardiopathy. Diabetologia 1979;16:207–209.

103. Neubauer B. A quantitative study of peripheral arterial calcification and glucose tolerance in elderly diabetics and non-diabetics. Diabetologia 1971;7:409–413.

104. Hamet P, Sugimoto H, Umeda F, et al. Abnormalities of platelet-derived growth factors in insulin-dependent diabetes. Metabolism 1985;34:25–31.

105. Reaven GM, Chen YD, Jeppesen J, Maheux P, Krauss RM. Insulin resistance and hyperinsulinemia in individuals with small, dense low density lipoprotein particles. J Clin Invest 1993;92:141–146.

106. Howard BV. Insulin resistance and lipid metabolism. Am J Cardiol 1999;84:28J–32J.

107. Prisco D, Rogasi PG, Paniccia R, et al. Altered membrane fatty acid composition and increased thromboxane A2 generation in platelets from patients with diabetes. Prostaglandins Leukot Essent Fatty Acids 1989;35:15–23.

108. Matsuda Y, Hirata K, Inoue N, et al. High density lipoprotein reverses inhibitory effect of oxidized low density lipoprotein on endothelium-dependent arterial relaxation. Circ Res 1993;72:1103–1109.

109. Lacoste L, Lam JY, Hung J, Letchacovski G, Solymoss CB, Waters D. Hyperlipidemia and coronary disease. Correction of the increased thrombogenic potential with cholesterol reduction. Circulation 1995;92:3172–3177.

110. Hackman A, Abe Y, Insull W Jr, et al. Levels of soluble cell adhesion molecules in patients with dyslipidemia. Circulation 1996;93:1334–1338.

111. Sampietro T, Tuoni M, Ferdeghini M, et al. Plasma cholesterol regulates soluble cell adhesion molecule expression in familial hypercholesterolemia. Circulation 1997;96:1381–1385.

112. Nofer JR, Tepel M, Kehrel B, et al. Low-density lipoproteins inhibit the Na+/H+ antiport in human platelets. A novel mechanism enhancing platelet activity in hypercholesterolemia. Circulation 1997;95:1370–1377.

113. Vogel RA. Cholesterol lowering and endothelial function. Am J Med 1999;107:479–487.

114. Kugiyama K, Kerns SA, Morrisett JD, Roberts R, Henry PD. Impairment of endothelium-dependent arterial relaxation by lysolecithin in modified low-density lipoproteins. Nature 1990;344:160–162.

115. Creager MA, Gallagher SJ, Girerd XJ, Coleman SM, Dzau VJ, Cooke JP. L-arginine improves endothelium-dependent vasodilation in hypercholesterolemic humans. J Clin Invest 1992;90:1248–1253.

116. Chen LY, Mehta P, Mehta JL. Oxidized LDL decreases L-arginine uptake and nitric oxide synthase protein expression in human platelets: relevance of the effect of oxidized LDL on platelet function. Circulation 1996;93:1740–1746.

117. Chin JH, Azhar S, Hoffman BB. (1992) Inactivation of endothelial derived relaxing factor by oxidized lipoproteins. J Clin Invest 1992;89:10–18.

118. Quyyumi AA, Dakak N, Diodati JG, Gilligan DM, Panza JA, Cannon RO, 3rd Effect of L-arginine on human coronary endothelium-dependent and physiologic vasodilation. J Am Coll Cardiol 1997;30:1220–1227.

119. Small KW, Stefansson E, Hatchell DL. Retinal blood flow in normal and diabetic dogs. Invest Ophthalmol Vis Sci 1987;28:672–675.

120. Feke GT, Buzney SM, Ogasawara H, et al. Retinal circulatory abnormalities in type 1 diabetes. Invest Ophthalmol Vis Sci 1994;35:2968–2975.

121. Bursell SE, Clermont AC, Kinsley BT, Simonson DC, Aiello LM, Wolpert HA. Retinal blood flow changes in patients with insulin-dependent diabetes mellitus and no diabetic retinopathy. Invest Ophthalmol Vis Sci 1996;37:886–897.

122. Clermont AC, Brittis M, Shiba T, McGovern T, King GL, Bursell SE. Normalization of retinal blood flow in diabetic rats with primary intervention using insulin pumps. Invest Ophthalmol Vis Sci 1994;35:981–990.

123. Miyamoto K, Ogura Y, Nishiwaki H, et al. Evaluation of retinal microcirculatory alterations in the Goto-Kakizaki rat. A spontaneous model of non-insulin-dependent diabetes. Invest Ophthalmol Vis Sci 1996;37:898–905.

124. Takagi C, Bursell S E, Lin YW, et al. Regulation of retinal hemodynamics in diabetic rats by increased expression and action of endothelin-1. Invest Ophthalmol Vis Sci 1996;37:2504–2518.

125. Yokota T, Ma, RC, Park JY, et al. Role of protein kinase C on the expression of platelet-derived growth factor and endothelin-1 in the retina of diabetic rats and cultured retinal capillary pericytes. Diabetes 2003;52:838–845.

126. Aiello LP, Pierce EA, Foley ED, et al. Suppression of retinal neovascularization in vivo by inhibition of vascular endothelial growth factor (VEGF) using soluble VEGF-receptor chimeric proteins. Proc Natl Acad Sci USA 1995;92:10457–10461.

127. Tolentino MJ, Miller JW, Gragoudas ES, et al. Intravitreous injections of vascular endothelial growth factor produce retinal ischemia and microangiopathy in an adult primate. Ophthalmology 1996;103:1820–1828.

128. Ditzel J, Schwartz M. Abnormally increased glomerular filtration rate in short-term insulin-treated diabetic subjects. Diabetes 1967;16:264–267.

129. Christiansen JS, Gammelgaard J, Frandsen M, Parving HH. Increased kidney size, glomerular filtration rate and renal plasma flow in short-term insulin-dependent diabetics. Diabetologia 1981;20:451–456.

130. Hostetter TH, Troy JL, Brenner BM. Glomerular hemodynamics in experimental diabetes mellitus. Kidney Int 1981;19:410–415.

131. Viberti GC. Early functional and morphological changes in diabetic nephropathy. Clin Nephrol 1979;12:47–53.

132. Schambelan M, Blake S, Sraer J, Bens M, Nivez MP, Wahbe F. Increased prostaglandin production by glomeruli isolated from rats with streptozotocin-induced diabetes mellitus. J Clin Invest 1985;75:404–412.

133. Craven PA, Caines MA, DeRubertis FR. (1987) Sequential alterations in glomerular prostaglandin and thromboxane synthesis in diabetic rats: relationship to the hyperfiltration of early diabetes. Metabolism 1987;36:95–103.

134. Kamata K, Miyata N, Kasuya Y. (1989) Involvement of endothelial cells in relaxation and contraction responses of the aorta to isoproterenol in naive and streptozotocin-induced diabetic rats. J Pharmacol Exp Ther 1989;249:890–894.

135. Mayhan WG. (1989) Impairment of endothelium-dependent dilatation of cerebral arterioles during diabetes mellitus. Am J Physiol 1989;256:H621–625.

136. Tesfamariam B, Jakubowski JA, Cohen RA. Contraction of diabetic rabbit aorta caused by endothelium-derived PGH2-TxA2. Am J Physiol 1989;257: H1327–1333.

137. McVeigh GE, Brennan GM, Johnston GD, et al. Impaired endothelium-dependent and independent vasodilation in patients with type 2 (non-insulin-dependent) diabetes mellitus. Diabetologia 1992;35:771–776.

138. Ohara Y, Sayegh HS, Yamin JJ, Harrison DG. Regulation of endothelial constitutive nitric oxide synthase by protein kinase C. Hypertension 1995;25:415–420.

139. Williamson JR, Chang K, Tilton RG, et al. Increased vascular permeability in spontaneously diabetic BB/W rats and in rats with mild versus severe streptozocin-induced diabetes. Prevention by aldose reductase inhibitors and castration. Diabetes 1987;36:813–821.

140. Lynch JJ, Ferro TJ, Blumenstock FA, Brockenauer AM, Malik AB. Increased endothelial albumin permeability mediated by protein kinase C activation. J Clin Invest 1990;85:1991–1998.

141. Oliver JA. Adenylate cyclase and protein kinase C mediate opposite actions on endothelial junctions. J Cell Physiol 1990;145:536–542.

142. Wolf BA, Williamson JR, Easom RA, Chang K, Sherman WR, Turk J. Diacylglycerol accumulation and microvascular abnormalities induced by elevated glucose levels. J Clin Invest 1991;87:31–38.

143. Nagpala PG, Malik AB, Vuong PT, Lum H. Protein kinase C beta 1 overexpression augments phorbol ester-induced increase in endothelial permeability. J Cell Physiol 1996;166:249–255.

144. Aiello LP, Avery RL, Arrigg PG, et al. Vascular endothelial growth factor in ocular fluid of patients with diabetic retinopathy and other retinal disorders. N Engl J Med 1994;331:1480–1487.

145. Xia P, Aiello LP, Ishii H, et al. Characterization of vascular endothelial growth factor's effect on the activation of protein kinase C, its isoforms, and endothelial cell growth. J Clin Invest 1996;98:2018–2026.

146. Suzuma K, Takahara N, Suzuma I, et al. Characterization of protein kinase C beta isoform's action on retinoblastoma protein phosphorylation, vascular endothelial growth factor-induced endothelial cell proliferation, and retinal neovascularization. Proc Natl Acad Sci USA 2002;99:721–726.

147. Vasilets LA, Schwarz W. Structure-function relationships of cation binding in the Na+/K(+)-ATPase. Biochim Biophys Acta 1993;1154:201–222.
148. Winegrad AI. Banting lecture 1986. Does a common mechanism induce the diverse complications of diabetes? Diabetes 1987;36:396–406.
149. MacGregor LC, Matschinsky FM. Altered retinal metabolism in diabetes. II. Measurement of sodium-potassium ATPase and total sodium and potassium in individual retinal layers. J Biol Chem 1986;261:4052–4058.
150. Xia P, Kramer RM, King GL. Identification of the mechanism for the inhibition of Na+,K(+)-adenosine triphosphatase by hyperglycemia involving activation of protein kinase C and cytosolic phospholipase A2. J Clin Invest 1995;96:733–740.
151. Williamson JR, Kilo C. Extracellular matrix changes in diabetes mellitus. In: Scarpelli DG, Scarpelli GM, eds. Comparative Pathology of Major Age-Related Diseases. Alan R Liss, New York, 1984, pp. 269–288.
152. Scheinman JI, Fish AJ, Matas AJ, Michael AF. The immunohistopathology of glomerular antigens. II. The glomerular basement membrane, actomyosin, and fibroblast surface antigens in normal, diseased, and transplanted human kidneys. Am J Pathol 1978;90:71–88.
153. Bruneval P, Foidart JM, Nochy D, Camilleri JP, Bariety J. Glomerular matrix proteins in nodular glomerulosclerosis in association with light chain deposition disease and diabetes mellitus. Hum Pathol 1985;16:477–484.
154. Yamamoto T, Nakamura T, Noble NA, Ruoslahti E, Border WA. Expression of transforming growth factor beta is elevated in human and experimental diabetic nephropathy. Proc Natl Acad Sci USA 1993;90:1814–1818.
155. Sharma K, Jin Y, Guo J, Ziyadeh FN. Neutralization of TGF-beta by anti-TGF-beta antibody attenuates kidney hypertrophy and the enhanced extracellular matrix gene expression in STZ-induced diabetic mice. Diabetes 1996;45:522–530.
156. Ziyadeh FN, Sharma K, Ericksen M, Wolf G. Stimulation of collagen gene expression and protein synthesis in murine mesangial cells by high glucose is mediated by autocrine activation of transforming growth factor-beta. J Clin Invest 1994;93:536–542.
157. Bierman EL. George Lyman Duff Memorial Lecture. Atherogenesis in diabetes. Arterioscler Thromb 1992;12:647–656.
158. Sobel BE. Insulin resistance and thrombosis: a cardiologist's view. Am J Cardiol 1999;84:37J–41J.
159. Schneider DJ, Nordt TK, Sobel BE. Attenuated fibrinolysis and accelerated atherogenesis in type II diabetic patients. Diabetes 1993;42:1–7.
160. Feener EP, King GL. Vascular dysfunction in diabetes mellitus. Lancet 1997;350(Suppl 1):S19–S13.
161. Feener EP, Northrup JM, Aiello LP, King GL. Angiotensin II induces plasminogen activator inhibitor-1 and -2 expression in vascular endothelial and smooth muscle cells. J Clin Invest 1995;95:1353–1362.

3   Diabetes and Advanced Glycoxidation End-Products

Melpomeni Peppa, MD, Jaime Uribarri, MD, and Helen Vlassara, MD

INTRODUCTION

The incidence of diabetes, especially type 2 diabetes, is increasing at an alarming rate assuming epidemic proportions *(1)*. Worldwide, 124 million people had diabetes by 1997, although an estimated 221 million people will have diabetes by the year 2010 *(1)*.

Diabetic patients may suffer a number of debilitating complications such as retinopathy, nephropathy, neuropathy, and atherosclerosis resulting in cardiovascular, cerebrovascular, or peripheral vascular disease. These diabetic complications lead to huge economic and psychosocial consequences. Although the pathogenesis of type 1 diabetes is different from that of type 2 diabetes, the pathophysiology of vascular complications in the two conditions appears to be similar.

Two landmark clinical studies, the Diabetes Control and Complications Trial (DCCT) and the United Kingdom Prospective Diabetes Study, showed that intensive control of hyperglycemia could reduce the occurrence or progression of retinopathy, neuropathy and nephropathy in patients with type 1 and type 2 diabetes *(2,3)*. Although these studies reinforce the important role of hyperglycemia in the pathogenesis of diabetic complica-

From: *Contemporary Cardiology: Diabetes and Cardiovascular Disease, Second Edition*
Edited by: M. T. Johnstone and A. Veves © Humana Press Inc., Totowa, NJ

tions, the identification of the mechanisms by which hyperglycemia exerts these effects remains limited *(4)*.

It is well known that long-term hyperglycemia leads to the formation of advanced glycation or glycoxidation end-products (AGEs), which mediate most of the deleterious effects of hyperglycemia and seem to play a significant role in the pathogenesis of diabetic complications *(5,6)*. AGEs, together with the interrelated processes of oxidative stress and inflammation, may account for many of the complications of diabetes *(5,6)*. Evidence for this emerges not only from an increased number of in vitro and in vivo studies exploring the role of AGEs in different pathologies, but also from studies demonstrating significant improvement of features of diabetic complications by inhibitors of the glycoxidation process *(7–13)*.

In the following review we will provide a general overview of the nature, formation, and action of AGEs and recent evidence on their pathogenic potential in the initiation and progression of diabetic complications. We will conclude delineating possible therapeutic interventions based on this new knowledge.

ADVANCED GLYCOXIDATION END-PRODUCTS

Endogenous Advanced Glycoxidation End-Products Formation

It is now appreciated that normal living is associated with spontaneous chemical transformation of amine-containing molecules by reducing sugars in a process described since 1912 as the Maillard reaction. This process occurs constantly within the body and at an accelerated rate in diabetes *(5,6)*. Reducing sugars react in a nonenzymatic way with free amino groups of proteins, lipids, and guanyl nucleotides in DNA and form Schiff base adducts. These further rearrange to form Amadori products, which undergo rearrangement, dehydration, and condensation reactions leading to the formation of irreversible moieties called AGEs. Among all naturally occurring sugars, glucose exhibits the slowest glycation rate, although intracellular sugars such as fructose, threose, glucose-6-phosphate, and glyceraldehyde-3-phosphate form AGEs at a much faster rate *(5,6,14)*.

Faster and more efficient than the modification of proteins is the glycoxidation of lipids that contain free amines producing advanced lipoxidation end-products *(5,6,15)* (Fig. 1). AGEs such as εN-carboxymethyl-lisine (CML) can also form through autoxidation of glucose or ascorbate *(16,17)*. Metal-catalyzed autoxidation of glucose is accompanied by the generation of reactive oxygen species as superoxide radicals, which can undergo dismutation to hydrogen peroxides *(18)*. Physiological glycation processes also involve the modification of proteins by reactive oxoaldehydes that come from the degradation of glucose, Schiff base adducts, Amadori products, glycolytic intermediates, and lipid peroxidation. Among them, glyoxal, methylglyoxal (MG), and 3-deoxyglucosone have been more extensively studied. Under normal conditions, in vivo produced oxoaldehydes are metabolized and inactivated by enzymatic conversion to the corresponding aldonic acids and only a small portion proceeds to form AGEs *(5,6,19)*.

Despite the identification of numerous AGE compounds that exist in nature the elucidation of the structure of pathogenic AGEs remains elusive. Pentosidine, CML, and MG derivatives are among the well-characterized compounds *(5,6)* that are commonly used as AGE markers in many studies. AGEs are immunologically distinct, but can co-exist on the same carrier proteins such as albumin, hemoglobin, collagen, or lipoproteins at different stages of the glycation process, some more unstable than others. This adds to the challenges presented to chemists and biologists interested in their characterization.

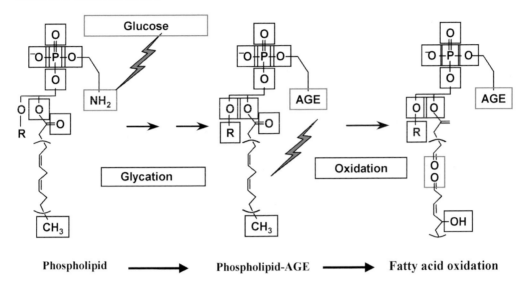

Fig. 1. Glycation and oxidation of lipids. Glycation of phospholipids containing a free amino group enhances the oxidation of the fatty acid chain (ref. *141*).

Exogenous Sources of Advanced Glycoxidation End-Products

AGEs can also be introduced in biological systems from exogenous sources. Methods of food processing (heating in particular) have a significant accelerating effect in the generation of diverse highly reactive α-β-dicarbonyl derivatives of glyco- and lipoxidation reactions that occur in complex mixtures of nutrients *(20–23)*.

About 10% of a single AGE-rich meal is absorbed into the body *(24,25)*. Food-derived AGEs, rich in MG, CML, and other derivatives, are potent inducers of oxidative stress and inflammatory processes. As with endogenous AGEs these processes can be blocked by antioxidants and anti-AGE agents *(26)*, pointing to many similarities (structural and biological) between exogenous and endogenous AGEs.

Animal studies have demonstrated the close relationship between increased dietary AGE intake and development and/or progression of many diabetes-related complications. Nephropathy, postinjury restenosis, accelerated atherosclerosis, and delayed wound healing were significantly inhibited by lowering dietary AGE intake *(27–30)*. Sebekova and associates demonstrated in the remnant-kidney rat model that feeding an AGE-rich diet for 6 weeks increases kidney weight and causes proteinuria, independent of changes in glomerular filtration rate, pointing to the detrimental effect of such diet on the kidney *(31)*. Of particular interest are studies showing that a low-glycotoxin environment can prevent or delay significantly autoimmune diabetes in successive generations of nonobese diabetic (NOD) mice *(32)* and to improve the insulin-resistant state in db/db (+/+) mice *(33)*. Reduction in exposure to exogenous AGEs of db/db (+/+) mice, lacking in leptin receptor and thus prone to insulin resistance and type 2 diabetes, led to amelioration of the insulin resistance and marked preservation of islet structure and function *(33)*.

Clinical studies have further confirmed the above laboratory data. Studies in diabetic patients with normal renal function and nondiabetic patients with chronic renal insufficiency, another condition with elevated serum AGE levels, demonstrated that lowering dietary AGE intake can significantly decrease circulating AGE levels followed by par-

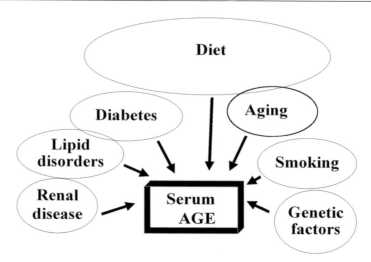

Fig. 2. Multifactorial influences determining circulating AGE levels.

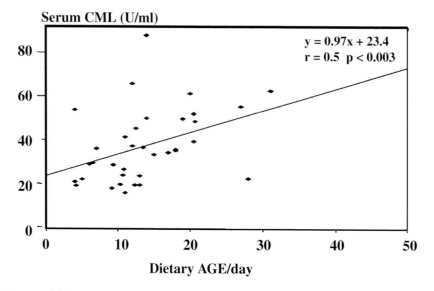

Fig. 3. Serum AGEs correlate with dietary AGE intake in humans. Association between daily dietary AGE content (assessed by dietary history) and serum AGE levels, measured as CML, in a large cross-section of chronic renal failure patients on dialysis (ref. *35*).

allel changes in circulating inflammatory markers such as C-reactive protein *(34–37)*. These preliminary but striking findings added further credence to the hypothesis that exogenous AGEs, in addition to being major determinants of the total AGE pool (Figs. 2 and 3), may be powerful modulators of the inflammatory state that is common in conditions such as chronic renal insufficiency (Fig. 4). This is highly relevant to human aging as it is associated with loss of renal function, often significant *(38)*.

Tobacco smoke is another exogenous source of AGE. Tobacco curing is essentially a Maillard "browning" reaction, as tobacco is processed in the presence of reducing sugars. Combustion of these adducts during smoking gives rise to reactive, toxic AGE formation

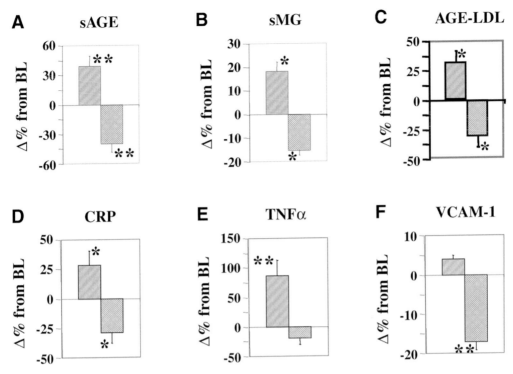

Fig. 4. Changes of circulating AGEs and markers of inflammation during dietary AGE modulation. Percent change of serum AGEs (CML, MG, and LDL-CML), C-reactive protein (CRP), tumor necrosis factor (TNF)-α and vascular adhesion molecule (VCAM)-1 in a group of stable diabetic patients fed either AGE-restricted or regular diet for up to 6 weeks (ref. *34*).

(39). Total serum AGE, or AGE-apolipoprotein (apo)-B levels have been found to be significantly higher in cigarette smokers than in nonsmokers. Smokers and especially diabetic smokers have high AGE levels in their arteries and ocular lenses *(40)*.

ADVANCED GLYCOXIDATION END-PRODUCTS METABOLISM

Steady-state serum AGE levels reflect the balance of oral intake, endogenous formation, and catabolism of AGEs. AGE catabolism is dependent on both tissue degradation and renal elimination.

Cells such as tissue macrophages can ingest and degrade AGEs via specific or nonspecific receptors *(5,6,41)*. Mesenchymal cells such as endothelial and mesangial cells seem to participate also in AGE elimination *(42)*. It has been postulated that insulin may accelerate macrophage scavenger receptor-mediated endocytic uptake of AGE proteins through the IRS/PI3 pathway *(43)*. Cellular removal of AGEs is processed largely through endocytosis and further intracellular degradation resulting in the formation of low-molecular-weight AGE peptides, which are released to the extracellular space and circulation *(5,41,44)*. These peptides undergo a variable degree of reabsorption and further catabolism in the proximal nephron and the rest is excreted in the urine. Therefore, effective AGE elimination is dependent on normal renal function *(5,41,44,45)*. We have recently found that diabetic patients with normal renal function have a significantly lower urinary AGE excretion than healthy controls. This impaired renal AGE clearance secondary to increased tubular reabsorption of AGE peptides may be a factor in the high-serum AGE levels obeserved in these patients (46).

Other intracellular protective systems also help to limit the accumulation of reactive AGE intermediates. Methylglyoxal is first converted by glyoxalase-I to S-D-lacto-ylglutathione in the presence of reduced glutathione as an essential cofactor, and then converted to D-lactate by glyoxalase-II. The significance of such systems is supported by studies in which overexpression of glyoxalase-I prevented hyperglycemia-induced AGE formation and increased macromolecular endocytosis (47). These systems, however, could still be overwhelmed by high AGE conditions such as diabetes, renal failure, or sustained excess dietary AGE intake.

ADVANCED GLYCOXIDATION END-PRODUCTS INTERACTIONS

AGEs can cause pathological changes in tissues by multiple receptor-dependent and receptor-independent processes. A characteristic of AGEs is their ability for covalent crosslink formation that leads to alterations of the structure and function of proteins (5,6,41). It is now clear that short- and long-lived molecules alike including circulating proteins, lipids, or intracellular proteins and nucleic acids can be modified (5,6,41,48). Glycation of one such molecule, low-density lipoprotein (LDL), leads to its delayed receptor-mediated clearance and subsequent deposition in the vessel wall, contributing to atherosclerosis and macrovascular disease (5,6,41,48).

Intracellular AGEs are reported to form at a rate up to 14-fold faster under high-glucose conditions, although the impact of intracellular glycation can be partially countered by the high turnover and short half-life of many cellular proteins (49).

Experimental work conducted over the last 15 years has led to the recognition of an AGE-receptor system and soluble AGE-binding proteins. The interaction of AGEs with these proteins leads either to endocytosis and degradation or to cellular activation (5,6,41). In addition to these receptor pathways, AGEs can also induce cellular activation via intracellularly generated glycoxidant derivatives or via free radical generation (5,6,41).

The first cell surface AGE-binding protein receptor identified was AGE-R1, with characteristic membrane-spanning and signal domains homologous to a 48kD component of the oligosaccharyltransferase complex-48 (5,41,50–52).This component has recently been shown to be linked to AGE removal and supression of undue oxidative stress and cell-activation events (53). An 80kD protein or AGE-R2, identical to a tyrosine-phosphorylated protein located largely within the plasma membrane was found involved in binding and forming complexes with adaptor molecules such as Shc and GRB-2. AGEs are highly efficient stimuli for AGE-R2 phosphorylation indicating its possible involvement in AGE-signaling (5,41,54–57). AGE-receptor-3 or Galectin-3, known as Mac-2 or carbohydrate-binding protein-35, is also known to interact with the β-galactoside residue of several cell surface and extracellular matrix (ECM) glycoproteins, via the carbohydrate recognition domain (5,41,54–58). AGE-R3 or Galectin-3 is only weakly detectable on cell surfaces under basal conditions, but becomes highly expressed with age and diabetes (55). AGE-R3 exhibits high-binding affinity for AGEs and appears to enhance AGE internalization and degradation in macrophages, astrocytes, and endothelial cells (5,41,54–57).

The expression of AGE receptors in mesangial cells and monocytes/macrophages in NOD mice and in diabetic patients was found to correlate with the severity of diabetic complications (5,41,52). AGE-receptor-3 knockout mice exhibited accelerated diabetic glomerulopathy, associated with marked renal/glomerular AGE accumulation implying a beneficial role for AGE-R3 in AGE clearance *(58)*. Recent in vitro studies imply a possible direct role of Galectin-3 in the pathogenesis of atherosclerosis and diabetic glomerulopathy *(5,41,57,58)*.

The receptor for advanced glycation end-products (RAGE), a well-characterized multiligand member of the immunoglobulin superfamily, is viewed as an AGE-binding intracellular signal-transducing peptide, which mediates diverse cellular responses rather than as a receptor involved in AGE endocytosis and turnover. Several other distinct ligands have been described for RAGE including amyloid, amphoterin, and S100/calgranulins *(5,41,59–62)*. RAGE is present at low levels in adult animals and humans, but is later upregulated regardless of diabetic vascular disease *(62)*. RAGE expression is increased in sites of increased AGE accumulation such as vasculature, neurons, lymphocytes, and tissue-invading mononuclear phagocytes. In the kidney, RAGE is expressed in glomerular visceral epithelial cells (podocytes) but not in mesangium or glomerular endothelium *(59)*. Diabetic RAGE-transgenic mice exhibit renal vascular changes characteristic of diabetic nephropathy *(60)*. In contrast, brief infusion of a soluble truncated RAGE is reported to intercept diverse processes such as endothelial leakage, atherosclerosis, and inflammatory bowel disease *(59)*.

Other well-studied AGE-binding molecules are the macrophage scavenger receptors, class A (MSR-A) and class B (MSR-B). MSR-A, better known as receptors for oxidized LDL may also play a role in endocytic uptake and degradation of AGE-proteins in vivo *(5,41,63,64)*. CD36, a member of MSR-B receptors, is a highly glycosylated 88-kD protein expressed on macrophages which, although not restricted to AGE uptake, may contribute to AGE-mediated foam cell formation *(65)*. The class B type I scavenger receptor (SR-BI) is also considered as an AGE-interactive molecule; it is suggested that it contributes to reverse cholesterol transport by suppressing selective uptake of high-density lipoprotein cholesterol efflux (HDL-CE) by liver and cholesterol efflux from peripheral cells to HDL *(66)*. Additionally, recently cloned LOX-1 and SREC, novel scavenger receptors expressed in vascular endothelial cells are awaiting studies to determine their affinity for AGE-proteins *(67)*.

Another molecule with significant AGE-binding affinity and intriguing anti-AGE properties is lysozyme. Lysozyme is a well-characterized natural host-defense protein thought to exert antibacterial effects through the catalytic degradation of the peptidoglycan component of the bacterial wall *(68)*. Lysozyme is found in saliva, nasal secretions, milk, mucus, serum, and in lysosomes of neutrophils and macrophages. Against all predictions, however, a novel AGE-binding site was mapped to a 17–18 amino acid hydrophilic domain (ABCD motif or AGE-binding cysteine-bounded domain), bounded on both sides by cysteines and located within one of the two lysozyme catalytic regions *(68)*. Lysozyme enhances the uptake and degradation of AGE proteins by macrophages, apparently via an AGE-specific receptor pathway not well defined thus far *(68)*. Lysozyme administration to diabetic mice, however, increases AGE clearance, suppresses macrophage and mesangial cell-specific gene activation in vitro, and improves albuminuria, thus presenting an unusual combination of advantages, which have stimulated interest in this native substance as a potential therapeutic target *(69)*. A novel receptor that mediates AGE-induced chemotaxis in rabbit smooth muscle cells has also been identified *(70)*.

The genomic organization, chromosomal location, and several prevalent gene polymorphisms of some of the AGE-R-related molecules have come to light in the past few years. For instance, a recent screening using single-strand conformational polymorphism analysis and direct sequencing of allelic polymerase chain reaction fragments in 48 type 1 diabetics with or without nephropathy showed variants of AGE receptors, mutations, and polymorphisms that correlated with the presence and the severity of complications, albeit only weakly *(71)*.

ADVANCED GLYCOXIDATION END-PRODUCTS AND DIABETIC MICROANGIOPATHY

Diabetic microangiopathy is a broad term that describes changes in microvascular beds in which endothelium and associated mural cells function are progressively disrupted, resulting in occlusion, ischemia, and organ damage. Although kidney and retina are most commonly affected, diabetic microangiopathy can occur in a wide range of tissues such as peripheral nerves and skin *(4)*. A large number of studies have supported the pathogenic role of AGE in diabetic microangiopathy *(4–6,41)*, even as their exact role is still under investigation.

Diabetic Nephropathy

The prevalence of diabetic nephropathy has increased dramatically and is now the first cause of end-stage renal disease requiring renal replacement therapy worldwide *(72)*. Although the genetic background is important in determining susceptibility to diabetic nephropathy, exposure to chronic hyperglycemia leading to the subsequent activation of multiple pathogenic pathways appears to be the main initiating factor *(2,3,4–6,41)*.

Diabetic nephropathy occurs in up to 30%–40% of diabetic patients. The initial abnormalities include glomerular hyperfiltration and hyperperfusion resulting in microalbuminuria, increased glomerular basement membrane thickening, and mesangial ECM deposition. These processes are followed by mesangial hypertrophy, diffuse and nodular glomerulosclerosis, tubulointerstitial fibrosis, and eventually progressive renal failure *(73)*.

In Vitro Data

The ability to culture cells that are affected by AGEs has provided an important insight into the mechanisms of action of these adducts, their receptors and the way they may contribute to tissue dysfunction in diabetes. In vitro, AGEs bind to renal mesangial cells through AGE receptors, which initiate overproduction of matrix proteins and changes in the expression of matrix metalloproteinases and proteinase inhibitors *(74,75)*. Exposure of rat mesangial cells to AGE-rich proteins results in mesangial oxidative stress and activation of RAGE or other processes, e.g., protein kinase C-β *(76)* or angiotensin II causing, for instance, in vitro inhibition of nephrin gene expression *(77)* or induction of apoptosis and secretion of vascular endothelin growth factor (VEGF) and monocyte chemotactic peptide-1 proteins, events that were prevented by *N*-acetylcysteine *(78)*. AGEs also stimulate production of collagen IV and fibronectin in glomerular endothelial cells *(79)*.

Animal Studies

Immunohistochemical studies of kidneys from normal and diabetic rats show that glomerular basement membrane, mesangium, podocytes, and renal tubular cells accumulate high levels of AGEs with AGE concentrations rising with age and more rapidly with diabetes *(80,81)*. Moreover, the intensity of CML immunostaining is greatest in the areas of extensive glomerular sclerosis characteristic of advanced diabetic nephropathy *(82)*.

Short-term exogenous AGE administration to normal, nondiabetic animals has reproduced some of the vascular defects associated with clinical diabetic nephropathy including induction of basement membrane components (e.g., α1-collagen IV) or transforming growth factor (TGF)-β *(82,83)*. Furthermore, chronic treatment of animals with AGE albumin can reproduce glomerular hypertrophy, basement membrane thickening, extracellular mesangial matrix expansion and albuminuria, all consistent with findings of diabetic nephropathy *(82,83)*.

The role of AGEs in the pathogenesis of diabetic nephropathy has been supported by studies in transgenic animals. RAGE overexpression in diabetic mice resulted in increased albuminuria, elevated serum creatinine, renal hypertrophy, mesangial expansion, and glomerulosclerosis *(60)*, although blockade of RAGE by soluble truncated RAGE suppressed structural and functional components associated with nephropathy in db/db mice *(58)*.

AGE inhibitors have been shown to prevent AGE accumulation in renal structures and diabetic nephropathy in diabetic animal models *(84–87)*. Aminoguanidine ameliorated overexpression of α1-type IV collagen, laminin B1, TGF-β, and platelet-derived growth factor, all associated with glomerular hypertrophy *(87)*. ORB-9195 administration to diabetic rats resulted in a reduction in the progression of diabetic nephropathy by blocking type IV collagen and overproduction of TGF-β and VEGF *(88)*. In the same context, the AGE-breaker, ALT-711, has also been shown to afford renoprotection to diabetic animals *(89)*.

HUMAN STUDIES

Biopsy samples from kidneys from diabetic subjects have demonstrated increased AGE deposition at AGE-specific binding sites throughout the renal cortex *(90,91)*. Specific AGE compounds (e.g., CML, pyralline, and pentosidine) have been identified in renal tissue of diabetics with or without end-stage renal disease; AGE accumulation appeared to parallel the severity of diabetic nephropathy *(92)*. Also, whereas low-level RAGE expression in normal control human subjects was restricted to podocytes, glomeruli of patients with diabetic nephropathy demonstrated diffuse upregulation of RAGE expression in podocytes, colocalizing with synaptopodin expression *(93)*. A recent study in kidney biopsies from patients with diabetic nephropathy showed significant reduction of nephrin, an important regulator of the glomerular filter integrity. In the same study, cultured podocytes showed significant downregulation in nephrin expression when glycated albumin was added *(77)*.

In a clinical study of type 1 diabetic patients serum levels of AGEs increased significantly as patients progressed from normal to microalbuminuria, clinical nephropathy and hemodialysis and correlated positively with urinary albumin excretion *(94)*.

Diabetic Retinopathy

Diabetic retinopathy occurs in three-fourths of all persons with diabetes for more than 15 years *(95)* and is the most common cause of blindness in the industrialized world *(96)*. It is primarily a disease of the intraretinal blood vessels, which become dysfunctional in response to hyperglycemia with progressive loss of retinal pericytes and eventually endothelial cells leading to capillary closure and widespread retinal ischemia *(97)*.

It has been shown that AGEs disturb retinal microvascular homeostasis by inducing pericyte apoptosis and VEGF overproduction *(98)*. In vitro work in bovine retinal endothelial cells showed that AGEs induced VEGF overproduction through generation of oxidative stress and downstream activation of the protein kinase C pathway *(99)*. In vitro studies in retinal organ cultures showed increased glyoxal-induced CML formation, a dose-dependent induction of apoptotic molecules and increased cell death, events that were prevented by anti-AGE agents and antioxidants *(100)*.

AGEs were found to retard the growth of pericytes and exert an acute toxicity to these cells *(98)*. In vitro, rat retinal vascular cells exposed to AGE show abnormal endothelial nitric oxide synthase expression, which may account for some of the vasoregulatory abnormalities observed in the diabetic vasculature *(101)*. In vitro studies in human donor eyes showed that vitreous collagen undergoes glycation as well as copper and iron glycoxidation, leading to structural and functional impairment and possibly retinopathy *(102)*.

Within a few months of diabetes, AGEs are already found to accumulate in vascular basement membrane and retinal pericytes of rats *(103)*.

When nondiabetic animals were infused with AGEs for several weeks, significant amounts of these adducts distributed around and within the pericytes, colocalized with AGE receptors and induced basement membrane thickening *(104)* leading to loss of retinal pericytes *(105)*. In contrast, the inhibition of AGE formation by aminoguanidine, a well known AGE inhibitor, prevented microaneurysm formation, endothelial proliferation, and pericyte loss *(97)*. A combination of antioxidants and AGE inhibitors has been shown to prevent AGE-induced apoptosis in primary (rat) retinal organ cultures *(100)*, although the administration of monoclonal antibodies, which recognize Amadori-modified glycated albumin, reduced the thickening of the retinal basement membrane in db/db mice, implying that even early glycated adducts may play a role in diabetic retinopathy *(104)*. More studies are needed to confirm these data, however.

A study comparing postmortem human retinas between diabetic subjects with diabetic retinopathy and nondiabetic subjects, found that CML and VEGF immunoreactivities, which were not evident in the control subjects, were distributed around blood vessels of diabetic retinas. Both VEGF and CML expression was greater in subjects with proliferative diabetic retinopathy *(106)*. These data suggest that CML could have a role in VEGF expression in diabetic retinopathy.

In a clinical study of type 1 diabetics (38 males and 47 females) a significant elevation of serum AGE levels was found associated with severe diabetic retinopathy. CML-AGE levels were also increased at the stage of simple diabetic retinopathy suggesting a possible role of CML in the early phases of this condition *(92)*.

Similarly, increased pentosidine levels were found in the majority of vitreous samples from diabetic patients with diabetic retinopathy compared to controls indicating that glycation occurs and is accelerated in human diabetic vitreous *(107)*. This was further confirmed in another clinical study which involved 72 type 2 diabetics, in which sugar-induced AGEs correlated with the severity of retinopathy *(108)*.

Diabetic Neuropathy

About half of all people with diabetes experience some degree of diabetic neuropathy, which can present either as polyneuropathy or mononeuropathy *(109)*. Diabetic neuropathy can also affect the central and the autonomic nervous systems. Level of hyperglycemia seems to determine the onset and progression of diabetic neuropathy *(110,111)*.

In vitro studies have shown that glycation of cytoskeletal proteins such as tubulin, actin, and neurofilament results in slow axonal transport, atrophy, and degeneration *(110)*. Additionally, glycation of laminin, an important constituent of Schwann cell basal laminae, impairs its ability to promote nerve fiber regeneration *(111)*. The process of glycation increases the permeability of proteins, albumin, nerve growth factor, and immunoglobulin G across the blood–nerve barrier *(112)* leading to protein accumulation in the central nervous system *(113)*.

Diabetic rats show reduction in sensory motor conduction velocities and nerve action potentials and reduction in peripheral nerve blood flow and all these abnormalities can be prevented by pretreatment with anti-AGE agents such as aminoguanidine *(114,115)*. Pentosidine content was increased in cytoskeletal proteins of the sciatic nerve of streptozotocin induced diabetic rats and decreased after islet transplantation *(111)*.

Pentosidine content was found elevated in cytoskeletal and myelin protein extracts of sural nerve from human subjects *(116)*. The sural and peroneal nerves of human diabetic subjects contain AGEs in the perineurium, endothelial cells, pericytes of endoneural microvessels, and in myelinated and unmyelinated fibers; a significant correlation has been observed between the intensity of CML accumulation and myelinated fiber loss *(117)*. At the submicroscopic level, AGE deposition appeared focally, as irregular aggregates in the cytoplasm of endothelial cells, pericytes, axoplasm and Schwan cells of both myelinated and unmyelinated fibers. Interstitial collagen and basement membrane of the perineurium also exhibited similar deposits. The excessive accumulation of intra and extracellular AGEs in human diabetic peripheral nerve supports the view of a causative role for these substances in the development of diabetic neuropathy *(117)*. Furthermore, AGE accumulation in the vasa nervorum could worsen wall thickening with occlusion and ischemia and secondarily segmental demyelination *(118)*.

Diabetic Dermopathy

Skin, like other tissues, accumulates glycoxidation products in diabetes *(119–121)*, which can account for alterations in physicochemical properties leading to the diabetic skin-related disorders *(61,122)*. AGE-related changes on diabetic skin are similar to those observed in aged skin and include altered tissue oxygen delivery *(123)*, growth factor activity *(124–127)*, vascular, skin, fibroblast, and inflammatory cell dysfunction *(128–131)*, increased metalloproteinase production *(132)*, and defective collagen remodeling *(122–130)*. In skin, inhibitors of AGE formation, such as aminoguanidine were shown to prevent AGE accumulation and subsequent collagen crosslinking, to improve angiogenesis and to restore the activity of various growth factors *(133–137)*.

From a pathogenic point of view, through the above described effects, AGEs could partially explain the delayed wound healing observed in diabetes. Recently, it has been showed that dietary AGEs can modify wound healing rate in db/db (+/+) mice by altering the total body AGE burden *(32)*. Another study has shown acceleration of wound healing in db/db mice by RAGE-receptor blockade further supporting a role for AGEs in the pathogenesis of delayed diabetic wound healing *(61)*.

ADVANCED GLYCOXIDATION END-PRODUCTS AND MACROANGIOPATHY

The two most frequent patterns of macrovascular disease are atherosclerosis, which leads to thickening of the intima, plaque formation, and eventual occlusion of the vascular lumen and stiffness of the arterial wall, which leads to ventricular hypertrophy. Based on the existing literature, AGEs play a significant role in the pathogenesis of both manifestations of cardiovascular disease (CVD).

In Vitro Studies

In vitro studies have shown that AGEs have complex properties that promote vascular disease including an ability to form chemically irreversible intra- and intermolecular crosslinks with matrix proteins in the vascular wall increasing arterial rigidity *(5,138)*. Also, the interaction of AGEs with endothelial cell receptors induces increased vascular permeability, increases procoagulant activity, migration of macrophages and T-lympho-cytes into the intima (initiating a subtle inflammatory response), and impairment of endothelium-dependent relaxation *(139)*. Impaired endothelial relaxation and endothe-lial migration of monocytes are generally considered to be among the first steps in atherogenesis. At the same time, AGE-induced activation of monocyte/macrophages leads to the release of a variety of inflammatory cytokines and growth factors, which induce over production of extracellular vascular wall matrix *(5,140)*.

Glycoxidation of LDL cholesterol makes this molecule less recognizable by the native LDL receptor, which results in delayed clearance, increased plasma levels and eventually enhanced uptake of cholesterol by the scavenger receptors on macrophages and vascular smooth muscle cells. This process, finally, results in lipid-laden foam cells formation in the arterial intima and atherosclerosis *(5,48,141)*. Glycated LDL has also been shown to stimulate production of plasminogen activator inhibitor-1 (PAI-1) and to reduce genera-tion of tissue plasminogen activator (tPA) in cultured human vascular endothelial cells *(142)*. These effects that could potentially increase thrombotic vascular complications in vivo were prevented by treatment with aminoguanidine.

Regarding HDL the net effect of glycation on this molecule is altered lipoprotein function and decreased ability to prevent monocyte adhesion to aortic endothelial cells, an important initial event in the development of atherosclerosis *(143)*. The physiological significance of this finding, however, remains to be further substantiated. Additionally, in vitro glycation of lipoprotein(a), an independent risk factor for CVD, has been shown to amplify lipoprotein(a)-induced production of PAI-1 and further reduced tPA genera-tion from vascular endothelial cells *(144,145)*.

More recently it has become apparent that the vascular wall also produces superoxide, mostly via enzymes similar to the neutrophil oxidase. All cell types in the vascular wall produce reactive oxygen species (ROS) derived from superoxide-generating protein complexes similar to the leukocyte nicotinamide adenine dinucleotide phosphate oxi-dase. AGE have been shown to enhance vascular oxidase activity *(146)* and increased vascular oxidase activity has been associated with diabetes *(147)*.

Animal Studies

Indirect evidence for AGE involvement in CVD emerges from histological studies that show increased AGE deposits in aortic atherosclerotic lesions, even in the absence of diabetes *(140,148)*. These AGE deposits correlate with the degree of atheroma *(146)*. In more direct experiments, prolonged intravenous infusion of glycated rabbit serum albu-min into nondiabetic rabbits promoted intimal thickening of the aorta *(149)*. Additional-ly, exogenous administration of AGE-modified albumin in healthy nondiabetic rats and rabbits was correlated with significantly increased AGE levels (approximately sixfold) in aortic tissue samples and increased vascular permeability together with markedly defective vasodilatory responses to acetylcholine and nitroglycerin. These abnormalities were prevented or reduced by the combined administration of aminoguanidine *(150)*. Infusion of diabetic red blood cells (carrying AGEs) into normal rats increased vascular

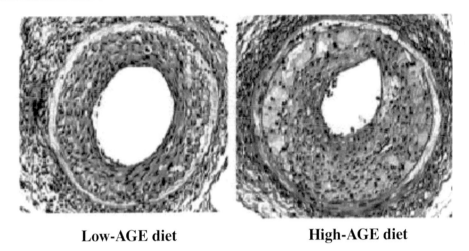

Low-AGE diet   **High-AGE diet**

Fig. 5. Dietary AGE restriction and neointimal proliferation in apolipoprotein E-deficient non-db mice. A, low AGE diet. B, regular AGE diet (ref. *28*).

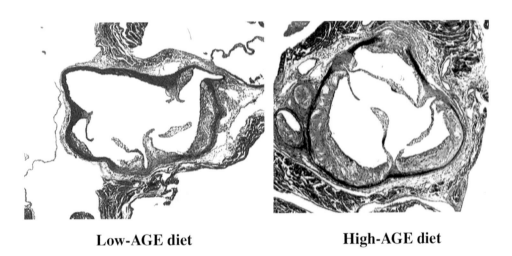

Low-AGE diet   **High-AGE diet**

Fig. 6. Dietary AGE restriction prevents atheroma formation in apoE knock out mice. A, low AGE diet. B, high AGE diet (ref. *29*).

permeability in these animals and this effect was prevented by blockade of RAGE *(151)*. Local application of AGEs to the vessel wall-enhanced intimal hyperplasia, independently of diabetes or hypercholesterolemia, in a model of atherosclerosis in the rabbit *(152)*.

In recent studies, dietary AGE restriction was associated with significant reduction in circulating AGE levels and a significant reduction in neointimal formation, 4 weeks after arterial injury in apo-E knockout mice (Fig. 5). This study also showed markedly decreased macrophage infiltration in the lesioned areas of the vessel wall *(28)*. Additionally, after 8 weeks on the low AGE diet, diabetic apo-E knockout mice showed significant suppression of atherosclerotic lesions accompanied by reduced circulating AGE levels and decreased expression of inflammatory molecules *(29)* (Fig. 6). These studies support the view that exogenous AGEs have a significant vasculotoxic effect.

Inhibition of AGE formation by aminoguanidine has been shown to lead to reduced atherosclerotic plaque formation in cholesterol-fed rabbits *(140,153)*. Aminoguanidine administration to rats has been shown to prevent diabetes-induced formation of fluorescent AGE and crosslinking of arterial wall connective tissue proteins *(153)*. Oral administration of 2-isopropylidenehydrazono-4-oxo-thiazolidin-5-ylacetanilide (OPB-9195), an inhibitor of both glycoxidation and lipoxidation reactions in rats, following balloon injury of the carotid artery, effectively prevented the intimal thickening that typically accompanies this injury *(7)*. These studies support a causative role for AGEs in atherosclerosis.

Treatment of apo-E deficient diabetic mice with the soluble extracellular domain of RAGE also suppressed diabetic atherosclerosis in a glycemia- and lipid-independent manner *(154)*.

Treatment of rats with streptozotocin-induced diabetes with the AGE-breaker ALT-711 for 1–3 weeks reversed the diabetes-induced increase of large artery stiffness as measured by systemic arterial compliance, aortic impedance, and carotid artery compliance and distensibility *(8)*. Administration of the same compound produced significant improvement of diabetes-induced myocardial structural changes in rats with streptozotocin-induced diabetes *(155)*. N-Phenylthiazolium bromide (PTB), another AGE breaker, has led to marked reduction in AGE-collagen from tail tendons in rats *(13)*. These findings support the role of AGE accumulation in causing arterial stiffness.

Treatment of diabetic rats with hydralazine and olmesartan showed equal renoprotective effect despite differential effect on the renin–angiotensin system. The fact that both drugs effectively suppress AGE formation suggests a critical role for AGEs in this nephropathy model *(156)*.

Human Studies

Currently, human studies provide only indirect support for a role of AGEs in initiating CVD. Long-term interventional trials will be able to prove this link. Highly suggestive of such role are the findings of AGE deposits in the atherosclerotic plaque of arteries from diabetic patients *(157,158)*, and chronic renal failure patients with or without diabetes *(159)*. An autopsy study showed increased colocalized deposition of AGE and apo-B in aortic atherosclerotic lesions in end-stage renal disease patients with or without diabetes compared to controls. These deposits correlated with the duration of hemodialysis, but not with the duration of diabetes *(160)*. A significant correlation between serum AGE-apo-B levels, tissue accumulation of AGE-collagen and severity of atherosclerotic lesions has been described in a group of nondiabetic patients with coronary artery occlusive disease requiring bypass surgery *(159)*. Histological sections of human aortas obtained from postpartem examination of diabetic subjects showed a correlation between AGE tissue accumulation and aortic stiffness *(161)*. A significant CML deposition in atherosclerotic plaques was also observed that correlated with the extent of the atherosclerotic changes. Moreover, AGE receptors were identified in the cellular components of the lesions with the same distribution pattern as AGE *(162)*.

A cross-sectional study showed that type 2 diabetic patients had increased serum AGE levels and impaired endothelium-dependent and endothelium-independent vasodilatation compared to healthy control subjects. Data analysis showed a significant inverse correlation between serum AGE levels and endothelium-dependent vasodilatation of the brachial artery, a well-established marker of early atherosclerosis. In multiple regression analysis, serum AGE levels were the only factors, which correlated independently with the endothelium-dependent vasodilatation *(163)*.

Administration of an AGE-restricted diet for several weeks in a group of diabetic patients was associated with significant reduction of serum levels of AGEs and vascular cell adhesion molecule-1, an indicator of endothelial dysfunction *(34)*. A recent abstract reported acute endothelial dysfunction in response to the ingestion of an AGE-rich beverage in diabetic subjects *(164)*. An obvious implication of these striking results is that a low AGE diet would reverse endothelial dysfunction among diabetes patients, but this remains to be further proven.

Arterial stiffness increases with duration of diabetes largely as the result of the effect of AGE on connective tissue and matrix components *(165)*. Oral administration of ALT-711, a novel nonenzymatic breaker of AGE crosslinks, significantly improved arterial compliance and decreased pulse pressure in older individuals with vascular stiffening compared to placebo *(9)*. These results strongly suggest that AGE have a pathogenic role in arterial stiffness.

ANTIADVANCED GLYCOXIDATION END-PRODUCT STRATEGIES

As the understanding of the biology of AGE has evolved, new strategies to forestall their adverse effects have developed. Several approaches seeking to decrease exogenous AGE intake, decrease or inhibit endogenous AGE formation, reduce AGE effects on cells, and break pre-existing AGE crosslinks have been explored.

Diet

As diet provides a significant source of exogenous AGE, recent work has focused on determining whether it represents a modifiable risk factor for the development of AGE-induced pathology. In vivo studies have demonstrated that the typical diabetes-related structural changes seen in experimental animals fed with standard AGE-enriched diets could be prevented by dietary AGE restriction *(27–30)*. A recent 6-week study in diabetic patients compared the effects of two nutritionally equivalent diets differing only by their AGE content and demonstrated 30%–50% reduction of serum AGE levels and a significant reduction in the levels of inflammatory factors in the subjects receiving the diet with low AGE content *(34)*. A significant reduction of circulating AGE levels was also observed in a study including nondiabetic renal failure patients undergoing peritoneal dialysis treatment *(35–37)*. These studies support the notion of a significant contribution of dietary AGE intake to the body pool of AGE and make evident that dietary AGE restriction is a feasible and safe strategy to decrease the body AGE burden.

Metabolic Factors

As hyperglycemia enhances AGE formation it is obvious that intensive treatment of hyperglycemia can modify the body AGE pool. Indeed, diabetic rats with good metabolic control exhibited lower levels of pentosidine, and lower intensity of collagen-linked fluorescence glycation and oxidation compared to rats with bad metabolic control *(166)*. Skin collagen glycation, glycoxidation, and crosslinking were lower in a large group of type 1 diabetic patients under long-term intensive vs conventional treatment, as was shown in a cohort of patients studied in the DCCT *(119)*.

Antioxidants

Several studies have proposed various antioxidants as anti-AGE agents, including vitamin E *(167)*, *N*-acetylcysteine *(168)*, taurine *(169)*, α-lipoic acid *(170)*, penicillamine *(171)*, and nicarnitine *(172)*. Also, pyruvate is a potent scavenger of ROS such as H_2O_2 and O_2^- that also minimizes the production of OH by the Haber-Weiss reaction. Additionally, it inhibits the initial reaction of glucose with free amino groups that results in Schiff base formation, as documented by in vitro data *(173,174)*. Despite the existing data, however, further studies are needed to establish the effectiveness of treatment with antioxidants as a strategy in reducing AGE levels.

Agents That Prevent Advanced Glycoxidation End-Products Formation

A large number of in vitro and in vivo studies have been conducted using agents that prevent AGE formation to modify diabetic complications. These agents act by inhibiting postAmadori advanced glycation reactions or by trapping carbonyl intermediates (glyoxal, methylglyoxal, 3-deoxyglucosone) and thus inhibiting both advanced glycation and lipoxidation reactions. Aminoguanidine *(11,13)*, ALT-946 *(11,175,176)*, 2-3-Diaminophenazine *(11,177)*, thiamine pyrophosphate *(178)*, benfotiamine *(179,180)*, and pyridoxamine *(181–183)* constitute known representatives of the first group of agents, although ORB-9195 is a derivative-representative of the second group of agents *(7,184–186)*.

Advanced Glycoxidation End-Product Crosslink Breakers

Recently, a promising therapeutic strategy has been to attack the irreversible intermolecular AGE crosslinks formed in biological systems providing prevention or reversal of various diabetes- and aging-related complications. This approach aims to "break" preaccumulated AGE and help renal elimination of resulting smaller peptides. PTB was originally studied *(187)* and more recently ALT-711 *(8,13,188)*. Long-term studies are in progress to establish the safety of this new category of anti-AGE agents

Advanced Glycoxidation End-Products Antibody (A717)

A monoclonal antibody that neutralizes the effects of excess glycated albumin has been studied and shown to offer significant primary or secondary prevention of diabetic nephropathy *(189,190)*.

Antihypertensive Agents

Recently, losartan and olmesartan, antihypertensive drugs known to act through angiotensin receptor inhibition, have been shown to decrease AGE formation *(191)*. Hydralazine, another antihypertensive agent whose effect does not involve the renin–angiotensin system, has AGE-inhibitory effects similar to those of low-dose olmesartan *(192)*. The renoprotective effects shown by these drugs suggest that they derive not only from the drugs effect on lowering blood pressure and blocking angiotensin but also from reduced AGE formation *(193)*.

CONCLUSIONS

An increasing body of evidence indicates that AGEs play a significant role in the pathogenesis of diabetic complications. Further studies, however, are still needed to elucidate the exact role of AGEs in this area. More importantly, as these studies progress, new approaches to therapy to reduce the life-threatening impact of these complications would develop. Dietary restriction of AGE intake appears as a novel and important intervention tool that deserves further development.

REFERENCES

1. Amos AF, McCarty DJ, Zimmet P. The rising global burden of diabetes and its complications estimates and projections to the year 2010. Diabet Med 1997;14(Suppl 5):S1–S85.
2. DCCT Research Group. The effect of intensive treatment of diabetes on the development and progression of long-term complications in insulin-dependent diabetes mellitus. N Engl J Med 1993;329:977.
3. Intensive blood-glucose control with sulphonylureas or insulin compared with conventional treatment and risk of complications in patients with type 2 diabetes (UKPDS 33). UK Prospective Diabetes Study (UKPDS) Group. Lancet 1998;352(9131):837–853.
4. Brownlee M. Biochemistry and molecular cell biology of diabetic complications. Nature 2001; 414(6865):813–820.
5. Vlassara H, Palace MR. Diabetes and advanced glycation endproducts. J Intern Med 2002;251(2):87–101.
6. Thorpe SR, Baynes JW. Role of the Maillard reaction in diabetes mellitus and diseases of aging. Drugs Aging 1996;9(2):69–77.
7. Miyata T, Ishikawa S, Asahi K, et al. 2-Isopropylidenehydrazono-4-oxo-thiazolidin-5-phenylacetanilide (OPB-9195) treatment inhibits the development of intimal thickening after balloon injury of rat carotid artery: role of glycoxidation and lipoxidation reactions in vascular tissue damage. FEBS Lett 1999;445(1):202–206.
8. Wolffenbuttel BH, Boulanger CM, Crijns FR, et al. Breakers of advanced glycation end products restore large artery properties in experimental diabetes. Proc Natl Acad Sci USA 1998;95(8):4630–4634.
9. Kass DA, Sapiro EP, Kawaguchi M, et al. Improved arterial compliance by a novel advanced glycation end-product crosslink breaker. Circulation 2001;104:1464–1470.
10. Nakayama M, Izumi G, Nemoto Y, et al. Suppression of N(epsilon)-(carboxymethyl)lysine generation by the antioxidant N-acetylcysteine. Perit Dial Int 1999;19(3):207–210.
11. Soulis T, Sastra S, Thallas V, et al. A novel inhibitor of advanced glycation end-product formation inhibits mesenteric vascular hypertrophy in experimental diabetes. Diabetologia 1999;42(4):472–479.
12. Asif M, Egan J, Vasan S, et al. An advanced glycation endproduct cross-link breaker can reverse age-related increases in myocardial stiffness. Proc Natl Acad Sci USA 2000;97(6):2809–2813.
13. Vasan S, Foiles PG, Founds, HW. Therapeutic potential of AGE inhibitors and breakers of AGE protein cross-links. Expert Opin Investig Drugs 2001;10(11):1977–1987.
14. Suarez G, Rajaram R, Oronsky AL, Gawinowicz MA. Nonenzymatic glycation of bovine serum albumin by fructose (fructation). Comparison with the Maillard reaction initiated by glucose. J Biol Chem 1989;264(7):3674–3679.
15. Fu MX, Requena JR, Jenkins AJ, Lyons TJ, Baynes JW, Thorpe SR. The advanced glycation end product, Nepsilon-(carboxymethyl)lysine, is a product of both lipid peroxidation and glycoxidation reactions. J Biol Chem 1996;271(17):9982.
16. Wolff SP, Dean RT. Glucose autoxidation and protein modification. The potential role of 'autoxidative glycosylation' in diabetes. Biochem J 1987;245(1):243–250.
17. Dunn JA, Ahmed MU, Murtiashaw MH, et al. Reaction of ascorbate with lysine and protein under autoxidizing conditions: formation of N epsilon-(carboxymethyl)lysine by reaction between lysine and products of autoxidation of ascorbate. Biochemistry 1990;29(49):10964–10970.
18. Hunt JV, Simpson JA, Dean RT. Hydroperoxide-mediated fragmentation of proteins. Biochem J 1988;250(1):87–93.
19. Thornalley PJ, Langborg A, Minhas HS. Formation of glyoxal, methylglyoxal and 3-deoxyglucosone in the glycation of proteins by glucose. Biochem J 1999;344(1):109–116.
20. Lee T, Kimiagar M, Pintauro SJ, Chichester CO. Physiological and safety aspects of Maillard browning of foods. Prog Food Nutr Sci 1981;5:243–256.
21. O'Brien J, Morrissey PA. Nutritional and toxicological aspects of the Maillard browning reaction in foods. Crit Rev Food Sci Nutr 1989;28:211–248.
22. Pellegrino L, Cattaneo S. Occurrence of galactosyl isomaltol and galactosyl beta-pyranone in commercial drinking milk. Nahrung 2001;45(3):195–200.
23. Henle T. A food chemist's view of advanced glycation end-products. Perit Dial Int 2001;21(Suppl 3):S125–S130.

24. Koschinsky T, He CJ, Mitsuhashi T, et al. Orally absorbed reactive advanced glycation end products (glycotoxins): an environmental risk factor in diabetic nephropathy. Proc Natl Acad Sci USA 1997;94:6474–6479.
25. He C, Sabol J, Mitsuhashi T, Vlassara H. Dietary glycotoxins: Inhibition of reactive products by aminoguanidine facilitates renal clearance and reduces tissue sequestration. Diabetes 1999;48:1308–1315.
26. Cai W, Cao Q, Zhu L, Peppa M, He C, Vlassara H. Oxidative stress-inducing carbonyl compounds from common foods: Novel mediators of cellular dysfunction. Mol Med 2002;8(7):337–346.
27. Zheng F, He C, Cai W, Hattori M, Steffes M, Vlassara H. Prevention of diabetic nephropathy in mice by a diet low in glycoxidation products. Diabetes Metab Res Rev 2002;18(3):224–237.
28. Lin RY, Reis ED, Dore AT, et al. Lowering of dietary advanced glycation endproducts (AGE) reduces neointimal formation after arterial injury in genetically hypercholesterolemic mice. Atherosclerosis 2002;163(2):303–311.
29. Lin RY, Choudhury RP, Cai W, et al. Dietary glycotoxins promote diabetic atherosclerosis in apolipoprotein E-deficient mice. Atherosclerosis 2003;168:213–220.
30. Peppa M, Brem H, Ehrlich P, et al. Adverse effects of dietary glycotoxins in genetically diabetic mice. Diabetes 2003;52:2805–2813.
31. Sebekova K, Faist V, Hofmann T, Schinzel R, Heidland A. Effects of a diet rich in advanced glycation end products in the rat remnant kidney model. Am J Kidney Dis 2003;41(3 Suppl 1):S48–S51
32. Peppa M, He C, Hattori M, et al. Fetal or neonatal low-glycotoxin environment prevents autoimmune diabetes in NOD mice. Diabetes 2003;52(6):1441–1448.
33. Hofmann SM, Dong HJ, Li Z, et al. Improved insulin sensitivity is associated with restricted intake of dietary glycoxidation products in the db/db mouse. Diabetes 2002;51(7):2082–2089.
34. Vlassara H, Cai W, Crandall J, et al. Inflammatory markers are induced by dietary glycotoxins: A pathway for accelerated atherosclerosis in diabetes. Proc Natl Acad Sci 2002;99(24):15,596–15,601.
35. Uribarri J, Peppa M, Cai W, et al. Dietary glycotoxins correlate with circulating advanced glycation end product levels in renal failure patients. J Am Kid Dis 2003;42(3):532–538.
36. Uribarri J, Peppa M, Cai W, et al. Restriction of dietary glycotoxins markedly reduces AGE toxins in renal failure patients. J Am Soc Nephrol 2003;14(3):728–731.
37. Peppa M, Uribarri J, Cai W, Lu M, Vlassara H. Glycoxidation and inflammation in renal failure patients. J Am Kid Dis 2004;43(4):690–696.
38. Swedko PJ, Clark HD, Paramsothy K, Akbari A. Serum creatinine is an inadequate screening test for renal failure in elderly patients. Arch Intern Med 2003;163:356–360.
39. Nicholl ID, Bucala R. Advanced glycation endproducts and cigarette smoking. Cell Mol Biol (Noisy-le-grand) 1998;44(7):1025–1033.
40. Nicholl ID, Stitt AW, Moore JE, et al. Increased levels of advanced glycation endproducts in the lenses and blood vessels of cigarette smokers. Mol Med 1998;4(9):594–601.
41. Vlassara H. The AGE-receptor in the pathogenesis of diabetic complications. Diabetes Metab Res Rev 2001;17(6):436–443.
42. Gardiner TA, Stitt AW, Archer DB. Retinal vascular endothelial cell endocytosis increases in early diabetes. Lab Invest 1995;72(4):439–444.
43. Sano H, Higashi T, Matsumoto K, et al. Insulin enhances macrophage scavenger receptor-mediated endocytic uptake of advanced glycation end products. J Biol Chem 1998;273(15):8630–8637.
44. Miyata T, Ueda Y, Shinzato T, et al. Accumulation of albumin-linked and free-form pentosidine in the circulation of uremic patients with end-stage renal failure: renal implications in the pathophysiology of pentosidine. J Am Soc Nephrol 1996;7(8):1198–1206.
45. Makita Z, Radoff S, Rayfield EJ, et al. Advanced glycosylation end products in patients with diabetic nephropathy. N Engl J Med 1991, 325(12):836–842.
46. Uribarri J, Cai W, Peppa M, Goldberg T, Vlassara H. Renal clearance of advanced glycoxidation end products (AGE) is markedly reduced in diabetic patients in the absence of impaired GFR. J Am Soc Nephrol 2003;14:394A.
47. Shinohara M, Thornalley PJ, Giardino I, et al. Overexpression of glyoxalase-I in bovine endothelial cells inhibits intracellular advanced glycation endproduct formation and prevents hyperglycemia-induced increases in macromolecular endocytosis. J Clin Invest 1998;101(5):1142–1147.
48. Bucala R, Mitchell R, Arnold K, Innerarity T, Vlassara H, Cerami A. Identification of the major site of apolipoprotein B modification by advanced glycosylation end products blocking uptake by the low density lipoprotein receptor. J Biol Chem 1995;270(18):10,828–10,832.

49. Giardino I, Edelstein D, Brownlee M. Nonenzymatic glycosylation in vitro and in bovine endothelial cells alters basic fibroblast growth factor activity. A model for intracellular glycosylation in diabetes. J Clin Invest 1994;94(1):110–117.

50. Li YM, Mitsuhashi T, Wojciechowicz D, et al. Molecular identity and cellular distribution of advanced glycation endproduct receptors: relationship of p60 to OST-48 and p90 to 80K-H membrane proteins. Proc Natl Acad Sci USA 1996;93(20):11,047–11,052.

51. He CJ, Koschinsky T, Buenting C, Vlassara H. Presence of diabetic complications in type 1 diabetic patients correlates with low expression of mononuclear cell AGE-receptor-1 and elevated serum AGE. Mol Med 2001;7(3):159–168.

52. He CJ, Zheng F, Stitt A, et al. Differential expression of renal AGE-receptor genes in NOD mice: possible role in nonobese diabetic renal disease. Kidney Int 2000;58(5):1931–1940.

53. Lu CY, He C, Cai W, Vlassara H. Overexpression of AGE-R1 inhibition AGE-induced MAPK and NF-kB activation in murine mesangial cells. Diabetes 2003;52(Suppl 1):A50.

54. Vlassara H, Li YM, Imani F, et al. Identification of galectin-3 as a high-affinity binding protein for advanced glycation end products (AGE): a new member of the AGE-receptor complex. Mol Med 1995;1(6):634–646.

55. Pugliese G, Pricci F, Leto G, et al. The diabetic milieu modulates the advanced glycation end product-receptor complex in the mesangium by inducing or upregulating galectin-3 expression. Diabetes 2000;49(7):1249–1257.

56. Zhu W, Sano H, Nagai R, Fukuhara K, Miyazaki A, Horiuchi S. The role of galectin-3 in endocytosis of advanced glycation end products and modified low density lipoproteins. Biochem Biophys Res Commun 2001;280(4):1183–1188.

57. Pricci F, Leto G, Amadio L, et al. Role of galectin-3 as a receptor for advanced glycosylation end products. Kidney Int 2000;Suppl 77:S31–S39.

58. Pugliese G, Pricci F, Iacobini C, et al. Accelerated diabetic glomerulopathy in galectin-3/AGE receptor 3 knockout mice. FASEB J 2001;15(13):2471–2479.

59. Schmidt AM, Yan SD, Wautier JL, Stern D. Activation of receptor for advanced glycation end products: a mechanism for chronic vascular dysfunction in diabetic vasculopathy and atherosclerosis. Circ Res 1999;84(5):489–497.

60. Yamamoto Y, Kato I, Doi T, et al. Development and prevention of advanced diabetic nephropathy in RAGE-overexpressing mice. J Clin Invest 2001;108(2):261–268.

61. Goova MT, Li J, Kislinger T, et al. Blockade of receptor for advanced glycation end-products restores effective wound healing in diabetic mice. Am J Pathol 2001;159(2):513–525.

62. Brett J, Schmidt AM, Yan SD, et al. Survey of the distribution of a newly characterized receptor for advanced glycation end products in tissues. Am J Pathol 1993;143(6):1699–1712.

63. Sano H, Nagai R, Matsumoto K, Horiuchi S. Receptors for proteins modified by advanced glycation endproducts (AGE)—their functional role in atherosclerosis. Mech Ageing 1999;107(3):333–346.

64. Ohgami N, Nagai R, Ikemoto M, et al. CD36, serves as a receptor for advanced glycation endproducts (AGE). J Diabetes Complications 2002;16(1):56–59.

65. Ohgami N, Nagai R, Miyazaki A, et al. Scavenger receptor class B type I-mediated reverse cholesterol transport is inhibited by advanced glycation end products. J Biol Chem 2001;276(16):13,348–13,355.

66. Sawamura T, Kume N, Aoyama T, et al. An endothelial receptor for oxidized low-density lipoprotein. Nature 1997;386(6620):73–77.

67. Dachi H, Tsujimoto M, Arai H, Inoue K. Expression cloning of a novel scavenger receptor from human endothelial cells. J Biol Chem 1997;272(50):31217–31220.

68. Li YM, Tan AX, Vlassara H. Antibacterial activity of lysozyme and lactoferrin is inhibited by binding of advanced glycation-modified proteins to a conserved motif. Nat Med 1995;1(10):1057–1061.

69. Zheng F, Cai W, Mitsuhashi T, Vlassara H. Lysozyme enhances renal excretion of advanced glycation endproducts in vivo and suppresses adverse age-mediated cellular effects in vitro: a potential AGE sequestration therapy for diabetic nephropathy? Mol Med 2001;7(11):737–747.

70. Higashi T, Sano H, Saishoji T, et al. The receptor for advanced glycation end products mediates the chemotaxis of rabbit smooth muscle cells. Diabetes 1997;46(3):463–472.

71. Poirier O, Nicaud V, Vionnet N, et al. Polymorphism screening of four genes encoding advanced glycation end-product putative receptors. Association study with nephropathy in type 1 diabetic patients. Diabetes 2001;50(5):1214–1218.

72. Ritz E, Rychlik I, Locatelli F, Halimi S. End-stage renal failure in type 2 diabetes: A medical catastrophe of worldwide dimensions. Am J Kidney Dis 1999;34(5):795–808.

73. Osterby R, Anderson MJF, Gundersen HJG, Jorgensen HE, Mogensen CE, Parving HH Quantitative study on glomerular ultrastructure in type I diabetes with incipient nephropathy. Diab Nephrop 1983;3:95–100.

74. Skolnik EY, Yang Z, Makita Z, et al. Human and rat mesangial cell receptors for glucose modified proteins: potential role in kidney tissue remodelling and diabetic nephropathy. J Exp Med 1991;174:931–939.

75. Doi T, Vlassara H, Kirstein M, Yamada Y Striker GE, Striker LJ. Receptor specific increase in extra-cellular matrix production in mouse mesangial cells by advanced glycosylation end products is mediated via platelet derived growth factor. Proc Natl Acad Sci USA 1992;89:2873–2877.

76. Scivittaro V, Ganz MB, Weiss MF. AGEs induce oxidative stress and activate protein kinase C-beta(II) in neonatal mesangial cells. Am J Physiol Renal Physiol 2000;278(4):F676–F683.

77. Doublier S, Salvidio G, Lupia E, et al. Nephrin expression is reduced in human diabetic nephropathy: evidence for a distinct role for glycated albumin and angiotensin II. Diabetes 2003;52(4):1023–1030.

78. Yamagishi S, Inagaki Y, Okamoto T, et al. Advanced glycation end product-induced apoptosis and overexpression of vascular endothelial growth factor and monocyte chemoattractant protein-1 in hu-man-cultured mesangial cells. J Biol Chem 2002;277(23):20309–20315.

79. Cohen MP, Wu VY, Cohen JA. Glycated albumin stimulates fibronectin and collagen IV production by glomerular endothelial cells under normoglycemic conditions. Biochem Biophys Res Commun 1997;239(1):91–94.

80. Bendayan M. Immunocytochemical detection of advanced glycated end products in rat renal tissue as a function of age and diabetes. Kidney Int 1998;54(2):438–447.

81. Gugliucci A, Bendayan M. Reaction of advanced glycation endproducts with renal tissue from normal and streptozotocin induced rats an ultrastructural study using colloidal gold cytochemistry. J Histochem. Cytochem 1995;43–6:591–600.

82. Yang CW, Vlassara H, Peten EP, He CJ, Striker GE, Striker LJ. Advanced glycation end products up-regulate gene expression found in diabetic glomerular disease. Proc Natl Acad Sci USA 1994;91(20): 9436–9440.

83. Vlassara H, Fuh H, Makita Z, Krungkrai S, Cerami A, Bucala R. Exogenous advanced glycosylation end products induce complex vascular dysfunction in normal animals: a model for diabetic and ageing complications. Proc Natl Acad Sci USA 1992;89:12043–12047.

84. Soulis T, Cooper ME, Vranes D, Bucala R, Jerums G. Effects of aminoguanidine in preventing experi-mental diabetic nephropathy are related to the duration of treatment. Kidney Int 1996;50–2:627–634.

85. Bach LA, Dean R, Youssef S, Cooper ME. Aminoguanidine ameliorates changes in the IGF system in experimental diabetic nephropathy. J Am Soc Nephrol 2001;12–10:2098–2107.

86. Osicka TM, Yu Y, Lee V, Panagiotopoulos S, Kemp BE, Jerums G. Aminoguanidine and ramipril prevent diabetes-induced increases in protein kinase C activity in glomeruli, retina and mesenteric artery. Clin Sci (Lond) 2001;100–3:249–257.

87. Kelly DJ, Gilbert RE, Cox AJ, Soulis T, Jerums G, Cooper ME. Aminoguanidine ameliorates overexpression of prosclerotic growth factors and collagen deposition in experimental diabetic nephr-opathy. J Am Soc Nephrol 2001;12(10):2098–2107.

88. Sharma K, Ziyadeh FN. Hyperglycemia and diabetic kidney disease. The case for transforming growth factor-beta as a key mediator. Diabetes 1995;44(10):1139–1146.

89. Forbes JM, Thallas V, Thomas MC, Jerums G, Cooper ME. Renoprotection is afforded by the advanced glycation end product (AGE) cross-link breaker, ALT-711. FASEB J 2003;17(12):1762–1764.

90. Schleicher ED, Wagner E, Nerlich AG. Increased accumulation of the glycoxidation product N(epsilon)-(carboxymethyl)lysine in human tissues in diabetes and aging. J Clin Invest 1997;99(3):457–468.

91. Horie K, Miyata T, Maeda K, et al. Immunohistochemical colocalization of glycoxidation products and lipid peroxidation products in diabetic renal glomerular lesions. Implication for glycoxidative stress in the pathogenesis of diabetic nephropathy. J Clin Invest 1997;100(12):2995–3004.

92. Sugiyama S, Miyata T, Horie K, et al. Advanced glycation end-products in diabetic nephropathy. Nephrol Dial Transplant.1996;11(Suppl 5):91–94.

93. Tanji N, Markowitz GS, Fu C, et al. Expression of advanced glycation end products and their cellular receptor RAGE in diabetic nephropathy and nondiabetic renal disease. J Am Soc Nephrol 2000;11(9): 1656–1666.

94. Miura J, Yamagishi S, Uchigata Y, et al. Serum levels of non-carboxymethyllysine advanced glycation endproducts are correlated to severity of microvascular complications in patients with Type 1 diabetes. J Diabetes Complications 2003;17(1):16–21.

95. Sheetz MJ, King GL. Molecular understanding of hyperglycemia's adverse effects for diabetic compli-cations. JAMA 2002;27;288(20):2579–2588.

96. Kahn HA, Moorhead HB. Statistics on blindness in the model reporting area 1969–1970 US. Department of Health, Education, and Welfare Publication No. (NIH) US. Government Printing Office, Washington, 1973, pp. 73–427.

97. Chappey O, Dosquet C, Wautier MP, Wautier JL. Advanced glycation end products, oxidant stress and vascular lesions. Eur J Clin Invest 1997;27(2):97–108.

98. Yamagishi S, Hsu CC, Taniguchi M, et al. Receptor-mediated toxicity to pericytes of advanced glycosylation end products: a possible mechanism of pericyte loss in diabetic microangiopathy. Biochem Biophys Res Commun 1995;213(2):681–687.

99. Mamputu JC, Renier G. Advanced glycation end products increase, through a protein kinase C-dependent pathway, vascular endothelial growth factor expression in retinal endothelial cells. Inhibitory effect of gliclazide. J Diabetes Complications 2002;16(4):284–293.

100. Reber F, Geffarth R, Kasper M, et al. Graded sensitiveness of the various retinal neuron populations on the glyoxal-mediated formation of advanced glycation end products and ways of protection. Graefes Arch Clin Exp Ophthalmol 2003;241(3):213–225.

101. Chakravarthy U, Hayes RG, Stitt AW, McAuley E, Archer DB. Constitutive nitric oxide synthase expression in retinal vascular endothelial cells is suppressed by high glucose and advanced glycation end products. Diabetes 1998;47:945–952.

102. Sulochana KN, Ramprasad S, Coral K, et al. Glycation and glycoxidation studies in vitro on isolated human vitreous collagen. Med Sci Monit 2003;9(6):BR219–BR223.

103. Stitt AW, Li YM, Gardiner TA, Bucala R, Archer DB, Vlassara H. Advanced glycation end products (AGEs) co-localize with AGE receptors in the retinal vasculature of diabetic and of AGE-infused rats. Am J Pathol 1997;150(2):523–531.

104. Clements RS Jr, Robison WG Jr, Cohen MP. Anti-glycated albumin therapy ameliorates early retinal microvascular pathology in db/db mice. J Diabetes Comp 1998;12:28–33.

105. Xu X, Li Z, Luo D, et al. Exogenous advanced glycosylation end products induce diabetes-like vascular dysfunction in normal rats: a factor in diabetic retinopathy. Graefes Arch Clin Exp Ophthalmol 2003;241(1):56–62.

106. Wautier MP, Massin P, Guillausseau PJ, et al. N(carboxymethyl)lysine as a biomarker for microvascular complications in type 2 diabetic patients. Diabetes Metab 2003;29(1):44–52.

107. Matsumoto Y, Takahashi M, Chikuda M, Arai K Levels of mature cross-links and advanced glycation end product cross-links in human vitreous. Jpn J Ophthalmol 2002;46(5):510–517.

108. Koga K, Yamagishi S, Okamoto T, et al. Serum levels of glucose-derived advanced glycation end products are associated with the severity of diabetic retinopathy in type 2 diabetic patients without renal dysfunction. Int J Clin Pharmacol Res 2002;22(1):13–17.

109. Dyck PJ, Kratz KM, Karnes JL, et al. The prevalence by staged severity of various types of diabetic neuropathy, retinopathy, and nephropathy in a population-based cohort: the Rochester Diabetic Neuropathy Study. Neurology 1993;43(4):817–824.

110. Dyck PJ, Giannini C. Pathologic alterations in the diabetic neuropathies of humans: a review. J Neuropathol Exp Neurol 1996;55(12):1181–1193.

111. Boel E, Selmer J, Flodgaard HJ, Jensen T. Diabetic late complications: will aldose reductase inhibitors or inhibitors of advanced glycosylation endproduct formation hold promise? J Diabetes Complications 1995;9(2):104–129.

112. Poduslo JF, Curran GL. Increased permeability across the blood-nerve barrier of albumin glycated in vitro and in vivo from patients with diabetic polyneuropathy. Proc Natl Acad Sci USA 1992;89(6):2218–2222.

113. Poduslo JF, Curran GL. Glycation increases the permeability of proteins across the blood-nerve and blood-brain barriers. Brain Res Mol Brain Res 1994;23(1–2):157–162.

114. Cullum NA, Mahon J, Stringer K, McLean WG. Glycation of rat sciatic nerve tubulin in experimental diabetes mellitus. Diabetologia 1991;34(6):387–389.

115. McLean WG. The role of axonal cytoskeleton in diabetic neuropathy. Neurochem Res 1997;22(8):951–956.

116. Graham AR, Johnson PC. Direct immunofluorescence findings in peripheral nerve from patients with diabetic neuropathy. Ann Neurol 1985;17(5):450–454.

117. Sugimoto K, Nishizawa Y, Horiuchi S, Yagihashi S. Localization in human diabetic peripheral nerve of N (epsilon)-carboxymethyllysine-protein adducts, an advanced glycation endproduct. Diabetologia 1997;40(12):1380–1387.

118. Vlassara H, Brownlee M, Cerami A. Nonenzymatic glycosylation of peripheral nerve protein in diabetes mellitus. Proc Natl Acad Sci USA 1981;78(8):5190–5192.

119. Monnier VM, Bautista O, Kenny D, et al. Skin collagen glycation, glycoxidation, and crosslinking are lower in subjects with long-term intensive versus conventional therapy of type 1 diabetes: relevance

of glycated collagen products versus HbA1c as markers of diabetic complications. DCCT Skin Collagen Ancillary Study Group. Diabetes Control and Complications Trial. Diabetes 1999;48(4):870–880.

120. Schleicher ED, Wagner E, Nerlich AG. Increased accumulation of the glycoxidation product N (epsilon)-(carboxymethyl)lysine in human tissues in diabetes and aging. J Clin Invest 1997;99(3):457–468.

121. Beisswenger PJ, Makita Z, Curphey TJ, et al. Formation of immunochemical advanced glycosylation end products precedes and correlates with early manifestations of renal and retinal disease in diabetes. Diabetes 1995;44(7):824–829.

122. Watala C, Golanski J, Witas H, Gurbiel R, Gwozdzinski K, Trojanowski Z. The effects of in vivo and in vitro non-enzymatic glycosylation and glycoxidation on physico-chemical properties of haemoglobin in control and diabetic patients. Int J Biochem Cell Biol 1996;28(12):1393–1403.

123. Duraisamy Y, Slevin M, Smith N, et al. Effect of glycation on basic fibroblast growth factor induced angiogenesis and activation of associated signal transduction pathways in vascular endothelial cells: possible relevance to wound healing in diabetes. Angiogenesis 2001;4(4):277–288.

124. Ido Y, Chang KC, Lejeune WS, et al. Vascular dysfunction induced by AGE is mediated by VEGF via mechanisms involving reactive oxygen species, guanylate cyclase, and protein kinase C. Microcirculation 2001;8(4):251–263.

125. Portero-Otin M, Pamplona R, Bellmunt MJ, et al. Advanced glycation end product precursors impair epidermal growth factor receptor signaling. Diabetes 2002;51(5):1535–1542.

126. Twigg SM, Joly AH, Chen MM, et al. Connective tissue growth factor/IGF-binding protein-related protein-2 is a mediator in the induction of fibronectin by advanced glycosylation end-products in human dermal fibroblasts. Endocrinology 2002;143(4):1260–1269.

127. Imani F, Horii Y, Suthanthiran M, et al. Advanced glycosylation endproduct-specific receptors on human and rat T-lymphocytes mediate synthesis of interferon gamma: role in tissue remodeling. J Exp Med 1993;178(6):2165–2172.

128. Collison KS, Parhar RS, Saleh SS, et al. RAGE-mediated neutrophil dysfunction is evoked by advanced glycation end products (AGEs). J Leukoc Biol 2002;71(3):433–444.

129. Bernheim J, Rashid G, Gavrieli R, Korzets Z, Wolach B. In vitro effect of advanced glycation end-products on human polymorphonuclear superoxide production. Eur J Clin Invest 2001;31(12):1064.

130. Abordo EA, Westwood ME, Thornalley PJ. Synthesis and secretion of macrophage colony stimulating factor by mature human monocytes and human monocytic THP-1 cells induced by human serum albumin derivatives modified with methylglyoxal and glucose-derived advanced glycation endproducts. Immunol Lett 1996;53(1):7–13.

131. Daoud S, Schinzel R, Neumann A, et al. Advanced glycation endproducts: activators of cardiac remodeling in primary fibroblasts from adult rat hearts. Mol Med 2001;7(8):543–551.

132. Brennan M. Changes in solubility, non-enzymatic glycation, and fluorescence of collagen in tail tendons from diabetic rats. J Biol Chem 1989;264(35):20947–20952.

133. Portero-Otin M, Pamplona R, Bellmunt MJ, et al. Advanced glycation end product precursors impair epidermal growth factor receptor signaling. Diabetes 2002;51(5):1535–1542.

134. Kochakian M, Manjula BN, Egan JJ. Chronic dosing with aminoguanidine and novel advanced glycosylation end product-formation inhibitors ameliorates cross-linking of tail tendon collagen in STZ-induced diabetic rats. Diabetes 1996;45(12):1694–1700.

135. Teixeira AS, Caliari MV, Rocha OA, Machado RD, Andrade SP. Aminoguanidine prevents impaired healing and deficient angiogenesis in diabetic rats. Inflammation 1999;23(6):569–581.

136. Teixeira AS, Andrade SP. Glucose-induced inhibition of angiogenesis in the rat sponge granuloma is prevented by aminoguanidine. Life Sci 1999;64(8):655–662.

137. Yavuz D, Tugteppe H, Kaya H, et al. Effects of aminoguanidine on wound healing in a diabetic rat model. (Abstract). Diabetes 2002;51 (Suppl 2):A256.

138. Eble AS, Thorpe SR, Baynes JW. Nonenzymatic glycosylation and glucose-dependent cross-linking of proteins. J Biol Chem 1983;258:9406–9412.

139. Bucala R, Tracey KJ, Cerami A. Advanced glycosylation products quench nitric oxide and mediate defective endothelium-dependent vasodilatation in experimental diabetes. J Clin Invest 1991;87:432–438.

140. Panagiotopoulos S, O'Brien RC, Bucala R, Cooper ME, Jerums G. Aminoguanidine has an anti-atherogenic effect in the cholesterol-fed rabbit. Atherosclerosis 1998;136:125–131.

141. Bucala R, Makita Z, Koschinsky T, Cerami A, Vlassara H. Lipid advanced glycosylation: pathway for lipid oxidation in vivo. Proc Natl Acad Sci 1993;90:6434–6438.

142. Zhang J, Ren S, Sun D, Shen GX. Influence of glycation on LDL-induced generation of fibrinolytic regulators in vascular endothelial cells. Arter Thromb Vasc Biol 1998;18:1140–1148.

143. Hedrick CC, Thorpe SR, Fu MX, et al. Glycation impairs high-density lipoprotein function. Diabetologia 2000;43:312–320.
144. Doucet C, Huby T, Ruiz J, Chapman MJ, Thillet J. Non-enzymatic glycation of lipoprotein(a) in vitro and in vivo. Atherosclerosis 1995;118:135–143.
145. Zhang J, Ren S, Shen GX. Glycation amplifies lipoprotein(a)-induced alterations in the generation of fibrinolytic regulators from human vascular endothelial cells. Atherosclerosis 2000;150:299–308.
146. Wautier MP, Chappey O, Corda S, Stern DM, Schmidt AM, Wautier JL. Activation of NADPH oxidase by AGE links oxidant stress to altered gene expression via RAGE. Am J Physiol Endocrinol Metab 2001;280(5):E685–E694.
147. Lassegue B, Clempus RE. Vascular NAD(P)H oxidases: specific features, expression, and regulation. Am J Physiol Regul Integr Comp Physiol 2003;285(2):R277–R297.
148. Palinski W, Koschinsky T, Butler SW, et al. Immunological evidence for the presence of advanced glycation end products in atherosclerotic lesions of euglycemic rabbits. Arter Thromb Vasc Biol 1995;15:571–582.
149. Vlassara H, Fuh H, Donnelly T, Cybulsky M. Advanced glycation endproducts promote adhesion molecule (VCAM-1, ICAM-1) expression and atheroma formation in normal rabbits. Mol Med 1995;1:447–456.
150. Vlassara H, Fuh H, Makita Z, Krungkrai S, Cerami A, Bucala R. Exogenous advanced glycosylation end products induce complex vascular dysfunction in normal animals: a model for diabetic and aging complications. Proc Natl Acad Sci USA 1992;89(24):12043–12047.
151. Wautier JL, Zoukourian C, Chappey O, et al. Receptor-mediated endothelial cell dysfunction in diabetic vasculopathy. Soluble receptor for advanced glycation end products blocks hyperpermeability in diabetic rats. J Clin Invest 1996;97:238–243.
152. Crauwels HM, Herman AG, Bult H. Local application of advanced glycation end products and intimal hyperplasia in the rabbit collared carotid artery. Cardiovasc Res 2000;40:173–182.
153. Brownlee M, Vlassara H, Kooney A, Ulrich P, Cerami A. Aminoguanidine prevents diabetes-induced arterial wall protein crosslinking. Science 1986;232:1629–1632.
154. Park I, Raman KG, Lee KJ, et al. Suppression of accelerated diabetic atherosclerosis by the soluble receptor for advanced glycation endproducts. Nat Med 1998;4:1025–1031.
155. Candido R, Forbes JM, Thomas MC, et al. A breaker of advanced glycation end products attenuates diabetes-induced myocardial structural changes. Circ Res 2003;92(7):785–792.
156. Nangaku M, Miyata T, Sada T, et al. Anti-hypertensive agents inhibit in vivo the formation of advanced glycation end products and improve renal damage in a type 2 diabetic nephropathy rat model. J Am Soc Nephrol 2003;14(5):1212–1222.
157. Nakamura Y, Horii Y, Nishino T, et al. Immunohistochemical localization of advanced glycosylation end products in coronary atheroma and cardiac tissue in diabetes mellitus. Am J Pathol 1993;143:1649–1656.
158. Schleicher ED, Wagner E, Nerlich AG. Increased accumulation of the glycoxidation product N(epsilon)-carboxymethyl)lysine in human tissues in diabetes and aging. J Clin Invest 1997;99:457–468.
159. Yamada K, Miyahara Y, Hamaguchi K, et al. Immunohistochemical study of human advanced glycation end-products in chronic renal failure. Clin Nephrol 1994;42:354–361.
160. Sakata N, Imanaga Y, Meng J, et al. Increased advanced glycation end products in atherosclerotic lesions of patients with end-stage renal disease. Atherosclerosis 1999;142:67–77.
161. Sims TJ, Rasmussen LM, Oxlund H, Bailey AJ. The role of glycation cross-links in diabetic vascular stiffening. Diabetologia 1996;39:946–951.
162. Stitt AW, He C, Friedman S, et al. Elevated AGE-modified apoB in sera of euglycemic, normolipidemic patients with atherosclerosis: relation to tissue AGE. Mol Med 1997;3:617–627.
163. Tan KC, Chow WS, Ai VH, Metz C, Bucala R, Lam KS. Advanced glycation end products and endothelial dysfunction in type 2 diabetes. Diabetes Care 2002;25(6):1055–1059.
164. Strirban A, Sander D, Buenting C, et al. Food advanced glycation end products (AGE) acutely impair endothelial function in patienst with diabetes mellitus (abstract). Diabetes 2003;52(Suppl 1):A19
165. Winer N, Sowers JR. Vascular compliance in diabetes. Curr Diab Rep 2003;3(3):230–234.
166. Odetti P, Traverso N, Cosso L, Noberasco G, Pronzato MA, Marinari UM. Good glycaemic control reduces oxidation and glycation end-products in collagen of diabetic rats. Diabetologia 1996;39(12):1440–1447.
167. Odetti P, Robaudo C, Valentini S, et al. Effect of a new vitamin E-coated membrane on glycoxidation during hemodialysis. Contrib Nephrol 1999;127:192–199.

168. Nakayama M, Izumi G, Nemoto Y, et al. Suppression of N(epsilon)-(carboxymethyl)lysine generation by the antioxidant N-acetylcysteine. Perit Dial Int 1999;19(3):207–210.

169. Trachtman H, Futterweit S, Prenner J, Hanon S. Antioxidants reverse the antiproliferative effect of high glucose and advanced glycosylation end products in cultured rat mesangial cells. Biochem Biophys Res Commun 1994;199(1):346–352.

170. Kunt T, Forst T, Wilhelm A, et al. Alpha-lipoic acid reduces expression of vascular cell adhesion molecule-1 and endothelial adhesion of human monocytes after stimulation with advanced glycation end products. Clin Sci (Lond) 1999;96(1):75–82.

171. Jakus V, Hrnciarova M, Carsky J, Krahulec B, Rietbrock N. Inhibition of nonenzymatic protein glycation and lipid peroxidation by drugs with antioxidant activity. Life Sci 1999; 65(18–19):1991–1993.

172. Hammes HP, Bartmann A, Engel L, Wulfroth P. Antioxidant treatment of experimental diabetic retinopathy in rats with nicanartine. Diabetologia 1997;40(6):629–634.

173. Zhao W, Devamanoharan PS, Varma SD. Fructose-mediated damage to lens alpha-crystallin: prevention by pyruvate. Biochim Biophys Acta 2000;1500(2):161–168.

174. Varma SD, Ramachandran S, Devamanoharan PS, Morris SM, Ali, AH. Prevention of oxidative damage to rat lens by pyruvate in vitro: possible attenuation in vivo. Curr Eye Res 1995;14(8):643–649.

175. Forbes JM, Soulis T, Thallas V, et al. Renoprotective effects of a novel inhibitor of advanced glycation. Diabetologia 2001;44(1):108–114.

176. Wilkinson-Berka JL, Kelly DJ, Koerner SM, et al. ALT-946 and aminoguanidine, inhibitors of advanced glycation, improve severe nephropathy in the diabetic transgenic (mREN-2)27 rat. Diabetes 2002;51(11):3283–3289.

177. Oturai PS, Christensen M, Rolin B, Pedersen KE, Mortensen SB, Boel E. Effects of advanced glycation end-product inhibition and cross-link breakage in diabetic rats. Metabolism 2000;49(8):996–1000.

178. Booth AA, Khalifah RG, Todd P, Hudson BG. In vitro kinetic studies of formation of antigenic advanced glycation end products (AGEs). Novel inhibition of post-Amadori glycation pathways. J Biol Chem 1997;272(9):5430–5437.

179. Pomero F, Molinar, Min A, et al. Benfotiamine is similar to thiamine in correcting endothelial cell defects induced by high glucose. Acta Diabetol 2001;38(3):135–138.

180. Stracke H, Hammes HP, Werkmann D, et al. Efficacy of benfotiamine versus thiamine on function and glycation products of peripheral nerves in diabetic rats. Exp Clin Endocrinol Diabetes 2001;109(6):330–336.

181. Onorato JM, Jenkins AJ, Thorpe SR, Baynes JW. Pyridoxamine, an inhibitor of advanced glycation reactions, also inhibits advanced lipoxidation reactions. Mechanism of action of pyridoxamine. J Biol Chem 2000;275(28):21177–21184.

182. Stitt A, Gardiner TA, Anderson NL, et al. The AGE inhibitor pyridoxamine inhibits development of retinopathy in experimental diabetes. Diabetes 2002;51(9):2826–2832.

183. Degenhardt TP, Alderson NL, Arrington DD, et al. Pyridoxamine inhibits early renal disease and dyslipidemia in the streptozotocin-diabetic rat. Kidney Int 2002;61(3):939–950.

184. Nakamura S, Makita Z, Ishikawa S, et al. Progression of nephropathy in spontaneous diabetic rats is prevented by OPB-9195, a novel inhibitor of advanced glycation. Diabetes 1997;46(5):895–899.

185. Wada R, Nishizawa Y, Yagihashi N, et al. Effects of OPB-9195, anti-glycation agent, on experimental diabetic neuropathy. Eur J Clin Invest 2001;31(6):513–520.

186. Mizutani K, Ikeda K, Tsuda K, Yamori Y. Inhibitor for advanced glycation end products formation attenuates hypertension and oxidative damage in genetic hypertensive rats. J Hypertens 2002;20(8):1607–1614.

187. Schwedler SB, Verbeke P, Bakala H, et al. N-phenacylthiazolium bromide decreases renal and increases urinary advanced glycation end products excretion without ameliorating diabetic nephropathy in C57BL/6 mice. Diabetes Obes Metab 2001;3(4):230–239.

188. Vaitkevicius PV, Lane M, Spurgeon H, et al. A cross-link breaker has sustained effects on arterial and ventricular properties in older rhesus monkeys. Proc Natl Acad Sci USA 2001;98(3):1171–1175.

189. Cohen MP, Clements RS, Cohen JA, Shearman CW. Prevention of decline in renal function in the diabetic db/db mouse. Diabetologia 1996;39(3):270–274.

190. Cohen MP, Sharma K, Jin Y, et al. Prevention of diabetic nephropathy in db/db mice with glycated albumin antagonists. A novel treatment strategy. J Clin Invest 1995;95(5):2338–2345.

191. Sebekova K, Schinzel R, Munch G, Krivosikova Z, Dzurik R, Heidland A. Advanced glycation end-product levels in subtotally nephrectomized rats: beneficial effects of angiotensin II receptor 1 antagonist losartan. Miner Electrolyte Metab 1999;25(4–6):380–383

192. Miyata T, van Y, persele de Strihou C, et al. Angiotensin II receptor antagonists and angiotensin-converting enzyme inhibitors lower in vitro the formation of advanced glycation end products: biochemical mechanisms. J Am Soc Nephrol 2002;13(10):2478–2487.

193. Parving HH, Hommel E, Jensen BR, Hansen HP. Long-term beneficial effect of ACE inhibition on diabetic nephropathy in normotensive type 1 diabetic patients. Kidney Int 2001;60(1):228–234.

4 The Renin–Angiotensin System in Diabetic Cardiovascular Complications

Edward P. Feener, PhD

CONTENTS

INTRODUCTION

The renin–angiotensin system (RAS) exerts a wide range of effects on cardiovascular homeostasis and blood pressure (BP) control. A large body of clinical evidence has demonstrated that inhibition of angiotensin II (Ang II, Asp1-Phe8) production by angiotensin-converting enzyme (ACE) inhibitors reduce the onset and/or progression of renal (1–7), retinal (8,9), and cardiovascular (5,9–12) complications of diabetes mellitus (DM). The majority of the BP-lowering effects and in vivo vascular effects of ACE inhibitors have been reproduced with angiotensin AT1 receptor antagonists (13–18), suggesting that the Ang II/AT1 receptor pathway mediates most of angiotensin's adverse cardiovascular effects in diabetes. Although inhibition of the RAS provides protective effects against both the microvascular and cardiovascular complications of DM, the actions and regulation of the RAS in diabetes remain incompletely understood. This chapter will review the interactions between the RAS and diabetes that have been associated with insulin resistance and cardiovascular disease (CVD).

EFFECT OF DIABETES ON THE RENIN–ANGIOTENSIN SYSTEM

Overview of the Renin–Angiotensin System: Angiotensinases, Peptides, and Receptors

The actions of the RAS are regulated both by angiotensinases in the extracellular milieu and by angiotensin receptor-coupled signaling networks. The precursor for angio-

From: *Contemporary Cardiology: Diabetes and Cardiovascular Disease, Second Edition*
Edited by: M. T. Johnstone and A. Veves © Humana Press Inc., Totowa, NJ

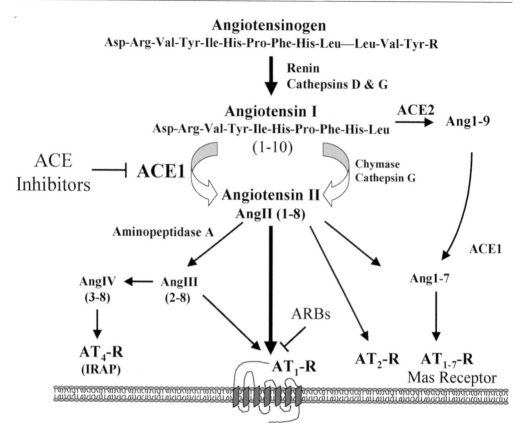

Fig. 1. Overview of the renin–angiotensin system. Angiotensinogen and angiotensin I-derived peptides are cleaved via a number of extracellular proteases resulting in at least four biologically active peptides, including Ang II, angiotensin II Asp1-Phe8, Ang III, Angiotensin Arg2-Phe8; Ang IV, Angiotensin Val3-Phe8; and Ang1-7, Angiotensin Asp1-Pro7. Angiotensin-converting enzyme 1 (ACE) generates Ang II and is the target of ACE inhibitors. ACE2 generates Ang1-9, Angiotensin Asp1-His9, which is further cleaved by ACE1 to generate Ang1-7. Angiotensin receptor blockers (ARBs) inhibit Ang II and Ang III signaling via the AT1 receptor.

tensin-derived peptides is angiotensinogen (AGT), a 452 amino acid protein in the serpin family that undergoes N-terminal proteolysis by renin to generate the decapeptide angiotensin I (Ang I) and des(Ang I)AGT (Fig. 1). Cathepsin G and cathepsin D also have renin-like activities, which may contribute substantially to Ang I production by vascular smooth muscle cells (VSMC) *(19)*. Once formed, Ang I is cleaved by ACE-1 (dipeptidyl carboxypeptidase 1), chymase, or cathepsin G to produce the octapeptide Ang II, which activates both angiotensin AT1 and AT2 receptor isotypes *(20–23)*. The relative contributions of ACE and alternative Ang I-processing pathways to Ang II generation appear to vary among specific tissues, and among species *(22)*. In the human heart in vivo, ACE appears to account for the majority of Ang II production *(24)*. Atherosclerotic plaques contain both ACE and chymase activity *(25–27)*, suggesting that both pathways contribute to local Ang II generation within vascular lesions. Ang I can also be cleaved by the carboxypeptidase ACE-2 to generate Ang 1-9 *(28)*, which results in decreased Ang II production. Targeted disruption of ACE-2 in mice results in elevated levels of Ang II and severe cardiac contractile dysfunction *(29)*. Thus, ACE-1 and ACE-2 appear to compete for Ang I substrate, such that ACE-2 diverts available angiotensin peptide away from the Ang II/AT1 pathway.

Ang II and Ang1-9 can undergo further proteolytic processing to generate additional biologically active peptides (Fig. 1). Conversion of Ang II to angiotensin Arg2-Phe8 (Ang III) occurs primarily via aminopeptidase A with Ang III retaining its ability to activate the AT1 receptor *(30,31)*. Ang III is a major effector peptide of the RAS in the brain in which it exerts neuronal effects on BP control *(32)*. Aminopeptidase or endopeptidase cleavage of Ang II can also generate angiotensin Val3-Phe8 (Ang IV), which appears to activate endothelial nitric oxide synthase (eNOS) activity and thereby increases blood flow *(33,34)*. Ang IV has been reported to bind insulin-regulated aminopeptidase, which may indirectly affect neuropeptide half-life *(35)*, however, a role of the AT1 receptor in mediating Ang IV action has also been reported *(36)*. C-terminal processing of Ang II by prolylcarboxypeptidase (angiotensinase C) or cleavage of Ang1-9 by ACE-1 generates angiotensin Asp1-Pro7 (Ang1-7) *(37)*, which binds the G protein-coupled Mas receptor and elicits inhibitory effects on VSMC growth and antihypertensive effects *(38–40)*.

Within the RAS, the AT1 receptor appears to mediate most of Ang II's growth promoting, metabolic, and gene-regulatory actions *(41,42)*. The phenotype of AT1 gene-deficient mice is virtually identical to that of angiotensinogen-deficient mice *(43,44)* and the pressor response to Ang II infusion is abolished in AT1 receptor null mice *(43)*. However, although Ang II is the major agonist for the AT1 receptor there is evidence that Ang III, Ang IV, and mechanical stress can also activate this receptor pathway *(31,36,45)*.

Expression of the Renin–Angiotensin System in Diabetes

The production and action of Ang II is regulated at multiple levels, including the availability of angiotensinogen, levels and activities of angiotensin-processing enzymes, angiotensin receptor isotype expression, and postreceptor signaling (Fig. 1). Although quantitation of Ang II levels would provide a direct measure of extracellular RAS activation, these measurements are complicated by the rapid degradation of this peptide *(46,47)* and its tissue-specific production *(26,27,48)*. Reports on the effects of diabetes on plasma and tissues Ang II levels are controversial. Studies of streptozotocin (STZ)-induced diabetes in rats have reported no effect of diabetes on Ang II levels in plasma, kidney, aorta, and heart *(49)*, reduced renal Ang II but normal levels in plasma Ang II *(50)*, and decreased plasma Ang II in diabetes *(51)*. Similar controversies appear for the effects of diabetes on changes in upstream components of the RAS. For example, recent studies have reported that plasma renin is normal *(52)* or reduced *(53)* in diabetes. Similarly, in experimental animal models of diabetes, plasma renin has been reported to be normal *(54,55)* or reduced *(56–60)* in STZ-induced diabetic rats, and reduced in Zucker diabetic fatty rats *(61)*. In addition to discrepancies on the changes of plasma renin levels, the significance of these changes is unclear. Although low-plasma renin may indicate suppression of the RAS it may also reflect autoregulation as a result of its renal activation. Ang II is a potent inhibitor of renal renin production *(62)*. Thus, low-plasma renin in diabetes may be the result, in part, of an increase in renal Ang II action. Increased renal perfusion response to AT1 antagonism suggests that increased intrarenal Ang II production and action may occur in type 2 diabetes even though plasma renin activity is reduced

(53). Acute hyperglycemia increases AGT expression in both liver and adipose tissue *(63)*, suggesting that diabetes may increase AGT substrate availability. High glucose increases Ang II release from cardiomyocytes *(64)* and AT1 receptor expression in VSMC *(65)*, suggesting that hyperglycemia may locally upregulate the RAS in vascular tissues.

Additional factors, including parasympathetic nervous activation, hypovolemia, and sodium resorption, may affect the regulation of the RAS in diabetes. Although changes in individual components of this system may affect overall RAS activity, interpretation of these changes is limited by the potential of downstream modulation of Ang II action or stability. Moreover, because the RAS appears to be locally regulated, it may not be appropriate to extrapolate changes in RAS component levels beyond the specific tissues and conditions studied.

AngII Sensitivity in Diabetes

Diabetes may increase RAS action in the vasculature by increasing its sensitivity to the effects of Ang II. Both increased systemic and renal sensitivity to the pressor effects of Ang II have been reported in diabetes *(66,67)*, and in diabetic patients with microvascular disease *(68,69)*. In cultured VSMCs, elevating extracellular glucose from 5 mM to 25 mM has been shown to exert additive and/or potentiating effects on Ang II-induced activation of the extracellular signal-regulated kinase (ERK) and the Janus kinase/signal transducer and activator of transcription (JAK/STAT) pathways *(70,71)*. The effects of diabetes on enhancing Ang II action could be mediated by increases in AT1 receptor expression, changes in postreceptor signaling mechanisms, and/or a reduction in cellular signals that suppress AT1 responses. STZ-induced diabetes upregulates AT1 receptor levels in the heart of rats *(55,56)* and within atherosclerotic lesions in apo-E deficient mice *(72)*. Elevated concentrations of extracellular glucose increase AT1 receptor expression in cultured VSMC *(65)*. Although these increases in AT1 expression may affect Ang II sensitivity and/or maximal effect in these vascular target tissues, physiological relevance of these changes in receptor levels as a rate limiting determinant in Ang II action have not yet been demonstrated. Additionally, the synergistic effects of Ang II and high glucose could be mediated by the convergence of these agonists on signaling pathways, such as protein kinase C and reduced form of nicotinamide adenine dinucleotide phosphate (NADPH) oxidase *(73)*.

A number of factors have been shown to attenuate AT1 signaling and action in the vasculature. The angiotensin AT2 receptor has been shown to inhibit or counteract many of the trophic effects of AT1 *(41)*. Thus, the relative expression of AT1 and AT2 receptors subtypes may be an important determinant in modulating the actions of the Ang II/AT1 signaling pathway. Additionally, other vascular hormones systems induce signals that oppose or interfere with AT1 signaling. Our laboratory and others have shown that cyclic *guanosine* monophosphate-coupled hormones, including nitric oxide (NO) and natriuretic factors, inhibit Ang II-induced plasminogen activator inhibitor-1 (PAI-1) gene expression in both vascular endothelial cells and VSMC *(74,75)*. NO donors have been shown to reduce Ang II-stimulated growth, migration, and gene expression in a variety of cultured vascular cells *(76–78)*. A role of NO in suppressing AT1 action is particularly intriguing because impaired NO action is a component of endothelial dysfunction in diabetes *(79,80)*. Thus NO generated from the endothelium may normally suppress or oppose AT1 action and the impairment of this endothelium function in diabetes may lead to the apparent sensitization of the Ang II/AT1 pathway.

ROLE OF THE RENIN–ANGIOTENSIN SYSTEM IN CARDIOVASCULAR DISEASE IN DIABETES

As reviewed elsewhere in this book, multiple factors, including hyperglycemia, insulin resistance, dyslipidemia, hypercoagulability, and inflammation contribute to the pathogenesis of atherosclerosis in DM. Although there is considerable evidence for a role of the RAS in vascular remodeling, inflammation, thrombosis, and atherogeneis *(81–83)*, the role of this system in atherosclerosis in the context of the other diabetes-associated cardiovascular risk factors is not fully understood. There is a growing body of evidence from both clinical studies and experiments in diabetic rodent models suggesting that the RAS contributes to CVD in both type 1 and type 2 diabetes.

Role of the Renin–Angiotensin Syndrome in Atherogenesis in Diabetic Animal Models

STZ-induced diabetes increases atherosclerotic plaque area by four- to fivefold in the aorta of apo-E deficient mice *(72,84,85)*. Treatment of diabetic apo-E -/- mice with the ACE inhibitor perindopril reduces lesion area, macrophage infiltration, and collagen content *(85)*. A similar reduction in aortic plaque area was observed in STZ-induced diabetic apo-E-deficient mice treated with the AT1 receptor antagonist Irbesartan *(72)*. Both ACE and AT1 receptor expression are increased in aortic lesions in the diabetic apo-E-deficient mice, suggesting that the Ang II/AT1 pathway is upregulated within the atherosclerotic plaque and contributing to the accelerated lesion formation in this model. Multiple factors may contribute to the increased expression of ACE and the AT1 receptor in athersclerotic lesions in diabetes. As previously mentioned, hyperglycemia can increase both Ang II production and AT1 expression *(64,65)*. Alternatively, the upregulation of AT1 receptor expression could be mediated by diabetes-induced inflammation. Elevated levels of C-reactive protein (CRP) have been associated with atherosclerosis in diabetic patients *(86)* and transgenic overexpression of CRP in apo-E-deficient mice induces a sixfold increase of AT1 receptor expression in atherosclerotic lesions *(87)*. Moreover, ACE inhibition, AT1 receptor antagonism, and genetic tissue ACE deficiency decrease atherosclerotic lesion area in apo-E-deficient mice in the absence of diabetes *(88,89)*, showing that the RAS promotes atherosclerosis in both the absence or presence of diabetes.

Effects of Renin–Angiotensin System Inhibition on Cardiovascular Disease Outcomes in Diabetic Patients

Meta-analyses of ACE inhibitor trials provide compelling evidence that ACE inhibitors reduce cardiovascular events and mortality related to acute myocardial infarction (MI) and heart failure *(90,91)*. Because diabetes is an independent risk factor for CVD *(92)* and the RAS and diabetes appear to interact at multiple levels, it is possible that diabetes may affect the efficacy of ACE inhibition on CVD. Several recent reports have provided retrospective analyses of data from diabetic subgroups, which participated in large ACE inhibitor trials. Although some of these trials were not designed to specifically address the effects of ACE inhibition in diabetes, comparison of the relative effects of ACE inhibition in the diabetic and nondiabetic subgroups may provide important insight into the role of the RAS in CVD in diabetes.

An underlying question regarding the vascular protective effects of antihypertensive therapies is whether these effects are mediated via the reduction in BP or whether these drugs may provide additional effects. This issue has been addressed in a number of studies. Comparisons of antihypertensive therapies on cardiovascular outcomes in hypertensive patients with type 2 diabetes have been performed in several trials. In the United Kingdom Prospective Diabetes Study, the effects of tight and less tight BP control by the ACE inhibitor captopril or the β-blocker atenolol were compared in patients with both hypertension and type 2 diabetes (9,93). This prospective study demonstrated that tight BP control was more effective than less tight control in reducing macrovascular endpoints, including stroke and deaths related to diabetes (9,93). Additionally, this study indicated that the ACE inhibitor and β-blocker were equally effective in reducing cardiovascular outcomes.

The Appropriate Blood Pressure Control in Diabetes trial compared the effects of moderate and intensive BP control using a dihydropyridine calcium channel blocker (CCB; nisoldipine) and an ACE inhibitor (enalapril) on hypertension in type 2 diabetic patients (94). Although these therapies were similarly effective in controlling BP for both the intensive- and moderate-treatment protocols, the incidence of MI were significantly greater in the CCB-treated group compared with the ACE inhibitor group (95). Although cardiovascular outcomes were a secondary endpoint, this study suggests that ACE inhibition may have protective effects against MI that go beyond BP lowering. Similar results were reported for hypertensive type 2 diabetic patients from the Fosinopril Versus Amlodipine Cardiovascular Events (FACET) randomized trial (12). The FACET trial showed that although ACE inhibition and calcium antagonism were similarly effective on BP reduction and certain biochemical parameters, the risk of major cardiovascular events was significantly lower in the ACE inhibitor-treated group.

The Microalbuminuria, Cardiovascular, and Renal Outcomes (MICRO)-Heart Outcomes Prevention Evaluation (HOPE) study was a placebo-controlled trial designed to evaluate the effects of the ACE inhibitor ramipril and vitamin E on the development of diabetic nephropathy and CVD in diabetic patients (5). The ACE inhibitor component of the HOPE trial was discontinued early, after 4.5 years, because there was clear evidence of a beneficial effect on cardiovascular endpoints in the ramipril-treated group (96). Analysis of the composite outcome including MI, stroke, or cardiovascular-related death, revealed that the protective effects associated with ACE inhibition were similar in the absence or presence of diabetes (96). The beneficial effects of ACE inhibition occurred in both type 1 and type 2 diabetic patients and were irrespective of hypertension (5). Interestingly, the results from this study demonstrated that ACE inhibition reduced cardiovascular endpoints beyond that which would be expected from its BP-lowering effects (5,96,97). Although it is likely that multiple mechanisms contribute to the reduction of cardiovascular endpoints following RAS inhibition, a substudy of the HOPE trial has shown that the ACE inhibitor-treated group had a reduced rate of progression in carotid intimal-medial thickness (98), which is consistent with a reduction in atherosclerosis.

A component of the Losartan Intervention for Endpoint reduction in hypertension (LIFE) study compared the effects of losartan and atenolol on diabetic patients with hypertension and signs of left-ventricular hypertrophy (99). Patients were followed for a mean of 4.7 years. This study reported the primary composite cardiovascular endpoint, including cardiovascular death, stroke, and MI, was lower in the patients assigned to the losartan treatment group (RR, 0.76, $p = 0.031$). Because similar reductions in BP were observed with losartan and atenolol, this study suggests that AT1 receptor antagonism could provide beneficial cardiovascular effects beyond BP control.

Effect of Angiotensin-Converting Enzyme Inhibition Following Acute Myocardial Infarction on Cardiovascular Outcomes in Diabetes

The GISSI-3 study examined the short-term effects of ACE inhibition when administered within 24 hours following an acute MI in a population of more than 18,000 patients, including 2790 patients who reported a history of diabetes *(10)*. Retrospective analysis of results from this study revealed that ACE inhibitor treatment provided greater protective effects against 6-week mortality in diabetic patients compared with nondiabetics. The overall risk reduction by ACE inhibitor treatment for the diabetic group was 32%, compared with a risk reduction of 5% for nondiabetic patients. Within the diabetic group, ACE inhibitor treatment reduced mortality rates for both insulin-dependent (IDDM) and noninsulin-dependent diabetes mellitus (NIDDM) patients by 49% and 27%, respectively. Although this report indicates that the benefit of ACE inhibitor treatment in the diabetic group was greater than that for the nondiabetic group, the basis for this difference is unclear. Although the baseline characteristics for the treated and untreated groups were closely matched, the overall diabetic group appeared to have worse baseline characteristics than the nondiabetic group. The subgroup analyses performed in this report did not reveal an association between ACE inhibitor effects and baseline characteristics or physiological responses. Characterization of the diabetic population did not include measures of glycemic control, duration of diabetes, renal function, or for IDDM, classification of type 1 vs type 2 diabetes. Thus, although this provocative study suggests that the ACE inhibition provided selective protective effects for the diabetic subgroup, the absence of information regarding glycemic control and renal function among treated and placebo groups limit the interpretation of these results.

A retrospective analysis of data from the Trandolapril Cardiac Evaluation study compared the effects of ACE inhibitor therapy in diabetic and nondiabetic patients with left-ventricular dysfunction following acute MI. In this study, ACE inhibitor was given 3 to 7 days after acute MI with a mean follow-up time of 26 months. This study revealed that ACE inhibition reduced progression to severe heart failure in diabetic patients by nearly 40% compared with a nonsignificant effect in the nondiabetic group *(11)*. ACE inhibitor treatment was associated with a trend for a greater relative risk reduction for cardiovascular and sudden death in the diabetic group compared with the nondiabetic group. As with the GISSI-3 study, the reason for the larger effects of ACE inhibitors for diabetics is unclear. Again, this could be related to worse baseline CVD in the diabetic group. Alternatively, differential responses for diabetic and nondiabetic groups may suggest that ACE inhibition normalizes or compensates for specific cardiovascular abnormalities associated with diabetes.

MECHANISMS OF RENIN–ANGIOTENSIN SYSTEM-INDUCED ATHEROGENESIS

Pressure and Hemodynamic Effects

The BP effects of Ang II are mediated via a combination of mechanisms including vasoconstriction, stimulation of renal tubular sodium resorption, and its effects on the central and sympathetic nervous tissues *(100,101)*. Because hypertension exacerbates diabetic vascular complications *(102)*, it is likely that the BP-lowering effects of ACE inhibitors are a major contributor to the reduction of vascular complications in diabetic patients with hypertension *(9,93)*. However, there is growing evidence that ACE inhibitors may also provide beneficial vascular effects in diabetes in the absence of systemic hypertension. Several large studies have demonstrated that ACE inhibition can reduce renal, retinal, and cardiovascular complications in normotensive diabetic patients *(1,5,8)*. Although a small reduction in systemic BP within the normotensive range may contribute to the vasoprotective effects of ACE inhibition, the magnitude of these effects is greater than that which would be predicted based on the magnitude of these BP-lowering effects alone. Local upregulation or sensitization of the RAS can result in tissue specific increases in Ang II action, which may not significantly affect systemic BP. These local changes in the RAS can affect hemodynamics and pressure within certain vascular structures, such as the renal glomerulus. RAS inhibition has been shown to alleviate glomerular capillary hypertension caused by efferent arteriolar vasoconstriction induced by diabetes *(103–106)*. Thus, in addition to systemic BP control, ACE inhibition can also affect local hemodynamics and pressure. Multiple mechanisms may mediate the detrimental vascular effects associated with mechanical stress caused by hypertension. Mechanical stretch stimulates cardiomyocytes to release Ang II, which induces an autocrine hypertrophic response *(107)*. A recent report has shown that mechanical stretch also induces Ang II-independent activation of the AT1 receptor *(45)*. Interestingly, this mechanical stretch response blocked the AT1 antagonist candesartan but not by the Ang II competitive inhibitor (Sar1,Ile8)-Ang. Additionally, increased shear stress and mechanical stretch can activate vascular calcium transport, transforming growth factor-β, and purinoceptors *(108–111)*.

Intravascular Actions of the Renin–Angiotensin System

In addition to its potent effects on vasoconstriction and BP control, Ang II also exerts a variety of effects on vascular biology, which are independent of vascular tone and pressure. AT1 receptors are expressed in most vascular cell types, including endothelial and VSMCs, cardiomyocytes, and cardiac fibroblasts *(23)*. Activation of these receptors affects a diverse array of vascular cell functions including growth, migration, oxidant production, and gene expression *(100)*. Overproduction of Ang II and/or increased Ang II sensitivity within the vasculature tissues may stimulate these cellular processes and thereby contribute to vascular remodeling, hypertrophy, fibrosis, thrombosis, and atherosclerosis. Consistent with this hypothesis, ACE inhibition and AT1 blockade have been shown to reduce perivascular fibrosis, PAI-1, and matrix metalloprotease expression in normotensive insulin-resistant diabetic rodents *(112,113)*. Additionally, AT1 antagonism has been shown to reduce neointimal thickening of balloon catheter-injured vessels in diabetic Wistar fatty rats *(114)*. Local activation of the RAS may have particular importance at sites of vascular injury or atherosclerosis, which have locally elevated ACE- and chymase-mediated Ang II production and upregulation of AT1 receptors *(26,27,48,115)*. Activation of AT1 receptors expressed on monocytes and macrophages may contribute to atherogenesis by increasing arterial thrombosis and inflammatory responses *(116–118)*. Given that components of Ang II generation and Ang II receptors (AT1 and AT2) are coexpressed in RAS target tissues, and the half-life of circulating Ang II is only 14 to 16 seconds *(46,47)*, it is likely that autocrine/paracrine actions of the RAS system play a major role in the BP-independent effects in vascular tissues.

Endothelium-Dependent Vasodilatation

Endothelial dysfunction associated with impaired production and/or stability of NO occurs in both type 1 and type 2 diabetics *(79,80)*, and in obese insulin-resistant subjects *(119)*. Multiple mechanisms contribute to the impairment in endothelium-dependent vasorelaxation in diabetes, including the oxidative inactivation of NO, reduced eNOS expression, reduced eNOS activity, vascular insulin resistance, elevation of circulating levels of asymmetric dimethylarginine (an endogenous NOS inhibitor), and a deficiency in tetrahydrobiopterin, a cofactor for eNOS *(120–126)*.

Both ACE inhibition and AT1 receptor antagonism improves acetylcholine-induced vasorelaxation in NIDDM subjects *(127,128)*. Treatment of normotensive type 1 diabetics with an ACE inhibitor has also been shown to increase acetylcholine-induced vasorelaxation in *(129,130)*. In these studies, no difference in vasodilatation induced by NO donors (sodium nitroprusside) was observed in diabetic vs control subjects, suggesting that the endothelium dysfunction was related to impairment in the generation of NO rather than an impaired response potential. ACE inhibition may improve endothelium-dependent relaxation by suppressing Ang II effects on vascular NADH/NADPH oxidase production of superoxide anions and/or vascular insulin signaling *(131–133)*. Although ACE inhibition improves endothelium-dependent vasorelaxation induced by acute aceylcholine infusion *(127,130)* it did not improve endothelial function in response to flow-mediated dilation *(134,135)*. Therefore, ACE inhibition appears to selectively affect endothelium response acetylcholine infusion in diabetes. Additional studies are needed to determine whether ACE inhibition affects endothelial functions in diabetes apart from its hemodynamic effects.

ROLE OF THE RENIN–ANGIOTENSIN SYSTEM ON GLYCEMIC CONTROL, INSULIN SENSITIVITY, AND DIABETES ONSET

Effect of Renin–Angiotensin System Inhibition on Glycemic Control and Insulin Sensitivity

There is growing evidence that inhibition of the RAS system by either ACE inhibition or AT1 receptor antagonism can increase insulin sensitivity and glucose utilization. Studies using euglycemic hyperinsulinemic clamps have shown that ACE inhibitor treatment improves insulin sensitivity in most *(136–140)*, but not all *(141,142)* individuals with hypertension, obesity, and/or type 2 diabetes. Similarly, although AT1 antagonism has been reported to improve muscle sympathetic nerve activity and insulin sensitivity in obese hypertensive subjects *(143)* and increase basal and insulin-stimulated glucose oxidation in normotensive individuals with type 1 diabetes *(144)*, other clinical studies have not observed improvement on insulin sensitivity and glucose homeostasis following treatment with AT1 receptor antagonists *(139,145,146)*.

In experimental rodent models, ACE inhibition has been shown to enhance glucose transport skeletal muscle and adipose tissue in insulin-resistant obese Zucker rats and spontaneously hypertensive rats *(147–150)*. Angiotensin AT1 receptor antagonism has been shown to improve insulin sensitivity and glucose uptake in skeletal muscle of normotensive diabetic KK-Ay mice *(151)*, partially reduce insulin resistance in Wistar fatty rats *(114)*, and increase 2DG uptake and GLUT-4 expression in skeletal muscle in obese Zucker rats *(152)*. Because insulin resistance and the metabolic syndrome accelerate CVD *(153)* inhibition of the RAS may improve cardiovascular outcomes, in part, by increasing insulin sensitivity and improving metabolic control.

Renin–Angiotensin System Inhibition and New-Onset Diabetes

Several large clinical studies have reported that ACE inhibitor treatment is associated with a reduction in the incidence of new-onset diabetes. The MICRO-HOPE study reported that the relative risk for new diagnosis of diabetes in the ramipril ACE inhibitor-treated group was 0.66 ($p < 0.001$) compared with the placebo-treated controls (96). The Captopril Prevention Project trial reported that the relative risk of developing diabetes in the ACE inhibitor treated group was 0.86 ($p = 0.039$) compared with the conventionally (diuretics, β-blockers) treatment group. Recently, the LIFE trial reported that AT1 receptor antagonism using Losartan was associated with a 25% lower incidence of new-onset diabetes compared with patients treated with atenolol, which were similarly matched for initial clinical characteristics and BP control (154). Consistent with the clinical finding on the effects of RAS inhibition on the onset of diabetes, experimental studies have also indicated that ACE inhibition delays the onset of noninsulin-dependent diabetes in Otsuka Long-Evans Tokushima fatty rats (155). Both ACE inhibition and AT1 receptor antagonism improve first-phase insulin secretion and histopathological changes in pancreatic islets from diabetic Zucker rats (156). These provocative findings suggest that inhibition of the RAS, by either ACE inhibition or AT1 antagonism, could provide protective effects against the onset of type 2 diabetes.

Effects of the Renin–Angiotensin System on Insulin Signaling

The effects of RAS inhibition on insulin action have been attributed to changes in both the inhibition of Ang II/ AT1 receptor signaling and enhancement of bradykinin/B2 receptor action. ACE, also called kininase II, degrades bradykinin 1-9 and thereby reduces bradykinin B2 receptor activation (Fig. 2). Several reports have shown that bradykinin B2-receptor antagonism blocks the decreases in insulin resistance and enhanced glucose uptake associated with ACE inhibition (148,149,157) and is mimicked by chronic bradykinin administration (158). Moreover, bradykinin B2 receptor deficient mice are insulin-resistant (159). Although the mechanisms responsible for the amelioration of insulin resistance by bradykinin are not fully understood, bradykinin has been shown to enhance insulin-stimulated insulin receptor substrate-1 (IRS-1) tyrosine phosphorylation and its subsequent association with Phosphatidylinositol 3'-kinase (PI3K) in skeletal muscle and liver (160,161), possibly by inhibiting insulin receptor dephosphorylation (162). Bradykinin has also been shown to increase GLUT-4 translocation to the plasma membrane, which may contribute to insulin-independent glucose uptake in the heart and skeletal muscle (163,164).

Although bradykinin appears to contribute to the effects of ACE inhibition on insulin sensitivity, there is also considerable evidence that Ang II can inhibit insulin signaling and induce insulin resistance. Infusion of Ang II during a hyperinsulinemic euglycemic clamp in anesthetized dogs results in increases in both plasma and interstitial insulin without a concomitant increase in glucose utilization, suggesting that Ang II induced insulin resistance at the cellular level (165). Increased Ang II production induced by transgenic over expression of renin in TG(mREN2)27 rats induces insulin-resistance compared with nontransgenic control rats (166). Infusion of Ang II in rats inhibits insulin-stimulated PI3K activation in the heart by reducing insulin-stimulated PI3K activity associated with IRS-1 without significantly impairing IRS-1 tyrosine phosphorylation or IRS-1/p85 P13K docking (132).

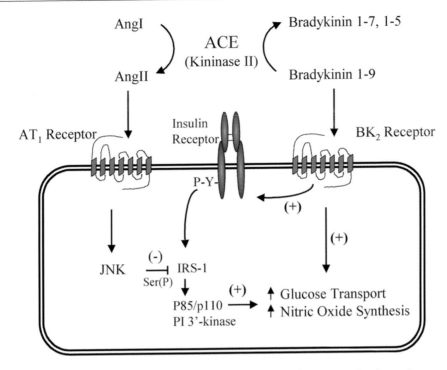

Fig. 2. Modulation of insulin signaling by the renin–angiotensin system. Angiotensin-converting enzyme (ACE) catalyses the conversion of Ang I to Ang II and degrades bradykinin 1-9 (BK2 receptor agonist). The Ang II/AT1 pathway stimulates serine phosphorylation of IRS-1, which reducing its tyrosine phosphorylation by activated insulin receptor thereby inhibiting insulin signaling. The Bradykinin BK2 receptor pathway increases insulin receptor phosphorylation resulting in enhanced insulin action. Both activated insulin receptor and BK2 receptor increase glucose transport and NO synthesis. JNK, Jun N-terminal kinase; IRS-1, insulin receptor substrate-1; PI3K, Phosphatidylinositol 3'-kinase; P-Ser, phosphoserine.

Our laboratory and others have shown that Ang II inhibits insulin stimulation of PI3K in both vascular cells and tissues. In cultured VSMCs, Ang II inhibits insulin-stimulated IRS-1 tyrosine phosphorylation, and its subsequent docking with the regulatory p85 subunit of PI3K *(131)*. Because Ang II did not alter insulin receptor autophosphorylation, the inhibitory effects of Ang II appear to occur subsequent to insulin receptor activation. Ang II-induced serine phosphorylation of IRS-1 correlated with impaired IRS-1 binding to activated insulin receptor, suggesting that Ang II-induced serine phosphorylation of IRS-1 prevents its ability to bind and become tyrosine phosphorylated by the insulin receptor (Fig. 2). Recent studies have shown that Ang II, via the AT1 receptor, increases IRS-1 phosphorylation at Ser312 and Ser616 via Jun NH(2)-terminal kinase (JNK) and ERK1/2, respectively, in human umbilical vein endothelial cells *(167)*. Additionally, activation of JNK has been shown to stimulate IRS-1 phosphorylation at Ser307 and inhibit insulin-stimulated tyrosine phosphorylation of IRS-1 *(168)*. These reports have begun to provide a biochemical basis for Ang II/insulin "crosstalk" at the signal transduction level in vascular cells. Although chronic AT1 antagonism has been associated with a 20% increase in GLUT-4 expression and increased glucose uptake in skeletal muscle *(151,152)*, the mechanisms that mediate these effects of AT1 receptor antagonists on insulin action in skeletal muscle have not yet been elucidated.

SUMMARY AND CONCLUSIONS

The RAS has emerged as a network of angiotensin peptides and receptors, whose production and activities are regulated at multiple levels. A growing number of clinical trials and experimental studies using diabetic animal models have shown that both ACE1 and the AT1 receptor contribute to cardiovascular dysfunctions and disease in diabetes. The cardiovascular effects of the RAS are results of a combination of its systemic and local/intravascular actions. The systemic actions of the RAS include BP control, and effects on insulin sensitivity, metabolic control, and circulating CVD risk factors, such as PAI-1. The intravascular RAS exerts additional effects on vascular remodeling, inflammation, oxidation, thrombosis, fibrosis, and endothelial functions including permeability and vasorelaxation. Although the RAS has emerged as a leading therapeutic target for diabetic microvascular and cardiovascular complications, additional factors associated with insulin resistance, metabolic control, and inflammation also play major roles in the excessive cardiovascular risk associated with diabetes. Further understanding of the interactions between RAS and diabetic vascular complications will provide new insight into the role of RAS inhibition in the treatment and management of CVD in diabetes.

ACKNOWLEDGMENTS

This work was supported in part by National Institutes of Health grant DK 48358.

REFERENCES

1. Lewis EJ, Hunsicker LG, Bain RP, Rohde RD. The effect of angiotensin-converting-enzyme inhibition on diabetic nephropathy. The Collaborative Study Group. N Engl J Med 1993;329:1456–1462.
2. Laffel L, McGill JB, Gan DJ. The beneficial effect of angiotensin-converting enzyme inhibition with captopril on diabetic nephropathy in normotensive IDDM patints with microalbuminuria. North Americn Microalbuminuria Study Group. Am J Med 1995;99:497–504.
3. Captopril reduces the risk of nephropathy in IDDM patients with microalbuminuria. The Microalbuminuria Captopril Study Group. Diabetologia 1996;39:587–593.
4. Mathiesen ER, Hommel E, Hansen HP, Smidt UM, Parving HH. Randomised controlled trial of long term efficacy of captopril on preservation of kidney function in normotensive patients with insulin dependent diabetes and microalbuminuria. BMJ 1999;319:24–25.
5. Effects of ramipril on cardiovascular and microvascular outcomes in people with diabetes mellitus: results of the HOPE study and MICRO-HOPE substudy. Heart Outcomes Prevention Evaluation Study Investigators. Lancet 2000;355(9200):253–259.
6. Randomised placebo-controlled trial of lisinopril in normotensive patients with insulin-dependent diabetes and normoalbuminuria or microalbuminuria. The EUCLID Study Group [see comments]. Lancet 1997;349:1787–1792.
7. Ravid M, Brosh D, Levi Z, Bar-Dayan Y, Ravid D, Rachmani R. Use of enalapril to attenuate decline in renal function in normotensive, normoalbuminuric patients with type 2 diabetes mellitus. A randomized, controlled trial. Ann Intern Med 1998;128:982–988.
8. Chaturvedi N, Sjolle AK, Stephenson JM, et al. Effect of lisinopril on progression of retinopathy in normotensive people with type 1 diabetes. Lancet 1998;351:28–31.
9. Tight blood pressure control and risk of macrovascular and microvascular complications in type 2 diabetes: UKPDS 38. UK Prospective Diabetes Study Group [published erratum appears in BMJ 1999;318(7175):29]. BMJ 1998;317:703–713.
10. Zuanetti G, Latini R, Maggioni AP, Franzosi MG, Santoro L, Tognoni G. Effect of the ACE inhibitor Lisinopril on mortality in diabetic patients with acute myocardial infarction data from the GISSI-3 study. Circulation 1997;96:4239–4245.
11. Gustafsson I, Torp-Pedersen C, Kober L, Gustafsson F, Hildebrandt P. Effect of the angiotensin-converting enzyme inhibitor trandolapril on mortality and morbidity in diabetic patients with left ventricular dysfunction after acute myocardial infarction. Trace Study Group. J Am Coll Cardiol 1999;34:83–89.

12. Tatti P, Pahor M, Byington RP, et al. Outcome results of the Fosinopril Versus Amlodipine Cardiovascular Events Randomized Trial (FACET) in patients with hypertension and NIDDM [see comments]. Diabetes Care 1998;21:597–603.

13. Brenner BM, Cooper ME, De Zeeuw D, et al. Effects of losartan on renal and cardiovascular outcomes in patients with type 2 diabetes and nephropathy. N Engl J Med 2001;345:861–869.

14. Black HR, Graff A, Shute D, et al. Valsartan, a new angiotensin II antagonist for the treatment of essential hypertension: efficacy, tolerability and safety compared to an angiotensin-converting enzyme inhibitor, lisinopril. J Hum Hypertens 1997;11:483–489.

15. McKelvie RS, Yusuf S, Pericak D, et al. Comparison of candesartan, enalapril, and their combination in congestive heart failure: randomized evaluation of strategies for left ventricular dysfunction (RESOLVD) pilot study. The RESOLVD Pilot Study Investigators [see comments]. Circulation 1999;100:1056–1064.

16. Kim S, Wanibuchi H, Hamaguchi A, Miura K, Yamanaka S, Iwao H. Angiotensin blockade improves cardiac and renal complications of type II diabetic rats. Hypertension 1997;30:1054–1061.

17. Hope S, Brecher P, Chobanian AV. Comparison of the effects of AT1 receptor blockade and angiotensin converting enzyme inhibition on atherosclerosis. Am J Hypertens 1999;12:28–34.

18. Horio N, Clermont AC, Abiko A, et al. Angiotensin AT(1) receptor antagonism normalizes retinal blood flow and acetylcholine-induced vasodilatation in normotensive diabetic rats. Diabetologia 2004;47:113–123.

19. Hu WY, Fukuda N, Ikeda Y, et al. Human-derived vascular smooth muscle cells produce angiotensin II by changing to the synthetic phenotype. J Cell Physiol 2003;196:284–292.

20. Urata H, Kinoshita A, Misono KS, Bumpus FM, Husain A. Identification of a highly specific chymase as the major angiotensin II- forming enzyme in the human heart [published erratum appears in J Biol Chem 1991;266(18):12114]. J Biol Chem 1990;265:22,348–22,357.

21. Owen CA, Campbell EJ. Angiotensin II generation at the cell surface of activated neutrophils: novel cathepsin G-mediated catalytic activity that is resistant to inhibition. J Immunol 1998;160:1436–1443.

22. Liao Y, Husain A. The chymase-angiotensin system in humans: biochemistry, molecular biology and potential role in cardiovascular diseases. Can J Cardiol 1995;11(Suppl F):13F–19F.

23. Ardaillou R. Angiotensin II receptors. JAm.Soc.Nephrol 1999;10(Suppl 11):S30–S39.

24. Zisman LS, Abraham WT, Meixell GE, et al. Angiotensin II Formation in the Intact Human Heart. JClin.Invest 1995;96:1490–1498.

25. Dzau VJ. Mechanism of protective effects of ACE inhibition on coronary artery disease. Eur Heart J 1998;19(Suppl J):J2–J6.

26. Takai S, Shiota N, Kobayashi S, Matsumura E, Miyazaki M. Induction of chymase that forms angiotensin II in the monkey atherosclerotic aorta. FEBS Lett 1997;412:86–90.

27. Song K, Shiota N, Takai S, et al. Induction of angiotensin converting enzyme and angiotensin II receptors in the atherosclerotic aorta of high-cholesterol fed Cynomolgus monkeys. Atherosclerosis 1998;138:171–182.

28. Donoghue M, Hsieh F, Baronas E, et al. A novel angiotensin-converting enzyme-related carboxypeptidase (ACE2) converts angiotensin I to angiotensin 1–9. Circ Res 2000;87:E1–E9.

29. Crackower MA, Sarao R, Oudit GY, et al. Angiotensin-converting enzyme 2 is an essential regulator of heart function. Nature 2002;417:822–828.

30. Healy DP, Song L. Kidney aminopeptidase A and hypertension, part I: spontaneously hypertensive rats. Hypertension 1999;33:740–745.

31. Chen HC, Bouchie JL, Perez AS, et al. Role of the angiotensin AT(1) receptor in rat aortic and cardiac PAI-1 gene expression. Arterioscler Thromb Vasc Biol 2000;20:2297–2302.

32. Reaux A, Fournie-Zaluski MC, David C, et al. Aminopeptidase A inhibitors as potential central antihypertensive agents. Proc Natl Acad Sci USA 1999;96:13,415–13,420.

33. Patel JM, Martens JR, Li YD, Gelband CH, Raizada MK, Block ER. Angiotensin IV receptor-mediated activation of lung endothelial NOS is associated with vasorelaxation. Am J Physiol 1998;275:L1061-L1068.

34. Coleman JK, Krebs LT, Hamilton TA, et al. Autoradiographic identification of kidney angiotensin IV binding sites and angiotensin IV-induced renal cortical blood flow changes in rats. Peptides 1998;19:269–277.

35. Albiston AL, McDowall SG, Matsacos D, et al. Evidence that the angiotensin IV (AT(4)) receptor is the enzyme insulin-regulated aminopeptidase. J Biol Chem 2001;276:48,623–48,626.

36. Lochard N, Thibault G, Silversides DW, Touyz RM, Reudelhuber TL. Chronic Production of Angiotensin IV in the Brain Leads to Hypertension that Is Reversible with an Angiotensin II AT1 Receptor Antagonist. Circ Res 2004;94:1451–1457.

37. Tan F, Morris PW, Skidgel RA, Erdos EG. Sequencing and cloning of human prolylcarboxypeptidase (angiotensinase C). Similarity to both serine carboxypeptidase and prolylendopeptidase families [published erratum appears in J Biol Chem 1993;268(34):26032]. J Biol Chem 1993;268:16,631–16,638.

38. Santos RA, Simoes e Silva AC, Maric C, et al. Angiotensin-(1–7) is an endogenous ligand for the G protein-coupled receptor Mas Proc Natl Acad Sci USA 2003;100:8258–8263.

39. Freeman EJ, Chisolm GM, Ferrario CM, Tallant EA. Angiotensin-(1–7) inhibits vascular smooth muscle cell growth. Hypertension 1996;28:104–108.

40. Benter IF, Ferrario CM, Morris M, Diz DI. Antihypertensive actions of angiotensin-(1–7) in spontaneously hypertensive rats. Am J Physiol 1995;269:H313–H319.

41. Horiuchi M, Akishita M, Dzau VJ. Recent progress in angiotensin II type 2 receptor research in the cardiovascular system. Hypertension 1999;33:613–621.

42. Unger T. Neurohormonal modulation in cardiovascular disease. Am Heart J 2000;139(Pt 2):S2–S8.

43. Oliverio MI, Kim HS, Ito M, Le T, Audoly L, Best CF, Hiller S, Kluckman K, Maeda N, Smithies O, Coffman TM. Reduced growth, abnormal kidney structure, and type 2 (AT2) angiotensin receptor-mediated blood pressure regulation in mice lacking both AT1A and AT1B receptors for angiotensin II. Proc Natl Acad Sci USA 1998;95:15,496–15,501.

44. Tsuchida S, Matsusaka T, Chen X, et al. Murine double nullizygotes of the angiotensin type 1A and 1B receptor genes duplicate severe abnormal phenotypes of angiotensinogen nullizygotes. J Clin Invest 1998;101:755–760.

45. Zou Y, Akazawa H, Qin Y, et al. Mechanical stress activates angiotensin II type 1 receptor without the involvement of angiotensin II. Nat Cell Biol 2004;6:499–506.

46. Al-Merani SA, Brooks DP, Chapman BJ, Munday KA. The half-lives of angiotensin II, angiotensin II-amide, angiotensin III, Sar1-Ala8-angiotensin II and renin in the circulatory system of the rat. J Physiol (Lond) 1978;278:471–90.

47. Chapman BJ, Brooks DP, Munday KA. Half-life of angiotensin II in the conscious and barbiturate-anaesthetized rat. Br J Anaesth 1980;52:389–393.

48. Diet F, Pratt RE, Berry GJ, Momose N, Gibbons GH, Dzau VJ. Increased accumulation of tissue ACE in human atherosclerotic coronary artery disease. Circulation 1996;94:2756–2767.

49. Campbell DJ, Kelly DJ, Wilkinson-Berka JL, Cooper ME, Skinner SL. Increased bradykinin and "normal" angiotensin peptide levels in diabetic Sprague-Dawley and transgenic (mRen-2)27 rats. Kidney Int 1999;56:211–221.

50. Vallon V, Wead LM, Blantz RC. Renal hemodynamics and plasma and kidney angiotensin II in established diabetes mellitus in rats: effect of sodium and salt restriction. J Am Soc Nephrol 1995;5:1761–1767.

51. Nakayama T, Izumi Y, Soma M, Kanmatsuse K. Adrenal renin-angiotensin-aldosterone system in streptozotocin-diabetic rats. Horm Metab Res 1998;30:12–15.

52. Cronin CC, Barry D, Crowley B, Ferriss JB. Reduced plasma aldosterone concentrations in randomly selected patients with insulin-dependent diabetes mellitus. Diabet Med 1995;12:809–815.

53. Price DA, Porter LE, Gordon M, et al. The paradox of the low-renin state in diabetic nephropathy. J Am Soc Nephrol 1999;10:2382–2391.

54. Anderson S, Jung FF, Inglefinger J. Renal renin-angiotensin system in diabetes: functional, immuno-histochemical, and molecular biological correlations. Am.JPhysiol 1993;265:F477–F486.

55. Brown L, Wall D, Marchant C, Sernia C. Tissue-specific changes in angiotensin II receptors in streptozotocin- diabetic rats. J Endocrinol 1997;154:355–362.

56. Sechi LA, Griffin CA, Schambelan M. The cardiac renin-angiotensin system in STZ-induced diabetes. Diabetes 1994;43:1180–1184.

57. Erman A, van Dyk DJ, Chen-Gal B, Giler ID, Rosenfeld JB, Boner G. Angiotensin converting enzyme activity in the serum, lung and kidney of diabetic rats. Eur J Clin Invest 1993;23:615–620.

58. Correa-Rotter R, Hostetter TH, Rosenberg ME. Renin and angiotensinogen gene expression in experimental diabetes mellitus. Kidney Int 1992;41:796–804.

59. Cassis LA. Downregulation of the renin-angiotensin system in streptozotocin- diabetic rats. Amer Physiol Soc 1992;262:E105–E109.

60. Jost-Vu E, Horton R, Antonipillai I. Altered regulation of renin secretion by insulinlike growth factors and angiotensin II in diabetic rats. Diabetes 1992;41:1100–1105.

61. Harker CT, O'Donnell MP, Kasiske BL, Keane WF, Katz SA. The renin-angiotensin system in the type II diabetic obese Zucker rat. J Am Soc Nephrol 1993;4:1354–1361.

62. Schunkert H, Ingelfinger JR, Jacob H, Jackson B, Bouyounes B, Dzau VJ. Reciprocal feedback regulation of kidney angiotensinogen and renin mRNA expressions by angiotensin II. Am J Physiol 1992;263:E863–E869.

63. Gabriely I, Yang XM, Cases JA, Ma XH, Rossetti L, Barzilai N. Hyperglycemia modulates angiotensinogen gene expression. Am J Physiol Regul Integr Comp Physiol 2001;281:R795–R802.
64. Malhotra A, Kang BP, Cheung S, Opawumi D, Meggs LG. Angiotensin II promotes glucose-induced activation of cardiac protein kinase C isozymes and phosphorylation of troponin I. Diabetes 2001;50:1918–1926.
65. Sodhi CP, Kanwar YS, Sahai A. Hypoxia and high glucose upregulate AT1 receptor expression and potentiate ANG II-induced proliferation in VSM cells. Am J Physiol Heart Circ Physiol 2003;284:H846–H852.
66. Drury PL, Smith GM, Ferriss JB. Increased vasopressor responsiveness to angiotensin II in type 1 (insulin-dependent) diabetic patients without complications. Diabetologia 1984;27:174–179.
67. Kennefick TM, Oyama TT, Thompson MM, Vora JP, Anderson S. Enhanced renal sensitivity to angiotensin actions in diabetes mellitus in the rat. Am J Physiol 1996;271:F595–F602.
68. Trevisan R, Bruttomesso D, Vedovato M, et al. Enhanced responsiveness of blood pressure to sodium intake and to angiotensin II is associated with insulin resistance in IDDM patients with microalbuminuria. Diabetes 1998;47:1347–1353.
69. Christlieb AR, Janka HU, Kraus B, et al. Vascular reactivity to angiotensin II and to norepinephrine in diabetic subjects. Diabetes 1976;25:268–274.
70. Natarajan R, Scott S, Bai W, Yerneni KK, Nadler J. Angiotensin II signaling in vascular smooth muscle cells under high glucose conditions. Hypertension 1999;33:378–384.
71. Amiri F, Venema VJ, Wang X, Ju H, Venema RC, Marrero MB. Hyperglycemia enhances angiotensin II-induced janus-activated kinase/STAT signaling in vascular smooth muscle cells. J Biol Chem 1999;274:32382–32386.
72. Candido R, Allen TJ, Lassila M, et al. Irbesartan but not amlodipine suppresses diabetes-associated atherosclerosis. Circulation 2004;109:1536–1542.
73. Shaw S, Wang X, Redd H, Alexander GD, Isales CM, Marrero MB. High glucose augments the angiotensin II-induced activation of JAK2 in vascular smooth muscle cells via the polyol pathway. J Biol Chem 2003;278:30634–30641.
74. Bouchie JL, Hansen H, Feener EP. Natriuretic factors and nitric oxide suppress plasminogen activator inhibitor-1 expression in vascular smooth muscle cells. Role of cGMP in the regulation of the plasminogen system. Arterioscler Thromb Vasc Biol 1998;18:1771–1779.
75. Yoshizumi M, Tsuji H, Nishimura H, et al. Atrial natriuretic peptide inhibits the expression of tissue factor and plasminogen activator inhibitor 1 induced by angiotensin II in cultured rat aortic endothelial cells. Thromb Haemost 1998;79:631–634.
76. Dubey RK, Jackson EK, Luscher TF. Nitric Oxide Inhibits Angiotensin II-induced Migration of Rat Aortic Smooth Muscle Cell. J Clin Invest 1995;96:141–149.
77. Pollman MJ, Yamada T, Horiuchi M, Gibbons GH. Vasoactive substances regulate vascular smooth muscle cell apoptosis. Countervailing influences of nitric oxide and angiotensin II. Circ Res 1996;79:748–756.
78. Takizawa T, Gu M, Chobanian AV, Brecher P. Effect of nitric oxide on DNA replication induced by angiotensin II in rat cardiac fibroblasts. Hypertension 1997;30:1035–1040.
79. Johnstone MT, Creager SJ, Scales KM, Cusco JA, Lee BK, Creager MA. Impaired endothelium-dependent vasodilation in patients with insulin- dependent diabetes mellitus [see comments]. Circulation 1993;88:2510–2516.
80. Williams SB, Cusco JA, Roddy M-A, Johnstone MT, Creager MA. Impaired nitric oxide-mediated vasodilation in patients with non-insulin-dependent diabetes mellitus. J Am Coll Cardiol 1996;27:567–574.
81. Dzau VJ. Theodore Cooper Lecture: Tissue angiotensin and pathobiology of vascular disease: a unifying hypothesis. Hypertension 2001;37:1047–1052.
82. Kon V, Jabs K. Angiotensin in atherosclerosis. Curr Opin Nephrol.Hypertens 2004;13:291–297.
83. Strawn WB, Ferrario CM. Mechanisms linking angiotensin II and atherogenesis. Curr Opin Lipidol 2002;13:505–512.
84. Park L, Raman KG, Lee KJ, et al. Suppression of accelerated diabetic atherosclerosis by the soluble receptor for advanced glycation endproducts. Nat.Med 1998;4:1025–1031.
85. Candido R, Jandeleit-Dahm KA, Cao Z, et al. Prevention of accelerated atherosclerosis by angiotensin-converting enzyme inhibition in diabetic apolipoprotein E-deficient mice. Circulation 2002;106:246–253.
86. Hayaishi-Okano R, Yamasaki Y, Katakami N, et al. Elevated C-reactive protein associates with early-stage carotid atherosclerosis in young subjects with type 1 diabetes. Diabetes Care 2002;25:1432–1438.
87. Paul A, Ko KW, Li L, et al. C-Reactive Protein Accelerates the Progression of Atherosclerosis in Apolipoprotein E-Deficient Mice. Circulation 2004;109:647–655.

88. Hayek T, Pavlotzky E, Hamoud S, et al. Tissue angiotensin-converting-enzyme (ACE) deficiency leads to a reduction in oxidative stress and in atherosclerosis: studies in ACE-knockout mice type 2. Arterioscler Thromb Vasc Biol 2003;23:2090–2096.

89. Hayek T, Attias J, Coleman R, et al. The angiotensin-converting enzyme inhibitor, fosinopril, and the angiotensin II receptor antagonist, losartan, inhibit LDL oxidation and attenuate atherosclerosis independent of lowering blood pressure in apolipoprotein E deficient mice. Cardiovasc Res 1999;44:579–587.

90. Domanski MJ, Exner DV, Borkowf CB, Geller NL, Rosenberg Y, Pfeffer MA. Effect of angiotensin converting enzyme inhibition on sudden cardiac death in patients following acute myocardial infarction. A meta-analysis of randomized clinical trials. J Am Coll Cardiol 1999;33:598–604.

91. Garg R, Yusuf S, for the Collaborative Group on ACE Inhibitor Trials. Overview of randomized trials of angiotensin-converting enzyme inhibitors on mortality and morbidity in patients with heart failure. JAMA 1995;273:1450–1456.

92. Diabetes mellitus: a major risk factor for cardiovascular disease. A joint editorial statement by the American Diabetes Association; The National Heart, Lung, and Blood Institute; The Juvenile Diabetes Foundation International; The National Institute of Diabetes and Digestive and Kidney Diseases; and The American Heart Association. [editorial; comment]. Circulation 1999;100:1132–1133.

93. Efficacy of atenolol and captopril in reducing risk of macrovascular and microvascular complications in type 2 diabetes: UKPDS 39. UK Prospective Diabetes Study Group [see comments]. BMJ 1998;317:713–720.

94. Estacio RO, Schrier RW. Antihypertensive therapy in type 2 diabetes: implications of the appropriate blood pressure control in diabetes (ABCD) trial. Am J Cardiol 1998;82:9R–14R.

95. Estacio RO, Jeffers BW, Hiatt WR, Biggerstaff SL, Gifford N, Schrier RW. The effect of nisoldipine as compared with enalapril on cardiovascular outcomes in patients with non-insulin-dependent diabetes and hypertension [see comments]. NEngl.JMed 1998;338:645–652.

96. Yusuf S, Sleight P, Pogue J, Bosch J, Davies R, Dagenais G. Effects of an angiotensin-converting-enzyme inhibitor, ramipril, on cardiovascular events in high-risk patients. The Heart Outcomes Prevention Evaluation Study Investigators [see comments] [published erratum appears in N Engl J Med 2000;342(10):748]. N Engl J Med 2000;342 (3):145–153.

97. Dagenais GR, Yusuf S, Bourassa MG, et al. Effects of ramipril on coronary events in high-risk persons: results of the Heart Outcomes Prevention Evaluation study. Circulation 2001;104:522–526.

98. Lonn E, Yusuf S, Dzavik V, et al. Effects of ramipril and vitamin E on atherosclerosis: the study to evaluate carotid ultrasound changes in patients treated with ramipril and vitamin E (SECURE). Circulation 2001;103:919–925.

99. Lindholm LH, Ibsen H, Dahlof B, et al. Cardiovascular morbidity and mortality in patients with diabetes in the Losartan Intervention For Endpoint reduction in hypertension study (LIFE): a randomised trial against atenolol. Lancet 2002;359:1004–1010.

100. Weir MR, Dzau VJ. The renin-angiotensin-aldosterone system: a specific target for hypertension management. Am J Hypertens 1999;12:205S–213S.

101. Fitzsimons JT. Angiotensin, thirst, and sodium appetite. Physiol Rev 1998;78:583–686.

102. Mehler PS, Jeffers BW, Estacio R, Schrier RW. Associations of hypertension and complications in non-insulin-dependent diabetes mellitus. Am J Hypertens 1997;10:152–161.

103. Zatz R, Dunn BR, Meyer TW, Anderson S, Rennke HG, Brenner BM. Prevention of diabetic glomerulopathy by pharmacological amelioration of glomerular capillary hypertension. J Clin Invest 1986;77:1925–1930.

104. Imanishi M, Yoshioka K, Konishi Y, et al. Glomerular hypertension as one cause of albuminuria in type II diabetic patients. Diabetologia 1999;42:999–1005.

105. Imanishi M, Yoshioka K, Okumura M, Konishi Y, Tanaka S, Fujii S, Kimura G. Mechanism of decreased albuminuria caused by angiotensin converting enzyme inhibitor in early diabetic nephropathy. Kidney Int Suppl 1997;63:S198–S200.

106. Anderson S, Rennke HG, Garcia DL, Brenner BM. Short and long term effects of antihypertensive therapy in the diabetic rat. Kidney Int 1989;36:526–536.

107. Sadoshima J, Xu Y, Slayter HS, Izumo S. Autocrine release of angiotensin II mediates stretch-induced hypertrophy of cardiac myocytes in vitro. Cell 1993;75:977–984.

108. Chen KD, Li YS, Kim M, et al. Mechanotransduction in response to shear stress. Roles of receptor tyrosine kinases, integrins, and Shc. J Biol Chem 1999;274:18393–18400.

109. Hoyer J, Kohler R, Haase W, Distler A. Up-regulation of pressure-activated Ca(2+)-permeable cation channel in intact vascular endothelium of hypertensive rats. Proc Natl Acad Sci USA 1996;93:11253–11258.

110. Hamada K, Takuwa N, Yokoyama K, Takuwa Y. Stretch activates Jun N-terminal kinase/stress-activated protein kinase in vascular smooth muscle cells through mechanisms involving autocrine ATP stimulation of purinoceptors. J Biol Chem 1998;273:6334–6340.

111. Ohno M, Cooke JP, Dzau VJ, Gibbons GH. Fluid shear stress induces endothelial transforming growth factor beta- 1 transcription and production. Modulation by potassium channel blockade. J Clin Invest 1995;95:1363–1369.

112. Jesmin S, Sakuma I, Hattori Y, Kitabatake A. Role of angiotensin II in altered expression of molecules responsible for coronary matrix remodeling in insulin-resistant diabetic rats. Arterioscler Thromb Vasc Biol 2003;23:2021–2026.

113. Zaman AK, Fujii S, Sawa H, et al. Angiotensin-converting enzyme inhibition attenuates hypofibrinolysis and reduces cardiac perivascular fibrosis in genetically obese diabetic mice. Circulation 2001;103:3123–3128.

114. Igarashi M, Hirata A, Yamaguchi H, et al. Candesartan inhibits carotid intimal thickening and ameliorates insulin resistance in balloon-injured diabetic rats. Hypertension 2001;38:1255–1259.

115. Yang BC, Phillips MI, Mohuczy D, et al. Increased angiotensin II type 1 receptor expression in hypercholesterolemic atherosclerosis in rabbits. Arterioscler Thromb Vasc Biol 1998;18:1433–1439.

116. Keidar S, Attias J, Heinrich R, Coleman R, Aviram M. Angiotensin II atherogenicity in apolipoprotein E deficient mice is associated with increased cellular cholesterol biosynthesis. Atherosclerosis 1999;146:249–257.

117. Napoleone E, Di Santo A, Camera M, Tremoli E, Lorenzet R. Angiotensin-converting enzyme inhibitors downregulate tissue factor synthesis in monocytes. Circ Res 2000;86(2):139–143.

118. Yanagitani Y, Rakugi H, Okamura A, et al. Angiotensin II type 1 receptor-mediated peroxide production in human macrophages. Hypertension 1999;33:335–339.

119. Steinberg HO, Chaker H, Leaming R, Johnson A, Brechtel G, Baron AD. Obesity/insulin resistance is associated with endothelial dysfunction. Implications for the syndrome of insulin resistance. J Clin Invest 1996;97:2601–2610.

120. Fard A, Tuck CH, Donis JA, et al. Acute elevations of plasma asymmetric dimethylarginine and impaired endothelial function in response to a high-fat meal in patients with type 2 diabetes. Arterioscler Thromb Vasc Biol 2000;20(9):2039–2044.

121. Jiang ZY, Lin YW, Clemont A, et al. Characterization of selective resistance to insulin signaling in the vasculature of obese Zucker (fa/fa) rats. J Clin Invest 1999;104:447–457.

122. Kuboki K, Jiang ZY, Takahara N, et al. Regulation of endothelial constitutive nitric oxide synthase gene expression in endothelial cells and in vivo : a specific vascular action of insulin. Circulation 2000;101:676–681.

123. Ting HH, Timimi FK, Boles KS, Creager SJ, Ganz P, Creager MA. Vitamin C improves endothelium-dependent vasodilation in patients with non-insulin-dependent diabetes mellitus. J Clin Invest 1996;97:22–28.

124. Zhao G, Zhang X, Smith CJ, et al. Reduced coronary NO production in conscious dogs after the development of alloxan-induced diabetes. Am J Physiol 1999;277:H268–H278.

125. Meininger CJ, Marinos RS, Hatakeyama K, et al. Impaired nitric oxide production in coronary endothelial cells of the spontaneously diabetic BB rat is due to tetrahydrobiopterin deficiency. Biochem J 2000;349(Pt 1):353–356.

126. Heitzer T, Krohn K, Albers S, Meinertz T. Tetrahydrobiopterin improves endothelium-dependent vasodilation by increasing nitric oxide activity in patients with Type II diabetes mellitus. Diabetologia 2000;43:1435–1438.

127. O'Driscoll G, Green D, Maiorana A, Stanton K, Colreavy F, Taylor R. Improvement in endothelial function by angiotensin-converting enzyme inhibition in non-insulin-dependent diabetes mellitus. J Am Coll Cardiol 1999;33:1506–1511.

128. Cheetham C, O'Driscoll G, Stanton K, Taylor R, Green D. Losartan, an angiotensin type I receptor antagonist, improves conduit vessel endothelial function in Type II diabetes. Clin Sci (Colch) 2001;100:13–17.

129. Arcaro G, Zenere BM, Saggiani F, et al. ACE inhibitors improve endothelial function in type 1 diabetic patients with normal arterial pressure and microalbuminuria. Diabetes Care 1999;22:1536–1542.

130. O'Driscoll G, Green D, Rankin J, Stanton K, Taylor R. Improvement in endothelial function by angiotensin converting enzyme inhibition in insulin-dependent diabetes mellitus. J Clin Invest 1997;100:678–684.

131. Folli F, Kahn CR, Hansen H, Bouchie JL, Feener EP. Angiotensin II inhibits insulin signaling in aortic smooth muscle cells at multiple levels. A potential role for serine phosphorylation in insulin/angiotensin II crosstalk. J Clin Invest 1997;100:2158–2169.

132. Velloso LA, Folli F, Sun XJ, White MF, Saad MJA, Kahn CR. Cross-talk between the insulin and angiotensin signaling systems. Proc.Natl.Acad.Sci.USA 1996;93:12,490–12,495.

133. Lang D, Mosfer SI, Shakesby A, Donaldson F, Lewis MJ. Coronary microvascular endothelial cell redox state in left ventricular hypertrophy : the role of angiotensin II. Circ Res 2000;86(4):463–469.

134. McFarlane R, McCredie RJ, Bonney MA, Molyneaux L, Zilkens R, Celermajer DS, Yue DK. Angiotensin converting enzyme inhibition and arterial endothelial function in adults with Type 1 diabetes mellitus. Diabet Med 1999;16:62–66.

135. Mullen MJ, Clarkson P, Donald AE, et al. Effect of enalapril on endothelial function in young insulin-dependent diabetic patients: a randomized, double-blind study. J Am Coll Cardiol 1998;31:1330–1335.

136. Torlone E, Britta M, Rambotti AM, Perriello G, Santeusanio F, Brunetti P, Bolli GB. Improved insulin action and glycemic control after long-term angiotensin-converting enzyme inhibition in subjects with arterial hypertension and type II diabetes. Diabetes Care 1993;16:1347–1355.

137. Valensi P, Derobert E, Genthon R, Riou JP. Effect of ramipril on insulin sensitivity in obese patients. Diabetes and Metabolism 1996;22:197–200.

138. Galletti F, Strazzullo P, Capaldo B, et al. Controlled study of the effect of angiotensin converting enzyme inhibition versus calcium-entry blockade on insulin sensitivity in overweight hypertensive patients: Trandolapril Italian Study (TRIS). J Hypertens 1999;17:439–445.

139. Fogari R, Zoppi A, Corradi L, Lazzari P, Mugellini A, Lusardi P. Comparative effects of lisinopril and losartan on insulin sensitivity in the treatment of non diabetic hypertensive patients. Br J Clin Pharmacol 1998;46:467–471.

140. Bonora E, Targher G, Alberiche M, et al. Effect of chronic treatment with lacidipine or lisinopril on intracellular partitioning of glucose metabolism in type 2 diabetes mellitus. J Clin Endocrinol Metab 1999;84:1544–1550.

141. Tillmann HC, Walker RJ, Lewis-Barned NJ, Edwards EA, Robertson MC. A long-term comparison between enalapril and captopril on insulin sensitivity in normotensive non-insulin dependent diabetic volunteers. J Clin Pharm Ther 1997;22:273–278.

142. New JP, Bilous RW, Walker M. Insulin sensitivity in hypertensive Type 2 diabetic patients after 1 and 19 days' treatment with trandolapril [In Process Citation]. Diabet Med 2000;17 (2):134–140.

143. Grassi G, Seravalle G, Dell'Oro R, et al. Comparative effects of candesartan and hydrochlorothiazide on blood pressure, insulin sensitivity, and sympathetic drive in obese hypertensive individuals: results of the CROSS study. J Hypertens 2003;21:1761–1769.

144. Nielsen S, Hove KY, Dollerup J, et al. Losartan modifies glomerular hyperfiltration and insulin sensitivity in type 1 diabetes. Diabetes Obes Metab 2001;3:463–471.

145. Trenkwalder P. Effects of candesartan cilexetil on glucose homeostasis. Multicenter Study Group. Basic.Res.Cardiol 1998;93(Suppl 2):140–144.

146. Trenkwalder P, Dahl K, Lehtovirta M, Mulder H. Antihypertensive treatment with candesartan cilexetil does not affect glucose homeostasis or serum lipid profile in patients with mild hypertension and type II diabetes. Blood Press 1998;7:170–175.

147. Henriksen EJ, Jacob S, Kinnick TR, Youngblood EB, Schmit MB, Dietze GJ. ACE inhibition and glucose transport in insulinresistant muscle: roles of bradykinin and nitric oxide. Am.JPhysiol 1999;277:R332–R336.

148. Henriksen EJ, Jacob S. Effects of captopril on glucose transport activity in skeletal muscle of obese Zucker rats. Metabolism 1995;44:267–272.

149. Caldiz CI, de Cingolani GE. Insulin resistance in adipocytes from spontaneously hypertensive rats: effect of long-term treatment with enalapril and losartan. Metabolism 1999;48:1041–1046.

150. Jacob S, Henriksen EJ, Fogt DL, Dietze GJ. Effects of trandolapril and verapamil on glucose transport in insulin- resistant rat skeletal muscle. Metabolism 1996;45:535–541.

151. Shiuchi T, Iwai M, Li HS, et al. Angiotensin II type-1 receptor blocker valsartan enhances insulin sensitivity in skeletal muscles of diabetic mice. Hypertension 2004;43:1003–1010.

152. Henriksen EJ, Jacob S, Kinnick TR, Teachey MK, Krekler M. Selective angiotensin II receptor receptor antagonism reduces insulin resistance in obese Zucker rats. Hypertension 2001;38:884–890.

153. Lakka HM, Laaksonen DE, Lakka TA, et al. The metabolic syndrome and total and cardiovascular disease mortality in middle-aged men. JAMA 2002;288:2709–2716.

154. Dahlof B, Devereux RB, Kjeldsen SE, et al. Cardiovascular morbidity and mortality in the Losartan Intervention For Endpoint reduction in hypertension study (LIFE): a randomised trial against atenolol. Lancet 2002;359:995–1003.

155. Uehara Y, Hirawa N, Numabe A, et al. Angiotensin-Converting Enzyme Inhibition Delays Onset of Glucosuria With Regression of Renal Injuries in Genetic Rat Model of Non-Insulin- Dependent Diabetes Mellitus. J Cardiovasc Pharmacol Ther 1998;3:327–336.

156. Tikellis C, Wookey PJ, Candido R, Andrikopoulos S, Thomas MC, Cooper ME. Improved islet morphology after blockade of the renin- angiotensin system in the ZDF rat. Diabetes 2004;53:989–997.

157. Shiuchi T, Cui TX, Wu L, et al. ACE inhibitor improves insulin resistance in diabetic mouse via bradykinin and NO. Hypertension 2002;40:329–334.

158. Henriksen EJ, Jacob S, Fogt DL, Dietze GJ. Effect of chronic bradykinin administration on insulin action in an animal model of insulin resistance. Am J Physiol 1998;275:R40–R45.

159. Duka I, Shenouda S, Johns C, Kintsurashvili E, Gavras I, Gavras H. Role of the B(2) receptor of bradykinin in insulin sensitivity. Hypertension 2001;38:1355–1360.

160. Carvalho CR, Thirone AC, Gontijo JA, Velloso LA, Saad MJ. Effect of captopril, losartan, and bradykinin on early steps of insulin action. Diabetes 1997;46:1950–1957.

161. Miyata T, Taguchi T, Uehara M, et al. Bradykinin potentiates insulin-stimulated glucose uptake and enhances insulin signal through the bradykinin B2 receptor in dog skeletal muscle and rat L6 myoblasts. Eur J Endocrinol 1998;138:344–352.

162. Motoshima H, Araki E, Nishiyama T, et al. Bradykinin enhances insulin receptor tyrosine kinase in 32D cells reconstituted with bradykinin and insulin signaling pathways. Diabetes Res Clin Pract 2000;48:155–170.

163. Rett K, Wicklmayr M, Dietze GJ, Haring HU. Insulin-induced glucose transporter (GLUT1 and GLUT4) translocation in cardiac muscle tissue is mimicked by bradykinin. Diabetes 1996;45 (Suppl 1):S66–S69.

164. Kishi K, Muromoto N, Nakaya Y, et al. Bradykinin directly triggers GLUT4 translocation via an insulin-independent pathway. Diabetes 1998;47:550–558.

165. Richey JM, Ader M, Moore D, Bergman RN. Angiotensin II induces insulin resistance independent of changes in interstitial insulin. Am J Physiol 1999;277:E920–E926.

166. Kinnick TR, Youngblood EB, O'Keefe MP, Saengsirisuwan V, Teachey MK, Henriksen EJ. Modulation of insulin resistance and hypertension by voluntary exercise training in the TG(mREN2)27 rat. J Appl Physiol 2002;93:805–812.

167. Andreozzi F, Laratta E, Sciacqua A, Perticone F, Sesti G. Angiotensin II impairs the insulin signaling pathway promoting production of NO by inducing phosphorylation of insulin receptor substrate-1 on Ser312 and Ser616 in human umbilical vein endothelial cells. Circ Res 2004;94:1211–1218.

168. Aguirre V, Uchida T, Yenush L, Davis R, White MF. The c-Jun NH(2)-terminal kinase promotes insulin resistance during association with insulin receptor substrate-1 and phosphorylation of Ser(307). J Biol Chem 2000;275(12):9047–9054.

5 PPARs and Their Emerging Role in Vascular Biology, Inflammation, and Atherosclerosis

Jorge Plutzky, MD

CONTENTS

INTRODUCTION

For many years, advances in understanding steroid hormone action typically proceeded through sequential stages that involved first identifying the role of a putative hormone, then isolating it, often from large quantities of body fluid, and ultimately identifying the nuclear receptor through which the cellular effects were being achieved *(1)*. More recently, this stepwise progression has been reversed by modern molecular biology techniques allowing rapid identification of many genes as encoding nuclear receptors based on structural motifs even without any information regarding the functional role of these so called orphan receptors. This process has been termed "reverse endocrinology" *(1)*. Peroxisome proliferator-activated receptors (PPARs) were examples of such orphan receptors, although their status changed through the serendipitous discovery of synthetic ligands that could bind to PPARs *(2)*. The fact that these synthetic agonists are now in clinical use for treating diabetes mellitus (DM) and dyslipidemia has helped draw attention to this nuclear receptor subfamily and its potential as a therapeutic target *(3)*. The identification of a possible role for PPARs in inflammation and atherosclerosis has only heightened this interest *(4)*.

From: *Contemporary Cardiology: Diabetes and Cardiovascular Disease, Second Edition*
Edited by: M. T. Johnstone and A. Veves © Humana Press Inc., Totowa, NJ

THE BASIC SCIENCE OF PEROXISOME PROLIFERATOR-ACTIVATED RECEPTOR BIOLOGY

Like all steroid hormone nuclear receptors, PPARs, including its three isotypes PPAR-α, PPAR-γ, and PPAR-δ, are ligand-activated transcription factors *(5)*. Also like other nuclear receptors, PPARs contain both ligand-binding and DNA-binding domains. In response to specific ligands, PPARs form a heterodimeric complex with another nuclear receptor-retinoic X receptor (RXR)—activated by its own ligand (9 *cis*-retinoic acid) *(2)*. This heterodimeric complex binds to defined PPAR-response elements in the promoters of specific target genes, determining their expression. Importantly, PPAR activation can either induce or repress the expression of different target genes. The mechanism through which PPAR repression occurs is not well understood but is thought to be indirect, for example influencing the critical inflammatory regulator nuclear factor κB (NF-κB) or controlling the small co-regulatory molecules (co-activators, co-repressors) that are central to transcriptional responses. Extensive studies over many years have defined specific metabolic roles for each PPAR isoform (Table 1). These individual characteristics provide a context for considering the potential role of each PPAR isoform in atherosclerosis and vascular biology.

Peroxisome Proliferator-Activated Receptor-γ: Key Regulator of Adipogenesis and Insulin Sensitivity

PPAR-γ was first identified as a part of a transcriptional complex essential for the differentiation of adipocytes, a cell type in which PPAR-γ is highly expressed and critically involved *(6)*. Homozygous PPAR-γ-deficient animals die at about day 10 *in utero* as a result of various abnormalities including cardiac malformations and absent white fat *(7–9)*. PPAR-γ is also involved in lipid metabolism, with target genes such as human menopausal gonadotropin coenzyme A synthetase and apolipoprotein (apo)-A-I *(10,11)*. Chemical screening and subsequent studies led to the serendipitous discovery that thiazolidinediones (TZDs) were insulin sensitizers that lower glucose by binding to PPAR-γ. Used clinically as antidiabetic agents, the TZD class includes pioglitazone (Actos) and rosiglitazone (formerly BRL49653, now Avandia) *(12,13)*. Troglitazone (ReZulin) was withdrawn from the market because of idiosyncratic liver failure. Naturally occurring PPAR-γ ligands have been proposed, although with more controversy, as discussed below. The fact that dominant negative mutations in PPAR-γ have been associated with severe insulin resistance and hypertension provides another argument for the importance of these receptors in human biology *(14,15)*.

Peroxisome Proliferator-Activated Receptor-α: Key Regulator of Fatty Acid Oxidation

PPAR-α is expressed in heart, liver, kidney, and skeletal muscle in which it plays a central role in the regulation of lipid, and especially fatty acid, metabolism *(16)*. PPAR-α target genes participate in the conversion of fatty acids to acyl-coenzyme A derivatives, peroxisome β-oxidation, and apolipoprotein expression (A1, AII, and CIII) *(10,17)*. Reminiscent of the story of PPAR-γ, fibrates in clinical use for lowering triglycerides and raising high-density lipoprotein (HDL), namely gemfibrozil (Lopid) and fenofibrate (TriCor), were found to be PPAR-α agonists *(18)*. Many insights into PPAR-α have come from the study of PPAR-α-deficient mice *(19)*. For example, these mice lack

Table 1
General Overview of Peroxisome Proliferator-Activated Receptor Isotypes

Isoform	PPAR-α	PPAR-γ	PPAR-δ
Major tissues	Liver Heart Muscle	Fat	Ubiquitous
Ligands	Fenofibrate Gemfibrozil WY14643*	Pioglitazone Rosiglitazone	Prostacarbacyclin
Biologic roles in metabolism	Fatty acid metabolism Lipid metabolism	Adipogenesis Insulin sensitivity Lipid metabolsim	Wound healing Lipid metabolism

Although peroxisome proliferator-activated receptor (PPAR) isoforms have a number of common attributes, they can also be distinguished by a number of unique characteristics. Perhaps most central to their different roles in metabolism, each PPAR is activated by different ligands, leading to regulation of specific target genes. A general overview utilizing illustrative examples for each PPAR isoform is listed to provide a general characterization. The evidence for PPAR expression and function in vascular and inflammatory responses is discussed elsewhere.

peroxisome proliferation in response to fibrates, confirming the connection between PPAR-α and peroxisome proliferation (20), a phenomenon that does not occur in humans (21). PPAR-α-deficient mice also manifest abnormal lipid profiles with increased total cholesterol, elevated apo-AI, and mildly increased total HDL levels, the latter as a result of apparent decreased HDL catabolism (22). Of note, PPAR-α activators do not lower triglycerides in PPAR-α null mice, implicating PPAR-α in the clinical effects of these drugs. Fibrates have been found to decrease cardiovascular events in patients with average low-density lipoprotein (LDL) levels and prior myocardial infarction (23). It remains unclear but of obvious interest if the vascular benefits of fibrates derive from their activation of PPAR-α. An expanding list of PPAR-α target genes that might underlie this is discussed further below.

Peroxisome Proliferator-Activated Receptor-δ: Widely Expressed, But Still Incompletely Understood

Although PPAR-δ is widely expressed in most cell types, its role has been less fully characterized. Recently, this has begun to change (24). PPAR-δ has been found to play an important part in wound healing and inflammatory responses in skin (25). PPAR-δ has also been implicated in cholesterol metabolism (26). One recent report suggested PPAR-δ activation might limit inflammation by sequestering the proinflammatory co-activator BCL-6 in macrophages (27). Perhaps one factor limiting research into PPAR-δ has been the absence of a ligand in clinical use. Given this, the main focus here will be on PPAR-γ and PPAR-α.

Peroxisome Proliferator-Activated Receptors in Vascular Biology and Atherosclerosis

The effects of PPAR agonists on vascular biology and atherosclerosis are an obvious issue given the patient populations that receive these drugs. Thiazolidinediones are used in patients with DM, and thus in patients with well-defined increased risk for cardiovascular events *(12)*. Fibrates are used to treat patients with increased triglycerides and low HDL, a profile with increased cardiovascular risk often seen among patients with insulin resistance if not frank diabetes *(18)*. Theoretically, PPAR agonists could have vascular benefits based on their various metabolic effects—improving insulin sensitivity, lowering glucose, and raising HDL. An alternative but not mutually exclusive hypothesis would be that if PPARs are expressed in vascular and inflammatory cells, then PPAR agonists could have direct effects that might influence atherosclerosis *(4)*. Indeed, this issue has become an area of considerable interest. All PPAR isoforms are now known to be expressed in endothelial cells (ECs), vascular smooth muscle cells (VSMCs), and monocytes/macrophages and T-lymphocytes *(28,29)*. An increasing amount of data continues to identify various PPAR-regulated target genes that are known to be involved in atherosclerosis. Moreover, this data is extending to in vivo studies in both rodents and humans.

Peroxisome Proliferator-Activated Receptor-γ in Inflammation, Vascular Biology, and Atherosclerosis

Early reports established not only that PPAR-γ was expressed in monocytes, macrophages, and human atherosclerosis, but also that PPAR-γ agonists could repress key proteins such as inflammatory cytokines and matrix metalloproteinases (MMPs) implicated in atherosclerosis and/or its complications *(30,31)*. These observations were countered by the finding that PPAR-γ agonists could also increase expression of CD36, a receptor mediating uptake of oxidized LDL *(32)*. Increased CD36 might be expected to promote foam cell formation. Subsequent studies identified coordinated induction by both PPAR-γ and PPAR-α of ABCA1, an important effector of cholesterol efflux *(33–35)*, an outcome that may offset potential pro-atherosclerotic effects of increased CD36. Interestingly, recent work establishes that TZDs have opposite effects on CD36 in vivo, decreasing their expression levels *(36)*. Aside from macrophages, PPAR-γ activation in VSMC decreases the proliferation and migration of these cells and their production of MMPs *(37,38)* and endothelin-1 *(39,40)*. The latter target suggests one possible mechanism accounting for the small but reproducible decrease in blood pressure seen with PPAR-γ agonists *(41)*.

Consistent with the effects seen in macrophages, PPAR-γ agonists repress inflammatory cytokine production in T-lymphocytes *(42)*. In ECs, PPAR-g may decrease adhesion molecule expression although the results are variable *(43,44)*, pointing out a limitation of a field that has depended heavily on synthetic agonists as experimental tools, with all the attendant concerns of pharmacological studies: physiological relevance, receptor dependence, dose dependence, and toxicity effects to name a few. One example of the potential complexities involved is evident in the relationship between PPAR-γ ligands and plasminogen activator inhibitor 1 (PAI-1) levels. Several reports indicate PPAR-γ ligands may increase expression of PAI-1, a pro-coagulant, pro-atherosclerotic response. Other laboratories find a PPAR-γ-mediated repression of PAI-1 *(45–47)*. Others report inhibition of PAI-1 expression *(48)*. In humans, PPAR-γ ligands clearly appear to decrease circulating PAI-1, although this may be a manifestation of improved glycemic control, less insulin resistance, or lower triglycerides *(41)*.

In vivo, PPAR-γ ligands have been given to various different mouse models of atherosclerosis. In general, these studies have all shown a decrease in the extent of atherosclerotic lesions *(31)*. Interestingly, in one study this decrease was not associated with a decrease in VCAM-1 expression *(49)*, potentially consistent with some in vitro work and again indicative of possible issues with in vitro vs in vivo findings. Regardless, the decrease in atherosclerosis is fairly consistent and in keeping with early surrogate marker studies in humans. For example, the PPAR-γ agonists in clinical use have been shown to lower levels of circulating MMP9 *(50,51)*, replicating the responses seen in vitro with VSMCs *(38)* and macrophages *(37)*. PPAR-γ agonists also decrease circulating levels of C-reactive protein (CRP) and levels of CD40 ligand (CD40L), both suggestive of an anti-inflammatory effect *(50)*. Several PPAR-γ agonists have been found to decrease carotid intimal-medial thickness, a parameter linked with cardiovascular risk *(52,53)*. These studies have all bolstered ongoing clinical trials examining the impact of PPAR ligands on cardiovascular endpoints. Independent of these direct effects on atherosclerosis, it remains possible that PPAR-γ agonists could limit atherosclerosis and/or inflammation indirectly by delaying or even preventing diabetes, as has been suggested in some studies *(54)*. Any such benefits must be gauged against any potential toxicity or adverse outcomes seen with TZDs. Edema and weight gain are two such issues that are receiving scrutiny given the occurrence of these side effects among patients taking TZDs *(55)*. The mechanism for these responses and the magnitude of the issue remain unclear but under study. Currently, TZDs are not recommended for individuals with low ejection fractions and known congestive heart failure *(55)*.

Peroxisome Proliferator-Activated Receptor-α in Vascular Biology, Inflammation, and Atherosclerosis

A similar but distinct picture as to one described for PPAR-γ has emerged for PPAR-α and its potential role in vascular responses. PPAR-α is also now known to be expressed throughout most vascular and inflammatory cells *(56)*. PPAR-α activation has been shown to favorably alter a number of well-established pathways strongly implicated in atherosclerosis. PPAR-α ligands clearly limit the inflammatory cytokine induction of adhesion molecules *(43,57)*. Importantly, this effect is absent when repeated in microvascular cells lacking PPAR-α *(58)*. The salutary benefits of fish oil may derive in part from PPAR-α activation with certain fatty acids limiting adhesion molecule expression and leukocyte adhesion in vivo in wild-type but not PPAR-α-deficient mice (Fig. 1) *(59)*. Interestingly, both omega-3 fatty acids and PPAR-α ligands can also limit expression of tissue factor, a protein found in macrophages and thought to be a major contributor to plaque thrombogenicity *(60,61)*. PPAR-α has also been found in VSMCs in which it represses the responses to inflammatory cytokines and, in limited data, decreased CRP levels *(62)*. Similar PPAR-α effects on CRP have been recently suggested in transgenic mice as well *(63,64)*. Like PPAR-γ, PPAR-α ligands have also been found to induce expression of the cholesterol efflux mediator ABCA1 *(35)*. In T-lymphocytes, PPAR-α ligands repress expression of inflammatory cytokines like interferon-γ, tumor necrosis factor-α, and interleukin-2, suggesting the potential for proximal upstream anti-inflammatory modulation *(42)*. One way in which PPAR-α activation may exert these effects is by limiting NF-κB activation.

The clinical trials using fibrates could be considered in some sense tests of the cardiovascular effects of PPAR-α agonists. In the Veterans Affairs HDL Intervention Trial, patients with a prior history of cardiovascular disease and a relatively average LDL, low HDL, and only modestly elevated triglycerides experienced fewer recurrent cardiac events in response to the fibrate gemfibrozil as compared to placebo *(23)*. It remains both

A

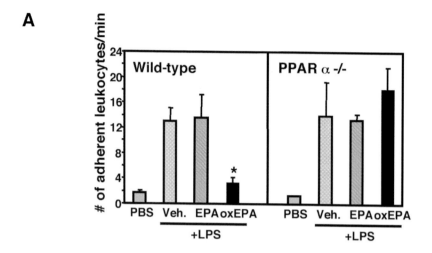

B

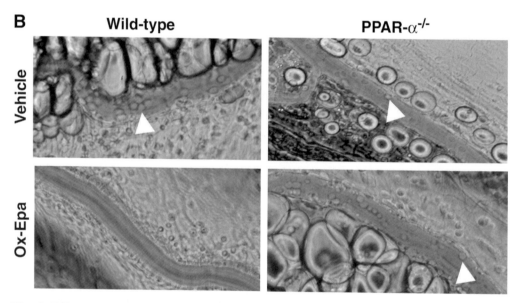

Fig. 1. Effect of oxidized EPA on leukocyte adhesion in mesenteric venules in wild-type and peroxisome proliferator-activated receptor-α-deficient mice. Several lines of in vitro and in vivo evidence suggest omega-3 fatty acids may exert their effects at least in part through PPAR-α activation. In the experiments shown here, wild-type or PPAR-α-deficient mice (PPARα–/–) were given an intraperitoneal injection of vehicle (Veh) alone; native EPA, or oxidized EPA (oxEPA), 1 hour prior to injection of a potent inflammatory stimulus (lipolysacharide). Five hours later, the adhesion of leukocytes to the gut microvasculature in anesthetized mice was examined using intravital microscopy. (**A**) Adherent leukocytes were determined ($n = 5$–7 for each group of mice). *$p < 0.03$ compared to Veh + LPS (wild-type) and oxidized EPA + LPS (PPAR-α –/–). Similar results were seen for leukocyte rolling. (**B**) Representative photographs of leukocytes interacting with the vessel wall (arrows) in LPS stimulated wild-type and PPARα–/– mice, after indicated treatments, are shown. The effects of oxidized EPA are abrogated in the genetic absence of PPAR-α *(59).*

unclear and challenging to establish that these clinical responses were a result of PPAR-α activation in metabolic pathways, like increased transcription of apo-A1, changes in inflammatory or vascular target genes, like repression of adhesion molecules or CRP, although this remains a plausible hypothesis. Perhaps studies with other more specific PPAR-α ligands in development might shed light on this possibility.

Endogenous Peroxisome Proliferator-Activated Receptor Activation: New Connections Between Fatty Acids, Lipid Metabolism, and Peroxisome Proliferator-Activated Receptor Responses

The metabolic benefits seen with synthetic PPAR agonists frame a key biological question: what does the body make to activate these receptors? Presumably, such molecules might replicate the effects of synthetic PPAR drugs, possibly protecting individuals from diabetes mellitus, dyslipidemia, and/or atherosclerosis. Early studies into endogenous PPAR agonists focused mainly on specific candidate molecules.

Oxidized linoleic acid in the form of 9 or 13 hydroxyoctadecanoic acid (HODE) appears to activate PPAR-γ (65), although it also has PPAR-α activity as well (58). The prostaglandin metabolite 15-deoxy-D12, 14-prostaglandin J2 (15d-PGJ2) (66,67) reportedly activates PPAR-γ agonist, although it can also act on IκB kinase and is of unclear physiologic significance (68,69). The greater biological effects seen with 15d-PGJ2 despite its lower PPAR-γ binding affinity may result from its PPAR-independent effects on IκB kinase (68,70). Oxidized linoleic acid (HODE) is generated by 15 lipoxygenase (71) and activates PPAR-γ and -α (32,58,72). Leukotriene B4 may be an endogenous PPAR-α ligand that terminates inflammation (73).

The identity of endogenous PPAR-α ligands has also been investigated. Early landmark experiments reported that certain fatty acids could activate PPARs, a great advance in the field (74–76). However, the physiological significance of those important observations was less clear, because the fatty acid effects seen required high concentrations of fatty acids (100–300 mM) and were not tested in vivo. Moreover, the link between endogenous lipid metabolism and subsequent PPAR activation remained obscure as did the mechanisms that might underlie selective PPAR isoform activation by natural ligands-like fatty acids. Given that PPAR isoforms are differentially regulated, it seems unlikely that endogenous PPAR activation is indiscriminate as to PPAR isotype. Recent work has continued to advance insight into endogenous PPAR activation. McIntyre and colleagues reported that lysophosphatidic acid could bind to and activate PPAR-γ (77). Very recently, oleylethanolamide, a fatty acid analogue, was found to regulate feeding by activating PPAR-α (78).

An alternative approach to understanding PPAR agonists is to investigate not specific candidate molecules but rather pathways that might lead to the generation of PPAR ligands. Through such studies, insight might be gained into PPAR function under more physiological conditions, connect pathways of lipid metabolism to PPAR activation, and perhaps account for selective PPAR responses. Recently, we and others have established that lipoprotein lipase (LPL), the primary enzyme in triglyceride metabolism, acts on triglyceride-rich lipoproteins like very low-density lipoprotein (VLDL) to generate PPAR ligands (79,80). These effects depended on intact LPL catalytic activity and were absent in response to LPL's known noncatalytic lipid uptake (79). Moreover, these studies revealed striking specificity in regards to lipid substrate (VLDL>>LDL>HDL) (Fig. 2). LPL hydrolysis may also explain selective PPAR activation, perhaps as a function of

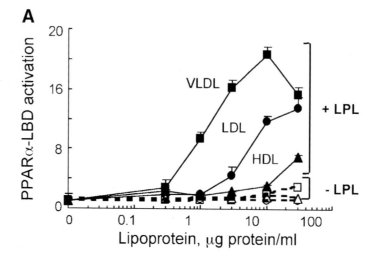

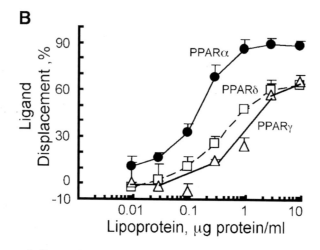

Fig. 2. Lipoprotein lipase (LPL) as a mechanism for peroxisome proliferator-activated receptor (PPAR) ligand generation. Endogenous PPAR agonists are generated through the action of LPL on triglyceride-rich lipoproteins *(79,80)*. **(A)** LPL treatment of various lipoproteins activates PPAR ligand-binding domains (LBDs) in an isoform specific manner. Concentration-dependent activation of PPAR-α-LBD by various lipoproteins in the presence or absence of LPL (30 U/mL) are shown. Endothelial cells (ECs) co-transfected with a PPAR-α-LBD, a luciferase reporter construct (pUASx4-TK-luc), and a β-galactosidase construct for normalization control and stimulated with increasing amounts of isolated human lipoproteins as shown; for comparison, PPAR-α-LBD activation by fenofibric acid (100 μM) was 16.2 ± 1.3-fold *(33)*. **(B)** The PPAR LBD assays shown in **(A)** demonstrate the presence of a PPAR activator but not a PPAR ligand (i.e., a molecule that binds directly to the receptor). Ligand status can be determined through the use of various other assays, including displacement of known high-affinity PPAR radioligands from expressed PPAR proteins. Such experiments establish LPL-mediated PPAR ligand generation as shown *(79)*. We find LPL action on very low-density lipoprotein preferentially generates PPAR-a ligands *(79)*, although cellular responses may vary depending on many factors, including levels of different PPAR isoforms in a given cell type *(80)*.

different cells and tissues. Although we observed LPL acted on VLDL to preferentially generate PPAR-α ligands, Evans and colleagues reported LPL-treatment of VLDL leads to PPAR-δ activation in macrophages *(80)*. Of note, mouse macrophages may have relatively low levels of PPAR-α, which may contribute to the greater PPAR-δ response seen *(81,82)*. Lipolytic PPAR activation may also be specific in regard to different lipases and specific fatty acids. For example, we found that other lipases, like phospholipases D, C, A2, failed to activate PPAR-α despite releasing equivalent amounts of fatty acids as LPL *(24)*. Presumably this is as a result of the release of different fatty acids, as determined by both the lipase and the composition of different lipoprotein substrates.

Interestingly, LPL action also replicated the effects of synthetic PPAR-α agonists on inflammation, decreasing VCAM-1 expression in a PPAR-α-dependent manner *(58,79)*. This data suggests a novel anti-inflammatory role for LPL, a mechanism that could explain the protection against atherosclerosis enjoyed by individuals with intact, efficient lipolytic pathways (i.e., individuals with normal triglyceride and higher HDL levels). Interestingly, extensive data establishes that patients with DM typically have elevated free fatty acids *(83)*. Other lines of well-done and carefully executed studies indicate that LPL overexpression in muscle induces insulin resistance *(84,85)*. Several possibilities might help reconcile these two sets of data. First, fatty acids are often referred to in a generic sense when, in fact, great differences exist between various fatty acids, for example ranging from the responses to omega-3 fatty acids, with their likely cardioprotective effects, to saturated fatty acids and their reported pro-atherosclerotic effects *(86,87)*. Thus, the elevated fatty acids in the circulation of patients with diabetes may differ from fatty acids produced by LPL, a significant percentage of which would be taken up by tissues as opposed to being present in the circulation. Moreover, these elevated fatty acids arise not out of the physiological function of LPL but rather abnormal metabolism. The DM seen in animal models overexpressing LPL in skeletal muscle is also associated with massive accumulation of triglycerides in these tissues *(88)*. Thus, the important observations from these experiments may not necessarily be a result of intact physiologic LPL action. Indeed, humans with LPL mutations that confer a gain of LPL function are associated with lower triglyceride levels, higher HDL, and apparent protection against atherosclerosis *(89)*. The exciting recent observations regarding the role of mitochondria as the main site of fatty acid oxidation in humans by Shulman and colleagues will only add new insight into the role of fatty acids in determining biological responses *(90–92)*.

CONCLUSION

The intense interest in PPARs as therapeutic targets is not surprising. PPARs are at the crossroads of metabolism, inflammation, and atherosclerosis, and suggest the possibility of modulating responses in all these pathways. The overwhelming impact abnormal metabolism—obesity, DM, dyslipidemia—is having in general, especially in terms of atherosclerosis, only heightens this interest. Moreover, PPARs, as transcription factors, raise the tantalizing prospect that PPAR ligands might achieve their effects by determining gene expression. Finally, the existence of PPAR ligands already in clinical use provides an established track that pharmaceutical and biotechnology concerns can hope to follow in bringing new agonists to market. Whether or not PPAR activation limits inflammation and atherosclerosis remains to be established; certainly the evidence to date supports the ongoing research examining the metabolic and cardiovascular effects of those PPAR agonists already approved and those in development.

REFERENCES

1. Kliewer SA, Lehmann JM, Willson TM. Orphan nuclear receptors: shifting endocrinology into reverse. Science 1999;284:757–760.
2. Willson TM, Brown PJ, Sternbach DD, Henke BR. The PPARs: from orphan receptors to drug discovery. J Med Chem 2000;43:527–550.
3. Moller DE. New drug targets for type 2 diabetes and the metabolic syndrome. Nature 2001;414:821–827.
4. Plutzky J. PPARs as therapeutic targets: reverse cardiology? Science 2003;302:406–407.
5. Willson TM, Wahli W. Peroxisome proliferator-activated receptor agonists. Curr Opin Chem Biol 1997;1:235–241.
6. Spiegelman BM. PPAR-gamma: adipogenic regulator and thiazolidinedione receptor. Diabetes 1998;47:507–514.
7. Rosen ED, Sarraf P, Troy AE, et al. PPAR-gamma is required for the differentiation of adipose tissue in vivo and in vitro. Mol Cell 1999;4:611–617.
8. Barak Y, Nelson MC, Ong ES, et al. PPAR gamma is required for placental, cardiac, and adipose tissue development. Mol Cell 1999;4:585–595.
9. Kubota N, Terauchi Y, Miki H, et al. PPAR gamma mediates high-fat diet-induced adipocyte hypertrophy and insulin resistance. Mol Cell 1999;4:597–609.
10. Auwerx J, Schoonjans K, Fruchart JC, Staels B. Regulation of triglyceride metabolism by PPARs: fibrates and thiazolidinediones have distinct effects. J Atheroscler Thromb 1996;3:81–89.
11. Latruffe N, Vamecq J. Peroxisome proliferators and peroxisome proliferator activated receptors (PPARs) as regulators for lipid metabolism. Biochimie 1997;79:81–94.
12. Henry RR. Thiazolidinediones. Endocrinol Metab Clin North Am 1997;26:553–573.
13. Schoonjans K, Auwerx J. Thiazolidinediones: an update. Lancet 2000;355:1008–1010.
14. Ristow M, Muller-Wieland D, Pfeiffer A, Krone W, Kahn CR. Obesity associated with a mutation in a genetic regulator of adipocyte differentiation. N Engl J Med 1998;339:953–959.
15. Barroso I, Gurnell M, Crowley VE, et al. Dominant negative mutations in human PPARgamma associated with severe insulin resistance, diabetes mellitus and hypertension [see comments]. Nature 1999;402:880–883.
16. Pineda Torra I, Gervois P, Staels B. Peroxisome proliferator-activated receptor alpha in metabolic disease, inflammation, atherosclerosis and aging. Curr Opin Lipidol 1999;10:151–159.
17. Forman BM, Chen J, Evans RM. The peroxisome proliferator-activated receptors: ligands and activators. Ann N Y Acad Sci 1996;804:266–275.
18. Staels B, Dallongeville J, Auwerx J, Schoonjans K, Leitersdorf E, Fruchart JC. Mechanism of action of fibrates on lipid and lipoprotein metabolism. Circulation 1998;98:2088–2093.
19. Lee SS, Pineau T, Drago J, et al. Targeted disruption of the alpha isoform of the peroxisome proliferator-activated receptor gene in mice results in abolishment of the pleiotropic effects of peroxisome proliferators. Mol Cell Biol 1995;15:3012–3022.
20. Lee SS, Gonzalez FJ. Targeted disruption of the peroxisome proliferator-activated receptor alpha gene, PPAR alpha. Ann N Y Acad Sci 1996;804:524–529.
21. Cattley RC, DeLuca J, Elcombe C, et al. Do peroxisome proliferating compounds pose a hepatocarcinogenic hazard to humans? Regul Toxicol Pharmacol 1998;27:47–60.
22. Peters JM, Hennuyer N, Staels B, et al. Alterations in lipoprotein metabolism in peroxisome proliferator-activated receptor alpha-deficient mice. J Biol Chem 1997;272:27,307–27,312.
23. Rubins HB, Robins SJ, Collins D, et al. Gemfibrozil for the secondary prevention of coronary heart disease in men with low levels of high-density lipoprotein cholesterol. Veterans Affairs High-Density Lipoprotein Cholesterol Intervention Trial Study Group. N Engl J Med 1999;341:410–408.
24. Lee CH, Olson P, Evans RM. Minireview: lipid metabolism, metabolic diseases, and peroxisome proliferator-activated receptors. Endocrinology 2003;144:2201–2207.
25. Tan NS, Michalik L, Noy N, et al. Critical roles of PPAR beta/delta in keratinocyte response to inflammation. Genes Dev 2001;15:3263–3277.
26. Michalik L, Desvergne B, Wahli W. Peroxisome proliferator-activated receptors beta/delta: emerging roles for a previously neglected third family member. Curr Opin Lipidol 2003;14:129–135.
27. Lee CH, Chawla A, Urbiztondo N, Liao D, Boisvert WA, Evans RM. Transcriptional Repression of Atherogenic Inflammation: Modulation by PPARδ. Science 2003;
28. Hsueh WA, Law R. The central role of fat and effect of peroxisome proliferator-activated receptor-gamma on progression of insulin resistance and cardiovascular disease. Am J Cardiol 2003;92:3J–9J.

29. Ziouzenkova O, Perrey S, Marx N, Bacqueville D, Plutzky J. Peroxisome Proliferator-activated Receptors. Curr Atheroscler Rep 2002;4:59–64.
30. Hsueh WA, Jackson S, Law RE. Control of vascular cell proliferation and migration by PPAR-gamma: a new approach to the macrovascular complications of diabetes. Diabetes Care 2001;24:392–397.
31. Beckman J, Raji A, Plutzky J. Peroxisome proliferator activated receptor gamma and its activation in the treatment of insulin resistance and atherosclerosis: issues and opportunities. Curr Opin Cardiol 2003;18:479–485.
32. Tontonoz P, Nagy L, Alvarez JG, Thomazy VA, Evans RM. PPARgamma promotes monocyte/macrophage differentiation and uptake of oxidized LDL. Cell 1998;93:241–252.
33. Chawla A, Barak Y, Nagy L, Liao D, Tontonoz P, Evans RM. PPAR-gamma dependent and independent effects on macrophage-gene expression in lipid metabolism and inflammation. Nat Med 2001;7:48–52.
34. Moore KJ, Rosen ED, Fitzgerald ML, et al. The role of PPAR-gamma in macrophage differentiation and cholesterol uptake. Nat Med 2001;7:41–47.
35. Chinetti G, Lestavel S, Bocher V, et al. PPAR-alpha and PPAR-gamma activators induce cholesterol removal from human macrophage foam cells through stimulation of the ABCA1 pathway. Nat Med 2001;7:53–58.
36. Liang CP, Han S, Okamoto H, Carnemolla R, Tabas I, Accili D, et al. Increased CD36 protein as a response to defective insulin signaling in macrophages. J Clin Invest 2004;113:764–773.
37. Ricote M, Li AC, Willson TM, Kelly CJ, Glass CK. The peroxisome proliferator-activated receptor-gamma is a negative regulator of macrophage activation. Nature 1998;391:79–82.
38. Marx N, Schonbeck U, Lazar MA, Libby P, Plutzky J. Peroxisome proliferator-activated receptor gamma activators inhibit gene expression and migration in human vascular smooth muscle cells. Circ Res 1998;83:1097–1103.
39. Iglarz M, Touyz RM, Amiri F, Lavoie MF, Diep QN, Schiffrin EL. Effect of peroxisome proliferator-activated receptor-alpha and -gamma activators on vascular remodeling in endothelin-dependent hypertension. Arterioscler Thromb Vasc Biol 2003;23:45–51.
40. Schiffrin EL, Amiri F, Benkirane K, Iglarz M, Diep QN. Peroxisome proliferator-activated receptors. Hypertension 2003;42(2):664–668.
41. Parulkar AA, Pendergrass ML, Granda-Ayala R, Lee TR, Fonseca VA. Nonhypoglycemic effects of thiazolidinediones. Ann Intern Med 2001;134:61–71.
42. Marx N, Kehrle B, Kohlhammer K, et al. PPAR activators as antiinflammatory mediators in human T lymphocytes: implications for atherosclerosis and transplantation-associated arteriosclerosis. Circ Res 2002;90:703–710.
43. Jackson SM, Parhami F, Xi XP, et al. Peroxisome proliferator-activated receptor activators target human endothelial cells to inhibit leukocyte-endothelial cell interaction. Arterioscler Thromb Vasc Biol 1999;19:2094–2104.
44. Pasceri V, Wu HD, Willerson JT, Yeh ET. Modulation of vascular inflammation in vitro and in vivo by peroxisome proliferator-activated receptor-gamma activators. Circulation 2000;101:235–238.
45. Marx N, Bourcier T, Sukhova GK, Libby P, Plutzky J. PPARgamma activation in human endothelial cells increases plasminogen activator inhibitor type-1 expression: PPARgamma as a potential mediator in vascular disease. Arterioscler Thromb Vasc Biol 1999;19:546–551.
46. Xin X, Yang S, Kowalski J, Gerritsen ME. Peroxisome proliferator-activated receptor gamma ligands are potent inhibitors of angiogenesis in vitro and in vivo. J Biol Chem 1999;274:9116–9121.
47. Ihara H, Urano T, Takada A, Loskutoff DJ. Induction of plasminogen activator inhibitor 1 gene expression in adipocytes by thiazolidinediones. Faseb J 2001;15:1233–1235.
48. Kato K, Satoh H, Endo Y, et al. Thiazolidinediones down-regulate plasminogen activator inhibitor type 1 expression in human vascular endothelial cells: A possible role for PPARgamma in endothelial function. Biochem Biophys Res Commun 1999;258:431–435.
49. Li AC, Brown KK, Silvestre MJ, Willson TM, Palinski W, Glass CK. Peroxisome proliferator-activated receptor gamma ligands inhibit development of atherosclerosis in LDL receptor-deficient mice. J Clin Invest 2000;106:523–531.
50. Haffner SM, Greenberg AS, Weston WM, Chen H, Williams K, Freed MI. Effect of rosiglitazone treatment on nontraditional markers of cardiovascular disease in patients with type 2 diabetes mellitus. Circulation 2002;106:679–684.
51. Marx N, Froehlich J, Siam L, et al. Antidiabetic PPAR gamma-activator rosiglitazone reduces MMP-9 serum levels in type 2 diabetic patients with coronary artery disease. Arterioscler Thromb Vasc Biol 2003;23:283–288.

52. Minamikawa J, Tanaka S, Yamauchi M, Inoue D, Koshiyama H. Potent inhibitory effect of troglitazone on carotid arterial wall thickness in type 2 diabetes. J Clin Endocrinol Metab 1998;83:1818–1820.

53. Koshiyama H, Shimono D, Kuwamura N, Minamikawa J, Nakamura Y. Rapid communication: inhibitory effect of pioglitazone on carotid arterial wall thickness in type 2 diabetes. J Clin Endocrinol Metab 2001;86:3452.

54. Buchanan TA, Xiang AH, Peters RK, et al. Preservation of pancreatic beta-cell function and prevention of type 2 diabetes by pharmacological treatment of insulin resistance in high-risk hispanic women. Diabetes 2002;51:2796–2803.

55. Nesto RW, Bell D, Bonow RO, et al. Thiazolidinedione use, fluid retention, and congestive heart failure: a consensus statement from the American Heart Association and American Diabetes Association. October 7, 2003. Circulation 2003;108:2941–2948.

56. Plutzky J. Peroxisome proliferator-activated receptors as therapeutic targets in inflammation. J Am Coll Cardiol 2003;42:1764–1766.

57. Marx N, Sukhova GK, Collins T, Libby P, Plutzky J. PPARalpha activators inhibit cytokine-induced vascular cell adhesion molecule-1 expression in human endothelial cells. Circulation 1999;99:3125–3131.

58. Ziouzenkova O, Asatryan L, Sahady D, et al. In peroxisome proliferation-activator receptor responses to electronegative low density lipoprotein. J Biol Chem 2003;278(41):39,874–39,881.

59. Sethi S, Ziouzenkova O, Ni H, Wagner DD, Plutzky J, Mayadas TN. Oxidized omega-3 fatty acids in fish oil inhibit leukocyte-endothelial interactions through activation of PPAR alpha. Blood 2002;100:1340–1346.

60. Marx N, Mackman N, Schonbeck U, et al. PPARalpha Activators Inhibit Tissue Factor Expression and Activity in Human Monocytes. Circulation 2001;103:213–219.

61. Neve BP, Corseaux D, Chinetti G, et al. PPARalpha Agonists Inhibit Tissue Factor Expression in Human Monocytes and Macrophages. Circulation 2001;103:207–212.

62. Staels B, Koenig W, Habib A, et al. Activation of human aortic smooth-muscle cells is inhibited by PPARalpha but not by PPARgamma activators. Nature 1998;393:790–793.

63. Kleemann R, Gervois PP, Verschuren L, Staels B, Princen HM, Kooistra T. Fibrates down-regulate IL-1-stimulated C-reactive protein gene expression in hepatocytes by reducing nuclear p50-NFkappa B-C/EBP-beta complex formation. Blood 2003;101:545–551.

64. Kleemann R, Verschuren L, De Rooij BJ, et al. Evidence for anti-inflammatory activity of statins and PPARα-activators in human C-reactive protein transgenic mice in vivo and in cultured human hepatocytes in vitro. Blood 2004;103(11):4188–4194.

65. Nagy L, Tontonoz P, Alvarez JG, Chen H, Evans RM. Oxidized LDL regulates macrophage gene expression through ligand activation of PPARgamma. Cell 1998;93:229–240.

66. Kliewer SA, Lenhard JM, Willson TM, Patel I, Morris DC, Lehmann JM. A prostaglandin J2 metabolite binds peroxisome proliferator-activated receptor gamma and promotes adipocyte differentiation. Cell 1995;83:813–819.

67. Forman BM, Tontonoz P, Chen J, Brun RP, Spiegelman BM, Evans RM. 15-Deoxy-delta 12, 14-prostaglandin J2 is a ligand for the adipocyte determination factor PPAR gamma. Cell 1995;83:803–812.

68. Rossi A, Kapahi P, Natoli G, et al. Anti-inflammatory cyclopentenone prostaglandins are direct inhibitors of IkappaB kinase. Nature 2000;403:103–108.

69. Bell-Parikh LC, Ide T, Lawson JA, McNamara P, Reilly M, FitzGerald GA. Biosynthesis of 15-deoxy-D12,14-PGJ2 and the ligation of PPARg. J Clin Invest 2003;112:945–955.

70. Straus DS, Pascual G, Li M, et al. 15-deoxy-delta 12,14-prostaglandin J2 inhibits multiple steps in the NF- kappa B signaling pathway. Proc Natl Acad Sci USA 2000;97:4844–4849.

71. Huang JT, Welch JS, Ricote M, et al. Interleukin-4-dependent production of PPAR-gamma ligands in macrophages by 12/15-lipoxygenase. Nature 1999;400:378–382.

72. Delerive P, Furman C, Teissier E, Fruchart J, Duriez P, Staels B. Oxidized phospholipids activate PPARalpha in a phospholipase A2- dependent manner. FEBS Lett 2000;471:34–38.

73. Devchand PR, Keller H, Peters JM, Vazquez M, Gonzalez FJ, Wahli W. The PPARalpha-leukotriene B4 pathway to inflammation control [see comments]. Nature 1996;384:39–43.

74. Keller H, Dreyer C, Medin J, Mahfoudi A, Ozato K, Wahli W. Fatty acids and retinoids control lipid metabolism through activation of peroxisome proliferator-activated receptor-retinoid X receptor heterodimers. Proc Natl Acad Sci USA 1993;90:2160–2164.

75. Forman BM, Chen J, Evans RM. Hypolipidemic drugs, polyunsaturated fatty acids, and eicosanoids are ligands for peroxisome proliferator-activated receptors alpha and delta. Proc Natl Acad Sci USA 1997;94:4312–4317.

76. Kliewer SA, Sundseth SS, Jones SA, et al. Fatty acids and eicosanoids regulate gene expression through direct interactions with peroxisome proliferator-activated receptors alpha and gamma. Proc Natl Acad Sci USA 1997;94:4318–4323.

77. McIntyre TM, Pontsler AV, Silva AR, et al. Identification of an intracellular receptor for lysophosphatidic acid (LPA): LPA is a transcellular PPARgamma agonist. Proc Natl Acad Sci USA 2003;100:131–136.

78. Fu J, Gaetani S, Oveisi F, et al. Oleylethanolamide regulates feeding and body weight through activation of the nuclear receptor PPAR-alpha. Nature 2003;425:90–93.

79. Ziouzenkova O, Perrey S, Asatryan L, et al. Lipolysis of triglyceride-rich lipoproteins generates PPAR ligands: evidence for an antiinflammatory role for lipoprotein lipase. Proc Natl Acad Sci USA 2003: 100(5):2730–2735.

80. Chawla A, Lee CH, Barak Y, et al. PPARdelta is a very low-density lipoprotein sensor in macrophages. Proc Natl Acad Sci USA 2003;100:1268–1273.

81. Welch JS, Ricote M, Akiyama TE, Gonzalez FJ, Glass CK. PPARgamma and PPARdelta negatively regulate specific subsets of lipopolysaccharide and IFN-gamma target genes in macrophages. Proc Natl Acad Sci USA 2003;100:6712–6717.

82. Glass C. PPARs in macrophage biology. Speech presented at Keystone Conference, DATE?, Keystone, Colorado.

83. Shulman GI. Cellular mechanisms of insulin resistance. J Clin Invest 2000;106:171–176.

84. Kim JK, Fillmore JJ, Chen Y, et al. Tissue-specific overexpression of lipoprotein lipase causes tissue-specific insulin resistance. Proc Natl Acad Sci USA 2001;98:7522–7527.

85. Ferreira LD, Pulawa LK, Jensen DR, Eckel RH. Overexpressing human lipoprotein lipase in mouse skeletal muscle is associated with insulin resistance. Diabetes 2001;50:1064–1068.

86. Jump DB. The biochemistry of n-3 polyunsaturated fatty acids. J Biol Chem 2002;277:8755–8758.

87. Kris-Etherton PM, Harris WS, Appel LJ. Fish consumption, fish oil, omega-3 fatty acids, and cardiovascular disease. Arterioscler Thromb Vasc Biol 2003;23:e20–e30.

88. Hegarty BD, Furler SM, Ye J, Cooney GJ, Kraegen EW. The role of intramuscular lipid in insulin resistance. Acta Physiol Scand 2003;178:373–383.

89. Hokanson JE. Functional variants in the lipoprotein lipase gene and risk cardiovascular disease. Curr Opin Lipidol 1999;10:393–399.

90. Petersen KF, Dufour S, Befroy D, Garcia R, Shulman GI. Impaired mitochondrial activity in the insulin-resistant offspring of patients with type 2 diabetes. N Engl J Med 2004;350:664–671.

91. Erol E, Kumar LS, Cline GW, Shulman GI, Kelly DP, Binas B. Liver fatty acid binding protein is required for high rates of hepatic fatty acid oxidation but not for the action of PPARalpha in fasting mice. Faseb J 2004;18:347–349.

92. Petersen KF, Befroy D, Dufour S, et al. Mitochondrial dysfunction in the elderly: possible role in insulin resistance. Science 2003;300:1140–1142.

6 Diabetes and Thrombosis

David J. Schneider, MD *and Burton E. Sobel,* MD

CONTENTS

DIABETES AND VASCULAR DISEASE

Complications of macrovascular disease are responsible for 50% of the deaths in patients with type 2 diabetes mellitus (DM), 27% of the deaths in patients with type 1 diabetes for 35 years or less, and 67% of the deaths in patients with type 1 diabetes for 40 years or more *(1,2)*. The rapid progression of macroangiopathy in patients with type 2 diabetes may reflect diverse phenomena; some intrinsic to the vessel wall; angiopathic factors such as elevated homocysteine and hyperlipidemia; deleterious effects of dysinsulinemia; and excessive or persistent microthrombi with consequent acceleration of vasculopathy secondary to clot-associated mitogens *(3,4)*. As a result of these phenomena, cardiovascular mortality is as high as 15% in the 10 years after the diagnosis of DM becomes established *(5)*. Because more than 90% of patients with diabetes have type 2 diabetes and because macrovascular disease is the cause of death in most patients with type 2 as opposed to type 1 (insulinopenic) diabetes, type 2 diabetes will be the focus of

From: *Contemporary Cardiology: Diabetes and Cardiovascular Disease, Second Edition*
Edited by: M. T. Johnstone and A. Veves © Humana Press Inc., Totowa, NJ

this chapter. In addition to coronary artery disease (CAD), patients with type 2 diabetes have a high prevalence and rapid progression of peripheral arterial disease (PAD), cerebral vascular disease, and complications of percutaneous coronary intervention including restenosis (6).

DM is associated with diverse derangements in platelet function, the coagulation, and the fibrinolytic system, all of which can contribute to prothrombotic state (Tables 1 and 2). Some are clearly related to metabolic derangements, particularly hyperglycemia. Others appear to be related to insulin resistance and hormonal derangements, particularly hyper(pro)insulinemia. In the material that follows, we will consider mechanisms exacerbating thrombosis as pivotal factors in the progression of atherosclerosis and their therapeutic implications.

THROMBOSIS AND ATHEROSCLEROSIS

Thrombosis appears to be a major determinant of the progression of atherosclerosis. In early atherosclerosis, microthrombi present on the luminal surface of vessels (7,8) can potentiate progression of atherosclerosis by exposing the vessel wall to clot-associated mitogens. In later stages of atherosclerosis, mural thrombosis is associated with growth of atherosclerotic plaques and progressive luminal occlusion.

The previously conventional view that high-grade occlusive, stenotic coronary lesions represent the final step in a continuum that begins with fatty streaks and culminates in high-grade stenosis has given way to a different paradigm because of evidence that thrombotic occlusion is frequently the result of repetitive rupture of minimally stenotic plaques. Thus, as many as two-thirds of lesions responsible for acute coronary syndromes (ACS) are minimally obstructive (less than 50% stenotic) at a time immediately before plaque rupture (9,10). Multiple episodes of disruption of lipid-rich plaques and subsequent thrombosis appear to be responsible for intermittent plaque growth that underlies occlusive coronary syndromes (11,12).

The extent of thrombosis in response to plaque rupture depends on factors potentiating thrombosis (prothrombotic factors), factors limiting thrombosis (anti-thrombotic factors), and the local capacity of the fibrinolytic system reflecting a balance between activity of plasminogen activators and their primary physiological inhibitor, plasminogen activator inhibitor type-1 (PAI-1). Activity of plasminogen activators leads to the generation of plasmin, an active serine proteinase, from plasminogen, an enzymatically inert circulating zymogen present in high concentration (~2 μM) in blood. The activity of plasmin is limited by inhibitors such as α2 antiplasmin.

When only limited thrombosis occurs because of active plasmin-dependent fibrinolysis at the time of rupture of a plaque, plaque growth may be clinically silent. When thrombosis is exuberant because of factors such as limited fibrinolysis, an occlusive thrombus can give rise to an ACS (acute myocardial infarction [MI], unstable angina, or sudden cardiac death).

The principle components of thrombi are fibrin and platelets. Other plasma proteins and white blood cells are incorporated to a variable extent. The rupture of an atherosclerotic plaque initiates coagulation and adhesion of platelets because of exposure to blood of surfaces denuded of endothelium and to constituents of the vessel wall such as collagen. Coagulation is initiated by tissue factor, a cell membrane-bound glycoprotein (13–15). Membrane-bound tissue factor binds circulating coagulation factor VII/VIIa to form the coagulation factor "tenase" complex that activates both circulating coagulation fac-

Table 1
Potential Impact of Insulin Resistance and Diabetes on Thrombosis

Factors predisposing to thrombosis
  Increased platelet mass
  Increased platelet activation
    • platelet aggregation
    • platelet degranulation
  Decreased platelet cAMP and cGMP
    • thromboxane synthesis
  Increased procoagulant capacity of platelets
  Elevated concentrations and activity of procoagulants
    • fibrinogen
    • von Willebrand factor and procoagulant activity
    • thrombin activity
    • factor VII coagulant activity
  Decreased concentration and activity of anti-thrombotic factors
    • anti-thrombin III activity
    • sulfation of endogenous heparin
    • protein C concentration

cAMP, cyclic adenosine monophosphate; cGMP, cyclic guanosine monophosphate. (Modified from ref. *4*.)

Table 2
Potential Impact of Insulin Resistance and Diabetes on Fibrinolysis

Factors attenuating fibrinolysis
  Decreased t-PA activity
  Increased PAI-1 synthesis and activity
    • directly increased by insulin
    • increased by hyperglycemia
    • increased by hypertriglyceridemia and increased FFA
    • synergistically increased by hyperinsulinemia combined with elevated triglycerides
      and FFA
  Increased concentrations of α2-antiplasmin

t-PA, tissue-type plasminogen activator; PAI-1, plasminogen activator inhibitor type-1; FFA, free fatty acid. (Modified from ref. *4*.)

tors IX and X expressed on activated macrophages, monocytes, fibroblasts, and endothelium in response to cytokines in the region of the ruptured plaque. Subsequent assembly of the "prothrombinase" complex on platelet and other phospholipid membranes leads to generation of thrombin. Availability of platelet factor Va is a key constituent of the initial prothrombinase complex. Subsequently, thrombin activates coagulation factor V in blood to form Va. Thrombin in turn cleaves fibrinogen to form fibrin. The generation of thrombin is sustained and amplified initially by its activation of circulating coagulation factors VIII and V. Thrombin generation is sustained by activation of other components in the intrinsic pathway including factor XI. Platelets are activated by thrombin, and activated platelets markedly amplify generation of thrombin.

A complex feedback system limits generation of thrombin. The tissue factor pathway becomes inhibited by tissue factor pathway inhibitor (TFPI) previously called lipoprotein-associated coagulation inhibitor (LACI). Furthermore, thrombin attenuates coagulation by binding to thrombomodulin on the surface of endothelial cells. The complex activates protein C (to yield protein Ca) that, in combination with protein S, cleaves (inactivates) coagulation factors Va and VIIIa.

Exposure of platelets to the subendothelium after plaque rupture leads to their adherence mediated by exposure to both collagen and multimers within the vessel wall of von Willebrand factor (16,17). The exposure of platelets to agonists including collagen, von Willebrand factor, adenosine diphosphate (ADP) (released by damaged red blood cells and activated platelets), and thrombin leads to further platelet activation. Activation is a complex process that entails shape change (pseudopod extension that increases the surface area of the platelet); activation of the surface glycoprotein (GP) IIb/IIIa; release of products from dense granules such as calcium, ADP, and serotonin and from α granules such as fibrinogen, factor V, growth factors and platelet factor 4 that inhibits heparin; and a change in the conformation of the platelet membrane that promotes binding to phospholipids and assembly of coagulation factors.

Activation of surface GP IIb/IIIa results in a conformational change that exposes a binding site for fibrinogen on the activated conformer (18). Each molecule of fibrinogen can bind two platelets, thereby leading to aggregation.

After activation, the plasma membranes of platelets express negatively charged phospholipids on the outer surface that facilitate the assembly of protein constituents and subsequently activity of the tenase and prothrombinase complexes (19). Thus, platelets participate in thrombosis by (a) forming a hemostatic plug (shape change, adherence to the vascular wall and aggregation); (b) supplying coagulation factors and calcium (release of α- and dense-granule contents); (c) providing a surface for the assembly of coagulation factor complexes; and (d) simulating vasoconstriction by releasing thromboxane and other vasoactive substances.

As noted previously, thrombosis complicating plaque rupture can occlude the lumen entirely or, when limited, contribute in a stepwise fashion over time to progressive stenosis. Mechanisms by which thrombi can contribute to plaque growth include incorporation of an organized thrombus into the vessel wall (20). Exposure of vessel wall constituents to clot-associated mitogens and cytokines can accelerate neointimalizaiton and migration and proliferation of vascular smooth muscle cells (VSMCs) in the media. Fibrin and fibrin-degradation products promote the migration of VSMCs and are chemotactic for monocytes (21). Thrombin itself and growth factors released from platelet α-granules such as platelet-derived growth factor and transforming growth factor-β activate smooth muscle cells (SMCs) potentiating their migration and proliferation (22–25). The powerful role of platelets has been demonstrated by a reduction in the proliferation of SMCs after mechanical arterial injury in thrombocytopenic rabbits with atherosclerosis (26).

Both local and systemic factors can influence the extent of thrombosis likely to occur in association with plaque rupture. The morphology and biochemical composition of the plaque influence thrombogenic potential. Atheromatous plaques with substantial lipid content are particularly prone to initiate thrombosis in contrast to the antithrombotic characteristics of the luminal surface of the normal vessel wall (27).

Both the severity of vascular injury and the extent of plaque rupture influence the extent to which blood is exposed to subendothelium and consequently to thrombogenicity.

The balances between the activity of prothrombotic factors and anti-thrombotic factors in blood and between thrombogenicity and fibrinolytic system capacity are important determinants of the nature and extent of a thrombotic response to plaque rupture. In subjects with type 2 diabetes, the balances between determinants are shifted toward potentiation and persistence of thrombosis and hence toward acceleration of atherosclerosis.

PLATELET FUNCTION IN SUBJECTS WITH DIABETES MELLITUS

The activation of platelets and their participation in a thrombotic response to rupture of an atherosclerotic plaque are critical determinants of the extent of thrombosis, incremental plaque growth, and the development of occlusive thrombi. Increased adherence of platelets to vessel walls manifesting early atherosclerotic changes and the release of growth factors from α-granules can exacerbate the evolution of atherosclerosis. Patients with diabetes, particularly those with macrovascular disease, have an increased circulating platelet mass secondary to increased ploidy of megakaryocytes (28). Activation of platelets is increased with type 2 diabetes. This is reflected by increased concentrations in urine of a metabolite of thromboxane A2, thromboxane B2, and by the spontaneous aggregation of platelets (29–31) in blood. The prevalence of spontaneous aggregation of platelets correlates with the extent of elevation of concentrations of hemoglobin (Hb)A1c (30). Stringent glycemic control decreases concentrations in urine of thromboxane B2 (29,31). Additionally, platelets isolated from the blood of subjects with diabetes exhibit impaired vasodilatory capacity (32), apparently mediated by release of a short-acting platelet-derived substance(s) that interferes with the ADP-induced dilatory response seen in normal vessels with intact endothelium (33).

EVIDENCE OF INCREASED PLATELET REACTIVITY

Platelets from subjects with both type 1 and 2 diabetes are hyperreactive (34–37). Platelet aggregometry performed with platelet-rich plasma and with suspensions of washed platelets in buffers from people with diabetes and control subjects has demonstrated increased aggregation of platelets in response to agonists such as ADP, epinephrine, collagen, arachidonic acid, and thrombin. Additionally, spontaneous (in the absence of added agonists) aggregation of platelets from subjects with diabetes is increased compared with aggregation of those from nondiabetic subjects (37).

Platelets from subjects with diabetes exhibit increased degranulation in response to diverse stimuli. The capacity to promote growth of SMCs in vitro is greater as shown by exposure of VSMCs to platelets from subjects with poorly controlled compared with well-controlled diabetes (38,39). Because α-granules contain growth factors, the enhanced growth-promoting activity of platelets from subjects with poorly controlled diabetes appears likely to be secondary to increased α-granule degranulation.

The threshold for induction of release of substances residing in dense granules in response to thrombin is lower in platelets from diabetic compared with nondiabetic subjects (40). Additionally, the procoagulant capacity of platelets from subjects with DM is increased (41,42). Thus, the generation of coagulation factor Xa and of thrombin is increased by three- to sevenfold in samples of blood containing platelets from diabetic compared with those from nondiabetic subjects (42).

In patients with diabetes, adhesion of platelets is increased because of increased surface expression of GP Ib-IX (43). The binding of von Willebrand factor multimers expressed on endothelial cells to GP Ib-IX mediates adherence and promotes subsequent activation of platelets. Adherence is promoted also by increased concentrations of and activity of von Willebrand factor *(43,44)*. Circulating von Willebrand factor stabilizes the coagulant activity of circulating coagulation factor VIIIa *(45)*.

An altered cellular distribution of guanine nucleotide-binding proteins (G proteins) appears to contribute to the increased reactivity of platelets in people with DM *(46)*. Platelet reactivity would be expected to be increased by the decreased concentrations of inhibitory G proteins that have been reported *(47)*. Additionally, platelet reactivity would be increased by the greater turnover of phosphoinositide and consequent intraplatelet release of calcium that have been seen *(48,49)*.

As noted above, activation of platelets leads to the expression of specific conformers of specific glycoproteins. Determination of the percentage of platelets expressing activation-dependent markers with flow cytometry can be used to delineate the extent of platelet activation that has occurred in vivo. Increased surface expression of CD63 (a marker of lysosomal degranulation), thrombospondin (a marker of α-granule degranulation), and CD62 (also called P-selectin), another marker of α-granule degranulation, has been observed with platelets isolated from patients with newly diagnosed diabetes and those with advanced diabetes regardless of whether or not overt macrovascular complications were present *(50,51)*. The increased PAI-1 in plasma *(see* Diabetes and Fibrinolysis) in patients with diabetes is associated with a paradoxically decreased platelet content of PAI-1 *(52)*, consistent with the possibility that release of PAI-1 from the platelets may contribute to the increased PAI-1 in blood.

Platelet survival is reduced in subjects with diabetes. The reduction is most pronounced in those with clinical evidence of vascular disease *(53)*. Thus, it appears to be more closely correlated with the severity of vascular disease *(54)* than with the presence of diabetes per se. Accordingly, the decreased survival of platelets may be both a marker of extensive vascular disease and a determinant of its severity.

Adherence of platelets to vessel walls early after injury resulting in de-endothelialization is similar in diabetic and nondiabetic animals *(55)*. By contrast, increased adherence of platelets to injured arterial segments 7 days after injury occurs in diabetic BB Wistar rats compared with that in control animals. A continued interaction of platelets with the vessel wall after injury is likely to be related to a decreased rate of healing and re-endothelialization in diabetic animals rather than to an increased propensity for adherence *per se (56)*. Regardless, continued interaction of platelets with the vessel wall and continued exposure of the vessel wall to growth factors released from α-granules of platelets are likely to accelerate and exacerbate atherosclerosis.

MECHANISMS RESPONSIBLE FOR HYPERREACTIVITY OF PLATELETS IN PEOPLE WITH DIABETES

Increased expression of the surface GPs Ib and IIb/IIIa has been observed in platelets from subjects with both type 1 and type 2 diabetes *(43)*. GP Ib-IX binds to von Willebrand factor in the subendothelium and is responsible for adherence of platelets at sites of vascular injury. Interaction between GP Ib-IX and von Willebrand factor leads to activation of platelets. Activation of GP IIb/IIIa leads to the binding of fibrinogen and aggregation of platelets. Thus, increased expression of either or both of these two surface glycoproteins is likely to contribute to the increased reactivity that has been observed platelets from people with diabetes.

Winocour and his colleagues have shown an association between decreased membrane fluidity and hypersensitivity of platelets to thrombin *(34)*. Reduced membrane fluidity may be a reflection of increased glycation of membrane proteins. A reduction in membrane fluidity occurs following incubation of platelets in media containing concentrations of glucose similar to those seen in blood from subjects with poorly controlled diabetes. Because membrane fluidity is likely to alter membrane receptor accessibility by ligands, reduced membrane fluidity may contribute to hypersensitivity of platelets. Accordingly, improved glycemic control would be expected to decrease glycation of membrane proteins, increase membrane fluidity, and decrease hypersensitivity.

Intracellular mobilization of calcium is critical in several steps involved in the activation of platelets. Platelets from subjects with type 2 diabetes exhibit increased basal concentrations of calcium *(57)*. Increased phosphoinositide turnover, increased inositide triphosphate production, and increased intracellular mobilization of calcium are evident in response to exposure to thrombin of platelets from subjects with type 2 diabetes *(58)*. The increased concentrations of several second messengers may contribute to the hypersensitivity seen in platelets from diabetic compared with nondiabetic subjects. Additionally, increased production of thromboxane A2 may contribute to the increased platelet reactivity *(31,34)*.

We have found that the osmotic effect of increased concentrations of glucose increase directly platelet reactivity *(59)*. Exposure of platelets in vitro to increased concentrations of glucose is associated with increased activation of platelets in the absence and presence of added agonist. Exposure of platelets to isotonic concentrations of glucose or mannitol increases platelet reactivity to a similar extent *(59)*. Thus, the osmotic effect of hyperglycemia on platelet reactivity may contribute to the greater risk of death and reinfarction that has been associated with hyperglycemia in patients with diabetes and MI *(60–62)*.

Insulin alters reactivity of platelets *(63)*. Exposure of platelets to insulin decreases platelet aggregation in part by increasing synthesis of nitric oxide (NO) that, in turn, increases intraplatelet concentrations of the cyclic nucleotides, cyclic guanosine monophosphate (cGMP), and cyclic adenosine monophosphate (cAMP). Both of these cyclic nucleotides are known to inhibit activation of platelets. Thus, it is not surprising that an insulin concentration-dependent increase in NO production exerts anti-aggregatory effects. Insulin deficiency typical of type 1 diabetes and seen in advanced stages of type 2 diabetes may contribute to increased platelet reactivity by decreasing the tonic inhibition of platelet reactivity otherwise induced by insulin. Furthermore, abnormal insulin signaling may contribute in subjects with type 2 diabetes. Accordingly, the increased resistance to insulin typical of type 2 diabetes may contribute to increased platelet reactivity by decreasing tonic inhibition of platelets that would have been induced otherwise by the high prevailing concentration of insulin.

Constitutive synthesis of NO is reduced in platelets from subjects with both type 1 and type 2 diabetes *(64)*. Thus, tonic inhibition of platelets and insulin-dependent suppression of reactivity may be reduced in subjects with diabetes.

ANTIPLATELET THERAPY AND DIABETES

Beneficial cardiovascular effects of aspirin are particularly prominent in people with diabetes. In the Physicians Health Study, prevention of MI was greater in those with compared with those without diabetes *(65)*. Treatment with aspirin decreased mortality in the Early Treatment Diabetic Retinopathy Study *(66)*. Because of the marked beneficial effects of aspirin, the American Diabetes Association has recommended treatment with aspirin of all patients with type 2 diabetes without specific contraindications.

Considered together, data acquired in vitro and in vivo suggest that platelets from subjects with diabetes are hypersensitive to diverse agonists. Unfortunately, currently available antiplatelet therapy does not restore normal responsiveness to platelets from subjects with diabetes. In animal preparations simulating selected aspects of diabetes, platelets remain hypersensitive to thrombin despite administration of aspirin *(67)*. This observation suggests that the hypersensitivity is not a reflection of generation of thromboxane A2, and that the treatment of subjects with diabetes with aspirin (as is being done often inferentially) is unlikely to decrease platelet reactivity to the level typical of that seen with platelets from nondiabetic subjects. Because hyperglycemia *per se* appears to increase platelet reactivity, improved glycemic control is a critical component of the antithrombotic regimen.

Therapy with abciximab (ReoPro), a GP IIb/IIIa inhibitor, reduces binding of fibrinogen and consequently the aggregation of platelets in response to agonists in vitro and has been shown to reduce the incidence of subsequent cardiac events in subjects underlying coronary angioplasty. Subjects with diabetes benefited, to some extent, from ReoPro. However, the subsequent incidence of cardiac events remained higher than that in nondiabetic subjects *(68)*. Perhaps of most importance, the need for target vessel revascularization was not decreased by therapy with ReoPro. These observations indicate that antiplatelet agents exert favorable effects and reduce the incidence of complications in patients with diabetes. However, currently available agents do not decrease the incidence of cardiac events to levels of incidence seen in nondiabetic subjects.

People with type 2 diabetes have a high incidence of overt cardiovascular and particularly CAD *(1,2,5)*. Thus, it appears likely that subclinical atherosclerosis is often present even in entirely asymptomatic subjects. Accordingly, many physicians believe the treatment guidelines such as those promulgated by the Adult Treatment Panel of the National Cholesterol Education Program *(69)* for subjects with known overt CAD should be applied to all people with type 2 diabetes, even those without signs or symptoms of cardiovascular disease (CVD). Based on this rationale, prophylaxis with daily aspirin is appropriate for all people with type 2 diabetes who have no specific contraindications (see Therapeutic Implications).

THE COAGULATION SYSTEM AND DIABETES MELLITUS

Activation of the coagulation system leads to the generation of thrombin and thrombin-mediated formation of fibrin from fibrinogen. The generation of thrombin depends on activation of procoagulant factors. It is limited by antithrombotic factors and inhibitors. Fibrinopeptide A (FPA) is released when fibrinogen is cleaved by thrombin. FPA has a very short half-life in the circulation and is cleared promptly by the kidneys. Elevated concentrations in blood are indicative of thrombin activity in vivo *(70)*. Subjects with DM (both types 1 and 2) have increased concentrations of FPA in blood and in urine compared with corresponding concentrations in nondiabetic subjects *(71–74)*. The highest concentrations are observed in patients with clinically manifest vascular disease *(72,74)*.

The increased concentrations of FPA seen in association with diabetes reflect an altered balance between prothrombotic and anti-thrombotic determinants in subjects with DM favoring thrombosis. This interpretation is consistent with other observations suggesting that generation of thrombin is increased with diabetes resulting in increased concentrations in blood of thrombin–anti-thrombin complexes *(75)*. The steady-state concentration of thrombin–anti-thrombin complexes in blood is a reflection of the rate of formation of thrombin being generated over time.

The increased generation of thrombin in people with diabetes is likely to be dependent on increased activity of factor Xa. This has been observed in patients with type 1 diabetes *(76)*. Factor Xa, a major component of the prothrombinase complex, is formed from components including circulating coagulation factor X assembled on phospholipid membranes in association with the tissue factor VIIa complex. Thrombin is generated by the prothrombinase complex comprising factors Xa, Va, and II assembled on phospholipid membranes. The activity of this complex is reflected by prevailing concentrations in blood of prothrombin fragment 1 + 2, a cleavage product of factor II (prothrombin). Increased concentrations of prothrombin fragment 1 + 2 in blood from patients with type 1 diabetes have been observed, consistent with the presence of a prothrombotic state.

MECHANISMS RESPONSIBLE FOR A PROTHROMBOTIC STATE ASSOCIATED WITH DIABETES

Patients with DM have increased concentrations in blood of the prothrombotic factors fibrinogen, von Willebrand factor, and factor VII coagulant activity *(77–79)*. Among the three coagulation factors, fibrinogen has been most strongly associated with the risk of development of CVD *(80)*. Although the mechanisms responsible for increased concentrations of fibrinogen and von Willebrand factor have not yet been fully elucidated, elevated concentrations in blood of insulin and proinsulin may be determinants in people with type 2 diabetes. This possibility is suggested by the close correlation between concentrations of fibrinogen with those of insulin and proinsulin in healthy subjects *(81)*. Because prediabetic subjects and people with early stages of diabetes have marked insulin resistance that leads to a compensatory increase in the concentrations in blood of insulin and proinsulin *(82–84)*, the hyper(pro)insulinemia of type 2 diabetes is likely to underlie, at least in part, the typically increased concentrations of fibrinogen. Improvement in metabolic control *per se* (euglycemia and amelioration of hyperlipidemia) has not been associated with normalization of the increased concentrations in blood of fibrinogen, von Willebrand factor, or factor VII coagulant activity *(79)*. By the same token, the extent of elevation of concentrations in blood of prothrombin fragment 1 + 2 is not closely correlated with the concentration of HbA1c, a marker of glycation of proteins *(85)*. First-degree nondiabetic relatives of subjects with type 2 diabetes exhibit increased concentrations of fibrinogen and factor VII coagulant activity in blood compared with values in age-matched controls *(86)*. Thus, the increases in fibrinogen and factor VII-coagulant activity are associated with other, presumably independent features of insulin resistance. Accordingly, increased concentrations of prothrombotic factors seen typically in subjects with type 2 DM are not reflections of the metabolic derangements typical of the diabetic state but instead appear to be dependent on insulin resistance and hyperinsulinemia. In fact, hormonal abnormalities, particularly insulin resistance and hyper(pro)insulinemia, appear to underlie the prothrombotic state *(81,86)*.

As mentioned in the preceding section on platelet function, procoagulant activity is increased in platelets from diabetic subjects. Procoagulant activity of monocytes is increased as well *(87)*. The negatively charged phospholipid surface of platelets and monocytes catalyzes both formation and activity of the tenase and prothrombinase complexes. Thus, increased procoagulant activity of platelets and monocytes can potentiate thrombosis.

Decreased activity of anti-thrombotic factors in blood can potentiate thrombosis. Of note, concentrations in blood of protein C and activity of anti-thrombin are decreased in diabetic subjects *(88–91)*, although not universally *(75)*. Unlike changes in concentrations of prothrombotic factors, altered concentrations and activity of anti-thrombotic factors appear to be reflections of the metabolic state typical of diabetes, either type 1 or type 2, especially hyperglycemia. Thus, decreased anti-thrombotic activity has been associated with nonenzymatic glycation of anti-thrombin.

To recapitulate, functional activity of the prothrombinase complex and of thrombin itself are increased consistently in blood of people with diabetes. The increased activity is likely to be a reflection of increased procoagulant activity of platelets and monocytes in association with increased concentrations of fibrinogen, von Willebrand factor , and factor VII. Diminished activity in blood of anti-thrombotic factors secondary to glycation of anti-thrombin and protein C may contribute to the prothrombotic state. To date, no anticoagulant pharmacological regimen has been identified that unequivocally decreases the intensity of the prothrombotic state in subjects with diabetes. To the extent that glycation of proteins contributes to a prothrombotic state, optimal glycemic control should attenuate it. Accordingly, the most effective mechanism available to attenuate a prothrombotic state is normalization of the hormonal and metabolic abnormalities in patients with diabetes. Results in the Diabetes Control and Complications Trial (DCCT) are consistent with this interpretation. Despite the fact that the DCCT focused on microvascular complications of diabetes, known to be influenced by hyperglycemia, a trend toward reduction of macrovascular events was seen with stringent and glycemic control *(92)*. This trend is consistent with reduction of the intensity of the prothrombotic state and hence attenuation of atherogenesis, determinants of its sequela, or both.

DIABETES AND FIBRINOLYSIS

Decreased fibrinolytic system capacity is observed consistently in blood from patients with DM, particularly those with type 2 diabetes *(93,94)*. It has been known for many years that obesity is associated with impaired fibrinolysis *(95)*; that elevated blood triglycerides and other hallmarks of hyperinsulinemia are associated with increased activity of PAI-1 *(96)*; and that elevated PAI-1 is a marker of increased risk of acute MI as judged from its presence in survivors compared with age-matched subjects who had not experienced any manifestations of overt CAD *(97)*. We found that impaired fibrinolysis in subjects with type 2 DM, not only under baseline conditions but also in response to physiological challenge, was attributable to augmented concentrations in blood of circulating PAI-1. Furthermore, obese diabetic subjects exhibited threefold elevations of PAI-1 in blood compared with values in nondiabetic subjects despite tissue-type plasminogen activator (t-PA) values that were virtually the same. The observation of an impairment of fibrinolysis not only under basal conditions but also in response to physiological stress implicates the pathophysiological import of the abnormality *(94)*. Subsequently, we found that precursors of insulin including proinsulin *(30,31)* and desproinsulin *(63,64)* induced time- and concentration-dependent elevation in expression of PAI-1 by human hepatoma cells in culture *(98)*. Additionally, we found that concentrations of PAI-1 can be elevated in blood in normal subjects rendered hyperglycemic, hyperinsulinemic, and hyperlipidemic *(99)*. Furthermore, women with the polycystic ovarian syndrome, known to be associated with hyperinsulinemia, have increased concentrations of PAI-1 in blood that can be reduced by administration of troglitazone, an insulin sensitizer *(100)*.

Thus, people with type 2 diabetes exhibit a decreased fibrinolytic system capacity secondary to increased PAI-1 in blood. Similar derangements are evident in association with other states of insulin resistance and compensatory hyperinsulinemia in conditions such as obesity (94,95), hypertension (101), and the polycystic ovarian syndrome (100,102,103).

Because the endogenous fibrinolytic system influences the evolution of thrombosis and the rapidity and extent of lysis of thrombi when vascular damage is repaired, overexpression of PAI-1 is likely to exacerbate development and the persistence of thrombi. Results in transgenic mice deficient in PAI-1 compared with wild type animals are consistent with this hypothesis. Thus, 24 hours after arterial injury, persistence of thrombosis and the residual thrombus burden were greater than in wild type mice that were not deficient in PAI-1 (104). Analogous observations have been obtained based on analysis of human tissues after fatal pulmonary embolism (105). Increased expression of PAI-1 in association with the pulmonary thromboembolism was evident. Thus, increased expression of PAI-1 typical of that seen in type 2 diabetes is likely to be a determinant of increased and persistent thrombosis.

MECHANISMS RESPONSIBLE FOR THE OVEREXPRESSION OF PAI-1 IN DIABETES

Increased expression of PAI-1 in diabetes is undoubtedly multifactorial. A direct effect of insulin on the expression of PAI-1 has been suggested by a positive correlation between the concentration of insulin and PAI-1 in vivo (93,94,96,100–103,106). Triglycerides and their constituents (fatty acids) appear to contribute to the overexpression of PAI-1 in view of the fact that both insulin and triglycerides independently increase expression of PAI-1 by human hepatoma cells in vitro (105,107–109). Liver steatosis is another determinant of elevated concentrations of PAI-1, perhaps indicative of the response of both to derangements in the tumor necrosis factor signaling pathway (110). Insulin and triglycerides exert a synergistic increase in accumulation of PAI-1 in conditioned media when both are present in pathophysiological concentrations (105). Analogous results are obtained with insulin in combination with very low-density lipoprotein-triglyceride, emulsified triglycerides, or albumin-bound free fatty acids (FFAs) (nonestrified). Thus, the combination of hyperinsulinemia and hypertriglyceridemia increases expression of PAI-1 consistent with the possibility that the combination is a determinant of the increased PAI-1 in people with diabetes in blood in vivo. Furthermore, because elevated concentrations of glucose increase expression of PAI-1 by endothelial cells and vascular smooth muscle cells in vitro (111,112), the metabolic state typical of diabetes may elevate concentrations of PAI-1 in blood-emanating release of PAI-1 from vessel wall cells.

A combination of hyperinsulinemia, hypertriglyceridemia, and hyperglycemia increases the concentration of PAI-1 in blood in normal subjects (99). Although neither the infusion of insulin with euglycemia maintained by euglycemic clamping nor the infusion of triglycerides without induction of hyperinsulinemia in normal subjects increases the concentration of PAI-1 in blood, the induction of hyperglycemia, hypertriglyceridemia, and hyperinsulinemia by infusion of glucose plus emulsified triglycerides plus heparin (to elevate blood FFAs) does increase concentrations of PAI-1 in blood. Of note, the infusion of insulin under euglycemic clamp conditions results in a marked decrease in the concentration of blood triglycerides and FFAs. Thus, results of the infusion studies demonstrate that the combination of hyperinsulinemia, hyperglycemia, and hypertriglyceridemia is sufficient to increase expression of PAI-1 in healthy subjects. However, results in these studies do not answer the question of whether, as in the case in vitro, insulin increases expression of PAI-1 when concentrations of glucose, triglycerides, and FFAs are all maintained within normal ranges. What is clear is that a combination of hormonal (hyperinsulinemia) and metabolic (particularly hypertriglyceridemia) derangements typical of type 2 DM elevate the concentration of PAI-1 in blood. The elevations of PAI-1 may subject people with diabetes to double jeopardy because the ratio of PAI-1 activity to the concentration of PAI-1 protein increases when the latter is high. This appears to reflect a slower rate of loss of PAI-1 activity associated with higher concentrations of PAI-1 protein (113).

Adipose tissue is another potential source of the increased blood PAI-1 in subjects with type 2 DM. Studies performed on genetically obese mice demonstrated that PAI-1 mRNA expression was increased four- to fivefold in mature adipocytes (114). The injection of insulin into lean mice increased expression of PAI-1 in adipocytes, an effect seen also with 3T3-L1 adipocytes in vitro. We have found that elaboration of PAI-1 from adipocytes is increased by transforming growth factor (TGF)-β, known to be released from activated platelets (115) secondary to increased transcription and furthermore, that caloric restriction per se lowers elevated PAI-1 in blood in obese, nondiabetic human subjects (116). Thus, the elevated concentrations of PAI-1 in blood seen in subjects with type 2 diabetes appear to be secondary to effects of hyperinsulinemia, particularly in combination with hypertriglyceridemia, and to effects of other mediators implicated in the prothrombotic state seen with diabetes on expression of PAI-1 by hepatic, arterial, and adipose tissue.

In addition to elevated PAI-1 in blood, expression of PAI-1 in vessel walls with subsequent elaboration into blood is increased by insulin (117). Pathophysiological concentrations of insulin increase the expression of PAI-1 by human arteries in vitro (117), an effect seen in both arterial segments that appear to be grossly normal and those that exhibit atherosclerotic changes. The increased PAI-1 expression is seen in arterial segments from subjects with or without insulin-resistant states. Augmented expression of PAI-1 is seen in response to insulin with VSMCs in culture (118) and with co-cultured endothelial cells and SMCs (117). Insulin increases expression of PAI-1 by vascular tissue in vivo. Local elaboration of PAI-1 follows perfusion with insulin in forearm vascular beds of healthy human subjects (119).

With the use of a co-culture system one mechanism by which insulin increases arterial wall expression of PAI-1 has been characterized (117). In vivo, insulin present in the luminal blood is known to be transported from the luminal to the abluminal surface of endothelial cells. In vitro, SMCs exposed to insulin have been shown to release a soluble factor(s) that increases endothelial cell expression of PAI-1. Thus, it appears likely that insulin in vivo alters expression of PAI-1 in arterial walls through a direct effect on VSMCs that, in turn, increases endothelial cell expression of PAI-1 in a paracrine fashion.

Therapy designed to reduce insulin resistance, the resultant hyperinsulinemia, or both have been shown to reduce PAI-1 in blood as well. Thus, treatment of women with the polycystic ovarian syndrome with metformin or troglitazone decreased concentrations in blood of insulin and of PAI-1 (100,103). Changes in the concentrations of PAI-1 in blood correlated significantly with those of insulin (100). The concordance supports the view that insulin contributes to the increased PAI-1 expression seen in vivo.

Human subjects who participate in relatively large amounts of leisure time physical activity have low levels of PAI-1 activity in blood (120). After adjustment for variables indicative of syndromes of insulin resistance such as high body mass index and waist to hip ratio in addition to advanced age and elevated concentrations of triglycerides, the association of PAI-1 activity with physical activity was no longer significant. This observation, particularly in combination with the results seen after therapy with troglitazone and metformin in women with the polycystic ovarian syndrome, demonstrates that interventions designed to attenuate insulin resistance will lower concentrations of PAI-1 in blood and increase fibrinolytic system capacity.

The exposure of human hepatoma cells to gemfibrozil decreases basal and insulin-stimulated secretion of PAI-1 (121). This inhibitory effect has been observed in vitro but not in vivo (122,123) despite reductions in vivo in the concentration of triglycerides in blood by 50% to 60%. No changes in insulin sensitivity or concentrations of insulin in the blood were seen after treatment of patients with gemfibrozil. Thus, unlike therapy with agents that reduce insulin resistance and lower concentrations of insulin, therapy with gemfibrozil that reduces triglycerides without affecting concentrations of insulin does not lower PAI-1 in vivo. These observations support the likelihood that insulin is the critical determinant of altered expression of PAI-1 in subjects with insulin resistance such as those with type 2 DM. As judged from results in studies in which human hepatoma cells were exposed to insulin and triglycerides in vitro, modest elevations in the concentrations of triglycerides and FFAs in the setting of hyperinsulinemia may be sufficient to augment expression of PAI-1. Thus, although the concentration of triglycerides in patients treated with gemfibrozil was decreased by 50%, the prevailing concentration of triglycerides may have been sufficient to lead to persistent elevation of PAI-1 in blood in the setting of hyperinsulinemia. Recent results in studies with several statins including atorvastatin fail to show concordant changes in PAI-1 in blood, consistent with this possibility (124).

FIBRINOLYSIS AND ARTERIAL MURAL PROTEOLYSIS

Results of recent work have highlighted the potential role of plasminogen activators and PAI-1 in the evolution of macroangiography in two compartments, blood in the arterial lumen (as described above) and in the arterial wall itself (125). Intramural plasminogen activators and PAI-1 influence proteolytic activity of matrix metalloproteinases (MMPs) that are activated from zymogens by plasmin. Cell surface plasmin-dependent proteolytic activation of MMPs promotes migration of SMCs and macrophages into the neointima and tunica media. Activation of MMPs appears to be a determinant of plaque rupture in complex atheroma and advanced atherosclerotic lesions, particularly in the vulnerable acellular shoulder regions of plaques (126).

Conversely, overexpression of PAI-1, by inhibiting intramural proteolysis and turnover of matrix, may contribute to accumulation of extracellular matrix (ECM) particularly in early atheromatous lesions. Overexpression of PAI-1 and the resultant accumulation of ECM have been implicated as a substrate for activation and migration of SMCs, chemotaxis of macrophages, and hence acceleration of early atherosclerosis. Analogously increased expression of PAI-1 has been observed in zones of early vessel wall injury after fatal pulmonary thromboembolism (127).

Taken together, these observations imply that an imbalance between the activity of plasminogen activators and the activity of PAI-1 can contribute to progression of atherosclerosis in diverse directions under diverse conditions. In early lesions, excess activity of PAI-1 may potentiate accumulation of matrix and its consequences. In complex lesions and late atherosclerosis, excess activity of plasminogen activators may exacerbate plaque rupture. Our observations regarding the relative amounts of plasminogen activators and of PAI-1 in association with the severity of atherosclerosis are consistent with both (128). The tissue content of PAI-1 is increased in early atherosclerotic lesions exemplified by fatty streaks. By contrast, the tissue content of plasminogen activators is increased in more complex lesions at a time when SMC proliferation is prominent.

The effects of PAI-1 in vessel wall repair have been clarified in animals genetically modified to be deficient in PAI-1 (PAI-1 knockout mice). Removal of noncellular debris and migration of SMCs are accelerated after mechanical or electrical injury of arteries in PAI-1-deficient mice (129). However, clot burden and persistence are increased. Thus, it appears likely that excess of either plasminogen activator or PAI-1 activity in the vessel wall may potentiate atherosclerosis. Excess PAI-1 may potentiate mural thickening secondary to accumulation of ECM and noncellular debris with diminished migration into the neointima of SMC during evolution of plaques destined to be vulnerable to rupture. Excess plasminogen activator activity may potentiate degradation of matrix and plaque rupture (125) in mature, vulnerable plaques. Consistent with this view, we have found increased immunoassayable PAI-1 and decreased urokinase plasminogen activator (u-PA) in atherectomy specimens from occlusive coronary lesions in patients with diabetes with or without restenosis compared with values in corresponding specimens from non-diabetic subjects (130). Conversely, immunoassayable urokinase in the atheroma was markedly diminished in association with diabetes.

It has been demonstrated that people with type 2 diabetes are remarkably prone not only to primary coronary lesions but also to restenosis after angioplasty (6,131,132). Our recent observations with extracted atheroma suggest that restenosis, especially that following iatrogenic injury to vessel walls associated with percutaneous coronary intervention (PCI), may develop, in part, because of increased expression of PAI-1. Although increased PAI-1 attenuates cell migration, it augments proliferation and inhibits apoptosis (133). Thus, restenosis may be exacerbated by increased PAI-1 resulting in increased proliferation and decreased apoptosis of SMCs within the arterial wall.

THERAPEUTIC IMPLICATIONS

Consideration of the derangements in platelet function, the coagulation system, and the fibrinolytic system and their contributions to exacerbation of macrovascular disease in type 2 diabetes gives rise to several therapeutic approaches. Empirical use of aspirin (160–325 mg per day in a single dose) seems appropriate in view of the high likelihood that covert CAD is present even in asymptomatic people with type 2 diabetes and the compelling evidence that prophylactic aspirin reduces the risk of heart attack when CAD is extant. Because many of the derangements contributing to a prothrombotic state in diabetes are caused by hyperglycemia, rigorous glycemic control is essential. Accordingly, the use of diet, exercise, oral hypoglycemic agents, insulin sensitizers, and if necessary insulin itself is appropriate to lower HbA1c to 7%. Because other derangements contributing to a prothrombotic state such as attenuation of fibrinolysis appear to be related to insulin resistance and hyper(pro)insulinemia, the use of insulin sensitizers as adjuncts to therapy with insulin or with other oral hypoglycemic agents is likely to be helpful.

Agents that enhance sensitivity to insulin and thereby promote glycemic control but limit hyperinsulinemia merit particular emphasis. Thiazolinediones lower elevated PAI-

1 in patients with hyperinsulinemia by attenuating insulin resistance, increasing peripheral glucose disposal, and modifying transcription of genes with protein products that are involved in carbohydrate and lipid metabolism and in fibrinolytic system activity. This class of agents exerts favorable effects on intimal medial thickness of carotid arteries in people with type 2 diabetes (134,135).

Use of metformin may attenuate abnormalities in the fibrinolytic system as well, although the primary mechanism of action of the drug differs from that of the glitazone. Metformin and its congeners decrease hepatic glucose output thereby normalizing carbohydrate and lipid metabolism and reducing requirements for insulin and lowering circulating endogenous insulin levels. Dosage should be initiated at 500 mg twice a day and gradually increased to a maximum of 2500 mg daily in three doses with meals. Optimal effects are generally seen with 1000 mg twice a day. Side effects are usually minor gastrointestinal disturbances, but lactic acidosis can be encountered particularly in patients with renal dysfunction, congestive heart failure, liver disease, or any condition predisposing to metabolic acidosis including diabetic ketoacidosis or excessive consumption of alcohol. Metformin should be discontinued temporarily when contrast agents are used (e.g., coronary angiography) to avoid lactic acidosis. In contrast to the glitazone, metformin can produce hypoglycemia, particularly when it is used with sulfonylureas.

The use of antiplatelet GP IIb/IIIa antagonists appears to be particularly beneficial in patients with symptomatic CAD and type 2 diabetes. The most cogent argument can be made for their use in patients who will be undergoing PCI. In one study of patients with diabetes who had sustained an ACS, the use of tirofiban reduced the incidence of the combined end-point of death or MI from 15.5% to 4.7% (136). The use of abciximab in patients with diabetes undergoing PCI reduced the 1-year mortality from 4.5% to 2.5% (137). GP IIb/IIIa inhibitors should be used for the treatment of people with diabetes with ACS including unstable angina and non-ST-segment elevation acute MI, especially in association with PCI.

Several complications and concomitants of diabetes can exacerbate a prothrombotic state and accelerate vascular disease. Thus, hypertriglyceridemia, hypertension, and hyperglycemia must be ameliorated. Lipid-lowering drugs should be used vigorously as is evident from results from studies such as the CARE trial in which the incidence of CAD was reduced by 27% in diabetic subjects to an extent comparable to that in nondiabetic subjects by administration of pravastatin over 5 years of follow-up (138).

Hypertension should be treated vigorously, generally with angiotensin-converting enzyme inhibitors because of the demonstrated reduction of progression of renal disease accompanying their use. An alternative may be angiotensin receptor blocking agents. Despite the ominous portent of macrovascular disease in type 2 diabetes, nephropathy continues to be a dominant life-threatening complication with an extraordinarily high incidence. Its occurrence is clearly related to hyperglycemia and may contribute to a prothrombotic state and acceleration of macrovascular disease through diverse mechanisms. Accordingly, rigorous glycemic control is essential.

Lifestyle modifications including implementation of a regular exercise program, reduction of obesity through dietary measures, and avoidance or cessation of cigarette smoking should be implemented to reduce the intensity of a prothrombotic state and the progression of macrovascular disease. Vitamin B_6 (1.7 mg per day) and folic acid (400 μg of dietary or 200 μg of supplemental folic acid per day) in recommended daily allowance (RDA) doses appear to be appropriate particularly because elevated homocysteine (139) and oxidative stress *(140)* associated with accelerated atherosclerosis are common in people with diabetes *(5)*. Elevated concentrations of homocysteine can be reduced readily with these doses of folic acid and vitamin B_6 in patients at risk of CAD whose homocysteine levels are in the upper percentiles of the normal range or only mildly elevated above normal. If concentrations of homocysteine are not normalized (to 14 μM) the likelihood of the subject being heterozygous for cystathionine β-synthase or homozygous for the thermolabile variant of the product of the methylene tetrahydrofolate reductase gene (MTHFR) is high in which case, 1 mg or more of folate per day may be needed to normalize concentrations of homocysteine. As a precaution, inclusion in supplements of vitamin B_{12} (1.2 μg per day, the RDA) is advisable when folic acid supplements are used to avoid potential neurological damage that can be induced by folate in the presence of occult B_{12} deficiency. Vitamin E (400 IU per day) has been more clearly implicated than vitamin C in reducing risk associated with oxidative stress although neither has been proved to be beneficial. It appears likely that increasing use of insulin sensitizers will retard the evolution of macrovascular disease as demonstrated already in the preliminary results of studies documenting favorable changes in carotid intimal-medial thickness accompanying their use *(134,135)*.

SUMMARY

Subjects with DM have a high prevalence and rapid progression of coronary artery, peripheral vascular, and cerebral vascular disease secondary in part to (a) increased platelet reactivity; (b) increased thrombotic activity reflecting increased concentrations and activity of coagulation factors and decreased activity of anti-thrombotic factors; and (c) decreased fibrinolytic system capacity resulting from overexpression of PAI-1 by hepatic, arterial, and adipose tissue in response to hyperinsulinemia, hypertriglyceridemia, and hyperglycemia. Additionally, macrovascular disease appears to be accelerated by an insulin-dependent imbalance in proteo(fibrino)lytic system activity within walls of arteries predisposing to accumulation of ECM and paucity of migration of SMCs during the evolution of atheroma predisposing toward the development of plaques vulnerable to rupture. Therapy designed to reduce insulin resistance decreases concentrations in blood not only of insulin but also of PAI-1. Thus, the treatment of subjects with diabetes, and particularly type 2 diabetes, should focus not only on improved metabolic control but also on reduction of insulin resistance and hyperinsulinemia. Treatment designed to address both the hormonal and metabolic abnormalities of diabetes is likely to reduce hyperactivity of platelets, decrease the intensity of the prothrombotic state, and normalize activity of the fibrinolytic system in blood and in vessel walls thereby reducing the rate of progression of macrovascular disease and its sequelae.

REFERENCES

1. Geiss LS, Herman WH, Smith PJ. Mortality in Non-Insulin-Dependent Diabetes. In: Harris MI, Cowie CC, Stern MP, Boyko, Reiber GE, Bennet PH, (eds). Diabetes in America. Washington, DC: U.S. Government Printing Office; DHHS NIH No. 95–1468, 1995, Chapter 11, pp. 233–257.
2. Portuese E, Orchard T. Mortality in Insulin-Dependent Diabetes. In: Harris MI, Cowie CC, Stern MP, Boyko, Reiber GE, Bennet PH, (eds). Diabetes in America. Washington, DC: U.S. Government Printing Office, DHHS NIH No 95–1468, 1995, Chapter 10, pp. 221–232.
3. Sobel BE. Coronary artery disease and fibrinolysis: From the blood to the vessel wall. Thromb Haemost 1999;82:8–13.

4. Schneider DJ, Sobel BE. Determinants of coronary vascular disease in patients with type II diabetes mellitus and their therapeutic implications. Clin Cardiol 1997;20:433–440.

5. Uusitupa MIJ, Niskanen LK, Siitonen O, Voutilainen E, Pyorala K. Ten-year cardiovascular mortality in relation to risk factors and abnormalities in lipoprotein composition in type 2 (non-insulin-dependent) diabetic and non-diabetic subjects. Diabetologia 1993;36:1175–1184.

6. Kornowski R, Mintz GS, Kent KM, et al. Increased restenosis in diabetes mellitus after coronary interventions is due to exaggerated intimal hyperplasia. Circulation 1997;95:1366–1369.

7. Velican C, Velican D. The precursors of coronary atherosclerotic plaques in subjects up to 40 years old. Atherosclerosis 1980;37:33–46.

8. Spurlock BO, Chandler AB. Adherent platelets and surface microthrombi of the human aorta and left coronary artery: a scanning electron microscopy feasibility study. Scanning Microsc 1987;1:1359–1365.

9. Ambrose JA, Tannenbaum AM, Alexpoulos D, et al. Angiographic progression of coronary artery disease and the development of myocardial infarction. J Am Coll Cardiol 1988;12:56–62.

10. Little WC, Constantinescu M, Applegate RJ, et al. Can coronary angiography predict the site of a subsequent myocardial infarction in patients with mild-to-moderate coronary artery disease? Circulation 1988;78:1157–1166.

11. Davies MJ, Richardson PD, Woolf N, Kratz DR, Mann J. Risk of thrombosis in human atherosclerotic plaques role of extracellular lipid, macrophage, and smooth muscle content. Br Heart J 1993;69:377–381.

12. Falk E, Shah PK, Fuster V. Coronary plaque disruption. Circulation 1995;92:657–671.

13. Nemerson Y. Tissue factor and hemostasis. Blood 1988;71:1–8.

14. Rand MD, Lock JB, Veer CV, Gaffney DP, Mann KG. Blood clotting in minimally altered whole blood. Blood 1996;88:3432–445.

15. Monroe DM, Roberts HR, Hoffman M. Platelet procoagulant complex assembly in a tissue factor-initiated system. Br J Haemotol 1994;88:364–371.

16. Staatz WD Rajpara SM, Wayner EA, Carter WG, Santoro SA. The membrane glycoprotein Ia-IIa (VLA-2) complex mediates the Mg+2-dependent adhesion of platelets to collagen. J Cell Biol 1989;108:1917–1921.

17. Kroll MH, Harris TS, Moake JL, Handin RI, Schafer AI. Von Willebrand Factor binding to platelet GP Ib initiates signals for platelet activation. J Clin Invest 1991;88:1568–1573.

18. Sims PJ, Ginsberg MH, Plow EF, Shattil SJ. Effect of platelet activation on the conformation of the plasma membrane glycoprotein IIb-IIIa complex. J Biol Chem 1991;266:7345–7352.

19. Monroe DM, Roberts HR, Hoffman M. Platelet procoagulant complex assembly in a tissue factor-initiated system. Br J Haemotol 1994;88:364–371.

20. Schwartz CJ, Valente AJ, Kelley JL, Sprague EA, Edwards EH. Thrombosis and the development of atherosclerosis: Roditansky revisited. Semin Thromb Hemost 1988;14:189–195.

21. Stirk CM, Kochhar A, Smith EB, Thompson WD. Presence of growth-stimulating fibrin-degradation products containing fragment E in human atherosclerotic plaques. Atherosclerosis 1993;103:159–169.

22. Ross R. The pathogenesis of atherosclerosis: A perspective for the 1990s. Nature 1993;362:801–809.

23. Scharf RE, Harker LA. Thrombosis and atherosclerosis: Regulatory role of interactions among blood components and endothelium. Blut 1987;55:131–144.

24. Bar-Shavit R, Hruska KA, Kahn AJ, Wilner GD. Hormone-like activity of human thrombin. Ann NY Acad Sci 1986;485:335–348.

25. Jawien A, Bowen-Pope DF, Lindner V, Schwartz SM, Clowes AW. Platelet-derived growth factor promotes smooth muscle migration and intimal thickening in a rat model of balloon angioplasty. J Clin Invest 1992;89:507–511.

26. Friedman RJ, Stemerman MB, Wenz B, et al. The effect of thrombocytopenia on experimental arteriosclerotic lesion formation in rabbits. Smooth muscle proliferation and re-endothelialization. J Clin Invest 1977;60:1191–1201.

27. Fernandez-Ortiz AJ, Badimon JJ, Falk E, Fuster V, Meyer B, Mailhac A, Weng D, Shah PK, Badimon LL. Characterization of relative thrombogenicity of atherosclerotic plaque components: Implications for consequences of plaque rupture. J Am Coll Cardiol 1994;23:1562–1569.

28. Brown AS, Hong Y, de Belder A, et al. Megakaryoctye ploidy and platelet changes in human diabetes and atherosclerosis. Arterioscl Thromb Vasc Biol 1997;17:802–807.

29. Mayfield RK, Halushka PV, Wohltmann HJ, et al. Platelet function during continuous insulin infusion treatment in insulin-dependent diabetic patients. Diabetes 1985;34:1127–1133.

30. Iwase E, Tawata M, Aida K, et al. A cross-sectional evaluation of spontaneous platelet aggregation in relation to complications in patients with type II diabetes mellitus. Metabolism 1998;47:699–705.

31. Davi G, Catalano I, Averna M, et al. Thromboxane biosynthesis and platelet function in type II diabetes mellitus. N Engl J Med 1990;322:1769–1774.
32. Oskarsson HJ, Hofmeyer TG. Platelets from patients with diabetes mellitus have impaired ability to mediate vasodilatation. J Am Coll Cardiol 1996;27:1464–1370.
33. Oskarsson HJ, Hofmeyer TG. Diabetic human platelets release a substance that inhibits platelet-mediated vasodilatation. Am J Physiol 1997;273:H371–H379.
34. Winocour PD, Watala C, Kinlough-Rathbone, RL. Membrane fluidity is related to the extent of glycation of proteins, but not to alterations in the cholesterol to phospholipid molar ratio in isolated platelet membranes from diabetic and control subjects. Thromb Haemostas 1992;67:567–571.
35. Ishii H, Umeda F, Nawata H. Platelet function in diabetes mellitus. Diabetes Metab Rev 1992;8:53–66.
36. Hendra T, Betteridge DJ. Platelet function, platelet prostanoids and vascular prostacyclin in diabetes. Prostaglandins Leukotrienes Essent Fatty Acids 1989;35:197–212.
37. Menys VS, Bhatnagar D, Mackness MI, Durrington PN. Spontaneous platelet aggregation in whole blood is increased in non-insulin-dependent diabetes mellitus and in female but not male patients with primary dyslipidemia. Atherosclerosis 1995;112:115–122.
38. Sugimoto H, Franks DJ, Lecavalier L, Chiasson JL, Hamet P. Therapeutic modulation of growth-promoting activity in platelets from diabetics. Diabetes 1987;36:667–672.
39. Koschinsky T, Bunting CR, Rutter R, Gries FA. Vascular growth factors and the development of macrovascular disease in diabetes mellitus. Diabete Metab 1987;13:318–325.
40. Winocour PD, Bryszewska M, Watala C, et al. Reduced membrane fluidity in platelets from diabetic patients. Diabetes 1990;39:241–244.
41. Rao AK, Goldberg RE, Walsh PN. Platelet coagulation activity in diabetes mellitus. Evidence for relationship between platelet coagulant hyeractivity and platelet volume. J Lab Clin Med 1984;103:82–92.
42. Lupu C, Calb M, Ionescu M, Lupu F. Enhanced prothrombin and intrinsic factor X activation on blood platelets from diabetic patients. Thromb Haemost 1993;70:579–583.
43. Tschoepe D, Roesen P, Kaufmann L, et al. Evidence for abnormal platelet glycoprotein expression in diabetes mellitus. Eur J Clin Invest 1990;20:166–170.
44. Romano M, Pomilio M, Vigneri S, et al. Endothelial perturbation in children and adolescents with type 1 diabetes: association with markers of the inflammatory reaction. Diabetes Care 2001;24:1674–1678.
45. Mann KG, Butenas S, Brummel K. The dynamics of thrombin formation. Arterioscler Thromb Vasc Biol 2003;23(1):17(Abstract).
46. Bastyr EJ 3rd, Lu J, Stowe R, Green A, Vinik AI. Low molecular weight GTP-binding proteins are altered in platelet hyperaggragation in IDDM. Oncogene 2003;8:515–518.
47. Livingstone C, McLellan AR, McGregor MA, et al. Altered G-protein expression and adenylate cyclase activity in platelets of non-insulin-dependent diabetic (NIDDM) male subjects. Biochim Biophys Acta 1991;1096:127–133.
48. Ishii H, Umeda F, Hashimoto T, Nawata H. Changes in phosphoinositide turnover, $Ca2+$ mobilization, and protein phosphorylation in platelets from NIDDM patients. Diabetes 1990;39:1561–1568.
49. Schaeffer G, Wascher TC, Kostner GM, Graier WF. Alterations in platelet $Ca2+$ signalling in diabetic patients is due to increased formation of superoxide anions and reduced nitric oxide production. Diabetologia 1999;42:167–176.
50. Tschoepe D, Roesen P, Esser J, et al. Large platelets circulate in an activated state in diabetes mellitus. Semin Thromb Hemostasis 1991;17:433–438.
51. Tschoepe D, Driesch E, Schwippert B, Nieuwenhuis K, Gries FA. Exposure of adhesion molecules on activated platelets in patients with newly diagnosed IDDM is not normalized by near-normoglycemia. Diabetes 1995;44:890–894.
52. Torr-Brown SR, Sobel BE. Plasminogen activator inhibitor is elevated in plasma and diminished in platelets in patients with diabetes mellitus. Thromb Res 1994;75:473–477.
53. Colwell JA. Vascular thrombosis in type II diabetes mellitus. Diabetes 1993;42:8–11.
54. Kinlough-Rathbone RL, Packham MA, Mustard JF. Vessel injury, platelet adherence, and platelet survival. Arteriosclerosis 1983;3:529–546.
55. Winocour PD, Richardson M, Kinlough-Rathbone RL. Continued platelet interaction with de-endothelialzed aortae of spontaneously diabetic BB Wistar rats is associated with slow re-endothelialiation and extensive intimal hyperplasia. Int J Exp Pathol 1993;74:603–613.
56. Winocour PD, Watala C, Perry DW, Kinlough-Rathbone RL. Reduced fluidity and increased glycation of membrane proteins of platelets from diabetic subjects are not associated wih increased platelet adherence to glycated collagen. J Lab Clin Med 1992;120:921–928.

57. Tschoepe D, Roesen P, Gries FA. Increase in the cytosolic concentration of calcium in platelets of diabetics tye II. Thromb Res 1991;62:421–438.
58. Ishi H. Umeda F, Hashimoto T, Nawata H. Changes in phosphoinositied turnover, Ca2+ mobilization, and protein phosphorylation in platelets from NIDDM patients. Diabetes 1990;39:1561–1568.
59. Keating FK, Sobel BE, Schneider DJ. Effects of increased concentrations of glucose on platelet reactivity in healthy subjects and in patients with and without diabetes. Am J Cardiol 2003;92:1362–1375.
60. Malmberg K, Norhammar A, Wedel H, Ryden L. Glycometabolic state at admission: important risk marker of mortality in conventionally treated patients with diabetes mellitus and acute myocardial infarction: long-term results from the Diabetes and Insulin-Glucose Infusion in Acute Myocardial Infarction (DIGAMI) study. Circulation 1999;99:2626–2632.
61. Fava S, Aquilina O, Azzopardi J, Agius Muscat H, Fenech FF. The prognostic value of blood glucose in diabetic patients with acute myocardial infarction. Diabet Med 1996;13:80–83.
62. Wahab NN, Cowden EA, Pearce NJ, Gardner MJ, Merry H, Cox JL. Is blood glucose an independent predictor of mortality in acute myocardial infarction in the thrombolytic era? J Am Coll Cardiol 2002;40:1748–1754.
63. Trovati M, Anfossi G, Massucco P, et al. Insulin stimulates nitric oxide synthesis in human platelets and, through nitric oxide, increases platelet concentrations of both guanosine-3',5'-cyclic monophosphate and adenosine-3',5'-cyclic monophosphate. Diabetes 1997;46:742–749.
64. Marina V, Bruno GA, Trucco F, et al. Platelet cNOS activity is reduced in patients with IDDM and NIDDM. Thromb Haemost 1998;79:520–522.
65. Final report on the aspirin component of the ongoing Physicians' Health Study. Steering Committee of the Physicians' Health Study Research Group. N Engl J Med 1989;321:129–135.
66. ETDRS Investigators. Aspirin effects on mortality and morbidity in patients with diabetes mellitus. Early Treatment Diabetic Retinopathy Study report 14. JAMA 1992;268:1292–1300.
67. Winocour PD, Kinlough-Rathbone RL, Mustard JF. Pathways responsible for platelet hypersensitivity in rats with diabetes. II. Spontaneous diabetes in BB Wistar rats. J Lab Clin Med 1986;109:154–158.
68. Kleiman NS, Lincoff M, Keriakes DJ, et al. Diabetes mellitus, glycoprotein IIB/IIIa blockade and heparin: evidence for a complex interaction in a multicenter trial. Circulation 1998;97:1912–1920.
69. Grundy SM, Bilheimer D, Chait A, et al. Summary of the Second Report of the National Cholesterol Education Program (NCEP) Expert Panel on Detection, Evaluation, and Treatment of High Blood Cholesterol in Adults (Adult Treatment Panel II). JAMA 1993;269:3015–3023.
70. Scharfstein JS, Abendschein DR, Eisenberg PR, et al for the TIMI-5 Investigators. Usefulness of fibrinogenolytic and procoagulant markers during thrombolytic therapy in predicting clinical outcomes in acute myocardial infarction. Am J Cardiol 1996;78:503–510.
71. Jones RL. Fibrinopeptide-A in diabetes mellitus. Relation to levels of blood glucose, fibrinogen disappearance, and hemodynamic changes. Diabetes 1985;34:836–843.
72. Librenti MC, D'Angelo A, Micossi P, Garimberti B, Mannucci PM, Pozza G. Beta-thromboglobulin and fibrinopeptide A in diabetes mellitus as markers of vascular damage. Acta Diabetol Lat 1985;22:39–45.
73. Marongiu F, Conti M, Mameli G, et al. Is the imbalance between thrombin and plasmin activity in diabetes related to the behaviour of antiplasmin activity. Thromb Res 1990;58:91–99.
74. Pszota HM, Kugler RK, Szigeti G. Fibrinopeptide-A as thrombotic risk marker in diabetic and atherosclerotic coronary vasculopathy. J Med 1992;23:93–100.
75. Morishita E, Asakura H, Jokaji H, et al. Hypercoagulability and high lipoprotein (a) levels in patients with type II diabetes mellitus. Atherosclerosis 1996;120:7–14.
76. Myrup B, Rossing P, Jensen T, Gram J, Kluft C, Jespersen J. Procoagulant activity and intimal dysfunction in IDDM. Diabetologia 1995;38:73–78.
77. Kannel WB, D'Agostino RB, Wilson PW, Belanger AJ, Gagnon DR. Diabetes, fibrinogen, and risk of cardiovascular disease: the Framingham experience. Am Heart J 1990;120:672–676.
78. Lufkin EG, Fass DN, O'Fallon WM, Bowie EJW. Increased von Willebrand factor in diabetes mellitus. Metabolism 1979;28:63–66.
79. Kannel WB, Wolf PA, Wilson PWF, D'Agostino RB. Fibrinogen and risk of cardiovasclarisease. JAMA 1987;258:1183–1186.
80. Knobl P, Schernthaner G, Schnack C, et al. Haemostatic abnormalities persist despite glycaemic improvement by insulin therapy in lean type 2 diabetic patients. Thromb Haemost 1994;71:692–697.
81. Eliasson M, Roder ME, Dinesen B, Evrin PE, Lindahl B. Proinsulin, intact insulin, and fibrinolytic variables and fibrinogen in healthy subjects. Diab Care 1997;20:1252–1255.

82. Warram JH, Martin BC, Krolewski AS, Soeldner JS, Kahn CR. Slow glucose removal rate and hyperinsulinemia precede the development of type II diabetes in the offspring of diabetic parents. Ann Int Med 1990;113:909–915.

83. Ward WK, LaCava EC, Paquette TL, Beard JC Wallum BJ, Porte D. Disproportionate elevation of immunoreactive proinsulin in type 2 (non-insulin-dependent) diabetes mellitus and in experimental insulin resistance. Diabetologia 1987;30:698–702.

84. Nagi DK, Hendra TJ, Ryle AJ, et al. The relationships of concentrations of insulin, intact proinsulin and 32–33 split proinsulin with cardiovascular risk factors in type 2 (non-insulin-dependent) diabetic subjects. Diabetologia 1990;33:532–537.

85. Marongiu F, Mascia F, Mameli G, Cirillo R, Balestrieri A. Prothromgin fragment F 1 + 2 levels are high in NIDDM patients independently of the Hb A1 c. Thromb Haemost 1995;74:805–806.

86. Mansfield MW, Heywood DM, Grant PJ. Circulating levels of factor VII, fibrinogen, and von Willebrand factor and features of insulin resistance in first-degree relatives of patients with NIDDM. Circulation 1996;94:2171–2176.

87. Jude B, Watel A, Fontaine O, Fontaine P, Cosson A. Distinctive features of procoagulant reponse of monocytes from diabetic patients. Haemostasis 1989;19:65–73.

88. Ceriello A, Russo PD, Zucotti C, Florio A, Nazzaro S, Pietrantuono C, Rosato GB. Decreased anti-thrombin III activity in diabetes may be due to non-enzymatic glycosylation: a preliminary report. Thromb Haemostas 1983;50:633–634.

89. Brownlee M, Vlassara H, Cerami A. Inhibition of heparin-catalyzed human antithrombin III activity by nonenzymatic glycosylation. Diabetes 1984;33:532–535.

90. Ceriello A, Giugliano D, Quatraro A, et al. Daily rapid blood glucose variations may condition anti-thrombin III biological activity but not its plasma concentration in insulin-dependent diabetes: a possible role for labile on-enzymatic glycation. Diabete Metab 1987;13:16–19.

91. Ceriello A, Quatraro A, Dello Russo P, et al. Protein C deficiency in insulin dependent diabetes: a hyperglycemia-related phenomenon. Thromb Haemostas 1990;65:104–107.

92. The Diabetes Control and Complications Trial Research Group. The effect of intensive treatment of diabetes on the development and progression of long-term complications in insulin-dependent diabetes mellitus. N Engl J Med 1993;329:977–986.

93. Auwerx J, Bouillon R, Collen D, Geboers J. Tissue-type plasminogen activator antigen and plasmino-gen activator inhibitor in diabetes mellitus. Arteriosclerosis 1988;8:68–72.

94. McGill JB, Schneider DJ, Arfken CL, Lucore CL, Sobel BE. Factors responsible for impaired fibrin-olysis in obese subjects and NIDDM patients. Diabetes 1994;43:104–109.

95. Vague P, Juhan-Vague I, Aillaud MF, et al. Correlation between blood fibrinolytic activity, plasmino-gen activator inhibitor level, plasma insulin level and relative body weight in normal and obese sub-jects. Metabolism 1986;35:250–253.

96. Juhan-Vague I, Vague P, Alessi MC, et al. Relationships between plasma insulin, triglyceride, body mass index, and plasminogen activator inhibitor 1. Diabete Metab 1987;13:331.

97. Keber I, Keber D. Increased plasminogen activator inhibitor activity in survivors of myocardial inf-arction is associated with metabolic risk factors of atherosclerosis. Haemostas 1992;22:187.

98. Nordt TK, Schneider DJ, Sobel BE. Augmentation of the synthesis of plasminogen activator inhibitor type-1 by precursors of insulin: A potential risk factor for vascular disease. Circulation 1994;89:321–330.

99. Calles-Escandon J, Mirza S, Sobel BE, Schneider DJ. Induction of hyperinsulinemia combined with hyperglycemia and hypertriglyceridemia increases plasminogen activator inhibitor type-1 (PAI-1) in blood in normal human subjects. Diabetes 1998;47:290–293.

100. Ehrmann DA, Schneider, DJ, Sobel BE, et al. Troglitazone improves defects in insulin action, insulin secretion, ovarian steroidogenesis, and fibrinolysis in women with polycystic ovary syndrome. J Clin Endocrinol Metabol 1997;82:2108–2116.

101. Jansson JH, Johansson B, Boman K, Nilsson TK. Hypo-fibrinolysis in patients with hypertension and elevated cholesterol. J Intern Med 1997;229:309–316.

102. Sampson M, Kong C, Patel A, Unwin R, Jacobs HS. Ambulatory blood pressure profiles and plasmi-nogen activator inhibitor (PAI-1) activity in lean women with and without the polycytic ovary syn-drome. Clin End 1996;45:623–629.

103. Velazquez EM, Mendoza SG, Wang P, Glueck CJ. Metformin therapy is associated with a decrease in plasma plasminogen activator inhibitor-1, lipoprotein (a), and immunoreactive insulin levels in pa-tients with the polycystic ovary syndrome. Metab Clin Exp 1997;46:454–457.

104. Farrehi PM, Ozaki CK, Carmeliet P, Fay WP. Regulation of arterial thrombolysis by plasminogen activator inhibitor-1 in mice. Circuation 1998;97:1002–1008.

105. Schneider DJ, Sobel BE. Synergistic augmentation of expression of PAI-1 induced by insulin, VLDL, and fatty acids. Coron Artery Dis 1996;7:813–817.

106. Pandolfi A, Giaccari A, Cilli C, et al. Acute hyperglycemia and actue hyperinsulinemia decrease plasma fibrinolytic activity and increase plasminogen activator inhibitor type 1 in the rat. Acta Diabetol 2001;38(2):71–76.

107. Chen Y, Billadello JJ, Schneider DJ. Identification and localization of a fatty acid response region in human plasminogen activator inhibitor-1 gene. Arterioscler Thrombos Vasc Biol 2000;20:2696–2701.

108. Chen Y, Sobel BE, Schneider DJ. Effect of fatty acid chain length and thioesterification on the augmentation of expression of plasminogen activator inhibitor-1. Nutr Metab Cardiovasc Dis 2002;12:325–330.

109. Chen Y, Schneider DJ. The independence of signaling pathways mediating increased expression of plasminogen activator inhibitor type 1 in HepG2 cells exposed to free fatty acids or triglycerides. Int J Exp Diabetes Res 2002;3:109–119.

110. Alessi M-C, Bastelica D, Mavri A, et al. Plasma PAI-1 levels are more strongly related to liver steatosis than to adipose tissue accumulation. Arterioscler Thromb Vasc Biol 2003;23:1262–1268.

111. Nordt TK, Klassen KJ, Schneider DJ, Sobel BE. Augmentation of synthesis of plasminogen activator inhibitor type-1 in arterial endothelial cells by glucose and its implications for local fibrinolysis. Arterioscler Thromb 1993;13:1822.

112. Chen YQ, Su M, Walia RR, Hao Q, Covington JW, Vaughan DE. Sp1 sites mediate activation of the plasminogen activaor inhibitor-1 promoter by glucose in vascular smooth muscle cells. J Biol Chem 1998;273:8225–8231.

113. Sobel BE, Neimane D, Mack WJ, Hodis HN, Buchanan TA. The ratio of plasminogen activator inhibitor type-1 activity to the concentration of plasminogen activator inhibitor type-1 protein in diabetes: adding insult to injury. Coron Artery Dis 2002;13:275–281.

114. Samad F, Loskutoff DJ. Tissue distribution and regulation of plasminogen activator inhibitor-1 in obese mice. Molec Medicine 1996;568–582.

115. Lundgren CH, Sawa H, Brown SL, Nordt T, Sobel BE, Fujii S. Elaboration of type-1 plasminogen activator inhibitor from adipocytes: A potential pathogenetic link between obesity and cardiovascular disease. Circulation 1996;93:106–110.

116. Calles-Escandon J, Ballor D, Harvey-Berino J, Ades P, Tracy R, Sobel BE. Amelioration of the inhibition of fibrinolysis in obese elderly subjects by moderate caloric restriction. Am J Clin Nutr 1996;64:7–11.

117. Schneider, DJ, Absher PM, Ricci MA. The Dependence of augmentation of arterial endothelial cell expression of plasminogen activator inhibitor type 1 by insulin on soluble factors released from vascular smooth muscle cells. Circulation 1997;96:2868–2876.

118. Pandolfi A, Iacoviello L, Capani F, Vitalonna E, Donati MB, Consoli A. Glucose and insulin independently reduce the fibrinolytic potential of human vascular smooth muscle cells in culture. Diabetologia 1996;39:1425–1431.

119. Carmassi F, Morale M, Ferrini L, et al. Local insulin infusion stimulates expression of plasminogen activator inhibitor-1 and tissue-type plasminogen activator in normal subjects. Am J Med 1999;107(4):344–350.

120. Eliasson M, Asplund K, Evrin PE. Regular leisure time physical activity predicts high activity of tissue plamsinogen activator: The northern Sweden MONICA study. Int J Epidemiol 1996;25:1182–1188.

121. Nordt TK, Kornas K, Peter K, et al. Attentuation by gemfibrozil of expression of plasminogen activator inhibitor type 1 induced by insulin and its precursors. Circulation 1997;95:677–683.

122. Broijersen A, Eriksson M, Wiman B, Angelin B, Hjemdahl P. Gemfibrozil treatment of combined hyperlipoproteinemia. No improvment of fibrinolysis despite marked reduction of plasma triglyceride levels. Arterioscl Thrombos Vasc Biol 1996;16:511–516.

123. Asplund-Carlson A. Effects of gemfibrozil therapy on glucose tolerance, insulin sensitivity and plasma plasminogen activator inhibitor activity in hypertriglyceridemia. J Cardiovasc Risk 1996;3:385–390.

124. Rosenson RS, Tangney CC. Antiatherothrombotic properties of statins. Implications for cardiovascular event reduction. JAMA 1998;279:1643–1650.

125. Sobel BE, Taatjes DJ, Schneider DJ. Intramural plasminogen activator inhibitor type-1 and coronary atherosclerosis. Arterioscler Thromb Vasc Biol 2003;23:1979–1989.

126. Libby P. Molecular bases of the acute coronary syndromes. Circulation 1995;91:2844–2850.

127. Lang IM, Moser KM, Schleef RR. Elevated expression of urokinase-like plasminogen activator and plasminogen activator inhibitor type 1 during the vascular remodeling associated with pulmonary thrmboembolism. Arterioscl Thromb Vasc Biol 1998;18:808–815.
128. Schneider D J, Ricci MA, Taatjes DJ, et al. Changes in arterial expression of fibrinolytic system proteins in atherogenesis. Arterioscler Thromb Vasc Biol 1997;17:3294–3301.
129. Carmeliet P, Moons L, Lijnen R, Janssens S, Lupu F, Collen D, Gerard RD. Inhibitory role of plasminogen inhibitor-1 in arterial wound healing and neointimal formation: a gene targeting and gene transfer study in mice. Circulation 1997;96:3180–3191.
130. Sobel BE, Woodcock-Mitchell J, Schneider DJ, Holt RE, Marutsuka K, Gold H. Increased plasminogen activator inhibitor type-1 in coronary artery atherectomy specimens from type 2 diabetic compared with nondiabetic patients: A potential factor predisposing to thrombosis and its persistence. Circulation 1998;17:2213–2221.
131. Sobel BE. Potentiation of vasculopathy by insulin: Implications from an NHLBI Clinical Alert. Circulation 1996;93:1613–1615.
132. Carrozza JP, Kuntz RE, Fishman RF, Baim DS. Restenosis after arterial injury caused by coronary stenting in patients with diabetes mellitus. Ann Intern Med 1993;118:344–349.
133. Chen Y, Kelm RJ Jr, Budd RC, Sobel BE, Schneider DJ. Inhibition of apoptosis and caspace-3 in vascular smooth muscle cells by plasminogen activator inhibitor type-1. J Cell Biochem 2004;92:178–188.
134. Minamikawa J, Tanaka S, Yamauchi M, Inoue D, Koshiyama H. Potent inhibitory effect of troglitazone on carotid arterial wall thickness in type 2 diabetes. J Clin Endocrinol Metab 1998;83:1818–1820.
135. Koshiyama H, Shimono D, Kuwamura N, Minamikawa J, Nakamura Y. Rapid communication: inhibitory effect of pioglitazone on carotid arterial wall thickness in type 2 diabetes. J Clin Endocrinol Metab 2001;86:3452–3456.
136. Theroux P, Alexander J Jr, Pharand C, Barr E, Snapinn S, Ghannam AF, Sax FL. Glycoprotein IIb/IIIa receptor blockade improves outcomes in diabetic patients presenting with unstable angina/non-ST-elevation myocardial infarction: results from the Platelet Receptor Inhibition in Ischemic Syndrome Management in Patients Limited by Unstable Signs and Symptoms (PRISM-PLUS) study. Circulation 2000;102:2466–2472.
137. Marso SP, Lincoff AM, Ellis SG, et al. Optimizing the percutaneous interventional outcomes for patients with diabetes mellitus: results of the EPISTENT (Evaluation of platelet IIb/IIIa inhibitor for stenting trial) diabetic substudy. Circulation 1999;100:2477–2484.
138. Otterstad JE, Hexeberg E, Holme I, Hjermann I. Cholesterol lowering therapy after myocardial infarction. Consequences of the CARE study. Tidsskr Nor Laegeforen 1997;117:2341–2344.
139. Colwell JA. Editorial: Elevated plasma homocysteine and diabetic vascular disease. Diabetes Care 1997;20:1805–1806.
140. Giugiano D, Ceriello A, Paolisso G. Oxidative stress and diabetic vascular complications. Diabetes Care 1996;19:257–267.

7 Role of Estrogens in Vascular Disease in Diabetes

Lessons Learned From the Polycystic Ovary Syndrome

Agathocles Tsatsoulis, MD, PhD, FRCP
and Panayiotis Economides, MD

CONTENTS

INTRODUCTION

Estrogen derives its name from the Greek word "oistros" that means to "drive mad with desire." More than a century ago, it was thought that peripheral vascular function could be influenced by the "evil effects" emanating from the female apparatus *(1)*. Thus, early beliefs regarding the effects of estrogens were shrouded in curiosity and fear. Even today, although estrogens are no longer considered to have an "evil" influence, their biological effects remain somewhat mysterious and controversial.

Epidemiological data suggest that premenopausal women are largely protected from coronary heat disease (CHD) compared with age-matched men *(2)*. This phenomenon, referred to as a "female advantage," is gradually lost after the menopause so that, by the sixth decade women and men have the same incidence of CHD. The disparity in the incidence of CHD between premenopausal women and men of similar age, and the rise in postmenopausal women, has been attributed to the cardioprotective effects of female sex hormones *(3)*. Indeed, estrogens are involved in many physiological processes that are known to be important for the cardiovascular health in women and were until very recently considered to protect women from cardiovascular disease (CVD). There is extensive evidence from epidemiological and observational studies to support this view,

From: *Contemporary Cardiology: Diabetes and Cardiovascular Disease, Second Edition*
Edited by: M. T. Johnstone and A. Veves © Humana Press Inc., Totowa, NJ

especially for heart disease *(4,5)*. Surprisingly, however, randomized clinical trials (RCTs) in postmenopausal women with or without existing CHD have found no benefits of combined hormone replacement therapy (HRT), casting doubt on the cardioprotective effect of estrogens in postmenopausal women *(6,7)*.

Evidence also suggests that diabetes abolishes the female advantage and eliminates the sex differences in cardiovascular risk in premenopausal women *(8)*. Exactly how diabetes obviates the cardiovascular protective effects of female sex hormones in premenopausal women is not well understood. Recently, it was suggested that the loss of "a healthy vascular endothelium" may prevent women from deriving cardioprotective benefits from endogenous or exogenous estrogens *(9)*.

According to this "healthy endothelium" hypothesis, the favorable anti-atherogenic and other vascular effects of estrogens are endothelium-dependent and receptor-mediated. Consequently, endothelial injury or decline in vascular estrogen receptor (ER) number can diminish the cardiovascular benefits of the reproductive hormones.

This concept may in part explain the disparity between the observational studies that supported the view of a cardioprotective effect of estrogens in healthy postmenopausal women and the recently published RCTs on secondary and primary prevention of CVD in postmenopausal women with HRT, which showed an opposite effect *(6,7)*. It may also explain the adverse impact of diabetes on the risk of CVD in premenopausal women.

In this chapter, we review the biological effects of estrogen on the vascular system and analyze recent data on the role of HRT on CVD in postmenopausal women. We discuss the effect of diabetes on CVD in women and the apparent loss of estrogen protection in premenopausal women with diabetes. We conclude that the likely role of estrogens is to contribute to the maintenance of a healthy vascular endothelium but in the presence of diseased vascular endothelium and atheromatous vascular wall, the use of HRT may be harmful.

BIOLOGICAL EFFECTS OF ESTROGENS RELATED TO THE CARDIOVASCULAR SYSTEM

Sources of Estrogens in Women

The estrogen compounds to which target tissues in women, including the vascular system, may be exposed are multiple and they arise from endogenous and exogenous sources. The naturally occuring estrogens 17 β-estradiol (E2), estrose (E1), and estriol (E2) are C18 steroids and are derived from cholesterol in steroidogenic cells. In the premenopausal women, the primary source of estrogens are the ovaries. E1 and E3 are primarily formed in the liver from E2 *(10)*. After menarche, when circulating E2 levels increase and begin to cycle, levels range from 10 to 80 pg/mL during the follicular phase to 600 pg/mL at midcycle. Following ovulation, progesterone is secreted from the luteinized cells during the luteal phase of the cycle. Progesterone has two main functions in the body, namely, transformation of the endometrium after estrogen priming (luteomimetic effect) and opposition to estrogen (anti-estrogenic effect), limiting proliferation of the endometrium.

After menopause, estrogen concentrations fall to levels that are equivalent to those in males (5–30 pg/mL), and most of the estrogen is formed by extragonadal conversion of testosterone through aromatization, mainly in adipose tissue. E1 is the predominant estrogen in these women. The level of estrogen synthesis in extragonadal tissues increases as a function of age and body weight *(10)*.

In the circulation, estrogen binds to sex hormone binding globulin (SHBG) produced in the liver and, with less affinity, to albumin *(11)*. Only about 2%–3% of estrogen is free. Changes in SHBG levels may influence the tissue availability of free estrogen and also free androgen because the latter also binds to SHBG. Estrogens themselves increase, whereas androgens and high insulin levels decrease SHBG levels. During the menopause, the drop of estradiol reduces SHBG levels, which in turn, results in decreased binding and an increased concentration of free androgens. Consequently, estrogens decrease to a greater extent than do androgens resulting in an increase of the androgen/estrogen ratio and a relative androgen excess in postmenopausal women. Some of the signs and symptoms observed after menopause and, in particular, changes in body composition are caused by this altered balance between estrogens and androgens *(12)*.

In addition to endogenously derived estrogens, there are other important exogenous sources in humans. Oral contraceptives usually contain a combination of ethinyl–estradiol and a synthetic progestogen. Estrogen replacement therapy (ERT) in postmenopausal women is usually in the form of conjugated equine estrogens (CEE) or other oral or transdermal forms of synthetic estrogens. To avoid the risk of endometrial hyperplasia and carcinoma associated with the use of unopposed estrogens, it is advised that women with an intact uterus use progestogen either cyclically or in a continuous combined regimen (HRT) *(13)*. Progestogens are derived from either progesterone itself (C21 progestogens) or testosterone (C19 progestogens) *(13)*.

A new synthetic steroid tibolone with a combination of weak estrogenic, progestogenic, and androgenic activity is also available for HRT *(14)*. Additionally, selective estrogen receptor modulators (SERMS), such as raloxifene are used for the treatment of osteoporosis and it is likely that vascular-specific SERMS will also soon be available *(15)*. Furthermore, phytoestrogens, a diverse group of compounds found in various plant-derived foods and beverages, can have both estrogenic and antiestrogenic effects *(16)*.

Estrogen Receptors and Molecular Actions

As mentioned above, sex steroids exert their actions by binding with high affinity to soluble proteins, the sex steroid receptors. For each of the sex steroid classes, specific receptors are present in target tissues. Androgen and progesterone receptors are encoded by a single gene although two different genes exist for ERs. Two ERs are currently known: ERα and ERβ, belonging to a superfamily of steroid hormone receptors *(17)*. The ER is situated in the nucleus of target cells in which it receives estrogens and other ligands transported into the cell by proteins. On binding of the ligand, the receptors act as gene-specific transcription factors: the liganded receptors can bind to genes that contain steroid-receptor sensitive regions within their regulatory deoxyribonucleic acid (DNA) sequences (promoter/enhancer region). These genes in turn are transcriptionally activated triggering the synthesis of proteins encoded by these regions and resulting in functional activity, in some settings stimulatory and others inhibitory. The altered cellular protein pattern changes the biochemical properties of the target cell *(10)*. Ligand-receptor complexes are affected by proteins called co-activators and co-repressors that modulate the process of DNA transcription. ERα is probably activated by a similar way to ERβ, although it is distributed differently within the tissues of the body and probably mediates different cell functions. Both types of receptors are found in the cells of the cardiovascular system *(18)*.

Overall, the specific nuclear actions of estrogens are determined by the structure of the hormone, the subtype or isoform of the ER involved, the characteristics of the target gene promoter, and the balance of co-activators and co-repressors that modulate the final transcriptional response to the complexes of estrogens and ERs *(10)*. Relevant to this is the fact that ER genes contain polymorphic sites that may modulate the hormone's transcriptional activity *(19)*. Additionally, the level of expression of ERα and ERβ in different vascular sites may differ in different situations. For example, fewer ERα receptors were found in women with atherosclerotic coronary arteries than in those with normal coronary arteries *(20)*. Finally, methylation of the promoter region of the ERα gene is associated with inactivation of gene transcription. Methylation-associated inactivation of the ER gene in vascular tissue may explain diminished ER expression in atheromatous vessels and thus, may contribute to the process of atherogenesis *(21)*.

The traditional estrogen-signaling pathway involving nuclear interaction takes minutes or hours to increase protein synthesis by transcriptional activation. Estrogens have other effects that cannot be explained by a transcriptional mechanism because of their rapid onset. These effects, known as nongenomic effects or, better, nontranscriptional effects, are the result of direct estrogenic action on cell membranes and are mediated by cell surface forms of ER, which resemble their intracellular counterparts *(10)*. Examples of effects mediated by this alternative pathway are the short-term vasodilation of coronary arteries and the rapid insulinotropic effects of estradiol on pancreatic β-cells *(22,23)*.

Vascular Effects of Estrogens

Blood vessels are complex structures with walls containing smooth muscle cells (SMCs) and an endothelial lining. Far from being only an anatomic barrier, the endothelium is a metabolically active organ system that maintains vascular homeostasis by modulating vascular tone, regulating local cellular growth and extracellular matrix deposition and also regulating the hemostatic, inflammatory, and reparative responses to local injury *(24)*.

Vasoregulation occurs as a balance between the release of relaxing and constricting factors. The predominant relaxing factor is nitric oxide (NO), which is synthesized from the amino acid L-arginine. NO release activates SMC guanylate cyclase, leading to increased cyclic guanosine monophosphate production and vascular relaxation *(25)*. Other relaxing factors include prostacyclin and hyperpolarizing factor, which act through cyclic adenosine monophosphate and potassium channels respectively. The major constricting factors are endothelin-1, thromboxane, and prostaglandin H2 *(24)*.

NO synthesis by endothelial cells is of paramount importance for the regulation of vascular tone and blood flow and for control of the hemostatic process. Furthermore, endothelium-derived NO is a potent anti-inflammatory and antiatherogenic factor, being able to prevent endothelial cell dysfunction that has been proposed as an early manifestation of atherosclerosis *(26,27)*.

Estrogen is widely regarded as beneficial to arterial wall function. The beneficial effects include changes in the biology of the endothelium, and the intima-media of the arterial wall. In the arterial endothelium, NO appears to be the primary vascular target of estrogens *(28)*.

Effects of Estrogen on Endothelial Function

Endothelial function is most commonly assessed as a vasodilatory response to pharmacological or mechanical stimuli. Increased blood-flow shear (flow-mediated) is a mechanical means to stimulate vasodilation through NO release *(29)*. The most commonly used clinical measure is high-frequency ultrasound assessed branchial artery diameter changes after blood pressure (BP) cuff-induced hyperemia *(30)*. An assessment of nonendothelium-dependent vasodilation by use of nitroglycerin or nitroprusside is usually performed concomitantly to assess nonspecific smooth muscle effects.

The onset of menopause provides a natural model of estrogen deprivation in which the effects of the endogenous hormone on vascular function can be evaluated. In studies of changes in branchial artery diameter after reactive hyperemia, responses were greater in premenopausal than in postmenopausal women *(31)*. Importantly, blood-flow responses to the NO donor glyceryl trinitrate (GTN) were similar in the two groups, indicating comparable vascular smooth muscle responses to NO. The responses in postmenopausal women were comparable to those observed in men *(31)*. In agreement with these findings, sex hormone deprivation after ovariectomy or premature ovarian failure, is associated with a decline in endothelial-dependent vasodilation, whereas the response to GTN is unaltered *(32,33)*. Another natural model of changes in estrogen levels is the menstrual cycle. In young women, endothelium-dependent vasodilation in the branchial artery paralleled serum estradiol levels, and furthermore, there was evidence of progesterone antagonism of this effect *(34,35)*.

ERT also provides insights into NO regulation by estrogen. Thus, endothelium-dependent vasodilation of the branchial and coronary arteries is enhanced after ERT in postmenopausal women and levels of plasma NO and NO metabolites are increased *(36,37)*. It is of interest that inclusion of progesterone in postmenopausal HRT may blunt the effects of estrogen on endothelial NO production *(38)*. Similar effects of enhanced endothelial function have been observed after ERT in young women with premature ovarian failure or following ovariectomy and in young women receiving oral contraception *(33,39)*. Furthermore, a case has been reported of a young man with nonfunctional ERα as a result of mutation of the ER gene *(40)*. The man was found to have impaired branchial endothelium-dependent relaxation and early coronary calcification supporting the view that ERα is important for endothelial NO release.

The mechanism by which estrogen exposure improves endothelial function is at least partially mediated by an enhancement of NO production by the endothelial isoform of nitric oxide synthase (eNOS) as a result of an increase in both eNOS expression and level of activation. The effects are primarily mediated at the level of gene transcription, and are dependent on ERs that classically serve as transcription factors *(28,41)*. Apart from the long-term effects of estrogen on the vasculature through gene expression (genomic effects), there is evidence that estrogen can cause short-term rapid vasodilation by both endothelium-dependent and endothelium-independent pathways *(41)*. These rapid effects do not appear to involve changes in gene expression (nongenomic or nontranscriptional effects). Thus, estrogen dilates coronary and branchial arteries within minutes when administered intravenously or intra-arterially to postmenopausal women *(42)*.

Recent studies suggest that the rapid effects of estrogen on vascular cells could be mediated by a subpopulation of ERα localized to caveolae in endothelial cells, in which they are coupled to eNOS in a functional signaling module, in a nongenomic manner *(22)*. These observations provide evidence for the existence of a steroid receptor fast-action complex in caveolae. Estrogen binding to ERα within caveolae leads to Gαi activation, which mediates downstream events. The downstream signaling includes activation of tyrosine kinase-mitogen-activated protein kinase and Akt/protein kinase B signaling, stimulation of heat shock protein-90 binding to eNOS, and changes in the local calcium environment, ultimately leading to eNOS stimulation *(43–45)*. Additional mechanisms for nongenomic estrogen-induced vasodilation are found in the potent and rapid regulation of Ca2+ mobilization and in the control of the cell membrane K+ channels in vascular smooth muscle cells (VSMCs), that produce vessel relaxation and increased blood flow *(46)*.

Other important factors released from the vascular endothelium include prostacyclin, a potent vasodilator and platelet inhibitor, and endothelin-1, a potent vasoconstrictor. Estrogen administration stimulates prostacyclin but inhibits production of endothelin in human vascular endothelial cells *(47)*. Estrogen also inhibits apoptosis of cultured human endothelial cells in an ER-dependent manner *(48)*. Additionally, estrogen directly inhibits the migration and proliferation of SMCs in vitro, and the expression of adhesion molecules by vascular cells *(49,50)*. Thus, estrogen contributes to long-term vascular health by inhibiting the proliferation of VSMC and accelerating the growth of endothelial cells.

Effects of Estrogen on Hemostatic Factors

Coagulation involves a series of enzymatic reactions leading to the conversion of soluble plasma fibrinogen to fibrin clots. Coagulation is limited to the site of vascular injury by inhibitors of coagulation and fibrinolysis (Fig. 1).

Hepatic expression of the genes for several coagulation and fibrinolytic proteins are regulated by estogen through ERs *(18)*. Elevated levels of fibrinogen, von Willebrand factor, and factor VII are thought to be important risk markers for ischemic heart disease. These factors have been reported to be increased in postmenopausal women *(51)*. Use of HRT in postmenopausal women has been shown to decrease fibrinogen levels but also to decrease plasma concentration of the anticoagulant protein anti-thrombin III and protein S, and to increase factor VII activity *(52)*.

On the other hand, reduced fibrinolytic activity is associated with atherosclerosis and has been attributed to increased levels of the antifibrinolytic factor plasminogen activator inhibitor-1 (PAI-1) *(53)*. Increased PAI-1 levels have been found in postmenopausal women, and a close relationship between low fibrinolytic activity, high PAI-1 and hyperinsulinemia has been observed in various populations *(54)*. Even small doses of oral ERT activate the fibrinolytic system via a marked reduction in PAI-1 levels, with the greatest reduction occurring in women with the highest PAI-1 levels. Combination with progestogen does not appear to diminish this beneficial effect. In contrast to oral therapy, transdermal therapy does not seem to change PAI-1 levels *(55,56)*. The activation of the fibrinolytic system by estrogens appears not to be dose-related, unlike the coagulatory activity that appears to be dose-dependent *(53)*. On balance, therefore, HRT at low dosages may affect fibrinolytic activity to a greater extent than coagulation activity, whereas the inverse trend holds at high estrogen doses.

It is currently unclear how these effects are brought about at the molecular level of the ER. It is likely that these effects at the cellular level are also under genetic control because the hemostatic system of some women appears to be more sensitive to the effect of estrogens than that of other women *(57)*.

Effects of Estrogen on Lipids and Lipoproteins

The effect of estrogens on lipid metabolism depends on many factors including the type of estrogen, whether it is used unopposed or in combination with progestogens, the type of progestogen, and the mode of delivery.

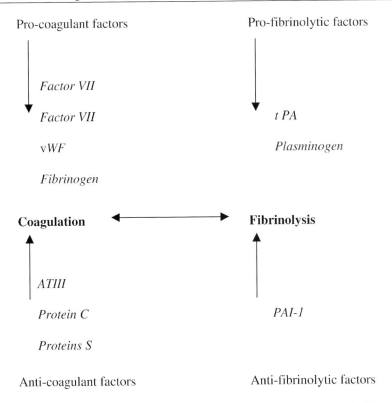

Fig. 1. Hemostatic balance. vWF, von Willebrand factor; ATIII, antithrombin III; t PA, tissue plasminogen activator; PAI-1, plasminogen activator inhibitor type 1.

Oral estrogen reduces plasma total and low-density lipoprotein (LDL) cholesterol by 5%–15%, increases high-density lipoprotein (HDL) cholesterol by 10% and reduces lipoprotein(a) [Lp(a)] levels. A potentially adverse effect of oral estrogen is an increase (20%–25%) in plasma triglycerides *(50)*. The mechanisms of estrogen actions involve enhanced catabolism and clearance of LDL by increasing the number of LDL (apo-B/E) receptors in hepatocytes, decreasing hepatic HDL receptors and reducing activity of hepatic lipase, thereby raising levels of HDL-cholesterol (HDL-C, mostly HDL-C2) and enhancing biliary excretion of cholesterol *(59,60)*. The overall effect, therefore, is to reduce cholesterol accumulation in peripheral tissues and to increase its biliary excretion.

In contrast to oral estrogens, the effects of transdermal preparations on serum lipids are negligible, probably related to the absence of a first-pass hepatic effect *(61)*. Progestogens, especially the more androgenic ones, tend to oppose the effect of estrogens on triglycerides and HDL levels, but they do not alter the effect on LDL and Lp(a) *(58)*.

Estradiol at physiological levels has an antioxidant capacity that is independent of its effects on serum lipid concentrations. Thus, administration of 17β-estradiol in postmenopausal women can decrease the oxidation of LDL cholesterol, which could enhance endothelial NO bioactivity *(62)*. This antioxidant effect may be as a result of ER-mediated changes in the expression of genes for enzymes that regulate the local production and degradation of superoxide.

Recent evidence suggests that remnant lipoprotein particles (RLPs) are the most athero-genic particles among the triglyceride-rich lipoproteins. In particular, RLPs appear to be associated with impaired endothelial function and with severity of atherosclerosis and were identified as an independent risk factor for CVD in women *(63)*. In this context, a recent randomized study demonstrates a favorable effect of HRT on lipoprotein remnant metabolism in postmenopausal women, without significantly affecting triglycerides *(64)*.

Effects of Estrogen on Inflammatory Markers

Evidence is accumulating to suggest a role for inflammation in the process of athero-genesis and plaque disruption. Among markers of low-grade systemic inflammation C-reactive protein (CRP) is the strongest independent predictor of cardiovascular events in apparently healthy women *(65,66)*.

Recent studies have indicated that oral estrogen therapy may increase levels of CRP in healthy postmenopausal women suggesting that estrogen may initiate or aggravate inflammation *(67,68)*. In contrast, animal studies failed to demonstrate such proinflam-matory effects of estrogen when given by subcutaneous implantation or injection *(69)*. In this regard, a recent study in postmenopausal women showed that oral but not transdermal estrogen therapy increased CRP by a first pass hepatic effect *(70)*. Addition-ally, although oral HRT may increase CRP it reduces other inflammatory markers includ-ing E-selectin vascular cell adhesion molecule-1, intercellular adhesion molecule (ICAM)-1, and soluble thrombomodulin *(71)*, indicating that the increase in CRP after oral HRT may be related to metabolic hepatic activation and not to an increased inflam-matory response. However, because CRP is a predictor of adverse cardiovascular prog-nosis and may be involved in the process of atherosclerosis, the route of administration may be an important consideration in minimizing this adverse effect of estrogen therapy on cardiovascular outcomes *(66)*. Further studies have also shown that oral HRT has divergent effects on serum markers of inflammation in women with coronary artery disease *(72)*. Thus, HRT significantly reduced serum levels of cell adhesion molecules that may reduce attachment of white blood cells to the vessel wall, but increased serum levels of metalloproteinase-9 (MMP-9). HRT may also reduce plasma levels of PAI-1, resulting in increased plasmin activity. Plasmin also activates MMPs by converting the inactive zymogen form of the enzyme to the active proteolytic form *(73)*. Accordingly, the combination of increased expression of MMP-9 and the potential for increased plas-min-mediated activation of MMP-9 in women with atheromatous plaques could result in the digestion of matrix proteins that comprise the fibrous cap, thus provoking thrombosis. The overall beneficial and adverse effects of estrogen on the vascular system are summa-rized in Table 1.

HORMONE REPLACEMENT THERAPY AND CARDIOVASCULAR DISEASE

CVD is the major cause of morbidity and mortality in Western societies. Although CVD is an uncommon cause of morbidity and mortality in premenopausal women, it is the most common cause of death among postmenopausal women *(74)*. The pathophysi-ology of CVD involves atherosclerotic plaque development, inflammation and plaque disruption with development of overlying thrombosis. This can lead to vessel occlusion and organ ischemia with clinical sequelae *(27,65)*.

Table 1
Effects of Estrogens on the Vascular System

Beneficial effects	
- Effects on endothelium	• ↑ NO generation
	• ↓ endothelin-1
	• ↓ adhesion molecules
- Smooth muscle effects	
	• ↓ proliferation / migration
	• ↓ vessel wall thickness
- Effects on lipids	• ↓ LDL cholesterol
	• ↑ HDL cholesterol
	• ↓ Lp(a)
	• ↓ oxidation of LDL
- Effects on hemostasis	• ↓ PAI-1, fibrinogen
Adverse effects	
- Lipids	• ↑ Triglycerides
- Proinflammatory	• ↑ CRP, MMP-9
- Procoagulant	• ↑ endogenous anticoagulants
	• ↑ coagulation activation

NO, nitric oxide; HDL, high-density lipoprotein; Lp(a), lipoprotein(a); LDL, low-density lipoprotein; PAI-1, plasminogen activator inhibitor-1; CRP, C-reactive protein; MMP-9, metalloproteinase-9.

An established approach to prevent this condition is comprehensive risk reduction including both lifestyle measures and pharmacological interventions. Over the last decades, HRT was thought to be among these therapies with potential to reduce vascular disease in postmenopausal women (75,76).

Observational Data

Extensive observational data indicate that exogenous estrogen therapy appears to be cardioprotective. Investigators in a review of population-based, case–control, cross-sectional and prospective studies of estrogen therapy (with most using conjugated estrogens) and CHD, calculated that estrogen use reduces the overall relative risk of CHD by approx 50% (4). Observational studies comparing current hormone users with nonusers have shown consistent reductions in CHD risk ranging from 35% to 50% (76,77). A recent updated report from the Nurses' Health Cohort Study with 70,533 postmenopausal women followed up for 20 years, noted that overall, current use of ERT was associated with a relative risk of major coronary events of 0.61 (confidence interval [CI], 0.52–0.71) when adjusted for age and the common cardiovascular risk factors (5). The findings from observational studies have been important in promoting the belief that HRT prevents CHD (77). Although the observational data are almost unanimously supportive of a beneficial effect of HRT on CHD in healthy postmenopausal women, a recent observational study in women with established coronary disease has suggested a deleterious effect of HRT. In this study, increased events were noted in women started on HRT after acute myocardial infarction (MI) (78).

Inherent to the design of all observational studies is the problem of bias. These studies compared women who had elected to take HRT with women who had either not considered it or elected not to take it (selection bias) *(79)*. These two groups of women may have differed with respect to education, socioeconomic status (SES), exercise and life style. HRT users were more likely to participate in preventive health measures than are women who do not use HRT *(80)*. Therefore, HRT users may be at lower risk of CVD compared to nonusers independent of HRT use (healthy user effect). However, adjustment for known confounding variables had little effect on the estimated relative risk of CVD. In the Nurse's Health Cohort Study, HRT also appeared protective despite similar educational level and SES in users and nonusers *(5)*.

Another potential difficulty with observational data is that most participants used unopposed estrogen rather than combined HRT. Progestogens may negate some of the cardiovascular effects of estrogens *(81)*. However, limited number of observational data with combined HRT suggest that the effect may not be substantial, although the progestogen regimen may be relevant *(82)*.

Although there are potential mechanisms that have been identified (discussed above) supporting the observational data, recently published clinical trials have suggested that the relationship between HRT in postmenopausal women and CVD is more complex and that the risk–benefit ratio may vary depending on various clinical and genetic factors.

Data From Randomized Clinical Trials

The first large clinical trial assessing HRT for secondary prevention in women with established coronary CHD was the Heart and Estrogen/Progestin Replacement Study (HERS) *(6)*. The HERS trial was a double-blind, placebo-controlled randomized study with combined continuous oral HRT (CEE 0.625 mg and medroxyprogesterone acetate [MPA] 2.5 mg daily) in almost 3000 postmenopausal women, mean age 66.7 years, with pre-existing CHD for more than 4.5 years. The study failed to demonstrate any overall differences in vascular events between the placebo and active treatment groups. There was an increase in the rate of coronary and thromboembolic events among HRT users in the first year of follow-up despite an improvement in lipid parameters. By the fourth year, the rate of vascular events in the HRT group was below that of the placebo group. However, recently published data from the extension of the HERS study to 6 years (HERS II) have shown that the trend toward reduction in cardiovascular events did not continue *(83)*. The HERS study confirmed the adverse effects of HRT on the hemostatic system with an increase in venous thrombosis. It was therefore suggested that the prothrombotic effects of HRT may negate possible atherosclerotic benefits in women with established CHD and pre-existing plaques, which are prone to rupture.

It has been argued that the apparent early thrombotic risk might have been attenuated by a lower dose of estrogen at the initiation of therapy. Thus, the possibility that lower doses of estrogen may preserve an atherogenic benefit without increasing thrombotic events is an attractive hypothesis. Another criticism was that the HERS study only investigated the effect of one HRT (CEE + MPA); therefore, it is not known whether these results are applicable to all HRT preparations. However, a report from the Papworth Hormone Replacement Therapy Atlerosclerosis Study showed no benefit from transdermal estradiol alone or in combination with norethisterone in reducing CHD events in women with pre-existing disease *(84)*.

In the second study, the Estrogen Replacement and Atherosclerosis (ERA) RCT evaluated progression of coronary artery changes in postmenopausal women with angiographically verified CHD at baseline *(85)*. After 3 years of follow-up, neither CEE alone nor combined CEE + MPA slowed the progression of coronary atherosclerosis as determined angiographically in these women with pre-existing disease. Given the results of the randomized clinical trials such as HERS and ERA, one cannot support the use of HRT for the sole purpose of secondary prevention of CHD. However, the results of these trials may not directly apply to the use of oral estrogen in healthy postmenopausal women.

To address this issue, a large randomized trial, the Women's Health Initiative (WHI) was designed to assess the role of HRT for primary prevention of CVD *(7,86)*. The WHI was a randomized controlled primary prevention trial in 16,608 healthy postmenopausal women aged 55–79 (mean age 63.7) years, based on oral combined continuous HRT (CCE 0.625 mg plus MPA 2.5 mg) daily compared with placebo. Another arm of the study, which is still continuing, addresses the effects of estrogen alone in women with previous hysterectomy. Although originally designed to run for 8.5 years, the study was stopped early, after 5.2 years follow-up, based on an assessment of greater risk than benefit. Although its primary outcome was nonfatal MI and coronary death, the trial was stopped as a result of a significant but small increased risk of invasive breast cancer (8 cases per 10,000 women), which exceeded the stopping boundaries. This excess risk increased with duration of treatment. For CVD there was an increased risk (7 cases per 10,000) of nonfatal MI and coronary death. This was seen early on within the first year of treatment, remaining neutral over the ensuing years. There was an excess risk of stroke (8 cases per 10,000) which persisted throughout the trial, and a doubling of risk for venous thromboembolism (18 cases per 10,000) This translates to an increased relative risk of 22% of an adverse outcome for CVD. The WHI study also showed evidence of benefit in terms of reduced incidence of hip fractures (8 cases per 10,000) and colorectal cancer (6 cases per 10,000). However, these outcomes did not result in an overall benefit over the 5.2 years of the trial. In conclusion, this large randomized trial does not support the use of this HRT regimen for the primary prevention of CHD in postmenopausal women.

The question regarding whether 17β-estradiol (the endogenous estrogen molecule) alone or administered sequentially with MPA can slow the progression of atherosclerosis was tested in the Women's Estrogen-Progestin Lipid lowering Hormone Atherosclerosis Regression Trial (WELL-HART), a randomized double-blind placebo-controlled trial *(87)*. The results of this trial showed that in older postmenopausal women with established coronary-artery atherosclerosis, 17 β-estradiol either alone or with sequentially administered MPA had no significant effect on the progression of atherosclerosis as assessed by quantitative coronary angiography.

The results of the WELL-HART study were strikingly different from those of the Estrogen in the Prevention of Atherosclerosis Trial (EPAT), a sister study that used similar protocols but in postmenopausal women without pre-existing disease *(88)*. The EPAT study found that relative to placebo, oral 17 β-estradiol alone slowed the progression of carotid intima-media thickness. The divergent outcomes of the two studies may be related to the timing of the intervention relative to the stage of atherosclerosis as is discussed next.

Interpreting the Divergent Data on Postmenopausal Hormone Replacement Therapy

The conclusions of the HERS and WHI trials were diametrically opposite to the overwhelming observational evidence that HRT could be cardioprotective in postmenopausal women, raising the question regarding in which the "clinical truth" is. Several explanations for this apparent discordance have seen suggested. Some discrepancies may be the result of methodological differences between the observational and clinical studies as discussed earlier. Other explanations may be biological, related to the complexity of the sex steroid actions, the vascular health status of the population under treatment, and various genetic factors.

The Complexity of Sex Steroid Actions

The mechanism of action of both estrogens and progestogens on the vascular system is diverse and complex. Some of the estrogen actions, including those on the atherogenic lipoproteins, antioxidant activity and enhancement of endothelial function are unequivocally antiatherogenic. Some of these effects, however, may be partly negated by certain synthetic progestogens used in conventional HRT. On the other hand, the net clinical effect of the prothrombotic vs fibrinolytic actions of estrogens may vary depending on dose, route of administration, the state of the vascular wall and genetic factors, so that in certain circumstances the prothrombotic effects may predominate resulting to thrombosis.

Finally, the divergent effects of estrogens on various inflammatory markers may be important in the later stages of atherosclerosis. Reduction in levels of vascular adhesion molecules could be atheroprotective by reducing the attachment of monocytes to the vessel wall. However, induction of CRP production in liver and increase in the expression of MMPs within the vessel wall could be detrimental because activation of the latter could digest and weaken fibrous caps of vulnerable plaques, thus provoking thrombosis (89,90).

It is interesting that estrogen-induced metalloproteinase expression may play a physiological role facilitating the rupture of the mature follicles during ovulation (91). However, this beneficial effect of estrogen during reproductive life may become the sword of Damocles by promoting plaque rupture in atheromatous vessels later in life.

The State of the Vascular Endothelium

Emerging experimental and clinical evidence suggest that the beneficial effects of estrogens are dependent on the integrity and functional status of the endothelium within the vascular system and the presence of atherosclerosis or its risk factors. The concept of "healthy endothelium" may explain in part the unfavorable findings of the HERS and WHI trials and guide future strategies in the use of HRT (9).

This concept is that many of the antiatherogenic effects of estrogens are receptor-mediated and endothelium-dependent. Consequently, endothelial injury or decline in vascular ER expression can diminish the anti-atherogenic properties of estrogen. In this context, experimental studies have looked at effects of endothelial damage induced by balloon catheter injury in rabbits and how estrogen affects progression of atherosclerosis. The studies reported that the direct anti-atherogenic effect of estrogen was present, absent or reversed, depending on the state of the arterial endothelium (92). In humans, nondiseased coronary-artery vessels dilate in response to the administration of estrogen, whereas diseased vessels do not respond (93). The lack of ER expression in the presence of atherosclerosis could result in a decreased ability of vascular tissue to respond to estrogen (20). This lack of ER expression may result from methylation of the promoter region of the gene for ERα, which occurs in aging and diseased vessels (21).

Support for this hypothesis also comes from randomized studies in oophorectomized cynomolgous monkeys. In monkeys assigned to conjugated estrogen (alone or in combination with MPA) begining 2 years (~ 6 human years) after oophorectomy and well after the establishment of atherosclerosis, HRT had no effect on the extent of coronary artery plaque. However, HRT resulted in 50% reduction in the extent of plaque when given to monkeys immediately after oophorectomy, during the early stages of atherosclerosis (94).

It appears that a woman's age and the number of years since menopause are potential factors modifying the influence of HRT on CHD. In this regard, in the Nurses' Health Cohort Study, the women ranged in age from 30 to 55 years at enrollment and almost 80%, commenced estrogen therapy within 2 years of menopause (5). In contrast, the mean age of participants was 63 years in the WHI and 67 years in HERS; thus, these women had on average been postmenopausal for 10 years at the time of enrollment. In light of the above observations it is possible that HRT could be beneficial in younger women, before plaque complications set in, but may not inhibit progression from complicated plaques to coronary events in older women.

HRT and Genetic Factors

Genetic variants that modify the effect of estrogens on various domains of estrogen action may account for the clinical heterogeneity in response to HRT.

Thus the estrogen associated risk for thrombosis may be increased in the presence of the prothrombin 20210 G→A variant, the factor V Leiden mutation or platelet antigen-2 polymorphisms (95–97). A common sequence variation of the ERβ gene is associated with the magnitude of the response of HDL cholesterol levels to HRT in women with coronary disease (19). The same ERβ genotype is also related to changes in the levels of SHBG, another index of estrogen action (95). It is also interesting that in the HERS trial high levels of Lp(a), which is largely genetically determined, were an independent risk factor for CHD events in the placebo group. HRT lowered Lp(a) levels and the cardiovascular benefit of HRT was significantly related to the initial Lp(a) levels and the magnitude of the reduction in the level (98). It appears therefore, that genetic factors may also contribute to the net clinical effect of HRT regarding CVD in postmenopausal women.

Alternative Therapies to Hormone Replacement Therapy

SERMs are nonsteroidal estrogenic compounds with both estrogenic agonist (on bone and lipoproteins) and estrogenic-antagonist (on breast and endometrium) effects in use for the treatment of osteoporosis. Although SERMs have shown beneficial effects on some surrogate markers of CVD it is not known whether this will translate into clinical benefit. The recent secondary analysis of the osteoporosis prevention study, the Multiple Outcomes of Raloxifene Evaluation (MORE) trial, suggested that there were no significant differences between raloxifene and placebo group regarding combined CHD and CVD events. Interestingly, however, in the subset with increased cardiovascular risk, the raloxifene group had a significantly lower risk of CVD events compared with placebo (99). The Raloxifene Use for the Heart Study is currently testing the impact of raloxifene on cardiovascular endpoints in postmenopausal women. The results of this trial will provide information on the net clinical cardiovascular benefits of SERMs.

Phytoestrogens are a group of natural compounds that have both estrogen agonist and antagonist properties and could be considered as natural SERMs. There is growing evidence from epidemiological and experimental studies that consumption of phytoestrogens has beneficial effects on the risk of CHD (100,101). Soy phytoestrogens have shown beneficial effects on endothelium-dependent vasodilation and the development of atherosclerosis in nonhuman primates (102,103). Some studies in postmenopausal women, but not all, have shown improvements on lipid profiles and endothelial function *(104)*. Clinical end-point data from randomized trials are not available to make recommendations regarding use of soy phytoestrogens for prevention of CVD.

Tibolone is a steroid hormone with a progestogen-like structure that is converted to estrogenic and androgenic derivatives in vivo. It improves menopausal symptoms and bone density and potentially has fewer side effects than conventional HRT. Limited human observational data on the cardiovascular effects of tibolone indicate that it reduces triglycerides and Lp(a) levels but also HDL and there is a suggestion that tibolone may not increase thrombotic risk *(105)*. We must await data from clinical trials on definite clinical end-points to establish the vascular effects of tibolone.

Conclusions and Future Directions

There are several plausible explanations for the divergent findings from the clinical trials and the observational studies regarding the effect of HRT on CVD in postmenopausal women. Some discrepancies may be methodological in nature and others may have a biological basis related to the pleiotropic effects of estrogens and the characteristics of the study population. The later may be related to age, time since menopause, state of the arterial endothelium and stage of atherogenesis. Genetic factors may also contribute to the heterogeneity of the population.

The cardiovascular effects of estrogen are certainly far more complex than was initially thought. Unraveling these effects remain a challenge for future research. Despite the disappointing outcomes from the clinical trials, there is considerable evidence to support the beneficial effects of estrogens in the early stages of atherogenesis (during the menopausal transition and the early years of postmenopause). In clinical practice it may not be safe to exploit these benefits with the conventional HRT regimens.

The possible use of lower doses of estrogen, novel estrogen agonists including vascular SERMs, combination of SERMs or phytoestrogens with low-dose estrogens are some future directions to explore. In short, using the words of an expert in this field 'the final chapter of this fascinating story has not yet been written" *(106)*. For the time being HRT is suspended for the primary or secondary prevention of CVD in postmenopausal women.

IMPACT OF DIABETES ON CARDIOVASCULAR DISEASE IN WOMEN

There is accumulating evidence that diabetes abolishes the female advantage in cardiovascular risk in premenopausal women. Indeed, population studies have shown that diabetes imposes a greater relative risk of CHD in women than in men and furthermore women with diabetes have a worse outcome for CHD than either men or women without diabetes. A recent metaanalysis of all prospective cohort studies that examined the risk of CHD among women and men with diabetes revealed that the relative risk of CHD death from diabetes was 2.58 (95% CI, 2.05–3.26) for women and 1.85 (1.47–2.33) for men *(8)*. It appears, therefore, that the presence of diabetes in women abrogates the cardioprotective effect of endogenous sex hormones.

Mechanisms

The mechanisms by which diabetes abolishes the cardiovascular protective effects of female sex hormones in premenopausal women are not well understood. In fact, the loss of the natural sex advantage in women with diabetes is independent of other diabetes-associated conventional risk factors. After adjusting for differences in hypertension, dyslipidemia, and obesity, the cardiovascular risk still remains higher in diabetic women than in men or women without diabetes *(8,107)*. This suggests that other mechanisms contribute to the increased cardiovascular risk in women with diabetes.

Given the central role of the endothelium in modulating vascular tone, lipid peroxidation, smooth muscle proliferation, and monocyte adhesion and the beneficial effects of estrogen in maintaining vascular health, it was hypothesized that diabetes may compromise the effects of estrogen on endothelial function, thereby increasing the potential for premature atherothrombosis. Indeed, recent clinical studies provide direct evidence that premenopausal women with diabetes have a significantly impaired regulation of vascular tone. In a recent study Di Carli and associates *(108)* demonstrated reduced coronary vasodilator function and impaired response of resistance vessels to increased sympathetic stimulation in premenopausal women with diabetes, similar to that observed in healthy postemenopausal women in whom the sex differential in cardiovascular risk is no longer present. Similar findings were reported in another study demonstrating impaired forearm and leg arterial vasoreactivity in premenopansal women with type 2 diabetes. Using Doppler flowmetry, Lim and associates *(109)* showed impaired cutaneous vasodilation in response to acetylcholine (endothelium-dependent) and sodium nitroprusside (endothelium-independent). The authors reported that the magnitude of endothelium-dependent forearm vasodilation in premenopausal women with diabetes was reduced by 52% compared with healthy premenopausal women, but it was similar to the vasodilator response in healthy postmenopausal women (not on HRT). Additionally they showed a 30% reduction in endothelium-independent vasodilation in premenopausal women with diabetes compared with the healthy premenopausal controls. Steinbeng and associates *(110)*, in an elegant study that included groups of lean, obese and type 2 diabetic women and age and body mass index-matched men reported that premenopausal normal women exhibit more robust endothelium-dependent vasodilation owing to higher rates of NO release than normal men. Given the potential vascular action of NO, this difference may partially explain the lower incidence of CVD in women. Diabetes causes impairment of endothelial function in premenopausal women, beyond that observed with obesity alone and leads to endothelial dysfunction similar to that observed in diabetic men. These findings indicate that type 2 diabetes abrogates the sex differences in endothelial function in premenopausal women.

The mechanisms for the enhanced NO-dependent endothelial vasodilation in normal premenopausal women in comparison to men, as shown by Steinberg and associates *(110)* are not known. It appears that female and male sex hormones exert differential effects on endothelial function. Thus in endothelial cell cultures, estrogen, the predominant female sex hormone, has been shown to stimulate NO synthesis *(111)*. Conversely, the male sex hormone testosterone may cause decreased NO production/release, as suggested by Herman and associates *(112)*.

Additionally, differences in insulin sensitivity between women and men may also explain the higher rates of NO production/release in women. Indeed, previous reports have indicated that women display higher insulin sensitivity than men of similar age and body mass index *(113)* suggesting that sex modulates the association between body fat distribution (central vs peripheral) and insulin sensitivity. Therefore, the enhanced endothelial function observed in women may be secondary to the higher insulin sensitivity in women than men. Type 2 diabetes with associated central obesity and insulin resistance may obviate this sex advantage in women.

The exact mechanism by which diabetes and its associated metabolic abnormalities negates the natural protective effects of endogenous estrogens on the vascular system in women are not well understood. As discussed earlier, estrogens modulate vascular tone by several mechanisms including direct and indirect actions on vascular endothelial and smooth muscle cells through activation of ERs in the vessel wall *(18)*. In endothelial cells estrogen increases the expression of eNOS, thereby controlling the tone of underlying smooth muscle cells and may also rapidly activate eNOS through ERα-mediated mechanisms not involving gene expression *(114)*. Conversely, estrogen blocks the synthesis of inducible NO synthase (iNOS) induced by inflammatory stimuli in SMCs and macrophages, probably through ERα downregulation, thus limiting potential proinflammatory effects *(115)*.

Diabetes-associated hyperglycemia and possibly other metabolic abnormalities may interfere with one or more of these mechanisms. Indeed, hyperglycemia decreases estradiol-mediated NO production from cultured endothelial cells *(116)*. Additionally, hyperglycemia may lead to increased formation of oxygen-derived free radicals that inactivate endothelium-derived NO and, thus, interfere with endothelium-dependent vasodilation. Further to this, a recent experimental study in cultured aortic smooth muscle cells from diabetic rats showed that iNOS response to inflammatory stimuli is less sensitive to estrogen inhibition probably on account of altered ERα/ERβ ratio in the diabetic environment *(117)*. It appears from this study that diabetes may also undermine the anti-inflammatory effects of estrogen on vascular wall, and this may provide another possible mechanism underlying the increased risk of macrovascular disease in diabetic premenopausal women.

Apart from the above considerations, diabetes may also affect the vascular system in women indirectly, through menstrual cycle irregularities and hypoestrogenemia. Indeed, previous epidemiological studies demonstrated that diabetic premenopausal women more frequently have menstrual irregularities, lower blood estrogen levels and higher androgen levels than nondiabetic women *(118)*. The reasons for these menstrual abnormalities and hypoestrogenemia in women with diabetes are not well known but may be hypothalamic in origin related to stress or poor metabolic control or may be related to insulin resistance and hyperinsulinemia *(119)*. Furthermore, in women with type 2 diabetes, low SHBG levels have been reported and this may contribute to relative hyperadrogenemia in these women, a condition frequently seen in women with polycystic ovary syndrome (PCOS) *(120)*. Low SHBG levels are believed to be a marker for future CVD in women *(121)*. Whatever the reason, the diabetes related-menstrual abnormalities and associated hypoestrogenemia may contribute to premature arteriosclerosis in premenopausal women with diabetes. Indeed studies have suggested that menstrual cycle irregularity and hypoestrogenemia of hypothalamic origin are significant predictors of CHD *(122,123)*.

In summary therefore, diabetes-related hyperglycemia and/or insulin resistance combined with diabetes-related estrogen insufficiency may explain the loss of the cardiovascular protective effects of estrogen in premenopausal women with diabetes and consequently the increased risk for premature atherosclerosis.

ROLE OF HORMONE REPLACEMENT THERAPY IN WOMEN WITH DIABETES

Healthy postmenopausal women undergo changes in lipoprotein and carbohydrate metabolism and in the pattern of body fat distribution similar to those of patients with diabetes. In fact, a picture resembling the metabolic syndrome emerges with the menopause *(12)*. Replacement therapy with estrogen can improve the adverse impact of menopause on lipid profile and bone mineral density, and there is evidence that estrogen may also improve carbohydrate metabolism and body fat distribution in healthy postmenopausal women *(124–126)*. The role of HRT in preventing CVD in postmenopausal women, as discussed in detail in the first part of this chapter, remains highly controversial, but there is strong evidence that it may be beneficial in the early postmenopausal period and early stages of atherosclerosis.

Postmenopausal women with diabetes are at risk of dyslipidemia, central obesity, hypertension, and accelerated atherosclerosis, all of which can contribute to an increased risk of CVD *(127)*. Thus, postmenopausal women with diabetes could benefit from a reduced risk of CVD with the use of HRT. However, whether HRT confers cardiovascular protection in postmenopausal women with diabetes is currently unknown and remains an issue for further clinical research.

An attempt is made in this section to shed some light in this issue based on current evidence. This is preceded by a brief review of the effects of estrogen on risk factors for diabetes and the metabolic syndrome in both nondiabetic and diabetic postmenopausal women.

Effects of Estrogen on Risk Factors for Diabetes

The changes in lipid metabolism that occur with the menopause, including increased total and LDLC, triglycerides and Lp(a), and decreased HDL-C, resemble those of type 2 diabetes and the metabolic syndrome *(12)*. Adverse changes in carbohydrate metabolism also emerge with the menopause including decreased insulin sensitivity and insulin secretion *(128)*. These together with increased central adiposity contribute to the increased risk of CVD in postmenopausal women.

The effects of estrogen on lipid parameters are discussed in detail in the first part of this chapter. A number of observational studies have also reported that estrogen improves insulin resistance in postmenopausal women, a factor that is predictive for the development of type 2 diabetes *(125,129)*. Estrogen therapy also appears to prevent central fat distribution, a factor that is strongly associated with insulin resistance *(126)*. Thus, estrogen can potentially prevent the insulin resistance associated with central obesity in postmenopausal women.

Another characteristic of postmenopausal women is androgenicity associated with low SHBG levels, which is also considered an important risk factor for insulin resistance and type 2 diabetes *(120)*. In the Rancho Bernardo Study, SHBG was found to be inversely correlated with type 2 diabetes and impaired glucose tolerance (IGT) in postmenopausal women *(130)*. In this regard, Andersson and associates *(131)* also reported that low SHBG levels were associated with type 2 diabetes in both men and women. Furthermore, they also reported that serum testosterone levels were positively correlated with the degree of insulin resistance in women. Estrogen, in contrast to androgens may increase SHBG levels. These increases in SHBG were associated with improved glucose homeostasis *(132)*. In this context, it is also interesting that the incidence of diabetes is higher in men than in women until women reach menopause *(133)*.

Given the evidence from the observational studies that estrogen improves insulin resistance and the other adverse factors associated with it, and the fact that insulin resistance is predictive for the development of type 2 diabetes one would expect a protective role of estrogen against the development of type 2 diabetes in postmenopausal women. In this regard, the Nurses' Health Cohort Study of 21,028 postmenopausal women aged 30 to 55 years showed that the use of HRT reduced slightly the relative risk (0.88, CI,

0.67–0.96) of developing type 2 diabetes after adjusting for age, body mass index and other confounding factors, although the duration of estrogen use was not associated with a decreased risk *(134)*. The Rancho Berdardo Study reported a linear trend toward a lower incidence of type 2 diabetes with current use of estrogen therapy (0.88, CI, 0.48–1.62), but the trend was reversed after adjusting for confounding factors *(135)*.

A recently published *post hoc* analysis from the HERS trial reported a lower risk for new-onset type 2 diabetes in postmenopausal women with heart disease receiving HRT *(136)*. At the start of the study the participants had fasting glucose levels measured and were categorized as having normal or impaired fasting glucose or having diabetes. Participants were followed up for the development of new cases of type 2 diabetes over 4 years. Daily treatment with 0.625 ng CEE plus 2.5 mg MPA resulted in a 35% lower risk for type 2 diabetes during the follow-up period. This reduction in risk was primarily as a result of the fact that women in the HRT group maintained a lower fasting glucose level than women in the placebo group. Thus, HRT prevented the increase in fasting glucose levels that was seen in the placebo group over time in this high-risk study population.

These data are encouraging and suggest important metabolic effects of hormone therapy. However, the results of this posthoc analysis of the HERS study are not definitive and require confirmation in a formal clinical trial. The authors do not recommend the use of HRT for diabetes prevention but encourage further study of the issue.

Effects of HRT on Carbohydrate Metabolism in Women With Diabetes

There is a degree of reluctance among health care professionals to prescribe HRT to women with diabetes. A community-based survey in London found that diabetic postmenopausal women were less than half as likely as the general population to be prescribed HRT *(137)*. Doctors and health care professionals perceive HRT as detrimental for diabetic women because of fear about glycemic control as is also the case with the oral contraceptive pill *(138)*. Yet there is no evidence that HRT results in deterioration of glycemic control in women with diabetes.

In general, the available data indicate that HRT either improves or has neutral effects on carbohydrate metabolism in women with diabetes depending on the estrogen and/or progestogen formulation used (Table 2).

Oral estradiol has been shown to improve glucose metabolism and insulin sensitivity in diabetic women *(132,139)*, whereas transdermal estradiol was found not to affect glycemic control *(140)*. The addition of norethisterone does not appear to adversely affect glycemic control, although it may reduce any benefit seen with oral 17β-estradiol alone. In women with IGT, Luotola and associates *(141)* reported that natural estrogen/progestogen substitution improved insulin sensitivity, as shown by decreased glucose levels on oral glucose tolerance test. In postmenopausal women with hyperinsulinemia, transdermal estradiol also decreased plasma insulin and improved insulin sensitivity with further improvement by the addition of dydrogesterone *(142)*. Regarding the effect of CEE in women with diabetes, limited work has shown either neutral effects on fasting blood glucose or insulin levels, or a reduction in HbA1c which was, however, attenuated when MPA was added to the regimen *(143,144)*. The mechanism of estrogen action on glucose metabolism is not clearly known. Brussaard and associates *(139)* showed that ERT enhanced insulin suppression of hepatic glucose production in postmenopausal women with diabetes. Interestingly, this suppression was enhanced only in women with normal triglyceride levels and not in those with hyperglyceridemia. On the other hand,

Table 2
Effects of Hormone Replacement Therapy on Carbohydrate Metabolism

Effects of Estrogens
-Estradiol improves insulin sensitivity
-Low-dose CEE does not affect insulin sensitivity
-High-dose CEE impairs glucose tolerance

Effects of progestogens
-MPA impairs glucose tolerance
-Norethisterone has neutral effects on insulin sensitivity
-Dydrogesterone improves insulin sensitivity

CEE, conjugated equine estrogen; MPA, medroxyprogesterone acetate.

Samaras and associates *(144)* suggested that estrogen effects on body composition and lipid metabolism may explain improvements in glycemic control; partitioning fatty acids away from the central abdominal depot to the gluteofemoral region reduces circulating fatty acid effects on insulin action *(145)*.

It is important also to note that in women with diabetes, the changes that accompany menopause may further deteriorate glycemic control and HRT may attenuate this effect. Indeed, in the studies conducted by Brussaard and associates *(139)* and Samaras and associates *(144)*, HbA1c detrimentally increased in the placebo groups in postmenopausal women with type 2 diabetes, whereas in the same reports, and in others, HbA1c was significantly reduced with ERT *(146)*.

It appears that regarding glycemic control, low-dose HRT can be used in women with type 2 diabetes without undue concern. The recent North American Menopause Society (NAMS) consensus paper *(147)* advised that if oral ERT is used in women with type 2 diabetes, then only low-dose formulations should be prescribed. Beneficial effects on insulin sensitivity may be observed with HRT, although more work is needed in the area.

Effects of HRT on Lipids in Women With Diabetes

Serum lipid parameters show an overall beneficial change on HRT in postmenopausal diabetic women. Unopposed oral estradiol increases HDL-C and reduces LDL-C, whereas the addition of norethisterone may not alter this beneficial effect *(132,148)*. Oral CEE 0.625 mg daily has been shown to reduce total and LDL-Cin women with diabetes, although increasing HDL-C *(149)*. In one study, the increase in HDL-C was less than among nondiabetic women *(150)*. Not all studies have shown an increase in triglycerides with oral CEE *(149)*, although one showed a greater increase among women with diabetes *(150)*. When MPA is added to the CEE regimen, the beneficial effect on HDL-C is attenuated *(149)*.

Transdermal estradiol combined with oral norethisterone significantly decreases total cholesterol and serum triglycerides without significantly affecting LDL-C and HDL-C *(151)*. A recent publication from the Third National Health and Nutrition Examination Survey (NHANES III) reported that, although HDL was found to be higher among nondiabetic women who were currently taking HRT than among never users of HRT, this finding was not observed among diabetic women. Total cholesterol and non-HDL-C, however, were significantly lower among diabetic women currently on HRT than among never or previous users. These findings were not observed in non diabetic women *(152)*. This divergent result may indicate differential effects of HRT on lipid metabolism in diabetic compared with nondiabetic women.

Regarding Lp(a), no significant differences were found among the groups studied in the NHANES III survey. However, in a randomized controlled study combined continuous HRT (CEE + MPA) has shown beneficial effects on Lp(a) in postmenopausal women with type 2 diabetes *(153)*. Also, a significant reduction in Lp(a) and triglycerides has been reported following treatment with tibolone *(154)*.

Overall, the use of HRT by women with type 2 diabetes appears to reduce total and LDL-C with variable effects on HDL-C and triglycerides. As a note of caution, diabetic women may already have mild hypertriglyceridemia and this could be exacerbated by HRT. A cross-sectional study reported that nearly 8% of diabetic women currently using HRT had triglyceride levels greater than 400 mg/dL, compared with 0.6% of nondiabetic users *(150)*. Additionally, severe exacerbation of hypertriglyceridemia can result when women with primary familial hypertriglyceridemia are given HRT (155). The researchers advised against using ERT in women with triglyceride levels greater than 750 mg/dL, to avoid pancreatitis *(155)*.

Whether the observed hypertriglyceridemia in diabetic women may be offset by improvement in other risk factors such as HDL and insulin sensitivity with HRT is not known. However, the hypertriglyceridemia associated with ERT/HRT appears to result from an increased production of large, triglyceride-rich, very LDL, which may be less atherogenic than smaller and denser particles *(150)*.

Additionally, it has been argued that the use of progestogens may also offset the unfavorable increase in triglycerides with estrogen. Indeed, a trend toward lower triglycerides with HRT has been reported *(156)*.

Oral HRT preparations, unlike transdermal estrogen, are subject to first-pass metabolism by the liver and the clinical differences in impact on lipid and carbohydrate metabolism may be secondary to this effect *(157)*. Oral preparations were also reported to have a more favorable influence on plasma lipoproteins and HbA1c in diabetic women *(158)*. At the same time, however, oral preparations increase triglycerides which may be detrimental to diabetic women. Thus, it has been recommended that, when oral ERT/HRT is prescribed to diabetic women, triglyceride levels should be monitored before and after treatment. If hypertriglyceridemia occurs or worsens, a transdermal preparation can be substituted.

Effects of HRT on Inflammatory and Thrombotic Factors in Women With Diabetes

In addition to beneficial effects on lipids, HRT has also been shown to improve other risk factors for atherothrombosis in diabetic women. CRP, a cardiovascular risk marker, is known to be increased in patients with type 2 diabetes. Sattar and associates *(159)* in a 6-month, double-blind, placebo-controlled study reported that transdermal estradiol in conjunction with continuous oral norethisterone significantly reduced CRP concentrations in postmenopausal women with type 2 diabetes. This is in contrast to what was reported for oral HRT formulations in nondiabetic postmenopausal women *(68)*. This beneficial effect on CRP is likely the result of the neutral effect of transdermal estradiol and the favorable effect of oral norethisterone. The same HRT regimen was also found to reduce factor VII activity and von Willebrand factor antigen levels. On the basis of these overall beneficial effects on inflammatory and thrombotic factors, the authors have suggested that HRT regimens based on 17β-estradiol and progestogen (norethisterone) may be more rational for women with diabetes than those based on synthetic or conjugated estrogens. Finally, in another randomized, double-blind, crossover trial investigating the effects of ERT/HRT on hemostasis, fibrinolytic activity improved in postmenopausal women with type 2 diabetes by decreasing the level of PAI-1, an important inhibitor of fibrinolysis that is increased in diabetic patients (161). A similar favorable effect on PAI-1 was reported by Brussard and associates (139), indicating that HRT is associated with increased fibrinolytic potential.

Finally fibrinogen levels were found to be significantly lower among current HRT users than in women who had never used HRT for both diabetic and non diabetic women in the NHANES III survey (152). This beneficial effect was also shown in a randomized-controlled study using combined continuous HRT (161) although no effect was reported in a similar study using transdermal 17β-estradiol combined with nonethisterone (160).

Effects of HRT on Endothelial Function in Postmenopausal Women With Diabetes

Endothelial dysfunction is the hallmark of diabetes and is regarded as an early manifestation of atherogenesis. In postmenopausal women with diabetes, multiple pathophysiological processes may contribute to endothelial dysfunction. These are diabetes- related, as a result of hyperglycemia and obesity/insulin resistance and menopause-related as a result of loss of the protective effect of estrogen, as discussed earlier.

Despite the importance of the endothelium, there is limited data on the effects of HRT on endothelial dysfunction in postmenopausal women with diabetes. In a recent study comparing healthy and diabetic postmenopausal women, Lim and associates (109) found that, although cutaneous vasodilation was impaired in postmenopausal women, it was able to be improved by HRT in nondiabetic subjects, but the improvement was less apparent in the diabetic cohort. However, the use of HRT in women with diabetes was associated with lower soluble ICAM levels, suggesting an attenuation in endothelial activation. There was a considerable variability in the HRT regimens used in this study and the number of participants small, so the study was unable to ascertain whether a particular form of HRT was superior in terms of improving endothelial function.

In a further study, Lee and associates (162) also confirmed that endothelial dysfunction was prominent in women with diabetes and significantly improved by estrogen (premarin 0.625 mg) but not reversed. These results suggest that other factors, in addition to estrogen deficiency, play a role in endothelial dysfunction in postmenopausal women with diabetes and they cannot be reversed by estrogen therapy alone.

An additional small study examined the vascular effects of CEE (0.625 mg) or placebo for 8 weeks in type 2 diabetic postmenopausal women in a randomized double-blinded, placebo-controlled crossover design. The authors concluded that the effects of estrogen on vascular dilatory function and vascular adhesion molecules were less apparent in type 2 diabetic postmenopausal women, despite a beneficial effect of estrogen on lipoprotein levels (163).

Taken together, the above findings suggest, that in regard to endothelial dysfunction, there is some resistance to HRT in diabetic postmenopausal women compared to healthy postmenopausal women. However, a more recent study challenges this suggestion. Perera and associates (164) examined endothelium-dependent and independent vascular relaxation in a small cohort of postmenopausal women with diabetes before and 6 months after transdermal 17β-estradiol (80 mg twice weekly) in combination with oral nonethisterone (1 mg daily). The authors concluded that this particular HRT regimen had potentially beneficial effects on vascular relaxation. Data were consistent with improvements in endothelial function, vascular smooth muscle function, or both. Abnormal responses to endothelium-independent agonists have been reported in type 2 diabetes by other workers (165) but there have been no previous reports of augmented endothelium-independent responses after HRT in women with or without type 2 diabetes.

Finally, despite evidence for a beneficial effect of HRT on indexes of arterial load and ambulatory BP, previously reported in normal subjects, a recent study reported no change in arterial stiffness and ambulatory BP in a small cohort of diabetic postmenopausal women (166). However, another study reported that ERT or HRT may produce beneficial effects on BP responses to psychological stress and on plasma renin activity in women with type 2 diabetes (167).

It appears, therefore, that data on the effect of HRT on endothelial function in postmenopausal women with diabetes are conflicting but the weight of evidence is that there may be a degree of resistance to HRT in diabetes.

HRT and Risk of Cardiovascular Disease in Women With Diabetes

CVD is the most common cause of death in type 2 diabetes. This increased risk is particularly apparent in women with diabetes in which the relative protection afforded by the female sex is lost (107). For women without diabetes, prospective cohort surveys such as the Nurse's Health Cohort Study, suggest that estrogen therapy decreases the risk of CHD in postmenopausal women who were initially healthy at the time of enrollment (5). However, data from the HERS and WHI clinical trials have questioned the validity of epidemiological evidence by reporting an increased risk of CHD among women assigned to HRT (6,7).

Little is known about the effect of HRT on CHD in women with diabetes. Secondary analyses among small subgroups of women with diabetes from case–control studies have been equivocal, some reporting a non significant reduced risk (168,169) and others nonsignificant increased risk of CHD with exposure to HRT (170). In a 3-year follow-up observational study of a cohort of 25,000 diabetic women aged 50 years and older from the Northern California Kaiser Permanente Registry, the risk of acute MI associated with current use of different hormone regimens was examined (171). The data revealed that current HRT use was associated with a significant 16% lower rate of fatal and nonfatal MIs. Lower risk of acute MI was observed among women using low or medium doses of estrogen (≤0.625 mg CEE) but not among those using a high dose. However, among women with a recent MI, current HRT use was associated with an 80% higher rate of recurrent acute MI, and the rate of recurrent events was fourfold higher during the first year of HRT (171). The observed decreased risk of acute MI associated with current HRT in diabetic women without a recent MI is reminiscent of the results from observational studies in nondiabetic women without CHD (74). On the other hand, the results among diabetic women who have had a recent MI, are consistent with those of the HERS trial (6) and a prospective , observational study of women with pre-existing CHD (172).

A recent large prospective observational study in Denmark, examined the association between HRT, based on a different regimen (17β-estradiol and norethisterone acetate) and ischemic heart disease (IHD), MI, and total number of deaths among a cohort of almost 20,000 Danish nurses aged 41 years and older *(173)*. The data showed that current users of HRT smoked more, consumed more alcohol, had lower self-rated health, but were slimmer and had a lower prevalence of diabetes than never users. In current users without diabetes, HRT had no protective effect on IHD or MI compared with never users. However current users with diabetes had an increased risk of death, IHD and MI compared with never users with diabetes. These findings suggest that HRT does not protect women against IHD. Rather the effect of treatment is modified by diabetes, with an increased risk among women with diabetes using HRT.

With respect to the effect of HRT on the progression of atherosclerosis, Dubuison and associates *(174)* conducted a cross-sectional analysis and found that the beneficial effect of ERT/HRT on carotid intima-media wall thickness—a common measure of subclinical atherosclerosis—was similar in diabetic and nondiabetic postmenopausal women. In the HERS trial, nearly 23% of the participants had diabetes. A *post hoc* subgroup analysis revealed that HRT imparted no treatment effect for patients with diabetes *(175)*. Similarly, the investigators of the WHI trial (4.4% of patients had diabetes) in a subgroup analysis demonstrated no increased risk among patients with diabetes taking HRT *(7)*. The findings of the above studies of a neutral or harmful effect of HRT among women with diabetes are in line with the previous observations that the cardioprotection associated with being female was lost in women with diabetes.

Although the biological mechanism for this lack of effect remains speculative it is consistent with the fact that estrogen does not improve the endothelium-dependent vasodilation in women with type 2 diabetes, previously reported *(109,162)*. One possible explanation is that HRT does not benefit the damaged endothelium and the proinflammatory and/or procoagulant effects of treatment may dominate when the endothelium is already damaged. However, data from controlled clinical trials in diabetic women are needed to understand the possible risks and benefits of HRT. The Raloxifene use for the Heart Study, an ongoing RCT that includes a large sample of women with diabetes, will add to our knowledge of the magnitude of the effect of the risks and benefits of HRT in women with diabetes *(176)*.

At present, the situation regarding the use of HRT for the prophylaxis or treatment of CVD in women with diabetes is unclear in the absence of data from randomized clinical studies. Women should be informed of the current uncertainty regarding HRT and CVD before initiating treatment for other reasons. However, this should not prevent women with diabetes from receiving HRT for menopausal symptoms or for treatment or prophylaxis of osteoporosis.

Polycystic Ovary Syndrome, Diabetes, and Cardivascular Disease

PCOS is the most common endocrinopathy that affects women of reproductive age *(177)*. Data on the exact prevalence are variable mostly because of the lack of well-accepted diagnostic criteria. At present, the diagnosis of PCOS is based on the presence of ovulatory dysfunction and clinical or biochemical evidence of hyperandrogenism. The diagnosis requires a complete evaluation for exclusion of other causes of hyperandrogenism such as nonclassic adrenal 21-hydroxylase deficiency and androgen secreting neoplasms. The presence of polycystic ovaries on ultrasound is not a criterion for diagnosis as this is commonly found in randomly selected women *(178)*. Although PCOS is known to be associated with reproductive morbidity and increased risk for endometrial cancer, diagnosis is especially important because PCOS is now thought to increase metabolic and cardiovascular risks *(179)*. These risks are strongly linked to insulin resistance which is present in both obese and lean women with PCOS.

Relationship to Insulin Resistance and Diabetes

Although the exact mechanisms that lead to the development of PCOS are not clear it has been shown that insulin resistance and compensatory hyperinsulinemia possess the central role in the pathophysiology of the syndrome. Women with PCOS have both basal and glucose-stimulated hyperinsulinemia compared with weight-matched women and the high levels of insulin are thought to mediate the development of hyperandrogenemia, anovulation, and infertility. At the same time, insulin resistance and compensatory hyperinsulinemia are responsible for the cardiovascular risk factors. The hyperinsulinism correlates with the hyperandrogenism and occurs independent of obesity *(180,181)*.

The insulin resistance in at least 50% of PCOS women appears to be related to excessive serine phosphorylation of the insulin receptor *(182)*. This abnormality is caused by a factor extrinsic to the insulin receptor, which is presumably a serine/threonine kinase. Serine phosphorylation appears to modulate the activity of P450c17, which is a key regulatory enzyme that regulates androgen biosynthesis explaining the hyperandrogenism. A second possible mechanism, perhaps in those who do not have the above defect, may be abnormal signaling at the receptor substrate-1 (IRS-1) level as a result of diminished activity of phosphatidylinositol-3 kinase (PI3K) *(183)*. It has also been suggested that women with PCOS have a deficiency of a chiroinositol containing phosphoglycan that mediates the action of insulin. Treatment with D-chiroinositol improved ovulatory function and decreased serum androgen concentrations, BP, and plasma triglyceride concentrations *(184)*.

Women with PCOS are at a greater risk for abnormal glucose tolerance and type 2 diabetes mellitus as compared with age- and weight-matched populations of women without PCOS. In a study that included 122 women with PCOS, glucose tolerance was abnormal in 45%: 35% had IGT and 10% had type 2 diabetes *(185)*. In a subset of 25 women that were re-studied 2.4 years after the initial evaluation it was shown that the conversion from IGT to diabetes mellitus was accelerated as compared to the women without PCOS. The increased risk for IGT and type 2 diabetes occurs at all weight levels and at a young age and additionally, PCOS itself may be a more important risk factor that ethnicity or race for glucose intolerance in young women *(186)*. Perimenopausal women with a history of PCOS are also at a higher risk for developing type 2 diabetes as compared to women without a history of PCOS *(187)*.

Women with PCOS should periodically have an oral glucose tolerance test and must be closely followed and monitored for the development of IGT or diabetes. The basal and 2 hour, glucose-stimulated levels rather than the fasting glucose levels alone are required for such screening *(188)*.

Polycystic Ovary Syndrome and Cardiovascular Risk

PCOS is associated with an increase in cardiovascular risk factors *(189)*. In addition to obesity that is commonly present and independently associated with increased cardiovascular risk, women with PCOS have dyslipedemia, hypertension and elevated PAI-1 levels. Obesity is a prominent feature in women with PCOS as about half of the patients are obese. Also, obesity appears to confer an additive and synergistic effect on the manifestations of the syndrome and additionally, it is one of the strongest risk factors for diabetes. The obesity is usually of the android type with an increased waist to hip ratio that may further contribute to diabetes risk.

Women with PCOS have higher serum triglycerides, total and LDL cholesterol and lower HDL cholesterol levels than weight-matched regularly menstruating women *(190)*. These findings however, vary and depend on the weight, diet and ethnic background. In a large study of non-Hispanic white women, elevated LDL-C was the predominant lipid abnormality in women with PCOS *(191)*. An additional parameter contributing to the elevated cardiovascular risk is hypertension. Obese women with PCOS have an increased incidence of hypertension and sustained hypertension is threefold more likely in later life in women with PCOS *(192)*. It is not clear whether this increase in hypertension is because of the PCOS status, obesity or both.

PAI-1 concentrations in blood are higher in women with PCOS as compared to those not affected. PAI-1 levels have been shown to be positively correlated with triglycerides, basal insulin and abdominal obesity *(193)*. It was shown that impaired fibrinolysis and particularly the high levels of PAI-1 in selected groups of patients with CHD, is not a consequence of the coronary disease itself but it is rather related to the metabolic risk factors of atherosclerosis *(194)*.

PCOS has also been associated with endothelial dysfunction. In the past several years it has been become evident that endothelial dysfunction may play the central pathogenetic role in the development of diabetes complications and CVDs. In a study that included 12 obese women with PCOS, endothelium-dependent vasodilation was found to be impaired *(195)*. Additionally, it was shown that endothelial dysfunction was associated with both elevated androgen levels and insulin resistance.

Furthermore, in women with PCOS, mean carotid intima-media wall thickness (IMT) was found to be greater as compared to age-matched women without PCOS *(196)*. Greater IMT is associated with an adverse cardiovascular risk profile that includes hyperlipidemia, central adiposity, hypertension and hyperinsulinemia, which is the profile of the dysmetabolic syndrome (syndrome X). Also, increases in the thickness of the carotid intima and media has been shown to be a reliable measure of atherosclerosis elsewhere and directly associated with increased risk of cerebrovascular events and MI in older adults *(197)*.

In addition to above, women with PCOS were found to have more extensive coronary artery disease *(198)*. This was shown in a study that examined patients that underwent coronary angiography for the assessment of chest pain or valvular disease. Polycystic ovaries were present in 42% of the women and coronary lesions were associated with hirsutism, previous hysterectomy, low HDL, higher free testosterone, triglycerides, and C-peptide levels.

Effect of Insulin Resistance Treatment on Polycystic Ovary Syndrome

WEIGHT LOSS

Weight reduction is of paramount importance and cornerstone of every therapeutic strategy in PCOS. Although obesity does not seem to be the primary insult in PCOS, many studies have demonstrated the beneficial impact of weight reduction on the manifestations of the syndrome and especially insulin sensitivity, risk for diabetes and adverse cardiovascular risk profile *(199)*. The effect of weight reduction by a hypocaloric low-fat diet on the metabolic and endocrine variables was studied in obese women with PCOS

(200). The insulin sensitivity was assessed by the euglycemic hyperinsulinemic clamp technique, which is the gold standard in evaluating insulin resistance. After the diet intervention, insulin sensitivity improved and did not differ significantly from the body mass index matched normo-ovulatory control women.

In another study, the effect of dietary intervention on insulin sensitivity and lipids, fibrinolysis and coagulation was examined also in obese women with PCOS *(201)*. Insulin sensitivity was assessed by the eyglycemic clamp technique before and after a very low-calorie, protein-rich diet for 4 weeks that was followed by a low-calorie, low-fat diet for 20 weeks. After the 24-week intervention, insulin sensitivity was significantly increased along with a significant reduction of total serum cholesterol and fasting triglyceride. Additionally, there was a significant reduction of fasting glucose and insulin. After the 20-week follow-up program, insulin sensitivity was still significantly increased and PAI-1 was significantly improved.

Weight reduction also decreases androgen levels and restores ovulation in women with PCOS *(202)*. Most of the studies suggest a significant reduction in total testosterone and a significant increase in SHBG, positively affecting the free testosterone levels. This effect is probably as a result of the improvement in hyperinsulinemia that directly affects ovarian androgen production.

THIAZOLIDINEDIONES

Thiazolidinediones (TZDs) are novel insulin-sensitizing agents that improve peripheral insulin resistance in adipose tissue and skeletal muscle and are currently widely used for the treatment of type 2 diabetes. Recent studies have shown that the TZD troglitazone, improves total body insulin action in PCOS resulting in lower circulating insulin levels without altering body weight and lowered circulating androgen, estrogen, and luteinizing hormone (LH) levels *(203)*. In addition to improving insulin resistance, troglitazone reduced PAI-1 levels *(204)* and was also shown to improve ovulation in a dose-related fashion *(205)*. More recently, troglitazone was shown to improve endothelial function in women with PCOS to near normal levels *(206)*. The latter agent was withdrawn from the market after reports of hepatotoxicity.

Rosiglitazone which is currently Food and Drug Administration (FDA)-approved for the treatment of type 2 diabetes is another insulin sensitizer that was shown to enhance both spontaneous and clomiphene- induced ovulation in overweight and obese women with PCOS *(207)*. Pioglitazone, also another FDA-approved insulin sensitizer, when added to metformin lowered insulin, glucose, insulin resistance, insulin secretion, and dehydroepiandrosterone sulfate, whereas it increased HDL-C and SHBG along with an improvement in menstrual regularity *(208)*.

METFORMIN

Metformin is an oral hypoglycemic agent that is extensively used for the treatment of type 2 diabetes mellitus. Its mechanism of action involves decreasing hepatic glucogenolysis that leads to a decrease in hepatic glucose output. To a lesser extent metformin increases peripheral glucose-mediated glucose uptake *(209)*.

Metformin (1500 mg), when administered daily for 4–8 weeks in obese women with PCOS, resulted in a decrease in insulin and free testosterone levels *(210)*. Metformin at the above dose improved insulin sensitivity, decreased serum LH and increased serum follicle-stimulating hormone and SHBG *(211)*. Higher plasma insulin, lower serum androstenedione and less severe menstrual abnormalities are baseline predictors of clinical response to metformin *(212)*. Metformin is also very useful in lean and normal weight women with PCOS *(213)*. In this population, metformin treatment for 4–6 weeks resulted in a decrease in fasting and glucose-stimulated insulin levels, decreased free testosterone concentrations, and increased SHBG.

One of the greatest challenges is whether metformin should be used in all women with PCOS to prevent or delay the development of type 2 diabetes. In the recently reported Diabetes Prevention Program, metformin therapy in nondiabetic persons with elevated fasting and postload plasma glucose concentrations, reduced the incidence of type 2 diabetes by 31% *(214)*. In nondiabetic women with PCOS, metfomin therapy throughout pregnancy was associated with a 10-fold decrease in the development of gestational diabetes *(215)*.

Women with PCOS very often require medications to induce ovulation. Metformin is very beneficial in ovulation induction when administered in combination with medications such as clomiphene citrate and this improves pregnancy rates *(216)*. Also, metformin, improved fertilization and pregnancy rates when administered to clomiphene-citrate-resistant women with PCOS who were undergoing in vitro fertilization *(217)*. Additionally, metformin administration during pregnancy reduced first-trimester pregnancy loss *(218)*. Metformin's beneficial reproductive effects are clearly attributed to amelirioration of hyperinsulinemic insulin resistance.

CONCLUSIONS

It has been established that HRT is beneficial in reducing osteoporosis and alleviating climacteric symptoms. HRT has also been shown to have beneficial effects on risk factors for CVD. However, data from recent clinical trials indicate that HRT, in the form of continuous combined CEE with MPA, has no cardioprotective effects and is not recommended for primary or secondary prevention of CVD in postmenopausal women.

Data on HRT in postmenopausal women with diabetes are scarce but are of major importance, because these women are characterized by hyperandrogenicity, insulin resistance, and dyslipidemia and are at a higher risk for developing CHD. Evidence from the available data suggest that short-term unopposed oral estradiol has a beneficial effect on glucose homeostasis, lipid profile, and other components of the metabolic syndrome, which may be compatible with a reduced risk of CHD. The addition of a progestogen may attenuate some of these favourable effects. On the other hand, HRT consisting of continuous combined transdermal 17β-estradiol and oral norethisterone, reduces plasma triglycerides and cholesterol concentrations, factor VII activity and von Willebrand factor antigen levels without concomitant changes in adiposity and glycemic control. These effects, allied with favorable effects on CRP and potential beneficial effects on vascular reactivity, suggest that this regimen may hold particular advantage for women with diabetes. Comparative studies are urgently needed to test this hypothesis.

On the basis of the current knowledge, NAMS has established consensus on the following issues: (a) controlling cardiovascular risk factors through pharmacological and nonpharmacological means can significantly decrease the risk for developing cardiovascular events, (b) a broad-based recommendation for ERT/HRT cannot be made; rather the benefits and risks must be weighted in the context of each woman's risk factors, (c) when ERT/HRT is recommended, the greatest benefits may be obtained from use of transdermal estrogen preparations, low doses of oral estrogens, progesterones instead of progestin, and/or nonandrogenic preparations, although more research is needed in this area, and (d) counseling can help maximize the patient's adherence to multiple medication regimens and increase her understanding of the potential benefits and risks of ERT/HRT *(147)*.

Thus, a century after the first description of the "evil effects" of the female sex hormones, their actual role in CVD remains controversial. However, as Marie Curie said "Nothing in life is to be feared, it is only to be understood" and so to this end, research is this area needs to continue.

REFERENCES

1. Mackenzie J. Irritation of the sexual apparatus as an etiological factor in the production of nasal disease. Ann J Med Sci 1884;87:360–365.
2. Barrett-Connor E. The 1995 Ancel Keys Lecture: Sex differences in coronary heart disease. Why are women so superior? Circulation 1997;95:252–264.
3. Sullivan JM, Fowlkes LP. The clinical aspects of estrogen and the cardiovascular system. Obstet Gynecol 1996;87:36S-43S.
4. Stampfer MJ, Colditz GA. Estrogen replacement therapy and coronary heart disease:a quantitave assesment of the epidemiologic evidence. Prev Med 1999;20:47–63.
5. Grodstein F, Manson JE, Colditz GA, et al. A prospective, observational study of postmenopausal hormone therapy and primary prevention of cardiovascular disease. Ann Intern Med 2000;133:933–934.
6. Hulley S, Grady D, Bush T, et al. Randomized trial of estrogen plus progestin for secondary prevention of coronary heart disease in postmenopausal women: Heart and Estrogen/Progestin Replacement Study (HERS) Research Group. JAMA 1998;280:605–613.
7. Manson JM, Hsia J, Johnson KC, et al. Estrogen plus progestin and the risk of coronary heart disease. N Engl J Med 2003;349:523–534.
8. Lee WL, Cheung AM, Cape D, Zinman B. Impact of diabets on coronary artery disease in women and men. Ann Rev Diabetes 2001;235–240.
9. Koh KK. Can a healthy endothelium influence the cardiovascular effects of hormone replacement therapy? Int J Cardiol 2003;87:1–8.
10. Gruber CJ, Tschugguel W, Schneeberger C, Huber J. Production and actions of estrogens. N Engl J Med 2002;346:340–351.
11. Selby C. Sex hormone binding globulin: origin, function and clinical significance. Ann Clin Biochem 1990;27:532–541.
12. Carr MC. The emergence of the metabolic syndrome with the menopause. J Clin Endocrinol Metab 2003;88:2404-2411.
13. Yen SSC, Jaffe RB, Barbieri RL. Reproductive Endocrinology, fourth ed. Philadelphia: Saunders, 1999, pp. 110–133,301–319,751–784.
14. Crook D. Cardiovascular risk assessment for postmenopausal hormone replacement therapies such as tibolone (Livial). In: Genazzani AR, (ed). Hormone Replacement Therapy and Cardiovascular Disease. New York: Parthenon, 2001, pp. 165–172.
15. Bryant HV, Dere WH. Selective estrogen receptor modulators: an alternative to hormone replacement therapy. Proc Soc Exp Biol Med 1998;217:45–52.
16. Knight DC, Eden JA. Plytoestrogens—a short review. Maturitas 1995;22:167–175.
17. Enmark E, Gustafsson J-A. Oestrogen receptors—an overview. J Int Med 1999;246:133–138.
18. Mendelsohn ME, Karas RH. Estrogen and the blood vessel wall. Curr Opin Cardiol 1994;9:619–626.
19. Herrington DM, Howard TD, Hawkins GA, et al. Estrogen-receptor polymorphisms and effects of estrogen replacement on high-density lipoprotein cholesterol in women with coronary disease. N Engl J Med 2002;346:967–974.
20. Losordo DW, Kearney M, Kim EA et al. Variable expression of the estrogen receptor in normal and atherosclerotic coronary arteries of premenopausal women. Circulation 1994;89:1501–1510.
21. Post WS, Goldschmidt-Clermont PJ, Wilbide CC et al. Methylation of the estrogen receptor gene is associated with aging and atherosclerosis in the cardiovascular system. Cardiovasc Res 1999;43:985–991.
22. Kim HP, Lee JY, Teong JK, Bae SW, Lee HK, Jo I. Nongenomic stimulation of nitric oxide release by estrogen is mediated by estrogen receptor localized in caveolae. Biochem Biophys Res Commun 1999;263:257–262.
23. Nadal A, Rovira JM, Laribi O, et al. Rapid insulinotropic effect of estradiol via a plasma membrane receptor. FASEB J 1998;12:1341–1348.

24. Rubanyi GM. The role of endothelium in cardiovascular hemeostasis and diseases. J Cardiovasc Pharmacol 1993;22:S1–S514.
25. Moncada S, Hiqqs A. The L-arginine-nitric oxide pathway. N Engl J Med 1993;329:2002–2012.
26. Liao JK. Endothelial nitric oxide and vascular inflammation. In: Panza JA, Cannon ROI, (eds). Endothelium, nitric oxide and atherosclerosis. Armonk NY: Futura, 1999, pp. 119–132.
27. Quyyumi AA. Endothelial function in health and disease: new insights into the genesis of cardiovascular disease. Am J Med 1998;105:325–395.
28. Kleinert H, Wallerath T, Euchenhofer C, Ihrig-Biedert I, Li H, Forstermann V. Estrogens increase transcription of the human endothelial NO synthase gene: analysis of the transcription factors involved. Hypertension 1998;32:588–592.
29. Nabel EL, Selwyn AP, Ganz P. Large coronary arteries in humans are responsive to changing blood flow: an endothelium dependent mechanism that fails in patients with atherosclerosis. J Am Coll Cardiol 1990;16: 349–356.
30. Celermajer DS, Sorensen KE, Gooch VM et al. Non-invasive detection of endothelial dysfunction in children and adults at risk of atherosclerosis. Lancet 1992;340:1111–1115.
31. Majmudar NG, Robson SC, Ford GA. Effects of menopause, gender, and estrogen replacement therapy on vascular nitric oxide activity. J Clin Endocrinol Metab 2000;85:1577–1583.
32. Pinto S, Virdis A, Chiadoni L, et al. Endogenus estrogen and acetycholine-induced vasodilation in normotensive women. Hypertention 1997;29:268–273.
33. Kalantaridou SN, Naka KK, Papanikolaou E, et al. Impaired endothelial function in young women with premature ovarian failure: normalization with hormone therapy. J Clin Endocrinol Metab 2004;89:3907–3913.
34. Kawano H, Motoyama T, Kugiyama K, et al. Menstrual cyclic variation of endothelium-dependent vasodilation of the branchial artery: possible role of estrogen and nitric oxide. Proc Assoc Am Physicians 1996;108:473–480.
35. English JL, Jacobs LO, Green G, Andrews TC. Effect of the menstrual cycle on endothelium-dependent vasodilation of the branchial artery in normal young women. Am J Cardiol 1998;82:256–258.
36. Lieberman EH, Gerhard MD, Uehata A, et al. Estrogen improves endothelium-dependent, flow-mediated vasodilation in postmenopausal women. Ann Intern Med 1994;121:936–941.
37. Best PJ, Berger PB, Miller VM, Lerman A. The effect of estrogen replacement therapy on plasma nitric oxide and endothelin-1 levels in postmenopausal women. Ann Intern Med 1998;128:285–288.
38. Sorensen KE, Dorup I, Hermann AP, Mosekilde L. Combined hormone replacement therapy does not protect women against the age-related decline in endothelium dependent vasomotor function. Circulation 1998;97:1234–1238.
39. John S, Jacobi J, Schlaich MP, Delles C, Schmieder RE. Effects of oral contraceptives on vascular endothelium in premenopausal women. Am J Obstet Gynecol 2000;183:28–33.
40. Sudhir K, Chou TM, Messina LM, et al. Endothelial dysfunction in a man with disruptive mutation in oestrogen-receptor gene. Lancet 1997;349:1146–1147.
41. Mendelsohn ME. Mechanisms of estrogen action in the cardiovascular system. J Steroid Biochem Mol Biol 2000;74:337–343.
42. Gilligan DM, Badar DM, Panza JA, Quyyumi AA, Cannon RO III. Acute vascular effects of estrogen in postmenopausal women. Circulation 1994;90:786–791.
43. Kato S, Erdoh H, Masuhiro Y et al. Activation of the estrogen receptor through phosphorylation by mitogen-activated protein kinase. Science 1995;270:1491–1494.
44. Haynes MP, Sinha D, Russel KS, et al. Membrane estrogen receptor engagement activates endothelial nitric oxide synthase via the PI3-kinase-Akt pathway in human endothelial cells. Circ Res 2000;87: 677–682.
45. Chen Z, Yuhama IS, Galcheva-Gargova ZI, Karas RH, Mendelsohn ME, Shaul PW. Estrogen receptor alpha mediates the nongenomic activation of endothelial nitric oxide synthase by estrogen. J Clin Invest 1999;103:401–406.
46. White RE. Estrogen and vascular function. Vasc Pharmacol 2002;38:73–80.
47. Mikkola T, Turunen P, Avela K, et al. 17-beta oestradiol stimulates prostacyclin but not endothelin-1 production in human vascular endothelial cells. J Clin Endocrinol Metab 1995;80:1832–1836.
48. Spyridopoulos I, Sullivan AB, Kearney M, Isner JM, Losordo DW. Estrogen-receptor-mediated inhibition of human endothelial cell apoptosis:estradiol as a survival factor. Circulation 1997;95:1505–1514.
49. Kolodgie FD, Jacob A, Wilson PS, et al. Estradiol attenuates directed migration of vascular smooth muscle cells in vitro. Am J Pathol 1996;148:969–976.

50. Caulin-Glaser T, Watson CA, Pardi R, Bender JR. Effect of 17Œ -estradiol on cytokine-induced endot-helial cell adhesion molecule expression. J Clin Invest 1996;98:36–42.
51. Meilahn EN, Kuller LH, Mathews KA, Kiss JE. Hemostatic factors according to menopausal status and use of hormone replacement therapy. Ann Epidemiol 1992;2:445–455.
52. Nabulsi AA, Folsom AR, White A, et al. Association of HRT with various cardiovascular risk factors in postmenopausal women. N Engl J Med 1993;328:1069–1075.
53. Winkler UH. Menopause, hormone replacement therapy and cardiovascular disease: a review of haemostaseological findings. Fibrinolysis 1992;6(Suppl 3):5–10.
54. Juhan-Vaque I, Alessi MC. Plasminogen activator inhibitor-1 and atherothrombosis. Thromb Haemostasis 1993;70:138–143.
55. Koh KK, Mincemoyer R, Bui MN, et al. Effects of hormone-replacement therapy on fibrinolysis in postmenopausal women. N Engl J Med 1997;336:683–690.
56. Kroon UB, Silverstolpe G, Tengborn I. The effects of transdermal estradiol and oral conjugated oestrogens on haemostasis variables. Thromb Haemost 1994 ; 71:420–421.
57. Rosendaal FR, Helmerhorst FM, Vandenbroucke JP. Female hormones and thrombosis. Arterioscler Thromb Vasc Biol 2002;22:201–210.
58. Godsland IF. Effects of postmenopausal hormone replacement therapy on lipid, lipoprotein and apolipoprotein (a) concentrations: analysis of studies published from 1974–2000. Fertil steril 2001;75:898–915.
59. Kovanen PT, Brown MS, Goldstein JL. Increased binding of low density lipoprotein to liver membranes from rats treated with 17β-ethinyl estradiol. J Biol Chem 1979;254:11,367–11,373.
60. Tikkanen MJ, Nikkia EA, Kuusi T, Sipinen S. High density lipoprotein-2 and hepatic lipase: reciprocal changes produced by estrogen and norgestrel. J Clin Endocrinol Metab 1982;54:1113–1117.
61. Crook D, Stevenson JC. Transdermal hormone replacement therapy, serum lipids and lipoproteins. Br J Clin Pract 1996; 86:17–21.
62. Sack NM, Rader DJ, O' Cannon R. Oesrtrogen and inhibition of oxidation of low-density lipoprotein in post-menopausal women. Lancet 1994;343;269–270.
63. McNamara JR, Shah PK, Nakajima K, et al. Remnant-like particle (RLPs) cholesterol is an independent cardiovascular disease risk factor in women: results from the Framingham heart study. Atherosclerosis 2001;154:229–236.
64. Ossewaarde ME, Dallinga, Thie GM, Bots ML, et al. Treatment with hormone replacement therapy lowers remnant lipoprotein particles in healthy postmenopausal women: results from a randomized trial. Eur J Clin Invest 2003;33:376–382.
65. Ross R. Atherosclerosis: an inflammatory disease. N Engl J Med 1999;340:115–126.
66. Ridker PM, Hennekens CH, Buring JE, et al. C-reactive protein and other markers of inflammation in the prediction of cardiovascular disease in women. N Engl J Med 2000; 342: 836–843.
67. Cushman M. Effects of hormone replacement therapy and estrogen receptor modulators on markers of inflammation and coagulation. Am J Cardiol 2002;90 (Suppl):7–10.
68. Cushman M, Leqault C, Barret-Connor E, et al. Effect of postmenopausal hormones on inflammation—sensitive proteins: the Postmenopausal Estrogen Progestin Interventions (PEPI) Study. Circulation 1999;100:717–722.
69. Nunomura W, Takakuwa Y, Higashi T. Changes in serum concentration and mRNA level of rat C-reactive protein. Bioch Bioph Acta 1994;1227:74–78.
70. Vongpatanasin W, Tuncel M, Wang Z, et al. Differential effects of oral versus transdermal estrogen replacement therapy on C—reactive protein in postmenopausal women. J Am Col Cardiol 2003;41:1358–1363
71. Silvestri A, Gebara O, Vitale C, et al. Increased levels of C—reactive protein after oral hormone replacement may not be related to an increased inflammatory response. Circulation 2003;107:3165–3169.
72. Zanger D, Yang B K, Addams J, Waclaviw M A, et al. Divergent effects of hormone therapy on serum markers of inflammation in postmenopausal women with coronary artery disease on appropriate medical management. J Am Coll Cardiol 2000, 36; 1797–1802.
73. Sperti G, Van Leeuwen RT, Guax PH, Maseri A, Kluft C. Cultured rat aortic vascular smooth muscle cells digest naturally produced extracellular matrix: involvement of plasminogen-dependent and plas-minogen-independent pathways. Circ Res 1992;71:385–392.
74. Colditz GA, Willett WC, Stampfer MJ, Rosner B, Speizer FE, Hennekens CH. Menopause and the risk of coronary heart disease in women. N Engl J Med1987; 316;1105–1110.

75. Mosca L. The role of hormone replacement therapy in the prevention of postmenopausal heart disease. Arch Intern Med 2000;160:2263–2272.

76. Grodstein F, Stampfer M. The epidemiology of coronary heart disease and estrogen replacement in postmenopausal women. Progress Cardiol 995;38:199–210.

77. Rackley CE. Estrogen and coronary artery disease in postmenopausal women. Am J Med 1995;99: 117–118.

78. Alexander KP, Newby LK, Hellkamp AS, et al. Initiation of hormone replacement therapy after acute myocardial infarction is associated with more cardiac events during follow-up. J Am Coll Cardiol 2001;38:1–7.

79. Hemminki E, Sihvo S. A review of postmenopausal hormone therapy recommendations: potential for selection bias. Obstet Gynecol 1993;82:1021–1028.

80. Barret-Connor E. Postmenopausal estrogen and prevention bias. Ann Intern Med 1991; 115 :455–456.

81. Adams MR, Register TC, Golden DK, Wagner JD, Williams JK. Medroxyprogesterone acetate antagonizes inhibitory effects of conjugated equine estrogens on coronary artery atherosclerosis. Arterioscler Thromb Vasc Biol 1997;17:217–221.

82. Grodstein F, Stampfer MJ, Manson JE et al. Postmenopausal estrogen and progestin use and the risk of cardiovascular disease. N Engl J Med 1996;335:413–461.

83. Grady D, Herrington D, Bittner V et al. Cardiovascular disease outcomes during 6.8 years of hormone therapy: Heart and Estrogen /progestin Replacement Study follow-up (HERS II) JAMA 2002;288:49–57.

84. Clarke SC, Kelleher T, Lloyd-Jones H, Slack M, Schofield PM. A study of hormone replacement therapy in postmenopausal women with ischaemic heart disease: the Papworth HRT atherosclerosis study. Br J Obstet Gynecol 2002;109:1056–1062.

85. Herrington DM, Reboussin DM, Brosnihan KB et al. Effects of estrogen replacement on the progression of coronary artery atherosclerosis. N Engl J Med 2000;343:522–529.

86. Writing Group for the Women's Health Initiative Investigators. Risks and benefits of estrogen plus progestin in healthy postmenopausal women: principal results from the Women's Health Initiative randomized controlled trial. JAMA 2002;288:321–333.

87. Hodis HN, Mack WJ, Azen SP, et al., for the Women's Estrogen-Progestin Lipid-Lowering Hormone Atherosclerosis Regression Trial Research Group. Hormone therapy and the progression of coronary-artery atherosclerosis in postmenopausal women. N Engl J Med 2003;349:535–545.

88. Hodis HN, Mack MJ, Lobo R A, et al. Estrogen in the prevention of atherosclerosis: a randomized double-blind, placebo-controlled trial. Ann Intern Med 2001;135:939–953.

89. Wingrove CS, Garr E, Godsland IF, Stevenson JC. 17beta oestradiol enhances release of matrix metalloproteinase-2 from human vascular smooth muscle cells. Biochim Biophys Acta 1998;1406: 169–174.

90. Galis ZS, Khatri JJ. Matrix metalloproteinases in vascular remodelling and atherogenesis: the good, the bad ,and the ugly. Circ Res 2002;90:251–262.

91. Curry TE Jr, Osteen KG. Cyclic changes in the matrix metalloproteinase system in the ovary and uterus. Biol Reprod 2001;64:1285–1296.

92. Holm P, Andersen HL, Andersen MR, et al. The direct antiatherogenic effect of estrogen is present, absent or reversed, depending on the state of the arterial endothelium. Circulation 1999;100:1727–1733.

93. Herrington DM, Espeland MA, Crouse JR, et al. Estrogen replacement and branchial artery flow—mediated vasodilation in older women. Arterioscler Thromb Vasc Biol 2001;21:1955–1961.

94. Mikkola TS, Clarkson TB. Estrogen replacement therapy, atherosclerosis, and vascular function.Cardiovasc Res 2002;53:605–619.

95. Psaty BM,Smith NL,Lemaitre RN, et al. Hormone replacement therapy, prothrombotic mutations, and the risk of incident non fatal myocardial infarction in postmenopausal women. JAMA 2001;285: 900–913.

96. Price DT, Ridker PM. Factor V leiden mutation and the risk for thromboembolic disease: a clinical perspective. Ann Intern Med 1997;127:895–903.

97. Weiss EJ, Bray PF, Tayback M, et al. A polymorphism of a platelet glycoprotein receptor as an inherited risk factor for coronary thrombosis. N Engl J Med 1996;334:1090–1094.

98. Shlipak MG, Simon JA, Vittinghoff E, et al. Estrogen and progestin, lipoprotein(a), and the risk of recurrent coronary heart disease events after menopause. JAMA 2000;283:1845–1852.

99. Barrett-Connor E, Grady D, Sashegyi A, et al. Raloxifene and cardiovascular events in osteoporotic postmenopausal women: four-year results from the MORE (Multiple Outcomes of Raloxifene Evaluation) randomized trial. JAMA 2002;287:847–857.

100. Vanharanta M, Voutilainen S, Lakka TA, van der Lee LM, Adlercreutz H, Salonen JT. Risk of acute coronary events according to serum concentrations of enterolactone: a prospective population-based case control study. Lancet 1999;354:2112–2115.

101. Anthony MS, Clarkson TB, Bullock BC, Wagner JD. Soy protein versus soy phytoestrogens in the prevention of diet-induced coronary artery atherosclerosis of male cynomolgus monkeys. Arterioscler Thromb Vasc Biol 1997;17:2524–2531.

102. Honore EK, Williams JK, Anthony MS, Clarkson JB. Soy isoflavones enhance coronary vascular reactivity in atherosclerotic female macaques. Fertil Steril 1997;67:148–154.

103. Nestel PJ, Jamashita T, Sasahara T, et al. Soy isoflavones improve systemic arterial compliance but not lipids in menopausal and perimenopausal women. Arterioscler Thromb Vasc Biol 1997;17:3392–3398.

104. Anderson JW, Johnstone BM, Cook -Newell ME. Metaanalysis of the effects of soy protein intake on serum lipids. N Engl J Med 1995; 333:276–282.

105. Bjarnason NH, Bjarnason K, Haarbo J, Bennink HJ, Christiansen C. Tibolone: influence on markers of cardiovascular disease. J Clin Endocrinol Metabol 1997; 82:1752–1756.

106. Herrington DM. Hormone replacement therapy and heart disease-Replacing dogma with data. Circulation 2003;107:2–4.

107. Barrett-Connor E, Cohn BA, Wingard DL, Edelstein SL. Why is diabetes mellitus a stronger factor for fatal ischemic heart disease in women than in men? The Rancho Bernardo Study. JAMA 1991;265: 627–631.

108. Di Carli MF, Afonso L, Campisi R, et al. Coronary vascular dysfunction in premenopausal women with diabetes mellitus. Am Heart J 2002;144:711–718.

109. Lim SC, Caballero AE, Arora S et al. The effect of hormonal replacement therapy on the vascular reactivity and endothelial function of healthy individuals and individuals with type 2 diabetes. J Clin Endocrinol Metab 1999;84:4159–4164.

110. Steinberg HO, Paradisi G, Cronin J, et al. Type II diabetes abrogates sex differences in endothelial function in premenopausal women. Circulation 2000;101:2040–2046.

111. Lantin-Hermoso RL, Rosenfeld CR, Yuhanna IS, German Z, Chen Z, Shaul PW. Estrogen acutely stimulates nitric oxide synthase activity in fetal pulmonary artery endothelium. Am J Physiol 1997; 273: L119–L126.

112. Herman SM, Robinson JTC, Mc Credie RJ, Adams MR, Boyer MJ. Androgen deprivation is associated with enhanced endothelium-dependent vasodilation in adult men. Arterioscler Thromb Vasc Biol 1997; 17:2004–2009.

113. Nuutila P, Knuuti MJ, Maki M, et al. Gender and insulin sensitivity in the heart and in skeletal muscles: studies using positron emission tomography. Diabetes 1995;44:31–36.

114. Mendelsohn ME. Nongenomic ER-mediated activation of endothelial nitric oxide synthase: how does it work? what does it mean? Circ Res 2000;87:956–960.

115. Zancan V, Santagati S, Bolego C et al. 17β-estradiol decreases nitric oxide synthase II synthesis in vascular smooth muscle cells. Endocrinology 1999;158:617–621.

116. Williams SB, Goldfine AB, Timini FK, et al. Acute hyperglycemia attenuates endothelium dependent vasodilation in humans in vivo. Circulation 1998:97:1695–1701.

117. Maggi A, Cignarella A, Brusadelli A, Bolego C, Pinna C, Duglisi L. Diabetes undermines estrogen control of inducible nitric oxide synthase function in rat aortic smooth muscle cells through over expression of estrogen receptor-α. Circulation 2003;108:211–217.

118. Montelango A, Lasuncion MA, Pallardo LF. Longitudinal study of plasma lipoproteins and hormones during pregnancy in normal and diabetic women. Diabetes 1992;41:1651–1659.

119. Weiss DJ, Charles MA, Dunaif A et al. Hyperinsulinemia is associated with menstrual irregularity and altered serum androgens in Pima Indian women. Metabolism 1994;43:803–807.

120. Lindstedt G, Lundberg P-A, Lapidus L, Lundgreen H, Bengtsson C, Bjorntorp P. Low sex-hormone-binding globulin concentration as independent risk factor for development of NIDDM. Diabetes 1991;40:123–128.

121. Lapidus L, Lindstedt G, Lundberg PA, Bengtsson C, Gredmark T. Concentrations of sex-hormone-binding-globulin and corticosteroid binding globulin in serum in relation to cardiovascular risk factors and to 12-year incidence of cardiovascular disease and overall mortality in postmenopausal women. Clin Chem 1986;32:146–152.

122. Merz CNB, Johnson D, Sharaf BL, et al (for the WISE Study Group). Hypoestrogenemia of hypothalamic origin and coronary artery disease in premenopausal women: a report from the NHLBI-Sponsored WISE study. J Am Coll Cardiol 2003;41:413–419.

123. Solomon CG, Hu FB, Dunaif A et al. Menstrual cycle irregularity and risk for future cardiovascular disease. J Clin Endocrinol Metab 2002;87:2013–2017.
124. Writing group for the PEPI trial. Effects of estrogen or estrogen/progestin regimens on heart disease risk factors in postmenopausal women. The postmenopausal Estrogen /Progestin Interventions (PEPI) trial. JAMA 1995;273:199–203.
125. Espeland MA, Hogan PE, Fireberg SE, et al. Effects of postmenopausal hormone therapy on glucose and insulin concentrations. Diabetes Care 1998;21:1584–1593.
126. Reubinoff BE, Wurtman J, Rojansky N, et al. Effects of hormone replacement therapy on weight, body composition, fat distribution, and food intake in early postmenopausal women: A prospective study. Fertil Steril 1995;64:963–967.
127. Sowers JR. Diabetes Mellitus and cardiovascular disease in women. Arch Intern Med 1998;158:617–621.
128. Walton C, Godsland IF, Proudler AJ, Wynn V, Stevenson JC. The effects of the menopause on insulin sensitivity, secretion and elimination in non-obese, healthy women. Eur J Clin Invest 1993;23:466–471.
129. Crook D, Godsland IF, Hull J, Stevenson JC. Hormone replacement therapy with dydrogesterone and 17-β-oestradiol: effects on serum lipoproteins and glucose tolerance during 24 month follow up. Br J Obstet Gynecol 1997;104:298–302.
130. Goodman-Gruen D, Barrett-Connor E. Sex hormone-binding-globulin and glucose tolerance in post-menopausal women. Diabetes Care 1997;10:645–649.
131. Andersson B, Marin P, Lissner L, Vermeulen A, Bjorntorp P. Testosterone concentrations in women and men with NIDDM. Diabetes Care 1994;17:405–409.
132. Andersson B, Mattsson L-A, Hahn L, et al. Estrogen replacement therapy decreases hyperadrogenicity and improves glucose homeostasis and plasma lipids in postmenopausal women with noninsulin-dependent diabetes mellitus. J Clin Endocrinol Metab 1997;82:638–642.
133. Sowers MR, La Pietra MT. Menopause: its epidemiology and potential association with chronic diseases. Epidemiol Rev 1995;17:287–291.
134. Manson JE, Rimm EB, Golditz GA, et al. A prospective study of postmenopausal estrogen therapy and subsequent incidence of non-insulin-dependent diabetes mellitus. Ann Epidemiol 1992;2:665–669.
135. Gabal LL, Godman-Gruen D, Barrett-Connor E. The effects of postmenopausal estrogen therapy on the risk of non-insulin-dependent diabetes mellitus. Am J Public Health 1997;87:443–447.
136. Kanaya AM, Herrington D, Vittinghoff E, et al. Glycemic effects of postmenopausal hormone therapy: The Heart and Estrogen/Progestin Replacement Study. Ann Intern Med 2003;138:1–9.
137. Feher MD, Issacs AJ. Is hormone replacement therapy prescribed for post-menopausal diabetic women? Br J Clin Pract 1996;50:431–432.
138. Davies PH, Barnett AH. Hormone replacement therapy in women with diabetes mellitus: a survey of knowledge of risks and benefits. Practical Diabetes Int 1998;15:78–80.
139. Brussaard HE, Gevers Leuven JA, Frolich M, Kluft C, Krans HMJ. Short-term oestrogen replacement therapy improves insulin resistance, lipids and fibrinolysis in post-menopausal women with NIDDM. Diabetologia 1997;40:843–847.
140. Anderson B, Mattsson L-A. The effect of transdermal estrogen replacement therapy on hyperandrogenicity and glucose homeostasis in postmenopausal women with NIDDM. Acta Obstet Gynecol Scand 1999;78:260–264.
141. Luotola H, Pyorala T, Loikkanen M. Effects of natural oestrgen/progestin substitution therapy on carbohydrate and lipid metabolism in postmenopausal women. Maturitas 1986;8:245–249.
142. Cucinelli F, Paparella P, Soranna L, et al. Differential effect of transdermal estrogen plus progestogen replacement therapy on insulin metabolism in postmenopausal women : Relation to their insulinemic secretion. Eur J Endocrinol 1999;140:215–219.
143. Friday K, Dong C, Fontent R. Conjugated equine estrogen improves glycemic control and blood lipoproteins in postmenopausal women with type 2 diabetes. J Clin Endocrinol Metab 2001;86:48–52.
144. Samaras K, Hayward CS, Sallivan D, Kelly RP, Campbell LV. Effects of postmenopausal hormone replacement therapy on central abdominal fat, glycemic control, lipid metabolism, and vascular factors in type 2 diabetes. Diabetes Care 1999;22:1401–1407.
145. Boden G. Role of fatty acids in the pathogenesis of insulin resistance and NIDDM. Diabetes 1997; 45:3–10.
146. Ferrara A, Karter AJ, Ackerson LM. Hormone replacement therapy is associated with better glycemic control in women with type 2 diabetes. Diabetes Care 2001;24:1144–1150.
147. Consensus opinion of the North American Menopause Society: Effects of menopause and estrogen replacement therapy or hormone replacement therapy in women with diabetes mellitus. Menopause 2000;7:87–95.

148. Brussaard HE, Gevers Leuven JA, Kluft C, et al. Effect of 17β-estradiol on plasma lipids and LDL oxidation in postmenopausal women with type II diabetes mellitus. Arterioscler Throm Vasc Biol 1997;17:324–330.

149. Manwaring P, Morfis L, Diamond T, Howeys LG. The effects of hormone replacement therapy on plasma lipids in type 2 diabetes. Maturitas 2000;34:239–247.

150. Robinson JG, Brancati FL, Folson AR, Cai J, Nabulsi AA, Watson R. Can postmenopausal hormone replacement improve plasma lipids in women with diabetes? Diabetes Care 1996;19:480–488.

151. Perera M, Sattar N, Petrie JR, et al. The effects of transdermal estradiol in combination with oral norethisterone on lipoproteins, coagulation , and endothelial markers in postmenopausal women with type 2 diabetes: randomized, placebo-controlled study. J Clin Endocrinol Metab 2001;86:1140–1143.

152. Crespo CJ, Smit E, Shelling A, Sempos CT, Andersen RE. Hormone replacement therapy and its relationship to lipid and glucose metabolism in diabetic and nondiabetic postmenopausal women: results from the Third National Health and Nutrition Examination Survey (NHANES III). Diabetes Care 2002;25:1675–1680.

153. Manning PT, Allum A, Jones S, Wayne HF, Sutherland F, Williams SM. The effect of hormone replacement therapy on cardiovascular risk factors in type 2 diabetes. Arch Intern Med 2001;161:1772–1776.

154. Feher MD, Coy A, Levy A, Mayne P, Lant AF. Short term blood pressure and metabolic effects of tibolone in postmenopausal women with non-insulin dependent diabetes. Br J Obstet Gynecol 1996; 103:281–283.

155. Glueck CJ, Lang J, Hamer T, Tracy T. Severe hypertriglyceridemia and pancreatitis when estrogen replacement therapy is given to hypertriglyceridemic women. J Lab Clin Med 1994;123:59–64.

156. Sattar N, Jaap AJ. Hormone replacement preparations and hypertriglyceridemia in women with NIDDM. Diabetes Care 1997;20:234–238.

157. Adami S, Rossini M, Zamberlan N, Bertoldo F, Dorizzi R, Lo Cascio V. Long-term effects of transdermal and oral estrogens on serum lipids and lipoproteins in postmenopausal women. Maturitas 1993;17:191–195.

158. Sattar n, Mckenzie J, MacCuish AC, Jaap AJ. Hormone replacement therapy in type 2 diabetes mellitus: A cardiovascular perspective. Diabetic Med 1998;15:631–632.

159. Sattar N, Perera M, Small M, Lumsden M-A. Hormone replacement therapy and sensitive C-reactive protein concentrations in women with type-2 diabetes. Lancet 1999;354:487–488.

160. Perera M, Sattar N, Petrie JR, et al. The effects of transdermal estradiol in combination with oral norethisterone on lipoproteins coagulation, and endothelial markers in postmenopausal women with type 2 diabetes: a randomized placebo-controlled study. J Clin Endocrinol Metab 2001;86:1140–1443.

161. Hahn L, Mattsson L-A, Anderson B, Tengborn L. The effects of oestrogen replacement therapy on haemostatic variables in postmenopausal women with non-insulin-dependent diabetes mellitus. Blood Coag Fibrinol 1999;10:81–85.

162. Lee SJ, Lee DW, Kim KS, Lee IK. Effect of estrogen on endothelial dysfunction in postmenopausal women with diabetes. Diabetes Res Clin Pract 2001;54 (Suppl 2):581–592.

163. Kon K, Kang MH, Jin DK, et al. Vascular effects of estrogen in type II diabetic postmenopausal women. J Am Coll Cardiol 2001;38:1409–1415.

164. Perera M, Petrie JR, Hillier C, et . Hormone replacement therapy can augment vascular relaxation in postmenopausal women with type 2 diabetes. Human Reprod 2002;17; 497–502.

165. Mc Veigh GE, Brennan GM, Johnston GD, et al. Impaired endothelium-dependent and independent vasodilation in patients with type 2 diabetes mellitus. Diabetologia 1992;35:771–776.

166. Hayward CS, Samaras K, Campbell L, Kelly RP. Effect of combination hormone replacement therapy on ambulatory blood pressure and arterial stiffness in diabetic postmenopausal women. Am J Hypert 2001;14:699–703.

167. Manwaring P, Phoon S, Diamond T, Howes LG. Effects of hormone replacement therapy on cardiovascular responses in postmenopausal women with and without type 2 diabetes. Maturitas 2002;43:157–164.

168. Kaplan RC, Heickbert SR, Weiss NS, et al. Postmenopausal estrogens and risk of myocardial infarction in diabetic women. Diabetes Care 1998;21:1117–1121.

169. Lawrenson RA, Leydon GM, Newson RB, et al. Coronary heart disease in women with diabetes: positive association with past hysterectomy and possible benefits of hormone replacement therapy. Diabetes Care 1999;22:856–857.

170. Petitti DB, Sidney S, Guesenberry CD. Hormone replacement therapy and the risk of myocardial infarction in women with coronary risk factors. Epidemiology 2000;11:603–606.

171. Ferrara A, Quesenberry, Karter AJ, et al. Current use of unopposed estrogen and estrogen plus progestin and the risk of acute myocardial infarction among women with diabetes. The Northern California Kaiser Rermanente Diabetes Registry, 1995–1998. Circulation 2003;107:43–48.

172. Grodstein F, Manson JE, Stampfer MJ. Postmenopausal hormone use and secondary prevention of coronary events in the Nurses Health Study: a prospective, observational study. Ann Intern Med 2001;135:1–8.

173. Lokkegaard E, Pedersen AJ, Heitmann BL, et al. Relation between hormone replacement therapy and ischaemic heart disease in women: prospective observational study BMJ 2003;326:1–5.

174. Dubuisson JT, Wagenknecht LE, D'Agostino RB Jr, et al. Association of hormone replacement therapy and carotid wall thickness in women with and without diabetes. Diabetes Care 1998;21:1790–1795.

175. Furberg CD, Wittinghoff E, Davidson M, et al. Subgroup interactions in the Heart and Estrogen/ progestin Replacement Study :lessons learned. Circulation 2002;105:917–922.

176. Barrett-Connor E, Wenger NK, Grady D, et al. Hormone and non-hormone therapy for the maintenance of postmenopausal health: the need for randomized controlled trials of estrogen and raloxifene. J Women's Health 1998;7:839–847.

177. Franks S. Polycystic ovary syndrome. N Engl J Med 1995;333:853–861.

178. Polson DW, Adams J, Wadsworth J, Franks S. Polycystic ovaries- a common finding in normal women. Lancet 1988;1:870–872.

179. Lobo RA, Carmina E. The importance of diagnosing the Polycystic ovary syndrome. Ann Intern Med 2000;132:989–993.

180. Burghen GA, Givens JR, Kitabchi AE. Correlation of hyperandrogenism with hyperinsulinism in polycystic ovarian disease. J Clin Endocrinol Metab 1980;50:113–116.

181. Chang RJ, Nakamura RM, Judd HL, Kaplan SA. Insulin resistance in non obese patients with polycystic ovarian disease. J Clin Endocrinol Metab 1983;57:356–359.

182. Dunaif A. Insulin resistance and the polycystic ovary syndrome: Mechanism and implications for pathogenesis. Endocrine Reviews 1997;18:774–800.

183. Amowitz LL, Sobel BE. Cardiovascular consequences of polycystic ovary syndrome. Endocrinol Metab Clin 1999;28:439–458.

184. Nestler JE, Jakubowicz DJ, Reamer P, Gunn RD, Allan G. Ovulatory and metabolic effects of D-chiro-inositol in the polycystic ovary syndrome. N Engl J Med 1999;340:1314–1320.

185. Ehrmann DA, Barnes RB, Rosenfield RL, Cavaghan MK, Imperial J. Prevalence of impaired glucose tolerance and diabetes in women with polycystic ovary syndrome. Diabetes Care 1999;22:141–146.

186. Legro RS, Kunselman AR, Dodson WC, Dunaif A. Prevalence and predictors of risk for type 2 diabetes mellitus and impaired glucose tolerance in polycystic ovary syndrome: a prospective, controlled study in 254 affected women. J Clin Endocrinol Metab 1999;84:165–169.

187. Cibula D, Cifkova R, Fanta M, Poledne R, Zivny J, Skibova J. Increased risk of non-insulin dependent diabetes mellitus, arterial hypertension and coronary artery disease in perimenopausal women with a history of the polycystic ovary syndrome. Hum Reprod 2000;15:785–789.

188. Legro RS. Diabetes prevalence and risk factors in polycystic ovary syndrome. Obstet Gynecol Clin North Am 2001;28:99–109.

189. Wild RA. Polycystic ovary syndrome: a risk for coronary artery disease? Am J Obstet Gynecol 2002;186:35–43.

190. Wild RA, Painter PC, Coulson PB, Carruth KB, Ranney GB. Lipoprotein lipid concentrations and cardiovascular risk in women with polycystic ovary syndrome. J Clin Endocrinol Metab 1985;61: 946–951.

191. Legro RS, Kunselman AR, Dunaif A. Prevalence and predictors of dyslipidemia in women with polycystic ovary syndrome. Am J Med 2001;111:607–613.

192. Dahlgren E, Johansson S, Lindstedt G, et al. Women with polycystic ovary syndrome wedge resected 1956 to 1965: a long term follow up focusing on natural history and circulating hormones. Fertil Steril 1992;57:505–513.

193. Dahlgren E, Janson PO, Johansson S, Lapidus L, Lindstedt G, Tengborn L. Hemostatic and metabolic variables in women with polycystic ovary syndrome. Fertil Steril 1994;61:455–460.

194. Keber I, Keber D. Increased plasminogen activator inhibitor activity in survivors of myocardial infarction is associated with metabolic risk factors of atherosclerosis. Haemostasis 1992;22:187–194.

195. Paradisi G, Steinberg HO, Hempfling A, et al. Polycystic ovary syndrome is associated with endothelial dysfunction. Circulation 2001;103:1410–1415.

196. Talbott EO, Guzick DS, Sutton-Tyrell K, et al. Evidence for an association between polycystic ovary syndrome and premature carotid atherosclerosis in middle-aged women. Arterioscler Thromb Vasc Biol 2000;20:2414–2421.

197. O'Leary DH, Polak JF, Kronmal RA, Manolio TA, Burke GL, Wolfson SK. Carotid-artery intima and media thickness as a risk factor for myocardial infarction and stroke in older adults. Cardiovascular Health Study Collaborative Research Group. N Engl J Med 1999;340:14–22.

198. Birdsall MA, Farquhar CM, White HD. Association between polycystic ovaries and extent of coronary artery disease in women having cardiac catheterization. Ann Intern Med 1997;126:32–35.

199. Hoeger K. Obesity and weight loss in polycystic ovary syndrome. Obstet Gynecol Clin North Am 2001;28: 85–97.

200. Holte J, Bergh T, Berne C, Wide L, Lithell H. Restored insulin sensitivity but persistently increased early insulin secretion after weight loss in obese women with polycystic ovary syndrome. J Clin Endocrinol Metab 1995;80:2586–2593.

201. Andersen P, Seljeflot I, Abdelnoor M, et al. Increased insulin sensitivity and fibrinolytic capacity after dietary intervention in obese women with polycystic ovary syndrome. Metabolism 1995;44:611–616.

202. Bates G, Whitworth MS. Effect of body weight reduction on plasma androgens in obese, infertile women. Fertil Steril 1982;38:406–409.

203. Dunaif A, Scott D, Finegood D, Quintana B, Whitcomb R. The insulin sensitizing agent troglitazone: a novel therapy for the polycystic ovary syndrome. J Clin Endocrinol Metab 1996;81:3299–3306.

204. Ehrmann DA, Schneider DJ, Sobel BE, et al. Troglitazone improves defects in insulin action, insulin secretion, ovarian steroidogenesis, and fibrinolysis in women with polycystic ovary syndrome. J Clin Endocrinol Metab 1997;82:2108–2116.

205. Azziz R, Ehrmann D, Legro RS, et al. Troglitazone improves ovulation and hirsutism in the polycystic ovary syndrome: a multicenter, double blind, placebo-controlled trial. J Clin Endocrinol Metab 2001;86:1626–1632.

206. Paradisi G, Steinberg HO, Shepard MK, Hook G, Baron AD. Troglitazone therapy improves endothelial function to near normal levels in women with polycystic ovary syndrome. J Clin Endocrinol Metab 2003;88:576–580.

207. Ghazeeri G, Kutteh WH, Bryer-Ash M, Haas D, Ke RW. Effect of rosiglitazone on spontaneous and clomiphene citrate-induced ovulation in women with polycystic ovary syndrome. Fertil Steril 2003;79:562–566.

208. Glueck CJ, Moreira A, Goldenberg N, Sieve L, Wang P. Pioglitazone and metformin in obese women with polycystic ovary syndrome not optimally responsive to metformin. Hum Reprod 2003;18:1618–1625.

209. DeFronzo RA, Barzilai N, Simonson DC. Mechanism of metformin action in obese and lean noninsulin-dependent diabetic subjects. J Clin Endocrinol Metab 1991;73:1294–1301.

210. Nestler JE, Jakubowicz DJ. Decreases in ovarian cytochrome p450c17alpha activity and serum free testosterone after reduction of insulin secretion in polycystic ovary syndrome. N Engl J Med 1996;335:617–623.

211. Velazquez EM, Mendoza S, Hamer T, Sosa F, Glueck CJ. Metformin therapy in polycystic ovary syndrome reduces hypernsulinemia, insulin resistance, hyperandrogenaemia, and systolic blood pressure, while facilitating normal menses and pregnancy. Metab Clin Exp 1994;43:647–654.

212. Moghetti P, Castello R, Negri C, et al. Metformin effects on clinical features, endocrine and metabolic profiles, and insulin sensitivity in polycystic ovary syndrome: a randomized, double-blind, placebo-controlled 6-month trial, followed by open, long-term clinical evaluation. J Clin Endocrinol Metab 2000;85:139–146.

213. Nestler JE, Jakubowicz DJ. Lean women with polycystic ovary syndrome respond to insulin reduction with decreases in ovarian p450c17alpha activity and serum androgens. J Clin Endocrinol Metab 1997;82:4075–4079.

214. Knowler WC, Barrett-Connor E, Fowler SE, Hamman RF, Lachin JM, Walker EA, Nathan DM; Diabetes Prevention Program Research Group. Reduction in the incidence of type 2 diabetes with lifestyle intervention or metformin. N Engl J Med 2002;346:393–403.

215. Glueck CJ, Wang P, Kobayashi S, Philips H, Sieve-Smith L. Metformin therapy throughout pregnancy reduces the development of gestational diabetes in women with polycystic ovary syndrome. Fertil Steril 2002;77:520–525.

216. Nestler JE, Jakubowicz DJ Evans WS, Pasquali R. Effects of metformin on spontaneous and clomiphene-induced ovulation in the polycystic ovary syndrome. N Engl J Med 1998;338:1876–1880.

217. Stadtmauer LA, Toma SK, Riehl RM, Talbert LM. Metformin treatment of patients with polycystic ovary syndrome undergoing in vitro fertilization improves outcomes and is associated with modulation of insulin- like growth factors. Fertil Steril 2001;75:505–509.
218. Jakubowicz DJ, Iuorno MJ, Jakubowicz S, Roberts KA, Nestler JE . Effects of metformin on early pregnancy loss in the polycystic ovary syndrome. J Clin Endocrinol Metab 2002;87:524–529.

8   Poly(ADP-Ribose) Polymerase Activation and Nitrosative Stress in the Development of Cardiovascular Disease in Diabetes

Pál Pacher, MD, PhD and Csaba Szabó, MD, PhD

CONTENTS

INTRODUCTION

Macro- and microvascular disease are the most common causes of morbidity and mortality in patients with diabetes mellitus (DM). Diabetic vascular dysfunction is a major clinical problem, which underlies the development of various severe complications including retinopathy, nephropathy, neuropathy, and increase the risk of stroke, hypertension, and myocardial infarction (MI). Hyperglycemic episodes, which complicate even well-controlled cases of diabetes, are closely associated with oxidative and nitrosative stress, which can trigger the development of cardiovascular disease. Recently, emerging experimental and clinical evidence indicates that high-circulating glucose in DM is able to induce oxidative and nitrosative stress in the cardiovascular system, with the concomitant activation of an abundant nuclear enzyme, poly(ADP-ribose) polymerase-1 (PARP) . This process results in acute loss of the ability of the endothelium to generate nitric oxide (NO; endothelial dysfunction) and also leads to a severe functional impairment of the diabetic heart (diabetic cardiomyopathy). Accordingly, neutralization of peroxynitrite or pharmacological inhibition of PARP protect against diabetic cardio-

From: *Contemporary Cardiology: Diabetes and Cardiovascular Disease, Second Edition*
Edited by: M. T. Johnstone and A. Veves © Humana Press Inc., Totowa, NJ

vascular dysfunction. The goal of this chapter is to summarize the recently emerging evidence supporting the concept that nitrosative stress and PARP activation play a role in the pathogenesis of diabetic endothelial dysfunction and cardiovascular complications.

POLY(ADP-RIBOSE) POLYMERASE: AN ABUNDANT NUCLEAR ENZYME WITH MULTIPLE REGULATORY FUNCTIONS

PARP-1 (EC 2.4.2.30) [also known as poly(ADP-ribose) synthetase and poly(ADP-ribose) transferase] is a member of the PARP enzyme family consisting of PARP-1 and an increasing number additional, recently identified poly(ADP-ribosylating) enzymes (minor PARP isoforms). PARP-1, the major PARP isoform, is one of the most abundant proteins in the nucleus. PARP-1 is a 116 kDa protein which consists of three main domains: the N-terminal deoxyribonucleic acid (DNA)-binding domain containing two zinc fingers, the automodification domain, and the C-terminal catalytic domain. The primary structure of the enzyme is highly conserved in eukaryotes (human and mouse enzyme have 92% homology at the level of amino acid sequence) with the catalytic domain showing the highest degree of homology between different species. Many differences between the various PARP isoenzymes have been demonstrated in domain structure, subcellular localization, tissue distribution and ability to bind to DNA (1). For the purpose of this chapter, it is important to note that PARP-1 is considered the major isoform of PARP in intact cells, and remains commonly termed as "PARP." This first isoform of PARP plays a crucial role in the pathophysiology of many diseases. PARP also has multiple physiological functions, which is a subject of several recent reviews and monographies (1–6). PARP-1 functions as a DNA damage sensor and signaling molecule binding to both single- and double-stranded DNA breaks. On binding to damaged DNA (mainly through the second zinc finger domain), PARP-1 forms homodimers and catalyzes the cleavage of NAD+ into nicotinamide and ADP-ribose and uses the latter to synthesize branched nucleic acid-like polymers poly(ADP-ribose) covalently attached to nuclear acceptor proteins. The size of the branched polymer varies from a few to 200 ADP-ribose units. As a result of its high-negative charge, covalently attached ADP-ribose polymer dramatically affects the function of target proteins. In vivo the most abundantly poly(ADP-ribosylated) protein is PARP-1 itself and auto-poly(ADP-ribosylation) represents a major regulatory mechanism for PARP-1 resulting in the downregulation of the enzyme activity. In addition to PARP-1, histones are also considered as major acceptors of poly(ADP-ribose). Poly(ADP-ribosylation) confers negative charge to histones leading to electrostatic repulsion between DNA and histones. This process has been implicated in chromatin remodeling, DNA repair, and transcriptional regulation. Several transcription factors, DNA replication factors and signaling molecules (NFκB, AP-1, Oct-1, YY1, TEF-1, DNA-PK, p53) have also been shown to become poly(ADP-ribosylated) by PARP-1. The effect of PARP-1 on the function of these proteins is carried out by noncovalent protein–protein interactions and by covalent poly(ADP-ribosylation). Poly(ADP-ribosylation) is a dynamic process as indicated by the short half life of the polymer. Two enzymes—poly(ADP-ribose) glycohydrolase (PARG) and ADP-ribosyl protein lyase—are involved in the catabolism of poly(ADP-ribose) with PARG-cleaving ribose–ribose bonds of both linear and branched portions of poly(ADP-ribose) and the lyase removing the protein proximal ADP-ribose monomer (7). PARP-1 plays an important role in DNA repair and maintenance of genomic integrity (8,9) and also regulates the expression of various proteins at the transcriptional level. Of special importance is the regulation by PARP-1 of the production of inflammatory mediators such as inducible NO synthase (iNOS), intercellular adhesion molecule-1 (ICAM-1) and major histocompatibility complex (MHC) class II *(10–14)*. Nuclear factor-κB (NF-κB) is a key transcription factor in the regulation of this set of proteins and PARP has been shown to act as a co-activator in the NF-κB-mediated transcription. Poly(ADP-ribosylation) can loosen up the chromatin structure thereby making genes more accessible for the transcriptional machinery *(15–20)*. Additionally, PARP-1 activation has been proposed to represent a cell elimination pathway whereby severely damaged cells are removed from tissues. PARP-1-mediated cell death occurs in the form of necrosis, which is probably the least desirable form of cell death. During necrotic cell death, the cellular content is released into the tissue-posing neighboring cells to harmful attacks by proteases and various proinflammatory intracellular factors. Recently, PARP can also serve as an emergency source of energy used by the base excision machinery to synthesize adenosine triphosphate (ATP) *(21)*. Furthermore, poly(ADP-ribose) may also serve as a signal for protein degradation in oxidatively injured cells *(22)*.

Poly(ADP-Ribose) Polymerase Mediates Oxidant-Induced Cell Dysfunction and Necrosis

Peroxynitrite, a reactive oxidant species, produced from the reaction of NO and superoxide free radicals, has been established as a pathophysiologically relevant endogenous trigger of DNA single strand breakage and PARP activation *(23,24)*. Additional endogenous triggers of DNA single strand breakage and PARP activation include hydrogen peroxide, hydroxyl radical, and nitroxyl anion, but not NO, superoxide, or hypochlorous acid *(25–29)*. Peroxynitrite is considered a key trigger of DNA strand breakage because (as opposed to hydroxyl radical, for instance) it can readily travel and cross cell membranes. When activated by DNA single-strand breaks, PARP initiates an energy-consuming cycle by transferring ADP ribose units from NAD+ to nuclear proteins. This process results in rapid depletion of the intracellular NAD+ and ATP pools, slowing the rate of glycolysis and mitochondrial respiration, eventually leading to cellular dysfunction and death *(1)*.

Poly(ADP-Ribose) Polymerase Regulates Gene Expression and Mononuclear Cell Recruitment

Using pharmacological inhibitors of PARP, it has been demonstrated (as briefly mentioned earlier) that the activity of PARP is required for the expression of the MHC class II gene, DNA methyltransferase gene, protein kinase C (PKC), collagenase, ICAM-1, and (iNOS) *(10–14)*. An oligonucleotide microarray analysis identified multiple genes that appear to be under the control of PARP-1 in resting cells *(14)* and even more genes are affected under conditions of immunostimulation *(30)*. A distinct mode of inhibition of the expression of pro-inflammatory mediators by inhibition of PARP relates to the regulation of NF-κB activation. It is unclear whether PARP catalytic activity vs PARP as a structural protein plays the most important role in its stimulatory role on NF-κB activation *(31,32)*, it may well be that both mechanisms can be involved under certain experimental conditions. Pharmacological evidence supports the view that PARP also regulates the *c-fos*—AP-1 transcription system and the activation of mitogen-activated protein kinase *(33,34)*. From the above experimental data it appears that PARP, via a not yet fully characterized mechanism, regulates the expression of a variety of genes, with the net result that PARP inhibition or PARP genetic inactivation results in the downregulation of a variety of important pro-inflammatory mediators and pathways.

The PARP-mediated pathway of cell necrosis and the PARP-mediated pathway of inflammatory signal transduction and gene expression may be interrelated in pathophysiological conditions. Oxidant stress can generate DNA single-strand breaks. DNA strand breaks then activate PARP, which in turn potentiates NF-κB activation and AP-1 expression, resulting in greater expression of the AP-1 and NF-κB-dependent genes, such as the gene for ICAM-1, and chemokines such as MIP-1α and cytokines such as tumor necrosis factor-α. Chemokine generation, in combination with increased endothelial expression of ICAM-1, recruits more activated leukocytes to inflammatory foci, producing greater oxidant stress. It is possible that a low-level, localized inflammatory response may be beneficial in recruiting mononuclear cells to an inflammatory site. However, in many pathophysiological states the above described feedback cycles amplify themselves beyond control.

Overactivation of PARP represents an important mechanism of tissue damage in various pathological conditions associated with oxidative and nitrosative stress, including myocardial reperfusion injury *(13,35)*, reperfusion injury after heart transplantation *(36)*, chronic heart failure *(37,38)*, stroke *(39)*, circulatory shock *(32,40–42)*, and the process of autoimmune β-cell destruction associated with DM *(43,44)*. Activation of PARP and beneficial effect of various PARP inhibitors have been demonstrated in various forms of endothelial dysfunction such as the one associated with circulatory shock, hypertension, atherosclerosis, preeclampsia, and aging *(40,45–48)*. Furthermore, recent evidence demonstrates that activation of PARP importantly contributes to the development of cardiac and endothelial dysfunction in various experimental models of diabetes and also in humans *(49–52)*. The following chapter will discuss this subject in detail.

THE ROLE OF OXIDATIVE AND NITROSATIVE STRESS IN THE PATHOGENESIS OF DIABETES-INDUCED CARDIOVASCULAR DYSFUNCTION

Oxidative and Nitrosative Stress in Diabetes-Induced Vascular Dysfunction

Various neurohumoral mediators and mechanical forces acting on the innermost layer of blood vessels, the endothelium, are involved in the regulation of the vascular tone. The main pathway of vasoregulation involves the activation of the constitutive, endothelial isoform of NO synthase (eNOS) resulting in NO production *(53)*. Endothelium-dependent vasodilatation is frequently used as a reproducible and accessible parameter to probe endothelial function in various pathophysiological conditions. It is well established that endothelial dysfunction, in many diseases, precedes, predicts, and predisposes for the subsequent, more severe vascular alterations. Endothelial dysfunction has been documented in various forms of diabetes, and even in prediabetic individuals *(52,54–58)*. The pathogenesis of this endothelial dysfunction involves many components including increased polyol pathway flux, altered cellular redox state, increased formation of diacylglycerol, and the subsequent activation of specific PKC isoforms, and accelerated nonenzymatic formation of advanced glycation end-products (AGE) *(59–61)*. Many of these pathways, in concert, trigger the production of oxygen- and nitrogen-derived oxidants and free radicals, such as superoxide anion and peroxynitrite, which play a significant role in the pathogenesis of the diabetes-associated endothelial dysfunction *(59,60,62)*.

The cellular sources of reactive oxygen species (ROS) such as superoxide anion are multiple and include AGEs, nicotinamide adenine dinucleotide phosphate (NADH/NADPH) oxidases, the mitochondrial respiratory chain, xanthine oxidase, the arachidonic acid cascade (lipoxygenase and cyclyoxygenase), and microsomal enzymes (60,63).

Superoxide anion may quench NO, thereby reducing the efficacy of a potent endothelium-derived vasodilator system that participates in the homeostatic regulation of the vasculature, and evidence suggests that during hyperglycemia, reduced NO availability exists (64). Hyperglycemia-induced superoxide generation contributes to the increased expression of NAD(P)H oxidase, which in turn generate more superoxide anion. Hyperglycemia also favors, through the activation of NF-κB an increased expression of iNOS, which may increase the generation of NO (65,66).

Superoxide anion interacts with NO, forming the strong oxidant peroxynitrite (ONOO-), which attacks various biomolecules, leading to—among other processes—the production of a modified amino acid, nitrotyrosine (67). Although nitrotyrosine was initially considered a specific marker of peroxynitrite generation, other pathways can also induce tyrosine nitration. Thus, nitrotyrosine is now generally considered a collective index of reactive nitrogen species, rather than a specific indicator of peroxynitrite formation (68,69). The possibility that diabetes is associated with increased nitrosative stress is supported by the recent detection of increased nitrotyrosine plasma levels in type 2 diabetic patients (70) and iNOS-dependent peroxynitrite production in diabetic platelets (71). Nitrotyrosine formation is detected in the artery wall of monkeys during hyperglycemia (72) and in diabetic patients during an increase of postprandial hyperglycemia (73). In a recent study we have demonstrated increased nitrotyrosine immunoreactivity in microvasculature of type 2 diabetic patients (52). In the same study significant correlations were observed between nitrotyrosine immunostaining intensity and fasting blood glucose, HbA1c, ICAM, and vascular cellular adhesion molecule (VCAM).

The toxic action of nitrotyrosine is supported by the evidence that increased apoptosis of endothelial cells, myocytes and fibroblasts in heart biopsies from diabetic patients (74), in hearts from streptozotocin (STZ)-induced diabetic rats (75), and in working hearts from rats during hyperglycemia (76), and the degree of cell death and/or dysfunction show a correlation with levels of nitrotyrosine found in those cells. There is also evidence that nitrotyrosine can also be directly harmful to endothelial cells (77). Additionally, high glucose-induced oxidative and nitrosative stress alters prostanoid profile in human endothelial cells (78,79). Recent studies have suggested that increased oxidative and nitrosative stress is involved in the pathogenesis of diabetic microvascular injury in retinopathy, nephropathy, and neuropathy (80–85).

Oxidative and Nitrosative Stress in Diabetic Cardiomyopathy

The development of myocardial dysfunction independent of coronary artery disease in DM has been well documented, both in humans and experimental studies in animals (86–90). Diabetic cardiomyopathy is characterized by complex changes in the mechanical, biochemical, structural, and electrical properties of the heart, which may be responsible for the development of an early diastolic dysfunction and increased incidence of cardiac arrhythmias in diabetic patients. The mechanism of diastolic dysfunction remains unknown but it does not appear to be as a result of changes in blood pressure, microvascular complications, or elevated circulating glycated hemoglobin levels (86–90).

There is circumstantial clinical and experimental evidence suggesting that increased sympathetic activity, activated cardiac renin–angiotensin system, myocardial ischemia/functional hypoxia, and elevated circulating levels of glucose result in oxidative and nitrosative stress in cardiovascular system of diabetic animals and humans. Oxidative stress associated with an impaired antioxidant defense status may play a critical role in subcellular remodeling, calcium-handling abnormalities, and subsequent diabetic cardiomyopathy *(75,89)*. Oxidative and nitrosative damage may be critical in the early onset of diabetic cardiomyopathy *(74,75)*. Consistent with this idea, significant nitrotyrosine formation was reported in cardiac myocytes from myocardial biopsy samples obtained from diabetic and diabetic-hypertensive patients *(74)* and in a mouse model of streptozotocin (STZ)-induced diabetes *(75)*. Perfusion of isolated hearts with high glucose caused a significant upregulation of iNOS, increased the coronary perfusion pressure and both NO and superoxide generation, a condition favoring the production of peroxynitrite, accompanied by the formation of nitrotyrosine and cardiac cell apoptosis *(76)*.

Peroxynitrite Neutralization Improves Cardiovascular Dysfunction in Diabetes

As mentioned above there is circumstantial evidence that nitrosative stress and peroxynitrite formation importantly contribute to the pathogenesis of diabetic cardiomyopathy both in animals and humans. We have tested a novel metalloporphyrin peroxynitrite decomposition catalyst, FP15, in murine models of diabetic cardiovascular complications *(92)*. We hypothesized that neutralization of peroxynitrite with FP15 would ameliorate the development of cardiovascular dysfunction in a STZ-induced murine model of diabetes. To ensure that the animals received the FP15 treatment at a time when islet cell destruction was already complete and hyperglycemia has stabilized the treatment was initiated 6 weeks after the injection of STZ. Although FP15 did not affect blood glucose levels, it provided a marked protection against the loss of endothelium-dependent relaxant ability of the blood vessels (Fig. 1A) and improved the depression of both diastolic (Fig. 1B) and systolic function of the heart *(92)*. The mechanism by which FP15 protects diabetic hearts from dysfunction may involve protection against vascular and myocardial tyrosine nitration, PARP activation, lipid peroxidation, and multiple other mechanisms, as all these mechanisms have previously been linked to diabetic cardiomyopathy and to peroxynitrite-induced cardiac injury. Additional mechanisms of peroxynitrite-mediated diabetic cardiac dysfunction may include inhibition of myofibrillar creatine kinase *(93)* and of succinyl-coenzyme A (CoA):3-oxoacid CoA-transferase *(94)* or activation of metalloproteinases *(95)*.

There are many pathophysiological conditions of the heart that are associated with peroxynitrite formation, including acute MI, chronic ischemic heart failure, doxorubicin-induced and diabetic cardiomyopathy *(93,94,96–98)*. It appears that peroxynitrite decomposition catalysts improve cardiac function and overall outcome in these models. For instance, FP15 reduced myocardial necrosis in our current rat model of acute MI *(95)* and in a recent porcine study *(98)*. Furthermore, FP15 significantly improved cardiac function in a doxorubicin-induced model of heart failure *(95)*. These observations—coupled with the recently reported protective effect of FP15 against diabetic cardiomyopathy—support the concept that peroxynitrite is a major mediator of myocardial injury in various pathophysiological conditions, and its effective neutralization can be of significant therapeutic benefit.

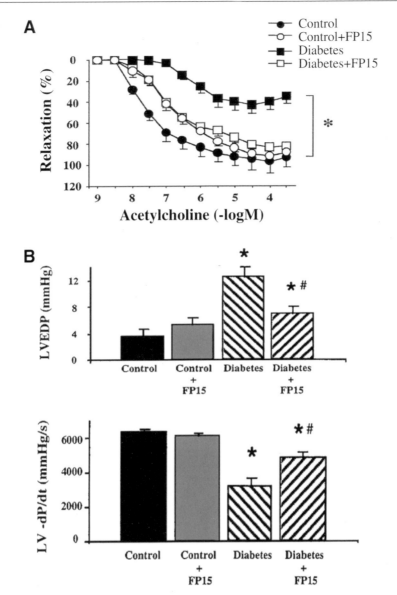

Fig. 1. (A) Reversal of diabetes-induced endothelial dysfunction by FP15 in vascular rings from STZ-diabetic mice. Acetylcholine (Ach) induced endothelium-dependent relaxation is impaired in rings from diabetic mice, which is markedly improved by FP15 treatment. Each point of the curve represents the mean ± SEM of five to seven pairs of experiments in vascular rings. *$p < 0.05$ in FP15-treated diabetic mice vs vehicle-treated diabetic mice. **(B)** Reversal of streptozotocin-evoked diabetes-induced diastolic cardiac dysfunction by FP15 in mice. Effect of diabetes (9–10 weeks) and FP15 treatment in diabetic mice on left ventricular end diastolic pressure (LVEDP) and left ventricular –dp/dt (LV –dp/dt). Results are mean ± SEM of seven experiments in each group. *$p < 0.05$ diabetic animals vs control; #$p < 0.05$ in FP15-treated diabetic mice vs vehicle-treated diabetic mice. (Reproduced with permission from ref. *92*.)

THE ROLE OF POLY(ADP-RIBOSE) POLYMERASE ACTIVATION IN THE PATHOGENESIS OF DIABETIC CARDIOVASCULAR DYSFUNCTION

The Role of Poly(ADP-Ribose) Polymerase Activation in Diabetic Vascular Dysfunction

POLY(ADP-RIBOSE) POLYMERASE-DEPENDENT ENDOTHELIAL DYSFUNCTION IN EXPERIMENTAL ANIMAL MODELS OF DIABETES

We have recently found that high glucose-induced oxidative and nitrosative stress leads to DNA single-strand breakage and PARP activation in murine and human endothelial cells (49) (Fig. 2). The involvement of oxyradicals and NO-derived reactive species in PARP activation and the evidence for nitrated tyrosine residues both suggested that peroxynitrite may be one of the final mediators responsible for single-strand breakage, and subsequent PARP activation (49). The role of hyperglycemia-induced oxidative stress in producing DNA damage is supported by the recent findings that increased amounts of 8-hydroxyguanine and 8-hydroxydeoxy guanosine (markers of oxidative damage to DNA) can be found in both the plasma and tissues of streptozotocin diabetic rats (99). Importantly, various forms of oxidant-induced DNA damage (base modifications and DNA strand breaks) have also been demonstrated in diabetic patients (100–104).

Pharmacological inhibition of PARP or genetic inactivation of PARP-1 protects against the development of the high glucose-induced endothelial dysfunction in vitro (49) (Fig. 3) by preventing glucose-induced severe suppression of cellular high-energy phosphate levels and by inhibiting the hyperglycemia-induced suppression of NAD+ and NADPH levels. Because eNOS is an NADPH-dependent enzyme, we proposed that the cellular depletion of NADPH in endothelial cells exposed to high glucose is directly responsible for the suppression of eNOS activity and the reduction in the diabetic vessels' endothelium-dependent relaxant ability. In support of this hypothesis, we have subsequently demonstrated that there is a PARP-dependent suppression of vascular NADPH levels in diabetic blood vessels in vivo (50).

Although most of the studies on the role of PARP in the pathogenesis of diabetic endothelial dysfunction, as discussed above, originated in macrovessels, there is circumstantial evidence that similar processes are operative for pathogenesis of diabetic microvascular injury (retinopathy, nephropathy). In fact, there is now evidence for PARP activation in the microvessels of the diabetic retina (105). Additionally, a study performed more than a decade ago demonstrated that the presence of glomerular depositions (mesangial distribution) of IgG was significantly reduced in STZ-diabetic rats treated with the PARP inhibitor nicotinamide for 6 months (106). In agreement with these results, we have recently provided evidence that PARP activation is present in the tubuli of STZ-induced diabetic rats. This PARP activation is attenuated by two unrelated PARP inhibitors, 3-aminobenzamide and 1,5-isoquinolinediol (ISO), which also counteract the overexpression of endothelin-1 and endothelin receptors in the renal cortex (107). It has recently been suggested that PARP activation may also play a key role in the development diabetic neuropathy: the progressive slowing of sensory and motor neuron conductance in diabetic rats and mice is preventable by PARP inhibition or PARP deficiency, and this is associated with maintained neuronal phosphocreatine levels, and improved endoneurial blood flow (108). Additional studies, utilizing potent and specific inhibitors of PARP are needed to further delineate the role of PARP in the pathogenesis of diabetic retinopathy, neuropathy, and nephropathy. It is important to emphasize that, although the above

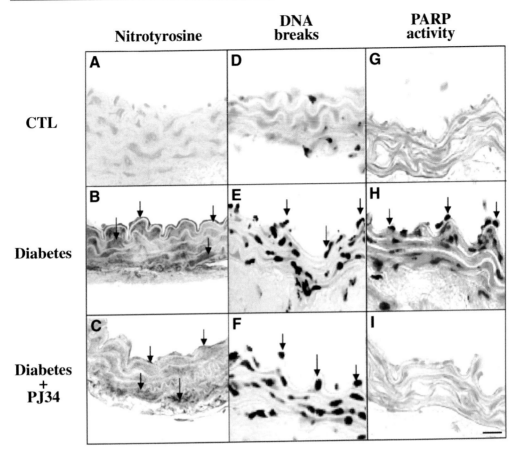

Fig. 2. Reactive nitrogen species generation, ssDNA breakage and poly(ADP-ribose) polymerase (PARP) activation in diabetic blood vessels. **(A–C)** Immunohistochemical staining for nitrotyrosine in control rings **(A)**, in rings from diabetic mice treated with vehicle at 8 weeks **(B)**, and in rings from diabetic mice treated with PJ34 **(C)**, **(D–F)** Terminal deoxyribonucleotidyl transferase-mediated dUTP nick-end labeling, an indicator of DNA strand breakage, in control rings **(D)**, in rings from diabetic mice treated with vehicle at 8 weeks **(E)**, and in rings from diabetic mice treated with PJ34 **(F)**, **(G–I)** Immunohistochemical staining for poly(ADP-ribose), an indicator of PARP activation, in control rings **(G)**, in rings from diabetic mice treated with vehicle at 8 weeks **(H)**, and in rings from diabetic mice treated with PJ34 **(I)**. (Reproduced with permission from ref. *49*.)

conditions are generally considered as separate pathophysiological entities, there is good evidence that, at least in part, they all develop on the basis of vascular (endothelial) dysfunction.

Pharmacological Inhibition of Poly(ADP-Ribose) Polymerase Improves Endothelial Dysfunction in Diabetes

In a mouse model of STZ-induced diabetes the time course of endothelial dysfunction was compared with that of the activation of PARP in the blood vessels. Intravascular PARP activation (seen in endothelial cells, and in vascular smooth muscle cells) was already apparent 2 weeks after the onset of diabetes and thus it slightly preceded the occurrence of the endothelial dysfunction, which developed between the second and the fourth weeks of diabetes (*49*; Fig. 3). Delayed treatment with the PARP inhibitor—starting at 1 week after STZ—ameliorated vascular poly(ADP-ribose) accumulation and

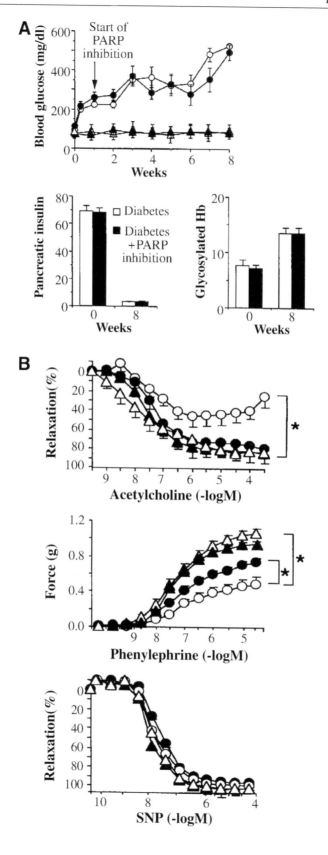

restored normal vascular function without altering systemic glucose levels, plasma-glycated hemoglobin levels, or pancreatic insulin content *(49,50)*. Furthermore, delayed treatment of the animals with the PARP inhibitor restored the established diabetic endothelial dysfunction (Fig. 4), and even in vitro incubation of diabetic dysfunctional blood vessels with PARP inhibitors of various structural classes (e.g., benzamide-, isoquinoline-, and phenanthridinone-derivatives) significantly enhanced the endothelium-dependent relaxant responsiveness *(49,50)* (Fig. 5A,B). The development of the endothelial dysfunction and its reversibility by pharmacological inhibition of PARP has recently also been demonstrated in an autoimmune model of diabetes, in the nonobese diabetic model in the mouse *(51)* (Fig. 6). The mode of PARP inhibitors protective action on endothelium likely involves a conservation of energetics, and a prevention of the upregulation of various pro-inflammatory pathways (cytokines, adhesion molecules (ICAM-1, VCAM-1 and E-selectin), mononuclear cell infiltration) triggered by hyperglycemia *(49,109,110)*. This latter mechanism may represent an important additional pathway whereby PARP activation can contribute to vascular dysfunction via the upregulation of adhesion molecules. As mentioned earlier, PARP regulates the activation of a variety of signal transduction pathways, and some of these pathways regulate the expression of cell surface and soluble adhesion molecules. Recent data indicate that pharmacological inhibition of PARP can suppress this process *(110)*. Intermittent high/low glucose induces a more pronounced expression of adhesion molecules that constant high glucose, and PARP inhibition suppresses NF-κB activation and the expression of adhesion molecules both under constant high glucose and under intermittent high/low glucose conditions in cultured endothelial cells in vitro *(110)*.

A recent in vitro study have demonstrated that the pharmacological inhibition of PARP completely blocks hyperglycemia-induced activation of multiple major pathways of vascular damage *(111)*. In cultured endothelial cells placed in high extracellular glucose, the development of DNA single-strand breaks, the activation of PARP and the depletion of intracellular NAD were all blocked by the cellular overexpression of uncoupling protein-1 (UCP-1), indicating that mitochondrial oxidant generation plays a key role in the activation of PARP in endothelial cells placed into high glucose. Incubation of bovine aortic endothelial cells in elevated glucose increased the membrane fraction of intracellular PKC activity, an effect which was also blocked by overexpression of UCP-1, consis-

---

Fig. 3. *(opposite page)* Reversal of diabetes-induced endothelial dysfunction by pharmacological inhibition of poly(ADP-ribose) polymerase (PARP). Symbols used for the respective groups: animals which received no streptozotocin injection (△), nondiabetic control animals at 8 weeks treated with PJ34 between week 1 and 8 (▲), diabetic animals at 8 weeks treated with vehicle (○), diabetic animals at 8 weeks treated with PJ34 between weeks 1 and 8 (●). (**A**) Blood glucose levels, pancreatic insulin content (ng insulin/mg pancreatic protein) and blood glycosylated hemoglobin (Hb) (expressed as % of total Hb) at 0–8 weeks in nondiabetic, control male BALB/c mice, and at 0–8 weeks after streptozotocin treatment (diabetic) in male BALB/c mice. PARP inhibitor treatment, starting at 1 week after streptozotocin and continuing until the end of week 8, is indicated by the arrow. Pancreatic insulin and Glycated hemoglobin levels content are shown at 8 weeks in vehicle-treated and streptozotocin-treated animals, in the presence or absence of PJ34 treatment. (**B**) acetylcholine-induced, endothelium-dependent relaxations, phenylephrine-induced contractions, and sodium nitroprusside-induced endothelium-independent relaxations.* $p < 0.05$ for vehicle-treated diabetic vs PJ34-treated diabetic mice ($n = 8$ per group). (Reproduced with permission from ref. *49*.)

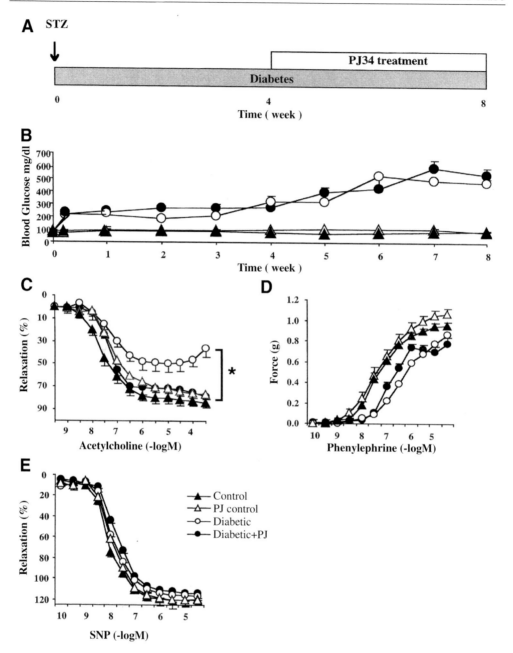

Fig. 4. Pharmacological inhibition of poly(ADP-ribose) polymerase (PARP) restores impaired endothelium-dependent relaxant ability of the diabetic vessels. Blood glucose levels and vascular responsiveness. Endothelium-dependent relaxations induced by acetylcholine, contractions induced by phenylephrine, and endothelium-independent relaxations induced by sodium nitroprusside (SNP) in control (nondiabetic) male Balb/c mice and 1, 4, and 8 weeks after streptozotocin (STZ)-induced diabetes. Vehicle or PARP inhibitor (PJ34, 10 mg/kg oral gavage once a day) treatment started at 4 weeks after STZ and continued until 8 weeks (the end of the experimental period). There was a marked and selective impairment of the endothelium-dependent relaxant ability of the vascular rings in diabetes at 4 and 8 weeks. Treatment with the PARP inhibitor between weeks 4 and 8 restored to normal the endothelium-dependent relaxant ability of the diabetic vessels despite the persistence of hyperglycemia. *$p < 0.05$ for differences between experimental groups, as indicated. $n = 8$ per group. (Reproduced with permission from ref. *50*.)

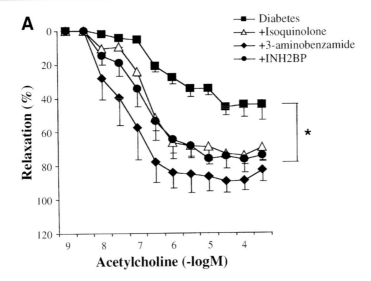

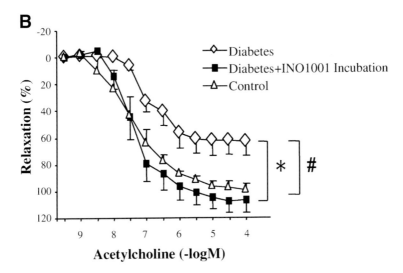

Fig. 5. In vitro treatment with all poly(ADP-ribose) polymerase (PARP) inhibitors improved the endothelium-dependent relaxant ability of the diabetic vessels. (**A**) Endothelium-dependent relaxations induced by acetylcholine in control (nondiabetic) male Balb/c mice and 4 weeks after streptozotocin (STZ)-induced diabetes. In a subgroup of the vascular rings, evaluation of vascular responsiveness was preceded by 1-hour incubation with three structurally different PARP inhibitors: 3-aminobenzamide (3 mmol/L), 5-iodo-6-amino-1,2-benzopyrone (100 µmol/L), or 1,5-dihydroxyisoquinoline (30 µmol/L). There was a marked and selective impairment of the endothelium-dependent relaxant ability of the vascular rings in diabetes at 4 weeks. In vitro treatment with all PARP inhibitors improved the endothelium-dependent relaxant ability of the diabetic vessels. *$p < 0.05$ for differences between experimental groups, as indicated. $n = 8$ per group. (Reproduced with permission from ref. *50*.) (**B**) Endothelium-dependent relaxations induced by acetylcholine in control (nondiabetic) male Balb/c mice and 6 weeks after STZ-induced diabetes. In a subgroup of the vascular rings, evaluation of vascular responsiveness was preceded by 1-hour incubation with the novel potent PARP inhibitor, INO1001 (3 µmol/L) *(112,113)*. There was a marked and selective impairment of the endothelium-dependent relaxant ability of the vascular rings in diabetes at 6 weeks. In vitro treatment with all PARP inhibitors improved the endothelium-dependent relaxant ability of the diabetic vessels. *$p < 0.05$ for differences between experimental groups, as indicated. $n = 8$ per group.

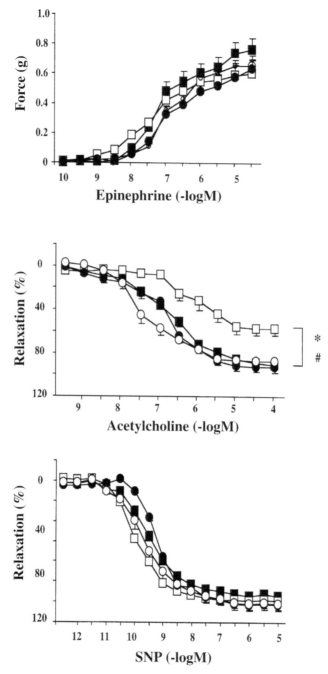

Fig. 6. Reversal of diabetes-induced endothelial dysfunction by pharmacological inhibition of poly(ADP-ribose) polymerase (PARP) in diabetic NOD mouse vascular rings. Epinephrine-induced contractions (upper panel), acetylcholine-induced endothelium-dependent relaxation (middle panel), and sodium nitroprusside-induced endothelium-independent relaxations (lower panel). Control (■); control + PJ34 (○); diabetes (□); diabetes + PJ34 (●). Each point of the curve represents the means ± SE of 5–8 experiments in vascular rings. *$p < 0.05$ vs C; #$p < 0.05$ vs D. (Reproduced with permission from ref. *51*.)

tently with an oxidant-mediated basis of PKC activation in endothelial cells subjected to hyperglycemia. Inhibition of PARP by PJ34 also completely prevented the activation of PKC by 30 mM glucose, indicative that the oxidant-mediated suppression of PKC activity in hyperglycemia involves the activation of PARP. Another key factor in the pathogenesis of hyperglycemia induced endothelial dysfunction is the inhibition of glyceraldehyde-3-phosphate dehydrogenase (GAPDH) activity. Recent studies demonstrated that this decrease in GAPDH activity is also dependent on PARP, and may be related to direct poly(ADP-ribosyl)ation, and consequent inhibition of GAPDH *(111)*.

POLY(ADP-RIBOSE) POLYMERASE ACTIVATION CONTRIBUTES TO THE VASCULAR DYSFUNCTION IN DIABETIC AND PREDIABETIC PATIENTS

A recent study extended our knowledge on the role of PARP activation in the development of diabetic endothelial dysfunction into the area of human investigations: in forearm skin biopsies from healthy subjects, healthy individuals with parental history of type 2 diabetes mellitus (T2DM), subjects with impaired glucose tolerance and a group of T2DM patients it was found that the percentage of PARP-positive endothelial nuclei was higher in the group of parental history of T2DM and diabetic patients when compared to the controls *(52)* (Fig. 7). Additionally, significant correlations were observed between the percentage of PARP-positive endothelial nuclei and fasting blood glucose, resting skin blood flow, maximal skin vasodilatory response to the iontopheresis of acetylcholine (which indicates endothelium-dependent vasodilation), and sodium nitroprusside (which indicates endothelium-independent vasodilation) and nitrotyrosine immunostaining intensity *(52)*. Nitrotyrosine immunoreactivity (a marker of reactive nitrogen species and peroxynitrite formation) was also higher in the diabetic patients when compared to all other groups *(52)*. Significant correlations were observed between nitrotyrosine immunostaining intensity and fasting blood glucose, HbA1c, ICAM, and VCAM. No differences in the expression of eNOS and receptor of advanced glycation end-products were found among all four groups. The polymorphism of the eNOS gene was also studied and was not found to influence eNOS expression or microvascular functional measurements. Thus, in humans, PARP activation is present in healthy subjects at risk of developing diabetes, and in established T2DM patients and it is associated with impairments in the vascular reactivity in the skin microcirculation *(52)*. It remains to be seen whether PARP activation in diabetic or prediabetic humans can be seen as a predictor or early marker for the development of diabetic vascular complications. It also remains to be studied whether various therapeutic interventions, which are known to have vascular protective effects in diabetes (antioxidant therapies, PPAR agonists, etc.), are able to suppress the activation of PARP in the cardiovascular system.

The Role of Poly(ADP-Ribose) Polymerase Activation in the Pathogenesis of Diabetic Cardiomyopathy

POLY(ADP-RIBOSE) POLYMERASE ACTIVATION IN DIABETIC MYOCARDIUM

The importance of the PARP pathway is well documented in various models of myocardial ischemia-reperfusion injury (a condition in which oxidative and nitrosative stress plays a key pathogenetic role) *(13,35,36)*. The PARP pathway also plays a role in the pathogenesis of diabetic cardiomyopathy *(51)* (Fig. 8). Cardiac dysfunction and PARP activation in the cardiac myocytes and coronary vasculature were noted both in the STZ-induced and genetic (nonobese diabetic) models of diabetes mellitus in rats and mice *(51)* (Figs. 8 and 9).

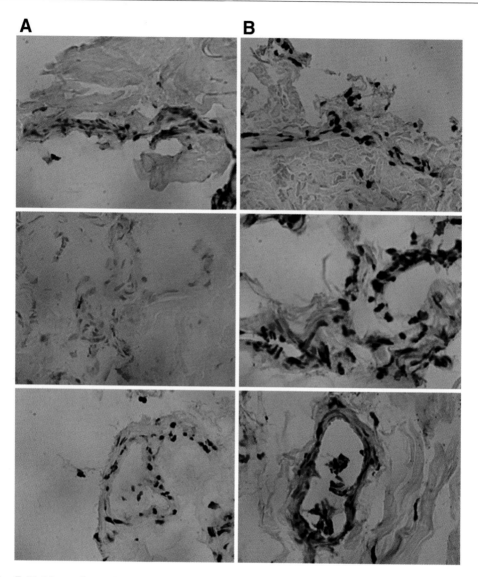

Fig. 7. Evidence for poly(ADP-ribose) polymerase (PARP) activation in diabetic skin vessels. Immunohistochemical staining for PARP formation, an indicator of PARP activation, in skin vessels from healthy subjects (**A**) and diabetic patients (**B**). PARP formation is localized in the nuclei of cells (shown in dark). Magnification ×400. (Reproduced with permission from ref. *52*.)

PHARMACOLOGICAL INHIBITION OF POLY(ADP-RIBOSE) POLYMERASE IMPROVES DIABETES-INDUCED CARDIAC DYSFUNCTION

Treatment with the phenanthridinone-based PARP inhibitor PJ34, starting 1 week after the onset of diabetes, restored normal vascular responsiveness and significantly improved cardiac function in diabetic mice and rats, despite the persistence of severe hyperglycemia *(51)* (Fig. 9A,B). The beneficial effect of PARP inhibition persisted even after several weeks of discontinuation of the PARP inhibitor treatment *(51)*. It is possible that the diabetic endothelial PARP pathway and the diabetic cardiomyopathy are interrelated: the impairment of the endothelial function may lead to global or regional myocardial ischemia, which may secondarily impair cardiac performance. The beneficial

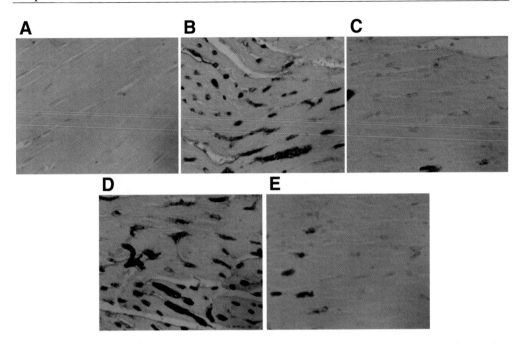

Fig. 8. Evidence for poly(ADP-ribose) polymerase (PARP) activation in diabetic rat hearts. Immunohistochemical staining for poly(ADP-ribose) formation, an indicator of PARP activation, in control (**A**), diabetic (**B,D**), and PJ34-treated diabetic (**C,E**) rat hearts. Panels B and D show poly(ADP-ribose) formation localized in the nuclei of myocytes in 5- and 10-week diabetic rat hearts, respectively. The evidence of poly(ADP-ribose) accumulation can be seen as dark, frequent, and widespread nuclear staining in panels B and D. Treatment with PJ34 for 4 weeks (**C**) markedly reduced PARP activation in diabetic (5-week) hearts. Notably, the PARP activation in diabetic hearts (10 weeks) was attenuated even after the discontinuation of the treatment with PJ34 (after 6 weeks) for an additional 3-week period (**E**). Similar immunohistochemical profiles were seen in $n = 4-5$ hearts per group. (Reproduced with permission from ref. *51*.)

effect of PARP inhibition on myocardial function, however, is not related to an anabolic effect because PJ34 treatment did not influence the body and heart weight loss in diabetic animals, although it dramatically improved cardiac function. It is noteworthy that the protective effect of PARP inhibition against diabetic cardiac dysfunction extended several weeks beyond the discontinuation of treatment; this observation may have important implications for the design of future clinical trials with PARP inhibitors. The prolonged protective effect may be related to the permanent interruption by the PARP inhibitor of positive feedback cycles of cardiac injury. Indeed, previous studies in various pathophysiological conditions have demonstrated that PARP inhibitors suppress positive feedback cycles of adhesion receptor expression and mononuclear cell infiltration, and cellular oxidant generation *(13,36,110)*. The mode of PARP inhibitors' cardioprotective action involves a conservation of myocardial energetics, and a prevention of the upregulation of various proinflammatory pathways (cytokines, adhesion receptors, mononuclear cell infiltration) triggered by ischemia and reperfusion *(13,36)*. It is conceivable that PARP inhibition exerts beneficial effects in experimental models of diabetic cardiomyopathy by affecting both above referenced pathways of injury, and also by suppressing positive feedback cycles initiated by them. Based on the results of the current study, we conclude that the ROS/reactive nitrogen species–DNA injury–PARP activation pathway plays a pathogenetic role in the development of diabetic cardiomyopathy.

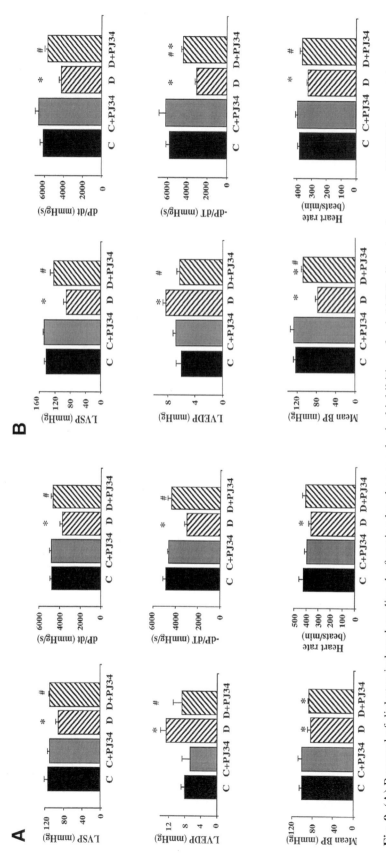

Fig. 9. (A) Reversal of diabetes-induced cardiac dysfunction by pharmacological inhibition of poly(ADP-ribose) polymerase (PARP) in an autoimmune mouse model of diabetes. Effect of diabetes and PJ34 on left ventricular systolic pressure (LVSP), left ventricular end-diastolic pressure (LVEDP), left ventricular +dP/dt, left ventricular −dP/dt, mean blood pressure (mean BP), and heart rate in NOD mice. C, control; D, diabetic; C + PJ34, control treated with PJ34 (for 4 weeks); D + PJ34, diabetic treated with PJ34 (for 4 weeks). Data are means ± SE. *$p < 0.05$ vs C; #$p < 0.05$ vs D (Reproduced with permission from ref. 51.) **(B)** Reversal of streptozotocin-evoked diabetes induced cardiac dysfunction by pharmacological inhibition of PARP in rats. Effect of diabetes (5 weeks) and PJ34 (4 weeks) on LVSP, LVEDP, left ventricular +dP/dt, left ventricular −dP/dt, mean mean BP, and heart rate in rats. C, control; D, diabetic (for 5 weeks); C + PJ34, control treated with PJ34 (for 4 weeks); D + PJ34, diabetic treated with PJ34 (treatment was started after 1 week of established diabetes for further 4 weeks). Data are means ± SE. *$p < 0.05$ vs C; #$p < 0.05$ vs D. (Reproduced with permission from ref. 51.)

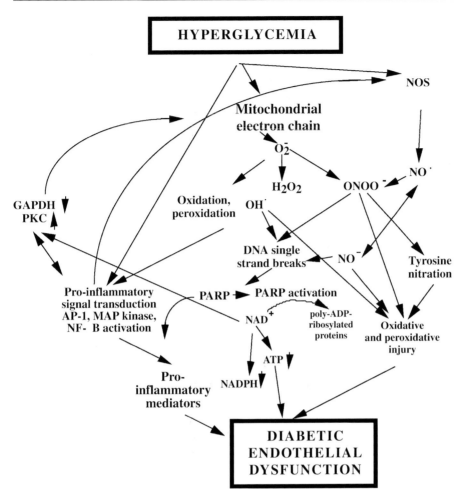

Fig. 10. Overview of the role of poly(ADP-ribose) polymerase (PARP) in regulating multiple component of hyperglycemia-induced endothelial dysfunction. High circulating glucose interacts with the vascular endothelium in which it triggers the release of oxidant mediators from the mitochondrial electron transport chain, and from NADH/NADPH oxidase and other sources. Nitric oxide (NO), in turn, combines with superoxide to yield peroxynitrite. Hydroxyl radical (produced from superoxide via the iron-catalyzed Haber-Weiss reaction) and peroxynitrite or peroxynitrous acid induce the development of DNA single-strand breakage, with consequent activation of PARP. Depletion of the cellular NAD+ leads to inhibition of cellular ATP-generating pathways leading to cellular dysfunction. The PARP-triggered depletion of cellular NADPH directly impairs the endothelium-dependent relaxations. The effects of elevated glucose are also exacerbated by increased aldose reductase activity leading to depletion of NADPH and generation of reactive oxidants. NO alone does not induce DNA single strand breakage, but may combine with superoxide (produced from the mitochondrial chain or from other cellular sources) to yield peroxynitrite. Under conditions of low-cellular L-arginine NOS may produce both superoxide and NO, which then can combine to form peroxynitrite. PARP activation, via a not yet characterized fashion, can promote the activation of nuclear factor kB, AP-1, mitogen-activated protein kinases, and the expression of proinflammatory mediators, adhesion molecules, and of iNOS. PARP activation contributes to the activation of protein kinase C. PARP activation also leads to the inhibition of cellular GAPDH activity, at least in part via the direct poly(ADP-ribosyl)ation of GAPDH. PARP-independent, parallel pathways of cellular metabolic inhibition can be activated by NO, hydroxyl radical, superoxide, and by peroxynitrite.

CONCLUSIONS AND IMPLICATIONS

The role of PARP activation in diabetes is not limited to the development of various forms of cardiovascular dysfunction. A vast body of evidence supports the role of nitrosative stress and PARP activation in the process of autoimmune islet cell death and in the process of islet regeneration *(1)*. In addition, PARP inhibitors exert beneficial effects in rodent models of diabetic neuropathy and retinopathy *(105,108)*. Taken together, multiple lines of evidence support the view that nitrosative stress and PARP activation play a crucial role in multiple interrelated aspects of the pathogenesis of diabetes and in the development of its complications (Fig. 10). PARP inhibition may emerge as a novel approach for the experimental therapy of diabetes, and for the prevention or reversal of its complications.

REFERENCES

1. Virag L, Szabo C. The therapeutic potential of poly(ADP-ribose) polymerase inhibitors. Pharmacol Rev 2002;54:375–429.
2. Szabó C, Dawson VL. Role of poly (ADP-ribose) synthetase activation in inflammation and reperfusion injury. Trends Pharmacol Sci 1998;19:287–298.
3. De Murcia G, Schreiber V, Molinete M, et al. Structure and function of poly(ADP-ribose) polymerase. Mol Cell Biochem 1994;138:15–24.
4. Le Rhun Y, Kirkland JB, Shah GM. Cellular responses to DNA damage in the absence of Poly(ADP-ribose) polymerase. Biochem Biophys Res Commun 1998;245:1–10.
5. Szabó C. Cell Death: the role of PARP. CRC Press, Boca Raton, FL: 2000.
6. De Murcia G, Shall S. (Eds.) From DNA damage and stress signaling to cell death; poly ADP-ribosylation reactions. Oxford University Press, Oxford, England, 2000.
7. Davidovic L, Vodenicharov M, Affar EB, Poirier GG. Importance of poly(ADP-ribose) glycohydrolase in the control of poly(ADP-ribose) metabolism. Exp Cell Res 2001;268:7–13.
8. Rudat V, Kupper JH, Weber KJ. Trans-dominant inhibition of poly(ADP-ribosyl)ation leads to decreased recovery from ionizing radiation-induced cell killing. Int J Radiat Biol 1998;73:325–330.
9. Menissier-de Murcia J, Niedergang C, Trucco C, et al. Requirement of poly(ADP-ribose) polymerase in recovery from DNA damage in mice and in cells. Proc Natl Acad Sci USA 1997;94:7303–7307.
10. Hiromatsu Y, Sato M, Yamada K, Nonaka K. Nicotinamide and 3-aminobenzamide inhibit recombinant human interferon-gamma-induced HLA-DR antigen expression, but not HLA-A, B, C antigen expression, on cultured human thyroid cells. Clin Endocrinol 1992;36:91–95.
11. Szabó C, Wong H, Bauer PI, et al. Regulation of components of the inflammatory response by 5-iodo-6-amino-1,2-benzopyrone, an inhibitor of poly (ADP-ribose) synthetase and pleiotropic modifier of cellular signal pathways. Int J Oncol 1997;10:1093–1104.
12. Ehrlich W, Huser H, Kroger H. Inhibition of the induction of collagenase by interleukin-1 beta in cultured rabbit synovial fibroblasts after treatment with the poly(ADP-ribose)-polymerase inhibitor 3-aminobenzamide. Rheumatol Int 1995;15:171–172.
13. Zingarelli B, Salzman AL, Szabó C. Genetic disruption of poly (ADP ribose) synthetase inhibits the expression of P-selectin and intercellular adhesion molecule-1 in myocardial ischemia-reperfusion injury. Circ Res 1998;83:85–94.
14. Simbulan-Rosenthal CM, Ly DH, et al. Misregulation of gene expression in primary fibroblasts lacking poly(ADP-ribose) polymerase. Proc Natl Acad Sci 2000;97:11,274–11,279.
15. Satoh MS, Lindahl T. Role of poly(ADP-ribose) formation in DNA repair. Nature 1992;356:356–358.
16. Oikawa A, Tohda H, Kanai M, Miwa M, Sugimura T. Inhibitors of poly(adenosine diphosphate ribose) polymerase induce sister chromatid exchanges. Biochem Biophys Res Commun 1980;97:1311–1316.
17. Park SD, Kim CG, Kim MG. Inhibitors of poly(ADP-ribose) polymerase enhance DNA strand breaks, excision repair, and sister chromatid exchanges induced by alkylating agents. Environ Mutagen 1983;5:515–525.
18. Herceg Z, Wang ZQ. Functions of poly(ADP-ribose) polymerase (PARP) in DNA repair, genomic integrity and cell death. Mutat Res 2001;477:97–110.
19. Poirier GG, de Murcia G, Jongstra-Bilen J, Niedergang C, Mandel P. Poly(ADP-ribosyl)ation of polynuclesomes causes relaxation of chromatin structure. Proc Natl Acad Sci 1982;79:3423–3427.

20. Lautier D, Lageux J, Thibodeau J, Ménard L, Poirier GG. Molecular and biochemical features of poly (ADP-ribose) metabolism. Mol Cell Biochem 1993;122:171–193.
21. Oei SL, Ziegler M. ATP for the DNA ligation step in base excision repair is generated from poly(ADP-ribose). J Biol Chem 2000; 28; 275:23,234–23,239.
22. Ullrich O, Ciftci O, Hass R. Proteasome activation by poly-ADP-ribose-polymerase in human myelomonocytic cells after oxidative stress. Free Radic Biol Med 2000;29:995–1004.
23. Szabó C, Zingarelli B, O'Connor M, Salzman AL. DNA strand breakage, activation of poly-ADP ribosyl synthetase, and cellular energy depletion are involved in the cytotoxicity in macrophages and smooth muscle cells exposed to peroxynitrite. Proc Natl Acad Sci USA 1996;93:1753–1758.
24. Szabó C, Virág L, Cuzzocrea S, et al. Protection against peroxynitrite-induced fibroblast injury and arthritis development by inhibition of poly(ADP-ribose) synthetase. Proc Natl Acad Sci USA 1998;95:3867–3872.
25. Schraufstatter IU, Hinshaw DB, Hyslop PA, Spragg RG, Cochrane CG. Oxidant injury of cells. DNA strand-breaks activate polyadenosine diphosphate-ribose polymerase and lead to depletion of nicotinamide adenine dinucleotide. J Clin Invest 1986;77:1312–1320.
26. Schraufstatter IU, Hyslop PA, Hinshaw DB, Spragg RG, Sklar LA, Cochrane CG. Hydrogen peroxide-induced injury of cells and its prevention by inhibitors of poly(ADP-ribose) polymerase. Proc Natl Acad Sci USA 1986;83:4908–4912.
27. Zhang J, Dawson VL, Dawson TM, Snyder SH. Nitric oxide activation of poly (ADP-ribose) synthetase in neurotoxicity. Science 1994;263:687–689.
28. Radons J, Heller B, Burkle A, et al. Nitric oxide toxicity in islet cells involves poly (ADP-ribose) polymerase activation and concomitant NAD depletion. Biochem Biophys Res Comm 1994;199:1270–1277.
29. Bai P, Bakondi E, Szabo EE, Gergely P, Szabo C, Virag L. Partial protection by poly(ADP-ribose) polymerase inhibitors from nitroxyl-induced cytotoxity in thymocytes. Free Radic Biol Med 2001;31:1616–1623
30. Ha HC, Hester LD, Snyder SH. Poly(ADP-ribose) polymerase-1 dependence of stress-induced transcription factors and associated gene expression in glia. Proc Natl Acad Sci USA 2002;99:3270–3275.
31. Hassa PO, Hottiger MO. A role of poly (ADP-ribose) polymerase in NF-kappaB transcriptional activation. Biol Chem 1999;380:953–959.
32. Oliver FJ, Menissier-de Murcia J, Nacci C, et al. Resistance to endotoxic shock as a consequence of defective NF-kappaB activation in poly (ADP-ribose) polymerase-1 deficient mice. EMBO J 1999;18:4446–4454 .
33. Amstad PA, Krupitza G, Cerutti PA. Mechanism of c-fos induction by active oxygen. Cancer Res 1992;52:3952–3960.
34. Roebuck KA, Rahman A, Lakshminarayanan V, Janakidevi K, Malik AB. H2O2 and tumor necrosis factor-alpha activate intercellular adhesion molecule 1 (ICAM-1) gene transcription through distinct cis-regulatory elements within the ICAM-1 promoter. J Biol Chem 1995;270:18,966–18,974.
35. Thiemermann C, Bowes J, Myint FP, Vane JR. Inhibition of the activity of poly(ADP ribose) synthetase reduces ischemia-reperfusion injury in the heart and skeletal muscle. Proc Natl Acad Sci USA 1997;94:679–683.
36. Szabo G, Bahrle S, Stumpf N, et al. Poly(ADP-Ribose) polymerase inhibition reduces reperfusion injury after heart transplantation. Circ Res 2002;90:100–106.
37. Pacher P, Liaudet L, Bai P, et al. Activation of poly(ADP-ribose) polymerase contributes to the development of doxorubicin-induced heart failure. J Pharmacol Exp Ther 2002;300:862–687.
38. Pacher P, Liaudet L, Mabley J, Komjati K, Szabo C. Pharmacologic inhibition of poly(adenosine diphosphate-ribose) polymerase may represent a novel therapeutic approach in chronic heart failure. J Am Coll Cardiol 2002;40:1006–1016.
39. Eliasson MJ, Sampei K, Mandir AS, et al. Poly(ADP-ribose) polymerase gene disruption renders mice resistant to cerebral ischemia. Nat Med 1997;3:1089–1095.
40. Szabo C, Cuzzocrea S, Zingarelli B, O'Connor M, Salzman AL. Endothelial dysfunction in a rat model of endotoxic shock: importance of the activation of poly (ADP-ribose) synthetase by peroxynitrite. J Clin Invest 1997;100:723–735.
41. Soriano FG, Liaudet L, Szabo E, et al. Resistance to acute septic peritonitis in poly(ADP-ribose) polymerase-1-deficient mice. Shock. 2002;17:286–292.
42. Pacher P, Cziraki A, Mabley JG, Liaudet L, Papp L, Szabo C. Role of poly(ADP-ribose) polymerase activation in endotoxin-induced cardiac collapse in rodents. Biochem Pharmacol. 2002;64:1785–1791.

43. Burkart V, Wang ZQ, Radons J, et al. Mice Lacking the Poly(ADP-Ribose) Polymerase Gene Are Resistant to Pancreatic Beta-Cell Destruction and Diabetes Development Induced by Streptozocin. Nat Med 1999;5:314–319.

44. Pieper AA, Brat DJ, Krug DK, et al. Poly(ADP-ribose) polymerase-deficient mice are protected from streptozotocin-induced diabetes. Proc Natl Acad Sci USA 1999;96:3059–3064.

45. Pacher P, Mabley JG, Soriano FG, Liaudet L, Komjati K, Szabo C. Endothelial dysfunction in aging animals: the role of poly(ADP-ribose) polymerase activation. Br J Pharmacol 2002;135:1347–1350.

46. Pacher P, Mabley JG, Soriano FG, Liaudet L, Szabo C. Activation of poly(ADP-ribose) polymerase contributes to the endothelial dysfunction associated with hypertension and aging. Int J Mol Med 2002;9:659–664.

47. Hung TH, Skepper JN, Charnock-Jones DS, Burton GJ. Hypoxia-reoxygenation: a potent inducer of apoptotic changes in the human placenta and possible etiological factor in preeclampsia. Circ Res 2002;90:1274–1281.

48. Martinet W, Knaapen MW, De Meyer GR, Herman AG, Kockx MM. Elevated levels of oxidative DNA damage and DNA repair enzymes in human atherosclerotic plaques. Circulation 2002;106:927–932.

49. Garcia Soriano F, Virág L, Jagtap P, et al. Diabetic endothelial dysfunction: the role of poly (ADP-ribose) polymerase activation. Nature Medicine 2001;7:108–113.

50. Soriano FG, Mabley JG, Pacher P, Liaudet L, Szabó C. Rapid reversal of the diabetic endothelial dysfunction by pharmacological inhibition of poly(ADP-ribose) polymerase. Circ Res 2001;89:684–691.

51. Pacher P, Liaudet L, Soriano FG, Mabley JG, Szabó É, Szabó C. The role of poly(ADP-ribose) polymerase in the development of myocardial and endothelial dysfunction in diabetes mellitus. Diabetes 2002;51:514–521.

52. Szabo C, Zanchi A, Komjati K, et al. Poly(ADP-Ribose) polymerase is activated in subjects at risk of developing type 2 diabetes and is associated with impaired vascular reactivity. Circulation. 2002;106:2680–2686.

53. Furchgott RF. Endothelium-derived relaxing factor: discovery, early studies, and identification as nitric oxide. Biosci Rep 1999;19:235–251.

54. Cai H, Harrison DG. Endothelial dysfunction in cardiovascular diseases: the role of oxidant stress. Circ Res 2000;87:840–844.

55. Caballero AE, Arora S, Saouaf R, et al. Microvascular and macrovascular reactivity is reduced in subjects at risk for type 2 diabetes. Diabetes 1999;48:1856–1862.

56. Ruderman NB, Williamson JR, Brownlee M. Glucose and diabetic vascular disease. FASEB J 1992;6:2905–2914.

57. Cosentino F, Luscher TF. Endothelial dysfunction in diabetes mellitus. J Cardiovasc Pharmacol 1998;32:S54–61.

58. Calles-Escandon J, Cipolla M. Diabetes and endothelial dysfunction: a clinical perspective. Endocr Rev 2001;22:36–52.

59. Guzik TJ, West NE, Black E, et al. Vascular superoxide production by NAD(P)H oxidase: association with endothelial dysfunction and clinical risk factors. Circ Res 2000;86:85–90.

60. De Vriese AS, Verbeuren TJ, Van de Voorde J, Lameire NH, Vanhoutte PM. Endothelial dysfunction in diabetes. Br J Pharmacol 2000;130:963–974.

61. Beckman JA. Inhibition of protein kinase Cbeta prevents impaired endothelium-dependent vasodilation caused by hyperglycemia in humans. Circ Res 2002;90:107–111.

62. Nishikawa T, Edelstein D, Du XL, et al. Normalizing mitochondrial superoxide production blocks three pathways of hyperglycaemic damage. Nature 2000;404:787–790.

63. Brownlee M. Biochemistry and molecular cell biology of diabetic complications. Nature 2001;414: 813–820.

64. Giugliano D, Ceriello A, Paolisso G. Oxidative stress and diabetic vascular complications. Diabetes Care 1996;19:257–267.

65. Spitaler MM, Graier WF. Vascular targets of redox signalling in diabetes mellitus. Diabetologia. 2002;45:476–494.

66. Cosentino F, Hishikawa K, Katusic ZS, Luscher TF. High glucose increases nitric oxide synthase expression and superoxide anion generation in human aortic endothelial cells. Circulation 1997;96:25–28.

67. Beckman JS, Koppenol WH. Nitric oxide, superoxide, and peroxynitrite: the good, the bad, and ugly. Am J Physiol. 1996;271:1424–1437.

68. Eiserich JP, Hristova M, Cross CE, et al. Formation of nitric oxide-derived inflammatory oxidants by myeloperoxidase in neutrophils. Nature 1998;391:393–397.

69. Halliwell B. What nitrates tyrosine? Is nitrotyrosine specific as a biomarker of peroxynitrite formation in vivo? FEBS Lett 1997;411:157–160.

70. Ceriello A, Mercuri F, Quagliaro L, Assaloni R, Motz E, Tonutti L, Taboga C. Detection of nitrotyrosine in the diabetic plasma: evidence of oxidative stress. Diabetologia. 2001;44:834–838.

71. Tannous M, Rabini RA, Vignini A, et al. Evidence for iNOS-dependent peroxynitrite production in diabetic platelets. Diabetologia 1999;42:539–544.

72. Pennathur S, Wagner JD, Leeuwenburgh C, Litwak KN, Heinecke JW. A hydroxyl radical-like species oxidizes cynomolgus monkey artery wall proteins in early diabetic vascular disease. J Clin Invest 2001;107:853–860.

73. Ceriello A, Quagliaro L, Catone B, et al. Role of hyperglycemia in nitrotyrosine postprandial generation. Diabetes Care 2002;25:1439–1443.

74. Frustaci A, Kajstura J, Chimenti C, et al. Myocardial cell death in human diabetes. Circ Res 2000;87:1123–1132.

75. Kajstura J, Fiordaliso F, Andreoli AM, et al. IGF-1 overexpression inhibits the development of diabetic cardiomyopathy and angiotensin II-mediated oxidative stress. Diabetes 2001;50:1414–1424.

76. Ceriello A, Quagliaro L, D'Amico M, et al. Acute hyperglycemia induces nitrotyrosine formation and apoptosis in perfused heart from rat. Diabetes 2002;51:1076–1082.

77. Mihm MJ, Jing L, Bauer JA. Nitrotyrosine causes selective vascular endothelial dysfunction and DNA damage. J Cardiovasc Pharmacol 2000;36:182–187.

78. Zou MH, Shi C, Cohen RA. High glucose via peroxynitrite causes tyrosine nitration and inactivation of prostacyclin synthase that is associated with thromboxane/prostaglandin H(2) receptor-mediated apoptosis and adhesion molecule expression in cultured human aortic endothelial cells. Diabetes 2002;51:198–203.

79. Cosentino F, Eto M, De Paolis P, et al. High glucose causes upregulation of cyclooxygenase-2 and alters prostanoid profile in human endothelial cells: role of protein kinase C and reactive oxygen species. Circulation. 2003;107:1017–1023.

80. Ellis EA, Guberski DL, Hutson B, Grant MB. Time course of NADH oxidase, inducible nitric oxide synthase and peroxynitrite in diabetic retinopathy in the BBZ/WOR rat. Nitric Oxide. 2002;6:295–304.

81. Du Y, Smith MA, Miller CM, Kern TS. Diabetes-induced nitrative stress in the retina, and correction by aminoguanidine. J Neurochem. 2002;80:771–779.

82. El-Remessy AB, Behzadian MA, Abou-Mohamed G, Franklin T, Caldwell RW, Caldwell RB. Experimental diabetes causes breakdown of the blood-retina barrier by a mechanism involving tyrosine nitration and increases in expression of vascular endothelial growth factor and urokinase plasminogen activator receptor. Am J Pathol. 2003;162:1995–2004.

83. Onozato ML, Tojo A, Goto A, Fujita T, Wilcox CS. Oxidative stress and nitric oxide synthase in rat diabetic nephropathy: effects of ACEI and ARB. Kidney Int 2002;61:186–194.

84. Coppey LJ, Gellett JS, Davidson EP, Dunlap JA, Lund DD, Yorek MA. Effect of antioxidant treatment of streptozotocin-induced diabetic rats on endoneurial blood flow, motor nerve conduction velocity, and vascular reactivity of epineurial arterioles of the sciatic nerve. Diabetes 2001;50:1927–1937.

85. Hoeldtke RD, Bryner KD, McNeill DR, et al. Nitrosative stress, uric Acid, and peripheral nerve function in early type 1 diabetes. Diabetes 2002;51:2817–2825.

86. Fein FS. Diabetic cardiomyopathy. Diabetes Care 1990;13:1169–1179.

87. Illan F, Valdes-Chavarri M, Tebar J, et al. Anatomical and functional cardiac abnormalities in type I diabetes. Clin Invest 1992;70:403–410.

88. Joffe II, Travers KE, Perreault-Micale CL, et al. Abnormal cardiac function in the streptozotocin-induced non-insulin-dependent diabetic rat: noninvasive assessment with doppler echocardiography and contribution of the nitric oxide pathway. J Am Coll Cardiol 1999;34:2111–2119.

89. Regan TJ, Ahmed S, Haider B, Moschos C, Weisse A. Diabetic cardiomyopathy: experimental and clinical observations. N Engl J Med 1994;91:776–778.

90. Bell DS. Diabetic cardiomyopathy: a unique entity or a complication of coronary artery disease? Diabetes Care 1995;18:708–714.

91. Dhalla NS, Liu X, Panagia V, Takeda N. Subcellular remodeling and heart dysfunction in chronic diabetes. Cardiovasc Res 1998;40:239–247.

92. Szabo C, Mabley JG, Moeller SM, et al. Soriano Part I: Pathogenetic Role of Peroxynitrite in the Development of Diabetes and Diabetic Vascular Complications: Studies With FP15, A Novel Potent Peroxynitrite Decomposition Catalyst. Mol Med. 2002;8:571–580.

93. Mihm MJ, Coyle CM, Schanbacher BL, Weinstein DM, Bauer JA. Peroxynitrite induced nitration and inactivation of myofibrillar creatine kinase in experimental heart failure. Cardiovasc Res 2001;49:798–807.

94. Turko IV, Marcondes S, Murad F. Diabetes-associated nitration of tyrosine and inactivation of succinyl-CoA:3-oxoacid CoA-transferase. Am J Physiol 2001; 281:2289–2294.

95. Pacher P, Liaudet L, Bai P, et al. Potent metalloporphyrin peroxynitrite decomposition catalyst protects against the development of doxorubicin-induced cardiac dysfunction. Circulation 2003;107:896–904.

96. Weinstein DM, Mihm MJ, Bauer JA. Cardiac peroxynitrite formation and left ventricular dysfunction following doxorubicin treatment in mice. J Pharmacol Exp Ther 2000;294:396–401.

97. Mihm MJ, Bauer JA. Peroxynitrite-induced inhibition and nitration of cardiac myofibrillar creatine kinase. Biochimie 2002; 84:1013–1019.

98. Bianchi C, Wakiyama H, Faro R, et al. A novel peroxynitrite decomposer catalyst (FP-15) reduces myocardial infarct size in an in vivo peroxynitrite decomposer and acute ischemia-reperfusion in pigs. Ann Thorac Surg 2002;74:1201–1207.

99. Park KS, Kim JH, Kim MS, et al. Effects of insulin and antioxidant on plasma 8-hydroxyguanine and tissue 8-hydroxydeoxyguanosine in streptozotocin-induced diabetic rats. Diabetes. 2001;50:2837–2841.

100. Lorenzi M, Montisano DF, Toledo S, Wong HC. Increased single strand breaks in DNA of lymphocytes from diabetic subjects. J Clin Invest 1987;79:653–656.

101. Anderson D, Yu TW, Wright J, Ioannides C. An examination of DNA strand breakage in the comet assay and antioxidant capacity in diabetic patients. Mutat Res 1998;398:151–161.

102. Astley S, Langrish-Smith A, Southon S, Sampson M. Vitamin E supplementation and oxidative damage to DNA and plasma LDL in type 1 diabetes. Diabetes Care 1999;22:1626–1631.

103. Sardas S, Yilmaz M, Oztok U, Cakir N, Karakaya AE. Assessment of DNA strand breakage by comet assay in diabetic patients and the role of antioxidant supplementation. Mutat Res 2001;490:123–129.

104. Dincer Y, Akcay T, Ilkova H, Alademir Z, Ozbay G. DNA damage and antioxidant defense in peripheral leukocytes of patients with Type I diabetes mellitus. Mutat Res 2003;527:49–55.

105. Szabó E, Kern TS, Virag L, Mabley J, Szabó C. Evidence for poly(ADP-ribose) polymerase activation in the diabetic retina. FASEB J 2001;15:A942.

106. Wahlberg G, Carlson LA, Wasserman J, Ljungqvist A. Protective effect of nicotinamide against nephropathy in diabetic rats. Diabetes Res 1985;2:307–312.

107. Minchenko AG, Stevens MJ, White L, et al. Diabetes-induced overexpression of endothelin-1 and endothelin receptors in the rat renal cortex is mediated via poly(ADP-ribose) polymerase activation. FASEB J 2003;11:1514–1516.

108. Obrosova IG, Li F, Abatan OI, et al. Role of poly(ADP-ribose) polymerase activation in diabetic neuropathy. Diabetes 2004;53(3):711–720.

109. Soriano FG, Virag L, Szabo C. Diabetic endothelial dysfunction: role of reactive oxygen and nitrogen species production and poly(ADP-ribose) polymerase activation. J Mol Med 2001;79:437–448.

110. Ceriello A, Piconi L, Quagliaro L, et al. Intermittent high glucose enhances ICAM-1, VCAM-1, E-selectin interleukin-6 expression in human umbilical endothelial cells in culture: the role of poly(ADP-ribose) polymerase. J Thromb Haemost 2004;8:1453–1459.

111. Du X, Martsumura T, Edelstein D, et al. Inhibition of GAPHH activity by poly(ADP-ribose) polymerase activates three major pathways of hyperglycemic damage in endothelial cells. J Clin Invest 2003;112:1049–1057.

112. Komjáti K, Jagtap P, Baloglu E, VanDuzer J, Salzman AL, Szabó C. Poly(ADP-ribose) polymerase inhibition in stroke: establishment of the therapeutic window of intervention and delineation of its role in the patgogenesis of white matter damage. FASEB J 2002;16:A599.

113. Shimoda K, Murakami K, Enkhbaatar P, et al. Effect of poly(ADP ribose) synthetase inhibition on burn and smoke inhalation injury in sheep. Am J Physiol Lung Cell Mol Physiol 2003;285:L240–249.

9 Adiponectin and the Cardiovascular System

Suketu Shah, MD, *Alina Gavrila,* MD,
and Christos S. Mantzoros, MD

CONTENTS

INTRODUCTION

Adiponectin, a recently discovered protein produced exclusively by adipocytes, is thought to be a possible mediator between obesity, insulin resistance, and cardiovascular disease (CVD). Although its function is not entirely known, body fat distribution, insulin, sex hormones, tumor necrosis factor (TNF)-α, and peroxisome proliferator-activated receptor (PPAR)-α may contribute to its regulation. Along with being associated with cardiovascular risk factors such as diabetes and dyslipidemia, deficiency in adiponectin may also directly compromise endothelial action and promote atherosclerosis.

Our understanding of the function of fat cells has changed dramatically with the realization of the endocrine function of adipose tissue. Initially thought to serve only as a repository for energy via storage of triglycerides, adipocytes are now known to secrete a variety of proteins with diverse metabolic functions. These proteins include leptin, TNF-α, plasminogen activator inhibitor-1, acylation-stimulating protein, resistin, and adiponectin *(1,2)*. Adiponectin has received much attention for its putative role in diabetes and CVD. Besides being associated with the development of diabetes, it may also have a direct role in modulating inflammation and atherosclerosis and thereby be one of the factors that links obesity to CVD.

From: *Contemporary Cardiology: Diabetes and Cardiovascular Disease, Second Edition*
Edited by: M. T. Johnstone and A. Veves © Humana Press Inc., Totowa, NJ

STRUCTURE OF ADIPONECTIN

In the mid-1990s, four different research groups, using either human or mouse-derived samples, concurrently discovered adiponectin, alternatively termed Acrp30, apM1 protein, adipoQ, and GBP28 *(3–6)*. Produced exclusively by differentiated adipocytes, adiponectin is a 30 kDa protein composed of 244 amino acids *(3,4)*. One of the most abundantly produced fat hormones, it comprises approx 0.01% of the plasma proteins in humans, with plasma levels ranging from 2 to 20 µg/mL *(7)*. Slightly increasing with age, adiponectin levels have a diurnal variation with nadir at night and peak in the morning *(8,9)*.

The adiponectin molecule has four distinct parts, with the amino terminal having two short regions consisting of a secretory signal sequence and a domain unlike any other known protein *(3–6)*. The next two regions, a collagen-like fibrous structure followed by a globular domain at the carboxy terminal, share homology with complement factor C1q and collagen VIII and X *(10)*. Despite different amino acid sequences, the overall tertiary structure of the globular domain has similarity to TNF-α, another protein secreted by adipocytes but having opposing actions *(11,12)*.

REGULATION OF ADIPONECTIN

Although its structure and source are known, the regulation of adiponectin remains to be determined. The various factors thought to be involved in controlling adiponectin production and secretion include obesity, nutritional status, hormones such as insulin, leptin, glucocorticoids, sex hormones, and catecholamines, TNF-α, and PPAR-α.

Obesity and Nutritional Intake

Obesity, in general, is associated with decreased adiponectin expression in adipose tissue and plasma levels *(7,13)*. In both men and women, overall obesity, assessed by parameters such as body mass index (BMI) and fat mass, is negatively correlated to adiponectin, although prolonged weight reduction leads to increased adiponectin levels *(7,14–17)*. Nutritional intake does not seem to explain this relationship. Although fasting decreases adiponectin messenger ribonucleic acid (mRNA) levels in mice, serum levels remain unchanged *(18)*. In humans, short-term fasting also does not change plasma levels of adiponectin, although prolonged caloric restriction does result in weight loss and increased adiponectin levels *(14,19)*. Additionally, daily caloric intake, macronutrient intake, or a high-fat meal is not related to any immediate change in circulating adiponectin levels in humans except possibly in obese individuals *(20–22)*.

Instead of food intake, the distribution of adipose tissue may be more closely associated with adiponectin. There is a strong inverse correlation between adiponectin levels and visceral or central fat, compared to subcutaneous fat *(9,19)*. In contrast to subcutaneous adipocytes, human omental adipose tissue had a significant negative correlation with BMI, and only it responded to insulin and PPAR-α agonist administration with increased adiponectin production *(23)*. These findings suggest that adipose tissue, particularly in the visceral distribution, may have an inhibitory mechanism for its own production of adiponectin, perhaps mediated by other factors produced by fat cells such as TNF-α *(13)*.

Hormone Regulation

Hormones have also been suggested to regulate adiponectin. Insulin likely has a role in regulating adiponectin, but its exact role remains controversial. In vitro studies have shown conflicting results on whether insulin has an inhibitory or stimulatory effect on adiponectin production and secretion *(23–25)*, whereas in an in vivo study involving humans, hyperinsulinemic euglycemic dosing for at least 2 hours led to a decrease in adiponectin levels *(26)*. Therefore, further studies would be helpful to resolve the relationship.

Sex hormones may also affect secretion of adiponectin, because women have higher plasma levels of adiponectin than men, independent of body composition *(14)*. Of the sex hormones, estrogen does not seem to account for the gender-related difference in adiponectin level, because premenopausal women have higher estrogen levels and lower adiponectin concentrations than postmenopausal females and estradiol levels actually have a strong negative correlation with serum adiponectin levels, females would be expected to have lower adiponectin concentrations than men *(19)*. Testosterone may lower adiponectin levels by possibly inhibiting its secretion, however. In mice, removal of the testes led to an increase in adiponectin, although administration of testosterone reduced adiponectin levels *(27)*. Although one study has demonstrated no association between adiponectin and free testosterone concentrations in women, this relationship remains to be explored in men *(19)*.

Leptin and glucocorticoids have also been thought to be involved in adiponectin regulation, because leptin is also secreted by adipose tissue and both hormones affect insulin sensitivity *(28,29)*. Although a cross-sectional study reported a strong inverse relationship between serum adiponectin and leptin levels *(30)*, leptin given exogenously to rodents or humans had no significant effect on the plasma concentration of adiponectin *(18,19)*. In vitro studies show that dexamethasone suppresses adiponectin gene expression *(24,25)*, but in human studies, cortisol was found to have no correlation with circulating levels of adiponectin *(19)*. Further studies are necessary to evaluate if glucocorticoids have a local effect on adiponectin production not reflected by their serum concentrations.

Catecholamines may also suppress expression of adiponectin, because β-adrenergic agonists reduced adiponectin gene expression in cultured mouse fat cells and human adipose tissue and decreased plasma levels in mice *(31)*. Stimulation of cultured adipocytes by isoproteronolol, a β1 and β2 agonist, leads to reduced expression of adiponectin, an effect that propranolol, a nonselective β-antagonist, can inhibit *(32)*. Another study in animals confirmed that peripheral injection of a β3-adrenergic agonist suppressed adiponectin mRNA expression in adipose tissue *(18)*.

TNF-α

As another factor produced by adipocytes, TNF-α may also be involved in the regulation of adiponectin. TNF-α and adiponectin inhibit each other's production in adipose tissue, in addition to having opposing actions. TNF-α decreases expression and secretion of adiponectin in mouse and human adipocytes *(25,33,34)* and adiponectin-knockout mice have elevated serum TNF-α levels that decrease with adiponectin administration *(35)*. Because these two molecules share, in part, similar tertiary structure, they may exert opposite actions by acting on the same cellular receptors *(11,13)*.

PPAR-α

PPAR-α is a transcription factor that enhances insulin sensitivity in adipose and other tissues *(36)*. In a randomized, double blind, placebo-controlled trial, patients with type 2 diabetes given 6 months of rosiglitazone, a PPAR-α agonist, had increased levels of adiponectin *(37)*, with a similar change being seen even in humans without insulin resistance *(38)*. PPAR-α agonists may mediate their effect by directly promoting adiponectin transcription or by inhibiting the actions of TNF-α *(34,39)*.

ADIPONECTIN AND CARDIOVASCULAR DISEASE RISK FACTORS

Although the role of adiponectin has not been definitively established, evidence is mounting that it is involved in insulin resistance, diabetes, inflammation, and atherosclerosis *(40)*. Because, among the various adipocytokines, it decreases with increasing body fat *(7)*, its low levels may lead to the development of pathological states associated with obesity such as insulin resistance and CVD.

Diabetes and Insulin Resistance

Adiponectin's involvement in CVD is likely multifactorial, but one of its main roles is likely in affecting traditional risk factors associated with coronary artery disease (CAD), particularly diabetes. As one of the diabetes susceptibility genes and the adiponectin gene both localize to 3q27, mutation at this locus has been associated with both type 2 diabetes and decreased adiponectin *(41)*.

The majority of data for animal studies thus far suggest that adiponectin acts as an insulin-sensitizing hormone. Adiponectin-knockout mice develop insulin resistance either independently of diet or only after high-fat and high-sucrose diet, and treating these mice with adiponectin ameliorates their insulin resistance *(35,42)*. The insulin resistance in adiponectin-deficient lipoatrophic and obese mice can partially be reversed via adiponectin administration and fully restored with both leptin and adiponectin supplementation *(29)*. Furthermore, in a longitudinal study analyzing the progression of type 2 diabetes in obese monkeys, decrease in adiponectin closely parallels the observed reduction in insulin sensitivity, and the obese monkeys with greater plasma levels of adiponectin had less severe insulin resistance *(43)*.

In humans, type 2 diabetes has been associated with decreased levels of adiponectin *(14)*. In several studies, adiponectin has a negative correlation with fasting glucose, insulin, and insulin resistance and a positive association with insulin sensitivity, independent of BMI *(9,14,44)*. One study demonstrated that adjusting for central obesity renders the negative correlation between adiponectin and insulin resistance no longer significant, suggesting that adiponectin may mediate the relationship between central obesity and insulin resistance *(19)*. In studies involving Pima Indians, Japanese people, and Europeans, subjects with lower adiponectin were more likely to develop type 2 diabetes, independent of adiposity parameters *(45–47)*. In contrast, type 1 diabetic patients have elevated adiponectin levels compared to nondiabetic individuals, and chronically administered insulin does not have an effect on adiponectin levels *(48)*.

Although not entirely known, the cellular and molecular mechanisms linking adiponectin to improved insulin sensitivity are also likely multifactorial. In rodents, adiponectin administration enhances insulin-stimulated glucose uptake into fat and skeletal muscle cells *(49–51)*. By increasing fatty acid oxidation, adiponectin can also lower circulating free fatty acids (FFAs), which may improve insulin action *(51,52)*. Another important function of adiponectin is enhancement of insulin-induced suppression of hepatic glucose production *(53,54)*. By generating nitric oxide (NO) formation, adiponectin may also augment vascular blood flow to promote glucose uptake *(55)*. Taken together, all these effects could explain why giving adiponectin to mice on a high-fat and high-sucrose diet will induce weight loss and reduction in FFA, triglycerides, and glucose levels *(56)*.

Adiponectin may also improve insulin sensitivity by promoting activation of the insulin-signaling system *(58)*. The main enzyme implicated in adiponectin's action is adenosine monophosphate-activated protein kinase (AMPK) *(49–51)*. A recent study demonstrates that binding of adiponectin to two distinct adiponectin receptors increases the levels of this enzyme *(57)*. AMPK prevents activation of other enzymes involved in gluconeogenesis and may stimulate enzymes contributing to fatty acid oxidation *(49,50,54,56)*.

Dyslipidemia

Besides diabetes and insulin resistance, adiponectin is also related to dyslipidemia, another risk factor for CVD. Adiponectin is a strong independent positive predictor of high-density lipoprotein levels and is negatively associated with serum triglycerides *(14,59,60)*. In contrast, low-density lipoprotein and total cholesterol do not have significant independent relationships to adiponectin levels *(19)*.

Adiponectin may lead to favorable lipid profiles by stimulating fatty acid oxidation. The administration of adiponectin to rodents has been associated with increased fatty acid oxidation in skeletal muscle, both in vitro and in vivo, an effect probably mediated by AMPK *(49,50,56)*. However, in one study, fatty acid oxidation in muscle cells was found to be increased in adiponectin-knockout mice *(61)*, and in a single cross-sectional study in humans, plasma levels of adiponectin did not have any correlation with lipid oxidation, as measured by energy expenditure and respiratory quotient *(62)*. Thus, further studies are needed to clarify adiponectin's effects on fatty acid oxidation in humans.

Hypertension

Adiponectin has also been associated with hypertension. In adiponectin-deficient mice, a high-fat and -sucrose diet led to increased blood pressure (BP) *(63)*. Although an initial study in humans reported that hypertensive males had increased plasma levels of adiponectin *(64)*, subsequent studies reported that BP has a negative correlation to adiponectin *(65–67)*. However, more recent data adjusting for insulin sensitivity did not show any significant correlation with hypertension and adiponectin, indicating that insulin resistance may mediate the potential association between adiponectin and BP *(68)*. However, adiponectin has been associated with a vasodilatory response *(63)*, with recent evidence suggesting that adiponectin increases NO formation through AMPK *(55)*. Further studies are needed to elucidate more completely adiponectin's role in regulating BP levels.

Cigarette Smoking

Smoking and even a history of smoking have been associated with decreased levels of circulating adiponectin. Among patients with heart disease, current and former smokers had lower adiponectin levels than nonsmokers, after adjusting for BMI and insulin resistance *(69)*. Possible explanations for this decrease include smoking inducing an increase in catecholamines that suppress adiponectin or consumption of adiponectin by endothelium injured by cigarette toxins *(69,70)*.

ADIPONECTIN'S DIRECT VASCULAR EFFECTS

Although development of insulin resistance and alterations in lipid profile may account for part of adiponectin's role in CVD, low adiponectin has also been associated with CAD independent of these risk factors, suggesting that it may have its own direct effect on the vascular system *(14,71,72)*.

Adiponectin might have a protective role against atherosclerosis, because increasing adiponectin levels of mice deficient in apolipoprotein (apo)-E slows the rate of atherosclerosis and reduces lipid accumulation in arterial plaques *(73)*. In adiponectin-knockout mice, injury induced to a femoral artery resulted in greater neointimal thickening compared to control, independent of degree of glucose intolerance *(42)*, but overexpression of adiponectin attenuated neointimal proliferation in these mice *(74)*.

Adiponectin's reduction of atherosclerosis may occur through its actions on inflammatory mediators, macrophages, smooth muscle cells, and endothelium *(40)*. With its association with inflammatory markers, lack of adiponectin may foster an inflammatory milieu related to developing atherosclerosis and diabetes *(75)*. In patients with or without CAD, serum C-reactive protein, an inflammatory marker, was inversely related to adiponectin *(75–77)*. Other inflammatory markers such as phospholipase A2, interleukin-6, and soluble E (SE)-selectin, are also negatively correlated with adiponectin in one study *(75)*.

As an anti-inflammatory agent, adiponectin may inhibit inflammatory mediators involved in atherosclerosis, particularly TNF-α. An in vivo study in mice demonstrated that administration of adiponectin decreased serum TNF-α levels *(35)*. Although no significant correlation occurred between adiponectin and serum TNF-α receptors 1 (sTNFR1) and 2 (sTNFR2), which are markers of activation of the TNF-α system, a study in humans found lower sTNFR2 in the highest quartile of circulating adiponectin, suggesting a threshold effect instead of a dose-dependent relationship *(78)*. A different study, however, found a significant negative correlation between plasma adiponectin and TNF-α mRNA expression *(13)*. Besides inhibiting the production of TNF-α, adiponectin may impede TNF-α's involvement in atherosclerosis by reducing TNF-α-induced expression of endothelial cell adhesion molecules such as vascular cell adhesion molecule-1, SE-selectin, and intracellular adhesion molecule-1, that otherwise recruit monocytes and macrophages involved in atherosclerosis development *(79,80)*. Through a cyclic adenosine monophosphate (cAMP)-dependent pathway, adiponectin may prevent TNF-α from inducing stimulation of nuclear factor κB, a transcriptional factor that promotes gene expression of endothelial adhesion molecules *(80)*.

The anti-inflammatory effects of adiponectin may also directly involve macrophages and monocytes, an integral aspect of atherosclerotic lesions. By decreasing the level of expression of class A scavenger receptors on macrophages, adiponectin suppressed macrophage-to-foam cell transformation *(81)*. It also attenuated the phagocytic action of macrophages and inhibited expression and secretion of TNF-α from macrophages *(82)*. Additionally, adiponectin may decrease proliferation of precursors of monocytes and macrophages by suppressing bone marrow production of these cells *(82)*.

In the pathogenesis of atherosclerosis, adiponectin may also affect the proliferation of smooth muscle cells in the vascular wall by inhibiting growth factors that promote hyperplasia. Adiponectin binds to and inhibits a subtype of platelet-derived growth factor produced by platelets and foam cells *(83)* and blocks the proliferative action of heparin-binding epidermal growth factor (HB-EGF)-like growth factor *(74)*. It also prevents TNF-α from inducing increase in HB-EGF mRNA production *(74)*.

Finally, adiponectin may mediate endothelial vasodilatation, because plasma adiponectin was independently correlated with peak forearm blood flow and vasodilator response to reactive hyperemia *(36,84)*, and stimulate production of the vasodilatory agent NO in vascular endothelial cells *(55)*.

FUTURE THERAPEUTIC DIRECTIONS

Because the adverse cardiovascular events associated with obesity may be related to the relative decrease in adiponectin, supplementing this protein exogenously, increasing endogenous production, or designing agonists for its receptor need to be tested in relation to cardiovascular outcomes. PPAR-α agonists have been shown to increase adiponectin levels in lean, obese, and diabetic humans (38). Because their ability to improve insulin resistance may be mediated by adiponectin, they may also prove to have an added indication for CVD. Angiotensin-converting enzyme inhibitors and angiotensin receptor blockers also may increase adiponectin (68), which may mediate in part their beneficial effects in insulin-resistant states including CVD. β-Adrenergic antagonists may also have similar use, as they prevent catecholamine-induced suppression of adiponectin production (32). Finally, with the discovery of adiponectin receptors, agonists at these sites may allow for targeted augmentation of adiponectin's effects in metabolically active tissues.

CONCLUSION

Obesity has long been associated with insulin resistance, hypertension, and CAD, but the mechanism has remained largely unknown. Adiponectin may be one of the factors that explains these associations. Because deficiencies in adiponectin may result in the development of these processes, increased endogenous production or exogenously administered adiponectin or its agonists may contribute to restoring insulin sensitivity and preventing atherosclerosis by increasing fatty acid oxidation and insulin-mediated glucose uptake, and decreasing the endothelial inflammatory process associated with atherosclerotic plaque development. Although animal studies have demonstrated benefits, clinical trials are needed to determine whether the beneficial effects of adiponectin can also be observed in humans and whether either adiponectin or adiponectin receptor agonists represent a novel treatment option for type II diabetes and CAD.

ACKNOWLEDGMENT

This chapter was supported by NIDDK grant DK 58785 and NIH grant K30 HL04095.

REFERENCES

1. Rajala MW, Scherer PE. Minireview: The adipocytes—at the crossroads of energy homeostasis, inflammation, and atherosclerosis. Endocrinology 2003;144:3765–3773.
2. Havel PJ. Control of energy homeostasis and insulin action by adipocyte hormones: leptin, acylation stimulating protein, and adiponectin. Curr Opin Lipidol 2002;13:51–59.
3. Scherer PE, Williams S, Fogliano M, Baldini G, Lodish HF. A novel serum protein similar to C1q, produced exclusively in adipocytes. J Biol Chem 1995;270:26,746–26,749.
4. Maeda K, Okubo K, Shimomura I, Funahashi T, Matsuzawa Y, Matsubara K. cDNA cloning and expression of a novel adipose specific collagen-like factor, apM1 (AdiPose Most abundant Gene transcript 1). Biochem Biophys Res Commun 1996;221:286–289.
5. Hu E, Liang P, Spiegelman BM. AdipoQ is a novel adipose-specific gene dysregulated in obesity. J Biol Chem 1996;271:10,697–10,703.
6. Nakano Y, Tobe T, Choi-Miura NH, Mazda T, Tomita M. Isolation and characterization of GBP28, a novel gelatin-binding protein purified from human plasma. J Biochem (Tokyo) 1996;120:803–812.
7. Arita Y, Kihara S, Ouchi N, et al. Paradoxical decrease of an adipose-specific protein, adiponectin, in obesity. Biochem Biophys Res Commun 1999;257:79–83.

8. Gavrila A, Peng CK, Chan JL, Mietus JE, Goldberger AL, Mantzoros CS. Diurnal and ultradian dynamics of serum adiponectin in healthy men: comparison with leptin, circulating soluble leptin receptor, and cortisol patterns. J Clin Endocrinol Metab 2003;88:2838–2843.

9. Cnop M, Havel PJ, Utzschneider KM, et al. Relationship of adiponectin to body fat distribution, insulin sensitivity and plasma lipoproteins: evidence for independent roles of age and sex. Diabetologia 2003;46:459–469.

10. Pajvani UB, Du X, Combs TP, et al. Structure-function studies of the adipocyte-secreted hormone Acrp30/adiponectin. Implications fpr metabolic regulation and bioactivity. J Biol Chem 2003;278:9073–9085.

11. Shapiro L, Scherer PE. The crystal structure of a complement-1q family protein suggests an evolutionary link to tumor necrosis factor. Curr Biol 1998;8:335–338.

12. Ruan H, Lodish HF. Insulin resistance in adipose tissue: direct and indirect effects of tumor necrosis factor-alpha. Cytokine Growth Factor Rev 2003;14:447–455.

13. Kern PA, Di Gregorio GB, Lu T, Rassouli N, Ranganathan G. Adiponectin expression from human adipose tissue: relation to obesity, insulin resistance, and tumor necrosis factor-alpha expression. Diabetes 2003;52:1779–1785.

14. Hotta K, Funahashi T, Arita Y, et al. Plasma concentrations of a novel, adipose-specific protein, adiponectin, in type 2 diabetic patients. Arterioscler Thromb Vasc Biol 2000;20:1595–1599.

15. Yang WS, Lee WJ, Funahashi T, et al. Weight reduction increases plasma levels of an adipose-derived anti-inflammatory protein, adiponectin. J Clin Endocrinol Metab 2001;86:3815–3819.

16. Faraj M, Havel PJ, Phelis S, Blank D, Sniderman AD, Cianflone K. Plasma acylation-stimulating protein, adiponectin, leptin, and ghrelin before and after weight loss induced by gastric bypass surgery in morbidly obese subjects. J Clin Endocrinol Metab 2003;88:1594–1602.

17. Esposito K, Pontillo A, Di Palo C, et al. Effect of weight loss and lifestyle changes on vascular inflammatory markers in obese women: a randomized trial. JAMA 2003;289:1799–1804.

18. Zhang Y, Matheny M, Zolotukhin S, Tumer N, Scarpace PJ. Regulation of adiponectin and leptin gene expression in white and brown adipose tissues: influence of beta3-adrenergic agonists, retinoic acid, leptin and fasting. Biochim Biophys Acta 2002;1584:115–122.

19. Gavrila A, Chan JL, Yiannakouris N, et al. Serum adiponectin levels are inversely associated with central fat distribution and estrogen levels but are not directly regulated by acute fasting or leptin administration in humans: cross-sectional and interventional studies. J Clin Endocrinol Metab 2003;88:4823–4831.

20. Yannakoulia M, Yiannakouris N, Bluher S, Matalas AL, Klimis-Zacas D, Mantzoros CS. Body fat mass and macronutrient intake in relation to circulating soluble leptin receptor, free leptin index, adiponectin, and resistin concentrations in healthy humans. J Clin Endocrinol Metab 2003;88:1730–1736.

21. Peake PW, Kriketos AD, Denyer GS, Campbell LV, Charlesworth JA. The postprandial response of adiponectin to a high-fat meal in normal and insulin-resistant subjects. Int J Obes Relat Metab Disord 2003;27:657–662.

22. English PJ, Coughlin SR, Hayden K, Malik IA, Wilding JP. Plasma adiponectin increases postprandially in obese, but not in lean, subjects. Obes Res 2003;11:839–844.

23. Motoshima H, Wu X, Sinha MK, et al. Differential regulation of adiponectin secretion from cultured human omental and subcutaneous adipocytes: effects of insulin and rosiglitazone. J Clin Endocrinol Metab 2002;87:5662–5667.

24. Halleux CM, Takahashi M, Delporte ML, et al. Secretion of adiponectin and regulation of apM1 gene expression in human visceral adipose tissue. Biochem Biophys Res Commun 2001;288:1102–1107.

25. Fasshauer M, Klein J, Neumann S, Eszlinger M, Paschke R. Hormonal regulation of adiponectin gene expression in 3T3-L1 adipocytes. Biochem Biophys Res Commun 2002;290:1084–1089.

26. Mohlig M, Wegewitz U, Osterhoff M, et al. Insulin decreases human adiponectin plasma levels. Horm Metab Res 2002;34:655–658.

27. Nishizawa H, Shimomura I, Kishida K, et al. Androgens decrease plasma adiponectin, an insulin-sensitizing adipocyte-derived protein. Diabetes 2002;51:2734–2741.

28. Olefsky JM, Kruszynska YT. Causes of insulin resistance. In: De Groot, L. (ed). De Groot's Textbook of Endocrinology, 4th ed. WB Saunders: Philadelphia, PA, 2001, pp. 780–782.

29. Yamauchi T, Kamon J, Waki H, et al. The fat-derived hormone adiponectin reverses insulin resistance associated with both lipoatrophy and obesity. Nat Med 2001;7:941–946.

30. Matsubara M, Maruoka S, Katayose S. Inverse relationship between plasma adiponectin and leptin concentrations in normal-weight and obese women. Eur J Endocrinol 2002;147:173–180.

31. Delporte ML, Funahashi T, Takahashi M, Matsuzawa Y, Brichard SM. Pre- and post-translational negative effect of beta-adrenoceptor agonists on adiponectin secretion: in vitro and in vivo studies. Biochem J 2002;367:677–685.

32. Fasshauer M, Klein J, Neumann S, Eszlinger M, Paschke R Adiponectin gene expression is inhibited by beta-adrenergic stimulation via protein kinase A in 3T3-L1 adipocytes. FEBS Lett 2001;507:142–146.

33. Bruun JM, Lihn AS, Verdich C, et al. Regulation of adiponectin by adipose tissue-derived cytokines: in vivo and in vitro investigations in humans. Am J Physiol Endocrinol Metab 2003;285:E527–E33.

34. Maeda N, Takahashi M, Funahashi T, et al. PPARgamma ligands increase expression and plasma concentrations of adiponectin, an adipose-derived protein. Diabetes 2001;50:2094–2099.

35. Maeda N, Shimomura I, Kishida K, et al. Diet-induced insulin resistance in mice lacking adiponectin/ACRP30. Nat Med 2002;8:731–737.

36. Hsueh WA, Law R. The central role of fat and effect of peroxisome proliferator-activated receptor-gamma on progression of insulin resistance and cardiovascular disease. Am J Cardiol 2003;92:3J–9J.

37. Yang WS, Jeng CY, Wu TJ, et al. Synthetic peroxisome proliferator-activated receptor-gamma agonist, rosiglitazone, increases plasma levels of adiponectin in type 2 diabetic patients. Diabetes Care 2002;25:376–380.

38. Yu JG, Javorschi S, Hevener AL, et al. The effect of thiazolidinediones on plasma adiponectin levels in normal, obese, and type 2 diabetic subjects. Diabetes 2002;51:2968–2974.

39. Iwaki M, Matsuda M, Maeda N, et al. Induction of adiponectin, a fat-derived antidiabetic and antiatherogenic factor, by nuclear receptors. Diabetes 2003;52:1655–1663.

40. Diez JJ, Iglesias P. The role of the novel adipocyte-derived hormone adiponectin in human disease. Eur J Endocrinol 2003;148:293–300.

41. Kondo H, Shimomura I, Matsukawa Y, et al. Association of adiponectin mutation with type 2 diabetes: a candidate gene for the insulin resistance syndrome. Diabetes 2002;51:2325–2328.

42. Kubota N, Terauchi Y, Yamauchi T, et al. Disruption of adiponectin causes insulin resistance and neointimal formation. J Biol Chem 2002;277:25,863–25,866.

43. Hotta K, Funahashi T, Bodkin NL, et al. Circulating concentrations of the adipocyte protein adiponectin are decreased in parallel with reduced insulin sensitivity during the progression to type 2 diabetes in rhesus monkeys. Diabetes 2001;50:1126–1133.

44. Weyer C, Funahashi T, Tanaka S, et al. Hypoadiponectinemia in obesity and type 2 diabetes: close association with insulin resistance and hyperinsulinemia. J Clin Endocrinol Metab 2001;86:1930–1935.

45. Lindsay RS, Funahashi T, Hanson RL, et al. Adiponectin and development of type 2 diabetes in the Pima Indian population. Lancet 2002;360:57–58.

46. Spranger J, Kroke A, Mohlig M, et al. Adiponectin and protection against type 2 diabetes mellitus. Lancet 2003;361:226–228.

47. Daimon M, Oizumi T, Saitoh T, et al. Decreased serum levels of adiponectin are a risk factor for the progression to type 2 diabetes in the Japanese Population: the Funagata study. Diabetes Care 2003;26:2015–2020.

48. Imagawa A, Funahashi T, Nakamura T, et al. Elevated serum concentration of adipose-derived factor, adiponectin, in patients with type 1 diabetes. Diabetes Care 2002;25:1665–1666.

49. Tomas E, Tsao TS, Saha AK, et al. Enhanced muscle fat oxidation and glucose transport by ACRP30 globular domain: acetyl-CoA carboxylase inhibition and AMP-activated protein kinase activation. Proc Natl Acad Sci USA 2002;99:16,309–16,313.

50. Yamauchi T, Kamon J, Minokoshi Y, et al. Adiponectin stimulates glucose utilization and fatty-acid oxidation by activating AMP-activated protein kinase. Nat Med 2002;8:1288–1295.

51. Wu X, Motoshima H, Mahadev K, Stalker TJ, Scalia R, Goldstein BJ. Involvement of AMP-activated protein kinase in glucose uptake stimulated by the globular domain of adiponectin in primary rat adipocytes. Diabetes 2003;52:1355–1363.

52. Boden G. Role of fatty acids in the pathogenesis of insulin resistance and NIDDM. Diabetes 1997; 46: 3–10.

53. Berg AH, Combs TP, Du X, Brownlee M, Scherer PE. The adipocyte-secreted protein Acrp30 enhances hepatic insulin action. Nat Med 2001;7:947–953.

54. Combs TP, Berg AH, Obici S, Scherer PE, Rossetti L. Endogenous glucose production is inhibited by the adipose-derived protein Acrp30. J Clin Invest 2001;108:1875–1881.

55. Chen H, Montagnani M, Funahashi T, Shimomura I, Quon MJ. Adiponectin stimulates production of nitric oxide in vascular endothelial cells. J Biol Chem 2003;278:45,021–45,026.

56. Fruebis J, Tsao TS, Javorschi S, et al. Proteolytic cleavage product of 30-kDa adipocyte complement-related protein increases fatty acid oxidation in muscle and causes weight loss in mice. Proc Natl Acad Sci USA 2001;98:2005–2010.

57. Yamauchi T, Kamon J, Ito Y, et al. Cloning of adiponectin receptors that mediate antidiabetic metabolic effects. Nature 2003;423:762–769.

58. Stefan N, Vozarova B, Funahashi T, et al. Plasma adiponectin concentration is associated with skeletal muscle insulin receptor tyrosine phosphorylation, and low plasma concentration precedes a decrease in whole-body insulin sensitivity in humans. Diabetes 2002;51:1884–1888.

59. Zietz B, Herfarth H, Paul G, et al. Adiponectin represents an independent cardiovascular risk factor predicting serum HDL-cholesterol levels in type 2 diabetes. FEBS Lett 2003;545:103–104.

60. Matsubara M, Maruoka S, Katayose S. Decreased plasma adiponectin concentrations in women with dyslipidemia. J Clin Endocrinol Metab 2002;87:2764–2769.

61. Ma K, Cabrero A, Saha PK, et al. Increased beta-oxidation but no insulin resistance or glucose intolerance in mice lacking adiponectin. J Biol Chem 2002;277:34658–34661.

62. Stefan N, Vozarova B, Funahashi T, et al. Plasma adiponectin levels are not associated with fat oxidation in humans. Obes Res 2002;10:1016–1020.

63. Ouchi N, Ohishi M, Kihara S, et al. Association of hypoadiponectinemia with impaired vasoreactivity. Hypertension 2003;42:231–234.

64. Mallamaci F, Zoccali C, Cuzzola F, et al. Adiponectin in essential hypertension. J Nephrol 2002;15:507–511.

65. Adamczak M, Wiecek A, Funahashi T, Chudek J, Kokot F, Matsuzawa Y. Decreased plasma adiponectin concentration in patients with essential hypertension. Am J Hypertens 2003;16:72–75.

66. Kazumi T, Kawaguchi A, Sakai K, Hirano T, Yoshino G. Young men with high-normal blood pressure have lower serum adiponectin, smaller LDL size, and higher elevated heart rate than those with optimal blood pressure. Diabetes Care 2002;25:971–976.

67. Huang KC, Chen CL, Chuang LM, Ho SR, Tai TY, Yang WS. Plasma adiponectin levels and blood pressures in nondiabetic adolescent females. J Clin Endocrinol Metab 2003;88:4130–4134.

68. Furuhashi M, Ura N, Higashiura K, et al. Blockade of the renin-angiotensin system increases adiponectin concentrations in patients with essential hypertension. Hypertension 2003;42:76–81.

69. Miyazaki T, Shimada K, Mokuno H, Daida H. Adipocyte derived plasma protein, adiponectin, is associated with smoking status in patients with coronary artery disease. Heart 2003;89:663.

70. Okamoto Y, Arita Y, Nishida M, et al. An adipocyte-derived plasma protein, adiponectin, adheres to injured vascular walls. Horm Metab Res 2000;32:47–50.

71. Zoccali C, Mallamaci F, Tripepi G, et al. Adiponectin, metabolic risk factors, and cardiovascular events among patients with end-stage renal disease. J Am Soc Nephrol 2002;13:134–141.

72. Kumada M, Kihara S, Sumitsuji S, et al., and the Osaka CAD Study Group. Association of hypoadiponectinemia with coronary artery disease in men. Arterioscler Thromb Vasc Biol 2003;23:85–89.

73. Okamoto Y, Kihara S, Ouchi N, et al. Adiponectin reduces atherosclerosis in apolipoprotein E-deficient mice. Circulation 2002;106:2767–2770.

74. Matsuda M, Shimomura I, Sata M, et al. Role of adiponectin in preventing vascular stenosis. The missing link of adipo-vascular axis. J Biol Chem 2002;277:37487–91.

75. Krakoff J, Funahashi T, Stehouwer CD, et al. Inflammatory markers, adiponectin, and risk of type 2 diabetes in the Pima Indian. Diabetes Care 2003;26:1745–1751.

76. Ouchi N, Kihara S, Funahashi T, et al. Reciprocal association of C-reactive protein with adiponectin in blood stream and adipose tissue. Circulation 2003;107:671–674.

77. Engeli S, Feldpausch M, Gorzelniak K, et al. Association between adiponectin and mediators of inflammation in obese women. Diabetes 2003;52:942–947.

78. Fernandez-Real JM, Lopez-Bermejo A, Casamitjana R, Ricart W. Novel interactions of adiponectin with the endocrine system and inflammatory parameters. J Clin Endocrinol Metab 2003;88:2714–2718.

79. Ouchi N, Kihara S, Arita Y, et al. Novel modulator for endothelial adhesion molecules: adipocyte-derived plasma protein adiponectin. Circulation 1999;100:2473–2476.

80. Ouchi N, Kihara S, Arita Y, et al. Adiponectin, an adipocyte-derived plasma protein, inhibits endothelial NF-kappaB signaling through a cAMP-dependent pathway. Circulation 2000;102:1296–1301.

81. Ouchi N, Kihara S, Arita Y, et al. Adipocyte-derived plasma protein, adiponectin, suppresses lipid accumulation and class A scavenger receptor expression in human monocyte-derived macrophages. Circulation 2001;103:1057–1063.

82. Yokota T, Oritani K, Takahashi I, et al. Adiponectin, a new member of the family of soluble defense collagens, negatively regulates the growth of myelomonocytic progenitors and the functions of macrophages. Blood 2000;96:1723–1732.

83. Arita Y, Kihara S, Ouchi N, et al. Adipocyte-derived plasma protein adiponectin acts as a platelet-derived growth factor-BB-binding protein and regulates growth factor-induced common postreceptor signal in vascular smooth muscle cell. Circulation 2002;105:2893–2898.

84. Shimabukuro M, Higa N, Asahi T, et al. Hypoadiponectinemia is closely linked to endothelial dysfunction in man. J Clin Endocrinol Metab 2003;88:3236–3240.

10 Nitric Oxide and Its Role in Diabetes Mellitus

Michael T. Johnstone, MD and Eli V. Gelfand, MD

INTRODUCTION

Diabetes mellitus (DM) is a major source of morbidity in the United States, affecting between 10 and 15 million people *(1)*. The cause of much of this morbidity and mortality is vascular disease, including both atherosclerosis and microangiopathy *(2-5)*. As discussed elsewhere in this text, atherosclerosis occurs earlier in diabetics than nondiabetics, its severity is often greater, and its distribution is more diffuse *(6,7)*. Vascular disease in diabetics affects not only large vessels but microvasculature as well, resulting in both diabetic retinopathy and nephropathy *(8,9)*.

Because diabetes is a vascular disease, much attention has been given to the vascular endothelium. It has a pivotal role in maintaining the homeostasis of the blood vessels. The endothelium's functions include modulating blood cell–vessel wall interaction and regulating blood fluidity, angiogenesis, lipoprotein metabolism, and vasomotion. One mediator that serves a significant function in maintaining vascular homeostasis is nitric oxide (NO), also known as endothelium-derived relaxing factor (EDRF). Alterations in its elaboration, activity, or degradation play an important role in the initiation and progression of vascular diseases.

From: *Contemporary Cardiology: Diabetes and Cardiovascular Disease, Second Edition*
Edited by: M. T. Johnstone and A. Veves © Humana Press Inc., Totowa, NJ

ENDOTHELIUM-DERIVED RELAXING FACTOR

In 1980, Furchgott discovered that the endothelium is responsible for the vasodilator action of acetylcholine *(10)*. This finding has fostered a great number of investigations on the role of the endothelium on the initiation and development of vascular disease and its subsequent clinical sequelae. Further research indicated that acetylcholine released a soluble factor from the endothelium termed EDRF and that this substance was released by other agents including bradykinin, substance P, serotonin, and adenosine triphosphate (ATP), and shear stress *(11)*. Ignarro used spectral analysis of hemoglobin to prove that EDRF was identical to NO *(12)*. Shortly thereafter, Palmer and colleagues concluded that NO was derived from the terminal guanidino nitrogen of the amino acid L-arginine. The production of NO is catalyzed by the family of enzymes known as NO synthase (NOS) *(13)*. Three isoforms of NOS have been identified: endothelial NOS (eNOS), neuronal NOS (nNOS), and cytokine-inducible NOS (iNOS) *(14)*. Although eNOS is expressed constitutively in endothelial cells, its activity can be modulated by many factors, including shear stress. Vascular smooth muscle responds to NO via stimulation of soluble guanylate cyclase and the formation of cyclic guanosine monophosphate (cGMP) *(12)*. cGMP activates cGMP-dependent protein kinases, which cause vascular smooth muscle relaxation by way of increased calcium extrusion from the cell and increased uptake into the sarcoplasmic reticulum *(15–17)* (Fig. 1). NO can affect systems that are cGMP independent, as well, including cytosolic adenosine 5'-diphosphate (ADP)-ribosobyl-transferase in the platelets, which catalyzes the transfer of ADP ribose to glyceraldehyde 3-phosphate dehydrogenase *(18)*.

NO appears to be released continuously in vivo because inhibition of NO synthesis results in vasoconstriction and hypertension *(19)*. Knockout mice, deficient in eNOS (-/-) develop hypertension, hyperlipidemia, and glucose intolerance *(20)*. Vascular disease may result in a chronic decrease in the tonic release of NO, and hypoxia reduces NO synthesis by inhibiting expression of eNOS *(21)*. Although NO synthesis occurs in a wide variety of cell types and tissues other than vascular endothelium including platelets, macrophages, and neuronal cells, the focus of this discussion is NO and the endothelium.

PHYSIOLOGIC EFFECTS OF NITRIC OXIDE ON THE VASCULAR SYSTEM

NO is released continuously by vascular endothelial cells through the action of eNOS, and this basal release regulates vascular tone. NO is important in the maintenance of resting vascular tone *(22)*, in particular the regulation of coronary resistance vessels as well as pulmonary, renal, and cerebral vascular resistance *(23,24)*. NO production is highest in the resistance vessels and may be important in the regulation of vascular tone of various vascular beds *(25)*, as well as blood pressure (BP) control. NO also modulates vascular tone by regulating the expression of various endothelial vasoconstrictors and growth factors, including platelet-derived growth factor-B and endothelin-1 (ET-1) *(26)*.

NO appears to be involved in the regulation of myocardial contractility by a cGMP-dependent mechanism. This regulation is possibly via the microvascular endothelium, which is in close proximity to cardiac myocytes. Increased iNOS in cardiac myocytes produces a level of NO that reduces myocardial contractility significantly *(27)*. NO can also modulate myocardial contractility by decreasing the intracellular levels of cyclic adenosine monophosphate in response to β-adrenergic stimulation *(28)*.

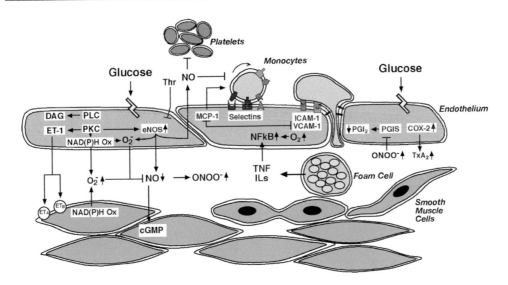

Fig. 1. Hyperglycemia and endothelium-derived vasocative substances. Hyperglycemia decreased the bioavailability of nitric oxide (NO) and prostacyclin (PGI₂) and increased the synthesis of vasoconstrictor prostanoids and endothelin (ET-1) via multiple mechanisms (*see* text). PLC, phospholipase C; DAG, diacylglycerol; PKC, protein kinase C; eNOS, endothelial nitric oxide synthase: Thr, thrombin; NAD(P)H Ox, nicotinamide adenine dinucleotide phosphate oxidase; O₂⁻, superoxide anion; OONO⁻, peroxynitrite; MCP, monocyte chemoattractant protein-1; NFκb, nuclear factor κ b; TNF, tumor necrosis factor; Ils, interleukins; COX-2, cyclooxygense-2. (Reproduced with permission from ref. *127*.)

NO also serves to maintain the integrity of the vascular endothelium through its interaction of both platelets and leukocytes with the vessel wall. Substances released during platelet activation (ADP), or the coagulation cascade (thrombin) stimulate NO production *(29)*. NO is then released from the endothelium into the vessel lumen, in which it interacts with platelets and disaggregates them via a cGMP-dependent mechanism *(30)*. NO also serves to attenuate leukocyte–vascular wall interactions. Inhibition of NO promotes leukocyte adhesion to the endothelium and causes a rapid increase in microvascular permeability and vascular leakage that is characteristic of an acute inflammatory response *(31)*.

In vitro *(32)* and in vivo *(33)* studies have demonstrated that NO can also attenuate vascular smooth muscle proliferation. Animal studies have shown that L-arginine, the substrate for NOS, impairs neointimal proliferation after vascular injury *(34)*.

NITRIC OXIDE AND THE DEVELOPMENT OF ATHEROSCLEROSIS

All the major cardiovascular risk factors (including hypertension, high levels of low-density lipoprotein [LDL] cholesterol, tobacco use, and hyperhomocysteinemia) are associated with decreased endothelium-dependent vasodilation prior to the development of clinically apparent vascular disease. This would suggest that the endothelial damage is implicated in the development of atherosclerosis *(35)*.

After endothelial injury, platelets aggregate in those areas of cell damage, releasing growth factors and cytokines. As a result, the endothelium is more permeable to lipoproteins and other macromolecules, resulting in subendothelial accumulation of LDL cholesterol, either directly or incorporated into macrophages. The LDL becomes oxidized, further promoting the development of atherosclerosis. This leads to vascular smooth muscle migration from the media to the intima and consequent intimal proliferation and extracellular matrix production.

NO plays a major role in preventing the development of atherosclerosis. Any decrease in NO production or level may result in the promotion of this process. The extent of atherosclerosis in both animal and human arteries correlates with the impairment of endothelium-dependent vasodilation (36). In experimental models in which there was chronic inhibition of NOS, the degree of atherosclerosis increased. Conversely, the addition of L-arginine, the substrate for NOS, the NOS gene, or the administration of a protein adduct of NO to hypercholesterolemic rabbits, not only increased the degree of endothelium-dependent vasodilation but also inhibited neointimal formation (37).

Specifically, NO inhibits the adhesion and migration of leukocytes including macrophages and monocytes, and the generation of proinflammatory cytokines including tumor necrosis factor (38). NO attenuates the expression of adhesion molecules such as E-selectin, which are necessary for leukocyte-endothelial cell interactions. NO also increases the production of IκBα, the inhibitor of nuclear factor (NF) κB, which reduces the inflammatory response (39–41). Finally, NO inhibits the proliferation and migration of vascular smooth muscle cells (32), resulting in vasodilation of the coronary vessels.

ENDOTHELIAL DYSFUNCTION AND DIABETES MELLITUS

Although the link between diabetes and cardiovascular disease is not well understood, endothelial dysfunction may be implicated in the pathogenesis of diabetic vascular disease. The evidence of endothelial dysfunction in diabetes comes largely from studies measuring the endothelial substances that mediate fibrinolysis and coagulation. Chapters 2 and 6 give detailed descriptions of these studies. For example, plasminogen activator inhibitor-1 levels are increased, whereas fibrinolytic activity and prostacyclin levels are decreased in both type 1 and 2 diabetes (42–45).

Endothelium-Dependent Vasodilation in Animal Models

Studies using different animal models of diabetes in several different vascular beds (46–49) suggest that there is a decrease in endothelium-dependent vasodilation in the diabetic state. In two such animal models of type 1 diabetes, rats are made diabetic with streptozocin or rabbits made diabetic with alloxan, pancreatic β-cells are destroyed, with a corresponding decrease in insulin secretion. Studies evaluating endothelium-dependent vasodilation in these animal models have demonstrated a decreased response to endothelial stimulators such as ADP, acetylcholine, or its analogue methacholine (47).

Similarly, in an animal model of type 2 diabetes, the Zucker rat, which is characterized by hyperglycemia because of insulin resistance, abnormal endothelium-dependent vasodilation is also seen (46). The early vascular dysfunction that occurs in type 1 diabetic animal models can be prevented by insulin therapy (50,51). The abnormal endothelial cell function that develops appears to be as a result of hyperglycemia rather than any other metabolic disturbance. This has been demonstrated by in vitro incubation experiments in which isolated arteries exposed to elevated glucose concentrations have similar decreases in endothelium-dependent vasodilation (52,53). This effect does not seem to be as a result of the hyperosmolarity because similar concentrations of mannitol have no effect on endothelium-dependent relaxation (52). The decreased endothelium-dependent vasodilation that occurs may be as a result of decreased synthesis or release of NO, decreased responsiveness of the smooth muscle to NO, the inactivation of NO by superoxide radicals, or the generation of endothelial vasoconstrictive factors. This will be discussed in greater detail later in this chapter.

Early in the course of experimental diabetes, there is a selective decrease in the response to those endothelium-dependent vasodilators that are mediated by endothelial cell receptors. The responsiveness of the endothelium to the direct endothelial vasodilator A23187, or the smooth muscle to nitrovasodilators, is preserved. Using a diabetic rabbit model, abnormal endothelium-dependent relaxation was also found *(54)* within 6 weeks of initiating the diabetic state. This may be explained by a decrease in the number of receptors, or in their function. These changes are specific to the diabetic state because these abnormal responses do not occur within 2 weeks after initiating the diabetic state and are not found in rabbits not made diabetic after alloxan treatment *(55)*. Yet after a longer duration of diabetes, several groups have demonstrated a decrease in smooth muscle cGMP, suggesting a decrease in NO release or action over time *(46,56)*.

Endothelial cell dysfunction in diabetes may be explained in part not only to perturbations in NO activity or levels but the effect of vasoconstrictor prostanoids. There is increased expression of cyclooxygenase-2 mRNA and proteins levels with hyperglycemia in cultured human aortic endothelial cells but not cyclooxygenase-1. Cohen's group noted that endothelium-dependent relaxation in arteries of diabetic animals could be restored by the administration of cyclo-oxygenase inhibitors or thromboxane A_2 receptor antagonists, suggesting the presence of vasoconstrictor prostanoids *(48,53)*. The responsiveness of smooth muscle to direct smooth muscle vasodilators is similar in both diabetic and normal animal models, suggesting that decreased responsiveness to NO is not affected *(47,48)*.

This is an increase in oxygen-derived free radicals *(57)*, either because of an increase in free radical production or because of a decrease in the free radical scavenger system. Furthermore, free radical scavengers have been shown to improve the abnormal endothelium-dependent vasodilation *(58,59)*, implying that such free radicals may contribute to the abnormal endothelium-dependent relaxations.

Human Studies of Endothelium-Dependent Vasodilation

INSULIN-DEPENDENT DIABETES MELLITUS

Human studies evaluating the effects of DM on endothelium-dependent vasodilation have yielded some conflicting results, although they generally corroborate those found in animal studies. Saenz de Tejada et al. *(60)* studied penile tissue excised from men with erectile dysfunction and found that endothelium-dependent relaxation is reduced in the corpus cavernosa of impotent men with diabetes relative to those who are nondiabetic.

However, in vivo studies involving human subjects with insulin-dependent diabetes have demonstrated both blunted and normal vasodilatory responses to acetylcholine, methacholine, or carbachol (the latter two being acetylcholine analogs) in forearm resistance vessels in patients with DM *(61–63)*. To evaluate in vivo endothelial function in these vessels, we and others have employed the venous occlusive plethysmography technique. Type 1 diabetic *(61)* individuals were shown to have impaired endothelium-dependent responses to methacholine in the forearm resistance vessels (Fig. 2A). The vasodilator response to both nitroprusside (Fig. 2B) and verapamil, both endothelium-independent, were preserved. In this study, all the patients were taking aspirin, making it unlikely that vasodilator prostanoids were responsible for the altered endothelium-dependent relaxation. The degree of attenuation of forearm blood flow (FBF) response

A

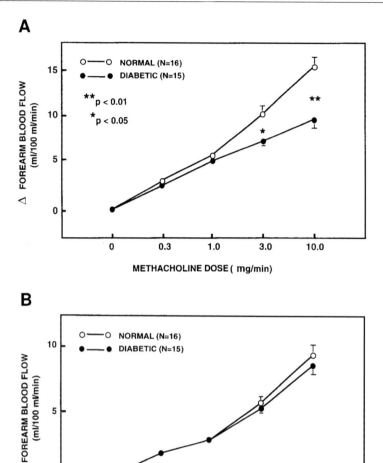

Fig. 2. Forearm blood flow (FBF) dose–response curves to intra-arterial (**A**) methacholine chloride and (**B**) in normal and insulin-dependent diabetic subjects. The cholinergic (**A**; endothelium-dependent) response in the diabetic patients is significantly lower than the normal group at the higher dosages, whereas the nitroprusside (**B**) response is not significantly different between the two groups (From ref. *63a*.)

to methacholine was inversely correlated with the serum insulin level, but it did not significantly correlate with serum glucose concentration, glycosylated hemoglobin, or duration of diabetes.

Calver et al. *(63)* reported a decrease in responsiveness of N-monomethyl-L-arginine (L-NMMA), an inhibitor of NOS, suggesting a decrease in the basal NO release from the endothelium. Conversely, Smits et al. *(62)* and Halkin et al. *(64)* did not detect any impairment in endothelium-dependent vasodilation with type 1 diabetes. Both flow-mediated relaxation and endothelium-independent responses have also been found to be impaired in nonatherosclerotic peripheral conduit arteries and in angiographically normal coronary vessels in diabetic subjects *(65,66)*.

The reason for these contradictory results is unclear and probably multifactorial. Closer examination of these reports reveals that the subject population was not uniform between the various groups. Variations included the presence or absence of macrovascular or microvascular complications and autonomic dysfunction, the gender studied (single sex vs mixed), the degree of long-term glycemic control, the serum glucose concentration, the presence or absence of microalbuminuria, and the serum insulin concentration. Microalbuminuria, an early marker of diabetic nephropathy and a predictor of coronary artery disease (CAD), may correlate with the severity of endothelial dysfunction. Endothelial function in insulin-dependent diabetic subjects was normal in those studies that excluded individuals with microalbuminuria *(62,64)* and abnormal in the study that included subjects with microalbuminuria *(63)*.

The degree of glucose control may, in part, explain the variation in the data *(61,63,67)*, because it has been established that glucose alone can alter endothelial function *(68)*. The serum insulin concentration was not routinely measured in most of these studies, although we found an inverse relationship between the serum insulin concentration and endothelial function *(61)*. Studies involving mixed genders might add further variation relative to studies with men alone because women appear to be protected against the adverse effects of risk factors of endothelium-dependent vasodilation compared with men *(69)*. Lastly, the presence of autonomic dysfunction in the study subjects may alter the response to the various agents administered.

NONINSULIN-DEPENDENT DIABETES MELLITUS

Two groups have demonstrated reduced endothelium-dependent and -independent vasodilation in noninsulin-dependent DM *(70,71)* (Fig. 3). These results would suggest that NO is inactivated by either oxygen-derived free radicals or an abnormality in the signal transduction of the guanylate cyclase pathway. Therefore, the mechanism of the impairment of vasodilation in type 2 diabetes is different from that of type 1. It is important to note that noninsulin-dependent diabetic patients are usually older and have other cardiovascular risk factors, including dyslipidemia and hypertension *(72)*, which in themselves can contribute to an impairment of endothelial function.

POSSIBLE MECHANISMS OF IMPAIRED ENDOTHELIUM-DEPENDENT VASODILATION

Although the data are conflicting, overwhelming evidence presently suggests that DM is associated with an impairment of endothelial vasodilation. The mechanism(s) for this impairment is even less well understood. The most likely initial insult is hyperglycemia. Tesfamarian and colleagues took normal rabbit aortic rings and exposed them to high concentrations of glucose (up to 800 mg/dL for 3 hours), resulting in a decrease in endothelium-dependent relaxation, in response to acetylcholine and ADP *(52,53)*. This effect appears to be both concentration and time dependent. As stated earlier, this effect does not appear to be a result of the hyperosmolar effects of glucose because mannitol did not cause any such endothelium-dependent vasodilation *(53)*. Bohlen and Lash *(73)* demonstrated that hyperglycemia at 300 and 500 mg/dL suppressed the vasodilatory response to acetylcholine but not to nitroprusside. Similarly, Williams and colleagues *(68)* found that acute hyperglycemia attenuated endothelium-dependent relaxation in forearm resistance vessels in healthy humans (Fig. 4). Akbari and colleagues *(74)* found that acute hyperglycemia resulted in similar degrees of impairment of endothelium-dependent vasodilation in the micro- and macrocirculation (Fig. 5).

A

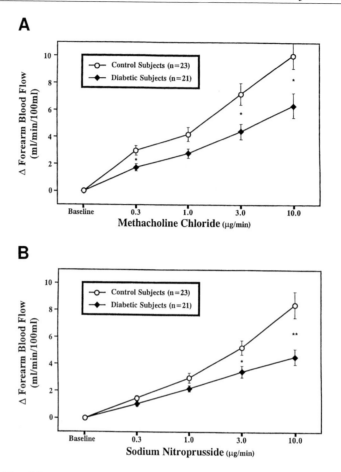

B

Fig. 3. Forearm blood flow (FBF) dose–response curves to intra-arterial (**A**) methacholine chloride and (**B**) nitroprusside in normal and noninsulin-dependent diabetic subjects. Both the cholinergic (**A**) and nitroprusside (**B**) responses in the diabetic patients are significantly lower than the normal age-matched control group at the higher dosages (From ref. *63a.*)

In contrast, Houben and coworkers *(75)* did not find that acute hyperglycemia resulted in an impairment of NO-mediated relaxation in the human forearm. This discrepancy may be explained by the fact that Williams and colleagues *(68)* used a hyperglycemic clamp to maintain the high-glucose level in the forearm along with infusion of octreotide, an inhibitor of insulin secretion. With increasing serum glucose, serum insulin level increases, which itself can result in vasodilation. By infusing octreotide, the confounding effect of increasing insulin levels is eliminated.

The proposed mechanisms by which glucose affects endothelial function may result from the decreased production of NO, the inactivation of NO by free radicals, increased circulating levels of free fatty acids (FAs), and/or the increased production of endothelium-derived contracting factors (Table 1).

IMPAIRED NITRIC OXIDE SYNTHESIS AND/OR SENSITIVITY

NO is continuously synthesized in endothelial cells by eNOS with L-arginine and oxygen, resulting in the formation of NO and L-citrulline (Fig. 1). Therefore, any alteration in this pathway will result in an impairment of NO synthesis. The production of NO

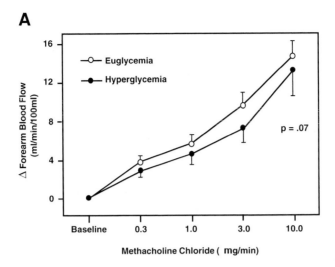

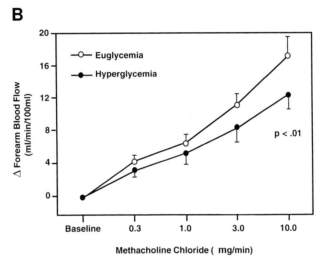

Fig. 4. Forearm blood flow (FBF) dose–response curves to intra-arterial methacholine chloride infusion before and during hyperglycemic clamping in normal subjects without (**A**) and with (**B**) octreotide (an inhibitor of pancreatic insulin secretion). As seen in A, there was a trend toward attenuated vasodilation during hyperglycemic clamping compared with euglycemia ($p = 0.07$). With coinfusion of octreotide (**B**), hyperglycemic clamping resulted in a significantly attenuated response to methacholine ($p < 0.01$) (From ref. *63a*.)

under normal physiological conditions is stimulated by various agonists that are mediated through a receptor-dependent Gi protein-mediated signal transduction *(76)*. Hypercholesterolemia results in an uncoupling of the receptor-Gi protein, resulting in a decrease in NO synthesis *(77)*. Although similar alterations have been reported in animal models of DM, Gi protein signal transduction was not altered in endothelial cells exposed to high levels of glucose *(78)*. Further research is necessary to determine whether any such receptor-Gi protein uncoupling occurs in diabetes.

Another explanation for a decrease in NO synthesis is the decreased availability of L-arginine, an important substrate for NO. There are conflicting reports as to whether depletion of L-arginine is an important factor in the modulation of vascular reactivity in

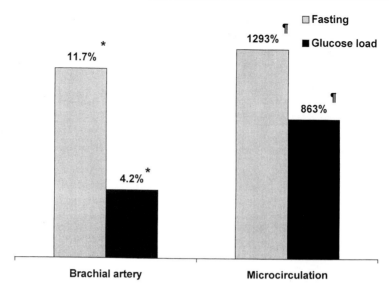

Fig. 5. Bar graph showing macrovascular and microvascular vasodilation before and after glucose ingestion. Macrovascular endothelium-dependent vasodilation is determined by the response to reactive hyperemia, as measured by the response to acetylcholine iontophoresis on erythrocytic flux. The endothelium-dependent vasodilation was reduced 60 minutes after the ingestion of 75 g of glucose (dark bars) compared with fasting conditions (light bars) at both the brachial artery ($p < 0.001$) and the microcirculation of the forearm ($p < 0.002$) (From ref. *63a.*)

Table 1
Possible Mechanisms for Decreased Endothelium-Dependent Vasodilation in Diabetes Mellitus

Impaired NO synthesis/sensitivity
  Decreased availability of L-arginine
  Altered Gi protein-controlled signaling transduction in endothelial cells
  Decreased availability of cofactors for NO synthesis (Ca^{2+}, calmodulin, tetrahydrobiopterin, NADPH)
Endogenous inhibitor of NO synthase (asymmetric dimehtylarginine [ADMA])
Increased NO inactivation and/or breakdown
  Increase in nonezymatic glycation products (AGE)
  Activation of the polyl pathway
  Activation of diacylglycerol (DAG)-protein kinase C (PKC)
  Uncoupling of eNOS
Increased production of endothelium-derived contracting factors
  Vasoconstrictor prostanoids

the diabetic state. Several studies involving hypercholesterolemic animals *(79,80)* and humans *(81,82)* have demonstrated an improvement in endothelium-dependent vasodilation with L-arginine supplementation. Studies using diabetic animal models have shown that supplementation with L-arginine increases NO activity *(83–85)*. However, studies with humans did not demonstrate any benefit with L-arginine supplementation *(86)* making L-arginine deficiency as a cause of impaired NO synthesis less likely. Giugliano et al. *(87)* gave L-arginine to healthy human volunteers who were hyperglycemic and found that L-arginine reversed the abnormal endothelium-dependent vasodilation caused by the hyperglycemia. Deanfield's group *(88)* found that L-arginine supplementation improved flow-mediated vasodilation in hypercholesterolemic or smoking individuals, but not those with insulin-dependent diabetes.

Whether this effect is caused by restoration of depleted L-arginine stores or an alternative mechanism is not known. An alternative explanation for the potential benefits of L-arginine on endothelial function is the reduction of endothelin-1 levels (89,90).

Another requirement for the synthesis of NO is the availability of cofactors, including oxygen, calcium, calmodulin, and reduced nicotinamide adenine dinucleotide phosphate (NAPDH) (91). Decreased availability of any of these cofactors would result in impaired synthesis of NO. One particular culprit that may be depleted in DM is NAPDH, which undergoes increased consumption in hyperglycemic states and is restored via the pentose phosphate pathway. However, hyperglycemia results in inhibition of this pathway, resulting in depletion of NAPDH (92). Further research is necessary to validate this possibility in vivo.

Endogenous Inhibitor of Nitric Oxide

Recently an endogenous inhibitor of NOS has been discovered, termed asymmetric dimethylarginine (ADMA) (93,94). This competitive antagonist of NOS acts by impairing the ability of dimethylarginine dimethylaminohydrolase to metabolize assymetric dimethylarginine. Plasma ADMA levels have been found to be elevated in patients with vascular disease, and with the risk factors for vascular disease (95). Intravenous infusions of ADMA can increase blood pressure in anesthetized guinea pigs, although intra-arterial infusion of ADMA in healthy volunteers reduced FBF by approx 30%. Also, ADMA-exposed endothelial cells increased the adhesiveness to monocytes in coculture (95). Significantly elevated levels of ADMA were found in animals with untreated diabetes, as compared to controls, and normalized after 8 weeks of intensive insulin treatment (96). In this study, elevation in serum ADMA was accompanied by endothelial dysfunction, as measured by the response of aortic rings to acetylcholine.

There is evidence that serum levels of ADMA appear to be dynamically regulated. One group reported that plasma ADMA increased with the administration of a high-fat diet in patients with type 2 DM (97). This was also associated with a temporally related impairment of endothelial vasodilation. Experimental hyperhomocysteinemia increases ADMA levels, and is associated with impairment of flow-mediated vasodilation (98). On the other hand, Paiva's group recently found that although higher plasma levels of ADMA were associated with lower glomerular filtration rate in subjects with type 2 diabetes, but, as a whole, diabetic subjects had lower plasma levels of ADMA than healthy controls (99). Hence, whether ADMA is a true pathological contributor to diabetic vasculopathy, or just a marker of vascular disease in this diverse patient population remains to be conclusively defined.

Increased Nitric Oxide Inactivation (Decreased Bioavailability) and/or Breakdown of Nitric Oxide

Interposed between the endothelium and the smooth muscle cells of the media is a layer of subendothelial collagen. The auto-oxidation of glucose results in a nonenzymatic glycosylation reaction between glucose and the amino groups of protein, termed advanced glycosylation end-products (AGEs). AGE-modified proteins interact with specific binding proteins, and trigger oxidation-enhancing reactions (see Chapter 3). Recent studies demonstrated an important role for AGEs in pathogenesis of diabetic vasculopathy. At concentrations similar to those found in plasma of diabetic subjects, AGEs have been shown both in vitro and in vivo to inhibit eNOS activity (100).

Bucala and coworkers demonstrated that AGE inactivated NO via a rapid chemical reaction both in vivo and in vitro (101). Diabetic rats were shown to have decreased endothelium-derived vasodilation over time, and insulin did not reverse this effect. However, aminoguanidine, an inhibitor of advanced glycosylation both in vivo and in vitro, slowed the development of vasodilatory impairment.

High glucose levels lead to increased NOS activity, making it likely that decreased NO bioavailability through either increased breakdown or other mechanisms is central to the overall decrease in NO activity in the diabetic state. One possible candidate that may modulate NO bioavailability is oxygen-derived free radicals (58,102). These increased free radicals are derived from either increased production or a decrease in the free radical scavenger system. In some animal models of diabetes, a decrease has been seen in levels of endogenous antioxidants including superoxide dismutase (SOD), catalase, and glutathionine peroxidase (103,104). If the aortas of diabetic rats are exposed to free radicals via xanthine and xanthine oxidase, endothelium-dependent relaxation is attenuated further (105). Furthermore, the addition of the free radical scavengers including SOD prevents the impairment of endothelium-dependent relaxation seen in aortic rings of diabetic rats (106). Normal rabbit aortas or mesenteric vessels incubated in hyperglycemic medium have an attenuated acetylcholine response that is restored by oxygen radical scavengers (59,73). These free radicals not only inactivate NO directly but also stimulate the production of contractile prostanoids in endothelial and smooth muscle cells through its formation of hydrogen peroxide (H_2O_2) and hydroxyl radicals (OH·) (107,108).

Prolonged hyperglycemia results in an alternative metabolism of glucose through the polyol pathway in which glucose is oxidized to sorbitol. This reaction is coupled with the oxidation of NADPH to $NADP^+$, generating free radicals. The second step is the oxidation of sorbitol to fructose, which is coupled with the reduction of NAD^+ to NADH (109,110). The increased cytolosic $NADH/NAD^+$ results in an altered redox state, which may alter the availability of tetrahydrobiopterin, an essential cofactor for NOS. If tetrahydrobiopterin is depleted, NO production is decreased (111,112). Tetrahydrobiopterin supplementation has been shown to improve impaired endothelium-dependent vasodilation in diabetic animals (113).

Elevated serum levels of glucose also result in the production of diacylglycerol (114) in many cell types, including endothelial cells. In turn, diacylglycerol activates protein kinase C (PKC), which results in an increase in the production of both oxygen-derived free radicals (115) and vasoconstrictor prostanoids (116,117).

Insulin Resistance and Nitric Oxide

Although hyperglycemia plays an essential role in the pathophysiology of DM, elevated serum insulin levels may also play an important role in atherogenesis, specifically in noninsulin DM. Furthermore, insulin resistance is a known cardiac risk factor.

Insulin mediates NO production through specific pathway, which includes insulin receptor tyrosine, phosphatidyl inositol 3-kinase and its downstream effector, akt (118,119). This increase in NO release, in turn, results in vasodilation (120). This endothelial-dependent relaxation is accompanied by an increase in glucose transport and metabolism (121,122) and may also potentially result in the removal of postprandial glucose. Therefore, endothelial dysfunction may lead to insulin resistance. This argument is further strengthened by the findings of Petrie and coworkers (123), which showed a correlation between basal endothelial function and insulin sensitivity in healthy controls. This relationship was not seen with either nitroprusside or acetylcholine, suggesting that this decreased sensitivity is not associated with a reduced ability of the vascular endothelium to synthesize NO when stimulated or with a reduction in sensitivity of vascular smooth muscle to NO released from the endothelium. Similar correlations between the degree of basal endothelial dysfunction and insulin sensitivity were seen in subjects with both hypertension and adult-onset DM (124), although this was not a consistent finding (125). However, Bursztyn and colleagues (126) demonstrated that inhibition of NO in an animal model did not result in glucose intolerance or hyperinsulinemia. These findings suggesting that endothelial function contributes to insulin sensitivity and, conversely, that insulin resistance is as a result of endothelial dysfunction) offer important new treatment options particularly in patients with adult-onset DM.

Free Fatty Acids and Nitric Oxide

Circulation free FAs may play a role in the impairment of endothelial function found in patients with DM. Such circulation free FAs are elevated in patients with DM because of excess liberation from adipose tissue and decreased uptake by skeletal muscle (127–129). Patients with type 2 DM have increased abdominal adipose tissue that is often more insulin resistant and tends to release more free FAs that adipose tissue from other locations. Infusion of free FAs have been shown to reduce endothelial-dependent vasodilation in both animal and human subjects (130).

The free FAs act to decrease endothelial function probably by several pathways including increased production of oxygen-derived free radicals, activation of PKC, and decrease insulin receptor substrate-1-associated phophatidylinositorl-3 kinase activity (131–133). This action may decrease NOSynthase activity via its effect on signal transduction.

Increased levles of free FAs causes increased very LDL production and cholesteryl ester synthesis. The resulting increased triglycerides found in diabetic subjects, coupled with the lower high-density lipoprotein (HDL), have also been associated with endothelial dysfunction (134,135).

OTHER RISK FACTORS IN DIABETIC ENDOTHELIAL DYSFUNCTION

Dyslipidemia

Dyslipidemia is a common problem affecting patients with DM. Much evidence shows that elevated total and LDL cholesterol levels are associated with impaired endothelial function, independent of the presence of other cardiac risk factors (136–140). Furthermore, it remains unclear whether the mechanism of the endothelial dysfunction associated with dyslipidemia is the same as or different from that of DM. Possible mechanisms include decreased NO availability (141,142), L-arginine deficiency (37,139), or increased NO inactivation via superoxide production (143). It is therefore difficult to determine accurately the relative contribution that dyslipidemia has on diabetic endothelial dysfunction.

The dyslipidemia frequently affecting type 2 diabetics is characterized by elevated levels of small dense LDLs and triglycerides with low levels of HDL. The degree of impairment of endothelium-dependent relaxation in type 2 diabetics is significantly correlated with the serum triglyceride level (144) and inversely correlated with LDL size (11,145,146). Skyrme-Jones and colleagues (147) have reported a similar deleterious effect of the small, dense LDLs and the reduced LDL vitamin E content on endothelium-dependent vasodilation in patients with type 1 diabetes. The diabetic state can result in the glycation of HDL, which may impair the protective effect of HDL on the endothelium (148).

Hypertension

Numerous animal and clinical studies have demonstrated that hypertension reduces endothelium-dependent relaxation (149–153). Two studies have shown that basal production or release of NO is decreased in hypertensive patients (63,154). The possible mechanisms underlying the endothelial vasodilator dysfunction associated with hypertension include L-arginine deficiency (155), decreased muscarinic receptor function (156,157) abnormalities in signal transduction (158), or NO inactivation by oxygen-derived free radicals (159–162).

As with dyslipidemia, hypertension is frequently associated with DM, making the relative contribution of either risk factor to the endothelial dysfunction found in the hypertensive diabetic person difficult to determine. Epidemiological studies have shown an association among obesity, insulin resistance, and hypertension (163,164). Further research has found that even lean individuals with essential hypertension are frequently insulin resistant. This finding led investigators to propose that insulin resistance and hyperinsulinemia may contribute to the pathogenesis of hypertension.

POTENTIAL PREVENTIVE AND THERAPEUTIC OPTIONS

Oral Hypoglycemic Agents

The cornerstone of DM therapy is optimal glycemic control, because hyperglycemia is the basis of all the metabolic disturbances that occurs in the disease. As shown previously, both in vivo and in vitro elevated glucose levels have been shown to cause abnormal endothelium-dependent relaxation. Lower glucose levels also result in a decrease in insulin levels, which consequently may also improve endothelial function. Therefore, therapy should be directed toward lowering glucose levels and increasing insulin sensitivity.

The effect of oral hypoglycemic agents on endothelial function is controversial and probably relates to the agent and model of diabetes being evaluated. Metformin has been shown to improve endothelium-dependent function in the mesenteric arteries of insulin-resistant rats in vitro (165), and the ATP-dependent potassium channel blocker gliclazide ameliorated endothelium-dependent relaxation of the aortas of (alloxan-induced) diabetic rabbits (166). However, clinical studies evaluating the effect of oral hypoglycemics on endothelial function have shown either no difference (167) or diminished reactivity to acetylcholine once the agent is discontinued (120).

Recent work has demonstrated that one of the thiazolidinediones, (a group of insulin-sensitizing agents), rosiglitazone, improved endothelial function and insulin resistance for patients with type 2 diabetic subjects, suggesting that therapy for insulin resistance may improve endothelial dysfunction (168).

Protein Kinase C Inhibitors

Hyperglycemia can activate PKC, which in turn increases oxidative stress. Inhibitors of PKC can restore vascular function and also increase mRNA expression of eNOS in aortic endothelial cells (143). Recently, an inhibitor of PKC, LY333531, has been developed; it normalizes retinal blood flow and glomerular filtration rate in parallel with inhibition of PKC activity (169). LY333531 is discussed in detail in Chapter 2. Beckman and colleagues (170) found that this inhibitor of PKCβ attenuated the impairment of endothelial-dependent vasodilation on healthy human subjects exposed to hyperglycemia.

Inhibitors of AGE Production

The production of AGE, as a result of prolonged exposure of proteins to chronic hyperglycemia, can result in direct quenching of NO and increasing the oxidative stress.

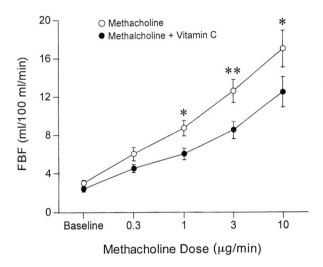

Fig. 6. Forearm blood flow (FBF) dose–response curves to intra-arterial methacholine chloride infusion before and during coinfusion of vitamin C in noninsulin-dependent diabetic subjects. The concomitant infusion of methacholine and vitamin C resulted in an improved endothelium-dependent vasodilation compared with methacholine alone ($p = 0.002$ by ANOVA). Comparisons of FBF at each methacholine dose before and during vitamin C administration were performed by paired t-tests adjusted with a Bonferoni correction for multiple comparison. $*p < 0.05$; $**p < 0.01$. (From ref. *63a*.)

An inhibitor of AGE production, aminoguanidine, has been shown both to reduce AGE and to improve endothelial function *(88,171)* in animal models.

Vitamins C and E

As discussed earlier, one possible mechanism of endothelial dysfunction in both type 1 and type 2 DM is the inactivation of NO by oxygen-derived free radicals. There is also a decrease in levels of endogenous antioxidants including superoxide dismutase and catalase in animal models of diabetes *(172)*. Furthermore, several clinical studies have reported a decrease in endogenous vitamin C *(173,174)* and E *(173,175)* levels in both type 2 and type 1 DM. Any means of decreasing the oxidative stress has the potential to improve endothelium-dependent vasodilation. Timimi et al. *(176)* and Ting and coworkers *(177)* (Fig. 6) found that intra-arterial infusion of vitamin C improved endothelium-dependent (but not endothelium-independent) relaxation in patients with type 1 and type 2 diabetes, respectively. Furthermore, the intra-artrial infusion of ascorbic acid restored the impaired endothelial vasodilation in healthy subjects exposed to hyperglycemic clamp *(178)*.

Tetrahydrobiopterin

Conversely, hyperglycemia, which increases oxidative stress, can convert even elevated levels of NO to peroxynitrite, which is deleterious to vascular function *(179)*. A decrease in oxidative stress can restore vascular function rather than increase the NO supply. Prolonged hyperglycemia and hypercholesterolemia both cause a depletion of tetrahydrobiopterin (BH_4), an essential cofactor for NOS, resulting in an uncoupling of eNOS and lowered production of NO *(180)*. Studies using both diabetic animal models *(113)* and hypercholesterolemic patients *(112)* have demonstrated that tetrahydrobiopterin supplementation restored endothelium-dependent vasodilation. This has yet to be confirmed in studies involving diabetic patients.

L-arginine

As stated earlier in this chapter, there are conflicting data as to whether L-arginine improves endothelial function in the diabetic state. Several studies using diabetic animal models *(83)* and healthy human volunteers who were made hyperglycemic *(87)* had improved endothelial-dependent vasodilation with L-arginine supplementation. However, Deanfield's group *(88)* found that L-arginine supplementation did not improve flow-mediated vasodilation in insulin-dependent diabetes.

Estrogen

The incidence of CAD in premenopausal women is less than in age-matched males *(181)*. One possible explanation is the effect of estrogen. Estrogen may have important effects on vascular function that are not totally explained on the basis of an improved lipoprotein profile *(182)*. Diabetic women have the same cardiovascular risk as nondiabetic men, suggesting that they are denied the cardiovascular protection of estrogen enjoyed by other premenopausal women *(182)*. Estrogen's possible beneficial effects include not only inhibition of platelet aggregation *(183)*, but also its antioxidative effect and antiproliferative effects on vascular smooth muscle. Several investigators have demonstrated that estrogen improves endothelium-dependent vasodilation in ovariectomized animals *(184,185)* and postmenopausal women *(186–188)*. The mechanism may be enhanced eNOS production *(188,189)* or, alternatively, suppression of a prostaglandin H synthase-dependent vasoconstrictor prostanoid *(190)*. Lim and colleagues *(191)* found that although hormonal replacement therapy (HRT) improved microvascular reactivity in postmenopausal healthy women, this effect was less apparent in type 2 diabetic women. However, HRT improved endothelial activation, as determined by soluble intracellular adhesion molecules, in these type 2 diabetic women.

Angiotensin-Converting Enzyme Inhibitors

Angiotensin-converting enzyme (ACE) inhibitors have been shown both to improve endothelial function and to reduce the development of atherosclerosis in various animal models of hypercholesterolemia *(192,193)*, independent of its BP-lowering effect. Similarly, the Heart Outcomes Prevention Evaluation (HOPE) study has demonstrated the utility of the ACE inhibitor ramipril in preventing cardiovascular events in diabetics *(194)* although the mechanism of this effect remains obscure. Clinical trials have demonstrated that the ACE inhibitor quinapril improved endothelial function in nondiabetic patients with CAD *(195)*. Studies evaluating the effect of ACE inhibitors on type 1 diabetic subjects have resulted in conflicting conclusions. Two studies have demonstrated that ACE inhibitors have no effect on vascular function in patients with type 1 DM, even after 6 months on the drug *(196,197)*. However, O'Driscoll and colleagues found improvement in endothelial function by ACE inhibition in insulin-dependent DM *(198)*. ACE inhibitors also improved both basal and stimulated NO-dependent endothelial function in patients with noninsulin-dependent (type 2) DM, including patients with both hypertension and diabetic nephropathy *(199)*. No effect, however, was seen with ACE inhibitors in patients with the insulin-resistance syndrome *(200)*.

ACE inhibitors may have a number of potential beneficial effects on vascular structure and function. In particular, it may enhance the bioavailability of NO. This latter effect may be as a result of attenuation of the angiotensin II-mediated production of superoxides *(167,201)* or through the inhibition of bradykinin degradation, a potent stimulus for NO release *(202,203)*.

HMG CoA Reductase Inhibitors

Large clinical trials have determined that hydroxymethylglutaryl-coenzyme A reductase inhibitors ("statins") significantly reduce cardiovascular morbidity and mortality. Furthermore, lipid-lowering therapy has been shown to improve endothelial function in several studies *(204,205)*. Attempts to ameliorate the impaired endothelium-dependent vascular relaxation that occurs in diabetic patients with dyslipidemia are few and the results mixed. Impaired endothelium-dependent vasodilation in patients with type 2 DM with dyslipidemia has been reported to improve with fibrate therapy *(206)* (which lowers the serum triglyceride level) but not with simvastatin *(206,207)*.

CONCLUSIONS

The normal endothelium plays an important role in the prevention of atherosclerosis and microvascular disease. DM is an important cause of both macro- and microvascular disease. Animal and clinical studies have demonstrated a decrease in endothelium-dependent vasodilation in both type 1 and type 2 DM. Possible mechanisms include abnormalities in signal transduction, reduced synthesis of NO, accelerated inactivation of NO, or production of vasoconstrictor prostanoids, probably through the relative increase of oxygen-derived free radicals (Table 1). The mediators of this abnormality include hyperinsulinemia, insulin resistance, or hyperglycemia. Improved glucose control, supplementation with either tetrahydrobiopterin, L-arginine, or vitamin C, or the addition of ACE inhibitors have been shown to improve endothelial function. Further research is required to determine whether restoring endothelial function in patients with either type 1 or type 2 diabetes will translate into an overall reduction in diabetic vascular disease.

REFERENCES

1. Cohen AM, Rosenmann E, Rosenthal T. The Cohen diabetic (non-insulin-dependent) hypertensive rat model. Description of the model and pathologic findings. Am J Hypertens 1993;6(12):989–995.
2. Kannel WB, McGee DL. Diabetes and cardiovascular disease. The Framingham study. JAMA 1979;241(19):2035–2038.
3. Garcia MJ, et al. Morbidity and mortality in diabetics in the Framingham population. Sixteen year follow-up study. Diabetes 1974;23(2):105–111.
4. Deckert T, et al. Natural history of diabetic complications: early detection and progression. Diabet Med 1991;8(Spec No):S33–S37.
5. Deckert T, et al. [Microalbuminuria as predictor of atherosclerotic cardiovascular disease in IDDM]. Ugeskr Laeger 1997;159(20):3010–3014.
6. Beach KW, Strandness DE Jr. Arteriosclerosis obliterans and associated risk factors in insulin-dependent and non-insulin-dependent diabetes. Diabetes 1980;29(11):882–888.
7. Keen H, Jarrett RJ. The WHO multinational study of vascular disease in diabetes: 2. Macrovascular disease prevalence. Diabetes Care 1979;2(2):187–195.
8. Zatz R, Brenner BM. Pathogenesis of diabetic microangiopathy. The hemodynamic view. Am J Med 1986;80(3):443–453.
9. Merimee TJ. Diabetic retinopathy. A synthesis of perspectives. N Engl J Med 1990;322(14):978–983.
10. Furchgott RF, Zawadzki JV. The obligatory role of endothelial cells in the relaxation of arterial smooth muscle by acetylcholine. Nature 1980;288(5789):373–376.
11. Furchgott RF, Vanhoutte PM. Endothelium-derived relaxing and contracting factors. Faseb J 1989;3(9):2007–2018.

12. Ignarro LJ, et al. Endothelium-derived relaxing factor produced and released from artery and vein is nitric oxide. Proc Natl Acad Sci USA 1987;84(24):9265–9269.

13. Palmer RM, Ferrige AG, Moncada S. Nitric oxide release accounts for the biological activity of endothelium-derived relaxing factor. Nature 1987;327(6122):524–526.

14. Forstermann U, et al. Nitric oxide synthase isozymes. Characterization, purification, molecular cloning, and functions. Hypertension 1994;23(6 Pt 2):1121–1131.

15. Dinerman JL, Lowenstein CJ, Snyder SH. Molecular mechanisms of nitric oxide regulation. Potential relevance to cardiovascular disease. Circ Res 1993;73(2):217–222.

16. Lincoln TM, Cornwell TL, Taylor AE. cGMP-dependent protein kinase mediates the reduction of Ca2+ by cAMP in vascular smooth muscle cells. Am J Physiol 1990;258(3 Pt 1):C399–C407.

17. Waldman SA, Murad F. Cyclic GMP synthesis and function. Pharmacol Rev 1987;39(3):163–196.

18. Dimmeler S, Lottspeich F, Brune B. Nitric oxide causes ADP-ribosylation and inhibition of glyceraldehyde-3-phosphate dehydrogenase. J Biol Chem 1992;267(24):16,771–16,774.

19. Rees DD, Palmer RM, Moncada S. Role of endothelium-derived nitric oxide in the regulation of blood pressure. Proc Natl Acad Sci USA 1989;86(9):3375–2278.

20. Duplain H, et al. Insulin resistance, hyperlipidemia, and hypertension in mice lacking endothelial nitric oxide synthase. Circulation 2001;104(3):342–245.

21. McQuillan LP, et al. Hypoxia inhibits expression of eNOS via transcriptional and posttranscriptional mechanisms. Am J Physiol 1994;267(5 Pt 2):H1921–H1027.

22. Griffith TM, et al. EDRF coordinates the behaviour of vascular resistance vessels. Nature 1987; 329(6138):442–445.

23. Stamler JS, et al. Nitric oxide regulates basal systemic and pulmonary vascular resistance in healthy humans. Circulation 1994;89(5):2035–2040.

24. Lowenstein CJ, Dinerman JL, Snyder SH. Nitric oxide: a physiologic messenger. Ann Intern Med 1994;120(3):227–237.

25. Ignarro LJ. Biological actions and properties of endothelium-derived nitric oxide formed and released from artery and vein. Circ Res 1989;65(1):1–21.

26. Kourembanas S, et al. Nitric oxide regulates the expression of vasoconstrictors and growth factors by vascular endothelium under both normoxia and hypoxia. J Clin Invest 1993;92(1):99–104.

27. Balligand JL, et al. Control of cardiac muscle cell function by an endogenous nitric oxide signaling system. Proc Natl Acad Sci USA 1993;90(1):347–351.

28. Joe EK, et al. Regulation of cardiac myocyte contractile function by inducible nitric oxide synthase (iNOS): mechanisms of contractile depression by nitric oxide. J Mol Cell Cardiol 1998;30(2):303–315.

29. Mellion BT, et al. Evidence for the inhibitory role of guanosine 3' 5'-monophosphate in ADP-induced human platelet aggregation in the presence of nitric oxide and related vasodilators. Blood 1981;57(5): 946–955.

30. Vallance P, Collier J, Moncada S. Effects of endothelium-derived nitric oxide on peripheral arteriolar tone in man. Lancet 1989;2(8670):997–1000.

31. Kubes P, Granger DN. Nitric oxide modulates microvascular permeability. Am J Physiol 1992;262(2 Pt 2):H611–H615.

32. Garg UC, Hassid A. Nitric oxide-generating vasodilators and 8-bromo-cyclic guanosine monophosphate inhibit mitogenesis and proliferation of cultured rat vascular smooth muscle cells. J Clin Invest 1989;83(5):1774–1777.

33. Marks DS, et al. Inhibition of neointimal proliferation in rabbits after vascular injury by a single treatment with a protein adduct of nitric oxide. J Clin Invest 1995;96(6):2630–2638.

34. Taguchi J, et al. L-arginine inhibits neointimal formation following balloon injury. Life Sci 1993;53(23):PL387–PL392.

35. Cohen RA. The role of nitric oxide and other endothelium-derived vasoactive substances in vascular disease. Prog Cardiovasc Dis 1995;38(2):105–128.

36. Bossaller C, et al. Impaired muscarinic endothelium-dependent relaxation and cyclic guanosine 5'-monophosphate formation in atherosclerotic human coronary artery and rabbit aorta. J Clin Invest 1987;79(1):170–174.

37. Cooke JP, et al. Antiatherogenic effects of L-arginine in the hypercholesterolemic rabbit. J Clin Invest 1992;90(3):1168–1172.

38. De Caterina R, et al. Nitric oxide decreases cytokine-induced endothelial activation. Nitric oxide selectively reduces endothelial expression of adhesion molecules and proinflammatory cytokines. J Clin Invest 1995;96(1):60–68.

39. Rajavashisth TB, et al. Induction of endothelial cell expression of granulocyte and macrophage colony-stimulating factors by modified low-density lipoproteins. Nature 1990;344(6263):254–257.

40. Collins T, et al. Transcriptional regulation of endothelial cell adhesion molecules: NF-kappa B and cytokine-inducible enhancers. Faseb J 1995;9(10):899–909.

41. Peng HB, Libby P, Liao JK. Induction and stabilization of I kappa B alpha by nitric oxide mediates inhibition of NF-kappa B. J Biol Chem 1995;270(23):14,214–14,219.

42. Almer LO, Pandolfi M, Aberg M. The plasminogen activator activity of arteries and veins in diabetes mellitus. Thromb Res 1975;6(2):177–182.

43. Auwerx J, et al. Tissue-type plasminogen activator antigen and plasminogen activator inhibitor in diabetes mellitus. Arteriosclerosis 1988;8(1):68–72.

44. Carreras LO, et al. Decreased vascular prostacyclin (PGI2) in diabetic rats. Stimulation of PGI2 release in normal and diabetic rats by the antithrombotic compound Bay g 6575. Thromb Res 1980;19(4–5):663–670.

45. Umeda F, Inoguchi T, Nawata H. Reduced stimulatory activity on prostacyclin production by cultured endothelial cells in serum from aged and diabetic patients. Atherosclerosis 1989;75(1):61–66.

46. Meraji S, et al. Endothelium-dependent relaxation in aorta of BB rat. Diabetes 1987;36(8):978–981.

47. Oyama Y, et al. Attenuation of endothelium-dependent relaxation in aorta from diabetic rats. Eur J Pharmacol 1986;132(1):75–78.

48. Mayhan WG, Simmons LK, Sharpe GM. Mechanism of impaired responses of cerebral arterioles during diabetes mellitus. Am J Physiol 1991;260(2 Pt 2):H319–H326.

49. Abiru T, et al. Decrease in endothelium-dependent relaxation and levels of cyclic nucleotides in aorta from rabbits with alloxan-induced diabetes. Res Commun Chem Pathol Pharmacol 1990;68(1):13–25.

50. Fortes ZB, Garcia Leme J, Scivoletto R. Vascular reactivity in diabetes mellitus: possible role of insulin on the endothelial cell. Br J Pharmacol 1984;83(3):635–643.

51. Taylor PD, et al. Prevention by insulin treatment of endothelial dysfunction but not enhanced noradrenaline-induced contractility in mesenteric resistance arteries from streptozotocin-induced diabetic rats. Br J Pharmacol 1994;111(1):35–41.

52. Tesfamariam B, et al. Elevated glucose promotes generation of endothelium-derived vasoconstrictor prostanoids in rabbit aorta. J Clin Invest 1990;85(3):929–932.

53. Tesfamariam B, Brown ML, Cohen RA. Elevated glucose impairs endothelium-dependent relaxation by activating protein kinase C. J Clin Invest 1991;87(5):1643–1648.

54. Tesfamariam B, Brown ML, Cohen RA. Aldose reductase and myo-inositol in endothelial cell dysfunction caused by elevated glucose. J Pharmacol Exp Ther 1992;263(1):153–157.

55. Cohen RA. Dysfunction of vascular endothelium in diabetes mellitus. Circulation 1993;87 (Suppl V):V67–V76.

56. Kamata K, et al. Functional changes in vascular smooth muscle and endothelium of arteries during diabetes mellitus. Life Sci 1992;50(19):1379–1387.

57. Wolff SP, Dean RT. Glucose autoxidation and protein modification. The potential role of 'autoxidative glycosylation' in diabetes. Biochem J 1987;245(1):243–250.

58. Tesfamariam B, Cohen RA. Free radicals mediate endothelial cell dysfunction caused by elevated glucose. Am J Physiol 1992;263(2 Pt 2):H321–H326.

59. Hattori Y, et al. Superoxide dismutase recovers altered endothelium-dependent relaxation in diabetic rat aorta. Am J Physiol 1991;261(4 Pt 2):H1086–H1094.

60. Saenz de Tejada I, et al. Impaired neurogenic and endothelium-mediated relaxation of penile smooth muscle from diabetic men with impotence. N Engl J Med 1989;320(16):1025–1030.

61. Johnstone MT, et al. Impaired endothelium-dependent vasodilation in patients with insulin-dependent diabetes mellitus. Circulation 1993;88(6):2510–2516.

62. Smits P, et al. Endothelium-dependent vascular relaxation in patients with type I diabetes. Diabetes 1993;42(1):148–153.

63. Calver A, Collier J, Vallance P. Inhibition and stimulation of nitric oxide synthesis in the human forearm arterial bed of patients with insulin-dependent diabetes. J Clin Invest 1992;90(6):2548–2554.

63a. Johnstone MT, Veves A. (Eds.) Diabetes and cardiovascular disease. Humana Press, Totowa, NJ:2001.

64. Halkin A, et al. Vascular responsiveness and cation exchange in insulin-dependent diabetes. Clin Sci (Lond) 1991;81(2):223–232.

65. Zenere BM, et al. Noninvasive detection of functional alterations of the arterial wall in IDDM patients with and without microalbuminuria. Diabetes Care 1995;18(7):975–982.

66. Clarkson P, et al. Impaired vascular reactivity in insulin-dependent diabetes mellitus is related to disease duration and low density lipoprotein cholesterol levels. J Am Coll Cardiol 1996;28(3):573–579.

67. Makimattila S, et al. Chronic hyperglycemia impairs endothelial function and insulin sensitivity via different mechanisms in insulin-dependent diabetes mellitus. Circulation 1996;94(6):1276–1282.

68. Williams SB, et al. Acute hyperglycemia attenuates endothelium-dependent vasodilation in humans in vivo. Circulation 1998;97(17):1695–1701.

69. Chowienczyk PJ, et al. Sex differences in endothelial function in normal and hypercholesterolaemic subjects. Lancet 1994;344(8918):305–306.

70. Williams SB, et al. Impaired nitric oxide-mediated vasodilation in patients with non- insulin-dependent diabetes mellitus. J Am Coll Cardiol 1996;27(3):567–574.

71. McVeigh GE, et al. Impaired endothelium-dependent and independent vasodilation in patients with type 2 (non-insulin-dependent) diabetes mellitus. Diabetologia 1992;35(8):771–776.

72. Cosentino F, Luscher TF. Endothelial dysfunction in diabetes mellitus. J Cardiovasc Pharmacol 1998;32(Suppl 3):S54–S61.

73. Bohlen HG, Lash JM. Topical hyperglycemia rapidly suppresses EDRF-mediated vasodilation of normal rat arterioles. Am J Physiol 1993;265(1 Pt 2):H219–H225.

74. Akbari CM, et al. Endothelium-dependent vasodilatation is impaired in both microcirculation and macrocirculation during acute hyperglycemia. J Vasc Surg 1998;28(4):687–694.

75. Houben AJ, et al. Local 24-h hyperglycemia does not affect endothelium-dependent or -independent vasoreactivity in humans. Am J Physiol 1996;270(6 Pt 2):H2014–H2020.

76. Davies MG, et al. The expression and function of G-proteins in experimental intimal hyperplasia. J Clin Invest 1994;94(4):1680–1689.

77. Gilligan DM, et al. Selective loss of microvascular endothelial function in human hypercholesterolemia. Circulation 1994;90(1):35–41.

78. Mancusi G, et al. High-glucose incubation of human umbilical-vein endothelial cells does not alter expression and function either of G-protein alpha-subunits or of endothelial NO synthase. Biochem J 1996;315 (Pt 1):281–287.

79. Cooke JP, et al. Arginine restores cholinergic relaxation of hypercholesterolemic rabbit thoracic aorta. Circulation 1991;83(3):1057–1062.

80. Boger RH, et al. Supplementation of hypercholesterolaemic rabbits with L-arginine reduces the vascular release of superoxide anions and restores NO production. Atherosclerosis 1995;117(2):273–284.

81. Boger RH, et al. Biochemical evidence for impaired nitric oxide synthesis in patients with peripheral arterial occlusive disease. Circulation 1997;95(8):2068–2074.

82. Drexler H, et al. Correction of endothelial dysfunction in coronary microcirculation of hypercholesterolaemic patients by L-arginine. Lancet 1991;338(8782–8783):1546–1550.

83. Pieper GM, Peltier BA. Amelioration by L-arginine of a dysfunctional arginine/nitric oxide pathway in diabetic endothelium. J Cardiovasc Pharmacol 1995;25(3):397–403.

84. Pieper GM, et al. Reversal by L-arginine of a dysfunctional arginine/nitric oxide pathway in the endothelium of the genetic diabetic BB rat. Diabetologia 1997;40(8):910–915.

85. Wu G, Meininger CJ. Impaired arginine metabolism and NO synthesis in coronary endothelial cells of the spontaneously diabetic BB rat. Am J Physiol 1995;269(4 Pt 2):H1312–H1318.

86. MacAllister RJ, et al. Vascular and hormonal responses to arginine: provision of substrate for nitric oxide or non-specific effect? Clin Sci (Lond) 1995;89(2):183–190.

87. Giugliano D, et al. Vascular effects of acute hyperglycemia in humans are reversed by L-arginine. Evidence for reduced availability of nitric oxide during hyperglycemia. Circulation 1997;95(7):1783–1790.

88. Thorne S, et al. Early endothelial dysfunction in adults at risk from atherosclerosis: different responses to L-arginine. J Am Coll Cardiol 1998;32(1):110–116.

89. Boulanger C, Luscher TF. Release of endothelin from the porcine aorta. Inhibition by endothelium-derived nitric oxide. J Clin Invest 1990;85(2):587–590.

90. Bell MR, et al. The changing in-hospital mortality of women undergoing percutaneous transluminal coronary angioplasty. JAMA 1993;269(16):2091–2095.

91. Knowles RG, Moncada S. Nitric oxide synthases in mammals. Biochem J 1994;298 (Pt 2):249–258.

92. Asahina T, et al. Impaired activation of glucose oxidation and NADPH supply in human endothelial cells exposed to H2O2 in high-glucose medium. Diabetes 1995;44(5):520–526.

93. Bode-Boger SM, et al. Elevated L-arginine/dimethylarginine ratio contributes to enhanced systemic NO production by dietary L-arginine in hypercholesterolemic rabbits. Biochem Biophys Res Commun 1996;219(2):598–603.

94. Lerman A, et al. Long-term L-arginine supplementation improves small-vessel coronary endothelial function in humans. Circulation 1998;97(21):2123–2128.

95. Cooke JP. Does ADMA cause endothelial dysfunction? Arterioscler Thromb Vasc Biol 2000;20(9):2032–2037.

96. Xiong Y, et al. Elevated levels of the serum endogenous inhibitor of nitric oxide synthase and metabolic control in rats with streptozotocin-induced diabetes. J Cardiovasc Pharmacol 2003;42(2):191–196.

97. Fard A, et al. Acute elevations of plasma asymmetric dimethylarginine and impaired endothelial function in response to a high-fat meal in patients with type 2 diabetes. Arterioscler Thromb Vasc Biol 2000;20(9):2039–2044.

98. Boger RH, et al. Elevation of asymmetrical dimethylarginine may mediate endothelial dysfunction during experimental hyperhomocyst(e)inaemia in humans. Clin Sci (Lond) 2001;100(2):161–167.

99. Paiva H, et al. Plasma concentrations of asymmetric-dimethyl-arginine in type 2 diabetes associate with glycemic control and glomerular filtration rate but not with risk factors of vasculopathy. Metabolism 2003;52(3):303–307.

100. Xu B, et al. Impairment of vascular endothelial nitric oxide synthase activity by advanced glycation end products. Faseb J 2003;17(10):1289–1291.

101. Bucala, R, Tracey KJ, Cerami A. Advanced glycosylation products quench nitric oxide and mediate defective endothelium-dependent vasodilatation in experimental diabetes. J Clin Invest 1991;87(2): 432–438.

102. Tesfamariam B. Free radicals in diabetic endothelial cell dysfunction. Free Radic Biol Med 1994;16(3):383–391.

103. Dohi T, et al. Alterations of the plasma selenium concentrations and the activities of tissue peroxide metabolism enzymes in streptozotocin-induced diabetic rats. Horm Metab Res 1988;20(11):671–675.

104. Wohaieb SA, Godin DV. Alterations in free radical tissue-defense mechanisms in streptozocin-induced diabetes in rat. Effects of insulin treatment. Diabetes 1987;36(9):1014–1018.

105. Pieper GM, Gross GJ. Oxygen free radicals abolish endothelium-dependent relaxation in diabetic rat aorta. Am J Physiol 1988;255(4 Pt 2):H825–H833.

106. Langenstroer P, Pieper GM. Regulation of spontaneous EDRF release in diabetic rat aorta by oxygen free radicals. Am J Physiol 1992;263(1 Pt 2):H257–H265.

107. Auch-Schwelk W, Katusic ZS, Vanhoutte PM. Contractions to oxygen-derived free radicals are augmented in aorta of the spontaneously hypertensive rat. Hypertension 1989;13(6 Pt 2):859–864.

108. Katusic ZS, et al. Endothelium-dependent contractions to oxygen-derived free radicals in the canine basilar artery. Am J Physiol 1993;264(3 Pt 2):H859–H864.

109. Ido Y, Kilo C, Williamson JR. Cytosolic NADH/NAD+, free radicals, and vascular dysfunction in early diabetes mellitus. Diabetologia 1997;40 Suppl 2:S115–S117.

110. Williamson JR, et al. Hyperglycemic pseudohypoxia and diabetic complications. Diabetes 1993;42(6): 801–813.

111. Schmidt K, et al. Tetrahydrobiopterin-dependent formation of endothelium-derived relaxing factor (nitric oxide) in aortic endothelial cells. Biochem J 1992;281 (Pt 2):297–300.

112. Cosentino F, Katusic ZS. Tetrahydrobiopterin and dysfunction of endothelial nitric oxide synthase in coronary arteries. Circulation 1995;91(1):139–144.

113. Pieper GM. Acute amelioration of diabetic endothelial dysfunction with a derivative of the nitric oxide synthase cofactor, tetrahydrobiopterin. J Cardiovasc Pharmacol 1997;29(1):8–15.

114. Lee TS, et al. Differential regulation of protein kinase C and (Na,K)-adenosine triphosphatase activities by elevated glucose levels in retinal capillary endothelial cells. J Clin Invest 1989;83(1):90–94.

115. Baynes JW, Thorpe SR. Role of oxidative stress in diabetic complications: a new perspective on an old paradigm. Diabetes 1999;48(1):1–9.

116. Craven PA, Patterson MC, DeRubertis FR. Role for protein kinase C in A23187 induced glomerular arachidonate release and PGE2 production. Biochem Biophys Res Commun 1987;149(2):658–664.

117. Fujita I, et al. Diacylglycerol 1-oleoyl-2-acetyl-glycerol, stimulates superoxide-generation from human neutrophils. Biochem Biophys Res Commun 1984;120(2):318–324.

118. Dunbar JC, et al. Mechanisms mediating insulin-induced hypotension in rats. A role for nitric oxide and autonomic mediators. Acta Diabetol 1996;33(4):263–268.

119. Zeng G, et al. Roles for insulin receptor, PI3-kinase, and Akt in insulin-signaling pathways related to production of nitric oxide in human vascular endothelial cells. Circulation 2000;101(13):1539–1545.

120. Steinberg HO, et al. Obesity/insulin resistance is associated with endothelial dysfunction. Implications for the syndrome of insulin resistance. J Clin Invest 1996;97(11):2601–2610.

121. Balon TW, Nadler JL. Evidence that nitric oxide increases glucose transport in skeletal muscle. J Appl Physiol 1997;82(1):359–363.

122. Young ME, Radda GK, Leighton B. Nitric oxide stimulates glucose transport and metabolism in rat skeletal muscle in vitro. Biochem J 1997;322 (Pt 1):223–228.

123. Petrie JR, et al. Endothelial nitric oxide production and insulin sensitivity. A physiological link with implications for pathogenesis of cardiovascular disease. Circulation 1996;93(7):1331–1333.

124. Cleland SJ, et al. Insulin action is associated with endothelial function in hypertension and type 2 diabetes. Hypertension 2000;35(1 Pt 2):507–511.

125. Utriainen T, et al. Dissociation between insulin sensitivity of glucose uptake and endothelial function in normal subjects. Diabetologia 1996;39(12):1477–1482.

126. Bursztyn M, et al. Effect of acute N-nitro-L-arginine methyl ester (L-NAME) hypertension on glucose tolerance, insulin levels, and [3H]-deoxyglucose muscle uptake. Am J Hypertens 1997;10(6):683–686.

127. Creager MA, Lusher T. Diabetes and vascular disease: pathophysiology, clinical consequences, and medical therapy: Part I. Circulation 2003;108:1527–1532.

128. Kelley DE, Simoneau JA. Impaired free fatty acid utilizaiton by skeletal muscle in non-insulin-dependent diabetes mellitus. J Clin Invest 1994;94:2349–2356.

129. Boden G. Free fatty acids, insulin resistance, and type 2 diabetes mellitus. Proc Assoc Am Physicians 1999;111:241–248.

130. Steinberg HO, Tarshoby M, Monestel R, et al. Elevated circulating free fatty acid levels impari endothelium-dependent vasodilation. J Clin Invest 1997;100:1230–1239.

131. Dresner A, Laurent D, Marcucci M, et al. Effects of free fatty acids on glucose transport and IRS-1-associated phosphatidylinositol 3-kinase activity. J Clin Invest 1999;103:253–259.

132. Dichtl W, Nilsson L, Goncalves I, et al. Very low-density lipoprotein activates nuclear factor-kappaB in endothelial cells. Circ Res 1999;84:1085–1094.

133. Inoguchi T, Li P, Umeda F, et al. High glucose level and free fatty acid stimulate reactive oxygen species production through protein kinase C-dependent activation of NAD(P)H oxidase in cultured vascular cells. Diabetes 2000;49:1939–1945.

134. de Man FH, Weverling-Rijnsburger AW, van der Laarse A, et al. Not acute but chronic hypertriglyceridemia is associated with impaired endothelium-dependent vasodilation: reversal after lipid-lowering therapy by atorvastatin. Arteroscler Thromb Vasc Biol 2000;20:744–750.

135. Kuhn FE, Mohler ER, Satler LF, et al. Effects of high-density lipoprotein on acetylcholine-induced coronary vasoreactivity. Am J Cardiol 1991;68:1425–1430.

136. Osborne JA, et al. Lack of endothelium-dependent relaxation in coronary resistance arteries of cholesterol-fed rabbits. Am J Physiol 1989;256(3 Pt 1):C591–C597.

137. Simon BC, Cunningham LD, Cohen RA. Oxidized low density lipoproteins cause contraction and inhibit endothelium-dependent relaxation in the pig coronary artery. J Clin Invest 1990;86(1):75–79.

138. Shimokawa H, Vanhoutte PM. Hypercholesterolemia causes generalized impairment of endothelium-dependent relaxation to aggregating platelets in porcine arteries. J Am Coll Cardiol 1989;13(6):1402–1408.

139. Creager MA, et al. L-arginine improves endothelium-dependent vasodilation in hypercholesterolemic humans. J Clin Invest 1992;90(4):1248–1253.

140. Chowienczyk PJ, et al. Impaired endothelium-dependent vasodilation of forearm resistance vessels in hypercholesterolaemia. Lancet 1992;340(8833):1430–1432.

141. Quyyumi AA, et al. Coronary vascular nitric oxide activity in hypertension and hypercholesterolemia. Comparison of acetylcholine and substance P. Circulation 1997;95(1):104–110.

142. Shiode N, et al. Nitric oxide production by coronary conductance and resistance vessels in hypercholesterolemia patients. Am Heart J 1996;131(6):1051–1057.

143. Ohara, Y, Peterson TE, Harrison DG. Hypercholesterolemia increases endothelial superoxide anion production. J Clin Invest 1993;91(6):2546–2551.

144. Makimattila S, et al. Impaired endothelium-dependent vasodilation in type 2 diabetes. Relation to LDL size, oxidized LDL, and antioxidants. Diabetes Care 1999;22(6):973–981.

145. Tan KC, et al. Influence of low density lipoprotein (LDL) subfraction profile and LDL oxidation on endothelium-dependent and independent vasodilation in patients with type 2 diabetes. J Clin Endocrinol Metab 1999;84(9):3212–3216.

146. O'Brien SF, et al. Low-density lipoprotein size, high-density lipoprotein concentration, and endothelial dysfunction in non-insulin-dependent diabetes. Diabet Med 1997;14(11):974–978.

147. Skyrme-Jones RA, et al. Endothelial vasodilator function is related to low-density lipoprotein particle size and low-density lipoprotein vitamin E content in type 1 diabetes. J Am Coll Cardiol 2000;35(2):292–299.

148. Hedrick CC, et al. Glycation impairs high-density lipoprotein function. Diabetologia 2000;43(3): 312–320.

149. Konishi M, Su C. Role of endothelium in dilator responses of spontaneously hypertensive rat arteries. Hypertension 1983;5(6):881–886.

150. Dohi Y, Criscione L, Luscher TF. Renovascular hypertension impairs formation of endothelium-derived relaxing factors and sensitivity to endothelin-1 in resistance arteries. Br J Pharmacol 1991;104(2):349–354.

151. Tuncer M, Vanhoutte PM. Response to the endothelium-dependent vasodilator acetylcholine in perfused kidneys of normotensive and spontaneously hypertensive rats. Blood Press 1993;2(3):217–220.

152. Bell DR. Vascular smooth muscle responses to endothelial autacoids in rats with chronic coarctation hypertension. J Hypertens 1993;11(1):65–74.

153. Vanhoutte PM, Boulanger CM. Endothelium-dependent responses in hypertension. Hypertens Res 1995;18(2):87–98.

154. Panza JA, et al. Role of endothelium-derived nitric oxide in the abnormal endothelium-dependent vascular relaxation of patients with essential hypertension. Circulation 1993;87(5):1468–1474.

155. Panza JA, et al. Effect of increased availability of endothelium-derived nitric oxide precursor on endothelium-dependent vascular relaxation in normal subjects and in patients with essential hypertension. Circulation 1993;87(5):1475–1481.

156. Panza JA, et al. Impaired endothelium-dependent vasodilation in patients with essential hypertension: evidence that the abnormality is not at the muscarinic receptor level. J Am Coll Cardiol 1994;23(7): 1610–1616.

157. Panza JA. Endothelial dysfunction in essential hypertension. Clin Cardiol 1997;20(11 Suppl 2):II-26–II-33.

158. Panza JA, et al. Impaired endothelium-dependent vasodilation in patients with essential hypertension. Evidence that nitric oxide abnormality is not localized to a single signal transduction pathway. Circulation 1995;91(6):1732–1738.

159. Wei EP, et al. Superoxide generation and reversal of acetylcholine-induced cerebral arteriolar dilation after acute hypertension. Circ Res 1985;57(5):781–787.

160. Nakazono K, et al. Does superoxide underlie the pathogenesis of hypertension? Proc Natl Acad Sci USA 1991;88(22):10,045–10,048.

161. Garcia CE, et al. Effect of copper-zinc superoxide dismutase on endothelium-dependent vasodilation in patients with essential hypertension. Hypertension 1995;26(6 Pt 1):863–868.

162. Cardillo C, et al. Xanthine oxidase inhibition with oxypurinol improves endothelial vasodilator function in hypercholesterolemic but not in hypertensive patients. Hypertension 1997;30(1 Pt 1):57–63.

163. Lucas CP, et al. Insulin and blood pressure in obesity. Hypertension 1985;7(5):702–706.

164. Modan M, et al. Hyperinsulinemia. A link between hypertension obesity and glucose intolerance. J Clin Invest 1985;75(3):809–817.

165. Katakam PV, et al. Metformin improves vascular function in insulin-resistant rats. Hypertension 2000;35(1 Pt 1):108–112.

166. Pagano PJ, et al. Vascular action of the hypoglycaemic agent gliclazide in diabetic rabbits. Diabetologia 1998;41(1):9–15.

167. Tack CJ, et al. Insulin-induced vasodilatation and endothelial function in obesity/insulin resistance. Effects of troglitazone. Diabetologia 1998;41(5):569–576.

168. Pistrosch F, et al. In type 2 diabetes, rosiglitazone therapy for insulin resistance ameliorates endothelial dysfunction independent of glucose control. Diabetes Care 2004;27(2):484–490.

169. Ishii H, et al. Amelioration of vascular dysfunctions in diabetic rats by an oral PKC beta inhibitor. Science 1996;272(5262):728–731.

170. Beckman JA, et al. Inhibition of protein kinase Cbeta prevents impaired endothelium-dependent vasodilation caused by hyperglycemia in humans. Circ Res 2002;90(1):107–111.

171. Vlassara H, et al. Exogenous advanced glycosylation end products induce complex vascular dysfunction in normal animals: a model for diabetic and aging complications. Proc Natl Acad Sci USA 1992;89(24):12,043–12,047.

172. Wohaieb SA, Godin DV. Alterations in tissue antioxidant systems in the spontaneously diabetic (BB Wistar) rat. Can J Physiol Pharmacol 1987;65(11):2191–2195.

173. Sundaram RK, et al. Antioxidant status and lipid peroxidation in type II diabetes mellitus with and without complications. Clin Sci (Lond) 1996;90(4):255–260.

174. Cunningham JJ, et al. Reduced mononuclear leukocyte ascorbic acid content in adults with insulin-dependent diabetes mellitus consuming adequate dietary vitamin C. Metabolism 1991;40(2):146–149.

175. Karpen CW, et al. Interrelation of platelet vitamin E and thromboxane synthesis in type I diabetes mellitus. Diabetes 1984;33(3):239–243.

176. Timimi FK, et al. Vitamin C improves endothelium-dependent vasodilation in patients with insulin-dependent diabetes mellitus. J Am Coll Cardiol 1998;31(3):552–557.

177. Ting HH, et al. Vitamin C improves endothelium-dependent vasodilation in patients with non-insulin-dependent diabetes mellitus. J Clin Invest 1996;97(1):22–28.

178. Beckman JA, et al. Ascorbate restores endothelium-dependent vasodilation impaired by acute hyperglycemia in humans. Circulation 2001;103(12):1618–1623.

179. Inoue S, Kawanishi S. Oxidative DNA damage induced by simultaneous generation of nitric oxide and superoxide. FEBS Lett 1995;371(1):86–88.

180. Stroes E, et al. Tetrahydrobiopterin restores endothelial function in hypercholesterolemia. J Clin Invest 1997;99(1):41–46.

181. Lerner DJ, Kannel WB. Patterns of coronary heart disease morbidity and mortality in the sexes: a 26-year follow-up of the Framingham population. Am Heart J 1986;111(2):383–390.

182. Barrett-Connor E, Bush TL. Estrogen and coronary heart disease in women. Jama 1991;265(14): 1861–1867.

183. Winocour PD. Platelet abnormalities in diabetes mellitus. Diabetes 1992;41 Suppl 2:26–31.

184. Keaney JF Jr, et al. 17 beta-estradiol preserves endothelial vasodilator function and limits low-density lipoprotein oxidation in hypercholesterolemic swine. Circulation 1994;89(5):2251–2259.

185. Gisclard V, Miller VM, Vanhoutte PM. Effect of 17 beta-estradiol on endothelium-dependent responses in the rabbit. J Pharmacol Exp Ther 1988;244(1):19–22.

186. Lieberman EH, et al. Estrogen improves endothelium-dependent, flow-mediated vasodilation in postmenopausal women. Ann Intern Med 1994;121(12):936–941.

187. Gilligan DM, et al. Acute vascular effects of estrogen in postmenopausal women. Circulation 1994;90(2):786–791.

188. Pinto S, et al. Endogenous estrogen and acetylcholine-induced vasodilation in normotensive women. Hypertension 1997;29(1 Pt 2):268–273.

189. Arora S, et al. Estrogen improves endothelial function. J Vasc Surg 1998;27(6):1141–1146; discussion 1147.

190. Davidge ST, Zhang Y. Estrogen replacement suppresses a prostaglandin H synthase-dependent vasoconstrictor in rat mesenteric arteries. Circ Res 1998;83(4):388–395.

191. Lim SC, et al. The effect of hormonal replacement therapy on the vascular reactivity and endothelial function of healthy individuals and individuals with type 2 diabetes. J Clin Endocrinol Metab 1999;84(11):4159–4164.

192. Chobanian AV, et al. Antiatherogenic effect of captopril in the Watanabe heritable hyperlipidemic rabbit. Hypertension 1990;15(3):327–331.

193. Becker RH, Wiemer G, Linz W. Preservation of endothelial function by ramipril in rabbits on a long-term atherogenic diet. J Cardiovasc Pharmacol 1991;18 (Suppl 2):S110–S115.

194. Effects of ramipril on cardiovascular and microvascular outcomes in people with diabetes mellitus: results of the HOPE study and MICRO-HOPE substudy. Heart Outcomes Prevention Evaluation Study Investigators. Lancet 2000;355(9200):253–259.

195. Mancini GB, et al. Angiotensin-converting enzyme inhibition with quinapril improves endothelial vasomotor dysfunction in patients with coronary artery disease. The TREND (Trial on Reversing ENdothelial Dysfunction) Study. Circulation 1996;94(3):258–265.

196. McFarlane R, et al. Angiotensin converting enzyme inhibition and arterial endothelial function in adults with Type 1 diabetes mellitus. Diabet Med 1999;16(1):62–66.

197. Mullen MJ, et al. Effect of enalapril on endothelial function in young insulin-dependent diabetic patients: a randomized, double-blind study. J Am Coll Cardiol 1998;31(6):1330–1335.

198. O'Driscoll G, et al. Improvement in endothelial function by angiotensin converting enzyme inhibition in insulin-dependent diabetes mellitus. J Clin Invest 1997;100(3):678–684.

199. Nielsen FS, et al. Lisinopril improves endothelial dysfunction in hypertensive NIDDM subjects with diabetic nephropathy. Scand J Clin Lab Invest 1997;57(5):427–434.

200. Bijlstra PJ, et al. Effect of long-term angiotensin-converting enzyme inhibition on endothelial function in patients with the insulin-resistance syndrome. J Cardiovasc Pharmacol 1995;25(4):658–664.

201. Griendling KK, et al. Angiotensin II stimulates NADH and NADPH oxidase activity in cultured vascular smooth muscle cells. Circ Res 1994;74(6):1141–1148.

202. Wiemer G, et al. Ramiprilat enhances endothelial autacoid formation by inhibiting breakdown of endothelium-derived bradykinin. Hypertension 1991;18(4):558–563.

203. Hornig B, Kohler C, Drexler H. Role of bradykinin in mediating vascular effects of angiotensin-converting enzyme inhibitors in humans. Circulation 1997;95(5):1115–1118.

204. Anderson TJ, et al. The effect of cholesterol-lowering and antioxidant therapy on endothelium-dependent coronary vasomotion. N Engl J Med 1995;332(8):488–493.

205. Treasure CB, et al. Beneficial effects of cholesterol-lowering therapy on the coronary endothelium in patients with coronary artery disease. N Engl J Med 1995;332(8):481–487.

206. Evans M, et al. Ciprofibrate therapy improves endothelial function and reduces postprandial lipemia and oxidative stress in type 2 diabetes mellitus. Circulation 2000;101(15):1773–1779.

207. Sheu WH, et al. Endothelial dysfunction is not reversed by simvastatin treatment in type 2 diabetic patients with hypercholesterolemia. Diabetes Care 1999;22(7):1224–1225.

11 Diabetes and Atherosclerosis

Maria F. Lopes-Virella, MD, PhD *and Gabriel Virella, MD, PhD*

INTRODUCTION

Macrovascular disease is the leading cause of mortality and morbidity in diabetes. The study of factors that may uniquely contribute to the accelerated development of atherosclerosis in diabetes has been an ongoing process for several years. However, the concepts behind both the pathogenic mechanisms of atherosclerosis and the trigger mechanisms that lead to acute clinical events have drastically changed in the last two decades. It is now fully accepted that arteriosclerosis is a chronic inflammatory process and not a degenerative process that inevitably progresses with age. Also accepted is the fact that plaque rupture or erosion not the degree of vessel obstruction is responsible for the majority of acute cardiovascular events. Diabetes most likely contributes to and enhances the chronic inflammatory process characteristic of arteriosclerosis and supporting this concept are the studies showing that atherectomy specimens from diabetic patients undergoing coronary atherectomy for symptomatic coronary artery disease (CAD) have a larger content of macrophages than specimens from patients without diabetes (1). In recent years, mechanisms that lead to plaque formation and to plaque erosion or rupture and the key event that precedes both, endothelial dysfunction, are being actively studied (Fig. 1).

The earliest atherosclerotic lesion is the fatty streak that, although not clinically significant on its own, plays a significant role in the events that lead to plaque progression and rupture. Formation of fatty streaks is induced by the transport of lipoproteins across the endothelium and their retention in the vessel wall. Schwenke and associates (2) have

From: *Contemporary Cardiology: Diabetes and Cardiovascular Disease, Second Edition*
Edited by: M. T. Johnstone and A. Veves © Humana Press Inc., Totowa, NJ

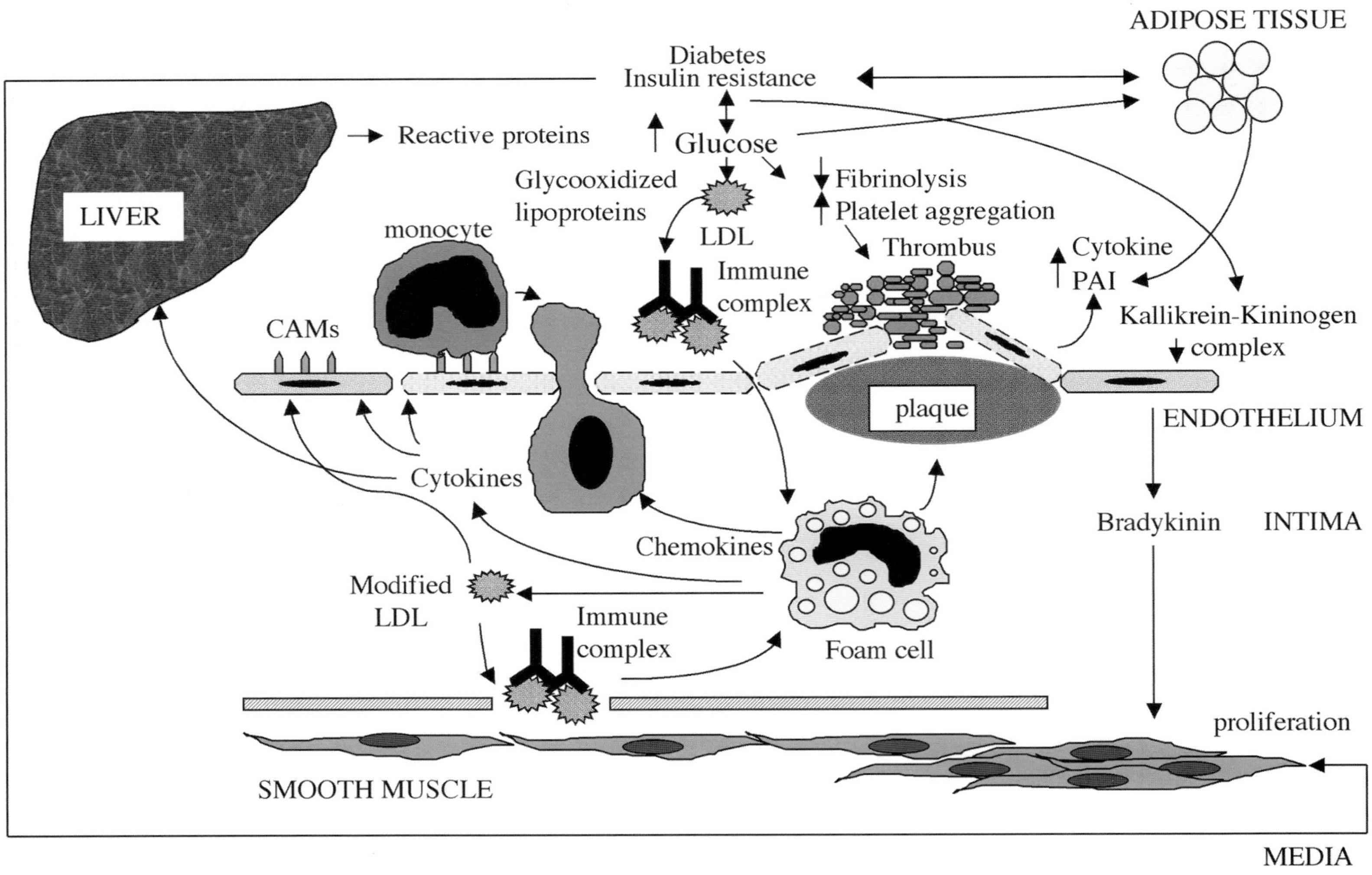
ADIPOSE TISSUE
Diabetes
Insulin resistance
Reactive proteins
Glucose
Glycooxidized
lipoproteins
Fibrinolysis
Platelet aggregation
LIVER
monocyte
LDL
Thrombus
Cytokine
PAI
Immune
complex
Kallikrein-Kininogen
complex
CAMs
plaque
ENDOTHELIUM
Cytokines
Bradykinin
INTIMA
Chemokines
Modified
LDL
Immune
complex
Foam cell
proliferation
SMOOTH MUSCLE
MEDIA

shown that for any given plasma lipoprotein concentration the degree of lipoprotein retention in the artery wall is more important than the rate of transport of the same lipoprotein into the artery wall. Frank and colleagues *(3)* demonstrated, using ultrastructural techniques, that low-density lipoprotein (LDL) can be rapidly transported across an intact endothelium and becomes trapped by the extracellular matrix (ECM) of the subendothelial space *(4)*. Once LDL is transported across the artery wall and binds to the ECM, lipid oxidation is initiated because microenvironment conditions excluding plasma soluble antioxidants are established *(5)*. With oxidation of LDL, endothelial cells are stimulated to release potent chemoattractants, such as monocyte-chemoattractant protein 1 *(4)*, monocyte-colony stimulating factor *(6)* and growth-related oncogene *(7)* and these chemoattractants promote the recruitment of monocytes into the subendothelial space. Recruitment of these cells, as a result of their enormous oxidative capacity, leads to further oxidation of LDL. Heavily modified LDL is cytotoxic to endothelial and smooth muscle cells *(8)* and it is no longer recognized by the LDL receptor. Heavily modified LDL is taken up by macrophage scavenger receptors leading to massive accumulation of cholesterol in macrophages and to their transformation into foam cells, the hallmark of the atherosclerotic process *(9)*. Besides promoting the transformation of macrophages into foam cells, oxidized LDL is a potent inducer of inflammatory molecules and stimulates the immune system. Stimulation of the immune system leads to the formation of antibodies and, as a consequence, to the formation of immune complexes that may play a crucial role in macrophage activation and therefore may contribute to the rupture of atheromatous plaques *(10,11)*.

Diabetes accelerates the sequence of events just described in many ways and in this chapter updated information concerning factors associated with the diabetic state that may accelerate the development of atherosclerosis and thrombosis and contribute to acute clinical events will be provided. Special emphasis will be placed on endothelial dysfunction, on abnormalities in platelet function, coagulation and fibrinolysis, and on

---

Fig. 1. *(opposite page)* Diagrammatic representation of the possible pathogenic mechanisms for the development of atherosclerosis in diabetes. Increased levels of glucose lead to decreased production of prostacyclin-stimulating factor (PSF), reduced nitric oxide activity, increased bradykinin in an injured endothelium and to multiple changes in lipoprotein metabolism and in cell–lipoprotein interactions. These changes contribute to the accelerated development of atherosclerosis in diabetic patients by reducing vasodilatation of the endothelium and, in the case of bradykinin promoting vasoconstriction and smooth muscle cell proliferation. Increased plasma glucose levels promotes also nonenzymatic glycation of lipoproteins and enhance their susceptibility to oxidative modification. These modified lipoproteins decrease fibrinolysis and increase platelet aggregation, which contributes to increased thrombosis. Modified lipoproteins may also stimulate the expression of cell adhesion molecules (CAMs). Monocyte adhesion to the endothelial cell layer and migration of these cells to the subendothelial space follow the expression of these molecules. Furthermore modified lipoproteins lead to a decrease in the release of nitric oxide by the endothelium and therefore to impaired vasodilatation. Glycated/oxidized lipoproteins in the intimal layer may be further modified by oxidative processes that result in the formation of glycoxidized lipoproteins that, in turn, stimulate the immune system to form antibodies. The resulting immune complexes are taken up by macrophages, and they stimulate the formation of cholesteryl ester-laden cells (foam cells) and the release of cytokines. Cytokines released during these processes will elicit release of reactive proteins by the liver (C-reactive protein) besides further injuring the endothelium and, thus, exacerbate the cycle.

qualitative and quantitative abnormalities of lipoproteins and their role in foam cell formation and in eliciting a humoral response with formation of antibodies and immune complexes.

ENDOTHELIAL DYSFUNCTION

The endothelium participates in a number of important homeostatic and cellular functions that are essential to preserve its functional integrity. Loss of functional integrity of the endothelium is responsible, not only for cell adhesion, the initial step in the atherosclerotic process, but also for the triggering of its final step: the formation of thrombi, which leads to vessel occlusion and to acute ischemic events.

The endothelium controls leukocyte adhesion, platelet reactivity, capillary permeability, the regulation of vascular smooth muscle cells (VSMC), and blood clotting. Regulation of smooth muscle cell tone is mediated by the endothelium through the release of potent vaso-relaxing agents (nitric oxide [NO], prostacyclin) and vasoconstrictor agents (thromboxane and endothelin).

Nitric Oxide

NO is synthesized from L-arginine by NO synthase (NOS) and it is an anti-thrombotic product of the endothelial cells. NO has been shown not only to mediate vasodilation but also to inhibit platelet aggregation and adhesion (12), prevent monocyte adherence to the endothelium (12), and prolong bleeding time (13). It has also been found to be responsible for reducing plasma fibrinogen levels (14) and to reduce platelet activation (15). Reduced NO bioavailability leads to impaired vasodilation, to abnormalities in the above functions and, as a consequence, enhances thrombotic events in humans (16).

Impairment of NO-mediated vasodilation has been shown in both type 1 and type 2 diabetes (17,18) and it may contribute to the accelerated development of macrovascular disease in diabetes. Recent studies using an inducible NO synthase (iNOS)-deficient mice shows that there is decreased response to acetylcholine in wild-type diabetic animals when compared to nondiabetic animals. No difference in response was, however, observed in the diabetic iNOS-deficient mice thus giving the first direct evidence that impairment of endothelium-dependent relaxation during diabetes is dependent on iNOS expression (19). Oxidized lipoproteins, which are present in increased levels in diabetes, may be behind the reduced NO activity in diabetes, as shown by several studies (20–22). Interestingly, NO may also influence lipoprotein oxidation. If cells are stimulated to express active NOS, their oxidative capability is lost (23). On the other hand, if conditions in the vessel wall favor the release of superoxide, NO can be converted to peroxynitrate, which is a powerful oxidant (24). Recently antioxidant status, lipid peroxidation and NO end-products were measured in a group of Asian-Indian patients with type 2 diabetes with and without nephropathy (25). This study confirmed that oxidative stress is increased and antioxidant defenses are compromised in patients with type 2 diabetes, and that these derangements are more severe in patients with nephropathy. Other possible factors behind reduced NO activity in diabetes include abnormalities in insulin and in the kallikrein/kinin pathway.

Insulin

Several clinical trials (26,27) clearly show that increased levels of insulin are frequently associated with increased risk for macrovascular disease and that led to the concept that administration of exogenous insulin would contribute to or enhance the development of macrovascular complications in diabetes. This concept has been clearly discredited by the data of two major trials *(28,29)*, one performed in type 1 and another in type 2 diabetic subjects (the Diabetes Control and Complications Trial [DCCT] and United Kingdom Prospective Diabetes Study trials). Both trials clearly show a reduction in cardiovascular events with intensive glycemic control and although the reduction did not reach statistical significance, it completely excluded the hypothesis that insulin administration would contribute to an increase in cardiovascular events.

However, although it is clear that administration of exogenous insulin do not lead to an increase in macrovascular disease, hyperinsulinemia syndromes like the insulin resistance syndrome, particularly when associated with central obesity, are definitively associated with accelerated development of macrovascular disease. Although the insulin resistance syndrome, characterized by glucose intolerance and hyperinsulinemia, is associated with several cardiovascular risk factors including dyslipidemia, hypertension, and dysfibrinolysis, the increased risk for macrovascular disease cannot be fully explained by the hypertension and dyslipidemia. It is likely that endothelial dysfunction, an important player in determining increased risk for macrovascular disease is involved.

Normal endothelial function is quite dependent on NO and insulin is a vasodilator and stimulates endothelial NO production *(30)*. Thus, reduction of NO production in insulin resistance states will lead to endothelial dysfunction and atherosclerosis. Baron and colleagues *(31)* have shown that insulin causes endothelial-derived NO-dependent vasodilatation and that inhibition of NO production with L-*NG*-monomethyl arginine (L-NMMA) causes complete abrogation of the insulin-induced vasodilatation. Interestingly the same authors *(31)* have also shown that insulin is unable to modulate endothelial-dependent vasodilatation in obese insulin-resistant subjects or in type 2 diabetic subjects. Therefore, although insulin levels are markedly elevated in these subjects, insulin action is reduced, NO-dependent vasodilatation usually induced by insulin is impaired and endothelial dysfunction occurs.

In conclusion, insulin-resistant states of obesity, hypertension, and non-insulin-dependent diabetes mellitus (NIDDM) exhibit blunted insulin-mediated vasodilatation and impaired endothelium-dependent vasodilatation, regardless of high levels of endogenous insulin. Thus, it appears that endothelial dysfunction is an integral aspect of the syndrome of insulin resistance, independent of hyperglycemia or hyperinsulinemia and this dysfunction of the endothelium may contribute to worsen insulin resistance and predispose to macrovascular disease.

Prostaglandins

PROSTACYCLIN

Prostacyclin (PGI2) is synthesized mainly by vascular endothelial cells and it is a potent vasodilator and an inhibitor of platelet adhesion and aggregation *(32)*. Previous studies summarized in a review article *(33)* have shown that the synthesis of PGI2 by the vasculature of diabetic patients is reduced. The expression of the prostacyclin-stimulating factor (PSF), assessed by immunostaining in smooth muscle cells (SMCs) of human coronary arteries, is markedly reduced in diabetic subjects with or without previous myocardial infarction (MI) and in nondiabetic subjects with prior MI *(34)*, strongly suggesting that the decreased production of prostacyclin, previously reported in diabetes, is likely a result of decreased production of PSF. Interestingly, it seems that the decreased expression of PSF is modulated by glucose levels and it is frankly diminished in presence of high glucose levels *(35)*, the usual milieu in diabetics when in poor glycemic control.

THROMBOXANE

The endothelium secrets not only vasorelaxing agents, but also vasoconstricting agents. Thromboxane A2, is one of the best studied vasoconstrictors and it is the physiological counteracting mediator for NO. Both thromboxane A2 and its precursor, prostaglandin H2, are synthesized by both platelets and vessel wall tissues. Thus, it is obvious that the increased activation of platelets in diabetics (36) contributes to the formation of thromboxane A2 and prostaglandin H2 in this disease state (37). Other factors that may equally contribute to the increased platelet biosynthesis of thromboxane A2 include cigarette smoking (38), hypercholesterolemia (39), and homozygous homocystinuria (40). The rate of thromboxane A2 biosynthesis appears to reflect the influence of co-existing disorders like diabetes, hypertension, and dyslipidemia on platelet biochemistry and function (41). Thus, enhanced thromboxane A2 biosynthesis may represent a common link between these cardiovascular risk factors and the thrombotic complication associated with macrovascular complications, specifically peripheral vascular disease, in diabetes.

The Kallikrein/Kinin Pathway

Bradykinin is generated by kallikreins from their precursor kininogens and it is a potent vasodilator that increases vascular permeability and plays a primary role in inflammation. In noninjured vessels, bradykinin causes relaxation of the VSMC through the synthesis and release of NO from the endothelium (42). In contrast, when the integrity of the endothelium is compromised, bradykinin will act directly in VSMCs promoting their vasoconstriction (43) and fibrosis. The direct action of bradykinin in VSMCs is mediated by its binding to its B2 receptors and subsequent activation and nuclear translocation of p42 and p44 mitogen-activated protein kinase (MAPK) that induces c-fos and c-jun mRNA levels and generation of reactive oxygen species (44,45). Activation of the MAPK pathway leads to an increase in ECM proteins, such as collagen I and fibronectin (45,46). Douillet and associates (46) have shown that activation of transforming growth factor (TGF)-β together with MAPK activation, mediates the increased production of collagen and tissue inhibitor of metalloproteinase (TIMP)-1 that contributes to the ECM accumulation induced by bradykinin.

Abnormalities in the kallikrein/kinin pathway have been found recently in the DCCT/Echo Dobutamine International Cooperative cohort of type 1 diabetes (47) and increased expression of B2-kinin receptors has been described in the vessel wall of diabetic animals (48). Interestingly hyperglycemia, which is known to induce endothelial dysfunction as a result of its ability to promote endothelial cell toxicity, has also been shown to up-regulate the expression of kinin receptors in VSMC (49). Thus, in diabetes, the abnormalities in the kallikrein/kinin system by modulating vascular fibrosis play an important role in the development of arteriosclerosis.

The Lipoxygenase Pathway

Several lines of evidence support the concept that lipoxygenases (LOs) and their products play an important role in the pathogenesis of arteriosclerosis. The LO pathway is one of the three major oxidative pathways able to metabolize arachidonic acid, leading to the formation of hydroperoxyeicosatetraenoic acids, hydroxyeicosatetraenoic acids (HETEs), and leukotrienes. All these products of the LO pathway have been shown to have potent inflammatory, growth, adhesive and chemoattractant effects in cells. They are also associated with oxidative stress and cellular apoptosis. The human and rabbit 15-LO enzymes and the leukocyte 12-LO enzymes have high homology and they have been classified as 12/15-LOs because they are able to lead to the formation of both 12(S) and 15 (S)-HETEs from arachidonic acid. 12(S) and 15(S)-HETEs have been detected in several vascular tissues and in cells including endothelial cells (50,51), monocytes (51) and SMCs (52). Interestingly, 12/15-LO has been found in rabbit arteriosclerotic regions co-localized with epitopes characteristic for oxidized LDL (53). Furthermore, analysis of the lipid oxidation products in human arteriosclerotic lesions revealed that oxidation of polyunsaturated fatty acids therein was mainly mediated by LOs (54). Several studies have shown that the 12/15-LO pathway is also able to mediate oxidative modification of LDL (55,56).

In diabetes, the importance of the LO pathway in the development of cardiovascular complications has also been supported by several studies. Endothelial cells cultured under hyperglycemic conditions produced increased amounts of HETEs that, in turn, mediate adhesion of monocytes to endothelial cells (57). Interestingly not only endothelial cells but also SMCs cultured under hyperglycemic conditions synthesized increased amounts of the cell-associated 12(S)-HETE (52) besides proliferating faster (58). 12-HETE leads also to a significant increase in fibronectin levels in the cells cultured under high-glucose conditions (59). Natarajan and Nadler (60) have also observed that treatment of VSMCs with advanced glycation end-products (AGE; which also mimic the diabetic milieu) was quite effective in increasing 12-LO activity

Recently, it was shown that the 12/15-LO pathway was activated in a swine model of hyperlipidemia and diabetes-induced accelerated atherosclerosis (61,62). Diabetes and hyperlipidemia on their own increased both monocyte-mediated oxidative stress and 12/15-LO expression in arteries, but the combination of these two risk factors not only led to a marked acceleration of atherosclerosis, but also to a synergistic increase in oxidative stress and 12/15-LO activation.

Endothelin-1

Endothelin-1 (ET-1) was first described in 1988 and since then a considerable amount of research has been performed to study this potent vasoconstrictor. Early studies suggested that ET-1 concentrations in the plasma of type 1 and type 2 diabetic patients were significantly elevated (approx 3.5-fold) compared to levels in nondiabetic patients (63) but no significant correlations between endothelin levels and complications were observed. In contrast, subsequent studies found a significant correlation between endothelin levels and both nephropathy (36,64) and retinopathy (65). The association between endothelin levels and macrovascular disease is, however, still controversial (66,67). Also, controversial are the factors that modulate plasma endothelin concentrations. Both insulin and glucose have been shown to stimulate the release of endothelin by culture cells including human endothelial cells (68), porcine and bovine aortic endothelial cells (69), and VSMCs (70). In vivo, however, the data is somewhat ambiguous. The levels of endothelin seem to be modulated by insulin in some in vivo studies (71,72) but not in others in which the relationship between endothelin and insulin was directly examined and found to be lacking (73). In conclusion, the relationship between diabetes and endothelin remains uncertain.

Von Willebrand Factor

It has been suggested that the plasma level of von Willebrand factor (vWF) may serve as a nonspecific marker of endothelial dysfunction (74). vWF is a complex glycoprotein synthesized by the vascular endothelium and megakaryocytes.

Several studies have shown an association between increased levels of vWF and diabetic complications, including macrovascular complications. The Munich General Practitioner Project, a 10-year study of macrovascular and overall mortality in 290 type 2 diabetic patients, concluded that vWF was a risk factor for death related to macrovascular disease *(75)*. Other studies performed in type 2 diabetic patients *(76)* also show that vWF is strongly related to the occurrence of cardiovascular events in these patients.

Interestingly, the concentration of vWF significantly decreases in patients who consume a diet high in monounsaturated fat *(77)*, although no changes were observed in patients placed on a high-carbohydrate diet. Whether or not the effects of monounsaturated fat are secondary to their ability to decrease susceptibility of LDL to oxidation in vitro and presumably in vivo is not known, but it should certainly be considered because of the numerous reports connecting oxidized LDL to endothelial dysfunction.

Cell Adhesion Molecules

Endothelial cells elaborate leukocyte-specific adhesion molecules, both constitutively and in response to cytokines and other mediators *(78,79)*. Circulating monocytes display receptors for these cell adhesion molecules. Vascular cell adhesion molecule (VCAM)-1 *(80,81)*, intercellular adhesion molecule (ICAM)-1 *(81,82)*, E-selectin *(81)*, and platelet endothelial cell adhesion molecule (CD31) *(81)*, are expressed in atherosclerotic lesions. Recent investigations have documented that soluble forms of these adhesion molecules are present in endothelial cell culture supernatants and human sera *(83–85)*. In diabetes, as earlier as 1994, increased levels of soluble cell adhesion molecules were found in plasma of type 1 and type 2 diabetic patients *(86–88)*. Recently increased levels of VCAM-1 and E-selectin were found not only in patients with type 2 diabetes but also in patients with impaired glucose tolerance *(89)*. The levels of these adhesion molecules were correlated with the levels of glucose and insulin obtained after a glucose tolerance test *(89)*. Similar results were obtained by another recent study by Matsumoto and associates *(90)* that shows that increased levels of VCAM-1 and E-selectin but not ICAM-1 are significantly increased in a group of type 2 diabetic patients with macroangiopathy and that the increase persisted after adjustment for age, sex, duration of diabetes, blood pressure, HbA1c, high-density lipoprotein (HDL)-cholesterol, and smoking status. In contrast, in a very small study of 28 diabetic patients without any complications at entry into the study and followed prospectively for 5 years, high baseline ICAM-1 levels were able to predict the development of macrovascular disease after adjusting for age, systolic blood pressure, creatinine, and glycemic control *(91)*.

Additionally, a positive correlation between plasma concentration of VCAM-1 and the thickness of the intimal plus medial layer of the carotid arteries was observed in type 2 diabetic patients *(88)*, suggesting that circulating VCAM-1 levels may be a marker of atherosclerotic lesions in type 2 patients with symptomatic and asymptomatic atherosclerosis. Increased levels of P-selectin *(92)* were also found to be significantly correlated in a group of 517 subjects (187 with type 2 diabetes) with arterial stiffness and arterial wall thickness and the later association was independent of other clinical factors.

Increased expression of adhesion molecules can be induced in vitro using cultured endothelial cells by exposure to either modified lipoproteins (oxidized, glycated, and AGE-LDL) or to cytokines *(93,94)*. Some lipoproteins, like AGE-LDL, on occupancy of macrophage receptors, induces the release of tumor necrosis factor, interleukin (IL)-1, platelet-derived growth factor (PDGF), and immunoglobin growth factor-1, and these mediators in turn promote the expression of adhesion molecules *(93)*. Infusion of AGE products in rabbits produced a variety of vascular changes. In endothelial cells, these included increased expression of VCAM-1 and ICAM-1: mainly in areas affected by atheroma *(93)*. Further supporting the significance of these interactions, it has been shown that blockade of receptor of advanced glycation end-products (RAGE) can inhibit AGE product-induced impairment of endothelial barrier function and consequent hyperpermeability. Inhibition of AGE product formation using antioxidants has a similar effect. More recently it has been shown that lesions from human coronary arteries from patients with diabetes when compared to lesions from nondiabetic patients, exhibit increased levels of an immunoreactive chemokine, fractalkine, that mediates firm adhesion of leukocytes *(95)*.

Modified lipoproteins also have the potential to induce the release of cytokines by yet another mechanism. They are immunogenic and therefore elicit production of antibodies and, as a consequence, the formation of immune complexes. These immune complexes containing modified LDL are able to stimulate macrophages and release increased amounts of tumor necrosis factor (TNF)-α and IL-1β *(94)*. The release of these cytokines leads to increased expression of adhesion molecules *(96,97)*.

Mechanisms of Foam Cell Formation

Foam cells are the hallmark of the arteriosclerotic process. Diabetes appears to enhance foam cell lesion formation in experimental animals and in humans. In animal models, type 1 diabetes induced by autoimmune-mediated β-cell destruction or by toxins, alloxan, or streptozotocin increases fatty streak formation *(98–100)*. Similarly, in human postmortem studies it has been shown that diabetes accelerates the formation of fatty streaks. The Pathobiological Determinants of Atherosclerosis in Youth study, a study in 3000 youths, ages 15 to 34 years, who died of trauma, showed that youths over 25 years of age with elevated levels of glycated hemoglobin (>8%), had significantly more fatty streaks in the right coronary artery than controls even when their lipid profiles were normal *(101,102)*. A recent high-resolution ultrasound in vivo study of common carotid arteries of 11-year-old children with type 1 diabetes showed that these children had an increased intima-media thickness (IMT) compared to a matched control group *(103)*. The increased IMT in children with type 1 diabetes did not appear to be the result of conventional risk factors, such as increased blood pressure, increased total and LDL cholesterol and triglycerides or low HDL levels *(103)*. Thus, these results indicate that diabetes, in the absence of conventional risk factors, accelerates arteriosclerosis in humans. The mechanisms behind such increase are not known but they may be related with the presence in diabetes of increased levels of modified lipoproteins or of lipoproteins of abnormal composition because the best-known mechanism leading to the transformation of macrophages into foam cells is the uptake of lipoproteins of abnormal composition by macrophages and the uptake of modified LDL by macrophages *(9)*. Another mechanism, not as well known but even more efficient in inducing foam cell formation, is the uptake of oxidized LDL immune complexes by Fcγ receptor I *(104,105)*.

QUANTITATIVE/QUALITATIVE ABNORMALITIES OF LIPOPROTEINS

In poorly controlled diabetic patients, plasma LDL, intermediate density lipoproteins and very low-density lipoprotein (VLDL) levels are elevated *(106–110)*. The increase in

VLDL levels has been attributed to increased hepatic production or decreased clearance of VLDL *(111)* and may be very significant in the development of arteriosclerosis in diabetes and in women *(112)*. HDL levels in diabetes vary with the type of diabetes and, in some groups, with glycemic control. In type 2 diabetic patients, HDL levels are usually low and do not necessarily increase with improved metabolic control *(107,110,113)*. The low HDL levels are secondary to an increased clearance rate by hepatic triglyceride lipase *(114)*. In type 1 diabetic patients it has been shown that HDL cholesterol levels are low during poor glycemic control and increase to normal or above normal when adequate control is attained *(108,110,115)*. Changes with improved glycemic control are less marked in women than in men *(108)*. In type 1 black diabetic women, little association is observed between plasma lipid levels and glycemic control *(115)*.

Besides quantitative abnormalities, diabetic patients are known to have significant qualitative lipoprotein abnormalities, which can be located either in the protein or in the lipid moiety of the lipoproteins. Apolipoprotein (apo)-E facilitates the uptake of triglyceride-rich lipoprotein remnants by the liver and plays a role in the recognition of VLDL by human macrophages *(116)*. In contrast, apo-CIII inhibits the uptake of remnants *(117,118)*. We found in some groups of diabetic patients that the ratio of apo-C/apo-E was decreased *(119,120)*. This might be expected to enhance hepatic clearance of remnants, but it will also favor the uptake of remnants by macrophages and cholesteryl ester (CE) accumulation in these cells.

Abnormalities in LDL lipid composition may also lead to altered lipoprotein metabolism and intracellular accumulation of cholesterol in the vessel wall. We have demonstrated, several years ago, that LDL isolated from patients with insulin-dependent diabetes mellitus (IDDM) in poor metabolic control was taken up and degraded less efficiently than normal LDL by human fibroblasts *(121)*. We have also shown that this same LDL was enriched in triglycerides. Hiramatsu and colleagues *(122)* confirmed our studies and demonstrated that triglyceride-enriched LDL isolated from both diabetic and nondiabetic subjects with hypertriglyceridemia was poorly recognized by fibroblasts. Lipoprotein surface lipid composition may also be abnormal even in "normolipemic" type 1 diabetic patients. Bagdade and colleagues *(123)* demonstrated altered free cholesterol/lecithin ratios in LDL and VLDL fractions, and these may result in altered lipoprotein metabolism. Similar observations were made in type 2 diabetic patients, and, like in type 1 diabetic patients, the abnormalities did not respond to improved glycemic control *(124)*. Finally, high levels of small, dense LDL have been described in patients with type 1 and type 2 diabetes, when in poor metabolic control *(125,126)* and that may contribute to enhance the atherogenicity of diabetic plasma. It may also explain why levels of apolipoprotein B in diabetics are often higher than expected for a given LDL cholesterol level.

HDL composition can also be markedly affected by diabetes, and this may impair reverse cholesterol transport *(127)*. Fielding and associates *(128,129)* observed that cholesterol efflux from normal fibroblasts was inhibited when the cells were incubated with plasma from poorly controlled type 2 diabetic patients compared with normal plasma. A spontaneous transfer of free cholesterol from VLDL and LDL to HDL, induced by free cholesterol (and phospholipid) enrichment of both VLDL and LDL present in diabetic plasma caused the defect in cholesterol transport. An increase in the triglyceride content of HDL has also been noted in type 2 diabetic patients with hypertriglyceridemia and low levels of HDL cholesterol *(124,130,131)* and cannot be fully corrected by improved glycemic control *(124)*. As with VLDL and LDL, the composition of surface lipids in

HDL is abnormal in diabetes and, at least in HDL3, remains so despite improvements in glycemic control *(124)*. Alterations in the apoprotein content of HDL in diabetes have also been described. Plasma apolipoprotein A-I levels are increased in diabetic patients *(110)*, and consequently the HDL cholesterol/apo-A-I ratio is reduced *(132)*, diminishing the anti-atherogenic potential of HDL.

Lipoprotein Glycation, Oxidation, and Glyco-Oxidation

In diabetes, increased nonenzymatic glycosylation affects any protein exposed to elevated levels of glucose. Glucose is covalently bound, mainly to lysine residues in protein molecules forming fructose-lysine. Subsequently, further reactions occur, mainly in long-lived proteins, leading to the development of unreactive end-products, many of which are cross-linked, brown or fluorescent *(133)*. The most common description for these end-products is AGE. Only a few are well-recognized structures such as carboxymethyllsine *(134)* and pentosidine *(135)*. Others have been identified in model systems and by immunological techniques in vivo, such as pyrraline *(136)* and crosslines *(137)*. The formation of these end products and the accompanying increase in protein fluorescence are mediated by free radical oxidation *(138)*. Thus, because glycation and oxidation are involved, the products are also called "glyco-oxidation products." Recently, it has been recognized that some of the AGEs are derived from oxidation of lipids *(139)*. Oxidation of unsaturated fatty acid side chains yields reactive carbonyl-containing fragments (glyoxal, 4-HNE, malondialdehyde [MDA]), which in turn may react with aminogroups, mainly lysine residues *(140)*. Some of the lipoxidation products are similar to glyco-oxidation products *(139)*. Thus, oxidative stress may damage carbohydrates, lipids, or glycated residues already present in proteins, leading to the formation of carbonyl-containing intermediates. These carbonyl-containing intermediates may not only modify proteins but also phospholipids *(141)* and nucleotides *(142)*.

It has been postulated that enhanced glycation, oxidation, and glyco-oxidation of lipoproteins may underlie the development of macrovascular disease in diabetes. This is quite an attractive hypothesis because it would explain the individual variation in the development of complications in diabetes. Regardless of the similarity in glycemic control and cardiovascular risk factors, the development of complications would also depend on differences in oxidative stress and variations in the antioxidant defenses and in differences in the immune response to the modified lipoproteins. A short summary of the large body of evidence showing that modified lipoproteins may be relevant to the accelerated development of atherosclerosis in diabetes is presented next.

Lipoprotein Glycation

Schleicher and associates *(143)* were the first investigators to demonstrate that human lipoproteins (LDL and HDL) undergo increased glycation when exposed to elevated glucose concentrations and to postulate that increased glycation of lipoproteins in vivo might have significant metabolic consequences. Their initial studies showed that the extent of incorporation of glucose into HDL and LDL apolipoproteins (apo-A-I, -A-II, -B, -C, and -E) was directly proportional to the time of incubation and to the concentration of glucose. Subsequent studies by our group built on these observations. We demonstrated that the extent of glycation of LDL correlates well with other short- and medium-term indicators of glycemic control (mean plasma glucose, plasma protein glycation, and HbA1c), and that increased LDL glycation is present even in normolipidemic diabetic patients in satisfactory glycemic control *(144)*.

Studies performed by a number of investigators who have prospectively treated IDDM patients with intensive insulin regimens to achieve euglycemia have reported decreases in LDL levels of 5 to 27% *(145–147)*. That decrease in LDL levels may be related to the decrease in LDL glycation induced by the intensive insulin therapy and subsequent increase in LDL clearance.

LDL clearance is mediated primarily by the LDL-receptor mediated pathway and, as mentioned before, glucose is covalently bound to the lysine residues of apo-B. These residues, as shown by Weisgraber and associates *(148)* are critical for the specific recognition of LDL by the LDL receptor. The degree of inhibition of LDL binding is proportional to the extent of lysine modification and can be observed even when only as few as 3% of the lysine residues of apo-B are modified. Studies *(149–150)* aimed at investigating the metabolism of glycated LDL in cultured human fibroblasts have shown that in normal human fibroblasts, which possess the classical LDL receptor, there was impaired binding and degradation of glycated compared to control LDL, the impairment being proportional to the extent of glycation. Modification of as few as 2 to 5% lysine residues of LDL led to a 5 to 25% decrease in LDL catabolism by human fibroblasts *(150)*.

The above studies were confirmed by our laboratory, using LDL isolated from diabetic subjects and sex, age, and race-matched control subjects. We have shown that recognition by human fibroblasts of LDL isolated from diabetic patients is markedly impaired *(121)*. Interestingly, unlike fibroblasts, human monocyte-derived macrophages recognized LDL glycated in vitro to a greater extent than native LDL, fourfold over control LDL values *(151)*. A separate, low-affinity, high-capacity receptor pathway by which glycated LDL gains entry into the macrophage was identified.

Other studies performed in our laboratory *(152)* further support the enhanced atherogenicity of glycated LDL in diabetes. In these studies we isolated, using a boronate affinity chromatography column that binds fructose-lysine adducts, two fractions of LDL from type 1 diabetic patients and compared their metabolic behavior. The glycated LDL fraction that binds to the column before elution was poorly taken up and degraded by fibroblasts when compared to the nonbound (nonglycated) LDL fraction. The impairment was directly related to the degree of glycation of the fraction. In human monocyte-macrophages, uptake of the bound (glycated) LDL was twofold greater than that of the nonbound (nonglycated) LDL fraction. The uptake, however, was not mediated by the LDL receptor pathway, but by a high-capacity, low-affinity receptor pathway. From the above studies, we concluded that "in vitro" glycated LDL and LDL from diabetic patients are poorly recognized by the classical LDL receptor but they are preferentially recognized by a distinct receptor pathway present in human macrophages. The recognition of glycated LDL by this alternate pathway leads to intracellular accumulation of cholesteryl esters and may thereby contribute to the accelerated development of atherosclerosis in diabetes.

Glycated LDL also affects platelet aggregation. Compared to LDL from control subjects, LDL from type 1 diabetic patients is a more potent stimulator of thromboxane B2 release and thrombin-induced platelet aggregation *(153)*.

Lipoprotein Oxidation and Glyco-Oxidation

Glycation of LDL under hyperglycemic conditions is likely to result in increased formation of oxidized LDL *(154)*. Several mechanisms have been proposed to explain the increased oxidation of lipoproteins in diabetes. One of them involves the auto-oxidation of simple monosaccharides *(155,156)*, such as glucose, and of fructose-lysine

(155,156,157), the first Amadori rearrangement product, under physiological conditions and in the presence of trace amounts of metal ions. Auto-oxidation of these compounds generates superoxide radicals and lipid peroxidation occurs. Another mechanism possibly responsible for increased oxidation of LDL in diabetes is the impaired clearance of glycated LDL that leads to an increase in the lipoprotein circulation time and facilitates its exposure to oxidative stress. In damaged vessel walls, trapping of LDL as a result of covalent glucose-derived crosslinking of LDL to glycated structural proteins may be yet another mechanism contributing to increased LDL oxidation in diabetes.

Several studies support the above mechanisms. Brownlee and associates *(158)* have reported an increase in LDL-collagen crosslinking when the lipoprotein is exposed to modified collagen (containing browning products), compared to control collagen. Some studies have shown that glycated LDL is more susceptible to oxidation than nonglycated LDL and that increased oxidative modification of LDL occurs in presence of high glucose levels *(155,157)*. Tsai and associates *(159)* showed that in poorly controlled IDDM patients without macrovascular disease, the lag phase of conjugated diene formation after initiation of LDL oxidation by the addition of copper was shorter than in normal control subjects. That increase in susceptibility to oxidation was not associated with an increase of small dense LDL in the diabetic population, but with a decrease in the total peroxyl radical trapping potential of plasma (TRAP) which was significantly decreased in the IDDM patients. The decrease in TRAP was secondary to a decrease in uric acid and vitamin A. Data from our own laboratory shows that, in contrast to what happens in poorly controlled diabetics, in IDDM without pre-existent complications and with normal lipid levels and good glycemic control, the susceptibility of LDL to oxidation is not enhanced *(160)*.

That oxidized or glyco-oxidized LDL indeed play an important role in the pathogenesis of atherosclerosis has been confirmed by several lines of evidence: the presence of oxidized lipoproteins in the vessel wall *(161,162)*, as demonstrated by immunochemical staining of lesions with antibodies recognizing oxidation-specific epitopes, and the demonstration that regression of lesions may occur in animals treated with antioxidants *(163)*. Recently, AGE epitopes have also been described in atherosclerotic lesions of euglycemic rabbits *(164)*. Interestingly, the AGE epitopes were found in similar locations as the epitopes generated during the modification of lipoproteins by oxidation. Other studies show that blockade of RAGE results in decreased inflammation in preformed lesions in streptozotocin diabetic apo-E-deficient mice *(165)*. Because RAGE binds to a large number of ligands, in addition to AGEs, it is not known if the effects of RAGE blockade in this study were as a result of decreased uptake of AGEs. In fact, RAGE blockade reduced atherosclerotic lesion size *(165)* and intimal thickening after arterial injury *(166)* in nondiabetic mice, suggesting that the role for RAGE ligands is not dependent on the diabetic state.

Several clinical studies further strengthened the morphological findings described above. Regnstrom and associates *(167)* have shown that the degree of susceptibility to oxidation of LDL isolated from 35 male survivors of MI was positively correlated with the severity of coronary atherosclerosis. Several other investigators described increased oxidizability of LDL in patients with coronary heart disease *(168)*, and patients with carotid or femoral atherosclerosis *(169)*.

In contrast with the pletora of information that exists concerning LDL oxidation very little is known concerning oxidation of other lipoproteins. Oxidation of VLDL has been shown to be cytotoxic *(170)* but very little is known concerning possible metabolic alterations that may result from the oxidation of this lipoprotein. Oxidative modification of HDL in vitro has been shown to remove the ability of HDL to stimulate cholesterol efflux from foam cells *(171)*. Recently, Bowry and associates *(172)* reported that HDL is the major carrier of oxidized lipids in plasma and may be responsible for the hepatic clearance of oxidized lipids from plasma.

Modified LDL Antibodies and LDL-Containing Immunocomplexes

In addition to the interactions described above, modification of proteins, such as oxidation and AGE modification, may alter their structure sufficiently to render them immunogenic. The presence of antibodies to oxidized LDL and AGE-LDL has been described in the sera of several groups of patients and controls. The levels of oxidized LDL (oxLDL) antibodies have been repeatedly reported to correlate with different endpoints considered as evidence of atherosclerotic vascular disease, progression of carotid atherosclerosis, or risk for the future development of MI *(173–178)*. According to Maggi and associates, a significantly higher level of oxLDL antibodies are measured in patients with carotid atherosclerosis compared to normal controls and the highest levels were found in patients with associated hyperlipidemia and hypertension *(174)*. Salonen and associates *(175)* reported a direct relationship between the titer of auto-antibodies to MDA-LDL and the rate of progression of carotid atherosclerosis. Lehtimaki and associates reported higher levels of oxLDL antibodies in patients with angiographically verified CAD *(176)*. According to Erkkilä and co-workers, oxLDL antibody levels were significantly elevated in men with MI *(177)*. In type 2 diabetic patients, Bellomo and associates found higher levels of oxLDL and MDA-LDL antibodies compared to healthy controls *(178)*. Antibodies against 2-furoyl-4(5)-(2-furanyl)-1H-imidazole, a specific model compound of AGE, and to AGE-modified proteins have been detected in the sera of diabetic and euglycemic subjects *(164,179)*, but the levels of AGE-LDL antibodies were lower in diabetics than in controls in one of the studies *(179)*. It must be noted that several other studies have yielded contradictory data, showing either no correlation between modified LDL antibodies and end-points of atherosclerotic disease, or even showing inverse correlations *(180–188)*.

The inverse correlations between modified LDL antibody levels and atherosclerosis, together with data obtained in laboratory animals suggesting that modified LDL antibodies are predominantly of the noninflammatory immunoglobin (Ig)M isotype *(189)* and human studies claiming that IgM antibodies to modified LDL may predominate over IgG antibodies *(190)* and have a protective effect in relation to the development of atherosclerosis *(191)* have led to considerable speculation, including the possibility of "vaccination" against atherosclerosis *(192)*. This seems highly unwarranted, because of several other lines of evidence. First, the proposed protective murine IgM antibodies are predominantly reactive with oxidized phospholipids, although human antibodies reacting with modified lysine groups have been extensively characterized *(193,194)*. Second, when the isotype distribution of modified LDL antibodies has been studied under stringent conditions, using affinity chromatography-purified antibodies, the predominant isotypes are IgG1 and IgG3, followed by IgM *(193,194)*. Given the TH2 dependency and proinflammatory characteristics of these two IgG subclasses antibodies *(195)*, the postulated protective role of antimodified LDL antibodies becomes untenable. The balance between IgG and IgM LDL antibodies may have, however, some pathogenic relevance, as suggested by recent reports showing that common carotid and femoral IMT are directly related to the levels of IgG oxLDL antibodies and inversely related to the levels of IgM oxLDL antibodies (196). Also of interest is the fact that the levels of IgG oxLDL: and MDA-LDL antibodies are associated with the metabolic syndrome and smoking (197).

A clearer perspective about the pathogenic role of modified LDL antibodies seems to emerge when the levels of circulating antigen-antibody complexes (immune complexes [IC]) containing modified forms of LDL (LDL-IC) are measured (10,187,198–200). LDL-IC have been reported to be increased in patients with CAD (200) and in diabetic patients with nephropathy (200) or that developed CAD over an 8-year period (187). The composition of IC isolated from the sera of diabetic patients by precipitation with polyethlylene-glycol has demonstrated a significant enrichment in carboxymethyl lysine and MDA-lysine (194), suggesting that oxLDL and AGE-LDL are involved in IC formation. This is supported by the detection in the IC of significantly elevated concentrations of oxLDL and AGE-LDL IgG antibodies of higher affinity than those that remain free in the supernatant (10,194,200).

The advantages and disadvantages of the measurement of LDL-IC vs the measurement of serum modified LDL antibodies have been recently summarized in a previous publication (10), but it needs to be stressed that there is ample evidence showing that LDL-IC are proinflammatory, thus supporting the measurement of LDL-IC as more directly related to the pathogenic potential of LDL antibodies than the measurement of free circulating antibodies. The evidence supporting the proinflammatory characteristics of LDL-IC has been obtained in in vitro studies using both rabbit apo-B antibodies and purified human oxLDL antibodies to prepare oxLDL-IC. Using LDL-IC prepared with rabbit antibodies we demonstrated their ability to induce foam cell formation (104,201). The transformation of human monocyte-derived macrophages into foam cells can be induced either by insoluble LDL-IC presented to the macrophages as large aggregates or as LDL-IC adsorbed to red blood cells (RBCs). Both types of LDL-IC may be formed in vivo. Subendothelial LDL deposits are likely to include LDL-IC formed in situ, and these are probably large insoluble aggregates. Soluble LDL-IC present in circulation are likely to be adsorbed to RBCs via C3b receptors and other nonspecific interactions. Once absorbed to RBC, LDL–IC are transported to organs rich in tissue macrophages in which the LDL-IC can be transferred to phagocytic cells expressing Fc receptors (11,195).

In vitro, both insoluble and soluble (RBC adsorbed) LDL-IC prepared with rabbit apo-B antibodies induce profound alterations in lipoprotein metabolism and in the cholesterol homeostasis of monocyte-derived macrophages (104,201). These observations were recently reproduced using LDL-IC prepared with human copper-oxLDL and purified human oxLDL antibodies (11). The increased accumulation of CE in human macrophages exposed to LDL-IC is secondary to an increased uptake of the LDL complexed with antibody, followed by altered intracellular metabolism of the particle (105). In the initial stages the intracellular accumulation of CE reflects the accumulation of intact LDL; in later stages the cell accumulates CEs generated by de novo esterification of the free cholesterol released during lysosomal hydrolysis of LDL and a foam cell is formed. LDL-IC are taken up by macrophages as a consequence of their interaction with the FcγI receptor (202). Surprisingly, although inducing foam cell formation, the LDL-IC also stimulates a considerable increase (approx 20-fold) in LDL receptor activity (201,203). The increase in LDL-receptor activity seems to be specifically induced by LDL-IC and not by other types of immune complexes (105,201).

Macrophage Activation

RELEASE OF CYTOKINES AND GROWTH FACTORS BY MODIFIED LIPOPROTEINS AND LDL-IMMUNE COMPLEXES

AGE product–receptor interactions in macrophages may induce release of cytokines, TNF and IL-1 *(204)* and these cytokines may mediate growth and remodeling and accelerate the atherosclerotic process. Vlassara and associates *(205)* identified a specific receptor for AGE products on monocyte/macrophages. Macrophages expressing this receptor may phagocytose proteins and even entire cells expressing glyco-oxidation products *(206)*. Consistent with this, AGE products in vessel walls have been localized immunologically to intracellular locations in macrophages, SMCs, and in foam cells derived from these cells. Other modified lipoproteins, such as oxLDL, have also been described as stimulating the release of cytokines but the data is somewhat conflicting.

Release of cytokines by macrophages can also be induced by exposure of the cells to immune complexes containing modified LDL. Exposure of macrophages to LDL-containing immune complexes has been shown to upregulate LDL and scavenger receptor expression, and to lead to the release of IL-1 and TNF-α and of oxygen active radicals *(11,207)*. Actually, in a large number of experiments carried out in our laboratory, incubation of human macrophages with LDL-IC in concentrations known to induce intracellular accumulation of CEs and foam cell formation stimulated both the cytokine release and the respiratory burst more efficiently than any other type of immune complexes. Time-course studies of cytokine release and mRNA expression suggest that the synthesis and release of these two cytokines is under independent control *(207)*. TNF-α was released almost immediately after addition of LDL-IC to the macrophages, coinciding with early expression of TNF-α mRNA, detectable 30 minutes after stimulation. In contrast, IL-1β was only detected in macrophage supernatants 8 hours after exposure to LDL-IC, and the onset of expression of IL-1β mRNA was also delayed in comparison to that of TNF-α mRNA. We noted wide variations in the amounts of TNF-α released by monocyte-derived macrophages from different donors.

The release of cytokines is a common event observed with immune complex-activated macrophages and is considered to be a key step in the pathway leading to inflammation as a result of the scavenging of immune complexes in tissues. Additionally, the release of cytokines has special significance from the point of view of the pathogenesis of atherosclerosis, because cytokines can contribute to atherogenesis by a variety of mechanisms. IL-1, for example, has been reported to stimulate the synthesis and cell surface expression of procoagulant activity and platelet-activating factor by endothelial cells *(208,209)*, the later of which can result in enhanced interactions with granulocytes, increased vascular permeability *(210)*, induction of IL-1 release from endothelial cells by a positive feedback mechanism *(211)*, and induction of PDGF-AA which can be indirectly responsible for fibroblast and SMC proliferation through an autocrine growth-regulating mechanism *(212)*. TNF-α can induce cellular responses similar to those of IL-1 such as cell surface expression of procoagulant activity *(213)* and production of IL-1 by endothelial cells *(214)*. Both TNF-α and IL-1 can enhance the expression of VCAMs on endothelial cells *(81,96,97)*, promoting the adherence of monocytes, which, if activated as a consequence of the interaction with endothelial cells or as a consequence of other stimulatory signals (such as interaction with RBC-bound IC) can cause or aggravate endothelial cell damage *(215)* probably through the release of superoxide radicals.

In addition to IL-1 and TNF-α, activated monocytes and macrophages have been shown to secrete other products such as interferon (IFN)-α, growth factors such as fibroblast growth factor and PDGF-BB *(216–218)*, TGF *(219)*, modulatory substances such as prostaglandin E2 *(220)*, proteases *(221)*, collagenases *(222)*, and oxygen radicals *(223)*. Several of these mediators have been shown to have effects that could be directly related to the development of atherosclerosis. PDGF-BB, released by monocytes/macrophages, besides playing a role in stimulating SMC proliferation, can also increase endocytosis, cholesterol synthesis, and LDL receptor expression in mononuclear cells. TGF-β stimulates matrix production by SMCs. Besides cytokines and growth factors, activated macrophages over express CD40, an important modulator of the inflammatory response in the vessel wall, on interaction with CD40 ligand. It is well known that in acute coronary syndromes (ACS), the levels of CD40 ligand are elevated and recently increased levels of CD40 ligand were also found in a group of 39 patients with diabetes and angiographically documented CAD *(224)*. Treatment with rosiglitazone but not with placebo was able to significantly decrease the levels of CD40 ligand in the same patients *(224)*.

Expression of Metalloproteinases Induced by Modified Lipoproteins and Modified LDL-ICs.

ROLE IN PLAQUE RUPTURE

In recent years, angiographic studies on patients with acute MI led to the surprising finding that, frequently, the atherosclerotic lesion that gave rise to the occlusive thrombus did not have high-grade stenosis *(225–227)*. These studies led to the concept that the composition of atherosclerotic plaques is more important than their size in triggering plaque rupture and acute vascular events.

The thickness and collagen content of the fibrous cap and the size of the lipid core are the most important elements in determining plaque vulnerability. Vulnerable plaques that are prone to rupture have a thin fibrous cap, as a result of a marked decrease in collagen content, and their lipid core usually occupies more than 40% of the plaque area. Thus, mechanisms that contribute to decrease the collagen content of plaques have been the focus of considerable attention in recent years.

Collagens are synthesized and assembled by VSMC and degraded by collagenases. Thus, both decreased production of collagen by SMCs, and enhanced degradation of collagen by collagenases, can contribute to plaque vulnerability *(228)*. It has been shown that the expression of collagens in SMCs is regulated by cytokines and growth factors *(229)*. TGF-β and PDGF stimulate the synthesis of collagen type I and III, whereas IFN-γ markedly decreases collagen biosynthesis *(229)*. Studies examining the pathology of atherosclerotic lesions and studies with cell culture systems indicated that IFN-γ, which is released by activated T cells, inhibits SMC proliferation and collagen expression in SMCs *(230,231)*. IFN-γ also promotes apoptosis of SMCs *(232)*. These findings provided important evidence for understanding the relative paucity of SMCs in vulnerable regions of atherosclerotic plaques. Decreased synthesis of collagen is not, however, the only mechanism leading to the decreased collagen content in vulnerable atherosclerotic plaques. As mentioned before, increased degradation of collagen by collagenases is also an important factor. Most of the collagen (50–75%) in a normal artery is type I collagen *(233–234)*. Interstitial collagenase, or metalloproteinase (MMP-1), is an important proteinase specialized in the initial cleavage of collagens, mainly type I. Other metalloproteinases, such as MMP-2 and -9, catalyze further the breakdown of collagen fragments or activate MMP-3 and -10 and other members of MMP family, promoting the degradation of a broad spectrum of matrix constituents, such as proteoglycans and elastin. MMP activity is also regulated by TIMPs *(235)*. MMP-1 has been found in vulnerable regions of atherosclerotic plaques, suggesting that this collagenase plays a role in plaque destabilization *(236)*. We have recently shown that oxidized LDL and oxLDL-IC stimulate the expression of MMP-1 in human vascular endothelial cells at transcriptional level. That increased expression is associated with a marked increase in collagenase activity *(237–239)*.

A few studies have investigated MMP levels and activities in diabetes. Serum levels of MMP-2, MMP-8 and MMP-9 are increased in patients with type 2 diabetes *(240)* and MMP-9 levels and activity are increased in aortas from streptozotocin-diabetic rats compared to controls *(241)*.

Another group of proteases, the cathepsins, may also be involved in causing plaque rupture. The cathepsins are cysteine proteinases that degrade elastin and fibrillar collagen. Cathepsins K, L, and S all have potent elastolytic activity. Cathepsin S is the most potent elastase known *(242)*, whereas cathepsin K cleaves collagen I and III *(243)*. The cathepsins were originally thought to function only in acidic lysosomes, but recent research shows that they can be released by macrophages *(244)*. Macrophages in human lesions contain abundant immunoreactive cathepsin K and S *(245)*, and atherosclerotic lesions from apo-E-deficient mice express cathepsins B, D, L, and S *(246)*. Cathepsin B has even been suggested as a biomarker of vulnerable plaques *(247)*. Expression levels of cathepsins C and D are upregulated in aneurysms *(248)*, which also contain lower levels of the endogenous cysteine protease inhibitor cystatin C *(249)*. Furthermore, human SMCs in culture can be stimulated to secrete active cathepsin S by IL-1β or IFN-γ *(245)*. Together, these findings suggest that the cathepsins may be involved in causing plaque rupture or aneurysms. So far, the presence of cathepsins and cystatin C in lesions from patients with diabetes has not been studied.

Another possible mechanism of plaque rupture is increased cell death. Contrary to what was conventionally accepted, it has been shown recently that "apoptotic" cells can release cytokines and that, following apoptosis, an inflammatory response in the arterial wall induced by the over expression of Fas-associating death domain protein, one of the signaling molecules in the apoptotic pathway may occur *(250)*. Furthermore, apoptotic cells have a potent procoagulant activity as a result of the redistribution of phosphatidylserine (PS) on the cell surface during apoptosis, which leads to increased tissue factor activity, a key element in the initiation of coagulation. During cell apoptosis, shedding to the lipid core of membrane apoptotic microparticles rich in PS, which carry almost all tissue factor activity, is responsible for the procoagulant activity of the plaque *(251)*. Luminal endothelial-cell apoptosis is also likely responsible for thrombus formation on eroded plaques without rupture. The increased expression of tissue factor is not limited however to the plaque but it is also found in circulating monocytes in patients with ACS *(252)*. Whether or not diabetes enhances the expression of tissue factor in circulating monocytes or in plaques is not known.

Thrombus Formation

Thrombi may form in atherosclerotic vessels leading to tissue ischemia, tissue death, or both. Formation of thrombi starts with adhesion of platelets to areas of endothelial damage and, as a consequence, to local accumulation of platelets at sites of vascular injury. Platelet aggregation follows platelet adhesion as a result of the release of intraplatelet materials that may affect not only the clotting/fibrinolytic system but also lead to the formation of microemboli. Thus, to understand the formation of thrombi, the final step of an acute vascular event, it is essential to understand the functional abnormalities of platelets.

ABNORMALITIES IN PLATELET FUNCTION

Many alterations in platelet function are seen in diabetes mellitus. Several studies have shown that platelets from diabetic subjects are more sensitive to platelet aggregating agents and that synthesis of thromboxane B2 is increased (253,254). These findings have been shown both in diabetic patients immediately after the onset of the disease and in patients with vascular disease, suggesting that platelet damage may occur as a result of diabetic vascular disease and possibly contributing to the development of the process.

Dispersion of platelet aggregates, as a result of the lysis of the fibrin meshwork, may be the limiting process of thrombus growth when chronic platelet activation and aggregation is present, as may be the case in diabetes. Recently, substantial evidence has accumulated indicating the importance of intraplatelet proteins in platelet disaggregation. One of the proteins, plasminogen activator inhibitor (PAI)-1 is released from activated platelets and bound within the thrombus. The amount of the thrombus-bound PAI-1 determines the resistance of the thrombus to thrombolysis by the activated fibrinolytic system (255). Recent studies found enhanced platelet PAI-1 expression and release in patients with type 2 diabetes (256,257).

ABNORMALITIES IN COAGULATION

Activation of the coagulation system leads to fibrin formation. Experimental and clinical data suggest that primary fibrin deposits and mural thrombi lead to the initial endothelial lesion and may contribute to the development of macrovascular disease (258). There are multiple data to support a pathogenetic rather than consequential role of increased clotting tendency in the development of vascular disease in diabetes (195). General activation of blood coagulation seems to be present in diabetes. Moreover, most of the individual factors in both the intrinsic and the extrinsic coagulation pathway, and the inhibitors of coagulation, may be altered in diabetes.

Attention has been directed at fibrinogen levels and dynamics in diabetes for a variety of reasons. The most important one is the fact that the plasma level of fibrinogen has been shown to be an independent risk factor for thrombotic events in population-based studies (260–262). In diabetes, plasma fibrinogen levels are found to be elevated, particularly in patients with hyperglycemia (263–265). Insulin deficiency leads to an increase in fibrinogen synthesis in IDDM, and infusion of insulin will decrease the fibrinogen synthetic rate (266). Interestingly, fibrinogen survival is decreased in diabetes, and this abnormality can be reversed by administration of insulin or by administration of heparin, suggesting that intravascular fibrin formation may be taking place (262). Exercise may also affect plasma fibrinogen and it has been shown that exercise conditioning will lower plasma fibrinogen levels in NIDDM individuals (267). The above findings suggest that there may be increased fibrin formation in vivo in individuals with diabetes. Because fibrinogen to fibrin formation may be catalyzed by thrombin, investigations have centered on the regulation of thrombin activity in diabetes and on an in vivo index of thrombin activity, the fibrinopeptide A (FPA) (268).

Plasma FPA is cleaved from the α-chain of fibrinogen by the action of thrombin. This forms the first step in the conversion of fibrinogen to fibrin. FPA levels tend to be elevated in diabetes, especially when control is poor or vascular problems exist (269). Furthermore, recent studies have indicated that elevated FPA levels may be seen in diabetic individuals before the development of vascular complications (270). A relation between plasma and urinary FPA and hyperglycemia in diabetes has been reported (268).

Another marker of coagulation activation in vivo, the prothrombin activation fragment F1+2, has been recently identified (271). Fragment F1+2 is released from prothrombin during its conversion to thrombin by activated factor X. In type I diabetic patients, F1+2 levels have been found to be lower when compared to those found in control subjects (263). Interestingly, microalbuminuria, which is believed to be a manifestation of generalized angiopathy, has been shown to have a significant relation to F1+2 levels (263).

Another factor contributing to activation of the coagulation system in diabetes is a decrease in antithrombin III (ATIII). ATIII is the most important inhibitor of the coagulation system and its activity may be modulated by glucose both in vitro and in vivo. Hyperglycemia causes a decrease in ATIII activity in nondiabetic subjects, and activity returns to normal after the infusion of glucose is stopped (264). Depressed levels of ATIII activity have been found in adult type 1 diabetic subjects, and normoglycemia obtained after insulin infusion returns ATIII activity to normal (265).

Brownlee and associates (272) have shown that increased glycation of ATIII impairs its thrombin-inhibiting activity and could contribute to the accumulation of fibrin in diabetic tissues. More recently, Ceriello and associates (273) described an inverse correlation between ATIII activity and both HbA1c and plasma glucose, independent of plasma concentrations of ATIII. They proposed that ATIII activity is influenced by glycation

Another potent inhibitor of coagulation that is altered in diabetes is protein C. Activated protein C is a vitamin K-dependent plasma protein that acts at the level of factor V and VIII in the intrinsic coagulation scheme. Several investigators have reported decreased levels of protein C antigen and activity levels in type 1 diabetes (265,274), and a return to normal with treatment (265).

Recently, it has been shown that exposure of human macrophages and SMCs to oxLDL enhances their ability to support activity of two major complexes of the intrinsic pathway, Xase and prothrombinase, leading to a 10- to 20-fold increase in thrombin formation (275). The increase in the intrinsic procoagulant activity was related to formation of additional factor VIII binding sites as a result of increased translocation of PS to the outer membrane of oxLDL-treated cells and a fivefold higher affinity of interaction between components of the Xase complex, activated factors VIII and IX (275). Because oxLDL is present in higher levels in diabetes this may be also an important prothrombotic mechanism in diabetes.

ABNORMALITIES IN THE FIBRINOLYTIC SYSTEM

The fibrinolytic system controls the patency of the vascular tree and is likely a critical regulator of thrombosis. One hypothesis is that small amounts of fibrin are constantly deposited on the endothelium and that these fibrin deposits are continually dissolved, resulting in a dynamic balance between coagulation and fibrinolysis. The generation and activity of plasmin, the enzyme responsible for the degradation of fibrin deposits and thrombi, are regulated mainly by the production of two critical proteins by the vascular endothelium, tissue-plasminogen activator (t-PA) and the main inhibitor of t-PA, PAI-1. t-PA converts inactive plasminogen into plasmin at the site of fibrin formation.

Impaired fibrinolytic activity is characterized by low t-PA activity and high PAI-1 antigen and activity. Studies in man have shown that t-PA antigen concentration (associated with high PAI-1 and low basal or stimulated t-PA activity) may be high in subjects with preclinical atherosclerosis and a marker for the development of coronary and cerebrovascular events *(276,277)*. Furthermore, t-PA antigen has been found to have a higher predictive value for mortality in patients with established CAD than cholesterol, triglycerides, fibrinogen, blood pressure, diabetes, or smoking *(278)*. Like in nondiabetic subjects, impaired fibrinolysis is an independent risk factor for MI in diabetic subjects *(279,280)*.

Decreased fibrinolytic function in type 2 diabetes correlates with the presence and severity of angiopathies *(281)*. In patients with type 1 diabetes, increased PAI-1 activity has been observed in association with microalbuminuria *(282)*. Regulation of PAI-1 gene expression and protein synthesis in HepG2 cells seems to be controlled by insulin alone *(283,284)* or insulin in association with VLDL *(284)*. Increased concentrations of free fatty acids in diabetes may account for the insulin and VLDL-mediated augmentation of PAI-1 synthesis and therefore normalization of elevated concentrations of free fatty acids by improvement of glycemic control may normalize or near-normalize the fibrinolytic system activity in type 2 diabetes. Some studies examining this issue in vivo *(285)* confirmed this postulate *(286)*. This observation is consistent with the favorable effects induced by sulfonylureas, metformin, and the two in combination in normalizing the fibrinolytic system activity in type 2 diabetes *(287)*.

Lipoproteins are also able to regulate t-PA and PAI-1 release, as demonstrated by in vitro studies using cultured endothelial cells. VLDL isolated from normal individuals induce the release of t-PA and PAI-1 from cultured endothelial cells, whereas VLDLs from hypertriglyceridemic individuals are unable to do so *(288)*. Endothelial production of PAI-1 is also increased by incubation with VLDL obtained from hyperglycemic patients *(289)*. In vivo evidence to support the "in vitro" studies showing increased PAI-1 activity in type 2 diabetes was provided by studies showing an abnormal response to the administration of desmopressin acetate in type 2 diabetic patients with hypertriglyceridemia. Plasma t-PA activity was frankly decreased and PAI-1 activity frankly increased when compared to the activity levels obtained in normal controls *(290)*. Recently it has been reported that lipoprotein [Lp](a) also attenuates fibrinolysis as a result of the interaction of apo(a) with the ternary complex of t-PA, plasminogen and fibrin *(291)*. Lp(a) species containing smaller apo(a) isoforms bind more avidly to fibrin and are better inhibitors of plasminogen *(292)*.

Another well-recognized contributor to augmented activity of PAI-1 in diabetes is the adipocyte. PAI-1 may be released directly from an increased mass of adipose tissue, particularly visceral fat, and that may account, in part, for the association between obesity and impaired fibrinolysis *(293–295)*. However, abnormal concentrations of cytokines such as TGF-β and TNF-α, may also contribute to augment PAI-1 expression in adipocytes *(296)*. Other cytokines including IL-1 and -6 have also been implicated as agonists for PAI-1 synthesis *(297)*. Another factor likely to influence PAI-1 expression in diabetes is the renin–angiotensin system (RAS) because PAI-1 synthesis is augmented by the binding of angiotensin II to the AT1 receptor *(298)*. As earlier work has shown the RAS is activated in patients with type 2 diabetes. In fact, the American Diabetes Association has recommended the use of angiotensin receptor blockers alone or in combination with angiotensin-converting enzyme inhibitors in diabetes not only for treatment of hypertension but also to attenuate microalbuminuria. Angiotensin-converting enzyme inhibition has also the advantage of attenuating hypofibrinolysis not only in blood but also in tissues including the heart *(299)*.

REFERENCES

1. Moreno PR, Murcia AM, Palacios IM, et al. Coronary composition and macrophage infiltration in atherectomy specimens from patients with diabetes mellitus. Circulation 2000;102:2180–2184.
2. Schwenke DC, Carew TE. Initiation of atherosclerotic lesions in cholesterol-fed rabbits, II: selective retention of LDL vs. selective increases in LDL permeability in susceptible sites of arteries. Arteriosclerosis 1989:9:908–918.
3. Frank FS, Fogelman AM. Ultrastructure of the intima in WHHL and cholesterol-fed rabbit aortas prepared by ultra-rapid freezing and freeze-etching. J Lipid Res 1989;30:967–978.
4. Nievelstein PFEM, Fogelman AM, Frank FS, Mottino G. Lipid accumulation in rabbit aortic intima 2 hours after bolus infusion of LDL: a deep-etch and immunolocalization study of rapidly frozen tissue. Arterioscler Thromb 1991;11:1795–1805.
5. Navab M, Imes SS, Hama SY, Hough GP, Ross LA, Bork RW. Monocyte transmigration induced by modification of low density lipoprotein in co-cultures of human aortic wall cells is due to induction of monocyte chemotactic protein 1 synthesis and is abolished by high density lipoprotein. J Clin Invest 1991;88:2039–2046.
6. Rajavashisth TB, Andalibi A, Territo MD, et al. Induction of endothelial cell expression of granulocyte and macrophage colony-stimulating factors by modified low density lipoproteins. Nature 1990;344:254–257.
7. Schwartz D, Andalibi A, Chaverri-Almada L, et al. The role of the gro family of chemokines in monocyte adhesion to MM-LDL-stimulated endothelium. J Clin Invest 1994;94:1968–1973.
8. Hessler JR, Robertson Jr AL, Chisolm GM. LDL-induced cytotoxicity and its inhibition by HDL in human vascular smooth muscle and endothelial cells in culture. Atherosclerosis 1979;32:213–218.
9. Fogelman AM, Shechter I, Seager J, Hokom M, Child JS, Edwards PA. Malondialdehyde alteration of LDL leads to cholesterol ester accumulation in human monocytes/macrophages. Proc Natl Acad Sci USA 1980;77:2214–2218.
10. Virella G, Lopes-Virella MF. Lipoprotein autoantibodies: measurement and significance. Clin Diag Lab Immunol 2003;10:499–505.
11. Virella G, Atchley D, Koskinen S, Zheng D, Lopes-Virella MF, DCCT/EDIC Research Group. Pro-atherogenic and pro-inflammatory properties of immune complexes prepared with purified human oxLDL antibodies and human oxLDL. Clin Immunol 2002;105:81–92.
12. Moncada S, Palmer R, Higgs E. Nitric oxide: physiology, pathophysiology, and pharmacology. Pharmacol Rev 1991;43:109–142.
13. Hogman M, Frostell C, Arnberg H, Hedenstierna G. Bleeding time prolongation and NO inhalation. Lancet 1993;341:1664–1665.
14. Kawabata A. Evidence that endogenous nitric oxide modulates plasma fibrinogen levels in rat. Br J Pharmacol. 1996;117:236–237.
15. Huszka M, Kaplar M, Rejto L, et al. The association of reduced endothelium derived relaxing factor-NO production with endothelial damage and increased in vivo platelet activation in patients with diabetes mellitus. Thrombos Res 1997;86:173–180.
16. Freedman JE, Loscalzo J, Benoit SE, Valeri CR, Barnard MR, Michelson AD. Decreased platelet inhibition by nitric oxide in two brothers with a history of arterial thrombosis. J Clin Invest 1996;97:979–987.
17. Johnstone MT, Creager SJ, Scales KM, Cusco JA, Lee BK, Creager MA. Impaired endothelium-dependent vasodilation in patients with insulin-dependent diabetes mellitus. Circulation 1993;88:2510–2516.
18. McVeigh GE, Brennan GM, Johnston GD, et al. Impaired endothelium-dependent and independent vasodilation in patients with type 2 (non-insulin-dependent) diabetes mellitus. Diabetologia 1992;35:771–776.
19. Gunnett CA, Heistad DD, Faraci FM. Gene-targeted mice reveal a critical role for inducible nitric oxide synthase in vascular dysfunction during diabetes. Stroke 2003;34:2970–2974.

20. Chin JH, Azhar S, Hoffman BB. Inactivation of endothelial-derived relaxing factor by oxidized lipopro-
    teins. J Clin Invest 1992;89:10–18.
21. Blair A, Shaul PW, Yuhanna IS, Conrad PA, Smart EJ. Oxidized low density lipoprotein displaces
    endothelial nitric oxide synthase from plasmalemmal caveolae and impairs eNOS activation. J Biol
    Chem 1999;274:32,512–32,519.
22. Drab M, Verkade P, Elger M, et al. Loss of caveolae , vascular dysfunction and pulmonary defects in
    caveolin-1 gene disrupted mice. Science 2001;293:2449–2452.
23. Jessup W, Dean RT. Autoinhibitor of murine macrophage mediated oscidation of LDL by nitric oxide
    synthesis. Atherosclerosis 1993;101:145–155.
24. Ischiropoulos H, al Mehdi A. Peroxynitrate-mediated oxidative protein modifications. FEBS Lett
    1995;364:279–282.
25. Bhatia S, Shukla R, Venkata MS, Gambhir J, Madhava PK. Antioxidant status, lipid peroxidation and
    nitric oxide end prodicts in patients with type 2 diabetes mellitus with nephropathy. Clin Biochem
    2003;36:557–562.
26. Fontbonne AM, Eschwege EM. Insulin and cardiovascular disease. Paris prospective study. Diabetes
    Care 1991;14:461–469.
27. Despres JP, Lamarche B, Mauriege P, et al. Hyperinsulinemia as an independent risk factor for ischaemic
    heart disease. New Engl J Med 1996;334:952–957.
28. The Diabetes Control and Complications Trial Research Group. New Engl J Med 1993;329:997–1017.
29. UK Prospective Diabetes Study Group. Lancet 1998;353:854–865.
30. Scherrer U, Randin D, Vollenweider L, Nicod P. Nitric oxide release accounts for insulin's vascular
    effects in humans. J Clin Invest 1994;94:2511–2515.
31. Baron AD. Insulin and the Vasculature—Old Actors, New Roles. Journal of Investigative Medicine
    1996;44:406–412.
32. Moncada S. Biological importance of prostacyclin, Br J Pharmac 1982;76:3–31.
33. Colwell JA, Lopes-Virella MF, Winocour PD, Halushka PV. New concepts about the pathogenesis of
    atherosclerosis in diabetes mellitus. In: Levin ME, O'Neal LW, (eds). The diabetic foot, 4th ed, Mosby-
    Year Book, St. Louis, MO, 1988, pp. 51–70.
34. Sekiguchi N, Umeda F, Masakado M, Ono Y, Hashimoto T, Nawata H. Immunohistochemical study of
    prostacyclin-stimulating factor (PSF) in the diabetic and atherosclerotic human coronary artery. Diabe-
    tes 1997;46:1627–1632.
35. Umeda F, Masakado M, Takei A. Difference in serum-induced prostacyclin production by cultured
    aortic and capillary endothelial cells. Prostagl Leukotr Essen Fatty Acids 1997;56:51–55.
36. Colwell JA, Jokl R. Clotting disorders in diabetes. In: Porte D, Sherwin R, Rifkin H, (eds). Diabetes
    mellitus: theory and practice, 5th ed, Appleton and Lange, Norwalk, CT, 1997, pp. 1543–1557.
37. Colwell JA, Winocour PD, Lopes-Virella MF. Platelet function and platelet interactions in atheroscle-
    rosis and diabetes mellitus. In: Rifkin H, Porte D, (eds). Diabetes mellitus: theory and practice. Elsevier,
    New York, 1989, pp. 249–256.
38. Uedelhoven WM, Rutzel A, Meese CO, Weber PC. Smoking alters thromboxane metabolism in man.
    Biochem Biophys Acta 1991;108:197–201.
39. Davi G, Averna M, Catalano I, et al. Increased thromboxane biosynthesis in type II a) hypercholester-
    olemia. Circulation 1992;85:1792–1798.
40. Di Minno G, Davi G, Margaglione M, et al. Abnormally high thromboxane biosynthesis in homozygous
    homocystinuria: evidence for platelet involvement and probucol-sensitive mechanism. J Clin Invest
    1993;92:1400–1406.
41. Davi G, Gresele P, Violi F, Catalano M, et al. Diabetes mellitus, hypercholesterolemia and hypertension,
    but not vascular disease per se, are associated with persistent platelet activation in vivo: Evidence
    derived from the study of peripheral arterial disease. Circulation 1997;96:69–75.
42. Toda N, Bian K, Akiba T, Okamura T. Heterogeneity in mechanisms of bradykinin action in canine
    isolated blood vessels. Eur J Pharmacol 1987;135:321–329.
43. Briner VA, Tsai P, Schrier RW. Bradykinin: potential for vascular constriction in the presence of
    endothelial injury. Am J Physiol Renal Fluid Electrolyte Physiol 1993;264:F322–F327.
44. Greene EL, Velarde V, Jaffa AA. Role of reactive oxygen species in bradykinin induced mitogen-
    activated protein kinase and c-fos induction in vascular cells. Hypertension 2000;35:942–947.
45. Velarde V, Ullian ME, Mornelli TA, Mayfield RK, Jaffa AA. Mechanisms of MAPK activation by
    bradykinin in vascular smooth muscle cells. Am J Physiol Cell Physiol 1999;277:C253–C261.
46. Douillet CD, Velarde V, Christopher JT, Mayfield RK, Trojanowska ME, Jaffa AA. Mechanisms by
    which bradykinin promotes fibrosis in vascular smooth muscle cells: role of TGF-β and MAPK. Am J
    Physiol Heart Circ Physiol 2000;279:H2829–H2837.

47. Jaffa AA, Durazo-Arvizu R, Zheng D, Lackland DT, Srikanth S, Garvey TW, Schmaier AH, DCCT/ EDIC Study Group. Diabetes 2003;52:1215–1221.

48. Christopher J, Jaffa AA. Diabetes modulates the expression of glomerular kinin receptors. International Immunopharmacology 2002;2:1771–1779.

49. Christopher J, Velarde V, Zhang D, Mayfield D, Mayfield R, Jaffa AA. Regulation of B2 kinin receptors by glucose in vascular smooth muscle cells. Am J Physiol Heart Circ Physiol 2000;280:H1537-H1546.

50. Lee Y, Kuhn WH, Kaiser S, Hennig B, Daugherty A, Toborek M. Interleukin 4 induces transcription of the 15-lipoxygenase 1 gene in human endothelial cells. J.Lipid Res 2001;42:783–791.

51. Kim JA, Gu JL, Natarajan R, Berliner JA, Nadler J. A leukocyte type of 12-lipoxygenase is expressed in human vascular and mononuclear cells. Evidence for up-regulation by angiotensin II. Arterioscler Thromb Vas Biol 1995;15:942–948.

52. Natarajan R, Gu JL, Rossi J, Gonzales N, Lanting L, Xu L, Nadler J. Elevated glucose and angiotensin II increase 12-lipoxygenase activity and expression in porcine aortic smooth muscle cells. Proc Natl Acad Sci USA 1993;90:4947–4951.

53. Yla-Herttuala S, Rosenfeld ME, Parthasarathy S, et al. Co-localization of 15-lipoxygenase mRNA and protein with epitopes of oxidized low density lipoprotein in macrophage-rich area of atherosclerotic lesions. Proc Natl Acad Sci USA 1990;87:6959–6963.

54. Folcick VA, Nivar-Aristy RA, Krajewski LP, Cathcart MC. Lipoxygenase contributes to the oxidation of lipids in human atherosclerotic plaques. J Clin Invest 1995;504–510.

55. Benz D, Mol JM, Ezaki M, et al. Enhanced levels of lipoperoxides in low density lipoprotein incubated with murine fibroblasts expressing high levels of human 15-lipoxygenase. J Biol Chem 1995;270:5191–5197.

56. Scheidegger K, Butler JS, Witztum JL. Angiotensin II increases macrophage-mediated modification of low density lipoprotein via a lipoxygenase-dependent pathway. J Biol Chem 1997;272:21,609–21,615.

57. Patricia MK, Kim JA, Harper CM, et al. Lipoxygenase products incease monocyte adhesion to human aortic endothelial cells. Arterioscler Thromb VASC Biol 1999;19:2615–2622.

58. Natarajan R, Gonzalez N, Xu L, Nadler JL. Vascular smooth muscle cells exhibit increased growth in response to elevated glucose. Biochem Biophys Res Commun 1992;187:552–560.

59. Natarajan R, Gonzales N, Lanting L, Nadler JL. Role of the lipoxygenase pathway in angiotensin II-induced vascular smooth muscle cell hypertrophy. Herpertension 1994;23:1142–1147.

60. Natarajan R, Nadler JL. Lipoxygenases and Lipid Signaling in Vascular Cells in Diabetes. Frontiers in Bioscience 2003;8:s783-s795.

61. Natarajan R, Gerrity RG, Gu JL, Lanting L, Thomas L, Nadler JL. Role of 12-lipoxygenase and oxidant stress in hyperglycemia-induced acceleration of atherosclerosis in a diabetic pig model. Diabetologia 2002;45:125–133.

62. Gerrity RG, Natarajan R, Nadler JL, Kimsey T. Diabetes-induced accelerated atherosclerosis in swine. Diabetes 2001;50:1654–1665.

63. Takahashi K, Ghater MA, Lam HC, O'Halloran DJ, Bloom SR. Elevated plasma endothelin in patients with diabetes mellitus. Diabetologia 1990;33:306–350.

64. Shin SJ, Lee YJ, Tsai JH. The correlation of plasma and urine endothelin-1 with the severity of nephropathy in Chinese patients with type 2 diabetes. Scand J Clin Lab Invest 1996;56:571–576.

65. Letizia C, Iannaccone A, Cerci S, et al. Circulating endothelin 1 in NIDDM with retinopathy. Horm Metab Res 1997;29:247–251.

66. Guvener N, Aytemir K, Aksoyek S, Gedik O. Plasma endothelin-1 levels in non-insulin dependent diabetes mellitus patients with macrovascular disease, Coronary Artery Disease 1997;8:253–258.

67. Bertello P, Veglio F, Pinna G, et al. Plasma endothelin in NIDDM patients with and without complications, Diabetes Care 1994;17:574–577.

68. Metsarinne K, Saijonmaa O, Yki-Jarvinen H, Fyhrquist F. Insulin increases the release of endothelin in endothelial cell cultures in vitro but not in vivo. Metabolism 1994;43:878–882.

69. Hattori Y, Kasai K, Nakamura T, Emoto T, Shimoda S. Effects of glucose and insulin on immunoreactive endothelin-1 release from cultured porcine aortic endothelial cells. Metabolism 1991;40:165–169.

70. Anfossi G, Cavalot F, Massucco P, et al. Insulin influences immunoreactive endothelin release by human vascular smooth muscle cells. Metabolism 1993;42:1081–1083.

71. Ferri C, Bellini C, Desideri G, De Mattia G, Santucci A. Endogenous insulin modulates circulating endothelin-1 concentrations in humans. Diabetes Care 1996;19:504–506.

72. Piatti PM, Monti LD, Conti M, et al. Hypertriglyceridemia and hyperinsulinemia are potent inducers of endothelin-1 release in humans. Diabetes 1996;45:316–321.

73. Katsumori K, Wasada T, Saeki A, Naruse M, Omori Y. Lack of acute insulin effect on plasma endothelin-1 levels in humans. Diabet Res Clin Pract 1996;32:187–189.

74. Lip GY, Lann A. von Willebrand factor: A marker of endothelial dysfunction in vascular disorders? Cardiovasc Res 1997;34:255–265.

75. Standl E, Balletshofer B, Dahl B, et al. Predictors of 10-year macrovascular and overall mortality in patients with NIDDM: the Munich General Practitioner Project. Diabetologia 1996;39:1540–1545.

76. Stehouwer CDA, Nauta JJ, Zeldenrust GC, Hackeng WH, Donker AJ. Urinary albumin excretion, cardiovascular disease, and endothelial dysfunction in non-insulin dependent diabetes mellitus. Lancet 1992;340:319–323.

77. Thomsen C, Rasmussen OW, Ingerslev J, Hermansen K. Plasma levels of von Willebrand factor in non-insulin dependent diabetes mellitus are influenced by dietary monounsaturated fatty acids. Thromb Res 1995;77:347–356.

78. Carter AM, Grant PJ. Vascular homeostasis, adhesion molecules, and macrovascular disease in non-insulin dependent diabetes mellitus. Diab Med 1997;14:423–432.

79. De Meyer GR, Herman AG. Vascular endothelial dysfunction. Prog Cardiovasc Dis 1997;39:325–342.

80. O'Brien KD, Allen MD, McDonald TO, et al. Vascular cell adhesion molecule-1 is expressed in human coronary atherosclerotic plaques. J Clin Invest 1993;92:945–951.

81. Davies MJ, Gordon JL, Gearing AJ, Pigott R, Woolf N, Katz D, Kyriakopoulos A. The expression of the adhesion molecules ICAM-1, VCAM-1, PECAM, and E-selectin in human atherosclerosis. J Pathol 1993;171:223–229.

82. Poston RN, Haskard DO, Croucher JR, Gall NP, Johnson-Tidey RR. Expression of intercellular adhesion molecule-1 in atherosclerotic plaques. Am J Pathol 1992;140:665–673.

83. Seth R, Raymond FD, Makgoba MW. Circulating ICAM-1 isoforms: diagnostic prospects for inflammatory and immune disorders. Lancet 1991;338:83–84.

84. Pigott R, Dillon LP, Hemingway IH. Soluble forms of E-selectin, ICAM-1 and VCAM-1 are present in the supernatants of cytokine activated cultured endothelial cells. Biochem Biophys Res Commun 1992;187:584–589.

85. Gearing AJH, Hemingway I, Pigott R, Hughes J, Rees AJ, Cashman SJ. Soluble forms of vascular adhesion molecules, E-selectin, ICAM-1 and VCAM-1: pathological significance. Annals NY Acad Sci 1992;667:324–331.

86. Lampeter ER, Kishimoto TK, Rothlein R, et al. Elevated levels of circulating adhesion molecules in IDDM patients and in subjects at risk for IDDM. Diabetes 1992;41:1668–1671.

87. Steiner M, Reinhardt KM, Krammer B, Ernst B, Blann AD. Increased levels of soluble adhesion molecules in type 2 (non-insulin dependent) diabetes mellitus are independent of glycemic control. Thromb Haemostas 1994;72:979–984.

88. Otsuki M, Hashimoto K, Morimoto Y, Kishimoto T, Kasayama S. Circulating vascular cell adhesion molecule-1 (VCAM-1) in atherosclerotic NIDDM patients. Diabetes 1997;46:2096–2101.

89. Kowalska I, Straczkowski M, Szelachowska M, et al. Circulating E-selectin, vascular cell adhesion molecule-1, and intercellular adhesion molecule-1 in men with coronary artery disease assessed by angiography and disturbances of carbohydrate metabolism. Metabolism 2002;51:733–736.

90. Matsumoto K, Sera Y, Ueki Y, Inukai G, Niiro E, Miyake S. Comparison of serum concentrations of soluble adhesion molecules in diabetic microangiopathy and macroangiopathy. Diabet Med 2002;19:822–826.

91. Jude EB, Douglas JT, Anderson SG, Young MJ, Boulton AJ. Circulating cellular adhesion molecules ICAM-1, VCAM-1, P-and E-selectin in the prediction of cardiovascular disease in diabetes mellitus. Eur J Intern Med 2002;13:185–189.

92. Koyama H, Maeno T, Fukumoto S, et al. Platelet P-selectin expression is associated with atherosclerotic wall thickness in carotid artery in humans. Circulation 2003;108:524–529.

93. Vlassara H, Fuh H, Donnelly T, Cybulsky M. Advanced glycation endproducts promote adhesion molecule (VCAM-1, ICAM01) expression and atheroma formation in normal rabbits. Molecular Medicine 1995;1:447–456.

94. Virella G, Munoz Jose F, Galbraith Gillian MP, Gisinger C, Chassereau C, Virella MF. Activation of human monocyte-derived macrophages by immune complexes containing low density lipoprotein. Clin Immunology and Immunopathology 1995;75:179–189.

95. Wong BW, Wong D, McManus BM. Characterization of fractalkine (CX3CL1) and CX3CR1 in human coronary arteries with native atherosclerosis, diabetes mellitus, and transplant vascular disease. Cardiovasc Pathol 2202;11:332–338.

96. Beekhuizen H, van Furth R. Monocyte adherence to human vascular endothelium. Leukoc Biol 1993;54:363–378.

97. Pohlman TH, Staness KA, Beatty, PG, Oehs HD, Harlan JM. An endothelial cell surface factor(s) induced in vitro by lipopolysaccharide, interleukin 1, and tumor necrosis factor a increases neutrophil adherence by a CDw18-dependent mechanism. J Immunol 1986;136:4548–4553.

98. Dixon JL, Stoops JD, Parker JL, Laughlin MH, Weisman GA, Sturek M. Dyslipidemia and vascular dysfunction in diabetic pigs fed an atherogenic diet. Arterioscler Thromb Vasc Biol 1999;19:2981–2992.

99. Renard CB, Suzuki LA, Kramer F, et al. A new murine model of diabetes-accelerated atherosclerosis. Diabetes 2002;51(Suppl 2):724.

100. Simionescu MD, Popov A, Sima MH, et al. Pathobiochemistry of combined diabetes and atherosclerosis studied on a novel animal model. The hyperlipemic-hyperglycemic hamster. Am J Pathol 1996;148:997–1014.

101. McGill HC Jr, McMahan CA, Malcom GT, Oalmann MC, Strong JP. Relation of glycohemoglobin and adiposity to atherosclerosis in youth. Pathobiological Determinants of Atherosclerosis in Youth (PDAY) Research Group. Arterioscler Thromb Vasc Biol 1995;15:431–440.

102. McGill HC Jr, McMahan CA, Zieske AW, Malcom GT, Tracy RE, Strong J P. Effects of non-lipid risk factors on atherosclerosis in youth with a favorable lipid profile. Circulation 2001;103:1546–1550.

103. Jarvisalo MJ, Putto-Laurila A, Jartti L, et al. Carotid artery intima-media thickness in children with type 1 diabetes. Diabetes 2002;51:493–498.

104. Griffith RL, Virella GT, Stevenson HC, Lopes-Virella MF. LDL metabolism by macrophages activated with LDL immune complexes: A possible mechanism of foam cell formation. J Exp Med 1988;168:1041–1059.

105. Lopes-Virella MF, Griffith RL, Shunk KA, Virella GT. Enhanced uptake and impaired intracellular metabolism of low density lipoprotein complexed with anti-low density lipoprotein antibodies. Arteriosclerosis and Thrombosis 1991;11:1356–1367.

106. Laakso M, Pyorala K. Lipid and lipoprotein abnormalities in diabetic patients with peripheral vascular disease. Atherosclerosis 1988;74:55–63.

107. Lopes-Virella MF, Stone PG, Colwell JA. Serum high density lipoprotein in diabetes. Diabetologia 1977;13:285–291.

108. Lopes-Virella MF, Wohltmann HJ, Mayfield RK, Laodholt CB, Colwell JA. Effect of metabolic control on lipid, lipoprotein and apolipoprotein levels in 55 insulin-dependent diabetic patients: a longitudinal study. Diabetes 1983;32:20–25.

109. Sosenko JM, Breslow JL, Miettinen OS, Gabbay KH. Hyperglycemia and plasma lipid levels: a prospective study of young insulin-dependent diabetic patients. N Engl J Med 1980;302:650–654.

110. Joven J, Vilella E, Costa B, Turner PR, Richart C, Masana L. Concentrations of lipids and apolipoproteins in patients with clinically well-controlled insulin-dependent and non-insulin-dependent diabetes. Clin Chem 1989;35:813–816.

111. Reaven GM, Javorski WC, Reaven EP. Diabetic hypertriglyceridemia. Am J Med Sci 1975;269:382–389.

112. Uusitupa MI, Niskanen LK, Siitonen O, Voutilainen E, Pyorala K. 5-year incidence of atherosclerotic vascular disease in relation of general risk factors, insulin level, and abnormalities in lipoprotein composition in non-insulin-dependent diabetic and nondiabetic subjects. Circulation 1990;82:27–36.

113. Nikilla EA. High density lipoproteins in diabetes. Diabetes 1981;30:82–87.

114. Kasim SE, Tseng K, Jen KL, Khilnani S. Significance of hepatic triglyceride lipase activity in the regulation of serum high density lipoproteins in type II diabetes mellitus. J Clin Endocrinol Metab 1987;65:183–187.

115. Semenkovich CF, Ostlund RE Jr, Schechtman KB. Plasma lipids in patients with type I diabetes mellitus: influence of race, gender and plasma glucose control: lipids do not correlate with glucose control in black women. Arch Intern Med 1989;149:51–56.

116. Wang-Iverson P, Ginsberg HN, Peteanu LA, Le NA, Brown WV. Apo E-mediated uptake and degradation of normal very low density lipoproteins by human monocyte/macrophages: a saturable pathway distinct from the LDL receptor. Biochem Biophys Res Commun 1985;126:578–586.

117. Havel RJ, Chao Y, Windler EE, Kotite L, Guo LS. Isoprotein specificity in the hepatic uptake of apolipoprotein E and the pathogenesis of familial dysbetalipoproteinemia. Proc Natl Acad Sci USA 1980;77:4349–4353.

118. Witztum JL, Fisher M, Pietro T, Steinbrecher UP, Elam RL. Nonenzymatic glucosylation of high-density lipoprotein accelerates its catabolism in guinea pigs. Diabetes 1982;31:1029–1032.

119. Klein RL, Lyons TJ, Lopes-Virella MF. Metabolism of very low and low density lipoproteins isolated from normolipidaemic type II (non-insulin dependent) diabetic patients by human monocyte-derived macrophages. Diabetologia 1990;33:299–305.

120. Klein RL, Lyons TJ, Lopes-Virella MF. Interaction of VLDL isolated from type I diabetic subjects with human monocyte-derived macrophages. Metabolism 1989;38:1108–1114.

121. Lopes-Virella MF, Sherer GK, Lees AM, et al. Surface binding, internalization and degradation by cultured human fibroblasts of low density lipoproteins isolated from type I (insulin-dependent) diabetic patients: changes with metabolic control. Diabetologia 1982;22:430–436.

122. Hiramatsu K, Bierman EL, Chair A. Metabolism of LDL from patients with diabetic hypertriglyceridemia by cultured human skin fibroblasts. Diabetes 1985;34:8–14.

123. Bagdade JD, Subbaiah PV. Whole-plasma and high-density lipoprotein subfraction surface lipid composition in IDDM men. Diabetes 1989;38:1226–1230.

124. Bagdade JD, Buchanan WE, Kuusi T, Taskinen MR. Persistent abnormalities in lipoprotein composition in non-insulin dependent diabetes after intensive insulin therapy. Arteriosclerosis 1990;10:232–239.

125. James RW, Pometta D. The distribution profiles of very low and low density lipoproteins in poorly controlled male, type II (non-insulin dependent) diabetic patients. Diabetologia 1991; 34:246–252.

126. James RW, Pometta D. Differences in lipoprotein subfraction composition and distribution between type I diabetic men and control subjects. Diabetes 1990;39:1158–1164.

127. Stein Y, Glangeaud MC, Fainaru M, Stein O. The removal of cholesterol from aortic smooth muscle cells in culture and Landschutz ascites cell fractions of human high density apoproteins. Biochem Biophs Acta 1975;380:106–118.

128. Fielding DF, Reaven GM, Fielding PE. Human non-insulin dependent diabetes: Identification of a defect in plasma cholesterol transport normalized in vivo by insulin and in vitro by immunoabsorption of apolipoprotein E. Proc Natl Acad Sci USA 1982;79:6365–6369.

129. Fielding CJ, Reaven GM, Liu G, Fielding PE. Increased free cholesterol in plasma low and very low density lipoproteins in non-insulin dependent diabetes mellitus: its role in the inhibition of cholesteryl ester transfer. Proc Natl Acad Sci USA 1984;81:2512–2516.

130. Biesbroeck RC, Albers JJ, Wahl PW, Weinberg CR. Abnormal composition of high-density lipoproteins in non-insulin dependent diabetics. Diabetes 1982;31:126–131.

131. Uusitupa M, Siitonen O, Voutilainen E, et al. Serum lipids and lipoproteins in newly diagnosed non-insulin dependent (type II) diabetic patients, with special reference to factors influencing HDL-cholesterol and triglyceride levels. Diabetes Care 1986;9:17–22.

132. Ronnemaa T, Laakso M, Kallio V, Pyorala K, Marniemi J, Puukka P. Serum lipids, lipoproteins, and apolipoproteins and the excessive occurrence of coronary heart disease in non-insulin-dependent diabetic patients. Am J Epidemiol 1989;130:632–645.

133. Ledl F, Schleicher E. New aspects of the Maillard reaction in foods and in the human body. Angew Chem (Int Ed Engl) 1990;29:565–594.

134. Ahmed MU, Thorpe SR, Baynes JW. Identification of carboxymethyllysine as a degradation product of fructose-lysine in glycosylated protein. J Biol Chem 1986;261:4889–4994.

135. Sell DR, Monnier VM. Structure elucidation of a senescence cross-link from human extracellular matrix. Implication of pentoses in the aging process. JH Biol Chem 1989;264:21,597–21,602.

136. Hayase F, Nagaraj RH, Miyata S, Njoroge FG, Monnier VM. Aging of proteins: immunological detection of a glucose-derived pyrrole formed during Maillard reaction in vivo. J Biol Chem 1989;263:3758–3764.

137. Ienaga K, Nakamura K, Hochi T, et al. Crosslines, fluorophores in the AGE-related crosslinked proteins. Contrib Nephrol 1995;112:42–51.

138. Fu M-X, Wells-Knecht KJ, Blackledge JA, Lyons TJ, Thorpe ST, Baynes JW. Glycation, glycoxidation and cross-linking of collagen by glucose. Kinetics, mechanisms and inhibition of late stages. Diabetes 1994;43:676–683.

139. Fu MX, Requena JR, Jenkins AJ, Lyons TJ, Baynes JW, Thorpe SR. The advanced glycation end-product, N (carboxymethyl) lysine (CML), is a product of both lipid peroxidation and glycoxidation reactions. J Biol Chem 1996;271:9982–9986.

140. Requena JR, Fu MX, Ahmed MU, et al. Quantitation of malondialdehyde and 4-hydroxynonenal adducts to lysine residues in native and oxidized human LDL. Biochem J 1997;322:317–325.

141. Requena JR, Ahmed MU, Fountain CW, et al. N-(carboxymethyl) ethanolamine: a biomarker of phospholipid modification by the Maillard Reaction in vivo. J Biol Chem 1997;272:17,473–17,479.

142. Pushkarsky T, Rourke L, Spiegel LA, Seldin MF, Bucala R. Molecular characterization of a mouse genomic element mobilized by advanced glycation endproduct modified-DNA (AGE-DNA). Mol Med 1997;3:740–749.

143. Schleicher E, Deufel T, Wieland OH. Non-enzymatic glycation of human serum lipoproteins. FEBS Lett 1987;129:1–4.

144. Lyons TJ, Patrick JS, Baynes JW, Colwell JA, Lopes-Virella MF. Glycation of low density lipoprotein in patients with type 1 diabetes: Correlations with other parameters of glycemic control. Diabetologia 1986;29:685–689.

145. Pietri A, Dunn FL, Raskin P. The effect of improved diabetic control on plasma lipid and lipoprotein levels. A comparison of conventional therapy and subcutaneous insulin infusion. Diabetes 1980;29:1001–1005.

146. Abrams JJ, Ginsberg H, Grundy SM. Metabolism of cholesterol and plasma triglycerides in nonketotic diabetes mellitus. Diabetes 1982;31:903–910.

147. Dunn FL, Raskin P, Bilheimer DW. The effect of diabetic control on very low density lipoprotein-triglyceride metabolism in patients with type II diabetes mellitus and marked hypertriglyceridemia. Metabolism 1984;33:117–123.

148. Weisgraber KH, Innerarity TL, Mahley RW. Role of the lysine residues of plasma lipoproteins in high affinity binding to cell surface receptors on human fibroblasts. J Biol Chem 1978;253:9053–9062.

149. Sasaki J, Cottam GL. Glycation of LDL decreases its ability to interact with high-affinity receptors of human fibroblasts in vitro and decreases its clearance from rabbit plasma in vivo. Biochim Biophys Acta 1982;713:199–207.

150. Steinbrecher UP, Witztum JL. Glucosylation of low density lipoproteins to an extent comparable to that seen in diabetes slows their catabolism. Diabetes 1984;33:130–134.

151. Lopes-Virella MF, Klein RL, Lyons TJ, Stevenson HC, Witztum JL. Glycation of low-density lipoprotein enhances cholesteryl ester synthesis in human monocyte-derived macrophages. Diabetes 1988;37:550–557.

152. Klein RL, Laimins M, Lopes-Virella MF. Isolation, characterization and metabolism of the glycated and non-glycated subfractions of low density lipoproteins isolated from type I diabetic patients and non-diabetic subjects. Diabetes 1995;44:1093–1098.

153. Watanabe J, Wohltmann HJ, Klein RL, Colwell JA, Lopes-Virella MF. Enhancement of platelet aggregation by low density lipoproteins from IDDM patients. Diabetes 1988;37:1652–1657.

154. Bucala R, Makita Z, Koschinsky T, Cerami A, Vlassara H. Lipid advanced glycosylation: pathway for lipid oxidation in vivo. Proc Natl Acad Sci USA 1993;90:6434–6438.

155. Hunt JV, Smith CCT, Wolff SP. Autooxidative glycation and possible involvement of peroxides and free radicals in LDL modification by glucose. Diabetes 1990;39:1420–1424.

156. Kawamura M, Heinecke JW, Chait A. Pathophysiological concentrations of glucose promote oxidative modification of LDL by a superoxide-dependent pathway. J Clin Invest 1994;94:771–778.

157. Mullarkey CJ, Edelstein D, Brownlee M. Free radical generation by early glycation products: a mechanism for accelerated atherogenesis in diabetes. Biochem Biophys Res Commun 1990;173:932–939.

158. Brownlee M, Vlassara H, Cerami A. Nonenzymatic glycosylation products on collagen covalently trap low-density lipoprotein. Diabetes 1985;34:938–941.

159. Tsai EC, Hirsch IB, Brunzell JD, Chait A. Reduced plasma peroxyl radical trapping capacity and increased susceptibility of LDL to oxidation in poorly controlled IDDM. Diabetes 1994;1010–1014.

160. Jenkins AJ, Klein RL, Chassereau CH, Hermayer KL, Lopes-Virella MF. LDL from patients with well controlled IDDM is not more susceptible to in vitro oxidation. Diabetes 1996;45:762–767.

161. Haberland ME, Fong D, Cheng L. Malondialdehyde-altered protein occurs in atheroma of Watanabe heritable hyperlipidemic rabbits. Science 1988;241:215–218.

162. Rosenfeld ME, Palinski W, Yla-Herttula S, Butler S, Witztum JL. Distribution of oxidation specific lipid-protein adducts and apolipoprotein B in atherosclerotic lesions of varying severity from WHHL rabbits. Arteriosclerosis 1990;10:336–349.

163. Carew TE, Schwenke DC, Steinberg D. Antiatherogenic effect of probucol unrelated to its hypocholesterolemic effect: evidence that antioxidants in vivo can selectively inhibit low density lipoprotein degradation in macrophage-rich fatty streaks and slow the progression of atherosclerosis in the Watanabe heritable hyperlipidemic rabbit. Proc Natl Acad Sci USA 1987;84:7725–7729.

164. Palinski W, Koschinsky T, Butler S, et al. Immunological evidence for the presence of AGE in atherosclerotic lesions of euglycemic rabbits. Arterioscler Thromb Vasc Biol 1995;15:571–582.

165. Bucciarelli LG, Wendt T, Qu W, et al. RAGE blockade stabilizes established atherosclerosis in diabetic apolipoprotein E-null mice. Circulation 2002;106:2827–2835.

166. Sakaguchi T, Yan SF, Yan SD, et al. Central role of RAGE-dependent neointimal expansion in arterial restenosis. J Clin Invest 2003;111:959–972.
167. Regnstrom J, Nilsson J, Tornvall P, Landou C, Hamsten A. Susceptibility to LDL oxidation and coronary atherosclerosis in man. Lancet 1991:339:1183–1186.
168. Chiu HC, Jeng JR, Shieh SM. Increased oxidizability of plasma LDL from patients with coronary heart disease. Biochim Biophys Acta 1994;225:200–208.
169. Andrews B, Burnand K, Paganga G, et al. Oxidizability of LDL in patients with carotid or femoral artery atherosclerosis. Atherosclerosis 1995;112:77–84.
170. Penn MS, Chisolm GM. Oxidized lipoproteins, altered cell function and atherosclerosis. Atherosclerosis 1994;108:S21–S29.
171. Nagano Y, Arai H, Kita T. High density lipoprotein loses its effect to stimulate efflux of cholesterol from foam cells after oxidative modification. Proc Natl Acad Sci USA 1991;88:6457–6461.
172. Bowry VW, Stanley KK, Stocker R. High density lipoprotein is the major carrier of lipid hydroperoxides in human blood plasma from fasting donors. Proc Natl Acad Sci USA 1992;89:10,316–10,320.
173. Palinski W, Yla-Herttuala S, Rosenfeld ME, et al. Antisera and monoclonal antibodies specific for epitopes generated during oxidative modification of low density lipoprotein. Arteriosclerosis 1990:10,325–335.
174. Maggi E, Chiesa R, Melissano G, et al. LDL oxidation in patients with severe carotid atherosclerosis. A study of in vitro and in vivo oxidation markers. Arterioscler Thromb 1994;14:1892–1899.
175. Salonen JT, Yla-Herttuala S, Yamamoto R, et al. Autoantibody against oxidised LDL and progression of carotid atherosclerosis. Lancet 1992;339:883–887.
176. Lehtimaki T, Lehtinen S, Solakivi T, et al. Autoantibodies against oxidized low density lipoprotein in patients with angiographically verified coronary artery disease. Arterioscl Thromb Vasc Biol 1999;19:23–27.
177. Erkkilä AT, Närvänen O, Lehto S, Uusitupa MIJ, Ylä-Herttuala S. Autoantibodies against oxidized low-density lipoprotein and cardiolipin in patients with coronary heart disease. Arterioscl Thromb Vasc Biol 2000;20:204–209.
178. Bellomo G, Maggi E, Poli M, Agosta FG, Bollati P, Finardi G. Autoantibodies against oxidatively modified low-density lipoproteins in NIDDM. Diabetes 1995;44:60–66.
179. Turk Z, Ljubic S, Turk N, Benko B. Detection of autoantibodies against advanced glycation endproducts and AGE-immune complexes in serum of patients with diabetes mellitus. Clin Chim Acta 2001;303:105–115.
180. Virella G, Virella I, Leman RB, Pryor MB, Lopes-Virella MF. Anti-oxidized low-density lipoprotein antibodies in patients with coronary heart disease and normal healthy volunteers. Int J Clin Lab Res 1993;23:95–101.
181. Boullier A, Hamon M, Walters-Laporte E, et al. Detection of autoantibodies against oxidized low-density lipoproteins and of IgG-bound low density lipoproteins in patients with corocnary artery disease. Clin Chim Acta 1995;238:1–10.
182. Uusitupa MIJ, Niskanen L, Luoma J, Vilja, P. Rauramaa R, Ylä-Herttula S. Autoantibodies against oxidized LDL do not predict atherosclerosis vascular disease in non-insulin-dependent diabetes mellitus. Arterioscl Thromb Vasc Biol 1996;16:1236–1242.
183. van de Vijver LP, Steyger R, van Poppel G, et al. Autoantibodies against MDA-LDL in subjects with severe and minor atherosclerosis and healthy population controls. Atherosclerosis 1996;122:245–253.
184. Leinonen JS, Rantalaiho V, Laippala P, et al. The level of autoantibodies against oxidized LDL is not associated with the presence of coronary heart disease or diabetic kidney disease in patients with non-insulin-dependent diabetes mellitus. Free Radic Res 1998;29:137–141.
185. Festa A, Kopp HP, Schernthaner G, Menzel EJ. Autoantibodies to oxidised low density lipoproteins in IDDM are inversely related to metabolic control and microvascular complications. Diabetologia 1998;41:350–356.
186. Wu R, de Faire U, Lemne C, Witztum JL, Frostegard J. Autoantibodies to OxLDL are decreased in individuals with borderline hypertension. Hypertension 1999;33:53–59.
187. Lopes-Virella MF, Virella G, Orchard TJ, et al. Antibodies to oxidized LDL and LDL-containing immune complexes as risk factors for coronary artery disease in diabetes mellitus. Clin Immunol 1999;90:165–172.
188. Hulthe J, Wiklund O, Hurt-Camejo E, Bondjers G. Antibodies to oxidized LDL in relation to carotid atherosclerosis, cell adhesion molecules, and phospholipase A(2). Arterioscler Thromb Vasc Biol 2001;21:269–274.

189. Shaw PX, Horkko S, Chang MK, et al. Natural antibodies with the T15 idiotype may act in atherosclerosis, apoptotic clearance, and protective immunity J Clin Invest 2000;105:1731–1740.

190. Wu R, Lefvert AK. Autoantibodies against oxidized low density lipoproteins (oxLDL): characterization of antibody isotype, subclass, affinity and effect on the macrophage uptake of oxLDL. Clin Exp Immunol 1995;102:174–180.

191. Palinski W, Witztum JL. Immune responses to oxidative neoepitopes on LDL and phospholipids modulate the development of atherosclerosis J Intern Med 2000;247:371–380.

192. Hansson GK. Vaccination against atherosclerosis: science or fiction? Circulation 2002;106:1599–1601.

193. Virella G, Koskinen S, Krings G, Onorato JM, Thorpe SR, Lopes-Virella M. Immunochemical Characterization of Purified Human Oxidized Low-Density Lipoprotein Antibodies. Clin Immunol 2000;95:135–144.

194. Virella G, Thorpe, S, Alderson NL, et al., and the DCCT/EDIC Research Group. Autoimmune response to advanced glycosylation end-products of human low density lipoprotein. J. Lipid Research 2003;443:487–493.

195. Virella G, Tsokos G. Immune complex diseases. In: Virella G, (ed.). Medical Immunology, 5th edition. Marcel Dekker, NY, 2002, pp. 453–471.

196. Hulthe J, Bokemark L, Fagerberg B. Antibodies to oxidized LDL in relation to intima-media thickness in carotid and femoral arteries in 58-year-old subjectively clinically healthy men. Arterioscler Thromb Vasc Biol 2001;21:101–107.

197. Fagerberg B, Bokemark L, Hulthe J. The metabolic syndrome, smoking, and antibodies to oxidized LDL in 58-year-old clinically healthy men. Nutr Metab Cardiovasc Dis 2001;11:227–235.

198. Szondy E, Lengyel E, Mezey Z, Fust G, Gero S. Occurrence of anti-low-density lipoprotein antibodies and circulating immune complexes in aged subjects. Mechanisms of Aging and Development 1985;29:117–123.

199. Tertov VV, Orekhov AN, Kacharava AG, Sobenin IA, Perova NV, Smirnov VN. Low density lipoprotein-containing circulating immune complexes and coronary atherosclerosis. Experimental and Molecular Pathology 1990;52:300–308.

200. Atchley D, Lopes-Virella MF, Zheng D, Virella G and the DCCT/EDIC Research Group. Oxidized LDL—Anti-Oxidized LDL Immune Complexes and Diabetic Nephropathy. Diabetologia 2002;45: 1562–1571.

201. Gisinger C, Virella GT, Lopes-Virella MF. Erthrocyte-bound low density lipoprotein (LDL) immune complexes lead to cholesteryl ester accumulation in human monocyte derived macrophages. Clin Immunol Immunopath 1991;59:37–52.

202. Lopes-Virella MF, BinZafar N, Rackley S, Takei A, LaVia M, Virella G. The Uptake of LDL-IC by Human Macrophages: Predominant Involvement of the FcgR I. Atherosclerosis, 1997;135:161–170.

203. Huang Y, Ghosh MJ, Lopes-Virella MF. Transcriptional and Post-transcriptional Regulation of LDL Receptor Gene Expression in PMA-treated THP-1 Cells by LDL-Containing Immune Complexes. Journal of Lipid Research 1997;38:110–120.

204. Vlassara H, Brownlee M, Manogue KR, Dinarello CA, Pasagian A. Cachectin/TNF and IL-1 induced by glucose-modified proteins: role in normal tissue remodeling. Science 1988;240:1546–1548.

205. Vlassara H, Brownlee M, Cerami A. Novel macrophage receptor for glucose-modified proteins is distinct from previously described scavenger receptors. J Exp Med 1986;164:1301–1309.

206. Vlassara H, Valinsky J, Brownlee M, Cerami C, Nishimoto S, Cerami A. Advanced glycosylation end products on erythrocyte cell surface induce receptor-mediated phagocytosis by macrophages. A model for turnover of aging cells. J Exp Med 1987;166:539–49.

207. Virella G, Muñoz JF, Galbraith GMP, Gissinger C, Chassereau C, Lopes-Virella MF. Activation of human monocyte-derived macrophages by immune complexes containing low density lipoprotein. Clin Immunol Immunopath 1995;75:179–189.

208. Bevilacqua MP, Pober JS, Majeau GR, Cotran RS, Gimbrone MA Jr. Interleukin 1 induces biosynthesis and cell surface expression of procoagulant activity in human vascular endothelial cells. J Exp Med 1984;160:618–623.

209. Breviario F, Bertocchi F, Dejana E, Bussolino F. IL-1 induced adhesion of polymorphonuclear leukocytes to cultured human endothelial cells. Role of platelet-activating factor. J Immunol 1988;141:3391–3397.

210. Martin S, Maruta K, Burkart V, Gillis S, Kolb H. IL-1 and INF-γ increase vascular permeability. Immunology 1988;64:301–305.

211. Warner SJC, Auger KR, Libby P. Interleukin 1 induces interleukin 1. II. Recombinant human interleukin 1 induces interleukin 1 production by adult human vascular endothelial cells. J Immunol 1987;139: 1911–1917.

212. Raines EW, Dower SK, Ross R. Interleukin-1 mitogenic activity for fibroblasts and smooth muscle cells is due to PDGF-AA. Science 1989;243:393–396.

213. Hansson GK, Jonasson L, Seifert PS, Stemme S. Immune mechanisms in atherosclerosis. Arteriosclerosis 1989;9:567–578.

214. Nawroth PP, Bank I, Hadley D, Cassimeris J, Chess L, Stern D. Tumor necrosis factor/cachectin interacts with endothelial cell receptors to induce release of interleukin 1. J Exp Med 1986;165:1363–1375.

215. Kilpatrick JM, Hyman B, Virella G. Human endothelial cell damage induced by interactions between polymorphonuclear leukocytes and immune complex-coated erythrocytes. Clin. Immunol. Immunopath 1987;44:335–347.

216. Stevenson HC, Dekaban GA, Miller PJ, Benyajati C, Pearson ML. Analysis of human blood monocyte activation at the level of gene expression. J Exp Med 1985;161:503–513.

217. Nathan CF, Murray HW, Cohn ZA. Current concepts: the macrophage as an effector cell. N Eng J Med 1980;303:622–626.

218. Ross R, Masuda J, Raines EW, et al. Localization of PDGF-b protein in macrophages in all phases of atherogenesis. Science 1990;248:1009–1012.

219. Assoian RK, Fleurdelys BE, Stevenson HC, et al. Expression and secretion of type beta transforming growth factor by activated human macrophages. Proc Natl Acad Sci USA 1987;84:6020–6024.

220. Ferreri NR, Howland WC, Spiegelberg HL. Release of leukotrienes C4 and B4 and prostaglandin E2 from human monocytes stimulated with aggregated IgG, IgA, and IgE. J Immunol 1986;136:4188–4193.

221. Musson RA, Shafran H, Henson PM. Intracellular levels and stimulated release of lysosomal enzymes from human peripheral blood monocytes and monocyte-derived macrophages. J Reticuloendothelial Soc 1980;28:249–264.

222. Werb Z, Bonda MJ, Jones PA. Degradation of connective tissue matrices by macrophages: I. Proteolysis of elastin, glycoproteins, and collagens by proteinases isolated from macrophages. J Exp Med 1980;152:1340–1357.

223. Nakagawara A, Nathan CF, Cohn ZA. Hydrogen peroxide metabolism in human monocytes during differentiation in vitro. J Clin Invest 1981;68:1243–1252.

224. Marx N, Imhof A, Froehlich J, et al. Effect of rosiglitazone treatment on soluble CD40L in patients with type 2 diabetes and coronary heart disease. Circulation 2003;107:1954–1957

225. Falk E. (1992) Why do plaques rupture? Circulation 86(Suppl III):III-30–III-42.

226. Giroud D, Li JM, Urban P, Meier B, Rutishauser W. Relation of the site of acute myocardial infarction to the most severe coronary arterial stenosis at prior angiography. Am J Cardiol 1992;69:729–732.

227. Little WC, Constantinescu M, Applegate RJ, et al. Can coronary angiography predict the site of a subsequent myocardial infarction in patients with mild-moderate coronary artery disease? Circulation 1988;78:1157–1166.

228. Libby P. Molecular bases of the acute coronary syndromes. Circulation 1995;91:2844–2850.

229. Amento EP, Ehsani N, Palmer H, Libby L. Cytokine positively and negatively regulate interstitial collagen gene expression in human vascular smooth muscle cells. Arterioscler Thromb 1991;11:1223–1230.

230. Hansson GK, Holm J, Jonasson L. Detection of activated T lymphocytes in the human atherosclerotic plaques. Am J Pathol 1989;135:169–175.

231. van der Wal AC, Becker AE, van der Loos CM, Das PK. Site of intimal rupture or erosion of thrombosed coronary atherosclerotic plaques is characterized by an inflammatory process irrespective of the dominant plaque morphology. Circulation 1994;89:36–44.

232. Fuster V, Lewis A. Conner Memorial Lecture. Mechanisms leading to myocardial infarction: insights from studies of vascular biology. Circulation 1994;90:2126–2146.

233. Morton LF, Barnes MJ. Collagen polymorphism in the normal and diseased blood vessel wall. Investigation of collagens types I, III and V. Atherosclerosis 1982;42:41–51.

234. Hanson AN, Bentley JP. Quantitation of type I to type III collagen ratios in small samples of human tendon, blood vessels, and atherosclerotic plaques. Anal Biochem 1983;130:32–40.

235. Matrisian LM. The matrix-degrading metalloproteinases. BioEssays 1992;14:455–463.

236. Sukhova G, Schoenbeck U, Rabkin E, et al. Colocalization of the interstitial collagenase MMP-1 & MMP-13 with sites of cleaved collagen indicates their role in plaque destabilization. Circulation (Suppl) 1998;98:I-48.

237. Huang Y, Mironova M, Lopes-Virella MF. Oxidized LDL stimulates matrix metalloproteinase-1 expression in human vascular endothelial cells. Arterioscler Thromb Vasc Biol 1999;19:2640–2647.

238. Huang Y, Fleming AJ, Wu S, Virella G, Lopes-Virella MF. Fc-gamma receptor cross-linking by immune complexes induces matrix metalloproteinase-1 in U937 cells via mitogen-activated protein kinase. Arterioscler Thromb Vasc Biol 2000;20:2533–2538.

239. Huang Y, Song L, Wu S, Fan F, Lopes-Virella MF. Oxidized LDL differentially regulates MMP-1 and TIMP-1 expression in vascular endothelial cells. Atherosclerosis 2001;156:119–125.

240. Marx N, Froehlich J, Siam L, et al. Antidiabetic PPAR – activator rosiglitazone reduces MMP-9 serum levels in type 2 diabetic patients with coronary artery disease. Arterioscler Thromb Vasc Biol 2003;23:283–288.

241. Uemura S, Matushita H, Li W, et al. Diabetes mellitus enhances vascular matrix metalloproteinase activity: role of oxidative stress. Circ Res 2001;88:1291–1298.

242. Shi GP, Munger JS, Meara JP, Rich DH, Chapman HA. Molecular cloning and expression of human alveolar macrophage cathepsin S, an elastinolytic cysteine protease. J Biol Chem 1992;267:7258–7262.

243. Kafienah W, Bromme D, Buttle DJ, Croucher LJ, Hollander AP. Human Cathepsin K cleaves native type I and II collagens at the N-terminal end of the triple helix. Biochem J 1998;331:727–732.

244. Reddy VY, Zhang QY, Weiss SJ. Pericellular mobilization of the tissue-destructive cysteine protein-ases, cathepins B, L, and S, by human monocyte-derived macrophages. Proc Natl Acad Sci USA 1995;92:3849–3853.

245. Sukhova GK, Shi GP, Simon DI, Chapman HA, Libby P. Expression of the elastolytic cathepsins S and K in human atheroma and regulation of their production in smooth muscle cells. J Clin Invest 1998;102:576–583.

246. Jormsjo S, Wuttge DM, Sirsjo A, et al. Differential expression of cysteine and aspartic proteases during progression of atherosclerosis in apolipoprotein E-deficient mice. Am J Pathol 2002;161:939–945.

247. Chen J, Tung C-H, Mahmood U, et al. In vivo imaging of proteolytic activity in atherosclerosis. Circulation 2002;105:2766–2771.

248. Gacko M, Glowinski S. Cathepsin D and cathepsin L activities in aortic aneurysm wall and parietal thrombus. Clin Chem Lab Med 1998;36:449–452.

249. Shi GP, Sukhova GK, Grubb A, et al. Cystatin C deficiency in human atherosclerosis and aortic aneurysms. J Clin Invest 1999;104:1191–1197.

250. Schaub FJ, Han DK, Liles WC, et al. Fas/FADD-mediated activation of a specific program of inflam-matory gene expression in vascular smooth muscle cells. Nature Med 2000;6:790–796.

251. Tedgui A, Mallat Z. Apoptosis as a determinant of atherothrombosis. Thromb Haemost 2001,86:420–426.

252. Moons AH, Levi M, Peters RJ. Tissue factor and coronary heart disease. Cardiovasc Res 2002;53:313–325.

253. Colwell JA, Halushka PV. Platelet function in diabetes mellitus. Br J Haematol 1980;44:521–526.

254. Colwell JA. Antiplatelet drugs and prevention of macrovascular disease in diabetes mellitus. Metabo-lism 1992;41 (Suppl 1):7–10.

255. Stringer HA, van Swieten P, Heijnen HF, Sixma JJ, Pannekoek H. Plasminogen activator inhibitor-1 released from activated platelets plays a key role in thrombolysis resistance. Studies with thrombi generated in the Chandler loop. Arterioscler Thromb 1994;14:1452–1458.

256. Jokl R, Laimins M, Klein RL, Lyons TJ, Lopes-Virella MF, Colwell JA. Platelet plasminogen activator inhibitor 1 in patients with type II diabetes. Diabetes Care 1994;17:818–823.

257. Jokl R, Klein RL, Lopes-Virella MF, Colwell JA. Release of platelet plasminogen activator inhibitor 1 in whole blood is increased in patients with type II diabetes. Diabetes Care 1995;18:1150–1155.

258. Loscalzo J. The relation between atherosclerosis and thrombosis. Circulation 1992;86:Suppl III:95–99.

259. Fuller JH. Haemostatic variables associated with diabetes and its complications. Br Med J 1979;2:964–966.

260. Kannel WB, Wolf PA, Castelli WP, D'Agostino RB. Fibrinogen and risk of cardiovascular disease: the Framingham study. JAMA 1987;258:1183–1186.

261. Jones RL, Peterson CM. Reduced fibrinogen survival in diabetes mellitus. J Clin Invest 1979;63:485–493.

262. Jones RL, Jovanovic L, Forman S, Peterson CM. Time course of reversibility of accelerated fibrino-gen disappearance in diabetes mellitus: association with intravascular volume shifts. Blood 1984;63:22–30.

263. Leurs PB, van Oerle R, Wolffenbuttel BH, Hamulyak K. Increased tissue factor pathway inhibitor (TFPI) and coagulation in patients with insulin-dependent diabetes mellitus. Thromb Haemost 1997;77:472–476.

264. Ceriello A, Giugliano D, Quatraro A, et al. Induced hyperglycemia alters antithrombin III activity but not plasma concentration in healthy normal subjects. Diabetes 1987;36:320–323.

265. Ceriello A, Giugliano D, Quatraro A, Marchi E, Barbanti M, Lefebvre P. Evidence for a hyperglycemia-dependent decrease of antithrombin complex formation in humans. Diabetologia 1990;33: 163–167.

266. De Feo P, Gaisano MG, Haymond MW. Differential effects of insulin deficiency on albumin and fibrinogen synthesis in humans. J Clin Invest 1991;88:833–840.

267. Hornsby WG, Boggess KA, Lyons TJ, Barnwell WH, Lazarchick J, Colwell JA. Hemostatic alterations with exercise conditioning in NIDDM. Diabetes Care 1990;13:87–92.

268. Jones RL. Fibrinopeptide-A in diabetes mellitus. Diabetes 1985;34:836–843.

269. Rosove MH, Frank HJL, Harwing SSL. Plasma beta-thromboglobulin, platelet factor 4, fibrinopeptide A, and other hemostatic functions during improved, short-term glycemic control in diabetes mellitus. Diabetes Care 1984;7:174–179.

270. Ford I, Singh TP, Kitchen S, Makris M, Ward JD, Preston FE. Activation of coagulation in diabetes mellitus in relation to the presence of vascular complications. Diabetic Med 1991;8:322–329.

271. Marmur JD, Merlini PA, Sharma S, et al. Thrombin generation in human coronary arteries after percutaneous transluminal balloon angioplasty. J Am Coll Cardiol 1994;24:1484–1491.

272. Brownlee M, Vlassara H, Cerami A. Inhibition of heparin-catalyzed antithrombin III activity by non-enzymatic glycosylation: possible role in fibrin deposition in diabetes. Diabetes 1984;33:532–535.

273. Ceriello A, Giugliano D, Quatraro A, et al. Daily rapid blood glucose variations may condition antithrombin biological activity but not its plasma concentration in insulin dependent diabetes: a possible role for labile non-enzymatic glycation. Diabetes Metab 1987;13:16–19.

274. Vukovich TC, Schernthaner G. Decreased protein C levels in patients with insulin-dependent type I diabetes mellitus. Diabetes 1986;35:617–619.

275. Ananyeva NM, Kouiavskaia DV, Shima M, Saenko EL. Intrinsic pathway of blood coagulation contributes to thrombogenicity of atherosclerotic plaque. Blood 2002; 99:4475–4485.

276. Ridker PM, Vaughan DE, Stampfer MJ, Manson JE, Hennekens CH. Endogenous tissue-type activator and risk of myocardial infarction. Lancet 1993;341:1165–1168.

277. Ridker PM, Hennekens CH, Stampfer MJ, Manson JE, Vaughan DE. Prospective study of endogenous tissue plasminogen activator and risk of stroke. Lancet 1994;343:940–943.

278. Jansson JH, Olofsson BO, Nilsson TK. Predictive value of tissue plasminogen activator mass concentration on long-term mortality in patients with coronary artery disease. Circulation 1993;88:2030–2034.

279. Garcia Frade LJ, de la Calle H, Torrado MC, Lara JI, Cuellar L, Garcia Avello A. Hypofibrinolysis associated with vasculopathy in non-insulin dependent diabetes mellitus. Thromb Res 1990;59:51–59.

280. Huber K, Jorg M, Probst P, et al. A decrease in plasminogen activator inhibitor-1 activity after successful percutaneous transluminal coronary angioplasty is associated with a significantly reduced risk for coronary restenosis. Throm Haemos 1992;67:209–213.

281. Gray RP, Patterson DLH, Yudkin JS. Plasminogen activator inhibitor activity in diabetic and nondiabetic survivors of myocardial infarction. Arteriosclerosis 1993;13:415–420.

282. Gruden G, Cavallo-Perin P, Bazzan M, Stella S, Vuolo A, Pagano G. PAI-1 and factor VII activity are higher in IDDM patients with microalbuminuria. Diabetes 1994;43:426–429.

283. Grant PJ, Ruegg M, Medcalf RL. Basal expression and insulin-mediated induction of PAI-1 mRNA in Hep G2 cells. Fibrinolysis 1991;5:81–86.

284. Chen Y, Sobel BE, Schneider DJ. Effect of fatty acid chain length and thioesterification on the augmentation of expression of plasminogen activator inhibitor-1. Nutrition, Metabolism, and Cardiovascular Disease 2002;12:325–330.

285. Juhan-Vague I, Vague P, Poisson C, Aillaud MF, Mendez C, Collen D. Effect of 24 hours of normoglycemia on tissue-type plasminogen activator plasma levels in insulin-dependent diabetes, Thromb Haemost 1984;51:97–98.

286. Vague P. Insulin and the fibrinolytic system. IDF Bull 1991;36:15–17.

287. Cefalu WT, Carlson HE, Schneider DJ, Sobel BE. Effect of combination glipizide GITS/metformin on fibrinolytic and metabolic parameters in poorly controlled, type 2 diabetic subjects. Diabetes Care 2002;25:2123–2128.

288. Booyse FM, Bruce R, Gianturco SH, Bradley WA. Normal but not hypertriglyceridemic very low-density lipoprotein induces rapid release of tissue plasminogen activator from cultured human umbilical vein endothelial cells. Semin Thromb Hemost 1988;14:175–179.

289. Stiko-Rahm A, Wiman B, Hamsten A, Nilsson J. Secretion of plasminogen activator inhibitor 1 from cultured human umbilical vein endothelial cells is induced by very low density lipoprotein. Arterio-sclerosis 1990;10:1067–1073.

290. Brommer EJ, Gevers Leuven JA, Barrett-Bergshoeff MM. Response of fibrinolytic activity and factor VIII-related antigen to stimulation with desmopressin in hyperlipoproteinemia. J Lab Clin Med 1982;100:105–114.

291. Hancock MA, Boffa MB, Marcovina SM. Inhibition of plasminogen activation by lipoprotein (a): critical domains in apolipoprotein (a) and mechanisms of inhibition on fibrin and degraded fibrin surfaces. J Biol Chem 2003;287:23260–269.

292. Kang C, Dominguez M, Loyau S. Lp(a) particles mold fibrin-binding properties of apo(a) in size-dependent manner: a study with different length recombinant apo(a), native Lp(a) and monoclonal antibody. Arterioscler Thromb Vasc Biol 2002;22:1232–38.

293. Loskutoff DJ, Sawdey M, Mimuro J. Type 2 plasminogen activator inhibitor. In: Coller S, (ed). Progress in Hemostatis and Thrombosis. WB Saunders: Philadelphia, PA, 1989, pp. 87–115.

294. Juhan-Vague I, Alessi MC. Regulation of fibrinolysis in the development of atherothrombosis: role of adipose tissue. Thromb Haemost 1999;82,832–836.

295. Alessi MC, Peiretti F, Morange P, Henry M, Nalbone G, Juhan-Vague I. Production of plasminogen activator inhibitor 1 by human adipose tissue. Possible link between visceral fat accumulation and vascular disease. Diabetes 1997;46,860–867.

296. Sakamoto TJ, Woodcock-Mitchell K, Marutsuka JJ, Mitchell BE, Sobel, Fujii S. TNF-alpha and insulin. Alone and synergistically, induce plasminogen activator inhibitor-1 expression in adipocytes. Am J Physiol 1999;276:C1391–C1397.

297. Okada HJ, Woodcock-Mitchell J, Mitchell T, et al. Induction of plasminogen activator inhibitor type 1 and type 1 collagen expression in rat cardiac microvascular endothelial cells by interleukin-1 and its dependence on oxygen-centered free radicals. Circulation 1998;97:2175–2182.

298. Feener EP, Northup JM, Aiello LP, King GL. Angiotensin II induces plasminogen activator inhibitor-1 and –2 expression in vascular endothelial and smooth muscle cells. J Clin Invest 1995;95:1353–1362.

299. Zaman AKMT, Fujii S, Sawa H, et al. Angiotensin-converting enzyme inhibition attenuates hypofibrinolysis and reduces cardiac perivascular fibrosis in genetically obese diabetic mice. Circulation 2001;103:3123–3128.

12 The Use of Animal Models to Study Diabetes and Atherosclerosis and Potential Anti-Atherosclerotic Therapies

Peter D. Reaven, MD and Wulf Palinski, MD

CONTENTS

INTRODUCTION

Epidemiological studies have documented that individuals with diabetes mellitus (DM) and those with impaired glucose tolerance (IGT) have an increased prevalence of atherosclerosis and increased rates of coronary artery disease (CAD) *(1,2)*. However, the mechanisms by which these conditions enhance atherogenesis are poorly understood. Hyperglycemia, the defining metabolic change in diabetes, may contribute to the development of atherosclerosis. However, the specific contribution of hyperglycemia has been difficult to demonstrate in either population studies or in animal models *(1,3–6)*. Moreover, hyperglycemia per se is unlikely to play a role in the development of atherosclerosis in individuals with IGT who usually demonstrate only modest postprandial hyperglycemia. This is confirmed by recent data from the United Kingdom Prospective Diabetes Study demonstrating that improved glucose control reduces microvascular complications, but has modest or no effects on macrovascular disease and its clinical sequelae *(3)*. Many investigators have therefore suggested that other factors besides glucose levels

From: *Contemporary Cardiology: Diabetes and Cardiovascular Disease, Second Edition*
Edited by: M. T. Johnstone and A. Veves © Humana Press Inc., Totowa, NJ

Table 1
Factors Potentially Increasing CAD in Individuals With Insulin Resistance and
Diabetes

A) "Traditional" Risk Factors

High plasma cholesterol
Low plasma HDL
High plasma triglyceride
Hypertension

B) "Nontraditional" Risk Factors

Hyperglycemia
Hyperinsulinemia
C-reactive protein
Increased plasma PAI-1
Increased plasma fibrinogen
Decreased platelet function
Increased prevalence of small dense LDL and triglyceride rich lipoproteins
Increased AGE formation
Increased oxidative stress and enhanced lipoprotein susceptibility to oxidation
Endothelial cell dysfunction

contribute to the development of macrovascular disease in diabetes. On the other hand, insulin resistance, an essential component of type 2 diabetes, is frequently associated with a number of metabolic abnormalities such as hypercholesterolemia, hypertriglyceridemia, low high-density lipoprotein (HDL), and hypertension that are considered "traditional" risk factors for atherosclerosis. However, these risk factors explain only some, but not all of the increased risk for CAD in individuals with IGT or diabetes *(7,8)*. Thus, additional factors associated with insulin resistance and diabetes are likely to contribute to the development of atherosclerosis (Table 1).

The mechanisms by which these traditional and "nontraditional" risk factors may enhance atherosclerosis in DM have been extensively reviewed elsewhere *(4,8,9)*. Experimental verification of these potential mechanisms of atherogenesis has been greatly hindered by a lack of appropriate animal models. Additionally, many studies carried out in existing animal models of diabetes and atherosclerosis were not controlled for changes in cholesterol or triglyceride levels or other relevant cardiovascular factors (such as increased blood pressure), thereby limiting the conclusions that can be drawn regarding the importance of specific risk factors such as hyperglycemia, advanced glycation end-products (AGE) formation and hyperinsulinemia.

"Ideal" animal models of insulin resistance or diabetes and atherosclerosis should have the following essential characteristics. Animal models of insulin resistance should have elevated fasting and postprandial insulin levels and relatively normal glucose levels. Models of type 1 diabetes should have low insulin levels, although models of type 2 diabetes should have normal or slightly elevated plasma insulin. Both diabetes models should also have moderate to severe hyperglycemia and lipoprotein distribution and metabolism typical of that present in human diabetes. Atherosclerotic lesions in these models should have many of the morphological and cellular features characteristic of early and advanced human lesions. Finally, the models should fulfill several practical criteria for in vivo studies of atherosclerosis. Induction of diabetes and its consequences should not lead to markedly impaired health and reduced survival, nor large variation in the extent of lesion formation from animal to animal. Some existing models, such as nonhuman primates, require years to develop measurable differences in atherosclerosis and are prohibitively expensive. Therefore, "ideal" animal models should develop atherosclerotic lesions within a relatively short time that are sufficiently extensive and consistent to allow one to detect differences between experimental groups with limited animal numbers. This would also help reduce the costs of purchasing, feeding, and housing the animals.

EXISTING MODELS OF INSULIN RESISTANCE OR DIABETES AND ATHEROSCLEROSIS

There are currently several models of insulin resistance in animals. Most commonly, insulin resistance is induced by high-fructose diets. Although this approach has been used in dogs and hamsters, fructose-enriched diets are most frequently used to induce a hyperinsulinemic, euglycemic insulin-resistant condition in rats *(10,11)*. These diets also induce enhanced hepatic secretion of very low-density lipoprotein (VLDL), frequently resulting in moderate hypertriglyceridemia *(10,11)*. Certain strains of mice such as the ob/ob mouse often spontaneously develop insulin resistance, but this is usually accompanied by hyperglycemia *(12,13)*. Although the etiology of insulin resistance in these mice is not clear, development of insulin resistance in the ob/ob model is accompanied by substantial increases in body weight *(12)*, suggesting that obesity may be an essential pathogenic factor. Genetically altered mouse models have also been developed, such as the insulin receptor substrate (IRS)-1-deficient mouse *(14,15)*, that have clearly defined mechanisms of insulin resistance. Although all of these animal models have proven useful for studies of insulin resistance, they do not develop extensive atherosclerosis, presumably because of their naturally low plasma cholesterol levels and genetic resistance to diet-induced hypercholesterolemia. The IRS-2-deficient mouse, however, does demonstrate an increased propensity to neointimal formation in response to vessel injury, presumably related to its greater nonglycemic metabolic abnormalities *(16)*.

There are also several different animal models of diabetes and atherosclerosis. Nonhuman primates fed atherogenic diets have been used to model human atherosclerosis for many years *(17)*. For the most part, they have demonstrated lipoprotein profiles and atherosclerotic lesions that are fairly representative of those of humans *(18)*. However, in some instances, as in the squirrel monkey, the plasma cholesterol elevation that develops following increased dietary cholesterol exposure results from increases in β-VLDL rather than in low-density lipoprotein (LDL) *(18)*. The atherosclerotic lesions that develop in cynomologus monkeys are characteristically more fibrotic and more mineral-rich than those typically found in other macaques and cynomologus monkeys may therefore be the most useful model of human atherosclerosis *(18,19)*. Glucose intolerance and insulin resistance do develop spontaneously in some nonhuman primates, although the development of diabetes is much more rare than in humans *(18)*. Therefore, diabetes is most often induced artificially. However, chemically induced diabetes in nonhuman primates has been problematic as the degree of β cell damage and the need for insulin vary greatly. Moreover, maintaining stable hyperglycemia and good health in these animals for long term atherosclerosis studies requires intensive monitoring and care.

Despite these problems, several studies have been performed in nonhuman primates with chemically induced or spontaneously developing diabetes. Alloxan-treated squirrel monkeys that were fed cholesterol-enriched diets developed insulinopenic hyperglycemia and elevated LDL levels *(20)*. Atherosclerosis was more extensive in the diabetic group compared to a nondiabetic control group that had equally elevated plasma cholesterol. More recently, there has been increasing interest in the diabetic cynomologus monkey. In one longitudinal study, it was noted that after 13 or more years of age, many cynomologus monkeys spontaneously developed diabetes, increased plasma cholesterol ester transfer protein (CETP) activity and increased triglyceride rich lipoproteins *(21)*. These changes in CETP activity and lipoprotein composition resemble those that occur in human diabetes. Lipoproteins from diabetic cynomologus monkeys also demonstrated increased glycation, which correlated with the degree of hyperglycemia in the animals *(22)*. In a different study, diabetes was induced in cynomologus monkey by injection of streptozotocin and the animals were monitored for changes in plasma HDL and triglyceride levels *(23)*. As expected, streptozotocin (STZ)-induced hypoinsulinemia and decreased plasma postheparin lipoprotein lipase activity and mass. Plasma triglycerides and nonesterified fatty acids increased, whereas HDL decreased, similar to the lipoprotein changes that occur in human diabetes. In a subsequent study of cynomologus monkeys, the extent and progression of atherosclerosis was compared in nondiabetic monkeys and monkeys made diabetic by intravenous STZ injections *(24)*. Diabetic monkeys had significant increases in glycated hemoglobin and glycated LDL concentrations and modest increases in total plasma cholesterol. Arterial accumulation of LDL in femoral arteries and the aorta, but not in iliac or carotid arteries, was increased in diabetic animals compared to control animals. Diabetic monkeys also showed greater accumulation of arterial cholesterol in the femoral and abdominal aorta. Interestingly, there were no differences in formation of AGE in arterial collagen between the two groups. Unfortunately, the conclusions that can be drawn from this study were limited by the fact that the pretrial diets were not similar in all groups and that the diabetic group had moderately higher cholesterol levels at the end of the study.

The New Zealand White rabbit has been widely used as a model for atherosclerosis studies *(25)*. When fed high-cholesterol diets, these rabbits develop marked hypercholesterolemia (primarily as a result of elevation in β-VLDL) and extensive atherosclerosis. However, prolonged exposure to diets with more than 1% cholesterol leads to serious side effects and high mortality. Surprisingly, in studies by Nordestgaard and associates *(26)*, cholesterol-fed rabbits made diabetic by alloxan treatment developed less atherosclerosis compared to their nondiabetic controls. The investigators suggested that this apparent paradox may have been the result of a shift from the normal apo-E-rich β-VLDL particles to larger apo-E-depleted particles. The latter particles may be less able to enter and accumulate in the artery wall *(27,28)*. Rabbits lacking functional LDL receptors (Watanabe heritable hyperlipidemic [WHHL] rabbits) also develop marked hypercholesterolemia and extensive aortic lesions. In contrast to the New Zealand White rabbit model, this occurs on a normal chow diet, and the rabbits enjoy good health and live a normal life span. An additional advantage to the WHHL rabbits is that the major carrier of their plasma cholesterol is LDL, not β-VLDL. To our knowledge, WHHL rabbits have not been used for studies of diabetes and atherosclerosis. Given the high mortality of alloxan-treated rabbits this approach could be quite costly. Thus, to date, rabbits have not proven to be a useful model of diabetic atherosclerosis. However, infusion of AGE in mice and rabbits has been reported to increase expression of vascular cell adhesion molecule-1 *(29,30)*, one of the mechanisms by which diabetes may enhance atherogenesis. Moreover, infusing AGE in nondiabetic rabbits for 16 weeks also induced early atherosclerotic changes (30). These studies raise the possibility that if atherogenic lipid profiles could be achieved, as in the WHHL model, rabbits could be a useful species in which to illustrate the atherogenic effect of AGE formation. If this is indeed true, agents that prevent AGE formation or break their crosslinks should be useful for interventions in these animals.

Another animal commonly used for atherosclerosis studies is the hamster. Although HDL is the major lipoprotein carrying cholesterol in the hamster (as is true with most rodents), hamsters and humans have many other features of lipoprotein metabolism in common. Hamster's plasma contains CETP activity and LDL receptor regulation in the hamster is also similar to that in humans. Additionally, cholesterol enriched diets induce elevations in both VLDL and LDL in the hamster. However, despite these increases in pro-atherogenic lipoproteins, hamsters on cholesterol-enriched diets have been relatively resistant to the development of atherosclerosis, most likely because the diet also leads to a marked rise in HDL cholesterol. Hamsters have occasionally been used in studies of chemically induced diabetes. In studies by the Simionescu group (31,32), intraperitoneal injections of STZ induced variable responses in blood glucose, with some animals showing marked hyperglycemia, weight loss, and poor survival, whereas others developed only moderate hyperglycemia and demonstrated prolonged survival. Diabetic hamsters fed standard diets showed modest rises in total cholesterol (TC) and plasma thiobarbituric acid-reactive substances (TBARS), a measure of lipid peroxidation, whereas a high-cholesterol diet led to significant increases in TC, TBARS, glycated LDL, and albumin. Ultrastructural changes in the aortic origin and distal aorta consistent with atherosclerosis (including increased subendothelial matrix, aggregated lipoproteins, increased accumulation of macrophages, and calcification) developed more rapidly in the diabetic hyperlipidemic hamsters than in the hyperlipidemic or diabetic-only animals. These data support the concept that diabetes increases atherosclerosis and that the diabetic hamster may be a useful model to investigate mechanisms by which diabetes enhances atherosclerosis. However, the extent of atherosclerosis that develops in the diabetic hamster model is modest, and more information is needed on the changes in lipoprotein levels and composition that occur.

Several different strains of rats have been proposed as models of type 2 diabetes. These models were the result of naturally occurring mutations in laboratory animals and the recognition that some rats are uniquely susceptible to develop insulin resistance and diabetes on special diets. Rats homozygous for the "fatty" (fa) or "corpulent" (cp) genes are typically obese, hyperlipidemic, hyperinsulinemic, and insulin resistant (33). The "fatty" (Zucker) rat has been used primarily as a model of obesity. However, because of the accompanying hyperglycemia and insulin resistance it is also useful as a model of type 2 diabetes. As in most animal models of insulin resistance there is an increased VLDL secretion from the liver and increased plasma levels of cholesterol and triglycerides. These VLDL particles are enriched in apo-C and depleted of apo-E. Despite these changes in lipoproteins, there is no evidence of spontaneous arterial lesion formation in the Zucker rat and studies have not yet been performed to assess the effects of cholesterol-enriched diets on atherogenesis in this model.

In contrast, the corpulent (JCR:LA-cp) rat does develop cardiac lesions while on standard chow. Rats of this strain (particularly the males) have marked hyperinsulinemia that develops shortly after birth and persists throughout their lifetime (34,35). As glucose levels are only modestly elevated, this strain is generally considered a model of insulin resistance and impaired glucose tolerance. Similar to other insulin-resistant animal models, increased VLDL secretion is present, resulting in increased plasma cholesterol and triglyceride levels. Other abnormalities, including increased plasma activity of plasminogen activator inhibitor (PAI)-1 and reduced vascular relaxation in response to acetylcholine have been identified (36). It is not surprising, therefore, that these rats develop spontaneous arterial lesions that by electron and light microscopy examination resemble early atherosclerotic lesions in humans (34,35). Lesion formation in the JCR:LA-cp rat appears causally linked to hyperinsulinemia and insulin resistance, as therapies that reduce insulin resistance also reduce lesion formation (33,34). In contrast to the beneficial effects of lipid lowering in diabetic human subjects, therapies that only reduce plasma lipid levels in the JCR:LA-cp rat do not decrease the occurrence of atherosclerotic lesions. This suggests that different etiologies for lesion formation may exist in humans and the JCR:LA-cp rat.

Another recently described rat model of type 2 diabetes and atherosclerosis is the sand rat (*Psammomys Obesus*). When fed standard rat chow, which contains more calories, greater amounts of fat and less fiber then their normal vegetarian diets, the sand rat becomes obese, hyperglycemic, hyperinsulinemic, and insulin resistant (37–39). VLDL secretion is increased, whereas clearance is reduced, presumably accounting for their elevated plasma cholesterol levels. When made hypothyroid and fed a cholesterol-enriched diet they develop cardiovascular lesions that contain increased lipid deposits, glycosaminoglycans, and fibrosis (33). As with many of the other models described here, no studies were reported in which the development of lesion formation in the sand rat is compared to control animals with matching levels of lipids or other cardiovascular risk factors. Thus, it remains unknown whether factors other than raised cholesterol levels contribute to the development of atherosclerosis in the insulin-resistant diabetic sand rat.

Although a variety of animal models of diabetes and atherosclerosis have been studied, most of them suffer from one or more of the following problems. Models of type 1 diabetes are usually generated by administration of chemicals toxic to the pancreas and require insulin to avoid developing marked hyperglycemia, dehydration, and ketosis. Using low doses of insulin to avoid the above health problems while maintaining appropriate levels of hyperglycemia is difficult and time-consuming. Therefore, mortality rates are frequently high and the possibility that poor health may influence metabolic parameters and development of atherosclerosis always remains a concern. As noted above, a common limitation of many of the existing animal models of diabetes has been that they develop only very modest atherosclerosis. Some species, particularly the rat and most wild-type strains of mice (discussed later), are naturally resistant to developing atherosclerosis. Even on high-fat or cholesterol-enriched diets there is frequently insufficient elevation in lipid levels to induce significant lesion formation. Additionally, lipoprotein patterns or lipoprotein metabolism in some animal models are sufficiently different from those in humans to raise concerns about the relevance of risk factors identified in studies using these models. Finally, induction of diabetes is frequently associated with substantial changes in lipoprotein levels and patterns. Thus, it has been particularly difficult to tease out the role of glycemia from the many other metabolic abnormalities in diabetes. The complexity of this situation has further increased with appreciation of other metabolic alterations, such as diminished fibrinolysis and increased inflammation that accompany insulin resistance and diabetes (9,40,41).

MURINE MODELS OF ATHEROSCLEROSIS

More recently, there has been increasing interest in using murine models for investigations of atherosclerosis. Mice offer obvious logistic and cost advantages. Although most wild-type mice are resistant to diet-induced hypercholesterolemia and atherogenesis, early work by Paigen demonstrated that certain strains, such as the C57BL/6 mouse, develop limited atherosclerotic lesions, mostly in the aortic origin, in the vicinity of the aortic valves *(42,43)*. Because this area is subject to turbulent flow and substantial pressure oscillation, because induction of lesions requires the use of a proinflammatory agent, cholate, in the diet, and because lesions commonly consist only of intimal foam cell accumulations that do not progress to more advanced atheromas, the appropriateness of this models for investigation of human atherosclerosis has been questioned in the past. Fundamental skepticism on the nature of murine lesions was overcome by the development, through the use of "gene knockout" technique, of several murine strains, such as the apo-E deficient (apoE–/–) and LDL receptor deficient (LDLR–/–) mice that develop more advanced atherosclerotic lesions. Transgene overexpression has also been utilized in the generation of mouse models that express human apo-B and/or CETP *(44)*. As discussed later, these models may even more closely approximate human lipoprotein metabolism and atherosclerosis. For a detailed review of murine models of atherosclerosis *see* ref. *45.*

The apo-E–/– strains were developed independently by the groups of Breslow and Maeda *(46,47)*. Because they lack apo-E, hepatic clearance of lipoproteins via hepatic apo-E receptors is impaired, and they show marked elevation in plasma levels of chylomicrons, VLDL, and VLDL remnant particles. LDL levels are raised to a lesser extent (by increased conversion of VLDL/IDL to LDL). Even when fed a regular chow, these mice spontaneously develop plasma cholesterol levels of 600 mg/dL or more and extensive atherosclerosis throughout the aorta and its main branches, such as the brachiocephalic trunc, and in major coronary arteries. Further increases of TC to more than 1200 mg/dL are achieved by cholate-free diets with increased fat and cholesterol content (0.15% cholesterol), termed "Western diets" by Breslow and colleagues.

A second model developing extensive atherosclerosis is the LDLR–/– mouse *(48)*. Although these mice have the same type of genetic defect as humans with familial hypercholesterolemia and LDL receptor-deficient (WHHL) rabbits, LDLR–/– mice develop only "moderately" elevated plasma cholesterol levels (about 250 mg/dL) when fed regular mouse diet. However, levels of about 1200 mg/dL are easily achieved by high-fat, high-cholesterol diets *(48)*. Similar to the apo-E–/– model, these extreme cholesterol levels induce extensive atherosclerosis throughout the aorta *(48–50)* (Fig. 1). In contrast to the apo-E–/– mice, most of the plasma cholesterol is carried in the intermediate-density lipoprotein (IDL)/LDL fraction in LDLR–/– mice.

To obtain a more homogeneous genetic background and to reduce atherosclerosis-resistance traits derived from the 129/Sv mouse strain in which the "gene knockouts" were performed, apo-E–/– and LDLR–/– mice have been backcrossed with C57BL/6 mice for 10 generations (Jackson Laboratories). Both models have been widely used for studies on atherogenic mechanisms, for intervention studies with drugs, and to investigate the role of the immune system in atherosclerosis *(45)*. Lesions in apo-E–/– and LDLR–/– mice have been extensively characterized *(47,50–53)* and share many of the features found in human atherosclerosis. The earliest lesions consist mostly of macrophage/foam cells and are similar to those found in the aortic root of C57BL/6 mice

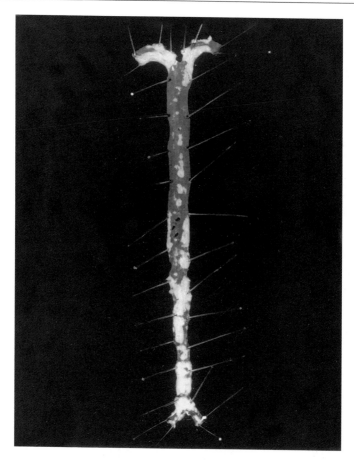

Fig. 1. An *en-face* preparation of an aorta from an LDLR–/– mouse fed an atherogenic diet for 6 months. Predilection sites of atherosclerotic lesions include the small curvature of the arch, branch sites of the brachiocephalic, the left common carotid, and subclavian arteries, several intercostal arteries, the abdominal aorta, and the iliac bifurcation.

not subjected to additional genetic alteration. In apo-E–/– and LDLR –/– mice, lesions in both the aorta and the aortic root then begin to form fibrous caps. These transitional lesions then progress toward classical atheromas. After prolonged exposure to high cholesterol levels, very large lesions can be found in the aortic origin that spread toward the aortic valve leaflets and often cause considerable stenosis. Lesions causing 50% or more stenosis can also be seen in some coronary arteries. Although apo-E–/– and LDLR–/– mice show elevated mortality, and electrocardiogram (ECG) changes of acute myocardial infarction were detected in at least one other murine model lacking the hepatic scavenger receptor B-1 *(54)*, it remains unclear to what degree murine models reflect the acute events associated with clinical manifestations in humans *(55,56)*. Both apo-E–/– and LDLR–/– mice have a high propensity to aortic aneurysm formation, and apo-E–/– mice in particular develop many signs of plaque vulnerability, i.e., rupture of fibrous caps, or at least deep erosions reaching necrotic core areas, associated with intraplaque bleeding. However, large intraluminal thrombi are rare *(57)*. The availability of models developing not just atherosclerosis, but progressing to clinical manifestations would be

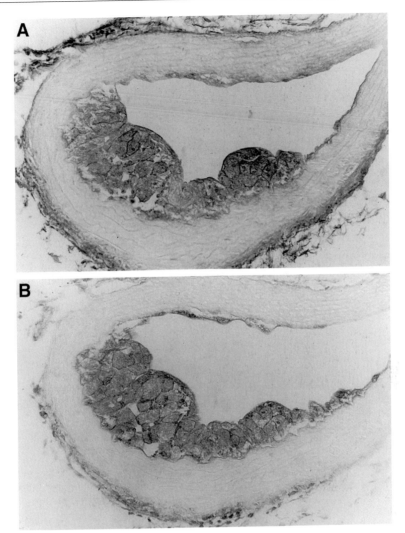

Fig. 2. Immunocytochemistry of atherosclerotic lesions from LDLR–/– mice. (**A**) Aortic section immunostained with MAL-2, a guinea-pig antiserum to an oxidation-specific epitope, MDA-lysine. (**B**) A serial section immunostained with an antiserum to mouse macrophages. As shown here, in early atherosclerotic lesions oxidation-specific epitopes (oxidized lipoproteins) mostly colocalize with intimal macrophages.

of value for diabetes research, because it is increasingly recognized from statin trials that changes of lesion composition, rather than lesion size, determine outcome *(55)*. In analogy, diabetic changes in the cellular composition and cytokine secretion patterns of intimal cells may contribute to increased coronary heart disease mortality, rather than to increased lesion size.

In addition to macrophages and some T cells *(58)*, early and advanced mouse lesions are rich in immunoglobulin (Ig)G and IgM *(49,53)*. Lesions also contain modified lipoproteins. Immunocytochemistry demonstrates that "oxidation-specific" epitopes, i.e., epitopes generated during the oxidation of LDL and other lipoproteins *(53,59,60)*, are also present in murine atheromas (Fig. 2A) and often colocalize with macrophages

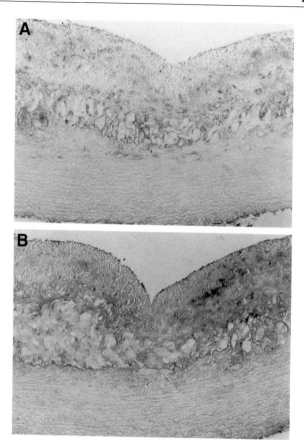

Fig. 3. Immunocytochemistry of atherosclerotic lesions from a Watanabe heritable hyperlipidemic rabbit with antibodies against oxidation-specific and AGE-specific epitopes. **(A)** Immunostaining with NA59, a monoclonal antibody against 4-hydroxynonenal-lysine epitopes. **(B)** Staining with FL-1, an AGE-specific antiserum. As shown in these representative sections, immunostaining for oxidation-specific epitopes (oxidized lipoproteins) colocalized with staining for AGE-epitopes. (Reprinted with permission from ref. *5a*.)

(Fig. 2B). Epitopes of proteins and lipoproteins modified by nonenzymatic glycation are also prevalent in advanced murine atherosclerotic lesions, even in euglycemic mice. We previously made a similar observation in euglycemic, but grossly hyperlipidemic, WHHL rabbits (Fig. 3A,B) *(61)*. In both nondiabetic rabbit and murine aortas, the formation of glycation-specific epitopes presumably results from increased lipid oxidation, through mutual interaction and enhancement of oxidation and glycation *(61)*. Epitopes of several putative AGE compounds, such as 4-furanyl-2-furoyl-[^{1}H]-imidazole (FFI), and epitopes of AGE formed by prolonged incubation of protein with reducing sugars occur even in "normal" apo-E–/– and LDLR–/– mice and colocalize with oxidation-specific epitopes *(5)*.

A disadvantage of murine models is the small size of the animal, which limits the amount of tissue and plasma samples available. However, reliable techniques have been developed to quantify atherosclerosis in cross-section through the aortic origin *(62)*. Palinski and colleagues have developed a method that allows one to determine atherosclerosis in the entire murine aorta, similar to the quantitation of human atherosclerosis

(50,53). In brief, the aorta is exposed from the heart to the iliac bifurcation and carefully dissected from the surrounding tissue. To obtain an *en-face* preparation the aorta is opened longitudinally while still attached to (and held in place by) the heart and the major branching arteries. The remaining branches of the major arteries are then cut off and the aorta is removed and pinned out on a black wax surface in a dissecting pan. The aortas are stained with Sudan IV and the extent of atherosclerosis is then quantitated by computer-assisted image analysis.

An important limitation to the use of murine models of atherosclerosis lies in the inherent difference in lipoprotein metabolism between mice and humans. As in most rodents, HDL is the major carrier of cholesterol in plasma of mice. Additionally, mice lack CETP; the HDL-associated enzyme that facilitates the exchange of HDL cholesterol with the triglycerides of VLDL. Other differences in lipoprotein metabolism, such as absence of plasma apo (a) have also been documented in the mouse *(63)*. Fortunately, mutant strains are being generated that overcome many of these deficiencies. For example, investigators have generated apo-A-I-deficient mice that have been crossbred with LDLR–/– mice *(64)*. These mice have substantially elevated LDL cholesterol levels and essentially no HDL particles. Another model of LDL cholesterol elevation is the transgenic mouse that over expresses human apo-B, generated by Dr. Young's laboratory *(65)*. These mice have markedly increased plasma LDL even on chow diets. When fed high-fat diets, plasma cholesterol levels nearly doubled in the transgenic mice compared to their chow fed counterparts. Most of the apo-B was found in LDL-sized particles. The extent of atherosclerosis that developed in the ascending aorta was substantially increased in the transgenic mice. These findings have subsequently been verified by other investigators *(66)*. In these later studies, the presence of the high-expressing apo-B transgene was associated with a several-fold increase in VLDL-LDL cholesterol and a 15-fold increase in proximal lesions compared with nontransgenic mice. Examination of aortas of mice expressing human apo-B demonstrated lesions along the entire length of the aorta and immunochemical analysis of the lesions revealed features characteristically seen in human lesions including the presence of oxidized lipoproteins, macrophages, and immunoglobulins

As noted above, mice expressing human apo-B-100 have also been developed and demonstrated modest to moderate elevations of cholesterol and triglyceride levels on chow diets. These increases in plasma lipids are primarily carried in LDL/IDL type particles, with little triglyceride or cholesterol in VLDL particles *(67)*. When placed on "Western" diets, substantial elevations in levels of these LDL/IDL particles occur and extensive atherosclerosis develops. To further approximate human patterns of plasma lipoproteins in diabetes, these investigators have also generated a mouse model that combines human apo-B and CETP overexpression with heterozygous lipoprotein lipase deficiency *(44)*. This combination of genetic mutations led to mice with mild to moderate elevations in plasma cholesterol and triglycerides and reduced levels of HDL cholesterol. Analysis of lipid distribution by fast protein liquid chromatography verified that the dyslipidemia present in this model closely reflects lipid patterns in humans with diabetes. Mice expressing human apo (a), and apo-A-I have also been generated *(68,69)*. Thus, genetically altered mice with lipoprotein metabolism similar to humans are now becoming available and as described below are beginning to be utilized to both enhance our understanding of atherosclerosis and to evaluate the efficacy of anti-atherogenic medications.

STUDIES ON THE EFFECTS OF INSULIN RESISTANCE
AND DIABETES ON ATHEROSCLEROSIS IN MICE

For the reasons outlined in the previous section, a very promising use of murine models is the study of atherogenesis in diabetes. To generate a murine model of diabetes that develops extensive atherosclerosis, several approaches are possible. Hyperlipidemic mice can be crossed with mice with a genetically determined predisposition to develop diabetes (70). Several strains of insulin-resistant and/or diabetes-prone mice have been identified. Most of these have occurred as a result of natural mutations of genes that play a role in the regulation of body weight. For example, the agouti, db/db, and ob/ob mouse strains are all characterized by marked obesity, insulin resistance, and moderate hyperglycemia (12). More recently, insulin-resistant mice have been generated through the targeted disruption of genes for proteins such as the insulin receptor, IRS-1 and -2, and Glut 4 (15,71–73). Although crossing LDLR–/– or apo-E–/– mice with these insulin-resistant or diabetes-prone mice would be a very useful approach, such mice are not currently available. The use of "Western" diets in some of these genetic models of insulin resistance and diabetes may accomplish similar goals, however. For example, feeding the db/db mouse a high-fat, high-cholesterol diet led to marked increases in cholesterol-containing particles in the size range of LDL (74). Although increases in large LDL particles occurred on this diet, these animals also retained their small LDL particles, a lipoprotein pattern found in human diabetes. However, these murine models still suffer from the lack of typical human levels of lipoprotein lipase and CETP. Moreover, variation in the age of onset and extent of hyperglycemia that results can be problematic in models with an inherited predisposition to develop diabetes.

Alternatively, diabetes may be achieved by injecting STZ in a hyperlipidemic, atherosclerosis-susceptible murine model (5). For this approach, the LDLR–/– mouse is a particularly attractive model. The pancreas of this mouse is readily susceptible to the toxic effects of STZ. Furthermore, the level of hypercholesterolemia in the LDLR–/– is easily altered by changes in the dietary fat and cholesterol content. This allows one to match the cholesterol levels of experimental groups and thus to determine potential atherogenic effects of diabetes independent of the modulation of cholesterol levels. In studies of type 1 diabetes by Reaven and colleagues, hyperglycemia was achieved in LDLR–/– mice by intraperitoneal injection of STZ (5). Providing small amounts of slow-release insulin moderated the extent of hyperglycemia. Insulin therapy also prevented the extreme hypertriglyceridemia and excess mortality frequently seen in other models of diabetes. Lipid profiles of diabetic mice were similar to those of poorly controlled diabetic patients, with increased VLDL levels and slightly reduced HDL levels (Fig. 4). Immunocytochemistry of lesions with an antiserum to model AGE epitopes, such as FFI-lysine, also demonstrated strikingly more staining in tissue of diabetic animals (Fig. 5A) than in nondiabetic controls (Fig. 5B). However, despite the presence of hyperglycemia, diabetic dyslipidemia, and enhanced formation of AGE in the vessel wall, diabetic mice did not show enhanced aortic atherosclerosis. Similar results were obtained in a study of mice overexpressing human apo-B that developed marked hypercholesterolemia while on an atherogenic diet (67). Effects on lipids, lipoproteins, and fatty streak formation were compared between a small number of these mice made severely hyperglycemic with STZ and their nondiabetic counterparts. Despite the tendency toward higher cholesterol levels (distributed in particles of VLDL and LDL size) in the male diabetic mice, no

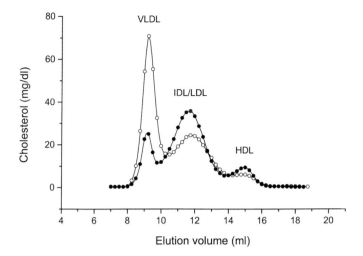

Fig. 4. Mean cholesterol content in lipoprotein fractions (mg/dL) in diabetic (○) and control (●) mice. Fast performance liquid chromatography was performed on plasma samples of mice using a Superose 6B column, and cholesterol content in each 250 mL fraction of eluate was determined. Lipoprotein peak identification was based on elution of standard mouse lipoprotein fractions isolated by density gradient ultracentrifugation. (Reprinted with permission from ref. *5a*.)

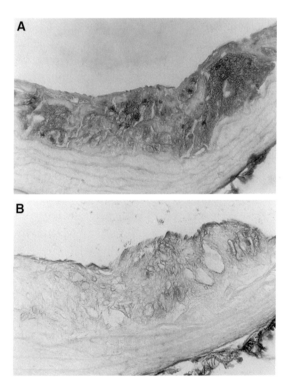

Fig. 5. Immunocytochemistry of atherosclerotic lesions from diabetic and control LDLR-/- mice with an antiserum to an AGE epitope. Aortic sections were obtained from diabetic and control mice with similar overall extent of atherosclerosis. Sections were then immunostained under identical conditions with FLI, a guinea-pig antiserum binding to FFI-lysine epitopes. As shown here, staining for this model epitope of AGE was strikingly more intense in lesions from diabetic animals (**A**) than in similar stage lesions of control mice (**B**). (Reprinted with permission from ref. *5a*.)

differences in fatty streak formation were detected. Moreover, diabetic female mice developed less atherosclerosis than their nondiabetic controls. Although the results from these two studies suggest a limited role for hyperglycemia and AGE formation in atherogenesis in these mice, it remains to be determined whether the effects of diabetes were overshadowed by the marked hypercholesterolemia (>1000 mg/dL) that developed during these experiments.

This latter concept was to a certain extent supported by results in a study using BALB/c mice in which plasma cholesterol levels were only modestly elevated (290 mg/dL) *(6)*. The investigators noted increased lesion formation in the aortic origin of mildly hypercholesterolemic diabetic BALB/c mice. However, in the same study, C57BL/6 mice with diabetes had similar levels of moderate hypercholesterolemia as their nondiabetic controls, yet did not have enhanced levels of fatty streak formation. This suggests that there may also be differences in the susceptibility to pro-atherogenic effects of diabetes between murine strains. Of importance, these initial mixed results regarding the importance of glycemia in animal models of atherosclerosis reflect the results to date in human studies. To further address this important question, several of the more recently described animal models of atherosclerosis have been studied in the setting of diabetes. To test whether the high levels of HDL typically present in murine models might overshadow the effects of hyperglycemia, Goldberg et al. compared the extent of atherosclerosis at 23 weeks in diabetic and nondiabetic combined LDLR–/– and apo-AI-deficient mice. Mice were made diabetic with STZ and both groups of mice were fed a high-cholesterol but low-fat diet. Although STZ-injected mice were markedly hyperglycemic (averaging 19.4 ± 6.5 mmol/L) and had similarly elevated levels of lipoproteins as the nondiabetic mice, measures of atherosclerosis were identical between the two groups *(64)*. In a separate study, several of these same investigators evaluated the effect of STZ-induced diabetes on atherosclerosis in the combined mutation model (described above) that consists of overexpression of human apo-B and CETP and a heterozygous deficiency in LPL. As noted above, these animals have moderate elevations in plasma TC (300–325 mg/dL on high-fat diets), increased VLDL and decreased HDL cholesterol, a pattern of dyslipidemia that is quite similar to that present in human type 2 diabetes. Fortunately, the levels of plasma lipids did not change with the onset of diabetes, thus allowing the investigators to specifically compare the effects of elevated levels of glucose on atherosclerosis. Despite glucose levels that were nearly twice as high in the diabetic mice, there were no differences in the extent of atherosclerosis between the diabetic and nondiabetic mice *(44)*. Although average plasma cholesterol levels were correlated with extent of atherosclerosis, average levels of glucose were not. Importantly, cholesterol levels were only moderately elevated in this model, making it unlikely that the pro-atherogenic effects of very high-cholesterol or triglyceride levels, as commonly occurs in apo-E–/– and LDLR–/– murine models, would overshadow the effects of hyperglycemia. Thus, in animal models of type 1 diabetes to date, there is little evidence that hyperglycemia by itself may substantially accelerate the development of atherosclerosis. The fact that infusion soluble receptors of advanced glycation end-products (sRAGE) has inhibited lesion formation in diabetic mice in several studies does not contradict this conclusion as it has subsequently been shown that sRAGE may have many direct and indirect anti-inflammatory effects, and may reduce atherosclerosis even in nondiabetic mice *(75)*.

Ideally, an animal model of type 1 diabetes and atherogenesis would not only reflect as closely as possible lipoprotein metabolism and atherogenesis of humans, but also the autoimmune mechanisms causing insulin deficiency. One possible approach would be to utilize a transgenic mouse that expresses a viral glycoprotein under control of the rat insulin promoter *(76,77)*. In these mice, infection with lymphocytic choriomeningitis virus triggers an immune response that destroys the pancreatic beta cells expressing the viral glycoprotein, and thus causes insulin deficiency and type I diabetes. These mice can be crossed into a model of atherosclerosis, such as the LDLR–/– mouse. A very recent study using this approach indicated that diabetes was sufficient to accelerate intimal macrophage accumulation and formation of early lesions *(78)*. However, in mice fed a hypercholesterolemic diet, diabetes did not increase the extent of advanced artherosclerosis, compared to nondiabetic mice with similar cholesterol levels *(78)*.

There have been fewer attempts to develop a murine model of type 2 diabetes and atherosclerosis. In a preliminary study from our laboratory, LDLR–/– mice were initially fed high-fat Western diets to induce insulin resistance, resulting in compensatory hyperinsulinemia and hyperlipidemia. They were then injected with low doses of STZ to modestly reduce pancreatic release of insulin. This normalized insulin levels and induced marked hyperglycemia. Because of the normal plasma insulin levels, these mice avoided progressive hyperglycemia, dehydration, and ketosis. Their long-term survival and general health were quite good and they did not appear to require more monitoring or care than do standard LDLR–/– mice. This model will likely prove useful for future investigations into the mechanisms of enhanced atherosclerosis in type 2 diabetes.

We also generated a model of insulin resistance in LDLR–/– mice *(79)*. Feeding a fructose-rich diet to LDLR–/– mice resulted in marked hypercholesterolemia, but in contrast to its effects in rats, failed to induce insulin resistance. Surprisingly, the fructose diet also enhanced atherosclerosis, compared to mice in which similar cholesterol levels had been induced by a Western diet. This may have been related in part to a fructose-induced increase in blood pressure. More importantly, the same study showed that the fat enriched Western diet not only induced hypercholesterolemia, but also insulin resistance and marked hyperinsulinemia in mice. This is consistent with earlier reports suggesting that high-fat diets may lead to insulin resistance in some rodent models *(80)*. Nevertheless, this is of considerable importance because the presence of insulin resistance in LDLR–/– mice fed standard Western diets may complicate the interpretation of many atherosclerosis studies using such diets.

A different approach was more recently tried by Lyngdorf and associates who injected apo-E–/– mice with gold thioglucose *(81)*. A single injection of this compound effectively destroys the satiety center and leads to extensive overeating, weight gain, hypertriglyceridemia, hyperinsulinemia, and hyperglycemia; a complex of metabolic abnormalities characteristic of type 2 diabetes. Levels of plasma lipids and lipoproteins were equal or higher in the mice injected with gold thioglucose and both glucose and insulin levels were higher in these mice. Surprisingly, despite these multiple metabolic abnormalities, mice injected with gold thioglucose developed less atherosclerosis after 4 months than did the control mice.

USE OF MURINE MODELS OF ATHEROSCLEROSIS TO TEST THE ANTI-ATHEROSCLEROTIC EFFECTS OF THIAZOLIDINEDIONES

Several recent studies have taken advantage of the above described models of insulin resistance and diabetes to determine whether peroxisome proliferator-activated receptor (PPAR)γ ligands may reduce fatty streak formation and whether this occurs through improvements in insulin resistance, hyperglycemia, or through direct anti-atherogenic activity in the vascular wall. These questions are of great clinical importance because patients with type 2 diabetes, who are at great risk of developing macrovascular disease, are taking these agents with increasing frequency to improve glycemic control.

Li and associates *(82)* fed high-fat diets with or without two structurally different PPARγ ligands (rosiglitazone or GW7845) to LDLR–/– mice and demonstrated that both PPARγ-specific agonists strongly inhibited atherosclerosis in male, but not female, mice. The anti-atherogenic effect in male mice was associated with improved insulin sensitivity and decreased aortic tissue expression of two proinflammatory factors, tumor necrosis factor (TNF)-α and gelatinase B. In contrast, female mice demonstrated less hyperinsulinemia on the high-fat diet, yet developed a similar degree of atherosclerosis. Female mice also demonstrated little if any change in insulin levels or expression of TNF-α and gelatinase B following PPARγ agonist treatment. These findings confirm that PPARγ-specific agonists may exert anti-atherogenic effects in animals that are presumably insulin-resistant; but do not demonstrate that reducing or preventing this condition *per se* is sufficient to inhibit development of atherosclerosis.

In a second study, hypercholesterolemia, hyperinsulinemia, and fasting hyperglycemia were induced by diets enriched in fructose or fat, respectively *(83)*. Interestingly, male LDLR–/– mice fed the fructose diet, which did not induce insulin resistance, developed significantly greater atherosclerosis than male mice receiving the high-fat diet. Troglitazone therapy decreased atherosclerosis in both groups of LDLR–/– mice, suggesting that it may have anti-atherogenic effects independent of its effects on insulin resistance. Chen and colleagues also showed that troglitazone reduces atherosclerosis in apo E–/– mice, demonstrating that the anti-atherogenic effect of these medications are not murine strain-specific *(84)*. Although insulin levels were reduced in the troglitazone-treated mice, there was no clear relationship between these changes and the extent of lesion formation. A more recent study by Levi and associates indicates that rosiglitazone reduces atherosclerosis significantly and equally in both diabetic and nondiabetic apo-E–/– mice, despite having no glucose-lowering effects *(85)*. As apo-E–/– mice in general have shown little tendency to develop insulin resistance and mice from this latter study were not provided a high-fat "Western" diet that might increase weight and insulin resistance, rosiglitazone-induced improvements in insulin sensitivity were also unlikely to explain the reported attenuation of atherosclerosis. These reports demonstrate that thiazolidinediones as a class consistently reduce atherosclerosis in animal models of insulin resistance and diabetes and even in animals with relatively normal glucose tolerance.

These effects are consistent with the results from the few short-term trials conducted to date in humans with diabetes *(86,87)*. However, their benefits in animal models cannot be directly linked to improvements in hyperglycemia or insulin resistance and thus they do not necessarily support a direct role for these abnormalities, independent of other metabolic alterations commonly associated with insulin resistance, in fatty streak formation. In fact, there is increasing evidence that reduced atherosclerosis in animal models treated with thiazolidinediones may be due, at least in part, to their anti-inflammatory effects *(82,88)*, to increased reverse cholesterol transport resulting from activation of the LXR/ABC-A1 pathway *(89)* and/or to other effects not yet identified. Down-regulation of inflammatory cytokines that control the intimal recruitment and secretory activity of monocytes and T cells, including interferon-α, interleukin (IL)-

1β, IL-6, TNFα, and chemokine receptor-CCR2 was indeed observed in cell cultures or in vivo *(82,90–92)*, but appears to be a common property of other classes of PPARs, such as PPARα and PPARβ/δ, some of which do not reduce atherogenesis in mice *(93)*. In particular, murine studies of PPARα yielded conflicting results. A study of PPARα-deficient apo-E–/– mice indicated a pro-atherogenic effect of PPARα *(94)*. However, the PPARα ligand fenofibrate exerted anti-atherogenic effects in apo-E–/– mice and apo-E–/– x human apo-AI mice *(95,96)*. We also saw a strong antiatherogenic effect in LDLR–/– mice treated with PPARα agonist, but in in PPARβ/δ agonist-treated mice that showed similar downregulation of inflammatory cytokines *(93)*. Furthermore, PPARs also upregulate the expression of the scavenger receptor, CD36, which is thought to be pro-atherogenic.

It will be a formidable challenge to determine which of these conflicting PPAR effects is/are actually responsible for the reduction of atherogenesis in mice, much less in humans. Similarly, the reasons for the gender differences in PPAR-treated mice remain unexplained, and it is not clear whether similar differences exist in humans.

CONCLUSIONS

As outlined above, a variety of animal models have been used to study the atherogenic effects of insulin resistance and diabetes. However, each model has its limitations. Compared to other animal models, lipoprotein metabolism and lesion morphology in nonhuman primates are the most similar to those in man. However, practical considerations severely reduce the usefulness of this model. In contrast, mice have become a valuable research tool for the study of diabetes and atherosclerosis because of their low cost and relative ease of genetic manipulation. In particular, atherogenesis in hypercholesterolemic LDLR–/– and apo-E–/– mice appears to more closely reflect many aspects of the atherogenic process in man. Initial studies in these mice have suggested that the relationships of insulin resistance and diabetes to atherosclerosis may be more complex than initially imagined, but have demonstrated that insulin resistance, type 1 and type 2 diabetes can be induced in these mice strains. However, to date, these studies have demonstrated that whereas diabetes associated dyslipidemia appears directly related to enhanced atherosclerosis, there is less evidence that hyperglycemia per se plays a major role in atherogenesis. Similar conclusions can be drawn from the results of studies using other animal models of diabetes and atherosclerosis. For example, the lipoprotein profile in the genetically modified mice that demonstrate overproduction of apo-B, expression of CETP and reduction of lipoprotein lipase is relatively similar to that in humans and thus this model appears particularly appropriate for studies of the mechanisms by which insulin resistance and diabetes may modulate atherogenesis. Yet, in this model as well, induction of hyperglycemia did not further accelerate atherosclerosis. It should be pointed out that these results are in fact consistent with studies in humans to date. In fact, the failure to clearly establish glucose as an important pathogenic factor in atherosclerosis in previous studies has led to the initiation of two multicenter center studies, the Action to Control Cardiovascular Risk in Diabetes and the Veterans Affairs Study of Glycemic Control and Complications in Type 2 Diabetes, that are specifically testing whether improvements in glycemic control alone in type 2 diabetes will be sufficient to reduce incident macrovascular disease events. Thus, the difficulty in establishing glycemia as an independent risk factor for atherosclerosis in animal models of diabetes suggests they may in fact correctly reflect the true complexity of atherogenesis and the relatively modest role that hyperglycemia may play in early lesion formation.

Although final conclusions regarding the value of PPARγ agonists in inhibition of atherogenesis in humans awaits results from several ongoing studies, murine models have proven invaluable in helping demonstrate their potential as anti-atherogenic agents and in elucidating their mechanisms of action.

ACKNOWLEDGMENTS

This review was supported by the office of Research and Development Medical Research Service, Department of Veterans Affairs, and NHLBI grant HL56989 (La Jolla Specialized Center of Research in Molecular Medicine and Atherosclerosis).

REFERENCES

1. Pyorälä K, Laakso M, Uusitupa M. Diabetes and atherosclerosis: an epidemiologic view. Diabetes Metab Rev 1987;3:463–524.
2. Uusitupa MI, Niskanen LK, Siitonen O, Voutilainen E, Pyorala K. Ten-year cardiovascular mortality in relation to risk factors and abnormalities in lipoprotein composition in type 2 (non- insulin-dependent) diabetic and non-diabetic subjects. Diabetologia 1993;36:1175–1184.
3. Prospective Diabetes Study (UKPDS) Group. Intensive blood-glucose control with sulphonylureas or insulin compared with conventional treatment and risk of complications in patients with type 2 diabetes (UKPDS 33). Lancet 1998;352:837–853.
4. Semenkovich CF, Heinecke JW. The mystery of diabetes and atherosclerosis: Time for a new plot. Diabetes 1997;46:327–334.
5. Reaven P, Merat S, Casanada F, Sutphin M, Palinski W. Effect of streptozotocin-induced hyperglycemia on lipid profiles, formation of advanced glycation endproducts in lesions, and extent of atherosclerosis in LDL receptor-deficient mice. Arterioscler Thromb Vasc Biol 1997;17:2250–2256.
5a. Johnstone MT, Veves A. (Eds.) Diabetes and Cardiovascular disease. Humana Press, Totowa, NJ:2001.
6. Kunjathoor VV, Wilson DL, LeBoeuf RC. Increased atherosclerosis in streptozotocin-induced diabetic mice. J Clin Invest 1996;97:1–8.
7. Uusitupa MI, Niskanen LK, Siitonen O, Voutilainen E, Pyorala K. 5-year incidence of atherosclerotic vascular disease in relation to general risk factors, insulin level, and abnormalities in lipoprotein composition in non-insulin-dependent diabetic and nondiabetic subjects. Circulation 1990;82:27–36.
8. Bierman EL. George Lyman Duff Memorial Lecture. Atherogenesis in diabetes. Arterioscler Thromb 1992;12:647–656.
9. Hayden JM, Reaven PD. Cardiovascular disease in diabetes mellitus type 2: a potential role for novel cardiovascular risk factors. Curr Opin Lipidol 2000;11:519–28.
10. Tobey TA, Mondon CE, Zavaroni I, Reaven GM. Mechanism of insulin resistance in fructose-fed rats. Metabolism 1982;31:608–612.
11. Hwang IS, Ho H, Hoffman BB, Reaven GM. Fructose-induced insulin resistance and hypertension in rats. Hypertension 1987;10:512–516.
12. Leibel RL, Chung WK, Streamson C, Chua J. The molecular genetics of rodent single gene obesities. J Biol Chem 1997;272:31,937–31,940.
13. Leibel RL. Single gene obesities in rodents: possible relevance to human obesity. J Nutr 1997;127: 1908S.
14. Tamemoto H, Kadowaki T, Tobe K, et al. Insulin resistance and growth retardation in mice lacking insulin receptor substrate-1. Nature 1994;372:182–186.
15. Araki E, Lipes MA, Patti ME, et al. Alternative pathway of insulin signalling in mice with targeted disruption of the IRS-1 gene. Nature 1994;372:186–190.
16. Kubota T, Kubota N, Moroi M, et al. Lack of insulin receptor substrate-2 causes progressive neointima formation in response to vessel injury. Circulation 2003;107:3073–80.
17. Armstrong ML, Trillo A, Pritchard RW. Naturally occurring and experimentally induced atherosclerosis in nonhuman primates. In: Kalter SS, (ed). The Use of Nonhuman Primates in Cardiovascular Disease. Austin, TX: University of Texas Press; 1979, pp. 58–101.
18. Clarkson TB, Koritnik DR, Weingand KW, Miller LC. Nonhuman primate models of atherosclerosis: potential for the study of diabetes mellitus and hyperinsulinemia. Metabolism 1985;34:51–59.

19. Wagner WD, St.Clair RW, Clarkson TB. Angiochemical and tissue cholesterol changes in Macaca fascicularis fed an atherogenic diet for three years. Exp Mol Pathol 1978;28:140–153.

20. Lehner ND, Clarkson TB, Lofland HB. The effect of insulin deficiency, hypothyroidism, and hypertension on artherosclerosis in the squirrel monkey. Exp Mol Pathol 1971;15(2):230–244.

21. Bagdade JD, Wagner JD, Rudel LL, Clarkson TB. Accelerated cholesteryl ester transfer and altered lipoprotein composition in diabetic cynomolgus monkeys. J Lipid Res 1995;36:759–766.

22. Wagner JD, Bagdade JD, Litwak KN, et al. Increased glycation of plasma lipoproteins in diabetic cynomolgus monkeys. Lab Anim Sci 1996;46:31–35.

23. Tsutsumi K, Iwamoto T, Hagi A, Kohri H.Streptozotocin-induced diabetic cynomologus monkey is a model of hypertriglyceridemia with low high density lipoprotein cholesterol. Biol Pharm Bul 1998;21: 693–697.

24. Litwak KN, Cefalu WT, Wagner JD. Chronic hyperglycemia increases arterial low-density lipoprotein metabolism and atherosclerosis in cynomolgus monkeys. Metabolism 1998;47:947–954.

25. Finking G, Hanke H. Nikolaj Nikolajewitsch Anitschkow (1885–1964) established the cholesterol-fed rabbit as a model for atherosclerosis research. Atherosclerosis 1997;135:1–7.

26. Nordestgaard BG, Stender S, Kjeldsen K. Reduced atherogenesis in cholesterol-fed diabetic rabbits. Giant lipoproteins do not enter the arterial wall. Arteriosclerosis 1998;8:421–428.

27. Nordestgaard BG, Wootton R, Lewis B. Selective retention of VLDL, IDL, and LDL in the arterial intima of genetically hyperlipidemic rabbits in vivo. Molecular size as a determinant of fractional loss from the intima-inner media. Arterioscler Thromb Vasc Biol 1995;15:534–542.

28. Nordestgaard BG, Zilversmit DB. Comparison of arterial intimal clearances of LDL from diabetic and nondiabetic cholesterol-fed rabbits. Differences in intimal clearance explained by size differences. Arteriosclerosis 1989;9:176–183.

29. Schmidt AM, Hori O, Chen JX, et al. Advanced glycation endproducts interacting with their endothelial receptor induce expression of vascular cell adhesion molecule-1 (VCAM-1) in cultured human endothelial cells and in mice. A potential mechanism for the accelerated vasculopathy of diabetes. J Clin Invest 1995;96:1395–1403.

30. Vlassara H, Fuh H, Donnelly T, Cybulsky M. Advanced Glycation Endproducts Promote Adhesion Molecule (VCAM-1,ICAM-1) Expression and Atheroma Formation in Normal Rabbits. Molecular Medicine 1995;1:447–456.

31. Simionescu M, Popov D, Sima A, et al. Pathobiochemistry of combined diabetes and atherosclerosis studied on a novel animal model. The hyperlipemic-hyperglycemic hamster. Am J Pathol 1996;148: 997–1014.

32. Sima A, Popov D, Starodub O, et al. Pathobiology of the heart in experimental diabetes: immunolocalization of lipoproteins, immunoglobulin G, and advanced glycation endproducts proteins in diabetic and/or hyperlipidemic hamster. Lab Invest 1997;77:3–18.

33. Mathe D. Dyslipidemia and diabetes: animal models. Diabete Metab 1995;21:106–111.

34. Richardson M, Schmidt AM, Graham SE, et al. Vasculopathy and insulin resistance in the JCR:LA-cp rat. Atherosclerosis 1998;138:135–146.

35. Russell JC, Amy RM. Early atherosclerotic lesions in a susceptible rat model. The LA/N-corpulent rat. Atherosclerosis 1986;60:119–129.

36. Schneider DJ, Absher PM, Neimane D, Russell JC, Sobel BE. Fibrinolysis and atherogenesis in the JCR:LA-cp rat in relation to insulin and triglyceride concentrations in blood. Diabetologia 1998;41: 141–147.

37. Ziv E, Kalman R, Hershkop K, Barash V, Shafrir E, Bar-on H. Insulin resistance in the NIDDM model Psammomys obesus in the normoglycaemic, normoinsulinaemic state. Diabetologia 1996;39:1269–1275.

38. Hilzenrat N, Sikuler E, Yaari A, Maislos M. Hemodynamic characterization of the diabetic Psammomys obesus—an animal model of type II diabetes mellitus. Isr J Med Sci 1996;32:1074–1078.

39. Kanety H, Moshe S, Shafrir E, Lunenfeld B, Karasik A. Hyperinsulinemia induces a reversible impairment in insulin receptor function leading to diabetes in the sand rat model of non-insulin-dependent diabetes mellitus. Proc Natl Acad Sci USA 1994;91:1853–1857.

40. Yudkin JS, Kumari M, Humphries SE, Mohamed-Ali V. Inflammation, obesity, stress and coronary heart disease: is interleukin-6 the link? Atherosclerosis 2000;148:209–214.

41. Shoelson SE, Lee J, Yuan M. Inflammation and the IKK beta/I kappa B/NF-kappa B axis in obesity- and diet-induced insulin resistance. Int J Obes Relat Metab Disord 2003;27(Suppl 3):S49–S52.

42. Paigen B, Mitchell D, Reue K, Morrow A, Lusis AJ, LeBoeuf RC. Ath-1, a gene determining atherosclerosis susceptibility and high density lipoprotein levels in mice. Proc Natl Acad Sci USA 1987;84: 3763–3767.

43. Paigen B, Ishida BY, Verstuyft J, Winters RB, Albee D. Atherosclerosis susceptibility differences among progenitors of recombinant inbred strains of mice. Arteriosclerosis 1990;10:316–323.

44. Kako Y, Masse M, Huang LS, Tall AR, Goldberg IJ. Lipoprotein lipase deficiency and CETP in streptozotocin-treated apoB-expressing mice. J Lipid Res 2002;43:872–7.

45. Palinski W, Napoli C, Reaven PD. Mouse models of atherosclerosis. In: Simons DI, Rogers C, eds. Vascular Disease and Injury: Preclinical Research. Humana Press, Inc., Totowa, NJ, 1999.

46. Plump AS, Smith JD, Hayek T, et al. Severe hypercholesterolemia and atherosclerosis in apolipoprotein E-deficient mice created by homologous recombination in ES cells. Cell 1992;71:343–353.

47. Zhang SH, Reddick RL, Piedrahita JA, Maeda N. Spontaneous hypercholesterolemia and arterial lesions in mice lacking apolipoprotein E. Science 1992;258:468–471.

48. Ishibashi S, Goldstein JL, Brown MS, Herz J, Burns DK. Massive xanthomatosis and atherosclerosis in cholesterol-fed low density lipoprotein receptor-negative mice. Clin Invest 1994;93:1885–1893.

49. Palinski W, Tangirala RK, Miller E, Young SG, Witztum JL. Increased autoantibody titers against epitopes of oxidized LDL in LDL receptor-deficient mice with increased atherosclerosis. Arterioscler Thromb Vasc Biol 1995;15:1569–1576.

50. Tangirala RK, Rubin EM, Palinski W. Quantitation of atherosclerosis in murine models: correlation between lesions in the aortic origin and in the entire aorta, and differences in the extent of lesions between sexes in LDL receptor-deficient and apolipoprotein E-deficient mice. J Lipid Res 1995;36:2320–2328.

51. Palinski W, Tangirala RK, Miller E, Young SG, Witztum JL. Increased autoantibody titers against epitopes of oxidized LDL in LDL receptor-deficient mice with increased atherosclerosis. Arterioscler Thromb Vasc Biol 1995;15:1569–1576.

52. Nakashima Y, Plump AS, Raines EW, Breslow JL, Ross R. ApoE-deficient mice develop lesions of all phases of atherosclerosis throughout the arterial tree. Arterioscler Thromb 1994;14:133–140.

53. Palinski W, Ord VA, Plump AS, Breslow JL, Steinberg D, Witztum JL. ApoE-deficient mice are a model of lipoprotein oxidation in atherogenesis. Demonstration of oxidation-specific epitopes in lesions and high titers of autoantibodies to malondialdehyde-lysine in serum. Arterioscler Thromb 1994;14:605–616.

54. Braun A, Trigatti BL, Post MJ, et al. Loss of SR-BI expression leads to the early onset of occlusive atherosclerotic coronary artery disease, spontaneous myocardial infarctions, severe cardiac dysfunction, and premature death in apolipoprotein E-deficient mice. Circ Res 2002;90:270–276.

55. Palinski W, Napoli C. Unraveling pleiotropic effects of statins on plaque rupture. Arterioscler Thromb Vasc Biol 2002;22:1745–1750.

56. Cullen P, Baetta R, Bellosta S, et al. Rupture of the atherosclerotic plaque: does a good animal model exist? Arterioscler Thromb Vasc Biol 2003;23:535–542.

57. Calara F, Silvestre M, Casanada F, Yuan N, Napoli C, Palinski W. Spontaneous plaque rupture and secondary thrombosis in apolipoprotein E-deficient and LDL receptor-deficient mice. J Pathol 2001;195:257–263.

58. Zhou X, Stemme S, Hansson GK. Evidence for a local immune response in atherosclerosis. CD4+ T cells infiltrate lesions of apolipoprotein-E-deficient mice. Am J Pathol 1996;149:359–366.

59. Palinski W, Rosenfeld ME, Yla-Herttuala S, et al. Low density lipoprotein undergoes oxidative modification in vivo. Proc Natl Acad Sci USA 1989;86:1372–1376.

60. Steinberg D. Low density lipoprotein oxidation and its pathobiological significance. J Biol Chem 1997;272:20,963–20,966.

61. Palinski W, Koschinsky T, Butler SW, et al. Immunological evidence for the presence of advanced glycosylation end products in atherosclerotic lesions of euglycemic rabbits. Arterioscler Thromb Vasc Biol 1995;15:571–582.

62. Paigen B, Morrow A, Holmes PA, Mitchell D, Williams RA. Quantitative assessment of atherosclerotic lesions in mice. Atherosclerosis 1987;68:231–240.

63. Gaw A, Hobbs HH. Molecular genetics of lipoprotein (a): new pieces to the puzzle. Curr Opin Lipidol 1994;5:149–155.

64. Goldberg IJ, Isaacs A, Sehayek E, Breslow JL, Huang LS. Effects of streptozotocin-induced diabetes in apolipoprotein AI deficient mice. Atherosclerosis 2004;172:47–53.

65. Purcell-Huynh D, Farese R, Johnson D, et al. Transgenic mice expressing high levels of human apolipoprotein B develop severe atherosclerotic lesions in response to a high-fat diet. J Clin Invest 1995;95:2246–2257.

66. Callow M, Verstuyft J, Tangirala RK, Palinski W, Rubin E. Atherogenesis in transgenic mice with human apolipoprotein B and lipoprotein (a). J Clin Invest 1995;96:1639–1646.

67. Kako Y, Huang L, Yang J, Katopodis T, Ramakrishnan R, Goldberg I. Streptozotocin-induced diabetes in human apolipoprotein B transgenic mice: effects on lipoproteins and atherosclerosis. Lipid Res 1999; 40:2185–2194.

68. Young SG. Using genetically modified mice to study apolipoprotein B. J Arterioscler Thromb 1996;3: 62–74.

69. Chiesa G, Parolini C, Canavesi M, et al. Human apolipoproteins A-I and A-II in cell cholesterol efflux: studies with transgenic mice. Arterioscler Thromb Vasc Biol 1998;18:1417–1423.

70. Nishina PM, Naggert JK, Verstuyft J, Paigen B. Athersclerosis in genetically obese mice: The mutants obese, diabetes, fat, tubby, and lethal yellow. Metabolism 1994;43:554–558.

71. Abe H, Yamada N, Kamata K, et al. Hypertension, hypertriglyceridemia, and impaired endothelium-dependent vascular relaxation in mice lacking insulin receptor substrate-1. J Clin Invest 1998;101:1784–1788.

72. Bruning JC, Winnay J, Bonner-Weir S, Taylor SI, Accili D, Kahn CR. Development of a novel polygenic model of NIDDM in mice heterozygous for IR and IRS-1 null alleles. Cell 1997;88:561–572.

73. Kadowaki T. Insights into insulin resistance and type 2 diabetes from knockout mouse models. J Clin Invest 2000;106:459–65.

74. Kobayashi K, Forte TM, Taniguchi S, Ishida BY, Oka K, Chan L. The db/db mouse, a model for diabetic dyslipidemia: molecular characterization and effects of Western diet feeding. Metabolism 2000;49:22–31.

75. Bucciarelli LG, Wendt T, Qu W, et al. RAGE blockade stabilizes established atherosclerosis in diabetic apolipoprotein E-null mice. Circulation 2002;106:2827–35.

76. Ohashi PS, Oehen S, Buerki K, et al. Ablation of "tolerance" and induction of diabetes by virus infection in viral antigen transgenic mice. Cell 1991;65:305–17.

77. Oldstone MB, Nerenberg M, Southern P, Price J, Lewicki H. Virus infection triggers insulin-dependent diabetes mellitus in a transgenic model: role of anti-self (virus) immune response. Cell 1991;65:319–31.

78. Renard CB, Kramer F, Johansson F, et al. Diabetes and diabetes-associated lipid abnormalities have distinct effects on initiation and progression of atherosclerotic lesions. J Clin Invest 2004;114:659–668.

79. Merat S, Casanada F, Sutphin M, Palinski W, Reaven P. Western-type diets induce insulin resistance and hyperinsulinemia in LDL receptor-deficient mice but do not increase aortic atherosclerosis, compared with normoinsulinemic mice in which similar plasma cholesterol levels are achieved by a fructose-rich diet. Arterioscler Thromb Vasc Biol 1999;19:1223–1230.

80. Surwit RS, Wang S, Petro AE, et al. Diet-induced changes in uncoupling proteins in obesity-prone and obesity-resistant strains of mice. Proc Natl Acad Sci USA 1998;95:4061–4065.

81. Lyngdorf LG, Gregersen S, Daugherty A, Falk E. Paradoxical reduction of atherosclerosis in apoE-deficient mice with obesity-related type 2 diabetes. Cardiovasc Res 2003;59:854–862.

82. Li AC, Brown KK, Silvestre MJ, Willson TM, Palinski W, Glass CK. Peroxisome proliferator-activated receptor gamma ligands inhibit development of atherosclerosis in LDL receptor-deficient mice. J Clin Invest 2000;106:523–531.

83. Collins AR, Meehan WP, Kintscher U, et al. Troglitazone inhibits formation of early atherosclerotic lesions in diabetic and nondiabetic low density lipoprotein receptor-deficient mice. Arterioscler Thromb Vasc Biol 2001;21:365–371.

84. Chen Z, Ishibashi S, Perrey S, et al. Troglitazone inhibits atherosclerosis in apolipoprotein E-knockout mice: pleiotropic effects on CD36 expression and HDL. Arterioscler Thromb Vasc Biol 2001;21:372–377.

85. Levi Z, Shaish A, Yacov N, et al. Rosiglitazone (PPARgamma-agonist) attenuates atherogenesis with no effect on hyperglycaemia in a combined diabetes-atherosclerosis mouse model. Diabetes Obes Metab 2003;5:45–50.

86. Minamikawa J, Tanaka S, Yamauchi M, Inoue D, Koshiyama H. Potent inhibitory effect of troglitazone on carotid arterial wall thickness in type 2 diabetes. J Clin Endocrinol Metab 1998;83:1818–1820.

87. Koshiyama H, Shimono D, Kuwamura N, Minamikawa J, Nakamura Y. Rapid communication: inhibitory effect of pioglitazone on carotid arterial wall thickness in type 2 diabetes. J Clin Endocrinol Metab 2001;86:3452–3456.

88. Hsueh WA, Bruemmer D. Peroxisome proliferator-activated receptor gamma: implications for cardiovascular disease. Hypertension 2004;43:297–305.

89. Chawla A, Boisvert WA, Lee CH, et al. A PPAR gamma-LXR-ABCA1 pathway in macrophages is involved in cholesterol efflux and atherogenesis. Mol Cell 2001;7:161–171.

90. Pasceri V, Wu HD, Willerson JT, Yeh ET. Modulation of vascular inflammation in vitro and in vivo by peroxisome proliferator-activated receptor-gamm activators. Circulation 2000;101:235–238.

91. Han KH, Chang MK, Boullier A, et al. Oxidized LDL reduces monocyte CCR2 expression through pathways involving peroxisome proliferator-activated receptor gamma. J Clin Invest 2000;106:793–802.
92. Marx N, Kehrle B, Kohlhammer K, et al. PPAR activators as antiinflammatory mediators in human T lymphocytes: implications for atherosclerosis and transplantation-associated arteriosclerosis. Circ Res 2002;90:703–710.
93. Li AC, Binder CJ, Gutierrez A, et al. Differential inhibition of macrophage foam-cell formation and atherosclerosis in mice by PPARalpha, beta/delta, and gamma. J Clin Invest 2004;114:1564–1576.
94. Tordjman K, Bernal-Mizrachi C, Zemany L, et al. PPARalpha deficiency reduces insulin resistance and atherosclerosis in apoE-null mice. J Clin Invest 2001;107:1025–34.
95. Duez H, Chao YS, Hernandez M, et al. Reduction of atherosclerosis by the peroxisome proliferator-activated receptor alpha agonist fenofibrate in mice. J Biol Chem 2002;277:48051–48057.
96. Claudel T, Leibowitz MD, Fievet C, et al. Reduction of atherosclerosis in apolipoprotein E knockout mice by activation of the retinoid X receptor. Proc Natl Acad Sci USA 2001;98:2610–2615.

II CLINICAL

A. Risk Factors

13 The Metabolic Syndrome and Vascular Disease

S. J. Creely, MD, Aresh J. Anwar, MD, MRCP, and Sudhesh Kumar, MD, FRCP

INTRODUCTION

The concept of the metabolic syndrome is perhaps the most significant development in the management of cardiovascular disease (CVD) in the last 15 years. Prior to this, physicians often treated diabetes, hypertension, or dyslipidaemia as separate diseases and did not really consider the impact of treatment of one of these conditions on the other co-existing conditions. Avogaro first described the syndrome more than 40 years ago *(1)*. The prevalence and importance of the concept to everyday clinical practice was, however, first highlighted in 1988 when Gerald Reaven drew attention to a constellation of features associated with coronary heart disease *(2)* (Table 1). Reavan gave the constellation the name Syndrome X *(3)*. He also suggested that insulin resistance played a central etiological role in providing a link between these components.

In the subsequent decade, it has become evident that Syndrome X encompasses far more complex alterations in metabolic profile than originally envisaged (Table 1). It is now known by numerous other terms including the "metabolic syndrome" and the "chronic cardiovascular risk factor syndrome," which perhaps describes the syndrome best (Table 2).

From: *Contemporary Cardiology: Diabetes and Cardiovascular Disease, Second Edition*
Edited by: M. T. Johnstone and A. Veves © Humana Press Inc., Totowa, NJ

Table 1
The Metabolic Syndrome: 1988 and 2003

Metabolic syndrome 1988	Metabolic syndrome 2003
Resistance to insulin-stimulated glucose uptake	Resistance to insulin-stimulated glucose uptake
Glucose intolerance	Glucose intolerance
Hyperinsulinemia	Hyperinsulinemia
Increased VLDL triglyceride	Increased VLDL triglyceride
Decreased HDL cholesterol	Decreased HDL cholesterol
Hypertension	Hypertension
	Central obesity
	Microalbuminuria
	High plasminogen activator inhibitor-1
	Hyperleptinemia
	Hyperuricemia
	Hypoadiponectinaemia
	Subclinical inflammation

VLDL, very low-density lipoprotein; HDL, high-density lipoprotein.

Table 2
Synonyms for the Metabolic Syndrome

Metabolic syndrome
Syndrome X
CHO syndrome
Reavans syndrome
Chronic cardiovascular risk factor syndrome
Insulin resistance syndrome

CHO syndrome, carbohydrate intolerance, hypertension, obesity syndrome.

In this chapter, we will outline the hypotheses proposed for pathogenesis of the syndrome, review evidence to validate its existence, and discuss some of the clinical and therapeutic implications that arise.

EPIDEMIOLOGICAL EVIDENCE FOR THE METABOLIC SYNDROME

There is now a considerable body of epidemiological evidence supporting the existence of a metabolic syndrome. Perhaps the most compelling evidence to support its existence is provided by the San Antonio Heart study *(4)*. It was found that a combination of three or more risk factors for coronary artery disease (CAD) in the same patient was more prevalent than either the presence of each risk factor in isolation or in combination with just one other (Table 3) *(4)*. This study also suggested that hyperinsulinemia might provide the common etiological link *(5)* (Table 4).

Second, the link with coronary heart disease (CHD) is well established. For example, a study of atherosclerotic lesions in autopsies carried out on 204 young persons aged 2 to 39 years, related arterial lesions to ante mortem risk factors for which data were available on 93 individuals. The study showed that the extent of fatty streak lesions in the

Table 3
Prevalence Rates of Risk Factors (Obesity, NIDDM, Impaired Glucose Tolerance,
Hypertension, Hypertriglyceridemia, and Hypercholesterolemia) in 2390 Subjects [a]

	Obesity	NIDDM	IGT	HBP	HTG	HCH
Overall	54.3	9.3	11.1	9.8	10.3	9.2
Isolated	29.1	1.3	1.8	1.0	1.8	
2 × 2 associations						
NIDDM	3.8 (5.1)					
IGT	4.6 (6.0)					
HBP	2.2 (5.3)	0.1 (0.9)	0.3 (1.1)			
HTg	3.0 (5.6)	0.2 (1.0)	0.2 (1.1)	0.1 (1.0)		
HCH	2.4 (5.0)	0.2 (0.9)	0.1 (1.0)	0.1 (0.9)	0.5 (1.0)	
Multiple associations (%)	17	40	37	56	51	45

[a]Entries are actual crude prevalence rates (in percent). The numbers in parentheses are expected prevalence rates of 2 × 2 associations, calculated as the product of the overall prevalence rates of the two members of the pair. The last line shows the percentage of all cases of each condition occurring in combinations of three or more with other conditions. NIDDM, non-insulin-dependent diabetes mellitus; IGT, imparied glucose tolerance; HBP, hypertension; HTG, hypertriglyceridemia; HCH, hypercholesterolemia. (From ref. 5).

Table 4
Eight-Year Incidence of Multiple Metabolic Disorders
According to First and Fourth Quartiles of Fasting Insulin at Baseline

Disorder	Baseline insulin		Relative risk	p value
	Low	High		
Hypertension	5.5%	11.4%	2.04	0.021
Hypertriglycerdemia	2.6%	8.9%	3.46%	0.001
Low HDL-C	16.2%	26.3%	1.63%	0.012
High LDL-C	16.4%	20.1%	1.23%	0.223
Type 2 diabetes	2.2%	12.3%	5.62%	0.001

HDL-C, high-density lipoprotein cholesterol; LDL-C, low-density lipoprotein cholesterol. (Reproduced with permission from ref. 4.)

coronary arteries was 8.5 times as great in persons with three or four risk factors compared with those with none (6). Earlier reports from this study had demonstrated clustering of risk factors even in the young (7).

It is important to emphasize, however, that although a common etiological thread may account for the association between the components of the syndrome there are large ethnic differences in the pattern of risk factors seen, and in how the syndrome is manifest. For example, based on the prevalence of obesity and hypertension, it was surprising that there were fewer cardiovascular deaths in North American Samoans, compared with Americans of European origin. Similarly low levels of cardiovascular risk factors are also reported in Nauruans and Pimas when compared to Caucasians based on obesity and frequency of non-insulin-dependent diabetes mellitus in these populations (8). In diabetic African Americans, serum high-density lipoprotein (HDL) cholesterol levels tend to be much higher and triglyceride levels much lower when compared to Caucasians and obesity appears to be better reflected by body mass index (BMI) in black women. This combination of protective factors may account for the reduced risk of CHD in individuals of African origin, while the increased prevalence of cerebrovascular disease is explained by the higher frequency and severity of hypertension in this population. In individuals of South Asian origin, the components of the syndrome are, however, of a far more classical nature and this is reflected by the increased incidence of ischemic heart disease in this population. Here, hyperinsulinemia, high plasma triglycerides, and low HDL cholesterol and diabetes rather than smoking, hypertension or altered hemostatic factors appear to account, at least in part, for the increased cardiovascular mortality. The pronounced tendency toward central adiposity in South Asians, despite similar BMIs to Europeans may, for example, help to explain this pattern of risk factors and increased mortality *(9)*.

ETIOLOGY

It is likely that both genetic and environmental factors are involved in development of the metabolic syndrome. Insulin resistance, to a degree similar to that seen in type 2 diabetes, is found in up to 25% of the general population *(2)*. The majority of studies and theories relating to its etiology have focused on the role of insulin resistance in the development of type 2 diabetes. Various hypotheses have been proposed.

Thrifty Genotype Hypothesis

More than 30 years ago, Neel proposed this hypothesis to explain the widespread prevalence of insulin resistance and type 2 diabetes in modern society. He suggested that despite its association with conditions detrimental to health and survival today, it must have provided a survival advantage to the human species during evolution for it to have such a high frequency within present-day populations *(10)*. Neel argued that hyperinsulinemia conferred a survival advantage to man when the regular food supply was lacking and cycles of "feast and famine" were common. He suggested that hyperinsulinemia provided a mechanism by which man could take maximal advantage of such a pattern of food supply, as it would minimize caloric loss during times of famine and facilitated fat storage during times of plenty. It has also been suggested that in the presence of selective insulin resistance in muscle and consequent hyperinsulinemia, energy would preferentially be stored in the liver and fat *(11)*. Although this would not be detrimental to health in a feast–famine environment, in an environment of persistent calorie excess these characteristics would predispose to obesity, diabetes, and the metabolic syndrome (Fig. 1).

Reaven/Cahill Hypothesis

Reaven, building on much of Cahills' experimental work, however, has interpreted the presence of such selective insulin resistance in a completely different manner *(12)*. Although the main thrust of Neels' hypothesis was efficient fuel storage providing the mechanism for survival, Cahill proposed that insulin resistance provided a mechanism by which protein breakdown (i.e., muscle breakdown) could be limited, thus allowing hunting to continue. This hypothesis is based on several assumptions. The first is that man has what Cahill described as a "hypertrophied" nervous system in constant need of substrate irrespective of overall nutritional state. The nutritional requirements of the brain can be overcome in two ways. First, nonesterified fatty acids (NEFA) released from

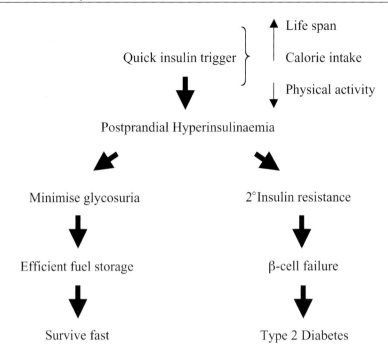

Fig. 1. The advantage of a quick insulin trigger to primitive man as suggested by Neel is seen on the left. The disadvantages of this phenotype to modern man and how it leads to type 2 diabetes is depicted on the right. (Reproduced with permission from ref. *12*.)

adipose tissue would serve as an energy source for the central nervous system following conversion to ketone bodies *(13,14)*. Second, enhanced quantities of glucose would be made available by reducing muscle glucose uptake. This is met by a physiological response, however, in the form of hyperinsulinemia, which while being ineffective in lowering plasma glucose because of insulin resistance would prevent the breakdown of muscle. Site-specific insulin resistance alone, however, is not enough and metabolic specificity in terms of insulin resistance is also required in that, although muscle must remain resistant to the actions of insulin in terms of glucose disposal, its antiproteolytic actions need to be maintained (Fig. 2).

Thrifty Phenotype Hypothesis

Some investigators have questioned the existence of a genetic component to the insulin resistance syndrome and suggest that insulin resistance, type 2 diabetes, and the metabolic syndrome seen in adulthood are the result of an adverse intra-uterine and neonatal environment (i.e., famine) and are therefore manifestations of a "thrifty phenotype." Using data from the county of Hertfordshire in England, where detailed records have been kept by the midwives since 1911, Barker showed that with increasing birth weight and weight at 1 year, the death rate from heart disease fell, while no similar trend could be shown in noncirculatory illness *(15)*. Further studies on this cohort of men looking specifically for the presence of Syndrome X (defined as 2-hour glucose 7.8 mmol/L, systolic blood pressure [SBP] > 160, triglycerides >1.4 mmol/L) showed that it reduces progressively from 30% to 6% as birth weight rose from less than 2.5 to more than 4.1 kg *(16)* (Table 5). Based on these findings, it has been proposed that the abnormalities

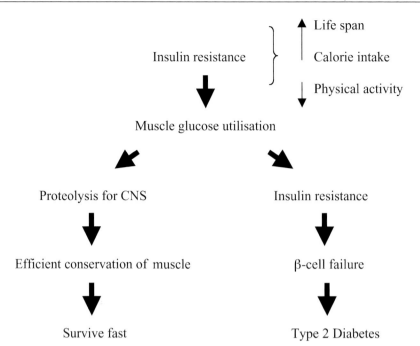

Fig. 2. An alternative view, based on the experimental studies by Cahill and colleagues. The survival advantage of muscle insulin resistance to primitive man as suggested by Neel is seen on the left. The disadvantages of this phenotype to modern man and how it leads to type 2 diabetes is depicted on the right. (Reproduced with permission from ref. *12*.)

Table 5
Percentage of Men in Hertfordshire, England With Syndrome X
According to Birth Weight

Birth weight (kg)	Total number of men	Percent (%) with Syndrome X	Odds ratio (95% confidence interval)
<2.5	20	6 (30)	18 (2.6–118)
–2.95	54	10 (19)	8.4 (1.5–49)
–3.41	114	19 (17)	8.5 (1.5–46)
–3.86	123	15 (12)	4.9 (0.9–27)
–4.31	64	4 (6)	2.2 (0.3–14)
>4.31	32	2 (6)	1.0
Total	407	56 (14)	

Reproduced with permission from ref. *16*.

that form Syndrome X co-exist because they share a common origin in the form of a suboptimal environment in early life. These studies are supported by data from several countries *(17–19)* including studies on twins discordant for type 2 diabetes, and do not seem to represent a purely British phenomenon *(20)* (Fig. 3). This hypothesis is, however, still unproven.

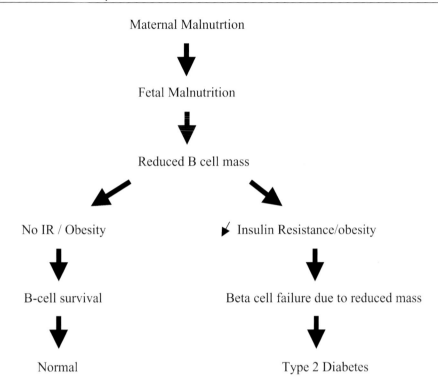

Maternal Malnutrtion

Fetal Malnutrition

Reduced B cell mass

No IR / Obesity   Insulin Resistance/obesity

B-cell survival   Beta cell failure due to reduced mass

Normal   Type 2 Diabetes

Fig. 3. Although this sequence demonstrates the mechanism by which reduced β-cell mass can in later life result in type 2 diabetes, Barker and colleagues have suggested that fetal malnutrition also results in abnormal vascular development and other metabolic derangements, which when combined with the above manifest as the metabolic syndrome.

The "Common Soil" Hypothesis

Stern suggested that although atherosclerosis is often considered to be a complication of diabetes, both share many of the same genetic and environmental antecedents and therefore both should be considered as consequences of the metabolic syndrome, i.e., spring from a "common soil" *(21)*. There is, in fact, a large body of evidence to suggest this may indeed be the case. In an excellent and extensive review, Stern has shown that if components of the metabolic syndrome are categorized (into four major categories: anthropometric variables, variables reflecting carbohydrate and lipid metabolism, and hemodynamic variables), usable mathematical predicting models, using representatives from each of the four categories, can be created to correctly predict the chances of developing diabetes *(22)*.

SUMMARY

Although all of the above hypotheses provide plausible frameworks with which to work, they generate more questions than they answer, and leave two major controversies. First, the debate continues regarding whether it is genetic or environmental factors, which play the major etiological role. Second, it has still not been resolved whether hyperinsulinemia or insulin resistance is the primary abnormality. It is likely that the metabolic syndrome results from a complex mixture with features of both insulin resistance and hyperinsulinemia *(23–27)*.

PATHOPHYSIOLOGY

Insulin Resistance and Coronary Heart Disease

The association of insulin with CHD can be considered at two levels. First, it appears to be the common link, in the form of resistance to its actions, between the components of the metabolic syndrome. The majority of these have well-documented pathogenetic roles in the development of CHD. Second, and far more contentiously, there is both experimental and epidemiological data suggesting a more direct role of insulin in the development of atheroma. We will review each of these in turn.

There is a substantial body of experimental in vitro and in vivo work studying the association of insulin and atherosclerosis *(28)*. The first indirect evidence was provided by Duff and McMillan *(29)*, who demonstrated that in alloxan-induced diabetic rabbits, a high-cholesterol diet would only induce arterial lesions comparable to those of the control rabbits when the diabetics were treated with insulin *(30–32)*. This was followed by experiments of Cruz and associates who caused unilateral femoral artery intimal and medial proliferation and lipid accumulation by infusing insulin into that artery for 28 weeks *(33)*. Other in vitro experiments have shown human smooth muscle cell proliferation *(34)*, increase in monocyte low-density lipoprotein (LDL) receptor activity *(35)*, reduction in fibroblast HDL activity *(36)*, and progression of arterial lipid lesions *(37)*, on incubation with insulin. Despite this wealth of experimental evidence extrapolations from in vitro data to in vivo situation has been fraught with difficulty. A number of large epidemiological studies, both cross-sectional and prospective, have examined the relationship between insulin and subsequent CHD. Although they have suggested a role for insulin (hyperinsulinemia) there has been variation both between studies and even within studies.

The Paris Prospective Study commenced with baseline examinations between 1968 and 1974 and has since reported at 5-year intervals, on results from 6093 male Parisian civil servants. Insulin levels were measured at fasting and at 2 hours after a 75 g oral glucose load. After 5 and 11 years, multivariate analysis suggested a significant association between fasting insulin levels and CHD mortality. By 15 years, this relationship only remained with the 2-hour insulin levels *(38–40)*. A complex model, however, had to be adopted with the relationship only holding if insulin was held to be categorical variable (i.e., last quintile of distribution? yes/no). Although fasting or 2-hour glucose levels at 5, 10, and 15 years were not related to the incidence of CHD, analysis at 20 years demonstrated that men in the upper 2.5% for fasting glucose had significantly higher risk of not only cardiovascular deaths but also all cause mortality.

Similarly, the Helsinki Policeman Study initiated in 1971, followed 982 male policeman aged 35 to 64, and reported after 5 and 9.5 years follow-up *(41,42)*. Measurements of insulin levels were made at fasting and at 1 and 2 hours after an oral glucose load based on body surface area. High 1- and 2-hour plasma insulin levels after an oral glucose load were associated with an increased risk of CHD. This independent association was maintained even with multivariate analysis and corrections for BMI, glucose, triglycerides, cholesterol, smoking, SBP, and exercise. Although a similar trend was seen with the fasting insulin levels, this did not reach statistical significance. As in the Paris Study, the association between CHD events and insulin was nonlinear with marked excess in CHD events (CHD deaths or nonfatal myocardial infarctions [MIs]) in the highest decile.

More recently, Despres and associates reported on a 5-year follow-up of 2103 men aged 45 to 76 recruited for the Quebec Cardiovascular Study *(43)*. In the 91 nondiabetic men who had their first ischemic event during this period, high-fasting insulin levels were an independent predictor for ischemic heart disease, even after multivariate analysis for plasma triglyceride, apolipoprotein (apo)-B, LDL cholesterol and HDL cholesterol. This is the only study in which fasting insulin has been shown to be an independent risk factor. Diabetes was, however, not vigorously excluded and it is possible that undiagnosed diabetes may explain the demonstrated association.

The insulin response to a standard oral glucose tolerance test and other anthropometric and biochemical risk factors for CHD were measured in a random sample of 107 Edinburgh men who were initially studied in 1976 when they were 40 and who were re-examined in 1988–1989 *(44)*. This study failed to identify insulin as a risk factor for CHD. The anthropometric measurements, which had been carried out, however, combined with the lipid analysis, did confirm a central role for abdominal obesity and low HDL cholesterol as a risk factor for ischemic heart disease.

This lack of an association was reconfirmed by a larger study looking at elderly men (born in 1913) born in Gothenburg. The 8-year incidence of CHD in 595 men, aged 67, was not significantly related to insulin levels. In fact, once all diabetic subjects were taken out of the analysis, the importance of hyperlipidemia was once again apparent with only triglycerides and cholesterol remaining as statistically significant risks *(45)*.

Rather surprisingly, only two studies have had females as part of their cohort. In the study by Welborn and colleagues, on the inhabitants of Busselton in Australia, 3,390 adults aged 21 to 70 years were examined as part of mass health screening with blood samples being taken following a 50 g oral glucose load *(46)*. Analysis of the results revealed a univariate association between insulin levels and CHD mortality only in men aged 60–69 years. Multivariate analysis at 13 years, however, failed to demonstrate any association between insulin levels and CHD mortality *(47)*. In a study by Ferrara and associates, once again no relationship was seen between the insulin and CHD in women *(48)*. This, as with the Gothenburg Study, may represent a survival bias as a result of the elderly nature of its subjects.

More recently, the results of two intervention trials quite clearly demonstrate a beneficial effect with therapeutic use of insulin. The 3-year follow up results of the Diabetes Mellitus Insulin Glucose Infusion in Acute Myocardial Infarction Study Group demonstrated that mortality in diabetic patients who have an MI is reduced by the immediate use of glucose and insulin infusion followed by a multidose insulin regimen *(49,50)*. Patients randomized to receive a glucose and insulin infusion showing an 11% reduction in mortality. This represents a reduction in relative risk of 0.72.

In the United Kingdom Prospective Diabetes Study, while treatment with insulin did not significantly ($p = 0.052$) decrease the risk of macrovascular disease, it did not result in an adverse effect *(51,52)*.

Thus, both the experimental and epidemiological evidence are somewhat contradictory and one cannot conclude that there is a direct link between insulin and atheromatous disease. Most importantly there is no evidence that therapeutic use of exogenous insulin has any detrimental effects on cardiovascular morbidity or mortality.

INSULIN AND CARDIOVASCULAR RISK FACTORS

Haffner recently called attention to the importance of the need to try and elucidate whether the major effect of insulin on atherosclerosis is a direct one as illustrated by experimental in vitro work, or mediated through its effect on other cardiovascular risk factors *(4)*. This has major implications in terms of interpretation of the epidemiological data (i.e., the need to interpret the results after multivariate analysis). In the next section, we will examine some of the evidence linking insulin resistance with other components of the metabolic syndrome.

Hypertension

Welborn and associates first noted this most controversial of associations in 1966 *(53)*. Although since then several large epidemiological studies have supported the association between insulin and hypertension, interethnic differences in the association and contradictory in vitro and in vivo data have cast doubt over its validity, as in the case of the association between insulin and atherosclerosis.

In one of the most significant studies, Modan, reporting on a study of 5711 people, demonstrated a significant association between elevated fasting and post-glucose insulin levels and hypertension in a subgroup of 1241 individuals *(54)*. This association was independent of glucose intolerance, obesity, age, and treatment for hypertension. In a similar study that Asch carried out on Californian subjects aged 50 to 93 (655 men and 784 women), significantly higher postload insulin levels were demonstrated. This association was lost, however, when the data was adjusted for obesity and glucose intolerance.

In a study confounded by the obese nature of its subjects (mean BMI 33 kg/m^2), Saad suggested that the association was one that was limited to the Europid population being absent in Pima Indians and blacks *(55)*. A study in black men of a leaner body composition (BMI = 23 kg/m^2), however, subsequently has also demonstrated a link between insulin resistance and hypertension in this population *(56)*.

A larger population study, however, carried out on 3528 subjects from three Pacific island populations (1067 Micronesians, Nauru; 1393 Polynesians, Western Samoa; 1068 Melanesians, New Caledonia) once again failed to demonstrate an association between the two *(57)*. In the San Antonio Heart Study, although fasting insulin was a univariate predictor of hypertension in an 8-year follow-up, the association was lost in multivariate analyses.

Experimentally, several theories have been proposed to provide a plausible mechanism for the association. Using euglycemic hyperinsulinemic clamps in young healthy subjects, DeFronzo and colleagues have demonstrated a decline in sodium excretion rate within 30 minutes and a nadir about 50% lower than the basal excretion rate. Both proximal and distal tubules appear to be affected both directly by insulin and indirectly by activation of the sympathetic nervous system *(58)* and augmentation of the angiotensin-induced aldosterone secretion *(59)*.

Activation and involvement of the sympathetic nervous system and its association with the syndrome is, in fact, far-reaching. Its activation is closely linked to changes in plasma insulin concentration, although clamp studies have shown a link with increased noradrenaline levels and increases in BP and pulse. In the Normative Aging Study, urinary noradrenaline and insulin were correlated significantly with BP *(60)*. Increase in myocardial contractility, and central venous constriction may also help contribute to increased BP *(61)*.

Critics of the association, however, cite evidence suggesting that this effect is only acute and that evidence from animal studies combined with more long-term observational data in humans do not justify the association. Certainly, insulin has a direct vasodilatory effect when given either systematically or locally with no elevation in BP despite the demonstration of elevated noradrenaline levels in clamp studies *(62–66)*. Furthermore, therapeutic use of exogenous insulin, clinical diagnosis of insulinoma, or the presence of an insulin-resistant disease process such as the polycystic ovary syndrome or one of the rarer insulin resistance syndromes are all free of such a close association with hypertension.

The renin–angiotensin axis may also be further implicated as a number of hormones involved in this pathway including angiotensinogen, renin, and angiotensin 2 have been discovered to be secreted by adipose tissue *(67,68)*. Recent studies have also established that angiotensinogen is not only elevated in obesity but also directly correlates with BP during weight loss *(69)*.

OBESITY AND DYSLIPIDAEMIA

There has been some controversy regarding not only the association of obesity with CVD *(70)*, but regarding whether or not it should be included as a feature of the metabolic syndrome. Although it undoubtedly is a common occurrence in those with other features of the syndrome, it is not a necessity. Obesity was not in fact a feature of the cohort originally defined by Reaven (all of whom had a BMI <26), which probably reflects the heterogeneity of the disorder with regional adiposity being more closely associated with morbidity and mortality than generalized obesity *(71)*. As a univariate predictor of cardiovascular mortality several large studies provide convincing evidence of the link between obesity *per se* and CHD. The American Cancer Society Study, detailing mortality data on 750,000 individuals, showed an increase in mortality from CHD as weight increased from less than 20% below to 40% above the average for the population as a whole *(72)*. A similar weight–cardiovascular mortality ratio was demonstrated when data from 4.2 million life insurance policyholders was analyzed in the Build Study *(73)*.

More recently, in the analysis of the Nurse's Study, a BMI of 25 to 28.9 was associated with a twofold increase in CVD, although the risk rose to almost fourfold once the BMI exceeded 2,974. Another important feature of adiposity highlighted in this study is the problems not simply of obesity but of weight gain from 18 years of age. An increase of between 8 and 10.9 kg being associated with a 1.6-fold increase in CVD. This has also been demonstrated in males in which an 86% increase in cardiovascular risk was associated with a 20% weight gain *(75)*.

It is important to note, however, that the association is not simply a direct one with CVD, but rather there is strong etiological association between obesity and other cardiovascular risk factors. This is particularly the case for diabetes in which up to 75% of patients with type 2 diabetes are reported as being obese and having a BMI of greater than 35 increases the risk of developing the disease by more than 93-fold *(76)*. There is also strong evidence now linking obesity with left ventricular hypertrophy, hypertension, alterations in hemostatic factors, as well as alterations in lipid profiles *(77)*.

Visceral Obesity

It is now well established that regional adiposity plays a greater role in the development of diabetes, impaired glucose tolerance , and atherosclerosis than generalized obesity. This concept is not entirely new: Vague first described it in 1956 *(78)*. Several epidemiological studies have demonstrated a clear relationship between central adiposity and insulin resistance/hyperinsulinemia. Larsson, in a study of 54-year-old Swedish men, demonstrated a significant association between waist-to-hip ratio (WHR) and incidence of CVD and cerebrovascular disease. Other measures of body fat distribution, in the form of BMI and skinfold measurements, did not demonstrate a similar statistically significant association and in fact, multivariate analysis eliminated the association *(79)*. A similar study in Swedish women, aged 38 to 60, demonstrated an association between the WHR and MI although on this occasion the association was independent of BMI and cholesterol *(80)*. Subscapular skinfold and waist circumference in men was also predictive of CVD over 22 years in the Framingham Study *(81)*.

This variation in regional adiposity partly reflects characteristic gender differences, which become more pronounced with increasing adiposity. The classic description of the "pear-shaped" female reflects the deposition of subcutaneous adipose tissue mainly in the gluteofemoral area, although the pattern of fat distribution in the nonobese male gradually changes from one of relatively uniform distribution to a more central accumulation in the obese male, with the resultant "apple shape" or upper body obesity. In the female with increasing adiposity there is increased deposition in the lower part of the abdominal wall and the gluteofemoral area *(82)*. This subcutaneous fat accounts for 80% of total adipose tissue yet, in vitro and in vivo studies suggest that it is the intraperitoneal fat, which accounts for 6% to 20% of total adipose tissue volume. The latter is the most metabolically active and deleterious to health and is strongly associated with insulin resistance. The mechanisms underlying visceral adiposity and also its links with insulin resistance are poorly understood. Insulin and glucocorticoids increase visceral adiposity and sex steroids and growth hormone appear to exert opposite effects. Visceral adipocytes not only express more glucocorticoid receptors, they also have higher 11-β-hydroxysteroid dehydrogenase type 1 isosenzyme activity *(83)*. As this enzyme is responsible for conversion of inactive cortisone to cortisol they have the ability to generate high local levels of active glucocorticoid, which is important for adipocyte differentiation. The reasons regarding why such a relatively small volume of fat should be so deleterious are probably multifactorial and are a reflection of both its functional properties and anatomical location.

Unfortunately, studies looking at the fundamental question of whether insulin resistance precedes and worsens during obesity *(84)*, or whether its a consequence of obesity *(85)*, are contradictory as there is conflicting epidemiological evidence even when the same population is studied *(86,87)*. At the cellular level, however, insulin resistance of visceral fat, combined with a number of other metabolic characteristics such as increased lipolytic response to catecholamines, results in an accelerated rate of lipolysis. This combined with the venous drainage of intraperitoneal fat, exposes the liver to high levels of NEFA and glycerol *(88)*. This results in increased secretion of very low-density lipoprotein (VLDL) triglyceride, as NEFAs are the major substrate for hepatic triglyceride production, and as VLDL secretion is normally under the tonic inhibitory influence of insulin and this is lost in the resistant state *(89)*. There is also reduced apo-B degradation, once again an insulin-regulated process *(90)*, with subsequent formation of small dense atherogenic LDL. This high flux also reduces hepatic insulin clearance with subsequent peripheral hyperinsulinemia and increases hepatic gluconeogenesis.

This situation is further exacerbated as adipose LPL, an insulin-responsive hormone that is normally responsible for triglyceride removal from VLDL, appears to be insulin resistant—a situation culminating in hypertriglyceridemia.

Innate Immunity, Adipokines, and the Metabolic Syndrome

It has been discovered that the previous belief that adipose tissue acts as just an energy store/insulatory and protective barrier is untrue, it also is an endocrine organ in its own right *(91)*. Many cytokines are produced by adipose tissue some, such as interleukin (IL)-6 and tumor necrosis factor (TNF)-α *(92)*, are found in other tissues and some are exclusive to adipose, such as adiponectin *(93–96)*. These factors are not only involved in insulin signaling pathways but are also products of, and initiators of, chronic inflammatory processes. These are termed the adipocytokines or adipokines.

It has been theorized that these inflammatory factors are fundamental to the development of insulin resistance *(97)*. There is considerable evidence linking these adipokines to the innate immune system and chronic inflammation within adipose tissue *(98,99)*.

The innate immune system is an evolutionary well-conserved acute inflammatory response mechanism, which acts as a first defense to infection by recognition of what could be termed antigens and activation of inflammatory mediators and the complement pathway. It is theorized that chronic activation of this system may lead to the long-term pathogenesis of type 2 diabetes as many of the adipokines are involved in the modulation of insulin signaling in both adipose tissue and throughout the body. There is also considerable epidemiological and biochemical evidence to support this *(100–102)*.

Leptin

The parabiosis experiments of the 1960s gave hope that there existed a possible "magic bullet" to help solve the problems of obesity *(104)*. The discovery of leptin, a 167-amino acid protein in 1994 *(105)*, which caused marked and rapid weight loss when administered to the ob/ob mouse (obese, leptin-deficient mouse), gave rise to hope that the magic bullet had finally been discovered *(106)*. Initially, it was thought that leptin, produced by adipose tissue, helped modulate body weight by a simple negative feedback loop reducing levels of hypothalamic hormone neuropeptide Y, which is known to increase food intake and appetite as adipose tissue mass increased *(107,108)*. Unfortunately, the story in man has not been as straightforward and leptin appears to play a far more complex role with both central and peripheral effects. There is increasing evidence linking it with the metabolic syndrome and insulin resistance.

In vitro experiments suggest that leptin reduces intracellular fatty acid and triglyceride stores *(109)* and hence has beneficial effects on insulin resistance, improves glucose homeostasis, for which there is in vivo data, and also affects β-cell function. The data here, unfortunately, is in conflict with other in vitro experiments showing that in primary cultured adipocytes leptin interferes with the insulin-signaling pathway *(110)*.

Like all features of the metabolic syndrome, however, the epidemiological data in respect to hyperleptinemia has been inconsistent and although several studies have shown an association *(111–113)* this has not been consistent across all ethnic groups *(114)*. As a novel and potentially therapeutically valuable signaling compound, it is under current scrutiny. However, recent studies on the effect of administration of leptin in lean and obese mouse and rodent models have shown little effect on weight loss in the obese subjects *(115)*. However, this may be the result of the presence of hyperleptinemia in these subjects already leading to an amelioration of the effects of exogenous leptin. Whether these conclusions will be borne out in human populations is difficult to say but some studies on human subjects have so far showed that administration of exogenous leptin to patients who were both in the obese and leptin-deficient/obese subpopulations showed a significant reduction in weight in the leptin-deficient patients with little effect in the obese population.

Plasminogen Activator Inhibitor-1

Activation of both the intrinsic and extrinsic clotting pathways culminates in the conversion of fibrinogen to fibrinolysis resistant crosslinked fibrin and subsequent thrombus formation. This is an extremely complex event being modulated not only by a series of natural inhibitors such as proteins C, S, and thrombomodulin but also by an equally complex lytic system, which in turn is modulated by its own inhibitors of which plasminogen activator inhibitor (PAI)-1 is one. It is not surprising, therefore, as MI requires not only plaque formation and rupture but thrombus formation, that these hemostatic factors have been under intense scrutiny. It appears that their involvement may not merely be confined to the manifestation of CHD (i.e., MI) but they may contribute to its development (i.e., plaque formation) *(116–119)*.

The association of PAI-1 with components of the metabolic syndrome, in particular associations with triglyceride and BMI *(120,121)*, and insulin are now well established through epidemiological, experimental, and interventional studies *(122–125)*. This association is, however, not only with insulin and other features of the metabolic syndrome but several large-scale prospective studies have shown a more direct link between PAI-1 and future CAD in both apparently healthy individuals and in patients with known CAD *(126)*. It is this wealth of evidence that has led to suggestions that it should be included as part of the syndrome, although the mechanism remains far from clear.

Experimentally, several cell lines have been shown to produce PAI-1 with stimulation of expression not only in the presence of insulin but with several other growth factors such as transforming growth factor-β, TNF-α, and the lipoproteins. It must be noted, however, that in vivo work has failed to demonstrate that acute modulation of insulin levels is accompanied by a rise in levels of PAI-1.

The greatest interest, however, has been sparked by the demonstration that not only rodent but human adipose tissue produces PAI-1 and that modulation in weight is matched by modulations in PAI-1 antigen levels. Furthermore, human omental tissue explants produced significantly more PAI-1 antigen than subcutaneous tissue from the same patient *(123)*. This finding suggests that in the patient with insulin resistance, visceral fat is an important site for PAI-1 production and provides a further mechanism by which this depot can contribute to the development of ischemic heart disease.

Tumor Necrosis Factor-α

It took a century before the toxin first shown by Coley to cause tumour regression was identified as the protein now known as TNF-α *(127,128)*. This protein forms part of the cytokine family and is not only produced by a number of cells but also has a variety of effects including insulin resistance, growth promotion, angiogenesis, and growth inhibition *(129)*. Increases in TNF-α levels associated with obesity, its production by adipose tissue, and the insulin resistance it causes, have resulted in interest in this molecule as a potential therapeutic target. This appears to be multifactorial in origin with TNF-α not only playing a part in determining adipose tissue distribution and mass through its effects on thermogenesis (possibly decreased in obese state), alterations in lipolytic pathway (lipogenesis ↓, lipolysis ↑) but also more directly through inhibition of insulin-receptor tyrosine kinase activity *(130)*. There also appears to be an effect on the expression of insulin receptors especially the GLUT-4 insulin-sensitive glucose transporter *(131,132)* and an interaction with other adipokines (IL-6 and leptin ↑ *(133,134)*, adiponectin and resistin ↓ *[135,136]*). Recent data collated on the use of thiazolidinediones (TZDs), which are activators of peroxisome proliferator-activated receptor (PPAR)γ, a transcription factor responsible for adipogenesis, which have the effect of reducing insulin resistance has further added to this evidence. The effects of TZDs are multifactorial with a reduction in TNF-α expression in adipocytes and an attenuation of the downregulatory effect that TNF-α has on insulin receptors *(137,138)*. The use of these drugs is leading to further understanding of the intracellular pathways of TNF-α signaling especially its involvement with the mediation of gene expression.

Interleukin 6

The initial description of IL-6 was as part of the cytokine pathway involved in macrophage and T cell-mediated immune responses. It has subsequently been found to be secreted from various tissues especially adipose tissue *(139)*. The picture with IL-6 is less clear than TNF-α and there is some contradictory evidence regarding its role. Like TNF-α, circulating levels are higher in obese individuals and correlate with BMI and central fat distribution *(140)*. It has also been shown that IL-6 levels are elevated in obesity then fall during weight loss with these individuals *(141)*.

One possible explanation for its action on insulin resistance is decreased expression of the GLUT-4 transporter by IL-6 treatment *(142)*. However, other studies have showed an increase in glucose uptake in adipocytes with similar treatment *(143)*. Therefore, it is thought that IL-6 is more likely to act by modulation of other proinflammatory cytokines and not by direct effects on the cells themselves. This is supported by the fact that adiponectin levels are inversely related to IL-6 *(144)* and that the levels of resistin are increased in the presence of raised IL-6 *(145)*.

There seems little doubt that IL-6 plays an important role in insulin resistance but as a result of the contradictory nature of some of the evidence the full pathways of its action are yet to be elucidated.

Adiponectin

Of all the adipokines discovered adiponectin is unique in that in all the major studies it appears to be reduced in obesity and insulin resistance states *(146)*. It was initially discovered in 1995 and is related in structure to complement factor C1q94. Its action is related to PPARγ activity and levels of adiponectin are upregulated by the use of glitazones with concomitant improvement in insulin resistance *(147)*. The effects of adiponectin are varied—it reduces glucose production *(148)*, increases fatty acid oxidation *(149)*, and increases cellular uptake of glucose *(149)*.

It has also been discovered that it may reduce atherogenesis *(150)* and that mice who are deficient for the gene have severe intimal thickening and smooth muscle proliferation in damaged arteries *(151)*. It has also been shown that adiponectin stimulates nitric oxide production in vascular endothelial cells allowing for increased vasodilatation *(152)*. There is also some evidence that it has an anti-inflammatory action on macrophages *(153)*.

TNF-α reduces the secretion and expression of adiponectin *(154,155)* and vice versa *(156)* it is therefore thought they may act as antagonists. Insulin has also been shown to reduce adiponectin expression in 3T3-L1 murine adipocytes *(154)*.

Glucocorticoids have also been shown to suppress levels of adiponectin *(154,157)*. Interestingly adiponectin levels are significantly lower in men than women and this is probably as a result of the inhibitory effect of testosterone on adiponectin secretion by adipocytes *(158)* and may be part of the explanation for the higher incidence of insulin resistance in the male population.

Therefore, there seem to be a number of ways that adiponectin is involved with insulin resistance and its full range of actions on the bodies metabolism are currently being researched

Resistin

This recently discovered molecule was first isolated in mice and was thought initially to be the missing link in the insulin-resistance story *(159)*. It was shown that treatment of obese mouse subjects with antiresistin antibody led to an improvement in insulin action and blood sugar and that treatment of normal mice lead to insulin resistance. In vitro it has been shown that PPARγ agonists downregulate the mRNA of resistin by 80% to 90%. This was confirmed in vivo mouse studies as well *(159)*.

The picture in humans is unfortunately less clear. Initially, several studies seemed to show that resistin was not related to insulin resistance and obesity in humans *(160,161)*. However, other in vitro studies have shown that there is a modest effect on glucose uptake in adipose and that the resistin expression was downregulated by use of PPARγ agonists *(162)*.

Resistin is not only secreted by adipose tissue but is also found in macrophages *(163)*, in pancreatic islets *(164)* and even in human placenta *(165)*. This expression in multiple tissues probably underlies a more complex role for resistin than first thought. Although resistin is not quite the missing link it does have effects on insulin resistance and its full role in the pathogenesis of the metabolic syndrome has yet to be discovered.

Clinical and Therapeutic Implications

The concept of the metabolic syndrome has been useful in clinical practice for the treatment and prevention of cardiovascular disease. First, patients with any one of the components of the syndrome are at risk of having the other conditions for which they should be screened. Second, reduction in cardiovascular risk in such a patient will require treatment of all risk factors and it is important to recognize that treatment of one may at times lead to detrimental changes in another (Table 6). For example, some antihypertensive agents may have deleterious effects on glucose and lipid metabolism. Third, obesity aggravates the syndrome and therefore the assessment of the patients should include an assessment of adiposity—in particular visceral adiposity. Several different techniques, including height, weight, skinfold thickness, and waist circumference have been employed in epidemiological studies to assess obesity. BMI (weight [kg]/height [m^2]) is currently the most frequently used parameter to assess and classify obesity. As already outlined, however, body fat distribution, in particular abdominal adiposity, provides better prognostic information. Several studies have used the relationship between skinfold thickness and WHR (waist circumference measured at a point halfway between the lower costal margin and the superior iliacs) to assess abdominal obesity although large interobserver error and lack of standardization has led to increasing use of the WHR alone as a measure of visceral obesity. Although many of the above techniques have been compared to abdominal computed tomography scanning as a means of measurement, Despres and colleagues have shown that waist circumference alone provides a good measurement of visceral fat and that metabolic complications may start to be observed with circumferences of 100 cm or more *(166)*.

Table 6
Treatment of Hypertension

	Glucose	Insulin resistance	Body weight	Cholesterol	Triglyceride	High-density lipoprotein	Impotence
Thiazides	↑	↑	0	↑	↑	↑	↑
β-Blockers	↑	↑	↑	0	↑	↑	↑
Angioensin-converting enzyme inhibitors	0/↓	↓	0	0	0	0	0
α-Blockers	0/↓	↓	0	↓	↓	↓	↓
Calcium channel blockers	0	0	0	0	0	0	↑
Centrally acting drugs	0	?	0	0	0	↑	↑
Vasodilators	0	?	0	0	0	0	↑

↓ = Improves; ↑ = Worsens.

Table 7
Diagnostic Criteria for the Metabolic Syndrome (WHO)

Impaired glucose regulation or diabetes
Insulin resistance (under hyperinsulinaemic, euglycaemic condtions, glucose uptake below
    lowest quartile for population under investigation)
Raised arterial pressure >140/90 mmHg
Raised plasma triglycerides (>1.7 mmol/L , 150 mg/dL) and/or low HDL cholesterol
    (<0.9 mmol/L, 35 mg/dL men, <1.0 mmol/L, 39 mg/dL women)
Central obesity (males waist to hip ratio >0.9; females waist-to-hip ratio >0.85)
    and /or BMI >30 kg/m^2
Microalbuminuria (urinary albumin excretion rate >20 μg/min or albumin creatinine
    ratio >30 mg/g

HDL, high-density lipoprotein; BMI, body mass index.

Diagnosis

The diagnosis of the metabolic syndrome has always been fraught with difficulties as there has been disagreement over the criteria that make up the syndrome. There have been several attempts to clarify guidelines with this regard. The first major attempt by the World Health Organization (WHO) in 1999 is described in the paper on definitions and treatment of diabetes mellitus (Table 7).

An alternative proposal for defining the metabolic syndrome by the National Cholesterol Education Panel Adult Treatment Panel III (ATP III) has important differences compared to the WHO criteria. It is based on clinical and biochemical parameters available to most clinicians (Table 8).

Treatment

Two important studies have shown not only the clustering of cardiovascular risk factors in the young, but also a direct correlation of these risk factors with the extent of underlying atherosclerotic lesions. As such it has been argued that intervention should

Table 8
Diagnostic Criteria for the Metabolic Syndrome
(National Cholesterol Education Panel ATP III)

Abdominal obesity (waist circumference >102 cm [40 in] in men, >88 cm [35 in] in women)
Hypertriglyceridemia ≥150 mg/dL)
Low HDL-C (<40 mg/dL in men, <50 mg/dL in women)
High blood pressure (≥130/85 mmHg)
Highfasting glucose (IGT [blood sugar ≥110 mg/dL and <126 mg/dL] without diabetes)

HDL-C, high-density lipoprotein cholesterol; IGT, impaired glucose intolerance

begin in childhood *(167)*. The lack of a specific therapy and the difficulties of both pharmacological and nonpharmacological intervention have led some to argue that the efficacy of intervention in childhood has yet to be proven, and that the risk– benefit ratio of intervention in childhood, in which the majority are at low cardiovascular risk, differs significantly from the adult population. The benefits of alterations in lifestyle, such as cessation of smoking, physical exercise, and attention to weight, however, are important interventions in both the young and adult populations.

Weight loss is associated with marked improvement in metabolic and physiological profiles even in patients who remain markedly heavier than their "ideal" body weight (Table 9). This has been defined by the Scottish Intercollegiate Guidelines Network (SIGN), an interdisciplinary clinical guidelines network in Scotland. The main obstacle, however, is achieving and sustaining this weight loss with pharmacological intervention being required in most patients. Fenfluramine and phenetramine have both been shown to help reduce body weight and improve the lipid profile of obese individuals. The latter may to some extent be independent of effects on weight. Concerns over the association of these drugs, especially when given in combination, with pulmonary hypertension and valvular heart defects has, however, led to their withdrawal.

The use of TZD antidiabetic agents has been increasing over recent years and the development and use in experimental models has greatly increased our understanding of the pathogenesis of insulin resistance especially in relation to the adipokines. They also provide the opportunity for prospective studies examining the effect of treating insulin resistance on features of the metabolic syndrome other than hyperglycemia. Metformin, another antidiabetic drug, has also been shown to decrease hepatic glucose production, reduce plasma insulin release, triglycerides, and cholesterol *(168)*. Intervention studies in the case of metformin have also shown that its can lead to a reduction in PAI-1 levels *(169)*.

Trials with newer classes of drugs in the form of pancreatic lipase inhibitors (Orlistat) and centrally acting serotonin and noradrenaline reuptake inhibitors (Sibutramine) have shown that both products produce modest (5%–10%) weight loss.

There are already several excellent and extensive reviews and many national and international guidelines on the management of hyperlipidemia and hypertension however when instituting these it is important to take note that often they involve unifactorial assessment and ignore the multiplicative rather than the additive nature of the presence of these disorders. As such, assessment and treatment must be based on the individual's absolute level of risk and must take account of several variables to allow appropriate assessment of their clinical significance *(170)*. The ability to make therapeutic decisions

Table 9
Benefits of 10 kg Weight Loss (SIGN 1996)

Mortality	>20% fall in mortality
	>30% fall in diabetes-related deaths
	>40% fall in obesity-related deaths
Blood pressure	Fall of 10 mmHg systolic
	Fall of 20 mmHg diastolic
Diabetes	Fall of 50% in fasting glucose
Lipids	Fall of 10% total cholesterol
	Fall of 15% low-density lipoprotein
	Fall of 30% triglycerides
	Increase of 8% high-density lipoprotein

based on the presence of such a complex mixture of metabolic and physical abnormalities can be enhanced by use of evidence-based predictive models of risk assessment such as those based on the Framingham Heart Study, and should result in optimal therapeutic intervention *(171)*.

CONCLUSIONS

The concept of a metabolic syndrome is now firmly established and has important pathological and therapeutic implications. Experimental and epidemiological research has failed, so far, to firmly establish the underlying etiology however it is likely to represent a pathological state secondary to a complex mixture with features of both insulin resistance and hyperinsulinemia. Currently, the main area of interest is that of adipokines and their involvement in the molecular control of metabolism and this area and research here may further elucidate the relationship between the various components of the metabolic syndrome.

Clinically, it provides an important concept for screening and aggressively treating patients for multiple cardiovascular risk factors with an increasing battery of drugs some of which now allow the treatment of insulin resistance itself.

REFERENCES

1. Avogaro P, Creapaldi G, Essential Hyperlipaemia, obesity and diabetes (abstract). Diabetologia 1965;1:137
2. Reaven GM. Banting lecture 1988: role of insulin in human disease. Diabetes 1988;37:1595–1607.
3. Laws A, Reaven GM. Insulin resistance and risk factors for coronary heart disease. Baillieres Clin Endocrinol Metab 1993;7(4):1063–1078.
4. Haffner SM, Mietinen H. Insulin resistance implications for type II diabetes mellitus and coronary heart disease. Am J Med 1997;103:152–159.
5. Ferranini E, Haffner SM, Mitschell BD, Stern MP. Hyperinsulinaemia: the key feature of a cardiovascular syndrome and metabolic syndrome. Diabetologia 1991;34:416–422.
6. Berenson GS, Srinivasan SR, Bao W, Newman WP, Tracy RE, Wattingney WA. Association between multiple cardiovascular risk factors and atherosclerosis in children and young adults. N Engl J Med 1998;338,23:1650–1656.
7. Bao W, Srinivasan SR, Wattingney WA, Berenson GS. Persistence of multiple cardiovascular risk clustering relating to syndrome X from childhood to adulthood: the Bogalusa Heart Study. Arch Intern Med 1994; 54:1842–1847.
8. Hodge AM, Zimmet PZ. The epidemiology of obesity. Baillieres Clin Endocrinol Metab 1994;8(3):577–599.

9. McKeigue PM. Insulin resistance and risk factors in different ethnic groups. In: Poulter N, Sever P, Thom S, (eds.). Cardiovascular Disease: Risk Factors and Intervention. Radcliffe Medical, Ltd.: Abingdon, UK, 1993, pp. 53–62.

10. Neel JV. Diabetes mellitus: a thrifty genotype rendered detrimental by "progress"? American Journal of Human Genetics 1962;14:353–362.

11. Wendorf M, Goldfine ID. Archaeology of NIDDM: excavation of the thrifty genotype. Diabetes 1991;40:161–165.

12. Reavan GM. Hypothesis: muscle insulin resistance is the ("not so") thrifty genotype. Diabetologia 1998;41(4):482–484.

13. Owen OE, Felig P, Morgan AP, Wahren J Cahill GF Jr. Liver and kidney metabolism during prolonged starvation. JCI 1969;48:574–583.

14. Owen OE, Morgan AP, Kemo HG, et al. Brain metabolism during prolonged starvation. JCI 1967;46;1589–1597.

15. Barker DJP. Intra-uterine origins of cardiovascular and obstructive lung disease in adult life. JR Coll Phys Lond 1991;25:129–133.

16. Barker DJP, Hales CN, et al. Type 2 (non-insulin dependent) diabetes mellitus, hypertension and hyperlipidaemia (syndrome X): relation to reduced foetal growth. Diabetologia 1993;36:62–67.

17. McCance DR, Pettitt DJ, Hanson RL, Jacobson LTH, Knowle WC, Bennett PH. Birth weight and non-insulin dependent diabetes: "thrifty genotype", "thrifty phenotype" or "surviving small baby genotype." Br Med J 1994;308:942–945.

18. Valdez R, Athens MA, Thompson GH, Bradshaw BS, Stern MP. Birth weight and adult outcomes in a diethnic population in the USA. Diabetologia 1994;37:624–631.

19. Lithell HO, Mckeigue PM, Berglund L, Mohsen R, Lithell U-B, Leon DA. Relation of size at birth to non-insulin dependent diabetes and insulin concentrations in men aged 50–60 years. Br Med J 1996;312:406–410

20. Poulsen P, Vaag AA, Kyvik KO, et al. Low birth weight is associated with NIDDM in discordant monozygotic and dizygotic twin pairs. Diabetologia 1997;40:439–446.

21. Stern MP. Diabetes and Cardiovascular Disease: The "Common Soil" Hypothesis. Diabetes 1995;44: 369–374.

22. Stern M. The Insulin Resistance Syndrome. In: Alberti KGMM, Zimmet P, DeFronzo R, Keen H, (eds.). International Textbook of Diabetes Mellitus. Wiley and Sons: New York, NY, 1997 pp. 255–283.

23. Hansen BC, Bodkin HL. Heterogeneity of insulin responses: phases leading to type II (non-insulin dependent) diabetes mellitus in the rhesus monkey. Diabetologia 1986;29:713–719.

24. Zimmet P. Kelly West Lecture 1991. Challenges in diabetes epidemiology-from west to the rest. Diabetes Care 1992;15(2):232–252.

25. Zimmet P, Dowse G, Bennet P. Hyperinsulinaemia is a predictor of non-insulin dependent diabetes mellitus. Diabetes Metab 1991;17:101–108.

26. Petit DJ, Moll PP, Kottke BA. Insulin resistance in apparently healthy children (Abstract). Diabetes 1990;339(Suppl 1):75A.

27. White K, Gracy M, Schumacher L, Spargo R, Kretchmer N. Hyperinsulinaemia and impaired glucose tolerance in young Australian Aborigines. Lancet 1990;2:735.

28. Stout RW. Insulin and Atheroma. Diabetes Care 1990;13(6):631–654.

29. Duff GL, McMillan GC. The effect of alloxan diabetes on experimental cholesterol atherosclerosis I. The inhibition of experimental cholesterol atherosclerosis in alloxan diabetes. II The effect of alloxan diabetes on the retrogression of experimental cholesterol atherosclerosis. Journal of Experimental Medicine 1949;89:611–629.

30. McGill HC Jr, Holman RL. The influence of alloxan diabetes on cholesterol atheromatosis in the rabbit. Proc Soc Exp Biol Med 1954;72:72–73.

31. Duff GL, Brechin DJH, Findelstein WE. The effect of alloxan diabetes on experimental cholesterol atherosclerosis in the rabbit.IV. The effect of insulin therapy on the inhibition of atherosclerosis in the alloxan-diabetic rabbit. J Exp Med 1954;100:371–80.

32. Norddestgaard BG, Zilversmit DB. Hyperglycaemia in normotriglyceridemic, hypercholestrolemic insulin treated diabetic rabbits does not accelerate atherogenesis. Atherosclerosis 1988;72:37–47.

33. Cruz AB Jr, Amatuzio DS, Grande F, Hay LJ. Effect of intra-arterial insulin on tissue cholesterol and fatty acids in alloxan-diabetic dogs. Circulation Research 1961;9:39–43.

34. Pfeilfle B, Ditschuneit H. Effect of insulin on growth of cultured arterial smooth muscle cells. Diabetologia 1981;20:155–158.

35. Krone W, Naegele H, Behnke B, Greten H. Opposite effects of insulin and catecholamines on LDL-receptor activity in human mononuclear leukocytes. Diabetes1988;37:1386–1391.
36. Oppenheimer MJ, Sundquist K, Bierman EL. Downregulation of high-density lipoprotein receptor in human fibroblasts by insulin and IGF-1. Diabetes 1989;38:117–122.
37. Elliot TG, Viberti G. Relationship between insulin resistance and the risk for coronary heart disease in diabetes mellitus and the general population: a critical appraisal. Baillieres Clin Endocrinol Metab 1993;7(4):1079–1103.
38. Duciemetiere P, Eschwege E, Papoz L, Richard JL, Claude JR. Relationship of plasma insulin levels to the incidence of myocardial infarction and coronary heart disease mortality in a middle aged population. Diabetologia 1980;19:205–210.
39. Eschwege E, Richard JL, Thibult N, et al. Coronary heart disease mortality in relation with diabetes, blood glucose and plasma insulin levels: the Paris prospective study, ten years later. Horm Metab Res 1985;15:41–46.
40. Fontbonne A, Charles MA, Thibult N, et al. Hyperinsulinaemia as a predictor of coronary heart disease mortality in a healthy population: the Paris prospective Study 15 year follow up. Diabetologia 1992;34: 356–361.
41. Pyorala K. Relationship of glucose tolerance and plasma insulin to the incidence of coronary heart disease: results from two population studies in Finland. Diabetes Care 1979;2:121–141.
42. Pyorala K, Savolainen E, Kaukola S, Haapakoski J. Plasma insulin as coronary heart disease risk factor: relationship to other risk factors and predictive value during 9.5 year follow-up of the Helsinki Police-man Study population. Acta Med Scad (Suppl) 1985;70:35–52.
43. Despres JP, Lamarche B, Mauriege P, Cantin B, Dagenais G, Moorajani S, Lupien PJ. Hyperinsulinaemia as an independent risk factor for ischaemic heart disease. N Engl J Med 1996;334(15):952–957.
44. Hargreaves AD, Logan RL, Elton RA, Buchanan KD, Oliver MF, Riemersma RA. Glucose tolerance, plasma insulin, HDL cholesterol and obesity: 12-year follow-up and development of coronary heart disease in Edinburgh men. Atherosclerosis 1992;94(1):61–69.
45. Welin L, Eriksson H, Larsson B, Ohlson LO, Svardsudd K, Tibblin G. Hyperinsulinaemia is not a major coronary risk factor in elderly men. The study of men born in 1913. Diabetologia 1992;35(8):766–770.
46. Welborn TA, Wearne K. Coronary heart disease incidence and cardiovascular mortality in Busselton with reference to glucose and insulin concentration. Diabetes Care 1979;21:154–160.
47. Cullen K, Stenhouse NS, Wearne KL, Welborne TA. Multiple regression analysis of risk factors for cardiovascular disease and cancer mortality in Busselton, Western Australia—3-year study. Journal of Chronic Diseases 1983;36:371–377.
48. Ferrara A, Barrett-Connor EL, Edelstein SL. Hyperinsulinaemia does not increase the risk of fatal cardiovascular disease in elderly men or women without diabetes: the Rancho Bernardo Study. 1984–1991. Am J Epidemiol 1994;140:857–869.
49. Nattrass M. Managing diabetes after myocardial infarction BMJ 1997;314:1497.
50. Malmberg K, for the DIGAMI study group. Prospective randomised study of intensive insulin treatment on long term survival after acute myocardial infarction in patients with diabetes mellitus. BMJ 1997;314:1512–1515.
51. UK Prospective Diabetes Study (UKPDS) Group. Intensive blood-glucose control with sulphonylureas or insulin compared with conventional treatment and risk of complications in patients with type 2 diabetes (UKPDS 33). Lancet 1998;12(352):837–853
52. Nathan D. Some answers, more controversy, from UKPDS. Lancet 1998;352:832–833.
53. Welborn TA, Breckenbridge A, Rubenstein AH, Dollery CT, Fraser TR. Serum insulin in essential hypertension and in peripheral vascular disease. Lancet 1996;1:1336–1337.
54. Modan M, Halkin H, Almog S, et al. Hyperinsulinemia: a link between hypertension, obesity and glucose intolerance. J Clin Inv.1985;75:809–817.
55. Saad MF, Lillioja S, Nyomba BL, et al. Racial differences in the relation between blood pressure and insulin resistance NEJM 1991;324:733–739.
56. Falkner B, Hulman S, Tannenbaum J, Kushner H. Insulin resistance and blood pressure in young black men. Hypertension 1990;16:706–711.
57. Collins VR, Dowse GK, Finch CFG, Zimmet PZ. An inconsistent relationship between insulin and blood pressure in three Pacific island populations. J Clin Epidemiol 1990;43:1369–1378.
58. Landsberg L, Krieger DR. Obesity, metabolism and the sympathetic nervous system. Am J Hyper 1989; 2:125S–132S.

59. Rocchini AP, Moorehead C, DeRemer S, Goodfriend TL, Ball DL Hyperinsulinaemia and the aldosterone and pressor responses to angiotensin II. Hypertension 1990;15:867–866.
60. Ward KD, Sparrow D, Landsberg L, Young JB, Weiss ST. The influence of obesity, insulin and the sympathetic nervous system activity on blood pressure. Clin Res 1993;41:168A.
61. DeFronzo RA, Ferrannini E. Insulin resistance: a multifaceted syndrome responsible for NIDDM, obesity, hypertension, dyslipidaemia and atherosclerotic cardiovascular disease. Diabetes Care 1991;14:173–194.
62. Laing C-S, Doherty JU, Faillace R, et al. Insulin infusion in conscious dogs: effects on systemic and coronary haemodynamics, regional blood flows and plasma catecholamines. J Clin Invest 1982;69:1321–1336.
63. Laakso M, Edelman SV, Brechtel G, Baron AD. Decreased effects of insulin to stimulate skeletal muscle blood flow in obese man: a novel mechanism for insulin resistance. J Clin Invest 1990;85:1844–1852.
64. Creagar MA, Liang C-S, Coffman JD. Beta-adrenergic-mediated vasodilator response to insulin in the human forearm. J Pharmacol Exp Ther 1985;235:709–714.
65. Anderson EA, Hoffman RP, Balon TW, Sinkey CA, Mark AL. Hyperinsulinaemia produces both sympathetic neural activation and vasodilation in normal humans. J Clin Invest 1991;87:2246–2252.
66. Berne C, Fagius J, Pollare T, Hjemdahl P. The sympathetic response to euglycaemic hyperinsulinaemia. Diabetologia 1992;35:873–879.
67. Karlson C, Lindell K, Ottosson M, et al. Huamn adipose tissue expresses angiotensinogen and enzymes necessary for its conversion to Angiotensin II. J Clin Endo Metab 1998;83:3925–3929.
68. Schling P, Mallow H, Trindl A, et al. Evidence for a local rennin angiotensin system in primary cultured pre-adipocytes. Int J Obes Relat Metab Disord 1999;23:336–341.
69. Eggena P, Sowers JR, Maxwell MH, Barrett JD, Golub MS. Hormonal correlates of weight loss associated with blood pressure reduction Clin Exp Hypertens A 1991;13(8):1447–1456.
70. Garrow J. Importance of obesity. BMJ 1991;303:704–706.
71. Kissebah AH, Krakower GR. Regional adiposity and morbidity. Physiological Reviews 1994;74:761–809.
72. Lew EA, Garfinkel L. Variations in mortality by weight among 750,000 men and women. J Chron Dis 1974;32:563–576.
73. Build study 1979. Chicago, IL: Society of Actuaries and Association of Life Insurance Medical Directors, 1980.
74. Willett WC, Manson JE, Stampfer MJ, et al. Weight, weight change and coronary heart disease in women. JAMA 1995:27:1461–1465.
75. Royal College of Physicians. Obesity. J Roy Coll Physicians Lond 1983;17:3–58.
76. Colditz GA, Willett WC, Rotnitzky A, Manson JE. Weight gain as risk factor for clinical diabetes mellitus in women Ann Int Med 1995;122:481–486.
77. Jung RT. Obesity as a disease. British medical Bulletin 1997;35(2):307–321.
78. Vague J. The degree of masculine differentiation of obesities, a factor determining predisposition to diabetes, atherosclerosis, gout and uric calculous disease. Am J Clin Nutr 1956;4:20–34.
79. Larsson B, Svardsudd K, Welin L, Wilhelmsen L, Bjorntorp P, Tibblin G. Abdominal adipose tissue distribution, obesity, and risk of cardiovascular disease and death: 12-year follow-up of participants in the study of men born in 1913. BMJ 1984;289:1401–1404.
80. Bengtsson C, Bjorkelund C, Lapidus L, Lissner L. Association of serum lipid concentration and obesity with mortality in women 20-year follow-up of participants in the prospective population study in Gothenburg Sweden. BMJ 1993:307(6916):1385–1388.
81. Stokes J, Garrison RJ, Kannek WB. The independent association of various indices of obesity to the 22-year incidence of coronary heart disease: the Framingham Heart Study. In: Vague J, Bjorntorp P, Guy-Grand B, Rebuffe-Scrive M, Vague P, (eds.). Proceedings of the international symposium on the metabolic complications of human obesities. Elservier: Marseilles, France, 1985, pp. 49–57.
82. Arner P. Regional adipocity in man. Journal of Endocrinology 1997;155:191–192.
83. Bujalska IJ, Kumar S, Stewart PM. does central obesity reflect Cushing's disease of the omentum. Lancet 1998;349:1210–1213.
84. Ludvil B, Nolan JJ, Bolago J, Sacks D, Olefsky J. Effects of obesity on insulin resistance in normal subjects and patients with NIDDM. Diabetes 1995;44:1121–1125.
85. Campbell PJ, Gerich JE. Impact of obesity on insulin action in volunteers with normal glucose tolerance: demonstration of threshold for the adverse effects of obesity. J Clin Endo Metab 1990,70:1114–1118.
86. Swinburn BA, Nyomba BL, Saad MF, et al. Insulin resistances associated with lower rates of weight gain in Pima Indians. JCI 1991,88:168–173.
87. Odeleeye OE, de Courten M, Ravussin E. Insulin resistance as a predictor of body weight gain in 5–10 year old Pima Indians. Diabetes 1995;44(Suppl 1):7a.

88. Bjorntorp P. Portal adipose tissue as a generator of risk factors for cardiovascular disease and diabetes Arteriosclerosis 1990;42:493–496.

89. Durrington PN, Newton RS, Weinstein DB, Steinberg D. Effects of insulin and glucose on VLDL triglyceride secretion by cultured rat hepatocytes. J Clin Invest 1982;70:63–73.

90. Jackson TW, Salhanick AI, Elvoson J, Deichman ML, Amaatruda JM. Insulin regulates apolipoprtein B turnover and phosphorylation in rat hepatocytes. J Clin Invest 1990;86:1746–1751.

91. Mohammed-Ali V, Goodrick S, Rawesh A, et al. Adipose tissue as an endocrine and paracrine organ. Int J of Obes and Rel Metab Disord 1998;22(12):1145–1158.

92. Funahashi T, Nakamura T, Shinmura K, et al. Role of adipocytokines on the pathogenesis of atherosclerosis in visceral obesity. Intern Med 1999;38:202–206.

93. Maeda K, Okubo K, Shimomura I, Funahashi T, Matsuzawa Y, Matsubara K. cDNA cloning and expression of a novel adipose specific collagen-like factor, apM1 (adipose most abundant Gene transcript 1) Biochem Biophys Res Commun 1996;221:286–296.

94. Scherer P.E, Williams S, Fogliano M Baldini G, Lodish HF. A novel serum protein similar to C1q, produced exclusively in adipocytes. J Biol Chem 1995;270:26,746–26,749.

95. Hu E, Liang P, Spiegelman BM. AdipoQ is novel adipose specific gene dysregulated in obesity. J Biol Chem 1996;271:10,697–10,703.

96. Nakano Y, Tobe T, Choi-Muira NH, Mazda T, Tomita M. Isolation and characterization OF gBP28, a novel gelatine-binding protein purified from human plasma. J .Biochem (Tokyo) 1991;120:802–812.

97. Pickup JC, Crook MA. Is type II diabetes a disease of the innate immune system? Diabetologia 1998;41(10):1241–1248.

98. Pickup JC, Mattock MB, Chusney GD, Burt D. NIDDM as a disease of the innate immune system: association of acute phase reactants and interleukin-6 with metabolic syndrome X. Diabetologia 1997;40:1286–1292.

99. Hotamisligil GS, Shargill NS, Spiegelman BM. Adipose expression of tumor necrosis factor-alpha: direct role in obestiy-linked insulin resistance. Science 1993;259(5091):87–91.

100. Kubaszek A, Pihlajamaki J, Komarovski V, et al. Promoter polymorphisms of the TNF-α(G-308A) and IL-6 (C174G) genes predict the conversion from impaired glucose tolerance to type 2 diabetes: the Finnish diabetes prevention study Diabetes 2003;52:1872–1876.

101. Hotamisligil GS, Budavari A, Murray D, Spiegelman BM. Reduced tyrosine kinase activity of the insulin receptor in obesity diabetes. Central role of TNF-α. J Clin Invest 1994;94:1543–1549.

102. Aljada A, Ghanim H, Assian E, Dandona P. Tumor necrosis factor-α inhibits insulin-induced increase in endothelial nitric oxide synthase and reduces insulin receptor content and phosphorylation in human aortic endothelial cells. Metabolism 2002;51:487–491.

103. Senn JJ, Klover PJ, Nowak IA, Mooney RA. Interleukin-6 induces cellular insulin resistance in hepatocytes. Diabetes 2002;51:3391–3399.

104. Coleman DL. Effects of parabiosis of obese with diabetic and normal mice. Diabetologia 1973;9:294–298.

105. Zhang Y, Proenca R, Maffei M, Barone M, Leopold L, Friedman JM. Positional cloning of the mouse obese gene and its human homologue. Nature 1994;372:425–432.

106. Halaas JL, Gajiwala KS, Maffei M, et al. Weight reducing effects of the plasma protein encoded by the obese gene. Science 1995;269:543–546.

107. Stephens TW, Basinski M, Bristow PK, et al. The role of neuropeptide Y in the antiobesity action of the obese gene product. Nature 1995;377:530–532.

108. Erickson JC, Clegg KE, Palmiter RD. Attenuation of the obesity syndrome of ob/ob mice by loss of neuropeptide Y. Science 1996;274:1704–1707.

109. Shimabukuro M, Koyama K, Chen G, et al. Direct antidiabetic effect of leptin through triglyceride depletion of tissues. Proc Natl Acad Sci USA 1997;94:4637–4641.

110. Muller G, Ertl J, Gerl M, Preibisch G. Leptin impairs metabolic actions of insulin in isolated rat adipocytes. J Biol Chem 1997;272:10,585–10,593.

111. Zimmet P, Hodge A, Nicholson M, et al. Serum leptin concentration, obesity and insulin resistance in Western Samoans: cross-sectional study. Br Med J 1996;313:965–969.

112. Larsson H, Elmstahl S, Ahren B. Plasma leptin levels correlate to islet function independently of body fat in post-menopausal women. Diabetes 1996;45:1580–1584.

113. Damani S, Gabriel M, Khan A, Boyadjian R, Kamadar V, Saad M. Adiposity and insulinaemia determine plasma leptin concentration (Abstract) Diabetes 1996;45(Suppl 1):41A.

114. Ramanchandran A, Snehalatha C, Vijay V, Satayavani K, Latha E, Haffner SM. Plasma leptin in nondiabetic Asian Indians. Association with abdominal obesity. Diabetic Med 1997;14:937–941.

115. Wilsey J, Zolotukhin S, Prima V, Scarpace PJ. Central leptin gene therapy fails to overcome leptin resistance associated with diet- induced obesity. Am J Physio Integr Comp Physiol 2003;285(5):R1011–R1020.

116. Carmeliet P, Schoonjans L, Kieckens L, et al. Physiological consequences of loss of plasminogen activator gene function in mice. Nature 1994;368:419–424.

117. Carmeliet P, Bouche A, De Clercq C, et al. Biological effects of disruption of the tissue-type plasminogen activator and plasminogen activator inhibitor-1 genes in mice Ann NY Acad Sci 1995;748:367–382.

118. Erickson LA, Fici Gj, Lund JE, Boyle TP, Polites HG, Marotti KR. Development of venous occlusions in mice transgenic for the PAI-1 gene. Nature 1990;346:74–76.

119. Schneiderman J, Sawdey MS, Keeton MR, et al. Increased type 1 Plasminogen activator inhibitor gene expression in atherosclerotic human arteries. Proc Natl Acad Sci 1992;89:6998–7002.

120. Eliasson M, Evrin PE, Lundblad D. Fibrinogen and fibrinolytic variables in relation to anthropometry, lipids and blood pressure. The Northern Sweden MONICA Study. J Clin Epidemiol 1994;47:513–524.

121. Sundell IB, Nilsson TK, Ranby M, Hallmans G, Hellsten G. Fibrinolytic variables are related to age, sex, blood pressure, and body build measurements: a cross-sectional study in Norsjo, Sweden. J Clin Epidemiol 1989;42:719–723.

122. Juhan-Vague I, Alessi MC. PAI-1, Obesity, Insulin resistance and risk of cardiovascular events. Thromb Haemostas 1997;78(1):656–660.

123. Eliasson M, Evrin PE, Lundblad D. Fibrinogen and fibrinolytic variables in relation to anthropometry, lipids and blood pressure. The Northern Sweden MONICA Study. J Clin Epidemiol 1994;47:513–524.

124. Sundell IB, Dahlgren S, Ranby M, Lundin E, Stenling R, Nilsson TK. Reduction of elevated plasminogen activator inhibitor levels during modest weight loss. Fibrinolysis 1989;3:51–53.

125. Gray RP, Panahloo A, Mohamed-Ali V, Patterson DL, Yudkin JS. Proinsulin-like molecules and plasminogen activator inhibitor type 1 (PAI-1) activity in diabetic subjects with and without myocardial infarction. Atherosclrerosis 1997;130:171–178.

126. Thompson SG, Kienast J, Pyke SDM, Haverkate F, van de Loo JCW. Haemostatic factors and the risk of myocardial infarction or sudden death in patients with angina pectoris N Engl J Med 1995;332:635.

127. Coley WB. The treatment of malignant tumours by repeated inoculations of erysipelas; with a report of ten original cases. Clin Orthop 1991;262:3–11.

128. Old LJ. Tumour necrosis factor (TNF) Science 1985;230:630–632.

129. Argiles JM, Lopez-Soriano J, Busquets S, Lopez-Soriano FJ. Journey from cachexia to obesity by TNF. FASEB 1997;11:743–751.

130. Hotamisligil GS, Peraldi P, Spiegelman BM. The molecular link between obesity and diabetes. Curr Opin Endocrinol Diabetes 1996;3:16–23.

131. Stephens JM, Pekela PH. Transcriptional reression of the GLUT4 and C/EBP genes in 3T3-L1 adipocytes by tumor necrosis factor-alpha. J Biol Chem 1191;266(32):21,839–21,845.

132. Hoffman C, Lorenz K, Braithwaite SS, et al. Altered gene expression for tumor necrosis factor-alpha and its receptors during drug and dietary modulation of insulin resistance. Endocrinology 1994;134(1):264–270.

133. FasshauerM, Klein J, Lossner U, Paschke R. Interleukin (IL)-6 expression is stimulated by insulin, tumor necrosis factor alpha, growth hormone and IL-6 in 3T3-L1 adipocytes. Horm Metab Res 2003;35(3):147–152.

134. Bullo M, Garcia-Lorda P, Peinado-Onsurbe J, et al. TNF-alpha expression of subcutaneous adipose tissue in obese and morbid obese females: relationship to adipocyte LPL activity and leptin synthesis. Int J Obes Relat Metab Disord 2002;26(5):652–658.

135. Kern PA, DiGregorio GB, Lu T, Rassouli N, Ranganathan G. Adiponectin expression from human adipose tissue: relation to obesity, insulin resistance and tumor necrosis factor-alpha expression. Diabetes 2003;57:1779–1785.

136. Shojima N, Sakoda H, Ogihara T, et al. Humoral Regulation of resistin expression in £T£-L! And mouse adipose cells. Diabetes 2002;51(6):1737–1744.

137. Peraldi P, Xu M, Speigelman BM. Thiiozolidinediones block tumor necrosis factor-alpha-induced inhibition of insulin signalling. J Clin Invest 1997;100(7):1863–1869.

138. Iwata M, Haruta T, Usui I, et al. Pioglitazone ameliorates tumor necrosis factor-alpha-induced insulin resistance by a mechanism independent of adipogenic activity of peroxisome proliferators-activated-receptor-gamma. Diabetes 2001;50(5):1083–1092.

139. Mohamed-Ali V, Goodrick S, Rawesh A, et al. Subcutaneous adipose tissue releases interleukin-6, but not TNF-α, in vivo. J Clin Endocrinol Metab 1997;82:4196–4200.

140. Vozarova B, Weyer C, Hanson K, Tataranni PA, Bogardus C, Pratley RE. Circulating interleukin in relation to adiposity, insulin action, and insulin secretion. Obes Res 2001;9:414–417.

141. Bastard J-P, Jardel C, Bruckert E, et al. Elevated levels of interleukin-6 are reduced in serum and subcutaneous adipose tissue of obese women after weight loss. J Clin Endocrin Metab 2000;85(9):338–342.

142. Rotter V, Nagaev I, Smith U. Interleukin-6 (IL-6) induces insulin resitance in 3T3-L1 adipocytes and is, like IL-8 and TNF-α, overexpressed in human fat cells form insulin resistant subjects. J Biol Chem 2003;278(46):45,777–45,784.

143. Stouthard JM, Oude Elferink RP, Sauerwein HP. Interleukin-6 enhances glucose transport in 3T3-L1 adipocytes. Biochem Biophys Res Commun 1996;220(2):241–245.

144. Engeli S, Feldpausch M, Gorzelniak K, et al. Association between adiponectin and mediators of inflammation in obese women. Diabetes 2003;52(4):942–947.

145. Kaser S, Kaser A, Sandhofer A, Ebenbichler CF, Tilg H, Patsch JR. Resistin messenger-RNA is increased by proinflammatory cytokines in vitro. Biochem Biophys Res Commun 2003;309(2):286–290.

146. Weyer C, Funahashi T, Tanaka S, et al. Hypoadiponectinaemia in obesity and type 2 diabetes. Close association with insulin resitance and hyperinsulinaemia. J Clin Endocrinol Metab 2001;86:1930–1935.

147. Yang WS, Jeng CY, Wu TJ, et al. Synthetic peroxisome proliferator-activated receptor-gamma agonist, rosiglitazone, increases plasma levels of adiponectin in type 2 diabetic patients Diabetes Care 2002;25(2):376–380.

148. Combs TP, Berg AH, Obicii S, Scherer PE, Rossetti L. Endogenous glucose production is inhibited by the adipose derived protein Arcp30. J Clin Invest 2001;108(12):1875–1881.

149. Fruebis J, Tsao TS, Javorschi S, et al. Proteolytic cleavage product of 30 kDa adipocyte complement related protein increases fatty acid oxidation in muscle and causes weight loss in mice. Proc Natl Acad Sci USA 2001;98(4):2005–2010.

150. Ouchi N, Kihara s, Arita Y, et al. Adiponectin, adipocyte-derived plasma protein inhibits NF-κB signalling through cAMP dependent pathway. Circulation 2000;102:1296–1301.

151. Kubota N, Teauchi Y, Yamauchi T, et al. Disruption of adiponectin causes insulin resistance and neointimal formation. Jour Biol Chem 2002;277:25,863–25,866.

152. Chen H, Montagnani M, Funahashi T, Shimomura I, Quon MJ. Adiponectin stimulates production of nitric oxide in vascular endothelial cells. J Biol Chem 2003;278(45):45,021–45,026.

153. Yokota T, Oritani K, Takahashi I, et al. Adiponectin, a new member of the family of soluble defense collagens, negatively regulates the growth of myelomonocytic progenitors and the functions of macrophages. Blood 2000;96:1723–1732.

154. Fasshauer M, Klein J, Neumann S, Eszlinger M, Paschke R. Hormonal regulation of adiponectin gene expression in 3T3-L1 adipocytes. Biochem Biophys Res Comm 2002; 290:1084–1089.

155. Kappes A, Loffler G. Influences of ionomycin, dibutyryl-cycloAMP and tumour necrosis factor-alpha on intracellular amount and secretion of apM1 in differentiating primary human preadipocytes. Horm Metab Res 2000;32:548–554.

156. Ouchi N, Kihara S, Arita Y, et al. Adipocyte-derived plasma protein, adiponectin, suppresses lipid accumulation and class A scavenger receptor expression in human monocyte-derived macrophages. Circulation 2001;103:1057–1063.

157. Halleux CM, Takahashi M, Delporte ML, et al. Secretion of adiponectin and regulation of apM1 gene expression in human visceral adipose tissue. Biochem Biophys Res Comm 2001;288:1102–1107.

158. Nishizawa H, Shimomura I, Kishida K, et al. Androgens decrease plasma adiponectin, an insulin-sensitizing adipocyte-derived protein. Diabetes 2002;51:2734–2741.

159. Steppan CM, Bailey ST, Bhat S, et al. The hormone resistin links obesity to diabetes. Nature 2001;409:307–312.

160. Lee JH, Chan JL, Yiannakouris N, et al. Circulating resistin levels are not associated with obesity or insulin resitance in humans and are not regulated by fasting or leptin administration: cross-sectional and interventional studies in normal, insulin resistant and diabetic subjects. J Clin Endocrin Metab 2003;88(10):4848–4856.

161. Janke J, Engeli S, Gorzelniak K, Luft FC, Sharma AM. Resistin gene expression in human adipocytes is not related to insulin resistance. Obes Res 2002;10(1):1–5.

162. McTernan PG, Fisher FM, Valsamakis G, et al. Resistin and type 2 diabetes: Regulation of Resistin Expression ny insulin and rosiglitazone and the effects of recombinant resistin on human differentiated adipocytes. Jour Clin Endocrin Metab 2003;88(12):6098–6106.

163. Patel L, Buckels AC, Kinghorn IJ, et al. Resistin is expressed in human macrophages and directly regulated by PPARgamma activtors. Biochem Biophys Res Commun 2003;300(2):472–476.

164. Minn AH, Patterson NB, Pack S, et al. Resistin is expressed in pancreatic islets. Biochem Biophys Res Commun 2003;310(2):641–645.

165. Yura S, Sagawa N, Itoh H, et al. Resistin is expressed in the human placenta. J Clin Endocrin Metab 2003;88(3):1394–1397.

166. Despres JP. Lipoprotein metabolism in visceral obesity International Journal of obesity 1991;2:5–15.

167. Gaziano JM. When should heart disease prevention begin. N Engl J Med 338;23:1690–1691.

168. De Fronzo RA, Varzilai N, Simonson DC. Mechanism of metformin action in obese and lean non-insulin dependent diabetic subjects. J Clin Endo Metab 991;73:1294–1301.

169. Vague P, Juhan-Vague I, Alessi MC, Badier C, Valadier J. Metformin decreases the high plasminogen activator inhibition capacity, plasma insulin and triglyceride levels in non diabetic obese subjects. Throm Haemostas 1987;57:326–328.

170. Wood D. European and American recommendations for coronary heart disease prevention. Eur Heart J 1998;19(Suppl A)A12–A19.

171. Jones AF, Game FL. Cardiovascular risk assessment. Mod Hyp Man 1999;1:10–13.

14 Diabetes and Hypertension

Samy I. McFarlane, MD, MPH,
Amal F. Farag, MD, David Gardner, MD,
and James R. Sowers, MD, FACP

CONTENTS

INTRODUCTION

Diabetes is a major public health problem that is rapidly approaching epidemic proportions in the United States and worldwide *(1–3)*. In the United States, more han 17 million persons currently have diabetes, a number that is expected to rise to 29 million by the year 2050 with a prevalence of 7.2% *(4)*. Furthermore, the economic burden of diabetes to the US economy is monumental. In the year 2002, diabetes cost the United States an estimated $132 billion in medical expenditure and lost productivity *(3)*. Cardiovascular disease (CVD) is by far the leading cause of death in people with diabetes accounting for up to 80% of mortality in this patient population *(5–8)*.

Risk factors for CVD that cluster in diabetes include hypertension, central obesity, dyslipidemia, microalbuminuria and coagulation abnormalities, and left ventricular hypertrophy (LVH) *(9)* (Table 1). Among those risk factors, hypertension is approximately as twice as frequent in patients with diabetes compared to those without the disease and accounts for up to 85% of the excess CVD risk. Conversely, patients with hypertension are more prone to have diabetes than are normotensive persons *(9)*. In a

From: *Contemporary Cardiology: Diabetes and Cardiovascular Disease, Second Edition*
Edited by: M. T. Johnstone and A. Veves © Humana Press Inc., Totowa, NJ

Table 1
Risk Factors for CVD That Cluster in Diabetes Mellitus

1. Hypertension
2. Central obesity
3. Microalbuminuria
4. Low high-density lipoprotein cholesterol levels
5. High triglycerides levels
6. Small, dense low-density lipoprotein cholesterol particles
7. Hyperinsulinemia
8. Endothelial dysfunction
9. Increased fibrinogen levels
10. Increased plasma activator inhibitor-1 levels
11. Increased C-reactive protein and other inflammatory markers
12. Absent nocturnal dipping of blood pressure and pulse
13. Left ventricular hypertrophy
14. Increased uric acid levels
15. Decreased renal function

large prospective study of 12,550 adults, the development of type 2 diabetes was almost 2.5 times as likely in patients with hypertension as in their normotensive counterparts after adjustment for age, sex, race, education, adiposity, family history with respect to diabetes, physical activity level and other health-related behaviors *(10)*.

EPIDEMILOGICAL ASPECTS OF HYPERTENSION IN DIABETICS AND THE METABOLIC SYNDROME

As a component of the metabolic syndrome, hypertension is much more common than diabetes. Data from the Third National Health and Nutrition Examination Survey (NHANES III) *(11)*, involving a representative sample of 8814 adult Americans and using the National Cholesterol Education Panel (NCEP) Adult Treatment Panel III (ATPIII) definition *(12)*, the prevalence of hypertension (as defined by blood pressure [BP] >130/85 mmHg, or the use of antihypertensive medications) was 34% compared to only 12.6% of those with hyperglycemia *(11)*. In this analysis, hypertension was the second most prevalent component of the metabolic syndrome, compared to central obesity, which was the most prevalent component (38.6%). Hypertension was followed in prevalence by low high-density lipoprotein (HDL) cholesterol (37.6%), hypertriglyceridemia (30%), and diabetes (12.6%) *(11)*. However, it is important to emphasize that although most patients with the metabolic syndrome do not have diabetes, the prevalence of this syndrome in the diabetic population is very high (86%) *(13,14)*. Furthermore, the prevalence of the metabolic syndrome in patients with impaired glucose tolerance (IGT) was 31% and 71% in those with impaired fasting glucose (IFG; >110 mmHg) *(13,14)*.

The overall prevalence of the NCEP-defined metabolic syndrome *(12)* among adults over the age of 20 years was 24% and above 40% in those over the age of 40 years *(11,13,14)*. The prevalence among women was 23.4% compared to 24% for men. However, there were significant ethnic differences as Mexican-American women had the highest prevalence of 35.6% compared to 22.8% for white women *(11)*. African-American men in this analysis had the lowest prevalence of the metabolic syndrome (16.4%) *(11)*. This could be explained by the use of separate lipid criteria as defined by NCEP (high triglycerides and low HDL-cholesterol), which likely offset the high prevalence of hypertension and hyperglycemia African-American population *(11,13)*. In fact, African-American men had highest prevalence of hypertension, as a component of the metabolic syndrome, of 49.9%, followed by African-American women (43.3%) and Mexican-American men (40.2) *(11)*.

Another analysis of NHANES data aiming to evaluate the risk of coronary heart disease (CHD), among people over the age of 50 years with the metabolic syndrome with and without diabetes showed that the overall prevalence of this syndrome is 44% *(15)*. In this analysis, which also used the NCEP definition *(12)*, the prevalence of diabetes was 17% for the entire population and 86% for those with the metabolic syndrome *(15)*. Hypertension was almost as twice as common in diabetic patients with the metabolic syndrome (82.7%), compared to diabetic patients without the syndrome (43%) *(15)*. These data underscore the common occurrence of diabetes and hypertension as components of the metabolic syndrome, particularly in the older population. Hypertension was the strongest predictor for the presence of CHD in patients over the age of 50, followed by low HDL cholesterol and diabetes. The odds ratio, 95% confidence interval was 1.87 (1.37–2.56), 1.74 (1.18–2.58), and 1.55 (1.07–2.25) for hypertension, low HDL cholesterol, and diabetes, respectively *(15)*.

A third analysis, from Europe *(16)*, using the World Heath Organization (WHO) definition *(17)*, was conducted to evaluate the prevalence and CVD risk associated with the metabolic syndrome. In this analysis, 4483 patients, age 35 to 70 years participating in a large study of type 2 diabetics in Finland and Sweden (the Botnia study) *(18)* were examined. The metabolic syndrome, as defined by the WHO, was present in 10% of those without diabetes compared to 50% of those with IFG/IGT, and 80% of those with diabetes *(16)*. The prevalence of the metabolic syndrome in diabetic patients in this European population, using the WHO definition, was close to that of the US population using the NCEP criteria (80% vs 86% respectively) *(15,16)*. Furthermore, hypertension occurred frequently in those with diabetes (59%), this prevalence increased with age and was 67% in those 60 to 69 years of age *(16)*. In this study hypertension was only second to microalbuminuria as the most potent predictor for CVD mortality *(16)*. These data from the United States and Europe, across different ethnic populations using the NCEP or WHO, consistently demonstrate the high prevalence of the metabolic syndrome that is approaching epidemic proportions in the United States and worldwide. These data also demonstrate the frequent occurrence of hypertension and diabetes mellitus as components of the metabolic syndrome conferring high risk for CVD in this patient population *(11,15,16)*.

HEMODYNAMIC AND METABOLIC CHARACTERISTICS OF HYPERTENSION IN DIABETICS

Hypertension in patients with diabetes, compared to those without diabetes, has unique features such as increased salt sensitivity, volume expansion, loss of nocturnal dipping of BP and pulse, increased propensity to proteinuria, orthostatic hypotension and, isolated systolic hypertension *(9)*. Most of these features are considered risk factors for CVD *(5)* and are particularly important for selecting the appropriate antihypertensive medication. For example, low-dose diuretics should be considered for the treatment of volume expansion, while angiotensin-converting enzyme (ACE) inhibitors or angiotensin receptor blockers (ARBs) used for those with proteinuria.

Loss of Nocturnal Decline of BP (Nondipping)

In normotensive individuals and most patients with hypertension, there is a reproducible circadian pattern to BP and heart rate during 24-hour ambulatory monitoring (19). Typically, the BP is highest while the patient is awake and lowest during sleep, a pattern called "dipping," in which BP decreases by 10% to 15%. Patients with loss of nocturnal decline in BP "nondippers" have less than 10% decline of BP during the night compared to daytime BP values (20). In patients with diabetes, and many of those with the cardiometabolic syndrome, there is a loss of nocturnal dipping as demonstrated by 24-hour ambulatory monitoring of BP. This is particularly important because the loss of nocturnal dipping conveys excessive risk for stroke and myocardial infarction (MI) (20–22). Indeed, ambulatory BP has been reported to be superior to office BP in predicting target organ involvement such as LVH and proteinuria (21,22). About 30% of MIs and 50% of strokes occur between 6AM and noon (23). This is especially important in deciding the optimal dosing strategies of antihypertensive medications where drugs that provide consistent and sustained 24-hour BP control will be advantageous (23). Indeed, nighttime BP control may be especially important in those diabetic patients with elevated nocturnal BP (9).

Volume Expansion and Salt Sensitivity

Alterations in sodium balance and extracellular fluid volume, have heterogeneous effects on BP in both normotensive and hypertensive subjects (24). Increased salt intake does not raise BP in all hypertensive subjects and sensitivity to dietary salt intake is greatest in the elderly, those with diabetes, obesity, renal insufficiency, low renin status and African Americans (25,26). Indeed salt sensitivity in normotensive subjects is associated with a greater age-related increase in BP (26). This is particularly important to consider in management of hypertension in patients with diabetes, especially elderly persons, because the prevalence of both diabetes and salt sensitivity also increases with age. Thus, a decreased salt intake along with other aspects of diet such as reduced fat and increased potassium are important to institute in these patients (9).

Microalbuminuria

There is considerable evidence that hypertension in type 1diabetes is a consequence, rather than a cause of renal disease and that nephropathy precedes the rise in BP (9). Persistent hypertension in patients with type 1 diabetes is often a manifestation of diabetic nephropathy as indicated by an elevation of the urinary albumin at diagnosis of diabetes (9,27). Both hypertension and nephropathy appear to exacerbate each other. In type 2 Diabetes, microalbuminuria is associated with insulin resistance (5,28), salt sensitivity, loss of nocturnal dipping, and other components of the metabolic syndrome (28,29). Elevated systolic BP (SBP) is a significant determining factor in the progression of microalbuminuria (29,30). Indeed, there is an increasing evidence that microalbuminuria is an integral component of the metabolic syndrome associated with hypertension (5,9,29). This concept is important to consider in selecting the pharmacological therapy for hypertension in patients with diabetes, as medications that decrease both proteinuria and BP, such as ACE inhibitors and ARBs, have evolved as increasingly important tools in reducing the progression of nephropathy in such patients. These agents also appear to improve insulin sensitivity *(9)*. Furthermore, aggressive BP lowering, often requiring several drugs, is very important in controlling the progressive course of diabetic renal disease. Other factors that are important include cholesterol and glycemic control and smoking cessation *(9)*.

Isolated Systolic Hypertension

With the progression of atherosclerosis in patients with diabetes, the larger arteries lose elasticity and become rigid and the SBP increases disproportionately because the arterial system is incapable of expansion for any given volume of blood ejected from the left ventricle leading to isolated systolic hypertension, which is more common and occurs at a relatively younger age in patients with diabetes *(9,31)*. Indeed, the relationship between systolic elevations in BP and micro/macrovascular disease is especially pronounced in patients with diabetes mellitus (DM) *(9)*.

Orthostatic Hypotension

Pooling of blood in dependent veins during rising from a recumbent position, normally leads to decrease in stroke volume and SBP with a concomitant sympathomimetic reflex-induced increase in systemic vascular resistance, diastolic BP (DBP), and heart rate. In patients with diabetes and autonomic dysfunction, excessive venous pooling and impaired baroreflex sensitivity can cause immediate or delayed orthostatic hypotension, and thus may result in a reduction in cerebral blood flow leading to intermittent lightheadedness, fatigue, unsteady gait, and syncope *(32–34)*. This is important to recognize in patients with diabetes and hypertension because it has several diagnostic and therapeutic implications. For example, discontinuation of diuretic therapy and peripheral vasodilators and volume repletion might be necessary for the treatment of chronic orthostasis. Also, in the subset of patients with "hyperadrenergic" orthostatic hypertension as manifested by excessive sweating and palpitation, the use of low-dose clonidine might be necessary to blunt an excess sympathetic response *(35)*. Furthermore, increased propensity for orthostatic hypertension in patients with diabetes renders peripheral α-adrenergic receptor blockers less desirable and second-line agents for these patients. Additionally, doses of all antihypertensive agents must be titrated more carefully in patients with diabetes who have greater propensity for orthostatic hypertension while having high supine BPs.

PATHOPHYSIOLOGY OF HYPERTENSION IN DIABETICS

The relation between hypertension, obesity, insulin resistance, and diabetes is complex. For example, hypertension is considerably more prevalent in diabetic patients than nondiabetics *(5,9)*. When matched to age, gender, ethnicity, adiposity, level of physical activity, and family history, hypertension is 2.5 times more likely to develop in type 2 diabetics than nondiabetics *(5,9)*. Possible reasons for the increased propensity to develop diabetes in persons with essential hypertension have been reviewed extensively *(5,9)*. These include an altered skeletal muscle tissue composition (i.e., more fat and less insulin-sensitive slow-twitch fibers), decreased blood flow to skeletal muscle tissue as a result of vascular hypertrophy, rarefaction and vasoconstriction and impaired postreceptor regulatory responses to insulin *(9)* (Table 2).

In type 1 diabetics, hypertension is uncommon in the absence of diabetic renal disease *(9)*. BP readings start to rise about 3 years after the onset of microalbuminuria *(5,9)*. In

Table 2
Pathophysiological Mechanisms of Insulin Resistance Associated
With Hypertension

Decreased delivery of insulin and glucose to skeletal muscles

1. Increased vasoconstriction
2. Vascular hypertrophy
3. Vascular refraction

Alteration of skeletal muscle fibers

1. Decreased insulin-sensitive slow-muscle twitch fibers
2. Increased fat interspersed with skeletal muscle fibers

Postreceptor insulin-signaling defect

1. Decreased PI3 kinase/AKT signaling responses to insulin
2. Decreased insulin-mediated glucose transport
3. Decreased glycogen synthase activity

contrast, in the Hypertension in Diabetes Study, 3648 patients recruited for the United Kingdom Prospective Diabetes Study (UKPDS) were examined; hypertension already existed in 39% of newly diagnosed type 2 diabetes cases *(37)*. In these patients, hypertension was often associated with other components of the metabolic syndrome such as obesity, elevated triglycerides, and elevated hyperinsemia. The prevalence of microalbuminuria in this hypertensive group was 24% *(37)*. These findings highlight differences in hypertension pathophysiology of types 1 and 2 diabetes, with hypertension in the latter being more closely linked to other components of the cardiometabolic syndrome *(9)*.

Microalbuminuria is often the first clinical sign of diabetic nephropathy. It is not only a risk factor for diabetic nephropathy, but also a risk factor of CVD morbidity and mortality in both diabetic and nondiabetic patients *(38)*. Microalbuminuria reflects generalized endothelial cell dysfunction including that occurring in renal glomeruli *(5,9)*. Hypertension and diabetic nephropathy exacerbate each other, and contribute to a cycle of progressive hypertension, nephropathy, and CVD. Several other renal-related factors contribute to the increased propensity to develop hypertension and subsequent complications in diabetic patients. Diabetic patients have an increased propensity to sodium retention and volume expansion *(39)*. Increased salt sensitivity in these patients involves multiple mechanisms including hyperglycemia-induced renal sodium reabsorption in the proximal renal tubule *(40)*, hyperinsulinemia, and renal abnormalities in renin–angiotensin–aldosterone system (RAAS) *(41)*. Thus, restriction of salt in the diet of these patients is important in the management of their hypertension *(9)*.

Insulin resistance and hyperinsulinemia increase sympathetic activity, which is associated with renal sodium retention, and predispose to increased vascular resistance *(5,9)*. Insulin normally enhances vasodilatation and increases muscle blood flow, which facilitates glucose utilization *(41–45)*. This effect is mediated, in part, by increased production of nitric oxide (NO) production *(44)*, as insulin increases endothelial NO synthase activity. Insulin fails to enhance muscle blood flow in both obese and diabetic patients as a result of decreased ability to stimulate NO *(45)*. Hyperinsulinemia and insulin resistance do not consistently lead to hypertension. Pima Indians have an increased incidence of obesity, insulin resistance, and hyperinsulinemia, but have a relatively low incidence of hypertension (2). These observations indicate that the relationship between insulin resistance and hypertension is complex, and dependent also on ethnic and environmental factors.

Obesity, especially central obesity, is a risk factor for both hypertension and diabetes (46,47). Central obesity, insulin resistance, hypertension, and diabetic dyslipidemia are parts of the cardiometabolic syndrome (5,9,48–61). There are other abnormalities found in the cardiometabolic syndrome such as microalbuminuria, increased coagulability, impaired fibrinolysis, and increased inflammatory status (5). Several definitions of the metabolic syndrome have been recently published; one by the WHO (15,16), and another by the NCEP- ATPIII in the United States (12). The cardiometabolic syndrome is a common disorder, the prevalence in the United States, using NCEP criteria, is 22% (15,16). The prevalence of this syndrome, and that of type 2 diabetes increases progressively with advancing age, obesity, and sedentary lifestyle (8,9).

The etiology of the cardiometabolic syndrome is complex, involving genetic and acquired abnormalities (5,9). Central obesity is a key element in the pathogenesis of this syndrome. It is characterized by a greater deposition of fat in the upper or central part of the body (visceral fat). Visceral adipocytes are more metabolically active and insulin - resistant than peripheral adipocytes (46). They release several cytokines like tumor necrosis factor α and interleukin-(IL)-6 that promote inflammation, dyslipidemia, hypertension, microalbuminuria, abnormal coagulability, and impaired fibrinolysis (46,47). Lipolysis of the abdominal fat releases free fatty acids, which are substrates for triglycerides production in the liver (45,52,56). The renin–angiotensin system (RAS) is also very active in the central adipocytes (47,57). Furthermore, adipocyte-derived peptides have a role in promoting the cardiometabolic syndrome. For example, leptin levels are high in obese patients, and elevated leptin levels may stimulate the sympathetic nervous system and may contribute to the pathogenesis of hypertension associated with obesity (46,47,54). Adiponectin has anti-inflammatory effects and its levels are low in insulin resistance conditions (47,52,56). Decreased adiponectin levels may be particularly important, given the role of adiponectin in enhancement of insulin-mediated vasodilatation and glucose transport activities (47,57). Finally, high concentrations of resistin (an adipocyte-derived peptide) in visceral fat are associated with both insulin resistance and obesity (58). This peptide, in contradistinction to adiponectin, inhibits insulin metabolic actions (46,47,58,60).

CARDIOVASCULAR EFFECTS OF INSULIN AND INSULIN-LIKE GROWTH FACTOR-1 IN THE NORMAL AND IN THE INSULIN-RESISTANT STATE

Insulin and its highly homologous peptide, insulin-like growth factor (IGF-1), both have important effects on vascular tone. Insulin is produced only in the pancreas (61). On the other hand, IGF-1 is an autocrine/paracrine peptide (59–69) produced by endothelial cells and vascular smooth muscle cells (VSMCs) following stimulation by insulin (61,62), angiotensin 2 (61,63), and mechanical stress (65,66). Furthermore, IGF-1 receptors are expressed to a greater extent than insulin receptors in VSMCs (60,61). IGF-1 has many important biological effects on the vasculature, including maintenance of the normal differentiated VSMC phenotype (67), glucose transport (68,69), and modulation of vascular tone *(61,64,68–81)*. IGF-1 and insulin normally attenuate vasoconstriction/enhance relaxation through a phosphatidylinositol 3-kinase (PI3K)-dependent stimulation of vascular NO synthase (NOS) enzyme *(61,68,69,71,76,78,80,81)* and Na+,K+-ATPase pump activity *(61,64,74,79,82,83)*. In animal models of obesity, insulin resistance and hypertension there is accumulating evidence that resistance to PI3K-signaling by IGF-1 and insulin plays an important role in the pathogenesis of hypertension *(61,75,78,84)*, impaired myocardial function *(61,80,85–93)*, and attenuated glucose transport *(67,83,86)*. Thus, alterations of cardiovascular and skeletal muscle IGF-2 and insulin signaling responses may explain the common co-existence of hypertension, insulin resistance and type 2 diabetes *(61,65,70)*.

Insulin and IGF-1 normally induce vasorelaxation, in part, by lowering VSMC intracellular calcium ([Ca2+]i) levels *(67,72,74,83)* and myosin light chain (MLC) phosphorylation/Ca2+ sensitization *(72,83)*. These actions involve activation of both vascular NOS and Na+,K+-ATPase pump activity *(64,68–74,78–83)*. Upon stimulation, the β-subunit of the insulin and IGF-1 receptor not only become phosphorylated on various tyrosine sites but also induce the phosphorylation of a number of accessory molecules *(60)*, such as insulin receptor substrate (IRS)-1, which serve as important docking sites for many kinases and phosphatases. Many insulin and IGF-1 metabolic effects are mediated by PI3K upon binding to IRS-1 through its regulatory subunit (p85) SH2 domain *(60)*. An important downstream target of IGF-1/insulin-stimulated PI3K is the serine-threonine kinase, Akt (protein kinase B) *(60,71,94,95)*. Akt interacts through its pleckstrin homology domain with the phospholipids produced by PI3K. Phosphorylation of Thr308 and Ser473 of Akt is important for its activation *(94,95)*. Akt is involved in insulin and IGF-1-regulated glucose transport and other cell functions *(94–100)*. A number of studies have demonstrated a critical role for Akt signaling in mediating the vascular actions of IGF-1/insulin *(71,79,98–103)*. Furthermore, it has been observed that angiotensin II (Ang II) inhibits IGF-1 signaling through the PI3K/Akt pathway resulting in less NOS/Na+, K+-ATPase activation in VSMCs *(80)*. Vascular relaxation in response to insulin and IGF-1 signaling is dependent, in part, on endothelial cells and VSMC production of NO and reductions in VSMC [Ca2+]i. The NO/cyclic guanosine monophosphate (cGMP) increase in response to insulin and IGF-1 stimulation results in inhibition of MLC phosphorylation/activation *(104)* by increasing the activity of the myosin-bound serine/threonine specific phosphatase (MBP) *(104–107)*. This effect of insulin and IGF-1 thus counterbalances the increase in [Ca2+]i and the Ca2+-MLC sensitization effects mediated by vasoconstrictor agonists such as Ang II *(108–111)*.

Accumulating evidence suggests that Ang II may antagonize the vasodilatory actions of insulin/IGF-1 through small-molecular-weight G protein-signaling mechanism *(108–112)*, increasing phosphorylation and activation of MLC *(109,110)*. Thus, there appears to be counterbalancing actions between insulin/IGF-1 and Ang II and other vasoconstrictors in the modulation of MLC-Ca2+ sensitization/vascular tone. Generation of vascular tissue reactive oxygen species appears to be an important mechanism by which Ang II inhibits the metabolic signaling pathways by insulin and IGF-1 *(113)*.

Insulin and IGF-1 also regulates vascular tone by increasing the VSMC Na+,K+-ATPase pump activity in VSMCs *(64,72,74,77)*, consequently elevating the transmembrane Na+ gradient that drives Ca2+ efflux via Na+/Ca2+ exchange *(64,72,74,82–84)*. Furthermore, insulin/IGF-1 may indirectly activate the Na+,K+-ATPase pump, and MBP, in VSMC by stimulating VSMC NO/cGMP *(113)*. Thus, in insulin-resistant

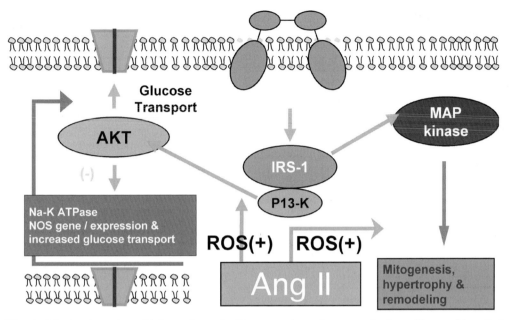

Fig. 1. Mechanisms by which angiotensin II antagonizes the vasorelaxing effects of insulin/ insulin-like growth factor-1.

states, including that associated with type 2 diabetes, there appears to exhibit vascular resistance to the vasodilatory actions of insulin and IGF-1 *(113–116)*. Increasingly, it appears that increased secretion of Ang II and consequent generation of reactive oxygen species *(71)* in vasculature contributes to this resistance *(71)* (Fig. 1).

TREATMENT GOALS AND PHARMACOLOGICAL THERAPY

The goal of lowering BP in persons with diabetes and hypertension is to prevent the inordinate hypertension-associated death and disability in this population *(9,117–124)*. Because of increased BP variability in these patients, more BP measurements over a longer period are needed to establish the "representative BP." Because of the greater propensity to orthostatic hypotension, standing BPs should be obtained on each office visit *(9,32–34)*. Therapy should begin with lifestyle modifications (Table 3) involving weight reduction, increased physical activity, and moderation of dietary salt and alcohol intake *(125)*.

Drug therapy should be initiated along with lifestyle modifications to lower BP to less than 130/80 mmHg in diabetic persons, a goal that is recommended by the American Diabetes Association and the Joint National Committee on Prevention, Detection, Evaluation, and Treatment of High Blood Pressure, seventh report (JNC 7) *(125)*. JNC 7 recommended four classes of drugs as effective first-line therapy in these patients *(120)*. Each drug class has potential advantages and disadvantages. Furthermore, most diabetic patients will need several different agents to lower BP adequately.

In diabetic patients, the benefit of tight BP control is well established *(9)*. The UKPDS trial *(118)* included 1148 hypertensive patients who were followed up for about 8.4 years. Tight BP control (<140/82 mmHg) compared to less tight control (<180/105 mmHg) was associated with a 24% reduction in diabetic-related endpoints, 32% in death related to diabetes, 44% in stroke, and a 37% reduction in microvascular complications. Interestingly, the relative benefits of strict BP control outweighed the benefits of tight blood glucose control.

Another major study, the Hypertension Optimal Trial, demonstrated a 51% reduction in major CVD events in the diabetic subgroup that was randomized to a DBP goal of less than 80 mmHg compared to a goal of less than 90 mmHg *(119)*. Other studies reported significant advantages of hypertension treatment in special categories of diabetic patient like the elderly and those with isolated systolic hypertension *(120,121)*. Based on the results of these clinical trials and on the data from epidemiological studies which suggested an increase in CVD events and mortality with BP more than 115/75 mmHg *(122)*, the currently recommended BP goal in diabetic patients is now less than 130/80 mmHg (Fig. 2) *(123–125)*.

Lifestyle Modifications in Management of Hypertension (Table 3)

Adaptation of a healthy lifestyle is an essential component of managing hypertension in patients with diabetes or the cardiometabolic syndrome *(123–125)*. These interventions include weight loss, dietary sodium reduction, increased aerobic physical activity, cigarette-smoking cessation, and moderation of alcohol intake (Table 1) *(125,126)*. The Dietary Approach to Stop Hypertension (DASH) diet, when combined with sodium reduction (2300 mg per day) is effective in lowering BP *(126)*. The DASH diet is rich in fiber, potassium, and calcium, low in cholesterol (150 mg per day), low in total and saturated fat (20% and 6% of daily calories, respectively), with 55% of daily calories coming from carbohydrates.

In addition to lowering BP, weight reduction and increased physical activity improve insulin resistance, serum glucose levels, and lipid profiles *(127)*. Exercise and weight reduction have also been shown to reduce the development of type 2 diabetes in patients with IGT *(128)*. The protective effects of physical activity have been demonstrated in prospective cohort studies *(128–132)*, where the development of type 2 diabetes was significantly lower in patients who exercise regularly even after adjustment for obesity, hypertension, and family history of diabetes. In these studies, the reduction in the development of type 2 diabetes was strongest among patients with hypertension and those with the highest risk for the development of diabetes *(128–130)*. More recently, the Finnish study and the US Diabetes Prevention Program *(130–132)* have shown that diet and exercise reduces the risk of development of type 2 diabetes, by more than 50% in high-risk patients with IGT. Therefore, these interventions are highly recommended in patients with hypertension who are at risk for the development of type 2 diabetes *(9)*.

Pharmacological Therapy for Hypertension in Patients With Diabetes

Diet and lifestyle modifications are usually the first step in the management of hypertension, but most diabetic patients will also require pharmacological treatment. In fact, most diabetic patients need more than one medication to maintain their BP within the target range of less than 130/80 *(123,125)*. Initiation of therapy with two drugs should be considered if BP is more than 20/10 mmHg above the goal i.e., less than or equal to 150/90 *(125)*. The optimal goal BP in patients with the cardiometabolic syndrome (without overt diabetes) is not known. However, because these patients are at high risk for CVD, it currently appears prudent to treat BP more aggressively than in the general population (i.e., same goal as in type 2 diabetic patients <130/80) *(5,9,125)*.

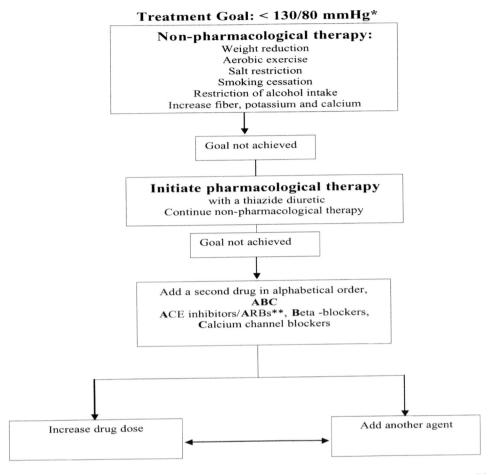

Fig. 2. Flow chart showing appropriate measures for lowering the blood pressure in patients with diabetes and hypertension.

THIAZIDE DIURETICS

Thiazides are an important component of hypertension treatment in almost all hypertension cases. They are inexpensive and effective, especially in treating systolic hypertension *(121)*. The Antihypertensive and Lipid Lowering treatment to prevent Heart Attack Trial (ALLHAT) included more than 33,000 patients aged 55 or older with at least one other CHD risk factor who were followed up for a mean period of 4.9 years *(133)*. The study showed that there was no difference between chlorthalidone (a thiazide), lisinopril (an ACE inhibitor), and amlodipine (a calcium channel blocker [CCB]) in preventing major coronary events or in their effects on overall survival. Chlorthalidone was associated with less combined CVD, stroke, and better BP control than lisinopril, especially in African Americans. Chlorthalidone, however, was associated with less heart failure incidence rate than both lisinopril and amlodipine *(133)*. It should be noted

Table 3
Lifestyle and Dietary Modification in Hypertension Management

1. Weight loss (maintain normal body weight [BMI, 18.5–24.9])
2. Exercise (aerobic physical activity) 30–45 minutes at least three times a week
3. Reduced sodium intake to 100 mmol (2.4 g) per day
4. Smoking cessation
5. Adequate intake of dietary potassium, calcium, and magnesium.
6. Reduced alcohol intake to <1 oz of ethanol (24 oz of beer) per day.
7. Diet rich in fruits and vegetables but low in fat

BMI, body mass index.

that the inability to use a diuretic in those patients randomized to lisinopril may have unmasked early heart failure. In clinical practice, the combination of ACE inhibitors and thiazide diuretics is a well-accepted treatment strategy in these patients (9).

The ALLHAT study, the largest hypertension trial to date, was not designed to prospectively assess the treatment effect in the diabetic patients. However, the diabetic cohort was predesigned for subgroup analysis. About 36% of ALLHAT participants had diabetes (134); the benefits of chlorthalidone were noticed in both diabetic and nondiabetic populations, however, for the diabetic patients, several points need to be made in order for the results of the ALLHAT trial to be viewed in the proper context:

1. Optimal control of BP in people with diabetes is difficult to achieve and requires multiple medications. Data from our investigative group showed that in a large diabetic cohort, with a mean age of 64.5 years (close to ALLHAT 66.6 mean age in the diabetic subgroup), a BP goal of 130/80 was achieved in only 25% of the patients. Furthermore, an average of 3.1 medications was required to achieve such a goal (135). The fact that diabetic patients require multiple antihypertensive medications for BP control is documented in all the major hypertension trials. This fact makes the issue of the initial antihypertensive therapy in people with diabetes less relevant.
2. The study clearly illustrates the importance of lowering BP to improve the CVD outcome. Therefore, efforts should be directed toward improving BP control that is currently suboptimal (135).
3. Although BP reduction was in favor of the diuretic group, there was a lack of difference in the primary outcome (fatal CHD or nonfatal MI) among treatment groups. Although ACE inhibitors have been shown to be beneficial in reducing mortality in heart failure patients (136), the observation that diuretic treatment is associated with less incidence of heart failure than ACE inhibitor treatment was likely the result, in part, of unmasking of early heart failure as a result of the inability to add a diuretic to the ACE inhibitor regimen. This also may be explained by the higher BP in the ACE inhibitor group, and in particular African-American subjects who may have less BP response to ACE inhibitors than whites. The efficacy of ACE inhibitors in diabetic nephropathy is well documented. Therefore, it is of major importance to know the results of the drug comparisons in the diabetic subjects involved in the study.
4. The ALLHAT, with its simple office-based design, did not offer information that is particularly relevant for the diabetic population such as the use of combination antihypertensive medications, or the treatment of diabetic patients with albuminuria or compromised renal function.

Furthermore, it is important to note that thiazide diuretics have been shown to increase insulin resistance *(9)* and have some adverse metabolic side effects; such as a small increase in serum blood sugar *(125)*, increased serum triglycerides, increased total cholesterol, increased serum uric acid, hyponatremia, hypokalemia, and hypomagnesemia. However, it is likely that some of these adverse effects can be minimized by using low doses of thiazides such as 12.5 mg of chlorthalidone or 25 mg of hydrochlorothiazide in combination with an ACE inhibitors or ARBs.

In using diuretics, it is important to avoid volume depletion and orthostatic hypotension. Diabetic patients with autonomic neuropathy, especially elderly people, are more prone to orthostatic hypotension with subsequent risk of falls *(9,32–34)*. This is particularly important in elderly diabetic patients who are often on multiple hypertensive medications *(9)*.

ACE INHIBITORS AND ARBS

The RAAS is linked to the pathophysiology of various conditions such as hypertension, dyslipidemia, insulin resistance, and inflammation. Ang II has two major types of receptors; ATI and ATII. ATI receptors are responsible for most the deleterious effects of Ang II including vasoconstriction and aldosterone release, and growth and remodeling *(135,136)* ACE inhibitors block the conversion of Ang I to Ang II. ARBs selectively block the binding of Ang II to (AT1) receptors. ACE is also a kininase, degrading bradykinin to nonactive products, thus ACE inhibitor treatment increases kinins levels *(135)*. Bradykinin is a vasodilator, which might be beneficial for hypertension, as it promotes endothelial production of NO *(9)*. However, it might be also responsible for the cough that some patients develop while taking ACE inhibitors.

Multiple clinical trials have provided cumulative evidence that using an antihypertensive agent that interrupts the RAS results in beneficial CVD and renal outcomes in hypertensive diabetic patients *(135–137)*. For example, the Heart Outcomes Prevention Evaluation (HOPE) study included 3577 diabetic patients who had also at least one other CVD risk factor. The participants were randomized to receive either ramipril (an ACE inhibitor) or placebo and were followed up for about 4.5 years. Compared to placebo, ramipril lowered the rates of MI, stroke, and all-cause mortality in diabetic patients by 22%, 33%, and 24%, respectively *(138)*. The CVD benefits of an ARB (losartan) were compared to a β-blocker (atenolol), in the Losartan Intervention For Endpoint reduction (LIFE) study. Losartan in diabetic hypertensive patients with LVH lowered the CVD mortality and total mortality by 37% and 39%, respectively *(139)*. In the HOPE trial, new-onset diabetes was decreased by 35%, and in the LIFE study, new-onset diabetes was decreased by 25% of those that began the study without evidence of clinical diabetes *(138,139)*. In the recent valsartan antihypertensive long-term use evaluation (VALUE) trial, new-onset diabetes was decreased in the valsartan group by 23% compared to the amlodipine treated patients *(140)*.

RAAS blockade has also been shown to reduce the risk for renal disease and renal disease progression in diabetes *(135)*. The benefits of ACE inhibitors in renal disease in type 2 appear promising, but there is a need for more investigation *(141)*. On the other hand, several major clinical trials—the Reduction of End-points in NIDDM with Angiotensin II Antagonist Losartan (RENAAL) trial *(142)*, the IRbesartan MicroAlbuminuria type II diabetes in hypertension patients (IRMA II) trial *(143)*, the Irbesartan in Diabetic Nephropathy Trial *(144)*, and the Microalbuminuria Reduction with VALsartan *(145)* demonstrated the renal protection effects of ARBs. Indeed, the mean BP was similar in the placebo and valsaratan-treated groups, indicating that ARBs renal protection effects are independent of BP reduction. In the RENAAL trial, which was done on diabetic patients with impaired renal function (creatinine 1.3–3 mg/dL) and proteinuria, losartan reduced the risk of the primary end-point (a composite of doubling of serum creatinine, end-stage renal disease [ESRD], and death from any cause) by 16%. The risk of doubling of serum creatinine and ESRD was reduced by 25% and 28%, respectively (142). Furthermore, the risk of the first hospitalization for congestive heart failure was reduced by 32%. Treatment with 300 mg of irbesartan in the IRMA II trial increased regression of microalbuminuria back to values within the normal range by 37% (143). The combination of an ACE inhibitor and an ARB in the Candesartan And Lisinopril Microalbuminuria trial was associated with significantly more reduction in urinary albumin to creatinine ratio (50%) than with either agent alone (24% for candesartan and 39% for lisinopril) (146).

ACE inhibitors are generally well tolerated by patients; they have no adverse effects on lipids or cation metabolism. Clinically important side effects are cough (up to 15%), hyperkalemia, and rarely angioedema. In patients with underlying renal disease or long-standing hypertension, initiation of ACE inhibitor therapy might cause a small increase in serum creatinine levels, which does not necessitate discontinuation of the agents. If creatinine levels rise to more than 30% or show progressive increase on repeated measurements, treatment should be stopped and volume status examined carefully (147). Many of these patients will be hypovolemic as a result of over treament with diuretics, and with the resumption of more normal volume status, the ACE inhibitors can be safely reinitiated. ACE inhibitors are relatively contraindicated in patients with bilateral renal artery stenosis or unilateral renal stenosis if they have one kidney as a result of a greater risk of these patients to develop acute renal failure. ARBs are very well tolerated, and the incidence rates of cough and angioedema are much lower than those of ACE inhibitor treatment (148,149). Both hyperkalemia and azotemia may be associated with ARB and ACE inhibitory therapy. The JNC 7 recommended the use of an ARB as one of several alternative first-line therapies for patients with hypertension who cannot tolerate or who do not respond to the recommended first-line medications (127). Additionally, ARBs were also recommended as an initial therapy for those who could not tolerate ACE inhibitors (usually because of cough) and in whom ACE inhibitors are recommended (127), such as patients with diabetes and proteinuria, heart failure, systolic dysfunction, post-MI and those with mild renal insufficiency.

The combination of ACE inhibitors/ARBs with thiazides helps to minimize the adverse effect on serum potassium levels. The interesting finding from HOPE and LIFE trials suggests that both ACE inhibitors and ARBs decrease the incidence of new-onset diabetes (138,139). Ongoing prospective studies are more definitely evaluating the potential of these agents to lessen the development of clinical diabetes in patients with essential hypertension and others with high risk for developing diabetes (128).

β-Blockers

β-Blockers are useful in the treatment of hypertensive diabetic patients with ischemic heart disease. There are some concerns regarding their metabolic adverse effects. In the Atherosclerosis Risk In Communities study, β-Blocker treatment was associated with 28% increased risk of developing diabetes compared to no-medication group (150). β-Blockers are a heterogeneous class of medications, having disparate metabolic and hemodynamic properties (150). Both selective β-1 blockers and nonselective β-blockers increase insulin resistance. In contrast, vasodilating β-blockers may improve insulin action *(151)*. In a study of 45 hypertensive diabetic patients who where treated with either carvedilol or atenolol, carvedilol was associated with 20% increase in glucose disposal (vs 10% decrease with atenolol), a 20% reduction in serum triglyceride levels (vs 12% elevation), and an 8% increase in serum HDL cholesterol (vs 12% decrease with atenolol) *(152)*. Further trials are needed to investigate the potential benefits of vasodilator β-blockers in diabetic patients. On the other hand, results from large clinical trials demonstrated the benefits of β-1 selective blockers in diabetic population, particularly in those with CHD. In the UKPDS study, atenolol was as effective as captopril in reducing microvascular and macrovascular events *(118)*.

CALCIUM CHANNEL BLOCKERS

CCBs are generally classified into two classes, dihydropyridines (DHP-CCBs; e.g., nifedipine and newer agents like amlodipine) and nondihydropyridines (NDHP-CCBs; e.g., verapamil and diltiazem). Long-acting DHP-CCBs and NDHP-CCBs are safe, effective, and have no adverse effects on serum lipids. They can be added to ACE inhibitors and diuretics in diabetic patients to achieve the BP target of 130/80 mmHg *(31)*. In the ALLHAT study, amlodipine had comparable effects to chlorthalidone on CHD, stroke, and all-cause mortality rate. Interestingly, noncardiovascular mortality rate was significantly lower and renal function better preserved in amlodipine group *(133)*. The ALLHAT study underscores the value of DHP-CCBs, as one of the antihypertensive drugs that are useful in treating the patients with diabetes and hypertension *(31,133)*. In the VALUE study *(140)*, amlodipine was associated with a more pronounced BP control, particularly early in the trial, compared to valsartan. However, despite BP differences, the primary composite cardiac endpoint was not different between the two treatment groups *(140)*.

Other Pharmacological Interventions to Treat Coronary Heart Disease Risk Factors

In addition to lifestyle modifications and antihypertensive medications, it is very important to address the other CVD risk factors, which are commonly found in hypertensive diabetic population. For example, the degree of hyperglycemia is associated epidemiologically with the incidence of microvascular and macrovascular disease. Controlling blood sugar significantly improves microvascular complications, but effects on macrovascular complications have not been proved *(153)*. On the other hand, statin therapy is highly beneficial for diabetic patients *(154–156)*. The beneficial effects of statins are independent of their classical actions on lipoproteins *(156)*. These effects include reductions in inflammation in the vasculature, kidney, and bone. Potential beneficial effects of these agents also include enhancement of NO production in vasculature and the kidney. These agents may improve insulin sensitivity and reduce the likelihood of persons progressing from IGT to type 2 diabetes *(156)*.

The low-density lipoprotein (LDL) cholesterol goal in diabetic patient, as generally recognized, is less than 100 mg /dL *(12)*, or lower. Furthermore, a non-HDL cholesterol of less than 130 mg/dL, in those with serum triglyceride levels greater than 200 mg/dL is increasingly recognized as an important target goal, as well *(12)*. Diabetes and hypertension associated with high risk for stroke. Using aspirin along with hypertension and lipid treatment significantly reduces the risk *(157)*.

Finally, it is important to emphasize that adequate lowering of BP in this high-risk group of patients with hypertension and diabetes often requires a minimum of three drugs, at least one of which should be an ACE inhibitor, if tolerated. Indeed, at least six clinical trials unequivocally demonstrate the substantial benefits of aggressive BP lowering in diabetic patients.

CONCLUSIONS

Hypertension is a common co-morbidity in people with diabetes. It substantially increases the risk of CVD in this patient population. The goal of treatment of hypertension in patients with diabetes is to prevent the hypertension-associated increase risk of CVD death and disability. Persons with DM often have more labile BPs, are more susceptible to postural hypotension, and often do not have a normal nocturnal "dip" of BPs. Thus, the level of BP and the diagnosis of hypertension should be based on multiple BP measurements obtained in a standardized fashion on at least three occasions. Because of the tendency to orthostatic hypotension, standing BPs should be measured at each office visit. Furthermore, because of the increased BP variability in these patients, ambulatory BP measurements or home BP monitoring may be very useful. The consensus BP goal in diabetic persons with hypertension is less than 130/80 mmHg. Pharmacological therapy should be initiated when lifestyle modifications do not lower BP to less than 130/80 mmHg in these patients. Combination therapy is usually necessary for adequate BP control. Recent data from several clinical studies, including the UKPDS emphasizes the importance of rigorous BP control, requiring several antihypertensive medications.

ACKNOWLEDGMENTS

This work was supported by grants from the National Institutes of Health (HL-63904–01), American Diabetes Association, and Veterans' Affairs Department to JRS and by a grant for the Diabetes Reduction Assessment with Ramipril and Rosiglitazone Medications (DREAM) study to SIM.

REFERENCES

1. Mokdad AH, Bowman BA, Ford ES, Vinicor F, Marks JS, Koplan JP. The continuing epidemics of obesity and diabetes in the United States. JAMA 2001;286:1195–1200.
2. Centers for Disease Control and Prevention. National Diabetes Fact Sheet: General Information and National Estimates on Diabetes in the United States 2000. Atlanta, GA: US Dept of Health and Human Services, Centers for Disease Control and Prevention, 2002.
3. American Diabetes Association. Economic Costs of Diabetes in the U.S. in 2002. Diabetes Care 2003;26:917–932.
4. Boyle JP, Honeycutt AA, Narayan KM, et al. Projection of diabetes burden through 2050: impact of changing demography and disease prevalence in the U.S. Diabetes Care 2001;24:1936–1940.
5. McFarlane SI, Banerji M, Sowers JR. Insulin resistance and cardiovascular disease. J Clin Endocrinol Metab 2001;86:713–718.
6. Grundy SM, Benjamin IJ, Burke GL, et al. Diabetes and cardiovascular disease: a statement for healthcare professionals from the American Heart Association. Circulation 1999;100:1134–1146.
7. Blendea MC, McFarlane SI, Isenovic ER, Gick G, Sowers JR. Heart disease in diabetic patients. Curr Diab Rep 2003;3:223–229.
8. Haffner SM, Lehto S, Ronnemaa T, Pyorala K, Laakso M. Mortality from coronary heart disease in subjects with type 2 diabetes and in nondiabetic subjects with and without prior myocardial infarction. N Engl J Med 1998;339:229–234.

9. Sowers JR, Epstein M, Frohlich ED. Diabetes, hypertension, and cardiovascular disease: an update. Hypertension 2001;37:1053–1059.

10. Gress TW, Nieto J, Shahar E, et al. Hypertension and antihypertensive therapy as risk factors for type 2 diabetes mellitus. N Engl J Med 2000;342:905–912.

11. Ford ES, Giles WH, Dietz WH. Prevalence of the metabolic syndrome among US adults: findings from the third National Health and Nutrition Examination Survey. JAMA 2002;287(3):356–359.

12. Third Report of the National Cholesterol Education Program (NCEP) Expert Panel on Detection, Evaluation, and Treatment of High Blood Cholesterol in Adults (Adult Treatment Panel III) final report. National Cholesterol Education Program (NCEP) Expert Panel on Detection, Evaluation, and Treatment of High Blood Cholesterol in Adults (Adult Treatment Panel III). Circulation 2002;106(25):3143–3421.

13. Haffner S, Taegtmeyer H. Epidemic obesity and the metabolic syndrome. Circulation 2003;108:1541–1545.

14. Kereiakes DJ, Willerson JT. Metabolic syndrome epidemic. Circulation 2003;108:1552–1553.

15. Alexander CM, Landsman PB, Teutsch SM, Haffner SM. NCEP-defined metabolic syndrome, diabetes, and prevalence of coronary heart disease among NHANES III participants age 50 years and older. Diabetes 2003;52:1210–1214.

16. Isomaa B, Almgren P, Tuomi T, et al. Cardiovascular morbidity and mortality associated with the metabolic syndrome. Diabetes Care 2001;24:683–689.

17. Alberti KG, Zimmet PZ.. Definition, diagnosis and classification of diabetes mellitus and its complications. Part 1: diagnosis and classification of diabetes mellitus provisional report of a WHO consultation. Diabet Med 1998;15(7):539–553.

18. Groop L, Forsblom C, Lehtovirta M, et al. Metabolic consequences of a family history of NIDDM (the Botnia study): evidence for sex-specific parental effects. Diabetes 1996;45:1585–1593.

19. Verdecchia P, Porcellati C, Schillaci G, et al. Ambulatory blood pressure. An independent predictor of prognosis in essential hypertension. Hypertension 1994;24:793–801.

20. Nakano S, Kitazawa M, Tsuda S, et al. INS resistance is associated with reduced nocturnal falls of blood pressure in normotensive, nonobese type 2 diabetic subjects. Clin Exp Hypertens 2002;24:65–73.

21. Nielsen FS, Hansen HP, Jacobsen P, et al. Increased sympathetic activity during sleep and nocturnal hypertension in Type 2 diabetic patients with diabetic nephropathy. Diabet Med 1999;16:555–562.

22. Ohkubo T, Hozawa A, Yamaguchi J, et al. Prognostic significance of the nocturnal decline in blood pressure in individuals with and without high 24-h blood pressure: the Ohasama study. J Hypertens 2002;20:2183–2189.

23. White WB. A chronotherapeutic approach to the management of hypertension. Am J Hypertens 1996;9:29S–33S.

24. Semplicini A, Ceolotto G, Massimino M, et al. Interactions between INS and sodium homeostasis in essential hypertension. Am J Med Sci 1994;307(Suppl 1):S43–S46.

25. Weinberger MH. Salt sensitive human hypertension. Endocr Res 1991;17:43–51.

26. Luft FC, Miller JZ, Grim CE, et al. Salt sensitivity and resistance of blood pressure. Age and race as factors in physiological responses. Hypertension 1991;17:I102–I108.

27. Arun CS, Stoddart J, Mackin P, MacLeod JM, New JP, Marshall SM. Significance of microalbuminuria in long-duration type 1 diabetes. Diabetes Care 2003;26:2144–2149.

28. Mitchell TH, Nolan B, Henry M, Cronin C, Baker H, Greely G. Microalbuminuria in patients with non-INS-dependent diabetes mellitus relates to nocturnal systolic blood pressure. Am J Med 1997;102:531–535.

29. Mogensen CE. Microalbuminuria and hypertension with focus on type 1 and type 2 diabetes. J Intern Med 2003;254:45–66.

30. Tagle R, Acevedo M, Vidt DG. Microalbuminuria: is it a valid predictor of cardiovascular risk? Cleve Clin J Med 2003;70:255–261.

31. McFarlane SI, Farag A, Sowers J. Calcium antagonists in patients with type 2 diabetes and hypertension. Cardiovasc Drug Rev 2003;21:105–118.

32. Streeten DH, Anderson GH, Jr. The role of delayed orthostatic hypotension in the pathogenesis of chronic fatigue. Clin Auton Res 1998;8:119–124.

33. Streeten DH, Auchincloss JH Jr, Anderson GH, Jr., Richardson RL, Thomas FD, Miller JW. Orthostatic hypertension. Pathogenetic studies. Hypertension 1985;7:196–203.

34. Jacob G, Costa F, Biaggioni I. Spectrum of autonomic cardiovascular neuropathy in diabetes. Diabetes Care 2003;26:2174–2180.

35. Streeten DH. Pathogenesis of hyperadrenergic orthostatic hypotension. Evidence of disordered venous innervation exclusively in the lower limbs. J Clin Invest 1990;86:1582–588.

36. Sowers JR, Bakris GL. Antihypertensive therapy and the risk of type 2 diabetes mellitus. N Engl J Med 2000;342(13):969–970.

37. Hypertension in Diabetes Study (HDS): I. Prevalence of hypertension in newly presenting type 2 diabetic patients and the association with risk factors for cardiovascular and diabetic complications. J Hypertens 1993;11(3):309–317.

38. Mattock MB, Morrish NJ, Viberti G, Keen H, Fitzgerald AP, Jackson G. Prospective study of microalbuminuria as predictor of mortality in NIDDM. Diabetes 1992;41(6):736–741.

39. Feldt-Rasmussen B, Mathiesen ER, Deckert T, et al. Central role for sodium in the pathogenesis of blood pressure changes independent of angiotensin, aldosterone and catecholamines in type 1 (INS-dependent) diabetes mellitus. Diabetologia 1987;30(8):610–617.

40. Sowers JR, Sowers PS, Peuler JD. Role of INS resistance and hyperINSemia in development of hypertension and atherosclerosis. J Lab Clin Med 1994;123(5):647–652.

41. Sowers JR. Effects of INS and IGF-I on vascular smooth muscle glucose and cation metabolism. Diabetes 1996;45(Suppl 3):S47–S51.

42. Sechi LA, Melis A, Tedde R. INS hypersecretion: a distinctive feature between essential and secondary hypertension. Metabolism 1992;41:1261–1266.

43. Frohlich ED. INS and INS resistance: impact on blood pressure and cardiovascular disease. Medical Clinics N Am 2004;88:63–82.

44. Steinberg HO, Brechtel G, Johnson A, Fineberg N, Baron AD. INS-mediated skeletal muscle vasodilation is nitric oxide dependent. A novel action of INS to increase nitric oxide release. J Clin Invest 1994;94(3):1172–1179.

45. Steinberg HO, Chaker H, Leaming R, Johnson A, Brechtel G, Baron AD. Obesity/INS resistance is associated with endothelial dysfunction. Implications for the syndrome of INS resistance. J Clin Invest 1996;97(11):2601–2610.

46. Sowers JR. Obesity and cardiovascular disease. Clin Chem 1998;44(8 Pt 2):1821–1825.

47. Sowers JR. Obesity as a cardiovascular risk factor. Am J Medicine 2003;115(8A): 375–415.

48. El-Atat F, Aneja A, McFarlane S, Sowers JR. Obesity and hypertension. Endocrinol Metab Clin N Amer 2003;32:823–854.

49. Jensen MD, Haymond MW, Rizza RA, Cryer PE, Miles JM. Influence of body fat distribution on free fatty acid metabolism in obesity. J Clin Invest 1989;83(4):1168–1173.

50. Janke J, Engeli S, Gorzelniak K, Luft FC, Sharma AM. Mature adipocytes inhibit in vitro differentiation of human preadipocytes via angiotensin type 1 receptors. Diabetes 2002;51(6):1699–1707.

51. Hall JE, Hildebrandt DA, Kuo J. Obesity hypertension: role of leptin and sympathetic nervous system. Am J Hypertens 2001;14(6 Pt 2):103S–115S.

52. Weyer C, Funahashi T, Tanaka S, et al. Hypoadiponectinemia in obesity and type 2 diabetes: close association with INS resistance and hyperINSemia. J Clin Endocrinol Metab 2001;86(5):1930–1935.

53. Ouchi N, Kihara S, Funahashi T, et al. Reciprocal association of C-reactive protein with adiponectin in blood stream and adipose tissue. Circulation 2003;107(5):671–674.

54. Shuldiner AR, Yang R, Gong DW. Resistin, obesity and INS resistance—the emerging role of the adipocyte as an endocrine organ. N Engl J Med 2001;345(18):1345.

55. Sowers JR, Ferdinand KC, Bakris GL, Douglas JG. Hypertension-related disease in African Americans. Factors underlying disparities in illness and its outcome. Postgrad Med 2002;112(4):24–26.

56. Sowers JR. Diabetic nephropathy and concomitant hypertension: a review of recent ADA recommendations. Am J Clin Proc 2002;3:27–33.

57. LeRoith D. INS-like growth factors. N Engl J Med 1998;336:633–640.

58. Sowers J. INS and INS-like growth factor in normal and pathological cardiovascular physiology. Hypertension 1997;29:691–699.

59. Standley PR, Zhang F, Sowers JR. IGF-1 regulation of Na^+-K^+-ATPase in rat arterial smooth muscle. Am J Physiol 1997;273:E113–E121.

60. Standley PR, Obards TJ, Martina CL. Cyclic stretch regulates autocrine IGF-1 in vascular smooth muscle cells: implications in vascular hyperplasia. Am J Physiol 1999;276:E697–E705.

61. Hayashi K, Saga H, Chimori Y, et al. Differentiated phenotype of smooth muscle cells depends on signaling pathways through INS-like growth factor and phosphatidylinositol 3-kinase. J Biol Chem 1998:273:28860–28867.

62. Sowers J. Effects of INS and IGF-1 on vascular smooth muscle glucose and cation metabolism. Diabetes 1996;45:S47–S51.

63. Walsh MF, Barazi M, Sowers JR. IGF-1 diminishes in vivo and in vitro vascular contractility: role of vascular nitric oxide. Endocrinology 1996;137:1798–1803.

64. Muniyappa R, Walsh MF, Sowers JR. INS-like growth factor-1 increases vascular smooth muscle nitric oxide production. Life Sciences 1997;61:925–933.

65. Wu HY, Jeng YY, Hsueh WA. Endothelial-dependent vascular effects of INS and INS-like growth factor I in the perfused rat mesenteric artery and aortic ring. Diabetes 1994;43:1027–1032.

66. Zeng G, Nystrom FH, Quon, MJ. Roles for INS receptor, PI3-kinase and Akt in INS-signaling pathways related to production of nitric oxide in human vascular endothelialc cells. Circulation 2000;101:1539–1545.

67. Sowers J. INS and INS-like growth factor-1 effects on CA2+ and nitric oxide in diabetes. In: Levin ER, Nadler JL, (eds.). Endocrinology of cardiovascular function. Kluwer Academic Publishers, Boston, Massachusetts, 1998, pp. 139–158.

68. Hasdai D, Rizza R, Holmes D, et al. INS and INS-like growth factor-1 cause coronary vasorelaxation in vitro. Hypertension 1998;32:228–234.

69. Li D, Sweeney G, Wang Q, Klip A. Participation of PI3K and atypical PKC in Na+,K+-pump stimulation by IGF-1 in VSMC. Am J Physiol 1999;276:H2109–H2116.

70. Inishi Y, Katoh T, Okada T. Modulation of renal hemodynamics by IGF-1 is absent in spontaneously hypertensive rats. Kidney Int 1997;52:165–170.

71. Isenovic ER, Muniyappa R, Sowers JR. Role of PI3-kinase in isoproterenol and IGF-1 induced ecNOS activity. BBRC 2001;285:954–958.

72. Walsh MF, Ali S. Sowers JR. Vascular INS/INS-like growth factor-1 resistance in female obese Zucker rats. Metabolism 2001;50:607–612.

73. Vecchione C, Colella S, Fratta L, et al. Impaired INS-like growth factor-1 vasorelaxant effects in hypertension. Hypertension 2001;37:1480–1485.

74. Isenovic ER, Jacobs DB, Kedees MH, et al. Angiotensin II regulation of the Na+ pump involves the phosphatidylinositol-3 kinase and p42/44 mitogen-activated protein kinase signaling pathways in vascular smooth muscle cells. Endocrinology 2004;145(3):1151–1160.

75. Sowers JR. INS resistance and hypertension. Am J Physiol Heart Circ Physiol 2004;286:H1597–1602.

76. Zeng G, Quon MJ. INS-stimulated production of nitric oxide is inhibited by wortmannin. Direct measurement in vascular endothelial cells. J Clin Invest 1996;15;98:894–898.

77. Tirupattur PR, Ram JL, Standley PR, Sowers JR. Regulation of Na+,K(+)-ATPase gene expression by INS in vascular smooth muscle cells. Am J Hypertens 1993;6:626–629.

78. Sowers JR, Draznin B. INS, cation metabolism and INS resistance. J Basic Clin Physiol Pharmacol 1998;9:223–233.

79. Sowers JR. Recommendations for special populations: diabetes mellitus and the metabolic syndrome. Am J Hypertens 2003;16:41S–45S.

80. Zemel MB, Peuler JD, Sowers JR. Hypertension in INS-resistant Zucker obese rats is independent of neural support. Am J Physiol 1992;262:E368–E371.

81. Henriksen EJ, Jacob S, Kinnick T, et al. Selective angiotensin II receptor antagonism reduces INS resistance in obese Zucker rats. Hypertension 2001;38:884–890.

82. Ouchi Y, Han S, Kim S, et al Augmented contractile function and abnormal Ca2+ handling in the aorta of Zucker obese rats with INS resistance. Diabetes 1996;45:S55–S58.

83. Kolter T, Uphues I, Eckel J. Molecular analysis of INS-resistance in isolated ventricular cardiomyocytes of obese Zucker rats. Am J Physiol 1997;36:E59–E67.

84. Ren J, Walsh MF, Sowers JR. Altered inotrophic response to IGF-1 in diabetic rat heart: influence of intracellular Ca2+ and NO. Am J Physiol 1998;275:H823–H830.

85. Leri A, Liu Y, Wang X, Kajstura J, et al. Overexpression of INS-like growth factor-1 attenuates the myocyte renin-angiotensin system in transgenic mice. Circ Res 1999;84:752–762.

86. Ren J, Jefferson L, Sowers JR. Influence of age on contractile response to INS-like growth factor 1 in ventricular myocytes from spontaneously hypertensive rats. Hypertension 1999;34:1215–1222.

87. Ren J, Samson WK, Sowers JR. INS-like growth factor I as a cardiac hormone: physiological and pathophysiological implications in heart disease. J Mol Cell Cardiol 1999;31:2049–2061.

88. Ren J, Sowers JR, Walsh MF, et al. Reduced contractile response to INS and IGF-I in ventricular myocytes from genetically obese Zucker rats. Am J Physiol 2000;279:H1708–H1714.

89. Hemmings BA. Akt signaling: linking membrane events to life and death situations. Science 1997;275:628–630.

90. Somwar R, Srimitani S, Klip A. Temporal activation of p70 S6 kinase and Akt1 by INS: PI3-kinase-dependent and –independent mechanisms. Am J Physiol 1998;38:E618–E625.

91. Begum N, Ragolia L, Rienzie J, et al. Regulation of mitogen-activated protein kinase phosphatase-1 induction by INS in vascular smooth muscle cells. J Biol Chem 1998;273:25164–25170.

92. Kaliman P, Canicio J, Begum N, et al. INS-like growth factor II, phosphatidylinositol 3-kinase, nuclear factor-KB and inducible nitric oxide synthase define a common myogenic signaling pathway. J Biol Chem 1999;274:17,437–17,444.

93. Dinmeter S, Fleming I, Fiss I, Thoder B, et al. Activation of nitric oxide synthase in endothelial cells by Akt-dependent phosphorylation. Nature 1999;399:601–605.

94. Luo Z, Fujio Y, Kureishi Y et al. Acute modulation of endothelial Akt/PKB activity alters nitric oxide-dependent vasomotor activity in vivo. J Clin Invest 2000;106:493–499.

95. Hermann C, Assmus B, Urbich C, et al. INS-mediated stimulation of protein kinase Akt: A potent survival signaling cascade for endothelial cells. Arterioscler Thromb Vasc Biol 2000;20:402–409.

96. Begum N, Song Y, Rienzie J, et al. Vascular smooth muscle cell growth and INS regulation of mitogen-activated protein kinase in hypertension. Am J Physiol 1998;275:C42–C49.

97. Villoso LA, Folli F, Sun XJ, et al. Cross-talk between the INS and angiotensin signaling systems. Proc Natl Acad Sci USA 1996;93:12,490–12,495.

98. Isenovic E, Walsh MF, Muniyappa R, Bard M, Diglio CA, Sowers JR. Phosphatidylinositol 3-kinase may mediate isoproterenol-induced vascular relaxation, in part through nitric oxide production. Metabolism 2002;51:380–386.

99. Lee MR, Li L, Kitazawa T. cGMP causes Ca2+ desensitization in vascular smooth muscle cells by activating the myosin light chain phosphatase. J Biol Chem 1997;272:5063–5068.

100. Begum N, Duddy N, Sandu OA, et al. Regulation of myosin bound protein phosphatase by INS in vascular smooth muscle cells. Evaluation of the role of Rho kinase and PI3-kinase dependent signaling pathways. Mol Endocrinol 2000;14:1365–1376.

101. Surks HK, Mochizuki N, Kasai Y, et al. Regulation of myosin phosphatase by a specific interaction with cGMP-dependent protein kinase 1alpha. Science 1999;286:1583–1587.

102. Sauzeau V, LeJeune H, Cario-Toumaniantz C, et al. Cyclic GMP-dependent protein kinase signaling pathway inhibits RhoA-induced Ca2+ sensitization of contraction in vascular smooth muscle. J Biol Chem 2000;275:21,722–21,729.

103. Kimura K, Ito M, Amano M, et al. Regulation of myosin phosphatase by Rho and Rho-associated kinase (Rho-kinase). Science 1996;273:245–248.

104. Uehata M, Ishizaki T, Satoh H, et al. Calcium sensitization of smooth muscle mediated by a Rho-associated protein kinase in hypertension. Nature 1997;389:990–994.

105. Yamakawa T, Tanaka A, Inagami T. Involvement of Rho-kinase in angiotensin II-induced hypertrophy of vascular smooth muscle cells. Hypertension 2000;35:313–318.

106. Kitazawa T, Eto M, Woodsome TP, Brautigan DL. Agonists trigger G protein-mediated activation of the CPI-17 inhibitor phosphoprotein of myosin light chain phosphatase to enhance vascular smooth muscle contractility. J Biol Chem 2000;275:9897–9900.

107. Kawano Y, Fukata Y, Oshiro N, et al. Phosphorylation of myosin-binding subunit (MBS) of myosin phosphatase by Rho-Kinase in vivo. J Cell Biol 1999;147:1023–1038.

108. Feng J, Ito M, Ichikawa K, et al. Inhibitory phosphorylation site for Rho-associated kinase on smooth muscle myosin phosphatase. J Biol Chem 1999;274:37385–7390.

109. Chibalin AV, Kovalenko MV, Ryder JW, et al. INS- and glucose-induced phosphorylation of the Na(+), K(+)-adenosine triphosphatase alpha-subunits in rat skeletal muscle. Endocrinology 2001;42:3474–3482.

110. Sandu OA, Ito M, Begum N. Selected Contribution: INS utilizes NO/cGMP pathway to activate myosin phosphatase via Rho inhibition in vascular smooth muscle. J Appl Physiol 2001;91:1475–482.

111. Berk B, Duff J, Marrero M. Angiotensin II signal transduction in vascular smooth muscle. In: Sowers JR, (ed.). Endocrinology of the Vasculature. Totowa, New Jersey, Humana Press, 1996, pp. 187–204.

112. Dzau VJ. Tissue angiotensin and pathobiology of vascular disease: a unifying hypothesis. Hypertension 2001;37:1047–1052.

113. Kureishi Y, Kobayashi S, Amano M, et al. Rho-associated kinase directly induces smooth muscle contraction through myosin light chain phosphorylation. J Biol Chem 1997;272:1257–12260.

114. Folli F, Kahn R, Hansen H, et al. Angiotensin II inhibits INS signaling in aortic smooth muscle cells at multiple levels. J Clin Invest 1997;100:2158–2169.

115. Clark E, King W, Brugge JS, et al. Integrin-mediated signals regulated by members of the Rho family of GTPases. J Cell Biol 1998;142:573–586.

116. Sandu O, Ragolia L, Begum N. Diabetes in the Goto-Kakizaki rat is accompanied by impaired INS-mediated myosin-bound phosphatase activation and vascular smooth muscle cell relaxation. Diabetes 2000;49:2178–2189.

117. Sowers JR. Insulin resistance and hypertension. Am J Physiol Heart Circ Physiol 2004;286:H1597–H1602.

118. Tight blood pressure control and risk of macrovascular and microvascular complications in type 2 diabetes: UKPDS 38. UK Prospective Diabetes Study Group. BMJ 1998;317(7160):703–713.

119. Hansson L, Zanchetti A, Carruthers SG, et al. Effects of intensive blood-pressure lowering and low-dose aspirin in patients with hypertension: principal results of the Hypertension Optimal Treatment (HOT) randomised trial. HOT Study Group. Lancet 1998;351(9118):1755–1762.

120. Tuomilehto J, Rastenyte D, Birkenhager WH, et al. Effects of calcium-channel blockade in older patients with diabetes and systolic hypertension. Systolic Hypertension in Europe Trial Investigators. N Engl J Med 1999;340(9):677–684.

121. Curb JD, Pressel SL, Cutler JA, et al. Effect of diuretic-based antihypertensive treatment on cardiovascular disease risk in older diabetic patients with isolated systolic hypertension. Systolic Hypertension in the Elderly Program Cooperative Research Group. JAMA 1996;276(23):1886–1892.

122. Lewington S, Clarke R, Qizilbash N, Peto R, Collins R, Prospective Studies Collaboration. Age-specific relevance of usual blood pressure to vascular mortality: a meta-analysis of individual data for one million adults in 61 prospective studies. Lancet 2002;360(9349):1903–1913.

123. Arauz-Pacheco C, Parrott MA, Raskin P, American Diabetes Association. Treatment of hypertension in adults with diabetes. Diabetes Care 2003;26(Suppl 1):S80–S82.

124. Sowers JR, Haffner S. Treatment of cardiovascular and renal risk factors in the diabetic hypertensive. Hypertension 2002;40:781–788.

125. Chobanian AV, Bakris GL, Black HR, et al., National Heart, Lung, and Blood Institute Joint National Committee on Prevention, Detection, Evaluation, and Treatment of High Blood Pressure, National High Blood Pressure Education Program Coordinating Committee. The Seventh Report of the Joint National Committee on Prevention, Detection, Evaluation, and Treatment of High Blood Pressure: the JNC 7 report. JAMA 2003;289(19):2560–2572.

126. Sacks FM, Svetkey LP, Vollmer WM, et al., DASH-Sodium Collaborative Research Group. Effects on blood pressure of reduced dietary sodium and the Dietary Approaches to Stop Hypertension (DASH) diet. DASH-Sodium Collaborative Research Group. N Engl J Med 2001;344(1):3–10.

127. Clinical Guidelines on the Identification, Evaluation, and Treatment of Overweight and Obesity in Adults—The Evidence Report. National Institutes of Health. Obes Res 1998;6(Suppl 2):51S–209S.

128. McFarlane SI, Shin JJ, Rundek T, Bigger JT. Prevention of type 2 diabetes. Curr Diab Rep 2003;3:235–241.

129. Eriksson KF, Lindgarde F. Prevention of type 2 (non-INS-dependent) diabetes mellitus by diet and physical exercise. The 6-year Malmo feasibility study. Diabetologia 1991;34:891–898.

130. Helmrich SP, Ragland DR, Leung RW, Paffenbarger RS, Jr. Physical activity and reduced occurrence of non-INS-dependent diabetes mellitus. N Engl J Med 1991;325:147–152.

131. Tuomilehto J, Lindstrom J, Eriksson JG, et al., Finnish Diabetes Prevention Study Group. Prevention of type 2 diabetes mellitus by changes in lifestyle among subjects with impaired glucose tolerance. N Engl J Med 2001;344(18):1343–1350.

132. Knowler WC, Barrett-Connor E, Fowler SE, et al. Reduction in the incidence of type 2 diabetes with lifestyle intervention or metformin. N Engl J Med 2002;346:393–403.

133. ALLHAT Officers and Coordinators for the ALLHAT Collaborative Research Group. The Antihypertensive and Lipid-Lowering Treatment to Prevent Heart Attack Trial. Major outcomes in high-risk hypertensive patients randomized to angiotensin-converting enzyme inhibitor or calcium channel blocker vs diuretic: the Antihypertensive and Lipid-Lowering Treatment to Prevent Heart Attack Trial (ALLHAT). JAMA 2002;288(23):2981–2997.

134. Barzilay JI, Jones CL, Davis BR, et al. Baseline characteristics of the diabetic participants in the Antihypertensive and Lipid-Lowering Treatment to Prevent Heart Attack Trial (ALLHAT). Diabetes Care 2001;24:654–658.

135. McFarlane SI, Jacober SJ, Winer N, et al. Control of cardiovascular risk factors in patients with diabetes and hypertension at urban academic medical centers. Diabetes Care 2002;25:718–723.

136. McFarlane SI, Kumar A, Sowers JR. Mechanisms by which angiotensin-converting enzyme inhibitors prevent diabetes and cardiovascular disease. Am J Cardiol 2003;91(12A):30H–37H.

137. Privratsky JR, Wold LE, Sowers JR, Quinn MT, Ren J. AT1 blockade prevents glucose-induced cardiac dysfunction in ventricular myocytes: role of the AT1 receptor and NADPH oxidase. Hypertension 2003;42(2):206–212.

138. Effects of ramipril on cardiovascular and microvascular outcomes in people with diabetes mellitus: results of the HOPE study and MICRO-HOPE substudy. Heart Outcomes Prevention Evaluation Study Investigators. Lancet 2000;22;355(9200):253–259.

139. Lindholm LH, Ibsen H, Dahlof B, et al., LIFE Study Group. Cardiovascular morbidity and mortality in patients with diabetes in the Losartan Intervention For Endpoint reduction in hypertension study (LIFE): a randomised trial against atenolol. Lancet 2002;359(9311):1004–1010.

140. Julius S, Kjeldsen SE, Weber M, et al. Outcomes in hypertensive patients at high cardiovascular risk treated with regimens based on valsartan or amlodipine: the VALUE randomised trial. Lancet 2004;363:2022–2031.

141. Bakris GL, Weir M. ACE inhibitors and protection against kidney disease progression in patients with type 2 diabetes: what's the evidence. J Clin Hypertens (Greenwich) 2002;4(6):420–423.

142. Brenner BM, Cooper ME, de Zeeuw D, et al., RENAAL Study Investigators. Effects of losartan on renal and cardiovascular outcomes in patients with type 2 diabetes and nephropathy. N Engl J Med 2001;345(12):861–869.

143. Parving HH, Lehnert H, Brochner-Mortensen J, Gomis R, Andersen S, Arner P, Irbesartan in Patients with Type 2 Diabetes and Microalbuminuria Study Group. The effect of irbesartan on the development of diabetic nephropathy in patients with type 2 diabetes. N Engl J Med 2001;345(12):870–878.

144. Lewis EJ, Hunsicker LG, Clarke WR, et al., Collaborative Study Group. effect of the angiotensin-receptor antagonist irbesartan in patients with nephropathy due to type 2 diabetes N Engl J Med 2001;345(12):851–860.

145. Viberti G, Wheeldon NM, MicroAlbuminuria Reduction With VALsartan (MARVAL) Study Investigators. Microalbuminuria reduction with valsartan in patients with type 2 diabetes mellitus: a blood pressure-independent effect. Circulation 2002;106(6):672–678.

146. Mogensen CE, Neldam S, Tikkanen I, et al. Randomized controlled trial of dual blockade of renin-angiotensin system in patients with hypertension, microalbuminuria, and non-INS dependent diabetes: the candesartan and lisinopril microalbuminuria (CALM) study. BMJ 2000;321(7274):1440–1444.

147. Palmer BF. Renal dysfunction complicating the treatment of hypertension.. N Engl J Med 2002;347(16):1256–1261.

148. Rake EC, Breeze E, Fletcher AE. Quality of life and cough on antihypertensive treatment: a randomized trial of eprosartan, enalapril and placebo. J Hum Hypertens 2001;15(12):863–867.

149. Gavras I, Gavras H. Are patients who develop angioedema with ACE inhibition at risk of the same problem with AT1 receptor blockers? Arch Intern Med 2003;27;163(2):240–241.

150. Kirpichnikov D, McFarlane SI, Sowers JR. Heart failure in diabetic patients: utility of beta-blockade. J Card Fail 2003;9(4):333–344.

151. Jacob S, Rett K, Wicklmayr M, Agrawal B, Augustin HJ, Dietze GJ. Differential effect of chronic treatment with two beta-blocking agents on INS sensitivity: the carvedilol-metoprolol study. J Hypertens 1996;14(4):489–494.

152. Giugliano D, Acampora R, Marfella R, et al. Metabolic and cardiovascular effects of carvedilol and atenolol in non-INS-dependent diabetes mellitus and hypertension. A randomized, controlled trial. Ann Intern Med 1997;126(12):955–959.

153. Intensive blood-glucose control with sulphonylureas or INS compared with conventional treatment and risk of complications in patients with type 2 diabetes (UKPDS 33). UK Prospective Diabetes Study (UKPDS) Group. Lancet 1998;352 (9131):837–853.

154. Heart Protection Study Collaborative Group. MRC/BHF Heart Protection Study of cholesterol lowering with simvastatin in 20,536 high-risk individuals: a randomised placebo-controlled trial. Lancet 2002;360(9326):7–22.

155. Goldberg RB, Mellies MJ, Sacks FM, et al. Cardiovascular events and their reduction with pravastatin in diabetic and glucose-intolerant myocardial infarction survivors with average cholesterol levels: subgroup analyses in the cholesterol and recurrent events (CARE) trial. The Care Investigators. Circulation 1998;98(23):2513–2519.

156. McFarlane SI, Muniyappa R, Francisco R, Sowers JR. Clinical review 145: Pleiotropic effects of statins: lipid reduction and beyond. J Clin Endocrinol Metab 2002;87:1451–1458.

157. Rolka DB, Fagot-Campagna A, Narayan KM. Aspirin use among adults with diabetes: estimates from the Third National Health and Nutrition Examination Survey. Diabetes Care 2001;24(2):197–201.

15 Diabetes and Dyslipidemia

Asha Thomas-Geevarghese, MD,
Catherine Tuck, MD, and Henry N. Ginsberg, MD

INTRODUCTION

Numerous prospective cohort studies have indicated that diabetes mellitus (DM) is associated with a three- to fourfold increase in risk for coronary artery disease (CAD) *(1–3)*. The increase in risk is particularly evident in both younger age groups and women. Females with type 2 DM appear to lose a great deal of the protection that characterizes nondiabetic females. Furthermore, patients with DM have a 50% greater in-hospital mortality, and a twofold increased rate of death within 2 years of surviving a myocardial infarction (MI). Overall, CAD is the leading cause of death in individuals with DM who are over the age of 35 years.

Although much of this increased risk is associated with the presence of well- characterized risk factors for CAD, a significant proportion remains unexplained. Patients with DM, particularly those with type 2 DM, have abnormalities of plasma lipids and lipoprotein concentrations that are less commonly present in nondiabetics *(4–7)*. This combination of lipid abnormalities has been called the diabetic dyslipidemia. Patients with poorly controlled type 1 DM can also have a dyslipidemic pattern. In this chapter, we will focus on approaches to the diabetic patient with significant dyslipidemia. Normal lipid and lipoprotein physiology will be reviewed briefly as a base from which we will examine the approach to treating the dyslipidemias commonly associated with diabetes.

From: *Contemporary Cardiology: Diabetes and Cardiovascular Disease, Second Edition*
Edited by: M. T. Johnstone and A. Veves © Humana Press Inc., Totowa, NJ

329

LIPOPROTEIN COMPOSITION

Lipoproteins are macromolecular complexes carrying various lipids and proteins in plasma (8). Several major classes of lipoproteins have been defined by their physical-chemical characteristics, particularly by their flotation characteristics during ultracentrifugation. However, lipoprotein particles actually form a continuum, varying in composition, size, density and function (Table 1). The lipids are mainly free and esterified cholesterol, triglycerides, and phospholipids. The hydrophobic triglyceride and cholesteryl esters (CEs) comprise the core of the lipoproteins, which is covered by a unilamellar surface containing mainly the amphipathic (both hydrophobic and hydrophilic) phospholipids, and smaller amounts of free cholesterol and proteins. Hundreds to thousands of triglyceride and CE molecules are carried in the core of different lipoproteins.

Apolipoproteins are the proteins on the surface of the lipoproteins. They not only help to solubilize the core lipids, but also play critical roles in the regulation of plasma lipid and lipoprotein transport. The major apolipoproteinss are described in Table 2. Apolipoprotein (apo)-B100 is required for the secretion of hepatic-derived very low-density lipoproteins (VLDL), intermediate density lipoproteins (IDL), and low-density lipoproteins (LDL). Apo-B48 is a truncated form of apo-B100 that is required for secretion of chylomicrons from the small intestine. Apo-A-I is the major structural protein in high-density lipoproteins (HDL). Apo-A-I is also an important activator of the plasma enzyme, lecithin cholesteryl-acyl transferase (LCAT), which plays a key role in reverse cholesterol transport. Other apolipoproteins will be discussed in the context of their roles in lipoprotein metabolism.

TRANSPORT OF DIETARY LIPIDS ON APO-B-48-CONTAINING LIPOPROTEINS IN DIABETES MELLITUS

After ingestion of a meal, dietary fat (triglyceride) and cholesterol are absorbed into the cells of the small intestine and are incorporated into the core of nascent chylomicrons. The newly formed chylomicrons are secreted into the lymphatic system and then enter the circulation via the superior vena cava. In the lymph and the blood, chylomicrons acquire apo-C-II, apo-C-III, and apo-E. In the capillary beds of adipose tissue and muscle, chylomicrons interact with the enzyme lipoprotein lipase (LPL), which is activated by apo-C-II, and the chylomicron core triglyceride is hydrolyzed. The lipolytic products, free fatty acids, can be taken up by fat cells and re-incorporated into triglyceride, or into muscle cells in which they can be used for energy. Apo-C-III can inhibit lipolysis, and the balance of apo-C-II and apo-C-III determines, in part, the efficiency with which LPL hydrolyzes chylomicron triglyceride. Chylomicron remnants, the product of this lipolytic process, have lost about 75% of the triglyceride and are relatively enriched in CEs (both from dietary sources and from HDL-derived CE, which has been transferred to the chylomicron). The chylomicron-remnants are also enriched in apo-E, and this protein is important for the interaction of chylomicron remnants with several pathways on hepatocytes that rapidly remove them from the circulation. Uptake of chylomicron remnants involves binding to the LDL receptor, the LDL receptor-related protein (LRP), hepatic lipase, and cell-surface proteoglycans (9).

Apo-E is thought to play a critical role in the hepatic uptake of chylomicron remnants, and some studies have indicated a role for the apo-E2 phenotype in the hyperlipidemia of diabetes. Apo-E2 is an allelic form of apo-E that is found in about 10% of the popu-

Table 1
Physical-Chemical Characteristics of the Major Lipoprotein Classes

Lipoprotein	Density	Molecular weight	Diameter	Lipid (%) Triglyceride	Cholesterol	PL
Chylomicrons	0.95	400×10^6	75–1200	80–95	2–7	3–9
VLDL	0.95–1.006	10–80×10^6	30–80	55–80	5–15	10–20
IDL	1.006–1.019	5–10×10^6	25–35	20–50	20–40	15–25
LDL	1.019–1.063	2.3×10^6	18–25	5–15	40–50	20–25
HDL	1.063–1.21	1.7–3.6×10^6	5–12	5–10	15–25	20–30

Density: g/dL

Molecular weight: daltons

Diameter: nm

Lipids (%): percent composition of lipids; apolipoproteins make up the rest.

VLDL, very low-density lipoprotein, IDL, intermediate density lipoproteins; LDL, low-density lipoprotein; HDL, high-density lipoprotein; PL, phospholipid.

Table 2
Characteristics of the Major Apolipoproteins

Apolipoprotein	Molecular weight	Lipoproteins	Metabolic functions
apo-A-I	28,016	HDL, chylomicrons	Structural component of HDL; LCAT activator
apo-A-II	17,414	HDL, chylomicrons	Unknown
apo-A-IV	46,465	HDL, chylomicrons	Unknown; possibly facilitates transfer of apos between HDL and chylomicrons
apo-B-48	264,000	Chylomicrons	Necessary for assembly and secretion of chylomicrons from the small intestine
apo-B-100	514,000	VLDL, IDL, LDL	Necessary for the assembly and secretion of VLDL from the liver; structural protein of VLDL, IDL and LDL; ligand for the LDL receptor
apo-C-I	6630	Chylomicrons, VLDL, IDL, HDL	May inhibit hepatic uptake of chylomicrons VLDL remnants
apo-C-II	8900	Chylomicrons, VLDL, IDL, HDL	Activator of lipoprotein lipase
apo-C-III	8800	Chylomicrons, VLDL, IDL, HDL	Inhibitor of lipoprotein lipase; inhibits hepatic uptake of chylomicron and VLDL remnants
apo-E	34,145	Chylomicrons, VLDL, IDL, HDL	Ligand for binding of several lipoproteins to the LDL receptor, LRP and proteoglycans
apo(a)	250,000 – 800,000	Lp(a)	Composed of LDL apo-B linked covalently to apo(a); function unknown but is an independent predictor of coronary artery disease

HDL, high-density lipoprotein; LCAT, lecithin cholesteryl-acyl transferase; apo, apolipoprotein; VLDL, very low-density lipoprotein; IDL, intermediate density lipoprotein; LDL, low-density lipoprotein; LRP, LDL receptor-related protein.

lation and is defective in binding to the LDL receptor. Hepatic triglyceride lipase (HTGL), which both hydrolyzes chylomicron- and VLDL-remnant triglyceride and acts on HDL triglyceride and phospholipids, may also plays a role in remnant removal (9). Deficiency of HTGL might, therefore, be associated with reduced remnant clearance. However, several studies (4) have indicated that HTGL is elevated in type 2 DM, and may be an important contributor to low HDL cholesterol levels in this disease.

Chylomicron and chylomicron-remnant metabolism can be altered significantly in diabetes *(4)*. In untreated type 1 DM, LPL will be low, and postprandial triglyceride levels will, in turn, be increased. Insulin therapy rapidly reverses this condition, resulting in improved clearance of chylomicron triglyceride from plasma. In chronically treated type 1 DM, LPL measured in post-heparin plasma (heparin releases LPL from the surface of endothelial cells in which it is usually found), and adipose tissue LPL, can be normal or increased, and chylomicron triglyceride clearance can be normal. In type 2 DM, metabolism of dietary lipids is complicated by co-existent obesity and the hypertriglyceridemia associated with insulin resistance. Defective removal of chylomicrons and chylomicron-remnants has been observed in type 2 DM *(4)*. However, LPL is normal or only slightly reduced in untreated patients *(5)*. Because both fasting hypertriglyceridemia and reduced plasma concentrations of HDL cholesterol are common in type 2 DM, and are correlated with increased postprandial triglyceride levels, it is difficult to identify a direct effect of type 2 DM on chylomicron metabolism.

TRANSPORT OF ENDOGENOUS LIPIDS ON APO-B-100-CONTAINING LIPOPROTEINS IN DIABETES MELLITUS

Very Low-Density Lipoprotein

VLDL is assembled in the endoplasmic reticulum of hepatocytes. VLDL triglyceride derives from the combination of glycerol with fatty acids that have either been taken up from plasma or newly synthesized in the liver. VLDL cholesterol is either synthesized in the liver from acetate or delivered to the liver by lipoproteins, mainly chylomicron remnants. Apo-B-100 and phospholipids form the surface of VLDL. Although some apo-C-I, apo-C-II, apo-C-III, and apo-E are present on the nascent VLDL particles as they are secreted from the hepatocyte, the majority of these molecules are probably added to VLDL after their entry into plasma. Regulation of the assembly and secretion of VLDL by the liver has not been completely defined. However, recent studies *(10)* in cultured liver cells indicate that a significant proportion of newly synthesized apo-B100 may be degraded before secretion, and that this degradation is inhibited when hepatic lipids are abundant *(11)*. There is evidence that high free fatty acid flux can stimulate high secretion rates of VLDL in individuals with insulin resistance and/or type 2 DM.

Once in the plasma, VLDL triglyceride is hydrolyzed by LPL (activated by apo-C-II), generating smaller and denser VLDL, and, subsequently IDL. IDL particles are similar to chylomicron remnants, but unlike chylomicron remnants, not all IDL are removed by the liver. IDL particles can also undergo further catabolism to become LDL. Some LPL activity appears necessary for normal functioning of the metabolic cascade from VLDL to IDL to LDL. It also appears that apo-E, HTGL, and LDL receptors play important roles in this process. Apo-B-100 is essentially the sole protein on the surface of LDL, and the lifetime of LDL in plasma appears to be mainly determined by the availability of LDL receptors. Overall, about 60% to 70% of LDL catabolism from plasma occurs via the LDL receptor pathway, although the remaining tissue uptake is by nonreceptor or alternative-receptor pathways *(8)*. One of these alternative pathways may recognize glycosylated and/or oxidatively modified lipoproteins, which can be present in increased amounts in the blood of patients with DM *(4,5)*.

Diabetic patients frequently have elevated plasma levels of VLDL triglyceride. In type 1 DM, triglyceride levels correlate closely with glycemic control, and marked hyperlipemia can be found in ketotic diabetics. The basis for increased VLDL levels in poorly controlled, but non ketotic type 1 DM subjects is usually overproduction of these lipo-proteins *(7)*. Reduced clearance plays a more significant role in severe cases of uncon-trolled diabetes. This results from a reduction of LPL, which returns to normal with adequate insulinization. Plasma triglyceride can actually be "low-normal" with intensive insulin treatment in type 1 DM, and lower than average production rates of VLDL have been observed in such instances. Several qualitative abnormalities in VLDL composition may persist, however, including enrichment in free- and esterified-cholesterol and an increase in the ratio of free cholesterol to lecithin. The latter may be an indication of increased risk for CHD.

Overproduction of VLDL, with increased secretion of both triglyceride and apo-B100, seems to be the central etiology of increased plasma VLDL levels in patients with type 2 DM *(12)*. Increased assembly and secretion of VLDL is probably a direct result of both insulin resistance (with loss of insulin's action to stimulate degradation of newly synthe-sized apo-B) and increased free fatty acid flux to the liver (with increased triglyceride synthesis). LPL levels have been reported to be reduced *(5)* in some type 2 diabetic patients, and this may contribute significantly to elevated triglyceride levels, particularly in severely hyperglycemic patients. Because obesity, insulin resistance, and concomitant familial forms of hyperlipidemia are common in type 2 DM, study of the pathophysiology is difficult. The interaction of these overlapping traits also makes therapy less effective. In contrast to type 1 DM, in which intensive insulin therapy normalizes (or even "super-normalizes") VLDL levels and metabolism, therapy of type 2 DM with either insulin or oral agents only partly corrects VLDL abnormalities in the majority of patients *(7)*. Some of the therapeutic choices available for the treatment of type 2 DM, such as metformin and the thiazolidinediones (TZDs), can lower plasma triglyceride concentrations 10% to 15% and 15% to 25%, respectively *(12)*. TZDs appear to improve peripheral insulin sensitivity, and this leads to inhibition of lipolysis in adipose tissue. Plasma levels of free fatty acids fall about 25% at the highest dose of both of the presently available TZDs, and such changes should lead to lower hepatic triglyceride synthesis and reduced VLDL secretion. Of interest, pioglitazone (Actos®) does lower plasma triglyceride levels but rosiglitazone (Avandia®) does not; the basis for this difference is unclear *(13)*.

Low-Density Lipoprotein

If glycemic control is good, LDL cholesterol levels and LDL metabolism is usually normal in patients with type 1 DM. In fact, with intensive insulin treatment, LDL produc-tion falls concomitant with reduced VLDL production *(7)*. The LDL receptor appears to be regulated to some extent by insulin, and severe insulin deficiency may lead to reduced catabolism of LDL. Patients with type 1 DM may have increased ratios of free cholesterol to lecithin even when glycemic control is adequate. Glycosylation of LDL does appear to occur in poorly controlled patients with DM, and reduced catabolism of LDL via the LDL receptor-pathway has been observed in some, but not all, in vitro studies using diabetic LDL and cultured fibroblasts.

In type 2 DM, regulation of plasma levels of LDL, like that of its precursor VLDL, is complex. In the presence of hypertriglyceridemia, dense, triglyceride-enriched LDL are present. Thus individuals with type 2 DM and mild to moderate hypertriglyceridemia may have the pattern B profile of LDL described by Austin and Krauss *(15)*. Patients with type 2 DM can be shown to have overproduction of LDL apo-B-100 even with mild degrees of hyperglycemia, particularly if there is concomitant elevation of VLDL. This situation is made more complex by the observation that there is both reduced VLDL conversion to LDL, and direct LDL entry into plasma in type 2 DM *(12)*.

Fractional removal of LDL, mainly via LDL receptor pathways, can be increased, normal, or reduced in type 2 DM. Increased LDL fractional catabolism is often seen in nondiabetics with significant hypertriglyceridemia, and although the basis for this is uncertain, elevated plasma triglyceride levels can probably increase LDL catabolism in patients with type 2 DM. Insulin seems to be required for normal LDL receptor function, and reduced LDL fractional removal from plasma has, therefore, been observed in more severe patients with type 2 DM. This could also be a consequence of glycosylation of LDL. These multiple potential effects on LDL metabolism make it difficult to predict what level of LDL will be present in any individual with type 2 DM. Overall, LDL elevations are not more commonly present in men with type 2 DM, although women with type 2 DM tend to have higher levels of LDL than women without diabetes. Insulin treatment tends to lower LDL, although sulfonylurea therapy has little or no effect *(14)*. Metformin has been observed to reduce LDL 5% to 10%, although TZDs either do not affect, or raise LDL by a similar degree. The metabolic basis for these changes has not been fully defined.

Some investigators have suggested that glycosylated LDL can be taken up by macrophage scavenger receptors, and contribute to foam cell formation *(16)*. Other studies indicate that LDL from patients with diabetes, particularly small, dense LDL, may be more susceptible to oxidative modification and catabolism via macrophage-scavenger receptors.

In summary, type 1 DM may be associated with elevations of VLDL triglyceride and LDL cholesterol if diabetic control is very poor or if the patient is actually ketotic. In contrast, type 2 DM is usually associated with lipid abnormalities, most common of which are high triglyceride, reduced HDL cholesterol levels, and the presence of smaller, CE-depleted LDL: the insulin resistance/diabetic dyslipidemia. Treatment of type 2 DM with hypoglycemic agents has a variable, drug-dependent effect on plasma lipid levels.

TRANSPORT OF APO-A-CONTAINING LIPOPROTEINS IN DIABETES MELLITUS

High-Density Lipoprotein

HDL may be the most complex of all the lipoprotein class. Subclasses of HDL, varying in size, density, lipid composition, and apolipoprotein components, have been isolated by a variety of physical-chemical techniques. The majority of HDL are formed by the apparent coalescence of individual phospholipid-apolipoprotein discs containing apo-A-I, apo-A-II, apo-A-VI, and possibly apo-E, together with two plasma proteins, LCAT and cholesteryl ester transfer protein (CETP). The small intestine does secrete some spherical HDL directly.

Nascent HDL was usually classified as HDL3, and was considered to be the main acceptors of cell membrane-free cholesterol. Recent studies *(17)* have identified even more primitive HDL forms called pre-β and pre-α HDL. These disc-like HDLs, particularly those with apo-A-I, appear to be the best acceptors of membrane-free cholesterol and may be the initial HDL particles involved in reverse cholesterol transport. The movement of cholesterol from cell membranes to these nascent HDL is mediated by a transport protein called ATP cassette binding protein A1 (ABCA1). When LCAT generates CE from the free cholesterol acquired, HDL3 are formed and further free cholesterol can be accepted. After adequate free cholesterol conversion to CE, HDL3 become HDL2. It appears that HDL2 can deliver their CE to the liver via a process called selective uptake (the CE enters the cells without uptake of the entire particle) or transfer their CEs to triglyceride-rich lipoproteins. The selective uptake of CEs from HDL to several organs, including the liver, results from the interaction of HDL with a receptor called scavenger receptor B (SRB)-1 *(18)*. It is not known if SRB-1 is affected by diabetes.

In humans, the CETP-mediated transfer of CE from HDL to triglyceride-rich lipoproteins (chylomicrons and VLDL in the fed and fasted states, respectively) appears to be another major pathway for movement of CE out of HDL2. The CEs can then be taken up by the liver, or other peripheral tissues, as chylomicron remnants, VLDL remnants or IDL, and finally LDL are removed from plasma. Individuals with hypertriglyceridemia and low plasma levels of HDL cholesterol have increased transfer of CE from HDL to triglyceride-rich lipoproteins, and this is probably true in decompensated type 1 DM and in almost all patients with type 2 DM. Low HDL levels in type 2 DM can be present in the absence of fasting hypertriglyceridemia, and the mechanism for this is undefined.

In type 1 DM, HDL cholesterol levels are often normal, and studies of the relationship between HDL cholesterol levels and degree of glycemic control in these patients have been inconsistent. HDL levels may actually be increased in individuals receiving intensive insulin therapy, and this may be linked to increased LPL activity and/or reduced HTGL activity. A recent report suggests that there were no differences in apo-A-I metabolism between patients with type 1 DM and nondiabetics when they are matched for a wide range of HDL cholesterol concentrations.

Reduced plasma HDL cholesterol levels do not seem to be related to control, or mode of treatment in patients with type 2 DM. Once again, however, understanding the metabolism of HDL in type 2 DM is complicated by the common presence of obesity and insulin resistance-associated dyslipidemias in this group. A consistent finding is the inverse relationship between plasma insulin (or C-peptide) concentrations, which are measures of insulin resistance, and HDL cholesterol levels. Fractional catabolism of apo-A-I is increased in type 2 DM with low HDL as it is in nondiabetics with similar lipoprotein profiles. Although apo-A-I levels are reduced consistently, correction of hypertriglyceridemia does not usually alter apo-A-I levels *(4)*.

It is very likely that the combination of insulin resistance, hyperinsulinemia, and increased free fatty acid flux in patients with type 2 DM is the underlying abnormality driving increased hepatic assembly and secretion of VLDL, IDL, and/or LDL particles (with or without absolute hypertriglyceridemia). In the presence of increased secretion of apo-B-containing lipoproteins, and concomitant hyperlipidemia, CETP-mediated transfer of HDL CE to those lipoproteins would result in lower levels of HDL cholesterol (and increased HDL triglyceride) in type 2 DM. This scheme, however, does not directly present a basis for the increased apo-A-I catabolism that have been observed. Studies have demonstrated, however, that apo-A-I may dissociate from triglyceride-enriched HDL and be cleared by the kidney *(19)*. Increased HTGL activity in type 2 DM, with increased hydrolysis of triglyceride and the generation of smaller HDL, may also play a role in this scheme.

Defective HDL3 mediated efflux of cellular free cholesterol, defective LCAT activity, increased selective delivery of HDL2 CE to hepatocytes, and increased direct hepatic uptake of apo-E-enriched HDL by the liver are other potential, but unproven, causes of low HDL in type 2 DM. The effect of diabetes on SRB-1 levels or function is also unknown. Glycosylation of HDL apo-C-II, apo-C-III and apo-E could also theoretically affect HDL metabolism. Finally, potential effects of diabetes and/or insulin resistance on ABCA1 must be defined.

Although control of hyperglycemia does not correlate well with HDL cholesterol levels in patients with type 2 DM, intensive insulin therapy has been shown to increase total HDL and HDL2 levels in some, but not all studies of patients with type 1 DM *(7)*. Therapy with sulfonylureas does not seem to increase HDL cholesterol concentrations *(4,5)*. On the other hand, modest increases in HDL levels, concomitant with modest decreases in triglyceride concentrations, have been observed with metformin therapy *(14)*. More recently, some of the TZDs, were shown to moderately reduce plasma triglyceride and raise HDL cholesterol levels in patients with type 2 DM *(14)*. The ability of these drugs to also lower plasma free fatty acids (FFAs) levels 25% to 30% is consistent with the hypothesis that increased FFA flux to the liver in type 2 DM drives VLDL secretion and the subsequent effects on HDL.

TREATMENT OF DIABETIC DYSLIPIDEMIA

Treatment Guidelines

The Adult Treatment Panel (ATP III) of the National Cholesterol Education Program (NCEP) *(32)* classified diabetes mellitus as a CHD equivalent, with the goal for LDL cholesterol of less than 100 mg/dL. More recently, the National Heart, Lung, and Blood Institute, the American College of Cardiology, and the American Heart Association revised recommendations with a lower LDL threshold based on a review of five major clinical trials of statin therapy conducted since the 2001 NCEP cholesterol guideline *(32a)*. Major updated recommendations include a lower LDL for very high-risk patients, those who have cardiovascular disease with either multiple risk factors (especially diabetes), severe and poorly controlled risk factors (e.g., continued smoking), or metabolic syndrome (a constellation of risk factors associated with obesity including high triglycerides and low HDL) *(32a)*. The update offers a new therapeutic option of treating LDL to under 70 mg/dL. For high-risk patients, the overall goal remains on LDL level of less than 100 mg/dL. The NCEP defines high-risk patients as those who have coronary heart disease or disease of the blood vessels of the brain or extremities, diabetes, or multiple (two or more) risk factors (e.g., smoking, hypertension) that give them a >20% chance of having a heart attack within 10 years *(32a)*. For high-risk patients, the update lowers the threshold for drug therapy to an LDL of 100 mg/dL or higher and recommends drug therapy for those high-risk patients whose LDL is 100–129 mg/dL. In contrast, ATP set the drug therapy threshold for high-risk patients at an LDL of 130 mg/dL or higher, and made drug treatment optional for LDL 100–129 mg/dL.

Dietary Therapy

The centerpiece of therapy for the treatment of diabetes is always diet, irrespective of the absence or presence of dyslipidemia *(20)*. However, the presence of dyslipidemia increases the rationale for intensive diet intervention. It is important to remember that improvements in plasma triglyceride and total cholesterol levels during dietary intervention can be observed even in the absence of weight loss. Thus, reductions in dietary saturated fat intake, along with reduced cholesterol consumption, can lower plasma triglyceride and LDL cholesterol levels even if caloric intake is unchanged.

Weight Loss

Weight reduction is an essential part of dietary therapy in individuals with type 2 DM. Weight loss has been shown not only to improve glycemic control and reduce insulin resistance, but to positively affect lipoprotein patterns as well. Several groups have shown that when weight reduction is achieved and maintained in type 2 DM patients, that there is a sustained decrease in triglyceride levels. Studies with weight loss in diabetic Pima Indians *(21)* revealed that there was decreased VLDL synthesis, although VLDL removal rate and LPL activity were unchanged. Most, but not all, studies show an increase in HDL cholesterol and an improvement in the ratio of total to HDL cholesterol in type 2 DM patients who lose weight.

The optimal weight loss diet in diabetics is controversial *(22)*. Most physicians would agree that a significant reduction in total calories is needed to achieve desirable body weight. This implies a restriction in all nutrients (i.e., fat, carbohydrate, and protein). It seems reasonable that because fats are more calorically dense than carbohydrates or proteins, a diet higher in carbohydrates (with high soluble fiber) and lower in fat (particularly saturated fat), as recommended by the American Diabetes Association (ADA) and the American Heart Association (AHA), would be a sound first approach. If this approach proved deleterious, with development of poor glycemic control and high levels of triglyceride, a higher-fat diet (low-saturated fat diet) as advocated by some authors, might then be attempted. A sustained, gradual weight loss is widely accepted as the best approach to prevent loss of muscle mass and precipitation of gallstones. Very low-calorie diets of about 600 kcal per day may be a reasonable short-term approach in patients who are morbidly obese and/or severely hypertriglyceridemic. Several studies of these diets, carried out under close physician observation, report improved glycemic control and decreased insulin resistance, and reduction in plasma triglyceride levels.

High-Carbohydrate vs High-Fat Diet

The recommendations of the ADA for the nutritional management of individuals with DM have varied over the past several decades, with shifting emphasis of carbohydrate vs fat restriction. The changes in diet recommendations have derived from concern about the balance of carbohydrate and fat in the diet. Thus, although there has been agreement for some time about the need to reduce dietary saturated fat intake and limit consumption of simple sugars, the issue of unsaturated fats vs "complex" carbohydrates has remained controversial. During the past decade, several investigators have suggested that a diet high in carbohydrate may in fact have a deleterious effect on both diabetic control and the dyslipidemia common in type 2 diabetic patients. Additionally, epidemiological evidence that diets high in fat but low in saturated fat (i.e., the "Mediterranean diet") are associated with low rates of heart disease was cited in support of an alternative approach. Studies have demonstrated that severely fat-restricted, very high-carbohydrate diets can raise plasma triglyceride levels in both hypertriglyceridemic individuals, and in individuals with normal levels of plasma triglyceride. In diabetics, diets that are high in carbohydrate have been shown to lead to higher postprandial glucose levels and high fasting triglyceride levels *(23,24)*. The etiology of higher triglyceride levels with high-carbohydrate diets has been linked to increased VLDL production by the liver. This diet-induced hypertriglyceridemia can, in turn, further decrease the already reduced levels of HDL cholesterol in patients with type 2 DM. However, higher carbohydrate, lower fat diets that are high in fiber (both soluble and insoluble) can be used without the deleterious effects on glucose and lipid levels (*see* below).

There is no evidence that low fat diets cause deterioration of diabetic control in patients with type 1 DM. Additionally, there are other studies demonstrating that diets high in carbohydrates can improve diabetic control and glucose tolerance in patients with type

2 DM. Inclusion of large quantities of soluble fiber in the high-carbohydrate diet abrogates many of the adverse effects on diabetic control and dyslipidemia (25,26). Not all patients with type 2 DM may benefit by increased dietary fiber, and there are certainly those patients who may not be able to tolerate high-fiber diets, especially if they have gastroparesis.

Based on all of the above information, the ADA recent dietary recommendations have focused on reductions of dietary saturated fat and cholesterol, and allowing for individualization of diet in terms of the optimal replacement for saturated fat (27). These guidelines are very similar to those recently published by the AHA (28). At the present time, it seems reasonable to recommend the diet approved by both the ADA and the AHA as a first approach to all diabetics irrespective of their plasma lipid concentrations. If there is then an adverse response to the recommended diet, such as worsening diabetic control or hypertriglyceridemia, a diet higher in monounsaturated fat (or polyunsaturated fat) could then be substituted. A cautionary note relevant to the use of high-monounsaturated fat diet: fat has more than twice the caloric density than carbohydrate (9 kcal/g vs 4 kcal/g). The use of high-fat diets may, therefore, predispose to weight gain.

Specific Types of Dietary Fat

The omega-3 fatty acids are unique polyunsaturated fatty acids that have aroused considerable interest (29). These fatty acids, found mostly in fatty fish, are comprised mainly of eicosapentaenoic acid and docosahexenoic acid. α-Linolenic acid, present in vegetables such as linseed, is also an omega-3 fatty acid. Fatty acids in this series have the ability to reduce platelet aggregability. Additionally, when consumed in large quantities (3–4 g per day), the omega-3 fatty acids appear to cause a profound decrease in plasma VLDL concentrations in subjects with severe (>1000 mg/dL) hypertriglyceridemia. In milder forms of hypertriglyceridemia, reductions in VLDL are often associated with increases in plasma LDL and apo-B levels. These responses to increased intake of omega-3 fatty acid, whether as fish or supplements, have been observed in both nondiabetics and diabetics. In early studies, worsening of diabetic control was observed during omega-3 fatty acid consumption; this has not been seen in larger, better designed trials. Several cohort studies and intervention trials suggest that diets high in omega-3 fatty acids are associated with reduced rates of CAD in high-risk populations (30). Although ingestion of increased quantities of fish should be recommended, use of omega-3 fatty acid supplements, at the level of 1 g per day, has also been recommended by the AHA for individuals with coronary heart disease (31).

Dietary Fiber

As noted above, diets high in fiber are beneficial to both type 1 and type 2 patients with diabetes (25–26). Most of the therapeutic effect comes from the nondigestable polysaccharide fractions of cell wall of plants. Consumption of either soluble or insoluble fiber slows glucose absorption, leading to improved glycemic control and increased insulin sensitivity although soluble fiber alone lowers cholesterol and triglyceride levels. Diets that are high in fiber have also been shown to promote weight loss and increase satiety in nondiabetic individuals, although few studies have been done with diabetics. It is recommended, therefore, that diabetics take in 20 to 30 g of fiber per 1000 kcal, and that one-third of this total be in the form of insoluble fiber. The fiber should be derived from dietary intake rather than supplements. However, this is five to six times the present fiber intake in the United States, and may not be attainable. In particular, diabetics with significant gastroparesis may not be able to tolerate a diet high in fiber.

Exercise

Exercise can increase glucose uptake by muscle as much as 20-fold, and as exercise continues, fat rather than carbohydrate becomes the predominant fuel that is burned. However, in glucose intolerant, nonobese hypertriglyceridemic males, exercise improved aerobic capacity and lowered insulin levels but did not improve either the abnormal response to an oral glucose load, or insulin sensitivity. Exercise alone without weight loss has variable effects on lipid profiles in type 2 diabetics.

Lipid Lowering

After an adequate trial of diabetic control, diet, weight loss, and exercise, drug therapy should be initiated for the treatment of dyslipidemia. Indeed, in the most recent report of the Adult Treatment Panel of the National Cholesterol Education Program *(32)*, DM was classified as a CAD equivalent, with the goal for LDL cholesterol of less than 100 mg/dL. Thus, the length of time taken in an attempt to have the patient make lifestyle changes should be minimized. In some patients, lifestyle and drug treatment should be started simultaneously. Patients with many correctable lifestyle habits and/or poorly controlled glycemia may require more time devoted to those problems prior to initiation of specific hypolipidemic drug treatment, but the "waiting period" should not be long. The severity of the dyslipidemia, independent of glycemic control, is an indicator of the presence of other genetic causes of lipid abnormalities, and this can also be taken into account when considering initiation of specific lipid-lowering therapy.

Bile Acid Binding

Cholestyramine and colestipol are resins that bind bile acids in the intestine, thus interrupting the enterohepatic recirculation of those molecules *(33)*. A fall in bile acids returning to the liver results in increased conversion of hepatic cholesterol to bile acids, which results in a diminution of a regulatory pool of hepatic cholesterol and upregulation of the gene for hepatic LDL receptors. All of these changes lead to increased LDL receptors on the surface of hepatoctyes and, therefore, decreased plasma LDL concentrations. Usual doses are 8 to 24 g per day for cholestyramine and 10 to 30 g per day for colestipol. Cholestyramine is mixed with sucrose, but there is a "light" form that is made with nutrasweet. Colestipol is also available in 1-g tablets. Bile acid-binding resins are not absorbed and, therefore, have no systemic toxicities. A drawback to the use of bile acid binding resin in diabetics is the increase in hepatic VLDL triglyceride production and plasma triglyceride levels commonly associated with their use. An additional major side effect of these agents is bloating and constipation, which may pose a significant problem in the diabetic with gastroparesis. The resins can also interfere with the absorption of other oral medications. Bile acid resins should therefore only be used alone in diabetics with pure elevations of total and LDL cholesterol. With the availability of 3-hydroxy-3-methylglutaryl-coenzyme-A (HMG-CoA) reductase inhibitors (see HMG-CoA Reductase Inhibitors) however, the need for resins has been markedly reduced.

A new agent in this class of drugs that is now available is colesevelam. It is a bile acid sequestrant polymer that has greater tolerability and few drug interactions than the other resins. It appears to have four to six times greater potency than the other bile acid sequestrants *(34)* and appears to work in a dose dependent manner. It is available in 625 mg tablets and is Food and Drug Administration-approved in the treatment of mild to moderate hypercholesterolemia, as monotherapy, and in conjunction with HMG-CoA reductase inhibitors, for therapy of more severe hypercholesterolemia. Gastrointestinal side effects seems to be significantly reduced compared to the older bile acid sequestrants.

Ezetimibe

A very recent addition to the drugs that can be used to lower LDL cholesterol is the inhibitor of intestinal cholesterol absorption, ezetimibe. This agent appears to interact with a receptor for cholesterol, as yet unidentified, in the brush border of enterocytes in the small intestine. At the single recommended dose of 10 mg per day, ezetimibe lowers LDL cholesterol between 15% and 20%. It has little effect on triglyceride or HDL cholesterol. Ezetimibe seems additive when used in combination with statins. There are no published data for ezetimibe in combination with other agents or as a therapy for patients with type 2 DM.

HMG-CoA Reductase Inhibitors

During the past decade, the treatment of hypercholesterolemia has undergone a revolution with the availability of potent, safe HMG-CoA reductase inhibitors, also known as statins *(35)*. Lovastatin, pravastatin, fluvastatin, simvastatin, atorvastatin, and rosuvastatin are available drugs in this category in the United States. They work to competitively inhibit HMG-CoA reductase, the rate-limiting enzyme in cholesterol synthesis, which results in both decreased hepatic production of apo-B-containing lipoproteins and upregulation of LDL receptors. The overall effect is a dramatic lowering of plasma levels of LDL cholesterol. VLDL triglyceride concentrations are also reduced in many subjects with moderate hypertriglyceridemia *(36)*. The reduction of triglyceride is directly related to the reduction of LDL cholesterol achieved. The most potent statins (simvastatin, atorvastatin, and rosuvastatin), at the highest doses, can lower LDL cholesterol by up to 45% to 60%, and decrease triglyceride 20% to 45% *(37)*. The reduction in triglyceride achieved at these high levels of LDL cholesterol reduction will depend on the starting triglyceride level. Reductase inhibitors can raise HDL cholesterol by up to 10%, but the more typical increase is about 5%. Statins should not be considered as first-line agents for individuals with very low HDL levels.

The main side effect associated with statin therapy is a myositis, characterized by diffuse severe muscle tenderness and weakness, and elevated levels of creatine phosphokinase (CPK) (usually >10,000 U). In severe cases, rhabdomyolysis and concomitant myoglobinemia can place the patients at risk for renal failure as a result of myoglobinuria. This is particularly a risk in diabetics who have pre-existing proteinuria. However, the incidence of myositis when statins are used as monotherapy is about 1 in 1000 patients, and careful instructions about the signs and symptoms, with advice to stop the medication and consume large volumes of liquids, should obviate more serious outcomes. Statins can also cause nonclinically significant elevations in liver function tests in 1% to 2% of patients, but only at the higher doses of each agent. The statins do not appear to affect diabetic control. Importantly, results from several clinical trials demonstrate reductions in CAD events and deaths type 2 diabetic patients treated with statins *(38,39)*. These agents are therefore, the first-line of approach to diabetic patients with isolated high levels of LDL cholesterol, with combined hyperlipidemia, or with moderate hypertriglyceridemia and an LDL cholesterol level that is above National Cholesterol Education Program (NCEP) goal. As discussed below, they can also be used in conjunction with other hypolipidemic agents under some circumstances.

The Heart Protection Study (HPS) prospectively evaluated 20,536 adults with CAD or diabetes randomized to receive simvastatin 40 mg or placebo over 5 years. The primary outcomes were mortality and fatal or nonfatal vascular events. All-cause mortality was significantly reduced as a result of the decrease in the coronary death rate in the simvastatin vs placebo groups (5.7% vs 6.9%, $p = 0.0005$). Relative reductions of most cardiovascular endpoints in the simvastatin group were in the range of 25%. There were almost 6000 patients with diabetes in HPS, and they had similar relative reductions in cardiovascular events when treated with simvastatin, albeit with higher absolute event rates than the nondiabetics. In HPS, the annual risk of myopathy was 0.01% and there were no significant increases in liver enzymes (40).

Fibric Acid Derivatives

Fenofibrate and gemfibrozil are the agents available in the United States at present. Several others are available in Europe and Canada. Fibric acid derivatives have potent lipid-altering effects that may be quite useful in diabetics. In general, fibrate use in patients with type 2 DM results in lowering of triglyceride from 20% to 35% and increases in HDL cholesterol from 10% to 20% (41). Although their mechanism of action is unclear, these agents appear to work by both decreasing hepatic VLDL production, and increasing the activity of LPL. Unfortunately, fibrates have modest and variable effects on LDL cholesterol in most patients with DM and may even raise LDL levels in patients who present with more significant hypertriglyceridemia and lower LDL cholesterol levels pretreatment. The basis for these variable outcomes is complex and has to do with the efficiency with which VLDL is converted to LDL, and how efficiently LDL is removed from plasma. The usual dose is 600 mg twice daily of gemfibrozil and 160 mg once daily for micronized fenofibrate. These agents are contraindicated in patients with gallstones, and because they are tightly bound to plasma proteins, levels of other drugs (e.g., coumadin) should be monitored carefully. Fibrates do not significantly affect glycemic control.

The rise in LDL cholesterol concentration that can accompany reduced triglyceride levels during fibrate therapy must be viewed in the context of clinical trials of fibrate therapy that included patients with DM. In the Helsinki Heart Study, the two groups with hypertriglyceridemia (with and without concomitant elevations in LDL cholesterol) had increases or no changes in LDL cholesterol levels during gemfibrozil therapy. Yet they achieved the same reduction in CAD events as did the group with isolated LDL elevations, in whom LDL cholesterol levels fell 10% to 12% with treatment (42). The two groups in which LDL changed little or not at all included the majority of the diabetic participants and a separate analysis of the Helsinki study demonstrated reductions in events among these patients taking gemfibrozil. In the Veterans Administration HDL Intervention Trial, gemfibrozil was efficacious in a group of men who had CAD and LDL cholesterol that was low (111 mg/dL) at baseline and did not change during the trial (43). The treated group did show a 7% increase in HDL cholesterol and a 25% reduction in triglyceride; these effects were associated with a 24% reduction in CAD events. Similarly, The Diabetes Atherosclerosis Intervention Study (DAIS) showed that treatment with fenofibrate was associated with lower triglyceride and higher HDL cholesterol levels, and decreases in focal CAD by angiography in subjects with type 2 diabetes (44).

When statins have been compared to fibrates in type 2 diabetic patients, the statins produced much greater reductions in LDL although the fibrates resulted in both greater d reductions in triglyceride and increases in HDL *(45)*. Several recent studies of combination treatment of patients with type 2 DM have shown the powerful, positive effects on the entire dyslipidemic pattern with this approach *(46)*. Of note, the combination of statins and fibrates may significantly increase the risk of myositis to about 1% to 2%. Recent studies have shown that gemfibrozil affects the formation of oxidative products and CYP3A4-mediated oxidative metabolites of simvastatin hydroxyacid, and markedly inhibiting the glucoronidation of oxidative products. Importantly, fenofibrate had a minimal effect on this glucoronidation pathway, suggesting that there may be a difference between fibrates in regard to their effects on statin concentrations in plasma. This hypothesis is supported by data showing that combinations of several statins with gemfibrozil was associated with increased blood levels of each of the statins *(47)*. More studies with fenofibrate are awaited, but preliminary results from the Lipid Diabetes Study (LDS), a study that used fenofibrate and cerivastatin alone or in combination are hopeful. The study was halted because cerivastatin was removed from the market after causing significantly more myositis and rhabdomyolysis than other statin. In LDS, there was one case of myositis among 1000 patients taking the combination of fenofibrate and cerivastatin; this was the same very low rate as seen in equal size groups taking cerivastatin alone, fenofibrate alone, or placebo.

Nicotinic Acid (Niacin)

The most common lipid abnormalities present in patients with DM are elevated triglyceride and low HDL cholesterol levels. Niacin, when used in pharmacological doses (1–3 g per day), has the ability to potently lower triglyceride (25%–40%) and raise HDL cholesterol (10%–25%). Niacin also lowers LDL cholesterol (15%–20%) and this adds to its potential efficacy in a high-risk population. The mechanism of action is generally thought to be through lowering hepatic VLDL apo-B production and increasing the synthesis of apo-A-I. Unfortunately, niacin has several side effects that often limit its utility in nondiabetics: Niacin produces a prostaglandin-mediated flush that occurs about 30 minutes after ingestion and can last as long as 1 hour; patients turn red and feel hot. Niacin can also cause gastric irritation and can exacerbate peptic ulcer disease; it has been associated with dry skin; it causes hyperuricemia and can precipitate gouty attacks, and its use is associated with elevations of hepatic transaminases in about 5% of patients. Rarely, niacin can also cause a clinically significant hepatitis. Most importantly, some studies have demonstrated that niacin therapy worsens diabetic control, likely by inducing insulin resistance *(48)*. This finding is interesting at a theoretical level, because niacin's ability to inhibit lipolysis and lower plasma FFA levels after a single dose of the drug might be expected to improve insulin sensitivity. Not all investigators believe that niacin is contraindicated in patients with diabetes and the availability of an intermediate-release form of niacin (Niaspan) has rekindled interest in its potential in this population *(49)*. A study of 148 diabetic patients randomized to placebo vs 1,000 mg or 1,500 mg of extended-release niacin showed statistically significant dose-dependent increases in HDL with both doses, and reduction in triglyceride with the 1500 mg dose (vs placebo) at 16 weeks. The glycosylated hemoglobin remained stable in the placebo and 1000 mg groups, but increased slightly in the 1500 mg group (7.2% and 7.5%, baseline and week 16 respectively, $p = 0.048$ vs placebo) *(50)*.

Hormone Replacement Therapy

For years, hormone replacement therapy (HRT) in women was used not only for the short-term benefit of alleviating postmenopausal symptoms, but also for the prevention of coronary heat disease. This was based on observational data and angiographic and autopsy data demonstrating an "anti-atherogenic property" of estrogen *(51–53)*. Recent data from the Women's Health Initiative (WHI) and the Heart and Estrogen/Progesterone Replacement Study (HERS I and II), however, have not confirmed the prior, indirect evidence of a protective effect of combined HRT on the heart. In fact, the data suggests that combined replacement therapy with estrogen and progestin may cause harm when used in primary or secondary prevention.

The WHI is an "umbrella structure" for a number of different trials in healthy post-menopausal women aged 50 to 79. WHI included two studies of HRT in its overall design. In one of the estrogen trials, 16,000 women were studied with continuous combined estrogen and progesterone vs placebo over 5.2 years. The study was stopped early as a result of an increased risk of stroke, CAD, venous thromboembolism, and breast cancer in the treated group. The treated group received 0.625 mg conjugated estrogen and 2.5 mg medroxyprogesterone acetate per day. The rate of CAD event increased by 29%, largely from nonfatal MIs, and this change persisted for the duration of the trial *(54)*. The WHI trial of unopposed estrogen vs placebo, in women who had prior hysterectomies, continues. Based on these findings and until further data are obtained, combined estrogen and progesterone cannot be recommended for primary prevention of CAD.

The proposed cardiovascular benefits of HRT were also called into question when results of the first randomized, placebo-controlled intervention trial, the HERS study, showed no benefit in women with prior MI who received combined equine conjugated estrogens (Premarin) plus continuous low-dose medroxyprogesterone (Provera) *(55)*. As noted earlier, it remains to be seen if estrogen replacement without progesterone will be protective, neutral, or detrimental in terms of cardiovascular risk in postmenopausal women.

Until the past few years, there were no published studies on the effects of HRT in women with DM. Reasons for the lack of interest may have included the knowledge that early oral contraceptives containing relatively large amounts of estrogen were associated with worsened glucose tolerance and increased risk of MI and stroke; and estrogen is known to increase triglyceride levels and diabetic women often have hypertrigly-ceridemia. Recent longitudinal data, however, show that the use of HRT does not increase the risk of developing diabetes later in life. Additionally, the results of three intervention trials have been published which assessed HRT in women with type 2 diabetes for periods of 6–12 weeks *(56–58)*. All three showed that isolated estrogen treatment lowered blood glucose levels and glycosylated hemoglobin levels without raising plasma insulin concentrations or causing insulin resistance. Lipid profiles were also improved, with lower LDL and higher HDL cholesterol levels, and with no significant rise in plasma triglyceride in two of the three studies. It is not known if combination therapy with estrogen and a progestin would have produced the same biochemical benefits. Interestingly, estrogen replacement therapy appears to improve postprandial lipemia in normal subjects despite its effect to raise fasting triglyceride levels. Oral estrogen given alone raises HDL levels by 10% to 20% by increasing apo-A-I synthesis and decreasing hepatic lipase activity. Estrogen alone also lowers LDL cholesterol about 20% by increasing LDL receptor number on cells, particularly in the liver. Another effect relates to the ability of estrogen to lower Lp(a) levels about 20% *(59)*. Some studies suggest that estrogen can improve endothelial function and nitric oxide synthesis, act as a vasodilator to decrease cardiac afterload, may act as a calcium blocking agent and an antioxidant, decrease both fibrinogen and plasminogen activator inhibitor-1 levels, and possibly lower plasma homocysteine levels. A potentially negative effect of estrogen administration is the increase in plasma triglyceride that occurs via increased hepatic secretion of VLDL. Severe hyperlipidemia, and pancreatitis, have been observed in women with pre-existing hypertriglyceridemia who were receiving oral estrogen treatment. More data is needed on unopposed estrogen treatment in this population.

SUMMARY

When rationally approached, the diabetic patient with hyperlipidemia can be well managed through both lifestyle interventions and pharmacotherapy. Close guidance and monitoring is needed, however, in choosing the proper approach. A variety of options are available to improve plasma lipids and thus reduce risk of CAD.

When specific lipid-altering therapy is indicated, the physician has effective and safe agents from which to choose. For the diabetic with isolated hypertriglyceridemia and low HDL cholesterol (with LDL cholesterol that is at or below goal, or at least no more than 120 mg/dL), fibric acid derivatives appear to be the first choice in most cases. In many cases, this will be all that is necessary. If the LDL cholesterol concentration is also above goal, or increased during treatment with the fibric acid agent, the physician has several choices. First, a bile acid binding resin could be added to the fibrate: this would lower LDL cholesterol without, in the presence of the fibrate, significantly effecting triglyceride levels. The second alternative would be to either switch to an HMG-CoA reductase inhibitor, this would be the logical choice if the triglyceride elevation (before or during fibrate treatment) was only moderate (<300 mg/dL), or to add the reductase inhibitor to the fibrate. The latter combination is very effective in correcting severe combined hyperlipidemia, but carries some increased risk of myositis, although the risk with fenofibrate plus statin may be significantly less than with gemfibrozil and statin. We believe that this combination can be used successfully, particularly if patients know clearly that they must stop the medications, drink large quantities of liquids, and call their physician if diffuse, severe muscle pain occurs. These patients should have liver function tests obtained regularly with use of fibrates or reductase inhibitors alone or in combination. A third choice would be the addition of ezetimibe, the new inhibitor of intestinal cholesterol absorption, which would be efficacious if the patients required no more than a 20% reduction in LDL to reach goal. The final choice, nicotinic acid, could be used in patients with severe, combined hyperlipidemia. Use of niacin should be limited, and may best be reserved for those diabetics with significant combined hyperlipidemia already on insulin.

In those patients who present with elevations of both LDL cholesterol and plasma triglyceride, an HMG-CoA reductase inhibitor is probably the most effective single agent. Again, niacin could also be used as a sole drug, with caution taken as described above. A fibric acid derivative can be added if triglyceride levels are not sufficiently reduced by either of those drugs alone. Alternatively, fibrates could be used initially with bile acid binding resins or ezetimibe.

Therapy for the diabetic patient with an isolated reduction in HDL cholesterol is not clearly defined. Fibrates have not been demonstrated to be very effective in raising HDL cholesterol levels in nondiabetics with isolated reductions in HDL, although no similar studies have been carried out in diabetics. Niacin may be more effective in elevating HDL cholesterol concentrations when they are the low in the absence of hypertriglyceridemia, but all of the caveats of niacin use in DM would apply here as well. An alternative to raising HDL in these subjects would be to more aggressively treat LDL cholesterol levels, with the goal of reducing them to well elow less than 100 mg/dL. It must be clear, however, that there are no endpoint trials supporting any approach to isolated reductions in HDL cholesterol either in nondiabetics or diabetics.

Finally, in those diabetics with isolated high levels of LDL cholesterol, bile acid resins, ezetimibe, or an HMG-CoA reductase inhibitor may be used primarily. The combination of a statin with one of the other two of these agents has been shown to be very effective in those individuals who have extremely high levels of LDL cholesterol, resistant to monotherapy. There are no published data for ezetimibe use in patients with diabetes. triglyceride levels need to be observed closely in those patients placed on resins.

REFERENCES

1. Kannel WB, D'Agostino RB, Wilson PWF, Bleanger AJ, Gagnon DR. Diabetes, fibrinogen, and risk of cardiovascular disease: the Framingham experience. Am Heart J 1990;120:672–676.
2. Haffner SM, Lehto S, Ronnemaa T, Pyorala K, Laakso M. Mortality from coronary heart disease in subjects with type 2 diabetes and in nondiabetic subjects with and without prior myocardial infarctions. N Engl J Med 1998;339:229–234.
3. Haffner SM. Management of dyslipidemia in adults with diabetes (Technical Review). Diabetes Care 1998;21:160–178.
4. Ginsberg HN. Lipoprotein Physiology in Nondiabetic and Diabetic States: relationship to Atherogenesis. Diabetes Care 1991;14:839–855.
5. Taskinen, M-R. Hyperlipidaemia in diabetes. Baillieres Clin Endocrinol Metab 1990;4(4):743–775.
6. Betteridge DJ. Diabetes, lipoprotein metabolism and atherosclerosis. British Medical Bulletin 1989;45:(1):285–311.
7. Dunn FL. Hyperlipidemia in diabetes mellitus. Diabetes/Metabolism Reviews 1990;6(1):47–61.
8. Ginsberg HN. Lipoprotein Physiology. In: Hoeg J, (ed.). Endocrinology and metabolism clinics of North America. WB Saunders Co., Philadelphia, Pennsylvania, 1998.
9. Cooper AD. Hepatic uptake of chylomicron remnants (Review). J Lipid Res 1997;38:2173–2192.
10. Davis RA. Cell and molecular biology of the assembly and secretion of apolipoprotein B-containing lipoproteins by the liver (Review). Biochim Biophys Acta 1999;1440:1–31.
11. Fisher EA, Ginsberg HN. Complexity in the Secretory Pathway: the Assembly and Secretion of Apolipoprotein B-containing Lipoproteins. The Journal of Biological Chemistry 2002;277:17,377–17,380.
12. Kissebah AH, Alfarsi S, Evans DJ, Adams PW. Integrated regulation of very low density lipoprotein triglyceride and apolipoprotein-B kinetics in non-insulin-dependent diabetes mellitus. Diabetes 1982;31:217–225.
13. Van Wijk JP, De Koning EJ, Martens EP, Rabelink TJ. Arterioscler Thromb Vasc Biol. Thiazolidinediones and Blood Lipids in Type 2 Diabetes. 2003;23(10):1744–1749.
14. Ginsberg HN, Plutzky J, Sobel BE. A review of metabolic and cardiovascular effects of oral antidiabetic agents: beyond glucose lowering. J. Cardiovasc Risk 1999;6:337–347.
15. Austin MA, Krauss RM. LDL density and atherosclerosis. JAMA 1995;273:115.
16. Lopes-Virella MF, Klein RL, Lyons TJ, Stevenson HC, Witztum JL. Glycosylation of low-density lipoprotein enhances cholesteryl ester synthesis in human monocyte-derived macrophages. Diabetes 1998;37:550–557.
17. Phillips MC, Gillotte KL, Haynes MP, Johnson WJ, Lund-Katz S, Rothblat GH. Mechanisms of high density lipoprotein-mediated efflux of cholesterol from cell plasma membranes. Atherosclerosis 1998;137(Suppl):S13–S17.
18. Trigatti B, Rigotti A, Krieger M. The role of the high-density lipoprotein receptor SR-BI in cholesterol metabolism. Curr Opin Lipidol 2000;11:123–131.
19. Horowitz BS, Goldberg IJ, Merab J, Vanni T, Ramakrishnan R, and Ginsberg HN. Increased plasma and renal clearance of an exchangeable pool of apolipoprotein A-I in subjects with low levels of high density lipoprotein cholesterol. J Clin Invest 1993;91:1743–1760.

20. Grundy SM. Dietary Therapy in Diabetes Mellitus. Diabetes Care 1991;14:796–808.

21. Howard BV. Diabetes and plasma lipoproteins in Native Americans. Studies of the Pima Indians. Diabetes Care 1993;16(1):284–291.

22. American Diabetes Association: nutrition recommendations and principles for people with diabetes mellitus (Position Statement). Diabetes Care 1990;22:S42–S45.

23. Garg A, Bantle JP, Henry RR, et al. Effects of varying carbohydrate content of diet in patients with non-insulin-dependent diabetes mellitus. JAMA 1994;271:1421–1428.

24. Garg A, Bonanome A, Grundy SM, Zhang Z, Unger RH. Comparison of a high-carbohydrate diet with a high-monounsaturated-fat diet in patients with non-insulin-dependent diabetes mellitus. N Engl J Med 1988;319:829–834.

25. Anderson JW, Gustafson NJ, Bryant CA, Tietyen-Clark CA. Dietary fiber and diabetes: a comprehensive review and practical application. J Amer Dietetic Assoc 1987;87:1189.

26. Anderson JW. Dietary fiber and diabetes: what else do we need to know? Diabetes Res Clin Pract 1992;17:71–73.

27. American Diabetes Association: evidence-based nutrition principles and recommendations for the treatment and prevention of diabetes and related complications. Diabetes Care 2003;26(Suppl 1):S51-S61.

28. Krauss RM, Eckel RH, Howard B, et al. AHA dietary guidelines: revision 2000: a statement for healthcare professionals from the nutrition committee of the American Heart Association. Circulation 2000;102: 2284–2299.

29. Harris WS. Dietary fish oil and blood lipids. Curr Opin Lipidol 1996;7(1):3–7.

30. Kris-Etherton P, Harris WS, Appel LJ. Fish consumption, fish oil, omega-3 fatty acids, and cardiovascular disease. Circulation 2002;106:2747–2757.

31. Kris-Etherton P, Harris WS, Appel LJ. Omega-3 fatty acids and cardiovascular disease: new recommendations from the American Heart Association. Arterio Thromb Vasc Biol 2003;23:151–152.

32. National Cholesterol Education Program. Third Report of the National Cholesterol Education Program (NCEP) Expert Panel on Detection, Evaluation, and Treatment of High Blood Cholesterol in Adults (Adult Treatment Panel III) final report. Circulation 2002;106:3143–3421.

32a. Grundy SM, Cleeman JI, Merz CN, et al. Implications of recent clinical trials for the National Cholesterol Education Program Adult Treatment Panel III guidelines. Circulation 2004;110:227–239.

33. Garg A, Grundy SM. Management of Dyslipidemia in NIDDM. Diabetes Care 1990;13:153–163.

34. Steinmetz KL. Colesevelam hydrochloride. Am J Health Syst Pharm 2002;59(10):932–939.

35. Ginsberg HN. Drug Therapy of Hypercholesterolemia. In: Rifkind B, (ed.). Cholesterol Lowering in High-Risk Individiuals and Populations. Marcel Dekker Inc, Publisher; New York, 1995, pp. 272–290.

36. Ginsberg HN. Effects of statins on triglyceride metabolism. Am J Cardiol 1998;81(4A):32B–35B.

37. Stein, EA, Lane MLaskarzewski P. Comparison of statins in hypertriglyceridemia. Am. J. Cardiol 1998;81(4A):66B–69B.

38. Pyorala K, Pedersen TR, Kjekshus JFaegerman O, Olsson AG, Thorgeirsson G. Cholesterol lowering with simvastatin improves prognosis of diabetic patients with coronary artery disease. A subgroup analysis of the Scandinavian Simvastatin Survival Study. Diabetes Care 1997;20:614–620.

39. Goldberg RB, Mellies MJ, Sacks FM, et al. Cardiovascular events and their reduction with pravastatin in diabetic and glucose intolerant myocardial infarction survivors with average cholesterol levels: subgroup analysis in the cholesterol and recurrent events (CARE) trial. Circ 1998;98:2513–2519.

40. Heart Protection Study Group. Heart Protection Study of cholesterol lowering with simvastatin in 20536 high-risk individuals: a randomized placebo-controlled trial. Lancet 2002;360:7–22.

41. Steiner G. Effects of Various Lipid-Lowering Treatments in Diabetes. J. Cardiovasc. Pharm 1990;16:S35–S38.

42. Frick MH, Elo H, Haapa K, et al. Helsinki Heart Study: primary prevention trial with gemfibrozil in middle-aged men with dyslipidemia. N Engl J Med 1987;317:1237–1245.

43. Rubins HB, Robbins SJ, Collins P, et al., for the Veterans Affairs High-Density Lipoprotein Cholesterol Intervention Trial Study group. Gemfibrozil for the secondary prevention of coronary heart disease in men with low levels of high-density lipoprotein cholesterol. N Engl J Med 1999;341:410–418.

44. Diabetes Atherosclerosis Intervention Study Investigators. Effect of fenofibrate on progression of coronary-artery disease in type 2 diabetes: the Diabetes Atherosclerosis Intervention Study, a randomized study. Lancet 2001;357:905–910.

45. Ooi TC, Heinonen T, Alaupovic P, et al. Efficacy and safety of a new hydroxymethylglutaryl-coenzyme A reductase inhibitor, atorvastatin, in patients with combined hyperlipidemia: comparison with fenofibrate. Arterioscler Thromb Vasc Biol 1997;17:1793–1799.

46. Tikkanen MJ, Laakso M, Ilmonen M, et al. Treatment of hypercholesterolemia and combined hyper-
    lipidemia with simvastatin and gemfibrozil in patients with NIDDM. A multicenter comparison study.
    Diabetes Care 1998;21:477–481.
47. Prueksaritanont T, Tang C, Qiu Y, Mu L, Subramanian R, Lin J. Effects of Fibrates on Metabolism of
    Statins in Human Hepatocytes. Drug Metabolism and Disposition 2002;30:1280–1287.
48. Garg A and Grundy SM. Nicotinic acid as therapy for dyslipidemia in non-insulin dependent diabetes
    mellitus. JAMA 1990;264:723–726.
49. Goldberg A, Alagona P, Capuzzi DM, et al. Multiple-dose efficacy and safety of an extended-release
    form of niacin in the management of Hyperlipidemia. Amer Jour of Card 2000;85:1100–1105.
50. Grundy SM, Vega GL, McGovern ME, et al. Efficacy, Safety and Tolerability of Once-Daily Niacin for
    the Treatment of Dyslipidemia Associated With Type 2 Diabetes 2002;162:1568–1576.
51. Manson JE, Martin KA. Clinical practice. Postmenopausal hormone-replacement therapy. N Engl J Med
    2001;345:34.
52. Bush TL, Barrett-Connor E, Cowan LD, et al. Cardiovascular mortality and noncontraceptive use of
    estrogen in women: results from three Lipid Research Clinics Program Follow-up Study. Circulation
    1987;75:1102.
53. Christian RC, Harrington S, Edwards WD, et al. Estrogen status correlates with the calcium content or
    coronary atherosclerotic plaques in women. J Clin Endocrinol Metab 2002;87:1062.
54. The Women's Health Initiative Study Group. Risks and benefits of estrogen plus progestin in healthy
    postmenopausal women: principal results from the Women's Health Initiative. JAMA 2002;288:321.
55. Hulley S, Grady D, Bush T, et al. Randomized trial of estrogen plus progestin for secondary prevention
    of coronary heart disease in postmenopausal women. Heart and Estrogen/progestin Replacement Study
    Research Group. JAMA 1998;280:605–613.
56. Andersson B, Mattsson, L-A, Hahn L, et al. Estrogen replacement therapy decreases hyperandrogenicity
    and improves glucose homeostasis and plasma lipids in postmenopausal women with noninsulin-depen-
    dent diabetes mellitus. J Clin Endocrinol Metab 1997;82:638–643.
57. Brussaard HE, Gevers Leuven JA, Kluft C, et al. Effect of 17 beta-estradiol on plasma lipids and LDL
    oxidation in postmenopausal women with type II diabetes mellitus. Arterioscler. Thromb. Vasc. Biol
    1997;17:324–330.
58. Friday KE. Estrogen replacement therapy improves glycemic control and high density lipoprotein
    cholesterol concentrations in post-menopausal type 2 diabetic women. Diabetes 1998;47:(Suppl 1):a357.
59. Tuck CH, Holleran S, Berglund L. Hormonal regulation of lipoprotein (a) levels: effects of estrogen
    replacement therapy on lipoprotein (a) and acute phase reactants in postmenopausal women. Arterioscler
    Thromb Vasc Biol 1997;17(9):1822–1829.

II Clinical

B. Microcirculation

16 Diabetic Retinopathy

Lloyd Paul Aiello, MD, PhD
and Jerry Cavallerano, OD, PhD

CONTENTS

INTRODUCTION

Diabetic retinopathy (DR) is a microvascular complication that eventually afflicts virtually all patients with diabetes mellitus (DM) *(1)*. Despite decades of research, there is presently no known cure or means of preventing DR, and DR remains the leading cause of new-onset blindness in working-aged Americans *(1)*. Several nationwide clinical trials have demonstrated that scatter (panretinal) laser photocoagulation reduces the 5-year risk of severe vision loss (i.e., best corrected visual acuity of 5/200 or worse) from proliferative DR from as high as 60% to less than 4%. Additionally, timely and appropriate focal laser photocoagulation for clinically significant diabetic macular edema (DME) reduces the risk of moderate vision loss (i.e., a doubling of the visual angle) from DME from nearly 30% to approx 12%. Vitrectomy surgery, with endolaser photocoagulation as indicated, can frequently prevent further vision loss or restore useful vision in eyes that have nonresolving vitreous hemorrhage or traction retinal detachment threatening central vision. Although numerous new therapies are under investigation with some already in phase 2 or 3 clinical trials, until a prevention or cure for diabetes is discovered, the keys to preventing vision loss from DR are regular eye examinations to determine the need for timely laser photocoagulation and rigorous control of blood glucose and any accompanying systemic medical conditions, such as hypertension, renal disease, and dyslipidemias.

From: *Contemporary Cardiology: Diabetes and Cardiovascular Disease, Second Edition*
Edited by: M. T. Johnstone and A. Veves © Humana Press Inc., Totowa, NJ

This chapter reviews the current understanding of the etiology and pathophysiology of DR, the clinical manifestations of the disease, and current guidelines for appropriate disease management and treatment strategies.

PATHOPHYSIOLOGY OF DIABETIC RETINOPATHY AND STRUCTURAL CHANGES OF RETINAL MICROCIRCULATION

Early Studies

Diabetic retinopathy (DR) is a highly specific retinal vascular complication of both type 1 and type 2 diabetes. Initial studies *(2–4)* of DR concentrated on retinal microaneurysms, an early clinical sign of retinal disease. Cogan, Toussaint, and Kuwabara pioneered many of these early investigations to elucidate the pathophysiology of DR *(2)*. Microaneurysms were shown to develop bordering areas of occluded capillaries with either normal or hyperplastic endothelial linings *(4)*. Additionally, a loss of mural cells in the diabetic vessels resulted in outpouchings of the capillary walls. The retinal microaneurysms appeared to develop from these areas that were deficient in mural cells.

The relative retinal ischemia common to DR and numerous other retinal vascular disorders is thought to underlie the development of retinal neovascularization (NV) and edema *(5,6)*. In 1948, Michaelson postulated that retinal ischemia initiated the release of a vasoproliferative factor *(5)*. This putative vasoproliferative factor resulted in new vessel growth at the optic disc and other areas of the retina and iris, and might account for the increased vascular permeability associated with these disorders. As discussed below, recent studies have greatly increased our understanding of these vasoproliferative factors.

Studies using experimentally induced diabetes in dogs demonstrated that hyperglycemia, characterized by deficient insulin activity, is capable of eliciting DR, even in animals that do not have hereditary forms of diabetes *(7–11)*. Engerman's studies of alloxan-induced diabetic dogs showed that progression of DR was related to the level of glycemic control, further underscoring the role of hyperglycemia as the underlying etiology of DR.

Present Understanding

More recent investigations of DR have focused on the biochemical basis of the disease *(12,13)*. Studies of numerous biochemical pathways, including the sorbitol pathway, advanced glycation end-products (AGE), and the protein kinase C (PKC) pathway demonstrate that biochemical changes occur in the retina long before clinically evident abnormalities are observed. These studies suggest that if appropriate novel therapeutic interventions can be identified, early intervention might prevent or reverse the microvascular abnormalities associated with DR.

Numerous studies have focused on the polyol pathway resulting from the increased flux through this pathway in the diabetic condition. Aldose reductase is present in the pericytes of the retinal capillaries and because damage to the pericytes occurs early in the evolution of DR, the role of aldose reductase in the pathogenesis of DR has been extensively evaluated. Furthermore, aldose reductase is present in nerve tissue and induces depletion of myoinositol, leading to a decrease in nerve conduction velocity in diabetic neuropathy. Inhibitors of aldose reductase have been effective in preventing damage to the lens, in preventing thickening of retinal capillary basement membranes in diabetic animals, and in improving nerve conduction velocity in patients with diabetic neuropathy. Thus, it has been postulated that aldose reductase inhibitors may also be able to prevent, delay, or halt the development or progression of DR. Unfortunately, clinical trials of the aldose reductase inhibitor sorbinil have not proved clinically effective in preventing the progression of DR *(14,15)*.

More recent studies have evaluated AGE. The presence of high concentrations of glucose can result in the glycation of numerous proteins, especially albumin. These glycated proteins adversely affect cellular and capillary function, structure, and metabolism. Exposure to glycated proteins induces changes in the glomerulus similar to those observed in diabetes, and changes in the nerves resembling diabetic neuropathy. The effect of AGE in the eye is being actively studied. AGE can affect both the neuronal and vascular components of the eye, and induce numerous growth factors. As such, it may play a role in the progression of DR.

Other studies have concentrated on the hyperglycemia-induced activation of PKC, which can affect a wide range of vascular functions including vascular permeability, contractility, retinal blood flow, and growth factor expression and signal transduction *(16,17)*. Hyperglycemia is known to increase the level of diacyglcerol (DAG), which is the physiological activator of PKC. Much of the vascular dysfunction associated with DM is thought to be mediated through this increased action of PKC. There are numerous isoforms of PKC; however, in the retina, PKCα, -β, and -ζ are primarily expressed. Numerous recent investigations have suggested that the β isoform of PKC is principally responsible for the pathology associated with the diabetic state *(16)*. In laboratory animals, PKCβ selective inhibitors have been shown to ameliorate renal dysfunction, retinal blood-flow abnormalities, vascular permeability *(17)*, and NV associated with DM and diabetes-like models *(18)*. Additionally, activation of PKC is involved in the expression of critical growth factors such as vascular endothelial growth factor (VEGF) *(19)*, which mediates much of the NV and vascular permeability in the eye. Furthermore, activation of the β isoform of PKC is required in order for VEGF to induce its actions within the cell. Thus, inhibition of PKC (especially the β isoform) is likely to block numerous pathological processes in the diabetic condition that result in the vascular dysfunction and ocular complications associated with diabetic retinopathy. Because a PKCβ-selective inhibitor has been shown to be well tolerated in animals and ameliorates many of the abnormalities associated with diabetes, these molecules are now under evaluation in clinical trial.

NATURAL HISTORY AND CLINICAL FEATURES OF DIABETIC RETINOPATHY

Epidemiology

Duration of diabetes is closely associated with the onset and severity of DR. DR is rare in prepubescent patients with type 1 diabetes, but nearly all patients with type 1 diabetes and more than 60% of patients with type 2 diabetes will develop some degree of retinopathy after 20 years *(1,20,21)*. In patients with type 2 diabetes, approx 20% will have retinopathy at the time of diabetes diagnosis, and most will develop some degree of retinopathy over subsequent decades. DR is the most frequent cause of new-onset blindness among Americans adults aged 20 to 74 years. In the Wisconsin Epidemiologic Study of Diabetic Retinopathy, approx 4% of younger-onset patients (aged <30 years at diabetes diagnosis) and nearly 2% of older-onset patients (aged >30 years at diabetes diagnosis) were legally blind. In the younger-onset group, 86% of blindness was attributable to DR. In the older-onset group, in which other eye diseases were also common, 33% of the cases of legal blindness were a result of DR *(20,21)*.

Level of glycemic control is another significant risk factor for the onset and progression of DR *(22–27)*. The Diabetes Control and Complications Trial (DCCT) demonstrated a clear relationship between hyperglycemia and diabetic microvascular complications in type 1 diabetes, including retinopathy, nephropathy, and neuropathy *(22–27)*. In the DCCT, 1,441 patients with type 1 diabetes who had either no retinopathy at baseline (primary prevention cohort) or minimal to moderate nonproliferative diabetic retinopathy (NPDR) (secondary progression cohort) were treated by either conventional diabetes therapy (i.e., one or two injections of insulin daily) or intensive diabetes management (i.e., three or more daily insulin injections or a continuous subcutaneous insulin infusion). The patients were followed for 4 to 9 years. The DCCT showed that intensive insulin therapy reduced or prevented the development of DR by 27% as compared with conventional therapy. Additionally, intensive therapy reduced the progression of DR by 34% to 76%, and had a substantial beneficial effect over the entire range of retinopathy. This improvement was achieved with an average 10% reduction in HbA1c from 8% to 7.2%. These results underscore that although intensive therapy does not prevent retinopathy completely, it reduces the risk of the development and progression of DR.

The United Kingdom Prospective Diabetes Study (UKPDS) found similar results for patients with type 2 diabetes. In the UKPDS, 4209 patients with newly diagnosed type 2 diabetes who had either no retinopathy at baseline (primary prevention cohort) or minimal to moderate NPDR (secondary progression cohort) were randomly assigned to conventional or intensive blood glucose control, using sulfonylureas and/or insulin. The UKPDS showed that intensive therapy reduced the risk of all microvascular endpoints, including vitreous hemorrhage, retinopathy requiring laser photocoagulation, and renal failure by 25%. Overall, intensive control resulted in a 29% reduction in need for laser photocoagulation, a 17% reduction in a two-step progression of DR, a 24% reduction in the need for cataract extraction, a 23% reduction in vitreous hemorrhage, and a 16% reduction in legal blindness. This improvement was achieved with an average 10% reduction in HbA1c from 7.9% to 7% *(81)*.

Renal disease, as manifested by microalbuminuria and proteinuria, is yet another significant risk factor for onset and progression of DR *(28,29)*. Similarly, hypertension is associated with proliferative DR and is an established risk factor for the development of DME *(30,82)*. Both renal retinopathy and hypertensive retinopathy can be superimposed on DR. Additionally, elevated serum lipid levels are associated with lipid in the retina (hard exudates) and visual loss *(31,83,84)* Thus, systemic control of blood pressure, renal disease, and serum lipids are critically important components in the management of DR *(85)*. Additionally, several studies suggest that pregnancy in patients with type 1 diabetes patients may aggravate retinopathy *(32–34)*.

Clinical Findings in Diabetic Retinopathy

Clinical findings associated with early and progressing DR include hemorrhages and/or microaneurysms (H/Ma), cotton wool spots (CWS), hard exudates (HE), intraretinal microvascular abnormalities (IRMA), and venous caliber abnormalities (VCAB), including venous loops, venous tortuosity, and venous beading. Microaneurysms are saccular outpouchings of the capillary walls. These microaneurysms can leak fluid, causing areas of hyperfluorescence on a fluorescein angiogram. Ruptured microaneurysms, leaking capillaries, and IRMAs result in intraretinal hemorrhages. These intraretinal hemorrhages can be "flame-shaped" or spot-like in appearance, reflecting the architecture of layer of the retina in which they occur. Flame-shaped hemorrhages are generally in the nerve fiber layer of the retina, which runs parallel to the retinal surface. Dot or pinpoint hemorrhages are deeper in the retina, reflecting cells that are arranged perpendicular to the retinal surface.

IRMAs are abnormal vessels located within the retina itself. They may represent either localized intraretinal new vessel growth or shunting vessels through areas of poor vascular perfusion. It is common for IRMAs to be found adjacent to CWS, which are feathery lesions in the nerve fiber layer of the retina resembling the fluffy appearance of cotton. CWS are caused by microinfarcts in the nerve fiber layer. CWS in a ring or partial ring surrounding the optic nerve head are frequently signs of severe renal disease or hypertension.

VCABs are a sign of severe retinal hypoxia. VCABs can be associated with any of the lesions of NPDR. However, in many cases of severe retinal hypoxia, distal retinal areas may be free of nonproliferative lesions resulting from the extensive vascular loss present. Such "lesion-free" areas are termed "featureless retina," and are a sign of severe retinal hypoxia.

Vision loss from DR generally results from persistent, nonclearing vitreous hemorrhage, traction retinal detachment, and/or DME. NV and contraction of the accompanying fibrous tissues can distort the retina and lead to traction retinal detachment. If a traction retinal detachment involves or threatens the macula, irreversible severe vision loss may result. Also, the new vessels may bleed, causing preretinal or vitreous hemorrhage. Pars plana vitrectomy can relieve the traction in cases in which vision is threatened and can remove persistent vitreous hemorrhage, often restoring useful vision. The most common cause of vision loss from diabetes, however, is macular disease and macular edema. Macular edema is more likely to occur in patients with type 2 diabetes, which represents 90% of the diabetic population. In diabetic macular disease, macular edema or nonperfusion of the capillaries in the macular area results in the loss of central vision.

Classification of Diabetic Retinopathy

Generally, DR progresses from mild nonproliferative disease, through moderate and severe nonproliferative disease, to proliferative diabetic retinopathy. Mild NPDR is characterized by microvascular abnormalities such as H/Ma, CWS, and increased vascular permeability. Moderate and severe NPDR are characterized by VCABs, IRMAs, and vascular closure. Proliferative diabetic retinopathy (PDR) is characterized by vasoproliferation on the retina and posterior surface of the vitreous. In elucidating the natural history of DR, the Early Treatment Diabetic Retinopathy Study (ETDRS) evaluated the risks of progression from no or minimal retinopathy to sight-threatening PDR. The ETDRS was a muilticentered, randomized clinical study designed to test (a) whether 650 mg of aspirin per day had any effect on the progression of DR, (b) whether focal laser photocoagulation for macular edema reduced the risk of moderate vision loss (i.e., a doubling of the visual angle; e.g., 20/20 reduced to 20/40), and (c) whether scatter laser photocoagulation was more beneficial in reducing the risk of severe vision loss (i.e., best corrected visual acuity of 5/200 or worse) when applied prior to the development of high-risk PDR, as defined below. The EDTSR enrolled 1377 patients at 22 centers nationwide and in Puerto Rico.

Major conclusions of the ETDRS are as follow: (a) a daily dose of 650 mg of aspirin did not prevent or retard the progression of DR and did not result in an increased risk of vitreous hemorrhage or greater need for cataract surgery, (b) focal laser photocoagulation for DME reduced the risk of moderate visual loss by at least 50%, and (c) both early scatter laser photocoagulation and photocoagulation at the time of reaching high-risk PDR resulted in significant reduction in the risk of severe visual loss, although some groups, including those with type 2 diabetes or type 1 diabetes of long duration, had a greater benefit of early treatment (74). Importantly, the ETDRS showed that certain nonproliferative lesions, particularly venous beading, IRMAs, and H/Mas were significant prognosticators for the development of proliferative disease within a 12-month period. Pregnancy, puberty, and cataract surgery can accelerate these changes.

DR is broadly classified as NPDR and PDR. As described above, the lesions of NPDR include dot and blot H/Mas, CWS, HEs, VCABs, and IRMAs. Based on the presence and extent of these retinal lesions, NPDR is further classified as mild, moderate, severe, or very severe NPDR (Table 1). PDR is characterized by new vessels on the optic disc (NVD), new vessels elsewhere on the retina (NVE), preretinal hemorrhage (PRH), vitreous hemorrhage (VH), and/or fibrous tissue proliferation (FP). Based on the presence or absence of proliferative lesions, their severity, and their location, PDR is classified as early PDR or high-risk PDR (Table 1). DME can be present with any level of DR and needs to be evaluated in addition to the level of DR. DME that involves or threatens the center of the macula is termed clinically significant macular edema (CSME) (Table 1). The level of NPDR establishes the risk of progression to sight-threatening retinopathy and appropriate clinical management as specifically detailed in Table 2.

In an effort to standardized classification of DR across international borders and among different health care providers, leaders from various groups and nations (the Global Diabetic Retinopathy Project Group) established and promulgated the Proposed International Classification of Diabetic Retinopathy (86) (Table 3). This classification identifies three levels of NPDR and one level of PDR. In regard to macular edema, two major categories—macular edema present and macular edema absent—are identified. If macular edema is present, three categories are defined: macular edema not threatening the center of the macula, macula edema threatening the center of the macula, and macula edema involving the center of the macula.

Treatment of Diabetic Retinopathy

OVERVIEW

Appropriate clinical management of DR has been defined by five major, randomized, multicentered clinical trials: the Diabetic Retinopathy Study (DRS) (35–48), the ETDRS (49–68), the Diabetic Retinopathy Vitrectomy Study (DRVS) (69–73), the DCCT (22–27), and the UKPDS (81). These studies have elucidated delivery and proper timing for laser photocoagulation surgery for the treatment of both DR and DME. They have also established guidelines for vitrectomy surgery. The DRS demonstrated that scatter (panretinal) laser photocoagulation was effective in reducing the risk of severe vision loss from PDR by 50% or more.

The ETDRS demonstrated that focal laser photocoagulation for clinically significant macular edema reduced the 5-year risk of moderate vision loss from nearly 30% to less than 15%. The study also demonstrated that scatter laser photocoagulation applied when an eye approaches or just reaches high-risk PDR reduces the risk of severe vision loss to less than 4%. The ETDRS also specifically evaluated the use of 650 mg of aspirin in patients with diabetes. The study conclusively demonstrated that the use of aspirin did not

Table 1
Levels of Diabetic Retinopathy[a]

Nonproliferative diabetic retinopathy (NPDR)	Characteristics
Mild NPDR	At least one microaneurysm
	Characteristics not met for more severe diabetic retinopathy (DR)
Moderate NPDR	Hemorrhages and/or microaneurysms (H/ma) of a moderate degree (i.e., $\geq$ Standard Photograph 2A[b])
	and/or
	Soft exudates (cotton wool spots), venous beading (VB), or intraretinal microvascular abnormalities (IRMAs) definitely present
	and
	Characteristics not met for more severe DR
Severe NPDR	One of the following:
	H/Ma $\geq$ standard 2A in four retinal quadrants
	Venous beading in more than two retinal quadrants (see standard photo 6B)
	IRMA in more than one retinal quadrant more than standard photo 8A
	Characteristics not met for more severe DR
Very severe NPDR	Two or more lesions of severe NPDR
	No retinal NV

Proliferative diabetic retinopathy (PDR)	Characteristics
Early PDR	New vessels definitely present
	Characteristics not met for more severe DR
High-risk PDR	One or more of the following:
	NV on the optic disc (NVD) greater than standard photo 10 A (i.e., $\geq$1/3 disc area)
	Any NVD with vitreous or preretinal hemorrhage
	NV elsewhere on the retina (NVE) greater than 1/2 disc area with vitreous or preretinal hemorrhage

Clinically Significant Macular Edema (CSME)

Any one of the following lesions:
   Retinal thickening at or within 500 μ (1/3 disc diameter) from the center of the macula
   Hard exudates at or within 500 μ from the center of the macula with thickening of the adjacent retina
   A zone or zones of retinal thickening greater than 1 disc area in size, any portion of which is at or within 1 disc diameter from the center of the macula

[a]Based on Early Treatment Diabetic Retinopathy Study definitions *(57)*.
[b]Standard photographs refer to the Modified Airlee House Classification of Diabetic Retinopathy (*see* ref. *61*).

Table 2
Recommended General Management of Diabetic Retinopathy

Level of DR	Risk of progression to		Evaluation		Laser treatment		Follow-up (months)
	PDR 1 yr	High risk PDR-5 years	Color photo	F.A.	Scatter laser (PRP)	Focal laser	
Mild NPDR	5%	15%					
• No ME			No	No	No	No	12
• ME			Yes	Occ	No	No	4–6
• CSME			Yes	Yes	No	Yes	2–4
Moderate NPDR	12-27%	33%					
• No ME			Yes	No	No	No	6–8
• ME			Yes	Occ	No	Occ	4–6
• CSME			Yes	Yes	No	Yes	2–4
Severe NPDR	52%	60%					
• No ME			Yes	No	Rarely	No	3–4
• ME			Yes	Occ	OccAF	Occ	2–3
• CSME			Yes	Yes	OccAF	Yes	2–3
Very Severe NPDR	75%	75%					
• No ME			Yes	No	Occ	No	2–3
• ME			Yes	Occ	OccAF	Occ	2–3
• CSME			Yes	Yes	OccAF	Yes	2–3
PDR less than high risk		75%					
• No ME			Yes	No	Occ	No	2–3
• ME			Yes	Occ	OccAF	Occ	2–3
• CSME			Yes	Yes	OccAF	Yes	2–3
High-risk PDR							
• No ME			Yes	No	Yes	No	2–3
• ME			Yes	Yes	Yes	Usually	1–2
• CSME			Yes	Yes	Yes	Yes	1–2

NPDR, Nonproliferative diabetic retinopathy; PDR, proliferative diabetic retinopathy; ME, macular edema; CSME, clinically significant macular edema; Occ, occasionally; OccAF, ocasionally after focal. (Copyright Lloyd M. Aiello, MD; used with permission.)

alter the course of DR and determined that aspirin use was not associated with increased risk of VH or PRH or stroke. Thus, patients who require the use of aspirin for optimum medical care should not be discontinued from treatment as a result of the presence of DR alone. The ETDRS has also clarified the natural history of DR and the risk of progression of retinopathy based on the baseline level of retinopathy (59–62) (Table 1). Finally, the ETDRS identified specific lesions that placed an eye at high-risk for visual loss (61). These lesions include H/Ma, VCABs, and IRMAs as detailed in Table 1 and discussed above. Consequently, proper diagnosis of the level of retinopathy (Table 2) determines appropriate timing of follow-up evaluation and when to initiate laser photocoagulation.

The DRVS demonstrated that early pars plana vitrectomy (PPV) was useful in restoring vision for some persons who have severe vision loss as a result of VH. Additionally, the DRVS demonstrated that persons with severe FP were more likely to obtain better vision, and less likely to have poor vision, when PPV was performed early. The DRVS demonstrated the value of PPV in restoring useful vision, particularly in patients with type 1 diabetes. The treatment benefits demonstrated in the DRVS, which was completed in 1989, are not totally applicable today as a result of dramatic advances in surgical

Table 3

Proposed International Clinical Diabetic Retinopathy (DR) and Diabetic Macular Edema (DME) Disease Severity Scales

Diabetic retinopathy disease severity

No apparent DR	No abnormalities
Mild NPDR	Ma only
Moderate NPDR	More than Ma only but less than severe NPDR
Severe NPDR	Any of the following and no PDR:
	a. More than 20 intraretinal hemorrhages in each four quadrants
	b. Definite VB in two or more quadrants
	c. Prominent IRMA in one quadrant
PDR	One or more of NV, VH, PRH

Diabetic macular edema disease severity

DME apparently absent	No apparent retinal thickening or HE in posterior pole
DME apparently present	Some apparent retinal thickening or HE in posterior pole

Mild DME—some retinal thickening or HE in posterior pole but distant from center of the macula

Moderate DME—Retinal thickening or HE approaching the center of the macula but not involving the center

Severe DME—Retinal thickening or HE involving the center of the macula

NPDR, nonproliferative diabetic retinopathy; ma, microaneurysm; VB, venous beading; IRMA, intraretinal microvascular abnormalities; PDR, proliferative diabetic retinopathy; NV, neovascularization; PRH, preretinal hemorrhage: HE, hard exudates. (Data from ref. *86.*)

techniques and the advent of laser endophotocoagulation that have occurred in the intervening years.

DR and DME are usually most amenable to laser surgery before any vision has been lost. Consequently, it is imperative that health care providers educate their patients regarding the natural course and effectiveness of treatment so as to motivate patients to seek regular eye examinations even in the absences of symptoms.

Scatter (Panretinal) Laser Photocoagulation for Proliferative Diabetic Retinopathy

Both the DRS and the ETDRS demonstrated the value of scatter (panretinal) laser photocoagulation for treating PDR. In scatter laser photocoagulation, 1200 to 1800 laser burns are applied to the peripheral retinal tissue, focused at the level of the retinal pigment epithelium. Large vessels are avoided, as are areas of PRH. The total treatment is usually applied in two or three sessions, spaced 1 to 2 weeks apart. Follow-up evaluation usually occurs at 3 months.

The response to scatter laser photocoagulation varies. The most desirable effect is to see a regression of the new vessels. In some cases, there may be a stabilization of the NV, with no further growth. This response may be acceptable, with careful clinical monitoring. In some cases, new vessels continue to proliferate, requiring additional scatter laser photocoagulation. In cases in which NV continues and does not respond to further laser photocoagulation, vitreous hemorrhage and/or traction retinal detachment may occur, possibly requiring surgical intervention with pars plana vitrectomy if vision is threatened. Eyes with high-risk PDR should receive prompt scatter laser photocoagulation. Eyes approaching high risk (i.e., eyes with PDR less than high risk, and eyes with severe or very severe NPDR) may also be candidates for scatter laser photocoagulation. Recent progression of the eye disease, status of the fellow eye, compliance with follow-up, concurrent health concerns such as hypertension or kidney disease, and other factors must be considered in determining if laser surgery should be performed in these patients. In particular, patients with type 2 diabetes should be considered for laser surgery of DR prior to the development of high-risk PDR because the risk of severe visual loss and the need for PPV can be reduced by 50% in these patients by early scatter treatment, especially when macular edema is present *(74)*.

Focal Laser Photocoagulation for Clinically Significant Macular Edema

Focal laser for CSME is effective in reducing the risk of moderate visual loss, as defined above. In focal laser photocoagulation, lesions from 300 µ to 3000 µfrom the center of the macula that are contributing to thickening of the macula area are directly photocoagulated. These lesions are generally identified by fluorescein angiography and consist primarily of leaking microaneurysms. Although fluorescein angiography is generally used to identify treatable lesions for focal laser photocoagulation, fluorescein angiography is not necessary for the diagnosis of clinically significant macular edema. Also, fluorescein angiography is generally not needed to identify lesions of PDR because these findings should be clinically evident in most cases.

Follow-up evaluation following focal laser surgery generally occurs after 3 months. In the cases in which macular edema persists, further treatment may be necessary. In the presence of macular edema, patients with severe or very severe NPDR should be considered for focal treatment of macular edema whether or not the macular edema is clinically significant because they are likely to require scatter laser photocoagulation in the near future and because scatter photocoagulation may exacerbate existing macular edema.

Vitrectomy for Advanced Proliferative Diabetic Retinopathy

As discussed earlier, in cases of advance PDR, or in cases that do not respond to scatter laser photocoagulation, PPV may be indicated to allow intraocular application of laser photocoagulation (endolaser), to remove nonclearing VH, or to relieve traction that involves or threatens the center of the macula.

Novel Treatments

Numerous recent advances in our understanding of the basic mechanisms underlying the progression of DR have raised the possibility of novel therapies against the progression of NPDR, PDR, and DME. Because the mainstay of DR treatment is laser photocoagulation surgery, which is an inherently destructive technique resulting in focal destruction of areas of the retina, a noninvasive and nondestructive therapy would be of great clinical importance. Significant advances have been made regarding the role of oxidative stress in the eye and the role of VEGF and PKC as discussed earlier. Increases in oxidative stress induced by the diabetic state are thought to promote ocular and other systemic abnormalities *(75)*. Thus, antioxidants such as vitamin E are being evaluated for their potential ameliorative effect on the progression of DR. Studies utilizing high-dose vitamin E in diabetic animals have demonstrated a normalization of retinal blood flow and amelioration of excessive PKC activity (76). Furthermore, initial studies utilizing high-dose vitamin E treatment in patients with recent-onset diabetes have demonstrated an amelioration of diabetes-associated retinal blood-flow abnormalities. Further studies will be necessary to determine if vitamin E might be able to slow the progression of diabetic retinopathy.

In the ETDRS, 650 mg of aspirin daily were compared to placebo to evaluate the effect of aspirin on progression of DR. In the ETDRS, there was no difference between the aspirin group and the placebo group on progression of retinopathy, risk of VH, or rate of cataract extraction (57). Although there was no measured beneficial effect of aspirin on progression of retinopathy at levels of disease enrolled in the ETDRS, studies of the effects of higher dose aspirin or other anti-inflammatory agents such as cyclooxygenase-2 (COX-2) inhibitors on early stages of disease have suggested possible benefit (87,88). Early clinical studies are currently underway to address the effect of COX-2 inhibitors on DME.

Numerous advances have been made in understanding the role of growth factors in DR. Growth factors mediate both the NV of PDR and the increased permeability associated with DME. One of the critical growth factors involved in these mechanisms is VEGF. Inhibitors of VEGF have been evaluated in animal models and shown to prevent ischemia-induced NV of the retina and iris (77–79). Furthermore, it has been demonstrated that PKCβ activation is essential for VEGF activity (19). PKC activation also increases the expression of VEGF. Finally, PKC activation itself also increases retinal vascular permeability (17). Thus, it would be predicted that an inhibitor of the β isoform of PKC would interrupt numerous diabetes-associated pathological processes that, if left unopposed, result in the complications of DR. PKCβ selective inhibitors have ameliorated the renal and retinal blood flow, retinal permeability, and retinal NV associated with diabetes and diabetes-like processes in animals (16,17). These results suggest that if such a molecule can be well tolerated in humans, an orally administered nondestructive novel therapy for DR would be available. PKCβ-selective inhibitor has been and continues to be evaluated in phase 3 clinical trials. Initial results suggest that this orally administered compound is well tolerated and has few side effects. The drug may have beneficial effects on DME in patients with mild to moderate NPDR especially when glycemic control is not poor at baseline. It also may reduce vision loss in patients with moderate to severe NPDR, but the results are not conclusive at this time and await findings from ongoing phase 3 clinical trials specifically addressing these endpoints.

The great need for rigorous and rapid evaluation of new treatment modalities for DR has prompted the formation of the Diabetic Retinopathy Clinical Research Network (DRCR.net), a National Eye Institute (NEI)-sponsored cooperative agreement dedicated to multicenter clinical trial research of DR, macular edema, and associated disorders. The network consist of numerous investigators across the country in both academic and community practices who all use the same certified procedures for patient evaluation and computer-assisted information recording. The DRCR.net is supported by a dedicated coordinating center, fundus photograph reading center and network chair office. This group has designed and implemented protocols evaluating less intense laser photocoagulation techniques and intravitreal steroid injections for DME. Additionally, surgical intervention trials and trials of novel biochemical agents are planned for future investigation.

CONCLUSIONS

Appropriate management of DR and diabetic eye disease requires a thorough knowledge of both DM and the findings of the key multicentered, randomized clinical trials such as the DRS, ETDRS, DRVS, DCCT, and UKPDS. Accurate diagnosis of retinopathy level is essential to determine appropriate follow-up schedules and to assess the need for timely laser photocoagulation for PDR and CSME. Because DR usually causes no symptoms when it is most amenable to treatment, strategies to reduce the risk of vision loss must stress the need for regular eye examination, even in patients with no ocular complaints (80) (Table 4). Currently, patients with type 1 diabetes 10 years of age and older are encouraged to have a comprehensive, dilated retinal eye examination within 3 to 5 years of diagnosis, and at least annually thereafter. Patients with type 2 diabetes are encouraged to have a comprehensive, dilated eye examination at the time of diagnosis, and at least annually thereafter. Patients contemplating pregnancy should have their eyes examined prior to conception whenever possible, and pregnant women should have their eyes examined early in the first trimester and each trimester thereafter. In all cases, abnormal findings may require accelerated examination schedules, and the presence of concurrent medical conditions such as hypertension and renal disease may also require more frequent ocular examination and should be aggressively controlled in conjunction with the patient's internist or diabetologist.

Our understanding of DR has expanded dramatically in the past 30 years. Treatment modalities that can substantially reduce visual loss have been developed and extensively validated. However, these therapies are not yet ideal and active research is continuing into methods of curing or preventing DR. Until these milestones are reached, current strategies must continue to address the critical need for regular eye examination and prompt, appropriate laser photocoagulation when indicated.

APPENDIX

American Diabetes Association Guidelines (80)

1. Patients less than 10 years of age with type 1 diabetes should have an initial dilated and comprehensive eye examination by an ophthalmologist or optometrist within 3 to 5 years after the onset of diabetes. In general, screening for diabetic eye disease is not necessary before 10 years of age. Patients with type 2 diabetes should have an initial dilated and comprehensive eye examination by an ophthalmologist or optometrist shortly after the diagnosis of diabetes is made.
2. Subsequent examinations for both type 1 and type 2 diabetic patients should be repeated annually by an ophthalmologist or optometrist who is knowledgeable and experienced in diagnosing the presence of diabetic retinopathy and is aware of its management. Examinations will be required more frequently if retinopathy is progressing.
3. When planning pregnancy, women with pre-existing diabetes should have a comprehensive eye examination and should be counseled on the risk of development and/or progression of diabetic retinopathy. Women with diabetes who become pregnant should have a comprehensive eye examination in the first trimester and close follow-up throughout pregnancy. This guideline does not apply to women who develop gestational diabetes because such individuals are not at increased risk for diabetic retinopathy.
4. Patients with any level of macular edema, severe NPDR, or any PDR require the prompt care of an ophthalmologist who is knowledgeable and experienced in the management and treatment of diabetic retinopathy. Referral to an ophthalmologist should not be delayed

Table 4
Suggested Frequency of Eye Examination

Type of diabetes mellitus (DM)	Recommended first examination	Routine minimal follow-up
Type 1 DM	Older than 10 years: 3–5 years after onset of diabetes or at puberty	Yearly
Type 2 DM	Upon diagnosis of diabetes	Yearly
During Pregnancy	• Prior to conception for counseling • Early in first trimester	• Each trimester • More frequently as indicated • 3–6 months postpartum

until PDR has developed in patients who are known to have severe nonproliferative or more advanced retinopathy. Early referral to an ophthalmologist is particularly important for patients with type 2 diabetes and severe NPDR, because laser treatment at this stage is associated with a 50% reduction in the risk of severe visual loss and vitrectomy.

5. Patients who experience vision loss from diabetes should be encouraged to pursue visual rehabilitation with an ophthalmologist or optometrist who is trained or experienced in low-vision care.

REFERENCES

1. Klein R, Klein BEK. Vision disorders in diabetes. National Institutes of Health: National Institute of Diabetes and Digestive and Kidney Diseases. NIH Publication No. 95–1468, 1995, p. 293.
2. Cogan DG, Toussaint D, Kuwabara T. Retinal vascular patterns: IV. Diabetic Retinopathy. Arch Ophthalmol 1961;66:366.
3. Cogan DG, Kuwabara T. Capillary shunts in the pathogenesis of diabetic retinopathy. Diabetes 1963;12:293.
4. Cogan DG, Kuwabara T. The mural cells in perspective. Arch Ophthalmol 1967;78:137.
5. Michaelson IC. The mode of development of the vascular system of the retina, with some observations on its significance for certain retinal diseases. Trans Ophthalmol Soc UK 1948;68:137–180.
6. Ashton N, Ward B, Supell G. Effect of oxygen on developing retinal vessels with particular reference to the problem of retrolental fibroplasia. Br J Ophthalmol 1954;38:397–432.
7. Engerman RI, Kern TS. Experimental galactosemia produces diabetic-like retinopathy. Diabetes 1984;33:97.
8. Engerman RI. Pathogenesis of diabetic retinopathy. Diabetes 1989;38:1203.
9. Engerman RI, Kern TS. Progression of incipient diabetic retinopathy during good glycemic control. Diabetes 1987;36:808.
10. Engerman RL, Kern TS. Is diabetic retinopathy preventable? International Ophthalmology Clinics 1987;27:225–229.
11. Engerman RI, Kern TS. Aldose reductase inhibition fails to prevent retinopathy in diabetic and galactosemic dogs. Diabetes 1993;42:820.
12. Kikkawa U, Nishizuka Y. The role of protein kinase C in transmembrane signaling. Ann Rev Cell Biol 1986;2:149.
13. Pu X, Aiello LP, Ishii H, et al. Characterization of vascular endothelial growth factor's effect on the activation of protein kinase C, its isoforms and endothelial growth. J Clin Invest 1996;98:2018–2026.
14. The Sorbinil Retinopathy Trial Research Group. A Randomized trial of sorbinil, an aldose reductase inhibitor in diabetic retinopathy. Arch Ophthalmol 1990;108:1234–1244.
15. The Sorbinil Retinopathy Trial Research Group. The sorbinil retinopathy trial: Neurology results. Neurology 1993;43:1141–1149.
16. Ishii H, Jirousek MR, Koya D, et al. Amelioration of vascular dysfunctions in diabetic rats by an oral PKC beta inhibitor. Science 1996;272:728–731.

17. Aiello LP, Bursell SE, Clermont A, et al. Vascular endothelial growth factor-induced retinal permeability is mediated by protein kinase C in vivo and suppressed by an orally effective beta-isoform-selective inhibitor. Diabetes 1997;46:1473–1480.

18. Danis Rp, Bingaman DP, Jirousek M, Yang Y. Inhibition of intraocular neovascularization caused by retinal ischemia in pigs by PKC beta inhibition with LY333531. Invest Ophthalmol Vis Sci 1998;39:171–179.

19. Xia P, Aiello LP, Ishii H, et al. Characterization of vascular endothelial growth factor's effect on the activation of protein kinase C, its isoforms, and endothelial cell growth. J Clin Invest 1996;98:2018–2026.

20. Klein R, Klein BEK, Moss SE, et al. The Wisconsin Epidemilogic Study of Diabetic Retinopathy. II. Prevalence and risk of diabetic retinopathy when age at diagnosis is less than 30 years. Arch Ophthalmol 1984;102:520–526.

21. Klein R, Klein BEK, Moss SE, et al. The Wisconsin Epidemilogic Study of Diabetic Retinopathy. III. Prevalence and risk of diabetic retinopathy when age at diagnosis is 30 or more years. Arch Ophthalmol 1984;102:527–532.

22. Diabetes Control and Complications Trial Research Group. Are continuing studies of metabolic control and microvascular complications in insulin-dependent diabetes mellitus justified? N Engl J Med 1988;318:246–250.

23. The Diabetes Control and Complications Trial Research Group. The relationship of glycemic exposure (HbA1c) to the risk of development and progression of retinopathy in the Diabetes Control and Complications Trial. Diabetes 1995;44:968–983.

24. The Diabetes Control and Complications Trial Research Group. Progression of retinopathy with intensive versus conventional treatment in the Diabetes Control and Complications Trial. Ophthalmology 1995;102:647–661.

25. The Diabetes Control and Complications Trial Research Group. Hypoglycemia in the Diabetes Control and Complications Trial. Diabetes 1997;46:271–286.

26. The Diabetes Control and Complications Trial Research Group. Lifetime benefits and costs of intensive therapy as practiced in the Diabetes Control and Complications Trial. JAMA 1996;276:1409–1415.

27. The Diabetes Control and Complications Trial Research Group The effect of intensive treatment of diabetes on the development and progression of long term complications in insulin dependent diabetes mellitus. N Engl J Med 1993;329:977–986.

28. Chase HP, Jackson WE, Hoops SL et al. Glucose control in the renal and retinal complications of insulin-dependent diabetes. JAMA 1989;261:1155–1160.

29. The Kroc Collaborative Study Group. Blood glucose control and the evolution of diabetic retinopathy and albuminuria. N Engl J Med 1984;311:365–372.

30. Krowlewski AS, Canessa M, Warram JH et al. Predisposition to hypertension and susceptibility to renal disease in insulin-dependent diabetes mellitus: N Engl J Med 1988;318:140–145.

31. Stern MP, Patterson JK, Haffner SM et al. Lack of awareness and treatment of hyperlipidemia in Type II diabetes in a community survey. JAMA 1989;262:360–364.

32. Moloney JEM, Drury MI. The effect of pregnancy on the natural course of diabetic retinopathy. Am J Ophthalmol 1982;93:745–756.

33. Serup L. Influence of pregnancy on diabetic retinopathy. Acta Endocrinol 1986; 277:122–124.

34. Phelps RL, Sakol P, Metzger BE et al. Changes in diabetic retinopathy during pregnancy: Correlations with regulation of hyperglycemia. Arch Ophthalmol 1986;104:1806–1810.

35. Diabetic Retinopathy Study Research Group. Preliminary report on effects of photocoagulation therapy. DRS Report No. 1. Am J Ophthalmol 1976;81:1–14.

36. Diabetic Retinopathy Study Research Group. Photocoagulation treatment of proliferative diabetic retinopathy. DRS Report No. 2. Ophthalmology 1978;85:82–106.

37. Diabetic Retinopathy Study Research Group. Four risk factors for severe visual loss in diabetic retinopathy. DRS Report No. 3. Arch Ophthalmol 1979;97:654–655.

38. Diabetic Retinopathy Study Research Group. A short report of long-term results. DRS Report No. 4. Proc 10th Congr Int Diabetes Fed. Vienna, September 9–14, 1979. North Holland: Excerpta Medica, 1980, pp. 789–794.

39. Diabetic Retinopathy Study Research Group. Photocoagulation treatment of proliferative diabetic retinopathy: relationship of adverse treatment effects to retinopathy severity. DRS Report No. 5. Dev Ophthalmol 1981;2:248–261.

40. Diabetic Retinopathy Study Research Group. Design methods and baseline results. DRS Report No. 6. Invest Ophthalmol 1981;21(1, Pt 2):149–209.

41. Diabetic Retinopathy Study Research Group. A modification of the Airlie House classification of diabetic retinopathy. DRS Report No. 7. Invest Ophthalmol 1981;21(1, Pt 2):210–226.
42. Diabetic Retinopathy Study Research Group. Photocoagulation treatment of proliferative diabetic retinopathy. Clinical applications of Diabetic Retinopathy Study (DRS) findings. DRS Report No. 8. Ophthalmology 1981;88:583–600.
43. Ederer F, Podgor MJ, DRS Research Group. Assessing possible late treatment effects in stopping a clinical trial early: a case study. DRS Report No. 9. Cont Clin Trials 1984;5:373–381.
44. Rand LI, Prud'homme GJ, Ederer F, Canner PL, DRS Research Group. Factors influencing the development of visual loss in advanced diabetic retinopathy. DRS Report No. 10. Invest Ophthalmol 1985;26:983–991.
45. Kaufman SC, Ferris F, Swartz M, DRS Research Group. Intraocular pressure following panretinal photocoagulation for diabetic retinopathy. DRS Report No. 11. Arch Ophthalmol 1987;102:807–809.
46. Diabetic Retinopathy Study Research Group. Macular edema in diabetic retinopathy study patients. DRS Report No. 12. Ophthalmology 1987;94:754–760.
47. Diabetic Retinopathy Study Report Number 13: Factors associated with visual outcome after photocoagulation for diabetic retinopathy. Invest Ophthalmol 1989;30:23–28.
48. Diabetic Retinopathy Study Research Group. Indications for photocoagulation treatment of diabetic retinopathy. DRS Report No. 14. Int Ophthalmol Clin 1987;27:239–253.
49. Early Treatment Diabetic Retinopathy Study Research Group. Photocoagulation for diabetic macular edema. ETDRS Report No. 1. Arch Ophthalmol 1985;103:1796–1806.
50. Early Treatment Diabetic Retinopathy Study Research Group. Treatment techniques and clinical guidelines for photocoagulation of diabetic macular edema. ETDRS Report No. 2. Ophthalmology 1987;96:761–774.
51. Early Treatment Diabetic Retinopathy Study Research Group. Techniques for scatter and local photocoagulation treatment of diabetic retinopathy. ETDRS Report No. 3. Int Ophthalmol Clin 1987;27:254–264.
52. Early Treatment Diabetic Retinopathy Study Research Group. Photocoagulation for diabetic macular edema. ETDRS Report No. 4. Int Ophthalmol Clin 1987;27:265–272.
53. Early Treatment Diabetic Retinopathy Study Research Group. Case reports to accompany early treatment diabetic retinopathy study reports Nos. 3 and 4. Int Ophthalmol Clin 1987;27:273–333.
54. Early Treatment Diabetic Retinopathy Study Research Group. Detection of diabetic macular edema: Ophthalmoscopy versus photography. ETDRS Report No. 5. Ophthalmology 1989;96:746–751.
55. Early Treatment Diabetic Retinopathy Study Research Group. C-peptide and the classification of diabetes patients in the Early Treatment Diabetic Retinopathy Study. ETDRS Report No. 6. Ann Epidemiol 1993;3:9–17.
56. Early Treatment Diabetic Retinopathy Study Research Group. Design and baseline patient characteristics. ETDRS Report No. 7. Ophthalmology 1991;98:741–756.
57. Early Treatment Diabetic Retinopathy Study Research Group. Effects of aspirin treatment on diabetic retinopathy. ETDRS Report No. 8. Ophthalmology 1991; 98:757–765.
58. Early Treatment Diabetic Retinopathy Study Research Group. Early photocoagulation for diabetic retinopathy. ETDRS Report No. 9. Ophthalmology 1991;98:766–785.
59. Early Treatment Diabetic Retinopathy Study Research Group. Grading diabetic retinopathy from stereoscopic color fundus photographs: an extension of the modified Airlie House classification. ETDRS Report No. 10. Ophthalmology 1991;98:786–806.
60. Early Treatment Diabetic Retinopathy Study Research Group. Classification of diabetic retinopathy from fluorescein angiograms. ETDRS Report No. 11. Ophthalmology 1991;98:807–822.
61. Early Treatment Diabetic Retinopathy Study Research Group. Fundus photographic risk factors for progression of diabetic retinopathy. ETDRS Report No. 12. Ophthalmology 1991;98:823–833.
62. Early Treatment Diabetic Retinopathy Study Research Group. Fluorescein angiographic risk factors for progression of diabetic retinopathy. ETDRS Report No. 13. Ophthalmology 1991;98:834–840.
63. Early Treatment Diabetic Retinopathy Study Research Group. Aspirin effects on mortality and morbidity in patients with diabetes mellitus. ETDRS Report No. 14. JAMA 1992;268:1292–1300.
64. Early Treatment Diabetic Retinopathy Study Research Group. Aspirin effects on the development of cataracts in patients with diabetes mellitus. ETDRS Report No. 16. Arch Ophthalmol 1992;110:339–342.
65. Early Treatment Diabetic Retinopathy Study Research Group. Pars plana vitrectomy in the early treatment diabetic retinopathy study. ETDRS Report No. 17. Ophthalmology 1992;99:1351–1357.

66. Early Treatment Diabetic Retinopathy Study Report Number 19. Focal photocoagulation treatment of diabetic macular edema: Relationship of treatment effect to fluorescein angiographic and other retinal characteristics at baseline. Arch Ophthalmol 1995;113:1144–1155.

67. Chew EY, Klein ML, Murphy RP, Remaley NA, Ferris FL III, ETDRS Research Group. Early Treatment Diabetic Retinopathy Study Report Number 20. Effects of aspirin on vitreous/preretinal hemorrhage in patients with diabetes mellitus. Arch Ophthalmol 1995;13:52–55.

68. Chew EY, Klein ML, Ferris FL III, Remaley NA, Murphy RP, Chantry K, Hoogwerf BJ, Miller D, ETDRS Research Group. Early Treatment Diabetic Retinopathy Study Report Number 22. Association of elevated serum lipid levels with retinal hard exudates in diabetic retinopathy. Arch Ophthalmol 1996;114:1079–1084.

69. Diabetic Retinopathy Vitrectomy Study Research Group. Two-year course of visual acuity in severe proliferative diabetic retinopathy with conventional management. DRVS Report No. 1. Ophthalmology 1985;92:492–502.

70. Diabetic Retinopathy Vitrectomy Study Research Group. Early vitrectomy for severe vitreous hemorrhage in diabetic retinopathy. Two year results of a randomized trial. DRVS Report No. 2. Arch Ophthalmol 1985;103:1644–1652.

71. Diabetic Retinopathy Vitrectomy Study Research Group. Early vitrectomy for severe proliferative diabetic retinopathy in eyes with useful vision. Results of a randomized trial. DRVS Report No. 3. Ophthalmology 1988;95:1307–1320.

72. Diabetic Retinopathy Vitrectomy Study Research Group. Early vitrectomy for severe proliferative diabetic retinopathy in eyes with useful vision. DRVS Report No. 4. Ophthalmology 1988;95:1321–1334.

73. Diabetic Retinopathy Vitrectomy Study Report Number 5: Early vitrectomy for severe vitreous hemorrhage in diabetic retinopathy. Four-year results of a randomized trial. Arch Ophthalmol 1990;108:958–964.

74. Ferris FL III. Early photocoagulation in patients with either Type I or Type II diabetes. Tr AM Ophth Soc 1996;94:505–537.

75. Baynes JW, Thorpe SR. Role of oxidative stress in diabetic complications. A new perspective on an old paradigm. Diabetes 1999;48:1–9.

76. Kunisaki M, Bursell SE, Clermont AC, Ishii H, Ballas LM, Jirousek MR et al. Vitamin E prevents diabetes-induced abnormal retinal blood flow via the diacylglycerol-protein kinase C pathway. Am J Physiol 1995;269:E239–E246.

77. Aiello LP, Pierce EA, Foley ED, Takagi H, Chen H, Riddle L et al. Suppression of retinal neovascularization in vivo by inhibition of vascular endothelial growth factor (VEGF) using soluble VEGF-recptor chimeric proteins. Proc Natl Acad Sci U S A 1995;92:10,457–10,461.

78. Robinson GS, Pierce EA, Rook SL, Foley E, Webb R, Smith LE. Oligodeoxynucleotides inhibit retinal neovascularization in a murine model of proliferative retinopathy. Proc Natl Acad Sci USA 1996;93:4851–4856.

79. Adamis AP, Shima DT, Tolentino MJ, Gragoudas ES, Ferrara N, Folkman J et al. Inhibition of vascular endothelial growth factor prevents retinal ischemia-assoociated iris neovasculrization in a nonhuman primate. Arch Ophthalmol 1996;114:66–71.

80. Position Statement: American Diabetes Association. Diabetic Retinopathy. Diabetes Care 2004;27:584–587.

81. Intensive blood-glucose control with sulphonylureas or insulin compared with conventional treatment and risk of complications in patients with type 2 diabetes (UKPDS 33). UK Prospective Diabetes Study (UKPDS) Group. Lancet 1998;352(9131):837–853 (Erratum in: Lancet 1999;354(9178):602).

82. Efficacy of atenolol and captopril in reducing risk of macrovascular and microvascular complications in type 2 diabetes: UKPDS 39. UK Prospective Diabetes Study Group. BMJ 1998;317(7160):713–720.

83. Chew EY, Klein ML, Ferris FL 3rd, et al. Association of elevated serum lipid levels with retinal hard exudate in diabetic retinopathy. Early Treatment Diabetic Retinopathy Study (ETDRS) Report 22. Arch Ophthalmol 1996;114(9):1079–1084.

84. Davis MD, Fisher MR, Gangnon RE, et al. Risk factors for high-risk proliferative diabetic retinopathy and severe visual loss: Early Treatment Diabetic Retinopathy Study Report #18. Invest Ophthalmol Vis Sci 1998;39(2):233–252.

85. Aiello LP, Cahill MT, Wong JS. Systemic considerations in the management of diabetic retinopathy. Am J Ophthalmol 2001;132(5):760–776.

86. Proposed international clinical diabetic retinopathy and diabetic macular edema disease severity scales. Ophthalmology 2003;110:1677–1682.

87. Kern TS, Engerman RL. Pharmacological inhibition of diabetic retinopathy: aminoguanidine and aspirin. Diabetes 2001;50:1636–1642.

88. Joussen AM, Poulaki V, Mitsiades N, Kirchhof B, Koizumi K, Dohmen S, Adamis AP. Nonsteroidal anti-inflammatory drugs prevent early diabetic retinopathy via TNF-alpha suppression. FASEB J 2002;16(3):438–440.

17 Diabetic Nephropathy

Richard J. Solomon, MD *and Bijan Roshan,* MD

CONTENTS

INTRODUCTION

Diabetic nephropathy is the leading cause of end-stage renal disease (ESRD) in the United States, accounting for nearly 40% of incident ESRD *(1)*. Diabetes mellitus (DM) is also an independent and strong risk factor for ESRD ascribed to causes other than diabetes *(2)*, such as hypertension, pyelonephritis, and other forms of glomerulopathies that can lead to chronic renal disease. Here we focus mainly on diabetic nephropathy as a major microvascular complication of both type 1 and type 2 diabetes.

Between 35% and 57% of type 1 diabetics *(3–5)* and 25% and 46% of type 2 patients with long-lasting diabetes *(4,6)*, develop clinically detectable nephropathy, indicated by proteinuria and/or renal insufficiency. In fact, the prevalence of proteinuria is the same in both types of diabetes, after adjustment for differences in diabetes duration *(4,7)*. Crossectional studies indicate that 20% of type 2 DM have microalbuminuria, many at the time diabetes is diagnosed. The prevalence increases to nearly 50% in those with advanced retinopathy *(8)*. Approximately 2–3% of patients with type 2 diabetes progress to overt proteinuria yearly *(9)*.

PATHOGENESIS

Recent large-scale intervention trials have provided compelling evidence for the role of hyperglycemia in the development and progression of nephropathy in type 1 and type 2 diabetes *(10,11)*. However the fact that only a proportion of individuals with diabetes develop nephropathy suggests that factors other than the hyperglycemic environment are involved in the pathogenesis of nephropathy. Genetic, ethnic, and familial factors may also play significant roles in the development of nephropathy. In the Diabetes Control and Complications Trial (DCCT) primary prevention cohort of type 1 patients without retinopathy, no familial concordance for development of diabetic retinopathy was found,

From: *Contemporary Cardiology: Diabetes and Cardiovascular Disease, Second Edition*
Edited by: M. T. Johnstone and A. Veves © Humana Press Inc., Totowa, NJ

whereas for nephropathy significant correlation was found *(12)*. On the other hand, analysis of the severity of nephropathy did not generally show familial correlation, although for the severity of retinopathy it was significant *(12)*.

Recent investigations have identified a number of candidate gene polymorphism that may contribute to diabetic nephropathy. The angiotensin-converting enzyme (ACE) gene variant with a deletion (D) of a 287 base pair sequence is one such polymorphism. This gene-deletion polymorphism is associated with elevated circulating and tissue activity of ACE *(13)* and increased risk of left ventricular hypertrophy *(14)*, ischemic heart disease *(15)*, and lacunar cerebrovascular accident *(16)*. A number of studies have found a positive association between the differential display phenotype and the prevalence and rate of progression of nephropathy *(17–19)*. Kunz and his colleagues in their meta-analysis conclude that diabetic nephropathy is not associated with the presence of the ACE-D allele in Caucasians with type I and type II diabetes, whereas the risk for nephropathy seemed to increase by 50% to 70% in type II Asian diabetics *(20)*. Additionally, the T allele of the AGT gene M235T polymorphism has been associated with increased risk of nephropathy *(21)* whereas the A14 allele of the NOS2 promoter has been associated with a decreased risk *(22)*.

Another basis for genetic/familial clustering of diabetic nephropathy is an increase in vitro sodium-lithium (Na-Li) countertransport activity, a biochemical marker of increased sodium reabsorptive capacity of the kidneys. Increased Na-Li countertransport activity has been found in some groups of patients with essential hypertension *(23)*. Abnormalities of this membrane countertransport system, which has an inheritable component *(24)*, have been found to be associated with diabetic nephropathy *(25,26)* and to predict the development of microalbuminuria in type 1 diabetes *(27)*. Recently, increased Na-Li countertransport has been identified with a splicing variant of the NHE1 exchanger that alters its affinity for lithium and eliminates its sensitivity to amiloride *(28)*.

How hyperglycemia causes nephropathy is multifactorial and is related to the stages of nephropathy.

Nephropathy Staging

Mogensen and his colleagues have developed a staging classification for the evolution of diabetic nephropathy *(29–32)* (Table 1). This staging pattern is more heterogeneous and possibly the pathogenesis is more complex in type 2 *(33)*, but overall similar patterns are seen in both type 1 and 2 patients *(34)*.

Early after diagnosis of diabetes in both type 1 *(35,36)* and type 2 *(37,38)*, glomerular filtration rate (GFR) increases. Nephromegaly and glomerular hypertrophy *(36,39)* accompany this glomerular hyperfiltration. More pronounced reduction in afferent compared to efferent arteriolar resistance may lead to elevated plasma flow in diabetics resulting in an increased GFR *(36)*. Additionally, total capillary surface area increases in early diabetics *(39)* and both elevated renal plasma flow and increased capillary surface area (that in turn increases glomerular ultrafiltration coefficient) contribute to increased GFR.

Hyperglycemia may directly increase the production of vasodilatory prostaglandins that can contribute to renal hyperperfusion, intraglomerular hypertension, and hyperfiltration. In experimental models, such as the streptozotocin-induced diabetic rat, glomeuli show increased production of vasodilatory prostaglandins *(40)*. Nitric oxide (NO) and atrial natriuretic peptide (ANP) are other vasodilator candidates for inducing hemodynamic changes leading to diabetic hyperfiltration. Elevated levels of ANP have been demonstrated in diabetic rats *(41)*, and a specific ANP receptor antagonist is capable of reducing

Table 1
Staging System for Diabetic Nephropathy

Stage 1	The earliest observation in development of nephropathy is an increase of up to 50% in the glomerular filtration rate (GFR). This is often present at diagnosis of diabetes and is frequently associated with increased kidney size and enlarged glomeruli.
Stage 2	Hyperfiltration may decrease to near normal levels of GFR and thickening of the glomerular capillary basement membrane (BM) is found histologically. Blood pressure and albumin excretion remain in normal range and clinically nephropathy remains undetectable at this stage.
Stage 3	Development of microalbuminuria (20–200 µg/minute or 30–300 mg/24 hours, not detectable by routine urine dipsticks) occurs after 6 to 15 years. Thickening of BM increases and mesangial matrix expansion appears. Incipient increases in blood pressure are seen in type 1. Type 2 diabetics may have hypertension even before development of nephropathy because of the genetic association of essential hypertension with type 2 diabetes. GFR may still be supranormal but declining.
Stage 4	Overt diabetic nephropathy and macroalbuminuria (>200 µg/minute or >300 mg/24 hours, that is detectable by routine dipsticks) with further development of structural changes. Usually takes 15 to 25 years to develop after appearance of diabetes mellitus. Increasing hypertension and more rapid fall in GFR (usually 10 mL/minute/year) without treatment are prominent features.
Stage 5	End-stage renal disease (ESRD) (usually 25–30 years after diagnosis) with glomerular closure and resultant decrease in proteinuria.

hyperfiltration in this experimental model *(42)*. Increased endothelial NO synthase mRNA *(43)* and increased sensitivity of peripheral and renal vascular circulation to endothelium-derived NO has also been found in experimental models *(44)*. Reversal of hyperfiltration with NO inhibition in experimental diabetes *(44,45)* indicates the potential importance of this mediator of diabetic hyperfiltration.

Indirectly, hyperglycemia may induce renal afferent vasodilation through activation of the tubuloglomerular feedback mechanism *(46)*. The increased filtration of glucose stimulates sodium reabsorption in the proximal tubules via Na-glucose transporters. This diminishes the amount of sodium reaching the early distal nephron in which the macula densa resides. The reduced sodium delivery to the macula densa results in a vasodilatory signal to the afferent arteriole supplying that nephron. The signal is mediated by NO and perhaps prostaglandins. The net effect is a decrease in afferent arteriole resistance and increase in renal blood flow *(47)*.

These metabolic and hemodynamic derangements may contribute to the initial structural changes in the early stages of diabetic nephropathy. Stretching of glomerular capillaries and mesangial cells as a result of glomerular hypertension, may be involved in increased basement membrane thickening and mesangial matrix formation, mediated by increased tissue production of angiotensin II. This is a potent promoter of increased local synthesis of transforming growth factor (TGF)-β. Changes in the level of TGF-β *(48)* and increased release of TGF-β (by glomerular endothelial, epithelial, and mesangial cells) may cause mesangial hypertrophy *(49)*. Increased and deranged production of basement membrane (BM) proteins, such as type IV collagen and fibronectin may contribute to structural changes. The effects of angiotensin II (Ang II) and glucose may be mediated by increased oxidative stress. Increased production of superoxide from endothelial nicotinamide adenine dinucleotide phosphate (NADPH) occurs as a result of both increased

Ang II and hyperglycemia. The superoxide ion can activate nuclear factor (NF)κB and induce a number of profibrotic genes including TGF-β and fibronectin *(43)*. Superoxide also scavenges NO, reducing its availability and leading to the formation of peroxynitrite. Peroxynitrite in turn oxidizes lipids and tyrosine residues.

Later in the course of diabetic nephropathy, hyperfiltration decreases and for many years the renal injury remains clinically undetectable with normal renal function and normal albumin secretion. In patients who later develop overt diabetic nephropathy, structural injury gradually becomes more prominent. Development of microalbuminuria is the earliest clinical sign to the presence of renal injury in diabetes. Both histological evidence of injury and increased mRNAs for profibrotic mediators are observed at this stage *(50)*. Still at this stage patients have normal or supranormal GFR. Other factors that cause urinary microalbuminuria, e.g., decompensated heart failure, acute febrile illness, urinary tract infection, metabolic decompensation, high-protein intake, heavy exercise *(51)*, and poorly controlled essential hypertension *(52)* should not be confused with true diabetic microalbuminuria *(51)*. For this reason, microalbuminuria measurements should be performed when control of these confounding conditions has been achieved and repeated measurements confirm the microalbuminuria is a persistent abnormality. Development of microalbuminuria is a strong predictor of progression to chronic renal insufficiency and ESRD in type 1 diabetes *(29–32,53)*. However, microalbuminuria at this stage can "regress" in association with glycemic control, normal levels of blood pressure (BP), cholesterol, and triglycerides *(54)*. This highlights the importance of screening early in the course of diabetes. In type 2, possibly the presence of essential hypertension and other comorbid confounding conditions, makes microalbuminuria a less strong predictive factor for the presence and progression of diabetic nephropathy *(34,35)*.

Prolonged hyperglycemia can also cause nonenzymatic glycosylation of proteins and lipids (advanced glycosylation end-products [AGEs]) *(56)*. As in other diabetic vascular complications, accumulation of AGEs in diabetic vasculature is believed to play an important role in pathogenesis of nephropathy *(56,57)*. Interaction of AGEs with a receptor on endothelial cells can cause increased expression of vascular cell adhesion molecule-1 *(58)*, increased vascular permeability *(59)* and increased production of reactive oxygen species *(60)*.

Long-term hyperglycemia can also increase the activity of another glucose-dependent pathway, the polyol pathway, which leads to accumulation of sorbitol in cells including the kidney and vasculature. This, in turn, depletes intracellular myoinositol, which interferes with cellular metabolism *(61)*.

Hyperglycemia also increases the activity of protein kinase C in diabetic rat glomeruli *(62)*. Hyperglycemia, perhaps through increased Ang II, upregulates plasminogen activator inhibitor type-1 (PAI-1) activity. PAI-1 inhibits not only fibrinolysis but proteolysis of extracellular matrix (ECM) *(63,64)*. This latter effects compounds the ECM accumulation resulting from increased production *(vide supra)* *(65)*.

Correlation of Microvascular Changes to Functional Tests and Screening for Nephropathy

Unfortunately, there is not a good test to identify the patients at the earliest stages (1 and 2). GFR measurements are notoriously inaccurate in the outpatient clinical setting and elevated levels must be confirmed and adjusted for body surface area. On the other hand, a normal GFR may indicate either the absence of hyperfiltration or decline in GFR after initial hyperfiltration and progression to overt nephropathy (stage 2).

Table 2
Recommendation for Screening for Microalbuminuria

World Health Organization	Urinary albumin excretion at least yearly for all patients with type 1 of more than 5 years duration and age above 12, and all patients with type 2 at the diagnosis until age 70. If abnormal it should be confirmed by repeat testing and repeated every 6 months.
National Kidney Foundation	At least a yearly urine albumin/creatinine ratio in first morning urine (or random urine). Positive result should be confirmed.

Other measurements in these early stages are also problematic. In a study of 36 type 1 diabetic adolescents without macroalbuminuria, Berg and associates found that an increased filtration fraction ([FF] = GFR/effective renal plasma flow) was predictive of structural changes including BM thickening and increased mesangial matrix *(66)*. They used clearance of inulin and para-amino hippuric acid during water diuresis to determine the GFR and effective renal plasma flow for calculating FF. They also found a direct correlation between epithelial foot process width and the log of urinary albumin excretion. Even if this correlation could be established by other studies, longitudinal determination of FF would be needed for developing temporal comparisons. Finally, such measurements are too complicated for routine clinical practice. Likewise, measurement of Na-Li countertransport activity, or determination of the ACE gene polymorphism or mRNA levels of profibrotic cytokines in renal tissue to stratify diabetic patients at risk for development of nephropathy is impractical at present.

The earliest clinical marker of diabetic nephropathy in both types 1 and 2 is the presence of microalbuminuria (*vide supra*). The presence of microalbuminuria identifies high-risk patients that will benefit from the therapeutic measures described below. Thus, several protocols exist for screening of diabetic patients for development of microalbuminuria. Table 2 summarizes the World Health Organization *(51)* and the National Kidney Foundation *(67)* screening recommendations for urinary albumin excretion (UAE):

It should be noted that not all albuminuric/proteinuria type 2 DM individuals have diabetic nephropathy. Other renal diseases have been found in 10% to 24% of these individuals *(68,69)* and 50% of those without retinopathy *(70)*. This is an important consideration because the rate of progression of renal disease in diabetes is generally greater than that seen with the other glomerulonephritides found in these patients *(71)*. The presence of other causes of renal disease might necessitate specific therapies and interventions.

TREATMENTS TO PREVENT OR DELAY PROGRESSION OF NEPHROPATHY

Long-term observational studies of cohorts of type 1 and type 2 DM have identified an number of modifiable promoters of nephropathy. These include arterial pressure, glucose control, serum cholesterol, and urinary protein *(72)*. A number of randomized prospective trials have documented the beneficial effects of targeting these promoters for both primary and secondary prevention of nephropathy.

Glycemic Control

The DCCT, United Kingdom Prospective Diabetes Study (UKPDS), *(33)* and Kumamoto trial *(11,73,74)* provide strong evidence in favor of the role of intensive glycemic control in preventing and decreasing the progression of diabetic nephropathy in type 1 and type 2 DM respectively. In the DCCT, intensive insulin therapy was associated with a 40% decrease in the incidence of new microalbuminuria *(10)*. In other observational studies, the lowest A1c levels were associated with the lowest incidence of developing microalbuminuria *(7)*. In the UKPDS, sulphonylureas and insulin produce equally good results with regards to diabetic microvascular complications *(11)*. The incidence of new microalbuminuria was decreased 34% with intensive control that resulted in a 1% lower A1c *(11)*. Progression from microalbuminuria to proteinuria was also diminished in type 1 diabetes *(10)* and the longer follow-up data from Epidemiology of Diabetes Interventions and Complications show that the early control of glycemia may have long-lasting benefits on the rate of development of microvascular complications *(75)*. Even in individuals with established nephropathy, observational studies suggest that the rate of loss of renal function is reduced in the presence of better glycemic control *(72,76)* although little effect was seen in some series *(77)*.

The use of thiazolidinedione (TZD) agents may also be of particular benefit in treating nephropathy. In a recent report, TZD compounds completely prevented the high-glucose-induced TGF-β promoter activity and elevation of c-Fos nuclear transcription factor *(78)*. Such actions might be expected to downregulate fibrosis and this has also been observed in animal studies. Activation of peroxisome proliferators-activated receptor-γ decreases type I collagen mRNA and protein *(79)*. Thus, is seems intriguing that TZDs may halt progression of nephropathy by mechanisms other than their hypoglycemic effect.

Smoking

Cigarette smoking, apart from its detrimental effects on macrovascular disease, has been implicated in progression of diabetic nephropathy in both types of diabetes in several studies *(80–82)*. With smoking cessation, the risk of progression of diabetic nephropathy can be reduced *(83)*.

Hypertension

The relationship between diabetes and hypertension has been discussed in detail in another chapter in this book. We focus on the role of hypertension in the pathogenesis of diabetic nephropathy and its importance as a target of therapy. More than two decades ago Mogensen showed that control of hypertension slows the progression of nephropathy *(84)*. BP control *per se* can reduce the amount of proteinuria in both types *(30,31,85)* and almost all antihypertensive medications can reduce proteinuria as a result of their BP-lowering effect. The seventh report of the Joint National Committee on prevention, detection, evaluation, and treatment of high BP, emphasizes the need for aggressive treatment of hypertension in the presence of diabetes, with an antihypertensive target of less than 130/80 mmHg *(86)*. Despite this consensus, less than one-third of patients with diabetes achieve these BP targets *(87)*. ACE inhibitors and angiotensin receptor blockers (ARBs) have an added effect on proteinuria that we will discuss later in more details.

The effect of many antihypertensive drugs in decreasing proteinuria and halting the progression of diabetic nephropathy has been compared to ACE inhibitors.

Table 3
Effect of Intensive Glycemic Control on Development of New Microalbuminuria (Primary Prevention) or Progression From Microalbuminuria to Proteinuria (Secondary Prevention) in Types 1 and 2 Diabetes

Study (reference)	N	Years follow-up	Diabetes mellitus type	Treatment	–A1C	Primary prevention	Secondary prevention
DCCT (10)	1441	9	1	Insulin	2%	39%	54%
Kumamoto (74)	110	8	2	Insulin	2%	74%	60%
UKPDS (11)	4209	9	2	Various	1%	24%	N/A

DCCT, Diabetes Control and Complications Trial; UKPDS, United Kingdom Prospective Diabetes Study; N/A: not applicable.

Nondihydropyridine calcium channel blockers (CCBs), verapamil and diltiazem, have been reported to have a beneficial effect comparable to that of ACE inhibitors (88,89). Short-acting dihydropyridine CCBs, on the other hand, do not have any added effect on proteinuria (90,91). Although, slow-release or long-acting newer dihydropyridines may reduce proteinuria (92,93), this needs further confirmation in larger trials. In the UKPDS, target BP control to less than 140/90 with either captopril or atenolol, in type 2 diabetes was equally effective in preventing macroalbuminuria and/or doubling of serum creatinine concentration (94).

Effects of ACE Inhibitors, ARBs, and Treatments Other Than Glycemic and Blood Pressure Control

ACE inhibitors and ARBs have an additional favorable effect on glomerular hemodynamics and proteinuria that are independent of BP changes (95–99). In contrast, reductions in proteinuria from other antihypertensive agents could be entirely explained by changes in BP. Even in normotensive diabetics with microalbuminuria or overt proteinuria, ACE inhibitors can decrease the rate of decline in GFR in both type 1 and 2 patients (100,101). The fact that ACE inhibitors can reduce the progression of microalbuminuria to macroalbuminuria in type 1 (102) and type 2 (101) patients and ARBs reduce progression in type 2 patients (96–99) underscores their efficacy at earlier stages of clinical nephropathy and provides an opportunity to halt the progression to ESRD (stage 5). Finally and perhaps most importantly, these agents reduce mortality in the more advanced stages of nephropathy (99,103). Thus, ACE inhibitors and ARBs have become the gold-standard treatment in diabetic patients with any stage of nephropathy. Based on evidence from clinical trials, the American Diabetes Association has recommended ACE inhibitors for type 1 patients with nephropathy and ARBs for type 2 patients with nephropathy (104). The dose required for the maximum antiproteinuric effect is generally greater than that for maximum antihypertensive effect. Some investigators have found that doses even greater than those approved by the Food and Drug Administration for BP control still have increasing antiproteinuric effects (104a).

The complex pathophysiology of hypertension in diabetic nephropathy usually demands two or more drugs for aggressive control of hypertension. The choice of a diuretic, CCB, β-blocker, or other antihypertensive agent is influenced by co-morbidities present in the individual patients. A diuretic will usually be needed in the presence of even mild reductions in GFR and should be accompanied by sodium restriction. Sodium restriction can potentiate the BP-lowering effects of most antihypertensive medications. In diabetic animals, salt restriction also reduced the hyperfiltration, albuminuria, and the kidney weight *(105)*. Salt restriction in man also improves the antiproteinuric effect of ACE inhibitors *(106)*.

Proteinuria

Numerous studies have documented that the amount of proteinuria is the best single predictor of disease progression *(107)*. Filtered proteins are taken up into proximal tubule cells in which they undergo degradation in lysosomes. This process when over-loaded generates profibrotic cytokines that accelerates nephron loss. Furthermore, the magnitude of the reduction in proteinuria with therapy is a predictor of renal preservation *(107a)*. For any degree of BP reduction, proteinuria is reduced more by ACE inhibitors and ARBs than other classes of antihypertensives. ACE inhibitors and ARBs reduce proteinuria through mechanisms independent of their BP-lowering effects. Tissue Ang II modulates the proteins comprising the slit diaphragm of the glomerular capillary wall. By affecting the distribution of nephrin *(108)* and other slit diaphragm proteins, the integrity of the slit diaphragm to macromolecules is maintained. Additionally, Ang II upregulates cytokines involved in the profibrotic process. These include TGF-β, fibronectin, and PAI-1 *(109)*. These cytokine effects may be mediated by increased oxygen radicals generated in response to Ang II effects on endothelial NADPH *(43)*.

The central role of the renin–angiotensin–aldosterone system in the pathogenesis of diabetic nephropathy has led to efforts to more completely inhibit this system. Trials in nondiabetic *(110)* and diabetic renal disease *(111–113)* with combinations of ACE inhibitors and ARBs have shown enhanced antiproteinuric effects. The addition of an inhibitor of aldosterone has also provided enhanced antiproteinuric effects *(114)*.

Dietary Interventions

Dietary protein restriction and its effect on progression of diabetic nephropathy has been a subject of controversy (as it is in nondiabetic renal disease). In the Modification of Diet in Renal Disease (MDRD) study a clear-cut benefit was not shown by protein restriction *(115)*. Although this was the largest prospective trial studying the effect of protein restriction, no patient in MDRD had type 1 diabetes and only 3% of the patients had type 2 diabetes. Furthermore, during the study few patients developed renal failure. In a rat model of diabetic nephropathy, protein restriction reduces hyperfiltration, intraglomerular pressure, and the rate of progression of renal disease *(116)*. In a recent meta-analysis of five smaller studies including type 1 diabetic patients, protein restriction ranging from 0.5 to 0.85 g/kg significantly reduced the rate of decline in GFR or creatinine clearance or the increase in UAE *(117)*. For type 2 diabetic nephropathy, compelling data is not available. At this time, a protein restriction of 0.8 g/kg for patients with evidence of nephropathy seems reasonable *(118)* and safe.

Dyslipidemia is common in both types of diabetes. The National Cholesterol Education Program advocates more aggressive control of cholesterol in diabetic patients with a target low-density lipoprotein of less than 100 mg/dL *(119)*. Dyslipidemia not only contributes to devastating macrovascular changes, but also is a risk factor for nephropathy *(120,121)*. Studies have shown the effect of correction of dyslipidemia with gemfibrozil *(122)* and lovastatin *(123)* in retarding the progression of diabetic nephropathy. A meta-analysis of 13 prospective controlled trials in patients with different types of chronic kidney disease has shown lipid reduction may preserve GFR and decrease proteinuria *(124)*. A large multicenter trial (Scottish Heart and Arterial Risk Prevention) is underway to further explore this aspect of therapy.

CONCLUSION

Nephropathy is a major microvascular complication of diabetes and in both types of diabetes it goes through similar pathophysiologic stages. Microalbuminuria is the earliest clinical marker for the presence of nephropathy, although it is a late manifestation of the pathophysiological process. Microalbuminuria is also a strong risk factor for development of macrovascular complications.

Tight glycemic control, aggressive BP control, use of ACE inhibitors and ARBs, smoking cessation, protein and salt restriction, and aggressive treatment of dyslipidemia can slow the progression of nephropathy to ESRD. An aggressive approach to the multiple risk factors for diabetic nephropathy can significantly reduce the risk of progression *(125)*.

REFERENCES

1. System USRD. USRDS 2002 Annual Data Report. Bethesda, MD, National Institutes of Health, 2002.
2. Brancati FL, Whelton PK, Randall BL, Neaton JD, Stamler J, Klag MJ. Risk of end-stage renal disease in diabetes mellitus: a prospective cohort study of men screened for MRFIT. JAMA 1997;278:2069–2074.
3. Andersen AR, Christiansen JS, Andersen JK, Kreiner S, Deckert T. Diabetic nephropathy in Type 1 (insulin-dependent) diabetes: an epidemiological study. Diabetologia 1983;25:496–501.
4. Hasslacher C, Ritz E, Wahl P, Michael C. Similar risks of nephropathy in patients with type I or type II diabetes mellitus. Nephrol Dial Transplant 1989;4:859–863.
5. Rossing P, Rossing K, Jacobsen P, Parving HH. Unchanged incidence of diabetic nephropathy in IDDM patients. Diabetes 1995;44:739–743.
6. Ballard DJ, Humphrey LL, Melton L Jr, et al. Epidemiology of persistent proteinuria in type II diabetes mellitus. Population-based study in Rochester, Minnesota. Diabetes 1988;37:405–412.
7. Stephenson JM, Kenny S, Stevens LK, Fuller JH, Lee E. Proteinuria and mortality in diabetes: the WHO Multinational Study of Vascular Disease in Diabetes. Diabet Med 1995;12:149–155.
8. Delcourt C, Villatte-Cathelineau B, Vauzzelle-Kervroedan F, Papoz L. Clinical correlates of advanced retinopthy in type II diabetes patients: implications for screening. J Clin Epidemiol 1996;49:679–685.
9. Adler AI, Stevens RJ, Manley SE, Bilous RW, Cull CA, Holman RR. Development and progression of nephropathy in type 2 diabetes. The United Kingdom Prospective Diabetes Study (UKPDS 64). Kidney Int 2003;63:225–232.
10. The effect of intensive treatment of diabetes on the development and progression of long-term complications in insulin-dependent diabetes mellitus. The Diabetes Control and Complications Trial Research Group. N Engl J Med 1993;329:977–986.
11. Intensive blood-glucose control with sulphonylureas or insulin compared with conventional treatment and risk of complications in patients with type 2 diabetes (UKPDS 33). UK Prospective Diabetes Study (UKPDS) Group. Lancet 1998;352:837–853.
12. Clustering of long-term complications in families with diabetes in the diabetes control and complications trial. The Diabetes Control and Complications Trial Research Group. Diabetes 1997;46:1829–1839.
13. Rigat B, Hubert C, Alhenc-Gelas F, Cambien F, Corvol P, Soubrier F. An insertion/deletion polymorphism in the angiotensin I-converting enzyme gene accounting for half the variance of serum enzyme levels. J Clin Invest 1990;86:1343–1346.
14. Shunkert H, Hense HW, Holmer SR, et al. Association between a deletion polymorphism of the angiotensin-converting-enzyme gene and left ventricular hypertrophy. N Engl J Med 1994;330:1634–1638.
15. Cambien F, Poirier O, Lecerf L, et al. Deletion polymorphism in the gene for angiotensin-converting enzyme is a potent risk factor for myocardial infarction. Nature 1992;359:641–644.

16. Markus HS, Barley J, Lunt R, et al. Angiotensin-converting enzyme gene deletion polymorphism. A new risk factor for lacunar stroke but not carotid atheroma. Stroke 1995;26:1329–1333.

17. Fujisawa T, Ikegami H, Kawaguchi Y, et al. Meta-analysis of association of insertion/deletion polymorphism of angiotensin I-converting enzyme gene with diabetic nephropathy and retinopathy. Diabetologia 1998;41:47–53.

18. Kimura H, Gejyo F, Suzuki Y, Suzuki S, Miyazaki R, Arakawa M. Polymorphisms of angiotensin converting enzyme and plasminogen activator inhibitor-1 genes in diabetes and macroangiopathy. Kidney Int 1998;54:1659–1669.

19. Yoshida H, Kuriyama S, Atsumi Y, et al. Angiotensin I converting enzyme gene polymorphism in non-insulin dependent diabetes mellitus. Kidney Int 1996;50:657–664.

20. Kunz R BJ, Fritsche L, Ringel J, Sharma, AM. Association between the angiotensin-converting enzyme-insertion/deletion polymorphism and diabetic nephropathy: methodologic appraisal and systemic review. J Am Soc Nephrol 1998;9:1653–1663.

21. Rogus JJ, Moczulski D, Freire MV, Yang Y, Warram JH, Krolewski AS. Diabetic nephropathy is associated with AGT polymorphism T235: results of family-based study. Hypertension 1998;31:627–631.

22. Johannesen J, Tarnow L, Parving HH, Nerup J, Pociot F. CCTTT-repeat polymorphism in the human NOS2-promoter confers low-risk of diabetic nephropathy in type 1 diabetic patients. Diabetes Care 2000;23:560–562.

23. Canessa M, Adragna N, Solomon HS, Connolly TM, Tosteson DC. Increased sodium-lithium countertransport in red cells of patients with essential hypertension. N Engl J Med 1980;302:772–776.

24. Hasstedt SJ, Wu LL, Ash KO, Kuida H, Williams RR. Hypertension and sodium-lithium countertransport in Utah pedigrees: evidence for major-locus inheritance. Am J Hum Genet 1988;43:14–22.

25. Krolewski AS, Canessa M, Warram JH, et al. Predisposition to hypertension and susceptibility to renal disease in insulin-dependent diabetes mellitus. N Engl J Med 1988;318:140–145.

26. Rutherford PA, Thomas TH, Carr SJ, Taylor R, Wilkinson R. Changes in erythrocyte sodium-lithium countertransport kinetics in diabetic nephropathy. Clin Sci (Lond) 1992;82:301–307.

27. Monciotti CG, Semplicini A, Morocutti A, et al. Elevated sodium-lithium countertransport activity in erythrocytes is predictive of the development of microalbuminuria in IDDM. Diabetologia 1997;40:654–661.

28. Zerbini G, Maestroni A, Breviario D, Mangili R, Casari G. Alternative splicing of NHEZ-1 mediates Na-Li countertranport and associates with activity rate. Diabetes 2003;52:1511–1518.

29. Mogensen CE, Christensen CK, Vittinghus E. The stages in diabetic renal disease. With emphasis on the stage of incipient diabetic nephropathy. Diabetes 1983;32 Suppl 2:64–78.

30. Mogensen CE, Hansen KW, Osterby R, Damsgaard EM. Blood pressure elevation versus abnormal albuminuria in the genesis and prediction of renal disease in diabetes. Diabetes Care 1992;15:1192–1204.

31. Mogensen CE. Systemic blood pressure and glomerular leakage with particular reference to diabetes and hypertension. J Intern Med 1994;235:297–316.

32. Mogensen CE. How to protect the kidney in diabetic patients: with special reference to IDDM. Diabetes 1997;46 Suppl 2:S104–S111.

33. Fioretto P, Mauer M, Brocco E, et al. Patterns of renal injury in NIDDM patients with microalbuminuria. Diabetologia 1996;39:1569–1576.

34. Nelson RG, Bennett PH, Beck GJ, et al. Development and progression of renal disease in Pima Indians with non-insulin-dependent diabetes mellitus. Diabetic Renal Disease Study Group. N Engl J Med 1996;335:1636–1642.

35. Ditzel J, Junker K. Abnormal glomerular filtration rate, renal plasma flow, and renal protein excretion in recent and short-term diabetics. Br Med J 1972;2:13–19.

36. Mogensen CE, Andersen MJ. Increased kidney size and glomerular filtration rate in untreated juvenile diabetes: normalization by insulin-treatment. Diabetologia 1975;11:221–224.

37. Myers BD, Nelson RG, Williams GW, et al. Glomerular function in Pima Indians with noninsulin-dependent diabetes mellitus of recent onset. J Clin Invest 1991;88:524–530.

38. Nowack R, Raum E, Blum W, Ritz E. Renal hemodynamics in recent-onset type II diabetes. Am J Kidney Dis 1992;20:342–347.

39. Kroustrup JP, Gundersen HJ, Osterby R. Glomerular size and structure in diabetes mellitus. III. Early enlargement of the capillary surface. Diabetologia 1977;13:207–210.

40. Schambelan M, Blake S, Sraer J, Bens M, Nivez MP, Wahbe F. Increased prostaglandin production by glomeruli isolated from rats with streptozotocin-induced diabetes mellitus. J Clin Invest 1985;75:404–412.

41. Ortola FV, Ballermann BJ, Anderson S, Mendez RE, Brenner BM. Elevated plasma atrial natriuretic peptide levels in diabetic rats. Potential mediator of hyperfiltration. J Clin Invest 1987;80:670–674.

42. Zhang PL, Mackenzie HS, Troy JL, Brenner BM. Effects of an atrial natriuretic peptide receptor antagonist on glomerular hyperfiltration in diabetic rats. J Am Soc Nephrol 1994;4:1564–1570.

43. Onozato ML, Tojo A, Goto A, Fujita T, Wilcox CS. Oxidative stress and nitric oxide synthase in rat diabetic nephropathy: effects of ACEI and ARB. Kidney Int 2002;61:186–194.
44. Komers R, Allen TJ, Cooper ME. Role of endothelium-derived nitric oxide in the pathogenesis of the renal hemodynamic changes of experimental diabetes. Diabetes 1994;43:1190–1197.
45. Tolinns J, Schultz, PJ, Raji L, et al. Abnormal renal hemodynamic response to reduced renal perfusion pressure in diabetic rats: role of NO. Am J Physiol 1993;265:F886-F895.
46. Vallon V, Richter K, Blantz RC, Thomson S, Osswald H. Glomerular hyperfiltration in experimental diabetes mellitus. J Am Soc Nephrol 1999;10:2569–2576.
47. Vallon V, Blantz RC, Thomson S. Glomerular hyperfiltration and the salt paradox in early Type 1 diabetes mellitus: a tubulo-centric view. J Am Soc Nephrol 2003;14:530–537.
48. Yasuda T, Kondo S, Homma T, et al. Mechanisms for accumulation of extracellular matrix in rat mesangial cells in response to stretch/relaxation. J Am Soc Nephrol 1994;5:834 (abstr).
49. Rocco MV, Chen Y, Goldfarb S, Ziyadeh FN. Elevated glucose stimulates TGF-beta gene expression and bioactivity in proximal tubule. Kidney Int 1992;41:107–114.
50. Adler SG, Kang SW, Feld S, et al. Glomerular mRNAs in human type 1 diabetes: biochemical evidence for microalbuminuria as a manifestation of diabetic nephropathy. Kidney Int 2001;60:2330–2336.
51. Prevention of diabetes mellitus. Report of a WHO Study Group. World Health Organ Tech Rep Ser 1994;844:1–100.
52. Parving HH, Mogensen CE, Jensen HA, Evrin PE. Increased urinary albumin-excretion rate in benign essential hypertension. Lancet 1974;1:1190–1192.
53. Almdal T, Norgaard K, Feldt-Rasmussen B, Deckert T. The predictive value of microalbuminuria in IDDM. A five-year follow-up study. Diabetes Care 1994;17:120–125.
54. Perkins BA, Ficociello LH, Silva KH, Finkelstein DM, Warram JH, Krolewski AS. Regression of microalbuminuria in Type 1 diabetes. N Engl J Med 2003;348:2285–2293.
55. Mogensen CE. Microalbuminuria predicts clinical proteinuria and early mortality in maturity-onset diabetes. N Engl J Med 1984;310:356–360.
56. Brownlee M, Cerami A, Valssara H. Advanced glycosylation endproducts in tissue and biochemical basis of diabetic complications. N Engl J Med 1988;318:1315–1320.
57. Brownlee M, Cerami A, Vlassara H. Advanced products of nonenzymatic glycosylation and the pathogenesis of diabetic vascular disease. Diabetes Metab Rev 1988;4:437–451.
58. Schmidt AM, Hori O, Chen JX, et al. Advanced glycation endproducts interacting with their endothelial receptor induce expression of vascular cell adhesion molecule-1 (VCAM-1) in cultured human endothelial cells and in mice. A potential mechanism for the accelerated vasculopathy of diabetes. J Clin Invest 1995;96:1395–1403.
59. Wautier JL, Zoukourian C, Chappey O, et al. Receptor-mediated endothelial cell dysfunction in diabetic vasculopathy. Soluble receptor for advanced glycation end products blocks hyperpermeability in diabetic rats. J Clin Invest 1996;97:238–243.
60. Vlasara H. The AGE-receptor in the pathogenesis of diabetic complications. Diabetes Metab Res Rev 2001;17:436–443.
61. Greene DA, Lattimer SA, Sima AA. Sorbitol, phosphoinositides, and sodium-potassium-ATPase in the pathogenesis of diabetic complications. N Engl J Med 1987;316:599–606.
62. Cravan PA, DeRubertis FR. Protein kinase C is activated in glomeruli from streptozotocin diabetic rats. Possible mediation by glucose. J Clin Invest 1989;83:1667–1675.
63. Bastard JP, Pieroni L, Hainque B. Relationship between plasma plasminogen activator inhibitor 1 and insulin resistance. Diabetes Metab Res Rev 2000;16:192–201.
64. Fogo AB, Vaughan DE. Compound interest: ACE and PAI-1 polymorphisms and risk of thrombosis and fibrosis. Kidney Int 1998;54 1765–1766.
65. Paueksakon P, Revelo MP, Ma LJ, Marcantoni C, Fogo AV. Microangiopathic injury and augmented PAI-1 in human diabetic nephropathy. Kidney Int 2002;61:2142–2148.
66. Berg UB, Torbjornsdotter TB, Jaremko G, Thalme B. Kidney morphological changes in relation to long-term renal function and metabolic control in adolescents with IDDM. Diabetologia 1998;41:1047–1056.
67. Bennett PH, Haffner S, Kasiske BL, et al. Screening and management of microalbuminuria in patients with diabetes mellitus: recommendations to the Scientific Advisory Board of the National Kidney Foundation from an ad hoc committee of the Council on Diabetes Mellitus of the National Kidney Foundation. Am J Kidney Dis 1995;25:107–112.
68. Schwartz MM, Lewis EJ, Leonard-Matin T, Breyer-Lewis J, Battle D. Renal pathology patterns in type II diabetes mellitus: relationship with retinopathy. Nephrol Dial Transplant 1998;13:2547–2552.
69. Parving HH, Gall MA, Skott P, et al. Prevalence and cause of albuminuria in non-insulin-dependent diabetic patients. Kidney Int 1992;41:758–762.

70. Ruggenenti P, Remuzzi A. The diagnosis of renal involvement in non-insulin-dependent diabetes mellitus. Curr Opin Nephrol Hypertens 1997;6:141–145.
71. Christensen PK, Gall M, Parving HH. Course of glomerular filtration rate in albuminuric type 2 diabetic patients with and without diabetic glomerulopathy. Diabetes Care 2000;23:B14-B20.
72. Hovind P, Rossing P, Tarnow L, Smidt UM, Parving HH. Progression of diabetic nephropathy. Kidney Int 2001;59:702–709.
73. Effect of intensive therapy on the development and progression of diabetic nephropathy in the Diabetes Control and Complications Trial. Diabetes Control and Complication Research Group. Kidney Int 1995;47:1703–1720.
74. Shichiri M, Kishikawa H, Ohkubo Y, Wake N. Long-term results of the Kumamoto study on optimal diabetes control in type 2 diabetic patients. Diabetes Care 2000;23 (suppl 2):B21-B29.
75. Writing team for the Diabetes Control and Complication Trial. Effect of intensive therapy on the microvascular complications of type 1 diabetes mellitus. JAMA 2002;287:2563–2569.
76. Mulec H, Blohme G, Grande B, Bjorck S. The effect of metabolic control on rate of decline in renal function in insulin-dependent diabetes mellitus with overt diabetic nephropathy. Nephrol Dial Transplant 1998;13:651–655.
77. Parving HH. Renoprotection in diabetes: genetic and non-genetic risk factors and treatment. Diabetologia 1998;41:745–759.
78. Weigert C, Brodbeck K, Bierhaus A, Haring HU, Schleicher ED. C-fos-driven transcriptional activation of transforming growth factor beta-1: inhibition of high glucose-induced promoter activity by thiazolidinediones. Biochem Biophys Res Commun 2003;304:301–307.
79. Zheng F, Fornoni A, Elliot SJ, et al. Upregulation of type I collagen by TGF-beta in mesangial cells is blocked by PPAR-gamma activation. Am J Physiol 2002;282:F639–648.
80. Christiansen JS. Cigarette smoking and prevalence of microangiopathy in juvenile-onset insulin-dependent diabetes mellitus. Diabetes Care 1978;1:146–149.
81. Chase HP, Garg SK, Marshall G, et al. Cigarette smoking increases the risk of albuminuria among subjects with type I diabetes. JAMA 1991;265:614–617.
82. Biesenbach G, Grafinger P, Janko O, Zazgornik J. Influence of cigarette-smoking on the progression of clinical diabetic nephropathy in type 2 diabetic patients. Clin Nephrol 1997;48:146–150.
83. Ritz E, Ogata H, Orth SR. Smoking: a factor promoting onset and progression of diabetic nephropathy. Diabetes Metab 2000;26 (Suppl 4):S54-S63.
84. Mogensen CE. Progression of nephropathy in long-term diabetics with proteinuria and effect of initial anti-hypertensive treatment. Scand J Clin Lab Invest 1976;36:383–388.
85. Parving HH, Andersen AR, Smidt UM, Hommel E, Mathiesen ER, Svendsen PA. Effect of antihypertensive treatment on kidney function in diabetic nephropathy. Br Med J (Clin Res Ed) 1987;294:1443–1447.
86. Chobanian AV, Bakris GL, Black HR, et al. The seventh report of the joint national committee on prevention, detection, evaluation, and treatment of high blood pressure. JAMA 2003;289:2560–2572.
87. McFarlane SI, Jacober SJ, Winer N, et al. Control of cardiovascular risk factors in patients with diabetes and hypertension at urban academic medical centers. Diabetes Care 2002;25:718–723.
88. Bakris GL. Effects of diltiazem or lisinopril on massive proteinuria associated with diabetes mellitus. Ann Intern Med 1990;112:707–708.
89. Demarie BK, Bakris GL. Effects of different calcium antagonists on proteinuria associated with diabetes mellitus. Ann Intern Med 1990;113:987–988.
90. Abbott K, Smith A, Bakris GL. Effects of dihydropyridine calcium antagonists on albuminuria in patients with diabetes. J Clin Pharmacol 1996;36:274–279.
91. Smith AC, Toto R, Bakris GL. Differential effects of calcium channel blockers on size selectivity of proteinuria in diabetic glomerulopathy. Kidney Int 1998;54:889–896.
92. Crepaldi G, Carta Q, Deferrari G, et al. Effects of lisinopril and nifedipine on the progression to overt albuminuria in IDDM patients with incipient nephropathy and normal blood pressure. The Italian Microalbuminuria Study Group in IDDM. Diabetes Care 1998;21:104–110.
93. Sumida Y, Yano Y, Murata K, et al. Effect of the calcium channel blocker nilvadipine on urinary albumin excretion in hypertensive microalbuminuric patients with non-insulin-dependent diabetes mellitus. J Int Med Res 1997;25:117–126.
94. Efficacy of atenolol and captopril in reducing risk of macrovascular and microvascular complications in type 2 diabetes: UKPDS 39. UK Prospective Diabetes Study Group. BMJ 1998;317:713–720.
95. Kasiske BL, Kalil RS, Ma JZ, Liao M, Keane WF. Effect of antihypertensive therapy on the kidney in patients with diabetes: a meta-regression analysis. Ann Intern Med 1993;118:129–138.

96. Viberti G, Wheeldon NM. Microalbuminuria reduction with valsartan in patients with type 2 diabetes mellitus: a blood pressure-independent effect. Circulation 2002;106:672–678.

97. Parving HH, Lehnert H, Brochner-Mortensen J, Gomis R, Andersen S, Arner P. The effect of irbesartan on the development of diabetic nephropathy in patients with type 2 diabetes. N Engl J Med 2001;345:870–878.

98. Lewis EJ, Hunsicker LC, Clark WR, et al. Renoprotective effect of the angiotensin-receptor antagonist irbesartan in patients with nephropathy due to type 2 diabetes. N Engl J Med 2001;345:851–860.

99. Brenner BM, Cooper ME, de Zeeuw D, et al. Effects of losartan on renal and cardiovascular outcomes in patients with type 2 diabetes and nephropathy. N Engl J Med 2001;345:861–869.

100. Parving HH, Hommel E, Damkjaer Nielsen M, Giese J. Effect of captopril on blood pressure and kidney function in normotensive insulin dependent diabetics with nephropathy. BMJ 1989;299:533–536.

101. Ravid M, Lang R, Rachmani R, Lishner M. Long-term renoprotective effect of angiotensin-converting enzyme inhibition in non-insulin-dependent diabetes mellitus. A 7-year follow-up study. Arch Intern Med 1996;156:286–289.

102. Viberti G, Mogensen CE, Groop LC, Pauls JF. Effect of captopril on progression to clinical proteinuria in patients with insulin-dependent diabetes mellitus and microalbuminuria. European Microalbuminuria Captopril Study Group. JAMA 1994;271:275–279.

103. Lewis EJ, Hunsicker LG, Bain RP, Rohde RD. The effect of angiotensin-converting-enzyme inhibition on diabetic nephropathy. The Collaborative Study Group. N Engl J Med 1993;329:1456–1462.

104. American Diabetes Association: Diabetic nephropathy (position statement). Diabetes Care 2003;26 (Suppl 1):S94-S98.

104a. Weinberg AJ, Zappe DH, Ashton M, Weinberg MS. Safety and tolerability of high-dose angiotensin receptor blocker therapy in patients with chronic kidney disease: a pilot study. Am J Nephrol 2004; 24(3):340–345.

105. Allen TJ, Waldron MJ, Casley D, Jerums G, Cooper ME. Salt restriction reduces hyperfiltration, renal enlargement, and albuminuria in experimental diabetes. Diabetes 1997;46:19–24.

106. Heeg JE, de Jong PE, van der Hem GK, de Zeeuw D. Efficacy and variability of the antiproteinuric effect of ACE inhibition by lisinopril. Kidney Int 1989;36:272–279.

107. Breyer JA, Bain RP, Evans JK, et al. Predictors of the progression of renal insufficiency in patients with insulin-dependent diabetes and overt diabetic nephropathy. Kidney Int 1996;1996:1651–1658.

107a. de Zeeuw D, Remuzzi G, Darving HH, Keane WF, Zhang Z, Shahinfar S. Proteinuria, a target for renoprotection in patients with type 2 diabetic nephropathy: lessons from RENAAL. Kidney Int 2004;65(6):2309–2320.

108. Benigni A, Tomasoni S, Gagliardini E, et al. Blocking angiotensin II synthesis/activity preserves glomerular nephrin in rats with severe nephrosis. J Am Soc Nephrol 2001;12:941–948.

109. Wolf G, Ziyadeh FN. The role of angiotensin II in diabetic nephropathy: emphasis on nonhemodynamic mechanisms. Am J Kidney Dis 1997;29:153–163.

110. Nakao N, Yoshimura A, Morita H, Takada M, Kayano T, Ideura T. Combination treatment of angiotensin II receptro blocker and angiotensin-converting enzyme inhibitor in non-diabetic renal disease (COOPERATE): a randomized controlled trial. Lancet 2003;361:117–124.

111. Kuriyama S, Tomonari H, Tokudome G. Antiproteinuric effects of combined antihypertensive therapies in patients with overt type 2 diabetic nephropathy. Hypertens Res 2002;25:849–855.

112. Jacobsen P, Andersen S, Jensen BR, Parving HH. Additive effect of ACE inhibition and angiotensin II receptor blockade in type 1 diabetes with diabetic nephropathy. J Am Soc Nephrol 2003;14:992–999.

113. Mogensen CE, Neldam S, Tikkanen I, et al. Randomised controlled trial of dual blockade of renin-angiotensin system in patients with hypertension, microalbuminuria, and non-insulin dependent diabetes: the candesartan and lisinopril microalbuminuria (CALM) study. BMJ 2000;321:1440–1444.

114. Sato A, Hayashi K, Naruse M, Saruto T. Effectiveness of aldosterone blockade in patients with diabetic nephropathy. Hypertension 2003;41:64–68.

115. Klahr S, Levey AS, Beck GJ, et al. The effects of dietary protein restriction and blood-pressure control on the progression of chronic renal disease. Modification of Diet in Renal Disease Study Group. N Engl J Med 1994;330:877–884.

116. Zatz R, Meyer TW, Rennke HG, Brenner BM. Predominance of hemodynamic rather than metabolic factors in the pathogenesis of diabetic glomerulopathy. Proc Natl Acad Sci U S A 1985;82:5963–5967.

117. Pedrini MT, Levey AS, Lau J, Chalmers TC, Wang PH. The effect of dietary protein restriction on the progression of diabetic and nondiabetic renal diseases: a meta-analysis. Ann Intern Med 1996;124: 627–632.

118. Franz MJ, Horton ES, Sr, Bantle JP, et al. Nutrition principles for the management of diabetes and related complications. Diabetes Care 1994;17:490–518.
119. Executive summary of the Third Report of the National Cholesterol Education Program (NCEP) Expert Panel on Detection, Evaluation, and Treatment of high blood cholesterol in adults. JAMA 2001;285:2486–2497.
120. Krolewski AS, Warram JH, Christlieb AR. Hypercholesterolemia—a determinant of renal function loss and deaths in IDDM patients with nephropathy. Kidney Int Suppl 1994;45:S125–131.
121. Ravid M, Brosh D, Ravid-Safran D, Levy Z, Rachmani R. Main risk factors for nephropathy in type 2 diabetes mellitus are plasma cholesterol levels, mean blood pressure, and hyperglycemia. Arch Intern Med 1998;158:998–1004.
122. Smulders YM, van Eeden AE, Stehouwer CD, Weijers RN, Slaats EH, Silberbusch J. Can reduction in hypertriglyceridaemia slow progression of microalbuminuria in patients with non-insulin-dependent diabetes mellitus? Eur J Clin Invest 1997;27:997–1002.
123. Lam KS, Cheng IK, Janus ED, Pang RW. Cholesterol-lowering therapy may retard the progression of diabetic nephropathy. Diabetologia 1995;38:604–609.
124. Fried LF, Orchard TJ, Kasiske BL. Effect of lipid reduction on the progression of renal disease: a meta-analysis. Kidney Int 2001;59:260–269.
125. Gaede P, Vedel P, Larsen N, Jensen GV, Parving HH. Multifactorial intervention and cardiovascular diseae in patients with type 2 diabetes. N Engl J Med 2003;348:383–393.

18 Diabetic Neuropathy

Rayaz A. Malik, MB.ChB, PhD
and Aristidis Veves, MD, DSc

CONTENTS

DEFINITIONS AND CLASSIFICATION

Dysfunction and damage of the somatic and autonomic nervous systems leads to diabetic neuropathy. Simply defined it is characterized by "The presence of symptoms and /or signs of peripheral nerve dysfunction in people with diabetes after the exclusion of other causes" *(1)*. For the practicing physician, a clinically relevant classification is preferred *(2)* (Table 1). However, to enable quantification for epidemiology and research, particularly for clinical trials, a more detailed definition that includes subclinical neur-

From: *Contemporary Cardiology: Diabetes and Cardiovascular Disease, Second Edition*
Edited by: M. T. Johnstone and A. Veves © Humana Press Inc., Totowa, NJ

Table 1
Clinical Classification of Diabetic Neuropathies

Polyneuropathy	Mononeuropathy
Sensory	Cranial
• Chronic sensorimotor	
• Acute sensory	
Autonomic	Isolated peripheral
Proximal motor	Mononeuritis multiplex
Truncal	

Adapted from ref. *1*.

opathy is required *(3,4)*. An established paradigm for use in clinical trials includes the following:

- Neuropathic symptoms (NSS: neuropathy symptom score).
- Neuropathic deficits (NIS: neuropathy impairment score).
- Motor/sensory nerve conduction velocity (MS:NCV).
- quantitative sensory testing (QST)
- Autonomic function testing (AFT).

The minimum criteria for the diagnosis of neuropathy require two or more abnormalities of the above, of which one should be based on electrophysiology. Patients are staged for severity as follows:

- N0 = No neuropathy: minimum criteria unfulfilled.
- N1 = asymptomatic neuropathy (NSS = 0).
- N2 = symptomatic neuropathy.
- N3 = disabling neuropathy.

To incorporate the full spectrum of abnormalities encountered in diabetic neuropathy, recent proposals have also included a detailed assessment of symptoms *(5)* and deficits in quantitative sensory testing *(6)*.

EPIDEMIOLOGY

The quality of epidemiological data on diabetic neuropathy remains poor *(4)*. Across Europe, clinic-based studies demonstrate an overall prevalence of symptomatic neuropathy between 22.5% and 28.5% *(7–9)*. Neuropathy may be present in 5% to 10% of type 2 diabetic patients at diagnosis as demonstrated by the Finnish prospective study *(10)* and the United Kingdom Prospective Diabetes Study *(11)*. Neuropathic deficits may occur in approx 50% of patients with type 2 diabetes *(3)*. In a comparative study of recently diagnosed (<5 years) patients with Latent Autoimmune Diabetes in Adults the prevalence of peripheral neuropathy was found to be similar to that in type 1 diabetes and much lower than in type 2 diabetes *(12)*. Autonomic neuropathy has been the subject of fewer epidemiological studies. In type 1 diabetes, the Pittsburgh epidemiology study demonstrated a relationship between abnormal autonomic function tests, female gender, hypertension and high low-density lipoprotein *(13)*, whereas in the Diabetes Control and Complications Trial, mixed results were obtained for the association with glycemic control *(14)*. In type 2 diabetes, the Finnish prospective neuropathy study found that fasting insulin and female gender related to the cumulative incidence of parasympathetic neuropathy, but neither predicted sympathetic neuropathy *(9)*. More recently in a French multicenter study, 24.5% of the patients had symptomatic autonomic neuropathy and 51% had cardiac autonomic neuropathy that related to body mass index, diabetes duration, and urinary albumin:creatinine ratio *(15)*.

CLINICAL FEATURES

Autonomic Neuropathy

Diabetic autonomic neuropathy forms an important, often misdiagnosed and poorly managed aspect of diabetic neuropathy, which has been reviewed extensively recently *(16)*. Vagal denervation leads to an initial increase in heart rate followed by sympathetic denervation causing a decrease in heart rate and finally a fixed heart rate supervenes, baring close similarity to the transplanted heart. Postural hypotension, defined as a 20 mmHg and 10 mmHg fall in the systolic and diastolic blood pressures, respectively, occurs as a consequence of impaired vasoconstriction in the splanchnic and cutaneous vascular beds as a result of efferent sympathetic denervation *(16)*. Autonomic neuropathy of the gastrointestinal system manifests as an abnormality in motility, secretion, and absorption through derangement of both extrinsic parasympathetic (vagus and spinal S2–S4) and sympathetic and intrinsic enteric innervation provided by Auerbach's plexus. Clinically, patients present with two major problems: diabetic gastroparesis manifest by nausea, postprandial vomiting, and alternating nocturnal diarrhea and constipation *(16)*. The absolute diagnosis and treatment of these abnormalities are a challenging clinical problem. Erectile dysfunction occurs secondary to disruption of cholinergic and noncholinergic noradrenergic neurotransmitters mediating erectile function. It is a frequent and under diagnosed problem that has a multifactorial etiology *(17)*. Neuropathy was the principal cause of erectile dysfunction (ED) in 27% of newly presenting patients with ED, and a contributory cause in a further 38% *(18)*. Other potential causes include vascular disease, concomitant medication, local problems such as Peyronies disease, and psychological factors. Bladder dysfunction is also well recognized as a consequence of autonomic neuropathy and leads to a reduction in bladder contraction, stasis and increased risk of urinary tract infection or more rarely, urinary incontinence.

Distal Sensory Neuropathy

Hyperglycemic neuropathy may occur in newly diagnosed patients, characterized by rapidly reversible abnormalities of nerve function and transient positive symptoms *(19)*. In those with established neuropathy symptoms are predominantly if not exclusively sensory and typically fall into a recognizable pattern of either being "positive" (burning pain, stabbing and shooting sensations, uncomfortable temperature sensations, paraesthesiae, hyperaesthesiae, and allodynia) or "negative" (decreased pain sensation, deadness, and numbness) *(19,20)*. Sensory loss occurs in a glove and stocking distribution, together with small muscle wasting, weakness, and loss of lower limb reflexes and may present with an insensitive foot ulcer *(19)*. A specific small-fiber neuropathy with neuropathic pain, sometimes together with autonomic dysfunction, but few signs have been described that share many similarities with acute sensory neuropathy, but symptoms tend to be more persistent *(19)*. These painful sensory neuropathies should not be confused with a rarer, acute sensory neuropathy with a rapid onset of painful symptoms but few clinical signs, following either a period of severe metabolic instability, or sudden improvement of glycemic control ("insulin neuritis") *(20)*.

The clinical features and management of the focal and multifocal neuropathies of diabetes have been reviewed extensively recently *(21)*.

PATHOPHYSIOLOGY

In patients with established diabetic neuropathy, both nerve conduction velocity and amplitude are reduced, suggestive of underlying demyelination and axonal degeneration *(22)*. Pathological studies of sural nerve biopsies confirm myelinated fiber demyelination and axonal degeneration with unmyelinated fiber degeneration and regeneration *(23–29)*, which is associated with an endoneurial microangiopathy *(30–35)*. However, the early pathological changes remain to be defined. While animal models of diabetic neuropathy replicate functional deficits such as a reduction in nerve conduction velocity and blood flow *(36)*, significant structural changes similar to those observed in established human diabetic neuropathy have not been observed *(37,38)*. Therefore, from a pathogenetic and translational view the limited data from patients with early diabetic neuropathy combined with a lack of a structural abnormality in animal models, limits our understanding of the initial processes that lead to and define nerve damage in diabetes.

PATHOGENESIS

Studies in animal models and cultured cells, provide a conceptual framework for the cause and treatment of diabetic neuropathy *(39)*. However, limited translational work in diabetic patients continues to generate much debate and controversy over the cause(s) of human diabetic neuropathy. To date we have no effective treatment.

HYPERGLYCEMIA

Longitudinal data from the Rochester cohort supports the contention that the duration and severity of exposure to hyperglycemia are related to the severity of neuropathy only *(40)*. However, recent studies in patients with impaired glucose tolerance (IGT) provide important insights into the relation between hyperglycemia and the development of neuropathy. Thus, in a study of patients with IGT the sural nerve amplitude, and myelinated fiber density did not differ significantly from those with normal glucose tolerance, suggestive of a glycemic threshold for the development of neuropathy *(41)*. Conversely, of 121 patients with a painful neuropathy and electrodiagnostic evidence of axonal injury together with epidermal nerve fiber abnormalities, 25% had impaired glucose tolerance *(42)*. The neuropathy associated with IGT is milder than the neuropathy associated with newly diagnosed diabetes and small nerve fiber involvement may be the earliest detectable sign of nerve damage *(43)*. With regard to intervention in patients with type 1 diabetes more intensive insulin therapy *(14)* or pancreatic transplantation *(44)* improves electrophysiological measures of neuropathy. However, in type 2 diabetes, the VA Cooperative Study on Type 2 Diabetes Mellitus failed to demonstrate a significant difference in the progression of either somatic or autonomic neuropathy despite a 2.07% difference in HbA1c over 2 years *(45)*.

POLYOL PATHWAY

Animal models of diabetes consistently demonstrate an association between increased flux through the polyol pathway and a reduction in nerve conduction velocity (NCV), both of which can be ameliorated with aldose reductase inhibitors (ARIs) *(46)*. The rationale for the continued investment in ARI programs is questionable as only early postmortem *(47)* and amputation *(48)* studies have demonstrated a significant activation of the polyol pathway. Whereas biopsy studies showed that sorbitol and fructose levels were increased in only one-third of sural nerve biopsies studied and could not be related to clinical, neurophysiological, or pathological severity of neuropathy *(49)*. Although, in a subsequent interventional study, a significant inverse correlation was observed between nerve sorbitol and myelinated fiber density *(50)*. In a recent study of patients with normal glucose tolerance, IGT, and type 2 diabetes only the diabetic patients demonstrated an elevation in nerve sorbitol, suggestive of a glycemic threshold for activation of this pathway *(41)*. The single measurement of whole-nerve sorbitol or fructose levels is clearly an oversimplification of a complex process with a polyol pathway in a constant state of changing flux that is known to be different amongst different cellular and structural compartments of the peripheral nerve. Furthermore, a recent study has demonstrated enhanced aldose reductase (AR) but minimal sorbitol dehydrogenase expression in the peripheral nerve of diabetic patients *(51)*. Moreover, it would appear that those at greatest risk of developing the complications are those with a higher set-point for AR activity *(52)*. To add to this complexity there may be a significant genetic determinant of polyol pathway flux and hence efficacy of ARIs as polymorphisms in the ARI promoter region leading to a highly significant decrease in the frequency of the Z+2 allele have been demonstrated in patients with overt neuropathy compared to those without neuropathy *(53)*.

Thus. it is not surprising that in a recent meta-analysis of all randomized controlled trials of ARIs only a small but statistically significant reduction in decline of median and peroneal motor nerve conduction velocity was observed *(54)*. Possible reasons for this marginal benefit may be related to the lack of a targeted approach identifying those most genetically susceptible to alterations in AR activity and thus those most likely to benefit from AR inhibition *(53)*. Furthermore, the degree of AR inhibition may determine the improvement observed. Thus in a randomized, placebo-controlled, double-blinded, multiple-dose, clinical trial with Zenarestat, dose-dependent increments in sural nerve sorbitol suppression were accompanied by significant improvement in NCV, and in doses producing greater than 80% sorbitol suppression there was a significant increase in the density of small-diameter myelinated fibers of the sural nerve *(55)*. More recently, Fidarestat, a potent ARI significantly improved median nerve F-wave conduction velocity (FCV) and minimal latency and symptoms of numbness, spontaneous pain, paraesthesiae and hyperaesthesia *(56)*.

GLYCATION

Hyperglycemia results in the formation of advanced glycation end-products (AGEs), which in turn act on specific receptors (RAGE) inducing monocytes and endothelial cells to increase the production of cytokines and adhesion molecules inducing endotheial dysfunction *(57)*. Glycation has also recently been shown to have an effect on matrix metalloproteinases (MMPs), in particular MMP-2, which degrades type IV collagen but also membrane type 1 MMP, tissue inhibitors of MMPs-1 and -2, and transforming growth factor (TGF)-β *(58)*. In experimental diabetes these changes can be prevented by AGE inhibitors such as the nucleophilic compounds pyridoxamine, tenilsetam, 2, 3-diaminophenazone or aminoguanidine *(59)* or alternatively the administration of recombinant RAGE hinders the AGE–RAGE interaction. The key question is, is this process relevant to the pathogenesis of human diabetic neuropathy, i.e., has this been observed in the peripheral nerve of diabetic patients. Human sural nerves obtained from diabetic and nondiabetic amputation specimens demonstrate normal furosine, an early reversible glycation product but significantly elevated pentosidine (AGE) levels in both cytoskeletal and myelin protein *(60)*. Furthermore, enhanced staining for carboxymethyllysine has been demonstrated in the sural nerve perineurium, endothelial cells and pericytes of endoneurial micro vessels and myelinated and unmyelinated fibers and has been related to a reduction in myelinated fiber density *(61)*. Pyrraline, an AGE is increased in post-mortem samples of optic nerve from diabetic patients *(62)*. In an early experimental study in streptozotocin (STZ)- diabetic rats treatment with aminoguanidine was associated with a 40% reduction in renal but not nerve AGE levels, an improvement in motor nerve conduction velocity but without alterations in myelinated nerve fiber morphology *(63)*. Ten months of aminoguanidine therapy failed to reduce the frequency of neuroaxonal dystrophy in the sympathetic ganglia of STZ-diabetic rats *(64)*. With regard to defining a mechanistic basis for a potential benefit of aminoguanidine therapy, paradoxically 16 weeks of intervention led to a reduction in endoneurial capillary luminal size and no effect on basement membrane thickening *(65)*. Furthermore, in a primate model of type 1 diabetes 3 years of treatment with aminoguanidine did not restore conduction velocity or autonomic dysfunction *(66)*. Thus it is not surprising that clinical intervention trials have focused on nephropathy *(67)* and no trial data are currently available for human diabetic neuropathy. Even in nephropathy there have been considerable problems in relation to drug toxicity. However, it is becoming increasingly apparent that many drugs that are currently used for other indications such as pioglitazone, metformin *(68)* and the angiotensin-converting enzyme (ACE) inhibitors and ATII antagonists *(69)* may act as powerful antiglycating agents. These findings provide a means of testing the glycation hypothesis effectively without having to develop new agents. Although whether or not a pharmaceutical company will invest in a clinical trial program, which does not necessarily produce future economic benefit is questionable.

OXIDATIVE STRESS

An increasing body of data supports the role of oxidative stress in the pathogenesis of diabetic neuropathy in animal models *(39)*. There is also emerging evidence that single-nucleotide polymorphisms of the genes for mitochondrial (SOD2) and extracellular (SOD3) superoxide dismutases may confer an increased risk for the development of neuropathy *(70)*. Benefits have been observed with α-lipoic acid (LA), a powerful anti-oxidant that scavenges hydroxyl radicals, superoxide and peroxyl radicals and regenerates glutathione. Thus, a series of well-conducted studies have shown benefit using both intravenous followed by oral LA *(71–73)*.

GROWTH FACTORS

Insulin-Like Growth Factors

A deficiency of insulin-like growth factors (IGFs) has been proposed to lead to cell death. Thus, in cultured Schwann cells and the STZ-diabetic rat, IGF-1 administration prevents apoptosis via PI3-kinase *(74)*. Neuroaxonal dystrophy (NAD) develops in nerve terminals of the prevertebral sympathetic ganglia and the distal portions of ileal mesenteric nerves in the STZ-diabetic and BB/W rat and has been related to hyperglycemia and a deficiency in circulating IGF-1 levels. In contrast, the Zucker Diabetic Fatty rat, an animal model of type 2 diabetes, develops hyperglycemia comparable to that in the STZ- and BB/W-diabetic rats but maintains normal levels of plasma IGF-1 and accordingly fails to demonstrate NAD *(75)*. To temper overenthusiastic translation to man both IGF-1 and IGF-1 receptor mRNA levels have not been shown to differ in the sural nerve of diabetic patients compared with control subjects *(76)*.

C-PEPTIDE

Impaired insulin/C-peptide action has emerged as a prominent factor in the pathogenesis of the microvascular complications in type 1 diabetes. Experimental studies have demonstrated a range of actions, which include effects on Na(+)/K(+)-ATPase activity, expression of neurotrophic factors, regulation of molecular species underlying the degeneration of the nodal apparatus, and DNA binding of transcription factors leading to modulation of apoptosis *(77)*. In the STZ rat, an improvement in nerve conduction velocity has been shown to be mediated via an improvement in nerve blood flow via enhanced activity of endothelial nitric oxide synthase (eNOS) *(78)*. These findings have recently been effectively translated into benefits in patients with type 1 diabetes with the demonstration of a significant improvement in sural sensory nerve conduction velocity and vibration perception but without a benefit in either cold or heat perception after 12 weeks of daily subcutaneous C-peptide treatment *(79)*.

VASCULAR ENDOTHELIAL GROWTH FACTOR

Vascular endothelial growth factor (VEGF) was originally discovered as an endothelial-specific growth factor with a predominant role in angiogenesis. However, recent observations indicate that VEGF also has direct effects on neurons and glial cells stimulating their growth, survival, and axonal outgrowth *(80)*. Thus, with its potential for a dual impact on both the vasculature and neurons it could represent an important therapeutic intervention in diabetic neuropathy. Although sciatic nerve and dorsal root ganglia from STZ-diabetic rats demonstrate intense VEGF staining in cell bodies and nerve fibers compared to no or very little VEGF in controls and animals treated with insulin or nerve growth factor (NGF) *(81)*. Both the STZ-diabetic rat and the alloxan-induced diabetic rabbit have demonstrated restoration of nerve vascularity, blood flow, and both large and small fiber dysfunction 4 weeks after intramuscular gene transfer of plasmid DNA encoding VEGF-1 or VEGF-2 *(82)*. Again, these findings should be tempered with the observation that endoneurial capillary density has not previously been shown to be reduced in either experimental *(37,38,65)* or human *(29–35)* studies. Thus, although there is an intrinsic capacity to upregulate VEGF, this appears insufficient and may require exogenous delivery possibly via gene therapy, but the mechanisms of its benefit require clarification. Nevertheless a phase I/II, single-site, dose-escalating, double-blind, placebo-controlled study to evaluate the safety and impact of phVEGF-1 *(65)* gene transfer on sensory neuropathy in patients with diabetes with or without macrovascular disease involving the lower extremities, is currently underway *(83)*.

NEUROTROPHINS

Neurotrophins promote the survival of specific neuronal populations by inducing morphological differentiation, enhancing nerve regeneration, stimulating neurotransmitter expression, and altering the physiological characteristics of neurons. Although the skin of diabetic patients with sensory fiber dysfunction demonstrates a depletion of NGF protein *(84)*, mRNA for both NGF *(85)* and neurotrophin (NT)-3 *(86)* are increased and sciatic nerve ciliary neurotrophic factor levels are normal *(87)*. *In situ* hybridization studies demonstrate an increased expression of trkA (high-affinity receptor for NGF), and trkC (receptor for NT-3) in the skin of diabetic patients. Curiously, the quest for a viable therapy in diabetic neuropathy has led investigators to interpret these observations as a compensatory upregulation rather than a tenuous link *(88)*. A phase II clinical trial of recombinant human nerve growth factor in 250 diabetic patients with symptomatic diabetic polyneuropathy demonstrated a significant improvement in the sensory component of the neurological examination, two quantitative sensory tests, and in a rather vague endpoint, "the clinical impression of most subjects that their neuropathy had improved" *(89)*. However, a phase III trial in 1019 diabetic patients with sensory polyneuropathy, failed to demonstrate a significant benefit *(90)*. These disappointing results led to much speculation regarding the reasons for failure of NGF specifically, with the hope that other neurotrophins may succeed where it had failed *(90)*. However, recently a randomized, double blind, placebo-controlled study of brain-derived neurotrophic factor in 30 diabetic patients demonstrated no significant improvement in nerve conduction, quantitative sensory and autonomic function tests, including the cutaneous axon-reflex *(91)*.

VASCULAR FACTORS

Some or all of the above factors may play a lesser or greater role in the development of a significant phenotypic change in neuronal function and structure in diabetic patients (Fig. 1). Two things are clear: (a) clinically relevant neuropathy only develops once myelinated and unmyelinated nerve fiber degeneration occurs; and (b) the maintenance of normal peripheral nerve function and structure demands an adequate vascular supply. Lesions, limiting adequate endoneurial oxygenation, may occur at any point from proximal arterial (aorta–iliac–femoral) segments to progressively more distal epineurial arterioles and terminal endoneurial capillaries. More than 100 years ago, Pryce described patchy areas of nerve degeneration in the posterior tibial nerve trunks as a consequence of proximal large vessel arteriosclerosis *(92)*. Woltman and Wilder attributed neuropathy to more distal arteriosclerosis of the vasa nervorum *(93)*. In day-to-day clinical practice, we have dramatic examples of the development of severe neurological deficits secondary to a significant reduction or complete abolition of nerve blood flow. Thus, diabetic amyotrophy is now considered to develop secondary to an epineurial vasculitis *(94)* and thrombotic occlusion and infarction of the oculomotor nerve results in third cranial nerve palsy *(95)*.

The symmetrical nature of distal, sensory polyneuropathy (DSPN) has been cited as evidence against the vascular hypothesis of nerve damage. However, autopsy studies in patients with DSPN demonstrate a focal loss of myelinated axons within the proximal lumbo-sacral trunk and posterior tibial nerve *(96)* in addition to proximal multifocal lesions *(97)* summating to produce more uniform fiber loss distally *(98)*. Furthermore, studies in nondiabetic patients with peripheral vascular disease confirm the occurrence of significant demyelination and axonal degeneration *(99,100)* together with an endoneurial microangiopathy *(101)*. Such studies provide support for the role of acute/ chronic ischemic injury resulting in neuronal death.

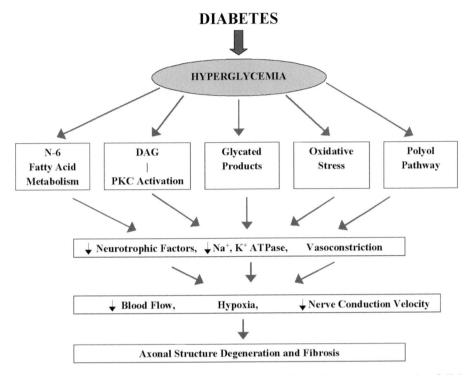

Fig. 1. Pathogenesis of diabetic neuropathy. Factors implicated in the pathogenesis of diabetic neuropathy include the activation of the polyol pathway, the activation of protein kinase C (PKC), increased oxidative stress, the impaired n-6 fatty acid metabolism, auto-oxidation of glucose and the formation of advanced glycation end-products (AGEs), and the reduced bioavailability of neurotrophic factors. All these mechanisms are interrelated and can potentiate each other's detrimental effects. Although the exact mechanisms of their action are not well understood, it is currently believed that these factors lead to reduced Na+, K+ ATPase activity and vasoconstriction, reduced endoneurial blood flow and nerve hypoxia. All these changes initially result in reduced nerve conduction velocities followed by axonal loss, and demyelination.

FUNCTIONAL ALTERATIONS

One of the principle components of the system controlling vascular function is nitric oxide (NO), which itself, responds to a variety of stimuli such as acetylcholine, histamine, bradykinin, angiotensin II, substance P, ischemia, and wall shear stress. Furthermore, the principle site of the arterial tree in which the majority of resistance to perturbations in pressure and flow are achieved is in the resistance vasculature (vessels 150–300 μm diameter). The resistance vasculature exists in a state of partial constriction, from which further contraction or dilatation can occur to regulate more distal capillary and hence tissue perfusion. A major determinant of this is pressure-dependent myogenic tone, so called because it is independent of neural and circulating constrictor or dilator influence. Resistance vessels of patients with type 2 diabetes demonstrate deficient endothelium-dependent relaxation to acetylcholine and bradykinin and remodeling with hypertrophy *(102)*. We have also recently demonstrated endothelial dysfunction and a highly significant loss of myogenic responsiveness leading to an increase in wall stress and vascular hypertrophy in resistance vessels of patients with type 2 diabetes *(103)*. This results in an increase in the wall/lumen ratio that is thought to offset and normalize the wall stress with increasing pressure. This is in accordance with the Laplace equation:

$$\text{Wall Stress} = \text{Pressure} \times \text{Radius/Wall Thickness}$$

Loss of the myogenic response has major consequences downstream as the increase in capillary pressure and blood flow and raised hydrostatic pressure may contribute to increased vessel wall permeability and stimulation of proliferative change in particular basement membrane thickening, in accordance with the hemodynamic hypothesis *(104)*. Retinal blood flow has been shown to be significantly increased in all grades of untreated diabetic retinopathy *(105)*. Similarly renal blood flow increases secondary to hyperglycemia and in diabetic subjects *(106)*. Paradoxically, renal interlobular artery resistance is increased in patients with type 2 diabetes *(107)*. Structural alterations comprised of a significant increase in the thickness of media and matrix of renal arterioles has been demonstrated in type 1 diabetic patients *(108)*, which are comparable to the alterations reported in gluteal resistance vessels of patients with type 2 diabetes *(102,103)*. However, it is important to consider the observation that a recent study in STZ rats has demonstrated markedly reduced renal cortical and medullary oxygenation despite apparently normal renal perfusion *(109)*.

Other factors that may contribute to basement membrane (BM) thickening include upregulation of the genes controlling expression of the extracellular matrix *(110)* and glycosylation *(57,59)*. Supporting the idea that capillary pressure and hence possibly also increased shear stress are important in the genesis of BM thickening are the findings that endothelial dysfunction *(111)* and dermal capillary BM thickening *(112)* is more prominent in the lower extremities of diabetic patients. Hypertension amplifies these abnormalities in type 2 diabetes *(102,113)*. The functional consequences of hyalinosis and BM thickening are a reduction in vascular distensibility *(114)* and hyperaemic response *(115)* demonstrated in the skin of type 1 diabetic patients.

Functionally, for a blood vessel a balance exists between the vasodilator and vasoconstrictor effectors to maintain optimal perfusion of tissues. This balance may be upset when either axis is altered. We and others have recently demonstrated a significant reduction in NO-mediated vasodilatation in patients with type 2 diabetes *(102,103)*. To date, two studies in diabetic patients with neuropathy demonstrate diminished intensity of staining of skin capillary eNOS *(116)* and actual levels of eNOS protein *(117)*. Although interestingly in the latter study both inducible nitric oxide synthase and eNOS protein levels were markedly increased in diabetic patients with severe neuropathy and foot ulceration *(117)*. Impaired NO-mediated vasodilation of epineurial arterioles is associated with an accumulation of superoxide, which can be ameliorated with the ARI sorbinil *(118)*, and the antioxidant α-LA *(119)*. Conversely, increased sensitivity and augmented epineurial arteriolar constriction to angiotensin II has been demonstrated in the sciatic nerve of diabetic rats, which responds to ACE inhibition *(120)*. In man intrabrachial norepinephrine infusion causes an exaggerated vasoconstrictor response in conjunction with a worsening of ulnar nerve latencies and sensory conduction velocity in patients with type 2 diabetes *(121)*. A structural consequence of these functional alterations is evidenced by the occurrence of epineurial arteriolar intimal hypertrophy and hyperplasia in diabetic patients with neuropathy *(122)*.

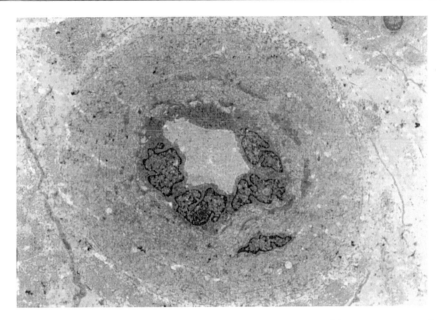

Fig. 2. Electronmicrograph of endoneurial capillary from a patient with severe neuropathy demonstrating basement membrane thickening (bm) and endothelial cell hyperplasia (ec) with an open lumen (l).

STRUCTURAL ALTERATIONS IN CAPILLARIES

In accordance with Pouiselle's Law, the rate of flow is proportional to the fourth power of the radius of a vessel. Thus, capillaries are particularly susceptible to episodes of low flow, which in the diabetic nerve will result in endoneurial hypoxia. Transperineurial capillaries in the sural nerve of diabetic patients with neuropathy, demonstrate endothelial cell hypertrophy and hyperplasia with a reduction in luminal size, which may reduce endoneurial blood flow *(123)*. Fagerberg (1959) *(124)* provided the first link between endoneurial capillary pathology and neuropathy with a detailed histopathological study demonstrating thickening and hyalinization of nerve vessel walls by a material staining positive with periodic acid Schiff. Many studies have now confirmed the presence of endoneurial microangiopathy, which is characterized by BM thickening, endothelial cell hyperplasia, and hypertrophy and pericyte cell degeneration in diabetic patients without clinically significant neuropathy *(125)* and with mild *(126)* and severe *(127–134)* neuropathy (Fig. 2). Such abnormalities have been localized to the sural nerve in which microangiopathy was found to be several-fold greater than in muscle or skin capillaries *(127)*. Moreover, more advanced microangiopathy has been observed in endoneurial capillaries (site of nerve fiber damage) compared to adjacent epineurial capillaries *(128)*. Furthermore, endoneurial, but not muscle, skin or epineurial capillary disease was related to the severity of neuropathy *(127,128)*. Endothelial cell hyperplasia has been found in endoneurial capillaries of diabetic patients with chronic sensorimotor neuropathy *(132)*, in some cases leading to complete occlusion of small vessels *(133)*. The frequency of closed endoneurial capillaries has been shown to be increased in patients with diabetic neuropathy and related to neuropathic severity employing semi-quantitative techniques

(134). However, this has not been confirmed by quantitative morphometry in diabetic patients with mild and severe neuropathy *(126,127,129)*. Thus a combination of epineurial arteriolar, transperineurial and endoneurial capillary abnormalities ultimately deprive the endoneurium of an adequate blood flow and hence oxygen. Hypoxia *per se* from chronic obstructive airway disease produces both neurophysiological and pathological abnormalities which are comparable with the changes found in mild diabetic neuropathy *(135)*.

In Vivo Studies

Endoneurial oxygen tension has been assessed by placing platinum microelectrodes within the sural nerve endoneurium and is significantly reduced in diabetic patients with neuropathy *(136)*. Furthermore, sural nerve epineurial oxygen saturation, employing a less invasive spectrophotometric probe, has also been shown to be significantly reduced in diabetic patients with neuropathy *(137)*. However, more recently the same group have demonstrated a significant increase in both epineurial oxygen saturation and blood flow in diabetic patients with painful neuropathy *(138)*. A laser Doppler study of human sural nerve in diabetic patients with mild neuropathy did not demonstrate a reduction in epineurial blood flow *(139)*. Although of interest a diabetic patient with lumbosacral plexopathy and those with vasculitic neuropathy did show a reduction in epineurial blood flow *(139)*. Elegant in vivo techniques of sural nerve photography and fluorescein angiography have demonstrated impaired nerve blood flow and the presence of active epineurial arterio-venous (A-V) shunts *(140)*. Diabetic patients with insulin neuritis show severe epineurial vessel arteriolar attenuation, venous distension and active A-V shunts and a fine network of blood vessels resembling the "new vessels" of the retina *(141)* (Fig. 3). Loss of sympathetic fibers could result in A-V shunting and this has been demonstrated in detailed electronmicroscopic studies assessing unmyelinated fiber counts in epineurial arterioles *(142)*. Another mechanism by which endoneurial perfusion may be impaired is by endoneurial edema, which has been demonstrated employing magnetic resonance spectroscopy in diabetic patients with and without neuropathy *(143)*. An earlier morphometric study has shown a progressive increase in mean fascicular area with increasing neuropathic severity *(127)*.

HEMORHEOLOGICAL STUDIES

Young and associates *(144)* demonstrated a good relationship between various hemorheological parameters and neuropathy. Furthermore, a number of key factors such as platelet aggregation and fibrinogen levels have been related to endoneurial microangiopathy and neuropathy *(145)*. More recently, a prospective study has demonstrated that raised levels of von Willebrand factor activity, a marker of endothelial cell dysfunction predicts the development of diabetic neuropathy *(146)*. A number of cell adhesion molecules have also been shown to predict the development and progression of neuropathy *(147)*.

VASCULAR THERAPIES

The most direct evidence that improving tissue blood flow may improve diabetic neuropathy is derived from large vessel revascularization studies that have shown an improvement in nerve conduction velocity in one *(148)* but not another study *(149)*. A longer term follow-up of the latter study did, however, show a prevention of worsening of peroneal nerve conduction velocity *(150)*. There are of course a number of pharmaco-

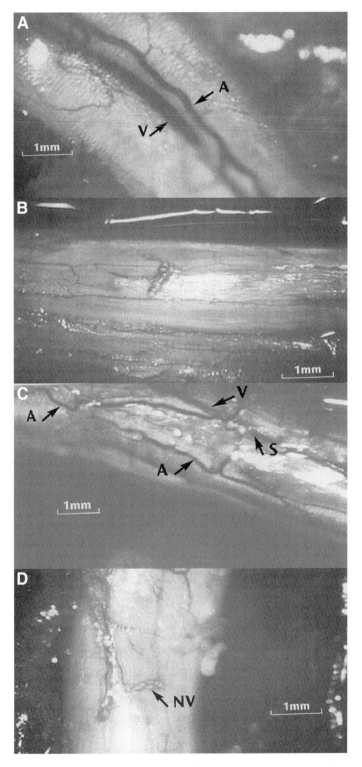

Fig. 3. Sural nerve surface photography demonstrating tortuous epineurial arterioles (A), distended venules (V), arterio-venous shunts (S), and new vessels (NV) in a patient with insulin neuritis.

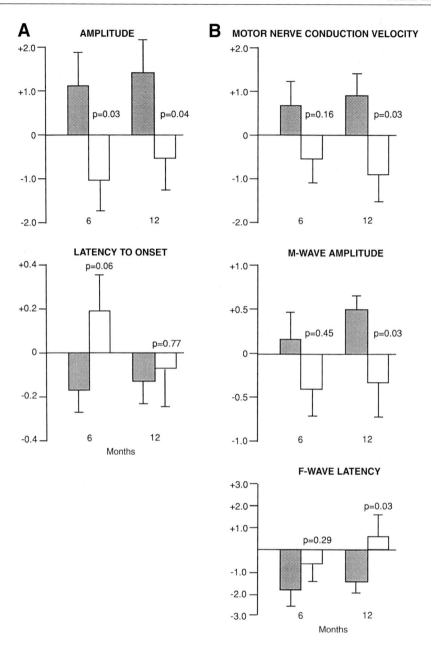

Fig. 4. Bar charts representing the change in sural (amplitude, latency to onset) and peroneal (conduction velocity, M-wave amplitude, F-wave latency) nerve electrophysiology, 6 and 12 months from baseline following treatment with the ACE inhibitor Trandolapril (solid bars) compared with placebo (open bars).

logical treatments that can achieve a similar effect. In a double-blind, placebo-controlled clinical trial of trandalopril over 12 months, peroneal motor nerve conduction velocity, M-wave amplitude, F-wave latency, and sural nerve amplitude improved significantly *(151)* (Fig. 4). Recently, the Appropriate Blood Pressure Control in Diabetes trial assessed the effects of intensive vs moderate blood pressure control with either nisoldipine or enalapril and surprisingly failed to prevent progression of diabetic nephropathy, retinopathy, and neuropathy *(152)*.

1, 2-diacylglycerol (DAG) induced activation pf protein kinase C (PKC); in particular PKCβ, has been proposed to play a major role in diabetic neuropathy *(153)*. However, even in nerve from diabetic animals a fall in DAG levels and a consistent pattern of change in PKC activity has not been observed *(154)*. Despite this, inhibition of PKCβ in diabetic rats appears to correct reduced nerve blood flow and nerve conduction velocity *(154)*. Based on the findings of a phase II clinical trial demonstrating some benefit in diabetic patients with neuropathy *(155)* multi-center, randomized, double-blind, placebo-controlled trials are underway, and are expected to be completed in 2006.

An increasing body of evidence suggests that conventional risk factors for macrovascular disease such as hypertension *(156)* and deranged lipids *(157)* are inde-pendent predictors for the development of human diabetic neuropathy. Recent studies show that hydroxymethylglutaryl coenzyme A reductase inhibitors may enhance endothelial cell NO bioavailabilty *(158)*, prevent AGE-induced NF-κb induced protein-1 activation and upregulation of VEGF mRNA *(158)* and thereby ameliorate experimental diabetic neuropathy *(159)*. Simvastatin has shown a trend toward slower progression of neuropathy measured by vibration perception threshold but no change in the status of clinical neuropathy *(160)*. As a cautionary note, recent observational data suggest a link between chronic statin use and an increased risk of peripheral neuropathy *(161)*.

REFERENCES

1. Boulton AJM, Gries FA, Jervell JA. Guidelines for the diagnosis and out-patient management of diabetic peripheral neuropathy. Diabetic Med 1998;15:508–514.
2. Thomas PK. Classification differential diagnosis and staging of diabetic peripheral neuropathy. Diabetes 1997;46(Suppl 2):S54–S57.
3. Dyck PJ, Kratz KM, Karnes JZ, et al. The prevalence by staged severity of various types of diabetic neuropathy, retinopathy and nephropathy in a population-based cohort: the Rochester Diabetic Neuropathy Study. Neurology 1993;43:817–824.
4. Dyck PJ, Melton J, O'Brien PC, et al. Approaches to improve epidemiological studies of diabetic neuropathy. Diabetes 1997;46(Suppl 2):55–58.
5. Apfel SC, Asbury AK, Bril V, et al. Positive neuropathic sensory symptoms as endpoints in diabetic neuropathy trials. J Neurol Sci 2001;189:3–5.
6. Shy ME, Frohman EM, So YT Arezzo JC, Cornblath DC, Giuliani MJ, the subcommittee of the American Academy of Neurology. Quantitative sensory testing. Neurology 2003;602:898–906.
7. Young MJ, Boulton AJM, McLeod AF, et al. A multicentre study of the prevalence of diabetic peripheral neuropathy in the UK hospital clinic population. Diabetologia 1993;36:150–154.
8. Tesfaye S, Stephens LK, Stephenson JM, et al. Prevalence of diabetic peripheral neuropathy and its relation to glycemic control and potential risk factors: the EURODIAB IDDM complications study. Diabetologia 1996;39:1377–1384.
9. Cabezas-Cerrato J. The prevalence of clinical diabetic neuropathy in Spain: a study in primary care and hospital clinic groups. Neuropathy Spanish study group of the Spanish Diabetes Society (SDS). Diabetologia 1998;41:1263–1269.
10. Partanen J, Niskanen L, Lehtinen J, et al. Natural history of peripheral neuropathy in patients with non-insulin dependent diabetes mellitus. N Engl J Med 1995;333:89–94.
11. UKPDS. Intensive blood glucose control with sulphonylureas or insulin compared with conventional treatment and risk of complications in patients with Type 2 diabetes. Lancet 1998;352:837–853.
12. Baum P, Hermann W, Verlohren HJ, Wagner A, Lohmann T, Grahmann F. Diabetic neuropathy in patients with "latent autoimmune diabetes of the adults" (LADA) compared with patients with type 1 and type 2 diabetes. J Neurol 2003;250:682–687.
13. Maser RE, Pfeifer MA, Dorman JS, et al. Diabetic autonomic neuropathy and cardiovascular risk: the Pittsburgh Epidemiology of Diabetic Complications Study III. Arch Int Med 1990;150:1218–1222.

14. DCCT Trial Research Group. The effect of intensive diabetes therapy on the development and progression of neuropathy. Ann Int Med 1995;122:561–568.
15. Valensi P, Paries J, Attali JR; French Group for Research and Study of Diabetic Neuropathy. Cardiac autonomic neuropathy in diabetic patients: influence of diabetes duration, obesity, and microangiopathic complications-the French multicentre study. Metabolism 2003;52:815–820.
16. Vinik AI, Maser RE, Mitchell BD, Freeman R. Diabetic autonomic neuropathy. Diabetes Care 2003;26:1553–1579.
17. Bacon CG, Hu FB, Giovannucci E, Glasser DB, Mittleman MA, Rimm EB Association of type and duration of diabetes with erectile dysfunction in a large cohort of men. Diabetes Care 2002;25:1458–1463.
18. Veves A, Webster L, Chen TF, et al. Aetiopathogenesis and management of impotence in diabetic males: four years' experience from a combined clinic. Diabetic Med 1995;12:77–82.
19. Malik RA. Current and future strategies for the management of diabetic neuropathy. Treat Endocrinol 2003;2:389–400.
20. Quattrini C, Tesfaye S. Understanding the impact of painful diabetic neuropathy. Diabetes Metab Res Rev 2003;19:S2–S8.
21. Malik RA. Focal and multifocal neuropathies. Curr Diab Rep 2002;2:489–494.
22. Valls-Canals J, Povedano M, Montero J, Pradas J. Diabetic polyneuropathy. Axonal or demyelinating? Electromyogr Clin Neurophysiol 2002;42:3–6.
23. Said G, Slama G, Selva J. Progressive centripetal degeneration of axons in small fibre type diabetic polyneuropathy. A clinical and pathologic study. Brain 1983;106:791–807.
24. Dyck PJ, Sherman WR, Hallcher LM, et al. Human diabetic endoneurial sorbitol, fructose and myoinositol related to sural nerve morphometry. Ann Neurol 1980;8:590–596.
25. Russell JW, Karnes JL, Dyck PJ. Sural nerve myelinated fiber density differences associated with meaningful changes in clinical and electrophysiological measurements. J Neurol Sci 1996;135:114–117.
26. Dyck PJ, Zimmerman BR, Vilen TH, et al. Nerve glucose, fructose, sorbitol, myo-inositol, and fibre degeneration and regeneration in diabetic neuropathy. N Engl J Med 1988;319:542–548.
27. Llewelyn JG, Gilbey SG, Thomas PK, King RH, Muddle JR, Watkins PJ. Sural nerve morphometry in diabetic autonomic and painful sensory neuropathy. A clinicopathological study. Brain 1991;114:867–892.
28. Brown MJ, Martin JR, Asbury AK. Painful diabetic neuropathy: a morphometric study. Arch of Neurol 1976;33:164–171.
29. Dyck PJ, Hansen S, Karnes J, O'Brien P, Yasuda H, Windebank A, Zimmerman B. Capillary number and percentage closed in human diabetic sural nerve. Proc Natl Acad Sci USA 1985;82:2513–2517.
30. Yasuda H, Dyck PJ. Abnormalities of endoneurial microvessels and sural nerve pathology in diabetic neuropathy. Neurology 1987;37:20–28.
31. Malik RA, Newrick PG, Sharma AK, et al. Microangiopathy in human diabetic neuropathy: relationship between capillary abnormalities and the severity of neuropathy. Diabetologia 1989;32:92–102.
32. Malik RA, Veves A, Masson EA, et al. Endoneurial capillary abnormalities in mild human diabetic neuropathy. J Neurol Neurosurg Psychiatry 1992;55:557–561.
33. Bradley J, Thomas PK, King RHM, Llewelyn JG, Muddle JR, Watkins PJ. Morphometry of endoneurial capillaries in diabetic sensory and autonomic neuropathy. Diabetologia 1990;33:611–618.
34. Britland ST, Young RJ, Sharma AK, Clarke BF. Relationship of endoneurial capillary abnormalities to type and severity of diabetic polyneuropathy. Diabetes 1990;39:909–913.
35. Sima AAF, Nathaniel V, Prashar A, Bril V, Greene DA. Endoneurial microvessels in human diabetic neuropathy. Endothelial cell dysjunction and lack of treatment effect by aldose reductase inhibitor. Diabetes 1991;40:1090–1099.
36. Cotter MA, Jack AM, Cameron NE. Effects of the protein kinase C inhibitor LY333531 on neural and vascular function in diabetic rats. Clin Sci 2002;103:311–321.
37. Walker D, Carrington A, Cannan SA, et al. Peripheral nerve structural abnormalities do not explain the reduction in nerve conduction velocity or nerve blood flow in the streptozotocin. Diabetic Rat J Anat 1999;195:419–427.
38. Walker D, Siddique I, Anderson H, et al. Peripheral Nerve pathology in the type 1 diabetic dog: effects of treatment with Sulindac. J Peripheral N System 2001;6:219–226.
39. Nishikawa T, Edelstein D, Du XL, et al. Normalizing mitochondrial superoxide production blocks three pathways of hyperglycemic damage. Nature 2000;404:787–790.
40. Dyck PJ, Davies JL, Wilson DM, Service FJ, Melton LJ 3rd, O'Brien PC. Risk factors for severity of diabetic polyneuropathy: intensive longitudinal assessment of the Rochester Diabetic Neuropathy Study cohort. Diabetes Care 1999;22:1479–1486.

41. Sundkvist G, Dahlin LB, Nilsson H, et al. Sorbitol and myo-inositol levels and morphology of sural nerve in relation to peripheral nerve function and clinical neuropathy in men with diabetic, impaired, and normal glucose tolerance. Diabetic Med 2000;17:259–268.

42. Smith AG, Ramachandran P, Tripp S, Singleton JR. Epidermal nerve innervation in impaired glucose tolerance and diabetes-associated neuropathy. Neurology 2001;13:1701–1704.

43. Sumner CJ, Sheth S, Griffin JW, Cornblath DR, Polydefkis M. The spectrum of neuropathy in diabetes and impaired glucose tolerance. Neurology 2003;60:108–111.

44. Navarro X, Sutherland DE, Kennedy WR. Long-term effects of pancreatic transplantation on diabetic neuropathy. Ann Neurol 1997;42:727–736.

45. Azad N, Emanuele NV, Abraira C, et al. The effects of intensive glycemic control on neuropathy in the VA cooperative study on type II diabetes mellitus (VA CSDM). J Diabetes Complications 1999;13:307–313.

46. Oates PJ. Polyol pathway and diabetic peripheral neuropathy. Int Rev Neurobiol 2002;50:325–392.

47. Mayhew JA, Gillon KR, Hawthorne JN. Free and lipid inositol, sorbitol and sugars in sciatic nerve obtained post-mortem from diabetic patients and control subjects. Diabetologia 1983;24:13–15.

48. Hale PJ, Nattrass M, Silverman SH, et al. Peripheral nerve concentrations of glucose, fructose, sorbitol and myoinositol in diabetic and non-diabetic patients. Diabetologia 1987;30:464–467.

49. Dyck PJ, Sherman WR, Hallcher LM, et al. Human diabetic endoneurial sorbitol, fructose, and myo-inositol related to sural nerve morphometry. Ann Neurol 1980;8:590–596.

50. Dyck PJ, Zimmerman BR, Vilen TH, et al. Nerve glucose, fructose, sorbitol, myo-inositol, and fiber degeneration and regeneration in diabetic neuropathy. N Engl J Med 1988;319:542–548.

51. Kasajima H, Yamagishi S, Sugai S, Yagihashi N, Yagihashi S. Enhanced in situ expression of aldose reductase in peripheral nerve and renal glomeruli in diabetic patients. Virchows Arch 2001;439:46–54.

52. Shimizu H, Ohtani KI, Tsuchiya T, et al. Aldose reductase mRNA expression is associated with rapid development of diabetic microangiopathy in Japanese Type 2 diabetic (T2DM) patients. Diabetes Nutr Metab 2000;13:75–79.

53. Demaine AG. Polymorphisms of the aldose reductase gene and susceptibility to diabetic microvascular complications. Curr Med Chem 2003;10:1389–1398.

54. Airey M, Bennett C, Nicolucci A, Williams R. Aldose reductase inhibitors for the prevention and treatment of diabetic peripheral neuropathy. Cochrane Database Syst Rev 2000;(2):CD002182.

55. Greene DA, Arezzo JC, Brown MB. Effect of aldose reductase inhibition on nerve conduction and morphometry in diabetic neuropathy. Zenarestat Study Group. Neurology 1999;53:580–591.

56. Hotta N, Toyota T, Matsuoka K, et al. The SNK-860 Diabetic Neuropathy Study Group. Clinical efficacy of fidarestat, a novel aldose reductase inhibitor, for diabetic peripheral neuropathy: a 52-week multicenter placebo-controlled double-blind parallel group study. Diabetes Care 2001;24:1776–1782.

57. King RH. The role of glycation in the pathogenesis of diabetic polyneuropathy. Mol Pathol 2001;54:400–408.

58. McLennan SV, Martell SK, Yue DK. Effects of mesangium glycation on matrix metalloproteinase activities: possible role in diabetic nephropathy. Diabetes 2002;51:2612–2618.

59. Vasan S, Foiles P, Founds H. Therapeutic potential of breakers of advanced glycation end product-protein crosslinks. Arch Biochem Biophys 2003;419:89–96.

60. Ryle C, Donaghy M. Non-enzymatic glycation of peripheral nerve proteins in human diabetics. J Neurol Sci 1995;129:62–68.

61. Sugimoto K, Nishizawa Y, Horiuchi S, Yagihashi S. Localization in human diabetic peripheral nerve of N (epsilon)-carboxymethyllysine-protein adducts, an advanced glycation end product. Diabetologia 1997;40:1380–1387.

62. Amano S, Kaji Y, Oshika T, et al. Advanced glycation end products in human optic nerve head. Br J Ophthalmol 2001;85:52–55.

63. Miyauchi Y, Shikama H, Takasu T, et al. Slowing of peripheral motor nerve conduction was ameliorated by aminoguanidine in streptozocin-induced diabetic rats. Eur J Endocrinol 1996;134:467–473.

64. Schmidt RE, Dorsey DA, Beaudet LN, Reiser KM, Williamson JR, Tilton RG. Effect of aminoguanidine on the frequency of neuroaxonal dystrophy in the superior mesenteric sympathetic autonomic ganglia of rats with streptozocin-induced diabetes. Diabetes 1996;45:284–290.

65. Sugimoto K, Yagihashi S. Effects of aminoguanidine on structural alterations of microvessels in peripheral nerve of streptozotocin diabetic rats. Microvasc Res 1997;53:105–112.

66. Birrell AM, Heffernan SJ, Ansselin AD, et al. Functional and structural abnormalities in the nerves of type I diabetic baboons: aminoguanidine treatment does not improve nerve function. Diabetologia 2000;43:110–116.

67. Kalousova M, Zima T, Tesar V, Stipek S, Sulkova S. Advanced Glycation End Products in Clinical Nephrology. Kidney Blood Press Res 2004;27:18–28.
68. Rahbar S, Natarajan R, Yerneni K, Scott S, Gonzales N, Nadler JL. Evidence that pioglitazone, metformin and pentoxifylline are inhibitors of glycation. Clin Chim Acta 2000;301:65–77.
69. Bui BV, Armitage JA, Tolcos M, Cooper ME, Vingrys AJ. ACE inhibition salvages the visual loss caused by diabetes. Diabetologia 2003;46:401–408.
70. Zotova EV, Chistiakov DA, Savost'ianov KV, et al. Association of the SOD2 Ala(-9)Val and SOD3 Arg213Gly polymorphisms with diabetic polyneuropathy in patients with diabetes mellitus type 1 Mol Biol (Mosk) 2003;37:404–408.
71. Reljanovic M, Reichel G, Rett K, et al. Treatment of diabetic polyneuropathy with the antioxidant thioctic acid (alpha-lipoic acid): a two year multicentre randomized double-blind placebo-controlled trial (ALADIN II). Free Radic Res 1999;31:171–179.
72. Ziegler D, Hanefeld M, Ruhnau KJ, et al. Treatment of symptomatic diabetic polyneuropathy with the antioxidant alpha-lipoic acid: a 7-month multicentre randomized controlled trial (ALADIN III Study). ALADIN III Study Group. Diabetes Care 1999;22:1296–1301.
73. Ametov AS, Barinov A, Dyck PJ, et al., SYDNEY Trial Study Group. The sensory symptoms of diabetic polyneuropathy are improved with alpha-lipoic acid: the SYDNEY trial. Diabetes Care 2003; 26:770–776.
74. Delaney CL, Russell JW, Cheng HL, Feldman EL. Insulin-like growth factor-I and over-expression of Bcl-xL prevent glucose-mediated apoptosis in Schwann cells. J Neuropathol Exp Neurol 2001;60: 147–160.
75. Schmidt RE, Dorsey DA, Beaudet LN, Peterson RG. Analysis of the Zucker Diabetic Fatty (ZDF) type 2 diabetic rat model suggests a neurotrophic role for insulin/IGF-I in diabetic autonomic neuropathy. Am J Pathol 2003;163:21–28.
76. Grandis M, Nobbio L, Abbruzzese M, et al. Insulin treatment enhances expression of IGF-I in sural nerves of diabetic patients. Muscle Nerve 2001;24:622–629.
77. Sima AA. C-peptide and diabetic neuropathy. Expert Opin Investig Drugs 2003;12:1471–1488.
78. Cotter MA, Ekberg K, Wahren J, Cameron NE. Effects of proinsulin C-peptide in experimental diabetic neuropathy: vascular actions and modulation by nitric oxide synthase inhibition. Diabetes 2003;52: 1812–1817.
79. Ekberg K, Brismar T, Johansson BL, Jonsson B, Lindstrom P, Wahren J. Amelioration of sensory nerve dysfunction by C-Peptide in patients with type 1 diabetes. Diabetes 2003;52:536–541.
80. Carmeliet P, Storkebaum E. Vascular and neuronal effects of VEGF in the nervous system: implications for neurological disorders. Semin Cell Dev Biol 2002;13:39–53.
81. Samii A, Unger J, Lange W. Vascular endothelial growth factor expression in peripheral nerves and dorsal root ganglia in diabetic neuropathy in rats. Neurosci Lett 1999;262:159–162.
82. Schratzberger P, Walter DH, Rittig K, et al. Reversal of experimental diabetic neuropathy by VEGF gene transfer. J Clin Invest 2001;107:1083–1092.
83. Isner JM, Ropper A, Hirst K. VEGF gene transfer for diabetic neuropathy. Hum Gene Ther 2001;12: 1593–1594.
84. Anand P, Terenghi G, Warner G, Kopelman P, Williams-Chestnut RE, Sinicropi DV. The role of endogenous nerve growth factor in human diabetic neuropathy. Nat Med 1996;2:703–707.
85. Diemel LT, Cai F, Anand P, et al. Increased nerve growth factor mRNA in lateral calf skin biopsies from diabetic patients. Diabetic Med 1999;16:113–118.
86. Kennedy AJ, Wellmer A, Facer P, et al. Neurotrophin-3 is increased in skin in human diabetic neuropathy. J Neurol Neurosurg Psychiatry 1998;65:393–395.
87. Lee DA, Gross L, Wittrock DA, Windebank AJ. Localization and expression of ciliary neurotrophic factor (CNTF) in postmortem sciatic nerve from patients with motor neuron disease and diabetic neuropathy. J Neuropathol Exp Neurol 1996;55:915–923.
88. Terenghi G, Mann D, Kopelman PG, Anand P. trkA and trkC expression is increased in human diabetic skin. Neurosci Lett 1997;228:33–36.
89. Apfel SC, Kessler JA, Adornato BT, Litchy WJ, Sanders C, Rask CA. Recombinant human nerve growth factor in the treatment of diabetic polyneuropathy. NGF Study Group. Neurology 1998;51:695–702.
90. Apfel SC, Schwartz S, Adornato BT, et al. Efficacy and safety of recombinant human nerve growth factor in patients with diabetic polyneuropathy: a randomized controlled trial. JAMA 2000;284:2215–2221.
91. Wellmer A, Misra VP, Sharief MK, Kopelman PG, Anand P. A double-blind placebo-controlled clinical trial of recombinant human brain-derived neurotrophic factor (rhBDNF) in diabetic polyneuropathy. J Peripher Nerv Syst 2001;6:204–210.

92. Pryce TD. On diabetic neuritis, with a clinical and pathological description of three cases of diabetic pseudo-tabes. Brain 1893;16:416.
93. Woltman HW, Wilder RM. Diabetes mellitus pathological changes in the spinal cord and peripheral nerves. Arch Intern Med 1929;44:576–603.
94. Said G, Goulon-Goeau C, Lacroix C, Moulonguet A. Nerve biopsy findings in different patterns of proximal diabetic neuropathy. Ann Neurol 1994;35:559–569.
95. Asbury AK. Focal and Multifocal neuropathies of diabetes. In: Dyck PJ, Thomas PK, Asbury AK, Winegrad AI, Porte D, (eds.). Diabetic Neuropathy. WB Saunders, Philadelphia, PA: 1987, pp. 45–55.
96. Johnson PC, Doll SC, Cromey DW. Pathogenesis of diabetic neuropathy. Ann Neurol 1986;19:450–457.
97. Dyck PJ, Karnes JL, O'Brien P, Okazaki H, Lias A, Engelstad J. The spatial distribution of fibre loss in diabetic polyneuropathy suggests ischaemia. Ann Neurol 1986;19:440–449.
98. Dyck PJ, Lais A, Karnes JL, O'Brien P, Rizza R. Fibre loss is primary and multifocal in sural nerves in diabetic polyneuropathy. Ann Neurol 1986;19:425–439.
99. Rodriguez-Sanchez C, Medina Sanchez M, Malik RA, Ah-See AK, Sharma AK. Morphological abnormalities in the sural nerve from patients with peripheral vascular disease. Histol Histopath 1991;6: 63–71.
100. Nukada H, van Rij AM, Packer SG, McMorran PD. Pathology of acute and chronic ischaemic neuropathy in atherosclerotic peripheral vascular disease. Brain 1996;119:1449–1460.
101. McKenzie D, Nukada H, van Rij AM, McMorran PD. Endoneurial microvascular abnormalities of sural nerve in non-diabetic chronic atherosclerotic occlusive disease. J Neurol Sci 1999;162:84–88.
102. Rizzoni D, Porteri E, Guelfi D, et al. Structural alterations in subcutaneous small arteries of normotensive and hypertensive patients with non-insulin-dependent diabetes mellitus. Circulation 2001;103: 1238–1244.
103. Schofield I, Malik RA, Izzard A, Austin C, Heagerty AM. Vascular structural and functional changes in type 2 diabetes mellitus: Evidence for the role of abnormal myogenic responsiveness and dyslipidemia. Circulation 2002;106:3037–3043.
104. Tooke JE. A pathophysiological framework for the pathogenesis of diabetic microangiopathy. In: Tooke JE, (ed.). Diabetic Angiopathy. Arnold: London, UK, 1999, pp. 187–194.
105. Patel V, Rassam S, Newsom R, Wiek J, Kohner E. Retinal blood flow in diabetic retinopathy. BMJ 1992;305:678–683.
106. Lansang MC, Hollenberg NK. Renal perfusion and the renal hemodynamic response to blocking the renin system in diabetes: are the forces leading to vasodilation and vasoconstriction linked? Diabetes 2002;51:2025–2028.
107. Taniwaki H, Ishimura E, Kawagishi T, Matsumoto N, Hosoi M, Emoto M, Shoji T, Shoji S, Nakatani T, Inaba M, Nishizawa Y. Intrarenal hemodynamic changes after captopril test in patients with type 2 diabetes: a duplex Doppler sonography study. Diabetes Care 2003;26:132–137.
108. Osterby R, Hartmann A, Bangstad HJ. Structural changes in renal arterioles in Type I diabetic patients. Diabetologia 2002;45:542–549.
109. Palm F, Cederberg J, Hansell P, Liss P, Carlsson PO. Reactive oxygen species cause diabetes-induced decrease in renal oxygen tension. Diabetologia 2003;46:1153–1160.
110. Cagliero E, Roth T, Roy S, Lorenzi M. Characteristics and mechanisms of high glucose induced overexpression of basement membrane components in cultured human endothelial cells. Diabetes 1991;40:102–109.
111. Arora S, Smakowski P, Frykberg RG, et al. Differences in foot and forearm skin microcirculation in diabetic patients with and without neuropathy. Diabetes Care 1998;21:1339–1344.
112. Walker D, Malik RA, Boulton AJM, Rayman G. Structural differences in skin between the arm and foot in normal subjects and diabetic patients. Diabetologia 1996;39:A266–A1011.
113. Khder Y, Briancon S, Petermann R, et al. Shear stress abnormalities contribute to endothelial dysfunction in hypertension but not in Type II diabetes. J Hypertens 1998;16:1619–1625.
114. Sorensen VB, Rossing P, Tarnow L, Parving H-H, Norgaard T, Kastrup J. Effects of Nisoldipine and lisinopril on microvascular dysfunction in hypertensive type I diabetes patients with nephropathy. Clin Sci 1998;95:709–717.
115. Rayman G, Malik RA, Sharma AK, Day JL. Microvascular response to tissue injury and capillary ultrastructure in the foot skin of type I diabetic patients. Clin Sci (Lond) 1995;89:467–474.
116. Veves A, Akbari CM, Primavera J, et al. Endothelial dysfunction and the expression of endothelial nitric oxide synthetase in diabetic neuropathy, vascular disease, and foot ulceration. Diabetes 1998;47:457–463.

117. Jude EB, Boulton AJM, Ferguson MWJ, Appleton I. The role of nitric oxide synthase isoforms and arginase in the pathogenesis of diabetic foot ulcers: possible modulatory effects by transforming growth beta 1. Diabetologia 1999;42:748–757.

118. Coppey LJ, Gellett JS, Davidson EP, Dunlap JA, Yorek MA. Effect of treating streptozotocin-induced diabetic rats with sorbinil, myo-inositol or aminoguanidine on endoneurial blood flow, motor nerve conduction velocity and vascular function of epineurial arterioles of the sciatic nerve. Int J Exp Diabetes Res 2002;3:21–36.

119. Coppey LJ, Gellett JS, Davidson EP, Dunlap JA, Lund DD, Yorek MA. Effect of antioxidant treatment of streptozotocin-induced diabetic rats on endoneurial blood flow, motor nerve conduction velocity, and vascular reactivity of epineurial arterioles of the sciatic nerve. Diabetes 2001;50:1927–1937.

120. Kihara M, Mitsui MK, Mitsui Y, et al. Altered vasoreactivity to angiotensin II in experimental diabetic neuropathy: Role of nitric oxide. Muscle and Nerve 1999;22:920–925.

121. Hogikyan RV, Wald JJ, Feldman EL, Greene DA, Halter JB, Supiano MA. Acute effects of adrenergic-mediated ischemia on nerve conduction in subjects with type 2 diabetes. Metabolism 1999;48:495–500.

122. Korthals JK, Gieron MA, Dyck PJ. Intima of epineurial arterioles is increased in diabetic polyneuropathy. Neurology 1988;38:1582–1586.

123. Malik RA, Tesfaye S, Thompson SD, et al. Transperineurial capillary abnormalities in the sural nerve of patients with diabetic neuropathy. Microvascular Res 1994;48:236–245.

124. Fagerberg SE. Diabetic neuropathy: a clinical and histological study on the significance of vascular affections. Acta Med Scand 1959;164:5–81.

125. Giannini C, Dyck PJ. Basement membrane reduplication and pericyte degeneration precede development of diabetic polyneuropathy and are associated with its severity. Ann Neurol 1995;37:498–504.

126. Malik RA, Veves A, Masson EA, et al. Endoneurial capillary abnormalities in mild human diabetic neuropathy. J Neurol Neurosurg Psychiatry 1992;55:557–561.

127. Malik RA, Newrick PG, Sharma AK, et al. Microangiopathy in human diabetic neuropathy: relationship between capillary abnormalities and the severity of neuropathy. Diabetologia 1989;32:92–102.

128. Malik RA, Tesfaye S, Thompson SD, et al. Endoneurial localisation of microvascular damage in human diabetic neuropathy. Diabetologia 1993;36:454–459.

129. Yasuda H, Dyck PJ. Abnormalities of endoneurial microvessels and sural nerve pathology in diabetic neuropathy Neurology 1987;37:20–28.

130. Britland ST, Young RJ, Sharma AK, Clarke BF. Relationship of endoneurial capillary abnormalities to type and severity of diabetic polyneuropathy. Diabetes 1990;39:909–913.

131. Dyck PJ, Giannini C. Pathologic alterations in the diabetic neuropathies of humans: A review. J Neuropathol Exp Neurol 1996;55:1181–1193.

132. Timperley WR, Boulton AJM, Davies Jones GAB, Jarrat JA, Ward JD. Small vessel disease in progressive diabetic neuropathy associated with good metabolic control. J Clin Pathol 1985;38:1030–1038.

133. Williams E, Timperly WR, Ward JD, Duckworth T. Electronmicroscopical studies of vessels in diabetic peripheral neuropathy. J Clin Pathol 1980;33:462–470.

134. Dyck PJ, Hansen S. Karnes J, et al. Capillary number and percentage closed in human diabetic sural nerve. Proc Nat Acad Sci (USA) 1985;82:2513–2517.

135. Malik RA, Masson EA, Sharma AK, et al. Hypoxic neuropathy: relevance to human diabetic neuropathy. Diabetologia 1990;33:311–318.

136. Newrick PG, Wilson AJ, Jakubowski J, Boulton AJM, Ward JD. Sural nerve oxygen tension in diabetes. BMJ 1986;293:1053–1054.

137. Ibrahim S, Harris ND, Radatz M, et al. A new minimally invasive technique to show nerve ischaemia in diabetic neuropathy. Diabetologia 1999;42:737–742.

138. Theriault M, Dort J, Sutherland G, et al. Local human sural nerve blood flow in diabetic and other polyneuropathies. Brain 1997;120:1131–1138.

139. Eaton SE, Harris ND, Ibrahim S, et al. Increased sural nerve epineurial blood flow in human subjects with painful diabetic neuropathy. Diabetologia 2003;46:934–939.

140. Tesfaye S, Harris N, Jakubowski J, et al. Impaired blood flow and arterio-venous shunting in human diabetic neuropathy: a novel technique of nerve photography and fluorescein angiography. Diabetologia 1993;36:1266–1274.

141. Tesfaye S, Malik R, Harris N, Jakubowski J, Mody C, Ward JD. Arterio-venous shunting and proliferating new vessels in acute painful neuropathy of rapid glycaemic control (insulin neuritis) Diabetologia 1996;39:329–335.

142. Beggs J, Johnson PC, Olafsen A, Watkins CL, Cleary C. Transperineurial arterioles in human sural nerve. J Neuropathol Exp Neurol 1991;6:704–718.

143. Eaton RP, Qualls C, Bicknell J, Sibbitt WL, King MK, Griffey RH. Structure-function relationships within peripheral nerves in diabetic neuropathy: the hydration hypothesis. Diabetologia 1996;39: 439–446.

144. Young MJ Bennett JL, Liderth SA, Veves A, Boulton AJM, Douglas JT. Rheological and microvascular parameters in diabetic peripheral neuropathy. Clin Sci 1996;90:183–187.

145. Ford I, Malik RA, Newrick PG, Preston EF, Ward JD, Greaves M. Relationship between haemostatic factors and capillary morphology in human diabetic neuropathy. Thrombosis and Haemostasis 1992; 68:628–633.

146. Plater ME, Ford I, Dent MT, Preston FE, Ward JD. Elevated von Willebrand factor antigen predicts deterioration in diabetic peripheral nerve function. Diabetologia 1996;39:336–343.

147. Jude E, Abbott CA, Young MJ, et al. Potential role of cell adhesion molecules in the pathogenesis of diabetic neuropathy. Diabetologia 1998;41:330–336.

148. Young MJ, Veves A, Walker MG, Boulton AJM. Correlations between nerve function and tissue oxygenation in diabetic patients: further clues to the aetiology of diabetic neuropathy? Diabetologia 1992;35:1146–1150.

149. Veves A, Donaghue VM, Sarnow MR, Giurini JM, Campbell DR, LoGerfo FW. The impact of reversal of hypoxia by revascularization on the peripheral nerve function of diabetic patients. Diabetologia 1996;39:344–348.

150. Akbari CM, Gibbons GW, Habershaw GM, LoGerfo FW, Veves A. The effect of arterial reconstruction on the natural history of diabetic neuropathy. Arch-Surg 1997;132:148–152.

151. Malik RA, Williamson S, Abbott CA, Carrington AL, Iqbal J, Schady W Boulton AJM. Effect of angiotensin-converting enzyme (ACE) inhibitor trandalopril on human diabetic neuropathy: randomised double-blind controlled trial. Lancet 1998;352:1978–1981.

152. Estacio RO, Jeffers BW, Gifford N, Schrier RW. Effect of blood pressure control on diabetic microvascular complications in patients with hypertension and type 2 diabetes. Diabetes Care 2000;23: B54–B64.

153. Eichberg J. Protein kinase C changes in diabetes: is the concept relevant to neuropathy? Int Rev Neurobiol 2002;50:61–82.

154. Cameron NE, Cotter MA. Effects of protein kinase C beta inhibition on neurovascular dysfunction in diabetic rats: interaction with oxidative stress and essential fatty acid dysmetabolism. Diabetes Metab Res Rev 2002;18:315–323.

155. Litchy W, Dyck PJ, Tesfaye S, Zhang D, Bastyr E, The MBBQ Study Group. Diabetic peripheral neuropathy (DPN) assessed by neurological examination (NE) and composite scores (CS) is improved with LY333531 treatment. Diabetes 2002;45(Suppl 2):197.

156. Forrest KY, Maser RE, Pambianco G, Becker DJ, Orchard TJ. Hypertension as a risk factor for diabetic neuropathy: a prospective study. Diabetes 1997;46:665–670.

157. The EURODIAB prospective complications study (PCS) group. Cardiovascular risk factors predict diabetic peripheral neuropathy in Type 1 subjects in Europe. Diabetologia 1999;42:A50–A181.

158. Okamoto T, Yamagishi SI, Inagaki Y, et al. Angiogenesis induced by advanced glycation end products and its prevention by cerivastatin. FASEB J 2002;16:1928–1930.

159. Nangle MR, Cotter MA, Cameron NE. Effects of rosuvastatin on nitric oxide-dependent function in aorta and corpus cavernosum of diabetic mice: relationship to cholesterol biosynthesis pathway inhibition and lipid lowering. Diabetes 2003;52:2396–2402.

160. Fried LF, Forrest KY, Ellis D, Chang Y, Silvers N, Orchard TJ. Lipid modulation in insulin-dependent diabetes mellitus: effect on microvascular outcomes. J Diabetes Complications 2001;15:113–119.

161. Backes JM, Howard PA. Association of HMG-CoA reductase inhibitors with neuropathy. Ann Pharmacother 2003;37:274–278.

19 Microcirculation of the Diabetic Foot

Chantel Hile, MD and Aristidis Veves, MD, DSc

CONTENTS

INTRODUCTION

Diabetic foot problems are major contributors to health care costs and hospitalizations. A complete understanding of how the disease process works is essential in learning how to best prevent and treat these complications. Abnormalities of the microcirculation are generally accepted as early changes in diabetes *(1–7)*. Eventual manifestations of altered microcirculation, such as retinopathy, nephropathy, and neuropathy, are related to the duration and severity of diabetes *(8–10)*. Intensive glycemic control was found in the Diabetes Control and Complications Trial to significantly delay the development and progression of these microvascular complications in type 1 diabetic patients, with similar results reported in type 2 diabetic patients *(10–13)*. The capillary microcirculation to foot skin is no exception and has shown signs of significant impairment in diabetic patients, especially when metabolic control is poor *(14)*. This chapter will focus on the changes that occur in the microcirculation of the diabetic foot and the different methods used for their evaluation.

The Concept of "Small Vessel Disease"

For the purpose of clarity in discussing microcirculation, the concept of "small vessel disease" must be eliminated. Early retrospective pathological studies in diabetic patients who underwent amputation led to the misconception that abnormalities in the microcirculation are occlusive in nature, so-called "small vessel disease" *(15)*. It was postulated that such occlusive small vessel disease occurs even in the absence of any macrovascular occlusive problem and causes ischemic lesions and impairment of wound healing *(15)*. This idea originated from the histological existence of periodic acid-Schiff-positive material occluding the medium-sized or small arteries in amputated limb specimens *(15)*.

From: *Contemporary Cardiology: Diabetes and Cardiovascular Disease, Second Edition*
Edited by: M. T. Johnstone and A. Veves © Humana Press Inc., Totowa, NJ

However, subsequent physiological studies *(16)* and other prospective staining and arterial casting studies *(17,18)* have demonstrated absence of such occlusive lesions. Thus, it is clear that the term "small vessel disease" initially referred to medium or small size arteries, not to the microcirculation. As it stands, the phrase creates confusion and should no longer be used.

STRUCTURAL CHANGES OF THE FOOT MICROCIRCULATION

Over the last two decades, it has become clear that metabolic alterations in diabetes cause both structural and functional changes in multiple areas within the arteriolar and capillary systems *(19–21)*. The most characteristic structural changes of the capillary circulation in diabetic patients are a reduction in the capillary size and thickening of basement membranes (BM) *(22,23)*. Skin capillary density in diabetics, on the other hand, does not differ from that of healthy subjects *(24)*. These changes in capillary size and BM thickness are more pronounced in the legs. This phenomenon is most likely the result of the higher hydrostatic pressure in the lower extremities *(25)*, especially in diabetic patients with poorly controlled blood sugar levels *(26)*. It is currently believed that increased hydrostatic pressure and shear force in the microcirculation evokes an injury response in the microvascular endothelium. This injury may result in increased elaboration of extravascular matrix proteins leading to capillary BM thickening and arteriolar hyalinosis *(27,28)*. Thickened membranes impair the migration of leukocytes and hamper the hyperemic response to injury, increasing the susceptibility of the diabetic foot to infection *(29,30)*. These structural modifications also decrease the elastic properties of the capillary vessel walls, limiting their capacity for vasodilatation, and may eventually result in a significant loss of the autoregulatory capacity *(31)*. It is of interest that these changes do not result in narrowing or occlusion of the capillary lumen; on the contrary, the arteriolar blood flow may be normal or even increased *(32)*.

Another factor that is most probably involved in the impaired vasodilatory capacity of diabetic patients is the increased stiffness of precapillary vessel walls as a result of increased glycosylation and formation of nonenzymatic advanced glycosylation endproducts (AGE). Irreversible chemical processes occur slowly as these compounds accumulate over time *(33)*. AGE receptors are found on both endothelial cells and monocytes *(34)*. It has been postulated that AGE contributes to the development of diabetic microangiopathy *(33)*, a hypothesis supported by the fact that diabetics have higher serum and arterial wall concentrations of AGE than healthy subjects. The difference was even more striking between diabetics with nephropathy as compared to healthy subjects *(35)*. A study of the effect of AGE on endothelial function in experimental animals showed that they inhibit endothelium-dependent vasodilatation, an effect that can be reversed by an AGE inhibitor *(36)*.

FUNCTIONAL CHANGES OF THE MICROCIRCULATION

In addition to the structural changes wrought by diabetes on the microcirculation, techniques that allow the measurement of skin blood flow have highlighted functional disturbances as well. Using these techniques, researchers have observed that diabetic patients have reduced maximal hyperemic response to heat, even in the early stages of the disease *(37)*. The idea that impaired capillary microcirculation could be a major contributing factor in the development of diabetic foot pathology has encouraged more in-depth research in this direction *(18,29,38)*. Further development of new techniques to evaluate

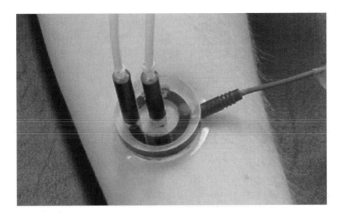

Fig. 1. Measurements of direct and indirect effect of vasoactive substance using single-point laser probes: One probe is used in direct contact with the iontophoresis solution chamber (colored ring) and measures the direct response. The center probe measures the indirect response (nerve-axon-related effect). A small quantity (<1 mL) of 1% acetylcholine chloride solution or 1% sodium nitroprusside solution is placed in the iontophoresis. A constant current of 200 mA is applied for 60 seconds achieving a dose of $6mC/cm^{-2}$ between the iontophoresis chamber and a second nonactive electrode placed 10 to 15 cm proximal to the chamber (black strap around the wrist). This current causes a movement of solution to be iontophorized toward the skin.

the microcirculation to peripheral tissues has expanded the understanding of these functional changes and their role in altering the microvascular blood flow. Before discussing the changes in vascular reactivity, it would be of particular importance to review the different techniques currently used for evaluating the microcirculation.

Methods of Evaluating the Microcirculation of the Feet

MEASUREMENTS OF CAPILLARY BLOOD FLOW USING LASER DOPPLER FLOWMETRY

Currently, this method is the most widely accepted technique for evaluating blood flow in the skin microcirculation. Basically, it measures the capillary flux, which is a combination of velocity and the number of moving red cells. This is achieved by employing red laser light that is transmitted to the skin through a fiber-optic cable. The frequency shift of light back-scattered from the moving red cells beneath the probe tip is computed to give a measure of the superficial microvascular perfusion *(39)*.

Either a single-point laser probe, which evaluates the microvascular blood flow at one point of the skin, or a real-time laser scanner, which evaluates the blood flow in an area of skin, can be used. The single-point laser probe is used mainly for evaluating the hyperemic response to a heat stimulus, or for evaluating the nerve-axon-related hyperemic response. To assess heat-related hyperemic response, the baseline blood-flow measurements are made first. The skin is then heated to 44°C for 20 minutes using a small brass heater, following which the maximum blood flow is measured to evaluate the magnitude of change from baseline. To measure nerve-axon-related hyperemic response, two single-point laser probes are applied (Fig. 1). One probe measures the blood flow to an area of skin, which is exposed directly to acetylcholine (Ach). The second probe, placed in close proximity (5 mm), measures the indirect effect of applied Ach. This indirect effect results from stimulation of C nociceptive nerve fibers in the area and reflects the integrity of the nerve-axon-related reactive hyperemia.

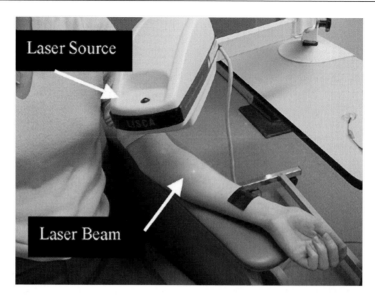

Fig. 2. Laser Doppler flowmetry: A helium-neon laser beam is emitted from the laser source to sequentially scan the circular hyperemic area (seen surrounding the laser beam) produced by the iontophorized vasoactive substance to a small area on the volar surface of the forearm.

The laser scanning method is also used for evaluating the endothelium-dependent microvascular reactivity (the magnitude of change in blood flow in response to Ach admitted to the skin through the iontophoresis technique), and the endothelium-independent microvascular reactivity (the magnitude of change in blood flow in response to sodium nitroprusside [SNP]).

The iontophoresis technique is used to apply these vasoactive substances to a localized area of the skin. In this technique, a delivery vehicle device is attached firmly to the skin with double-sided adhesive tape. The device contains two chambers that accommodate two single-point laser probes. A small quantity of (<1 mL) of 1% Ach solution or 1% of SNP solution is placed in the iontophoresis chamber and a constant current of 200 mA is applied for 60 seconds, achieving a dose of 6 mC/cm^{-2} between the iontophoresis chamber and a second nonactive electrode placed 10–15 cm proximal to the chamber. This current causes a movement of solution to be iontophoresed toward the skin, resulting in vasodilatation (Fig. 1).

After the adhesive device has been removed, the localized area exposed to either of the vasoactive substances is scanned. The laser Doppler perfusion imager employs a 1-mW helium-neon laser beam of 633-nm wavelength, which sequentially scans an area of skin (Fig. 2). The maximum number of measured spots is 4096, and the apparatus produces a color-coded image of skin erythrocyte flux on a computer monitor. The scanner is set up to scan up to 32 × 32 measurement points over an area approx 4 × 4 cm.

All laser measurements are expressed as volts and depend on the voltage difference created by the returned light to the computer. Higher blood flow at the skin level results in a higher amount of light picked by the single probe or the scanner and a higher voltage recorded by the computer. This technique is best suited for studying the relative changes in flow induced by variety of physiological maneuvers or pharmaceutical intervention procedures.

The technique has been validated against direct measurements of the capillary flow velocity *(40)*. The day-to-day reproducibility of the technique was evaluated in healthy subjects who were repeatedly tested at their foot and arm for 10 consecutive working days in our lab. The coefficient of variation (CV) for the baseline blood-flow measurement obtained with the laser probe evaluating the response to heat was 44%, although that for the maximal response to heat was 27.9%. The indirect response to Ach, measured by a single-point laser probe, had a CV of 60.6% for the baseline measurements and 35.2% for the maximal hyperemic response after the iontophoresis. The laser scanner had a significantly better reproducibility with the CV at the foot and forearm level being between 14% and 19%.

MEASUREMENTS OF TRANSCUTANEOUS OXYGEN TENSION

The technique of measuring oxygen tension transcutaneously is based on the fact that oxygen is capable of diffusing through tissue and skin. Although the rate of diffusion is very low at normal surface body temperature, the application of heat to a localized area sufficiently enhances the flow of oxygen through the dermis to allow noninvasive measurement of capillary oxygen level. The measurements are affected by the affinity of blood for oxygen and the tissue properties, and the change in skin temperature. These factors may influence, to some extent, the accuracy of these measurements.

Changes in Vascular Reactivity

The classic description of the diabetic neuropathic foot as warm and red with palpable pulses and distended veins points to a possibility of increased blood flow in the affected limb. Studies to explore this presentation found that the blood flow in the nutritional skin microcirculation is stable or even reduced *(41,42)*, indicating a functional ischemia of the skin microcirculation and maldistribution of blood flow to the foot *(14)*. It was also suggested that both structural and functional changes in the skin microcirculation result in a significant shifting of the blood flow away from nutritional capillaries to subpapillary arteriovenous shunts of a much lower resistance *(43)*. As these shunts are innervated by sympathetic nerves *(44)*, co-existing autonomic neuropathy and sympathetic denervation (such as occurs in diabetic patients with severe neuropathy) may lead to an opening of these shunts, augmentation of the maldistribution of blood between the nutritional capillaries and subpapillary vessels *(45,46)*, and consequent aggravation of microvascular ischemia. Studies using venous occlusion plethysmography, Doppler sonography, and venous oxygen tension measurements support this concept *(46,47)*. These disturbances in nutritive microcirculation may be of importance in the development of diabetic foot complications and may help explain why the diabetic foot is more susceptible to the effect of pressure and has an impaired ulcer-healing process.

FUNCTIONAL CHANGES

Using the new technique of measuring capillary blood flow by laser Doppler flowmetry has enabled researchers to evaluate endothelial function in diabetic limbs more precisely. Early application of this technique showed a reduced hyperemic response to heat stimulus and pointed to the role of endothelial dysfunction as the cause of the impaired vascular reactivity at microcirculatory level *(37)*. Such dysfunction was shown to occur early in the course of diabetes and may even predict diabetic micro- and macrovascular complications *(4,6,48,49)*. More recently, endothelial dysfunction was also reported in patients with impaired glucose tolerance and in relatives of type 2 diabetic patients *(50)*.

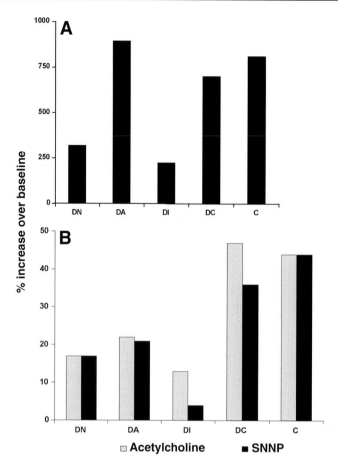

Fig. 3. (A) The maximal hyperemic response to heating of foot skin at 44°C for at least 20 min (expressed as the percentage of increase over baseline flow measured by a single-point laser probe) is reduced in the diabetic with neuropathy (DN) and in diabetic patients with neuropathy and peripheral vascular disease (DI) when compared with diabetic patients with Charcot arthropathy (DA), diabetic patients without complications (DC), and normal control subjects (C) ($p < 0.001$). **(B)** The response to iontophoresis of acetylcholine and sodium nitroprusside (SNP) (expressed as the percentage of increase over baseline flow measured by laser scanner). The response to acetylcholine is equally reduced in the DN, DI, and DA groups when compared with the DC and C groups ($p < 0.001$). The response to SNP was more pronounced in the DI group and also reduced in the DN and DA groups compared with the DC and C groups ($p < 0.001$).

To evaluate the relation between changes in microcirculation and neuropathy in the presence or absence of peripheral vascular disease, the skin microcirculation of foot was thoroughly investigated using both single-point laser imaging and laser scanning techniques in five groups *(51)*. The first group included diabetic patients with neuropathy (diabetic neuropathic [DN]), the second group included diabetic patients with both neuropathy and peripheral vascular disease (diabetic ischemic [DI]), the third group included diabetic patients with Charcot arthropathy (diabetic arthropathy [DA]), the fourth group included diabetic patients without complications (DC) and the fifth group included healthy control subjects (C). As seen in Fig. 3A, the percentage of increase in blood flow over baseline in response to heating the skin to 44°C was reduced in the DN and DI

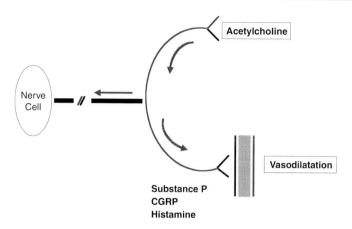

Fig. 4. Stimulation of the C-nociceptive nerve fibers leads to antidromic stimulation of the adjacent C fibers, which secrete substance P, calcitonin gene-related peptide (CGRP), and histamine that cause vasodilatation and increased blood flow.

patients, whereas no difference existed among the remaining three groups. On the other hand, the endothelium-dependent vasodilatation (response to iontophoresis of Ach) was reduced in DN, DI, and DA patients. The endothelium-independent vasodilatation (response to iontophoresis of SNP) was more severely reduced in the ischemic-neuropathic patients compared with other groups and was reduced in the neuropathic groups with or without Charcot disease compared to the controls (Fig. 3B). These findings pointed to the close association between diabetic neuropathy and microcirculatory impairment in the form of reduced endothelium-dependent and endothelium-independent vasodilation at the foot level even in the absence of large vessel peripheral vascular disease. They also implied that the presence of neuropathy may be an important contributing factor as the coexistence of neuropathy and peripheral vascular disease did not result in a greater decrease in endothelium-dependent vasodilation than that as a result of neuropathy alone.

The Role of the Nerve-Axon Reflex in Vasodilation

In healthy subjects, the ability to increase blood flow depends on the existence of normal neurogenic vascular response. The normal neurovascular response is conducted through the C nociceptive nerve fibers. Stimulation of these nerve fibers leads to antidromic stimulation of adjacent C fibers, which secrete substance P, calcitonin gene-related peptide and histamine, causing vasodilatation and increased blood flow to the injured tissues, thereby promoting wound healing (Lewis' triple-flare response) (Fig. 4). In cases of diabetic neuropathy, this neurovascular response is impaired, leading to a significant reduction of blood flow under conditions of stress (such as injury or infection) and increasing the vulnerability of the neuropathic limb to severe diabetic foot problems *(52,53)*.

Evidence that diabetic neuropathy contributes to vasodilatory impairment is provided by studies in our lab that used the previously described single-point laser probe technique to evaluate the nerve-axon-related vasodilatory response. We found that the indirect response to iontophoresis of Ach was significantly reduced in DN, DI, and DA patients, when compared with healthy subjects or DC patients *(54,55)* (Fig. 5). Further evidence is provided by a study designed to evaluate the role of the C-nociceptive nerve fibers in nerve-axon reflex-related vasodilation. In this study, nerve-axon reflex-related vasodi-

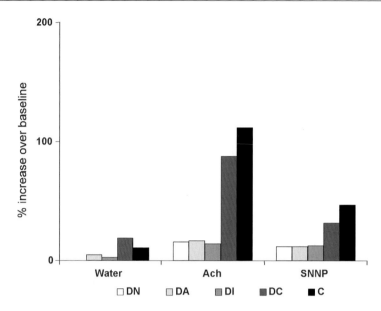

Fig. 5. The response of blood flow (expressed as the percentage of increase over baseline flow measured by a single-point laser probe) in a skin area adjacent to, but not in direct contact with, the iontophoresis solution. During the iontophoresis of deionized water, a mild response is observed in all groups. In contrast, during iontophoresis of acetylcholine (Ach), the response is reduced in diabetic patients with neuropathy (DN, first column), diabetic patients with neuropathy and peripheral vascular disease (DI, second column) and diabetic patients with Charcot arthropathy (DA, third column), when compared with diabetic patients without complications (DC, fourth column) and normal control subjects (C, fifth column) ($p < 0.001$). A similar response is observed during iontophoresis of sodium nitroprusside (SNP), but is less than half when compared with the response achieved with Ach.

lation was measured in three groups: DN, DC, and C. Measurements were first taken on the forearm and the foot of each subject. Then, after blocking the C-nociceptive nerve fibers with dermal anesthesia, measurements were repeated. A clear reduction in nerve-axon reflex-related vasodilation occurred in all three groups on the forearm but only in the two non-neuropathic groups on the foot, indicating that C-nociceptive fiber function is the main factor that influences nerve-axon reflex-related vasodilation *(56)* (Fig. 6).

The contribution of the nerve-axon reflex-related vasodilatation response to the total endothelium-dependent and endothelium-independent vasodilation was also studied in a group of diabetic patients vs a control group at both forearm and foot level *(57)*. The nerve-axon-related response in healthy subjects was found to be 35% of the total response at the forearm level and 29% at the foot level (Fig. 7). In contrast, the response to SNP, a substance that does not specifically excite the C-nociceptive fibers, was 13% and 12%, respectively, indicating that the presence of a nonspecific galvanic response may also be implicated (Fig. 8). In the presence of neuropathy the response significantly reduced, at a level of only 8% of the total response. These findings indicate that although the neurovascular response is an important factor in skin microcirculation function, it is not the sole or dominant pathway through which vasodilation is achieved *(52)*.

The abnormality in nerve-axon-related vascular reactivity is believed to further aggravate the abnormalities in the microcirculation and contribute to a vicious cycle of injury *(51)*. It becomes apparent that involvement of C-nociceptive fibers in diabetes not only

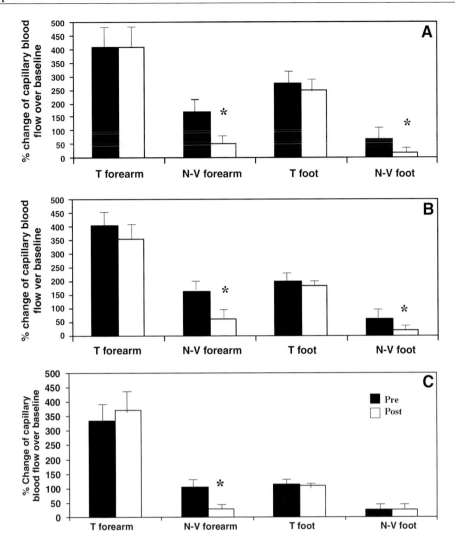

Fig. 6. Total and nerve-axon reflex-related vasodilatory response to acetylcholine before (black columns) and after (white columns) the application of local anesthesia in healthy subjects (**A**), nonneuropathic diabetic patients (**B**), and diabetic neuropathic patients (**C**).

leads to impaired pain perception but also to impaired vasodilation under condition of stress, such as injury or inflammation.

Differences Between Forearm and Foot Microcirculation

As mentioned previously, erect posture may lead to differences in the microcirculation at the foot level when compared to other parts of the body that are closer to the heart and therefore have a reduced hydrostatic pressure. In order to test this hypothesis, we have examined the differences in the foot and forearm skin microcirculation in diabetic patients with or without neuropathy and healthy subjects *(54)*. No differences were found in the maximal hyperemic response between forearm and foot level, although the response in the DN group was significantly lower at both levels in comparison to the DC and the C subjects (Fig. 9). The endothelium-dependent and endothelium-independent vasodilata-

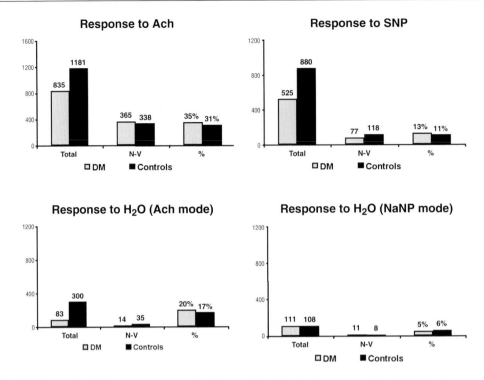

Fig. 7. The total and the nerve-axon-related vasodilatation in the upper extremities in response to acetylcholine (Ach), sodium nitroprusside (SNP) ,and deionized-water (H_2O) in a group of diabetic patients vs a control group of healthy subjects. The contribution of nerve-axon-related response to the total response to Ach is 35% in diabetic patients and 31% in control group ($p > 0.05$) and the contribution of nerve-axon-related response to the total response to SNP is 13% in diabetic patients and 11% in control group ($p > 0.05$).

tion was significantly lower at the foot level when compared to the forearm level in both Cs and in DNs and DCs (Fig. 10). Additionally, the DN group showed a significantly lower response at both forearm and foot levels when compared to the DC and C groups. Evaluation of the nerve-axon-mediated vasodilatation response also revealed a significantly lower response at the foot level vs the forearm level in the three groups (Fig. 9). These results indicate that the microcirculation at the foot level is compromised even in healthy subjects when compared to the forearm level. The presence of diabetes may further compromise the microcirculation to a level that creates a hypoxic environment and allows the development of neuropathic changes. These factors may also explain why neuropathy initially occurs in the lower extremities of diabetic patients *(58,59)*.

Expression of Endothelial Nitric Oxide Synthetase

One possible mechanism for impairment of endothelial functions in diabetic neuropathy is the reduction in the expression of the endothelial nitric oxide synthetase (eNOS) activity *(51)*. We have tested this hypothesis by evaluating the immunohistochemistry staining for eNOS of foot skin biopsies taken from diabetic neuropathic patients with or without peripheral vascular disease and healthy subjects *(51)*. The results showed reduced staining for the diabetic patients when compared to the healthy subjects. Similar results were reported by other investigators using immunohistochemistry and Western blotting techniques *(60)*.

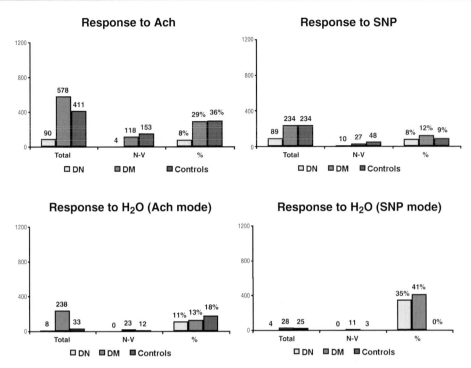

Fig. 8. The total and the nerve-axon related vasodilatation in the lower extremities in response to acetylcholine (Ach), sodium nitroprusside (SNP), and deionized-water (H₂O) in a group of diabetic patients with (DN) or without (DM) neuropathy vs a control group of healthy subjects. The contribution of nerve-axon-related response to the total response to Ach is 8% in DN, 29% in DM and 36% in the control group ($p < 0.001$ between DN and DM and controls) and the contribution of nerve-axon-related response to the total response to SNP is 8% in DN, 12% in DM and 9% in the control group ($p > 0.05$ between DN and DM and controls).

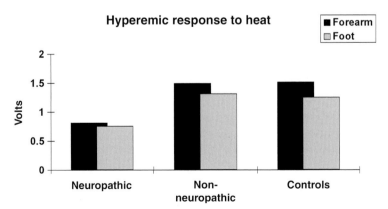

Fig. 9. The hyperemic response to heat stimulus (expressed as the percentage of increase over baseline flow measured by single-point laser probe) at forearm vs foot level in diabetic patients with or without neuropathy and in healthy control subjects. No difference was observed between the forearm and foot in any of the three groups. The response in neuropathic group is significantly lower compared with the other two groups at both forearm and foot level ($p < 0.001$).

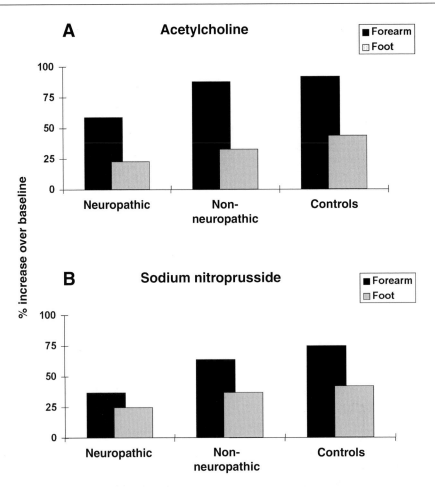

Fig. 10. The response to iontophoresis of acetylcholine **(A)** and sodium nitroprusside **(B)** (expressed as the percentage of increase over baseline flow measured by laser scanner) at forearm vs foot level in diabetic patients with or without neuropathy and in healthy control subjects. The response at the foot level is significantly lower than that of the forearm in all groups ($p < 0.01$). The response in neuropathic group is significantly lower compared with the other two groups at both forearm and foot level ($p < 0.05$).

Poly(ADP-Ribose) Polymerase Role in Impaired Vascular Reactivity

Recently, data has emerged showing poly(ADP-ribose) polymerase (PARP) to be involved in endothelial dysfunction as well. PARP is a nuclear enzyme that responds to oxidative DNA damage by activating an inefficient cellular metabolic cycle, leading to cell necrosis. In a study done in our unit, nondiabetic controls were compared to three groups: those with type 2 diabetes, those with glucose intolerance, and those with a family history of type 2 diabetes but no intolerance themselves. PARP activation was higher in all three diabetes-associated groups than in the healthy controls *(61)*. The activation of PARP was associated with changes in the vascular reactivity of the skin microcirculation in forearm biopsies taken from these subjects, supporting the hypothesis that PARP activation contributes to changes in microvascular reactivity. Further study is required to prove this association.

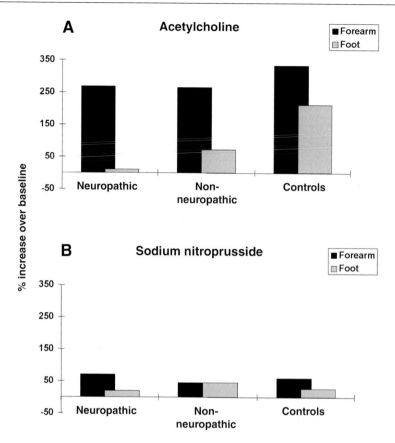

Fig. 11. The axon-reflex-mediated vasodilatation related to the C-nociceptive fibers (expressed as the percentage of increase over baseline flow measured by two single-point laser probe) at forearm vs foot level in diabetic patients with or without neuropathy and in healthy control subjects. The response to acetylcholine, which directly stimulates the C fibers, is lowest in the neuropathic group, but is also reduced in nonneuropathic group ($p < 0.001$), although no differences are found at the forearm level. A much smaller response is observed during the iontophoresis of sodium nitroprusside (nonspecific stimulus) at both foot and forearm level and is smaller in all three groups.

Microvascular Changes in Diabetic Foot With Charcot Arthropathy

The diagnosis of Charcot neuroarthropathy is made when gross destruction of the joints of the mid-foot results in significant foot deformity. The skin temperature of Charcot feet is usually higher as a result of increased blood flow in arterio-venous shunts. Although the endothelial-dependent and endothelial-independent vasodilatation is impaired in Charcot patients, the maximal hyperemic response to heat is preserved (Fig. 4). These findings indicate that the hyperemic response in Charcot disease is present but is probably unregulated and results in excessive bone resorption. The final results of these changes are complete joint destruction and gross deformity of the foot shape. These findings are consistent with clinical observations that the development of Charcot neuroarthropathy is extremely rare in the presence of peripheral vascular disease *(62)*. Poor blood flow to the extremity would prevent much of a hyperemic response, protecting the foot from bone resorption and deformation, although certainly contributing to other microcirculatory derangement.

CONCLUSIONS

Microcirculation to the diabetic foot suffers multiple significant structural and functional changes. Nerve-axon-related microvascular reactivity is clearly impaired in the diabetic population. There is a growing belief that both the failure of the dysfunctional vessels to dilate and the impairment of the nerve-axon reflex are major causes for impaired wound healing in diabetic patients. Further studies are required to clarify the precise etiology of observed endothelial dysfunction in diabetic patients and to identify the possible potential therapeutic interventions to prevent it or to retard its progression. Studies are also required to examine the vascular changes in the peripheral nerves, rather than in the skin.

Currently research is also ongoing in the connection of inflammatory states with both the development of vascular disease and diabetes. The hypothesis that inflammatory factors such as vascular cell adhesion molecule, interleukin-1, and tumor necrosis factor-α have a role in the development and progression of atherosclerosis is intriguing. These inflammatory factors are necessary in the cascade of wound healing, presenting a conflict of interest within the injured diabetic body. The factors required for healing a diabetic foot ulcer may actually worsen the atherosclerosis that is preventing adequate blood flow to heal the foot ulcer in the first place. An attempt to break the resulting cycle of wound, attempted healing, worsening circulation, worsening wound, is the next major focus in the field of diabetic microcirculation.

REFERENCES

1. Malik RA, Tesfaye S, Thompson SD, et al. Endothelial localization of microvascular damage in human diabetic neuropathy. Diabetologia 1993;36:454–459.
2. Tesfaye S, Harris N, Jakubowski JJ, et al. Impaired blood flow and arterio-venous shunting in human diabetic neuropathy: a novel technique of nerve photography and fluorescein angiography. Diabetologia 1993;36:1266–1274.
3. Tesfaye S, Malik R, Ward JD. Vascular factors in diabetic neuropathy. Diabetologia 1994;37:847–854.
4. Johnstone MT, Creager SJ, Scales KM, Cusco JA, Lee BK, Creager MA. Impaired endothelium-dependent vasodilation in patients with insulin-dependent diabetes mellitus. Circulation 1993;88:2510–2516.
5. Ross R. The pathogenesis of atherosclerosis: a perspective for the 1990s. Nature 1993;362:801–809.
6. Stevens MJ, Dananberg J, Feldman EL, et al. The linked roles of nitric oxide, aldose reductase and (Na + K+) - ATPase in the slowing of nerve conduction in the streptozotocin diabetic rat. J Clin Invest 1994;4: 853–859.
7. Stevens MJ, Feldman EL, Greene DA. The etiology of diabetic neuropathy: the combined roles of metabolic and vascular defects. Diabet Med 1995;12:566–579.
8. Pirart J. Diabetes mellitus and its degenerative complications: A prospective study of 4400 patients observed between 1947 and 1973. Diabetes Care 1978;1:168–188,252–261.
9. Palmberg P, Smith M, Waltman S, et al. The natural history of retinopathy in insulin-dependent juvenile-onset diabetes. Opthalmology 1981;88:613–618.
10. Diabetes Control and Complications Trial Research Group. The effect of intensive treatment of diabetes on the development and progression of long-term complications in insulin-dependent diabetes mellitus. N Engl J Med 1993;329:977–986.
11. Jaap AJ, Tooke JE. The pathophysiology of microvascular disease in type 2 diabetes. Clin Sci 1995;89: 3–12.
12. UK Prospective Diabetes Study (UKPDS) Group. Intensive blood-glucose control with sulphonylureas or insulin compared with conventional treatment and risk of complications in patients with type 2 diabetes (UKPDS 33). Lancet 1998;352(9131):837–53.
13. Ohkubo Y, Kishikawa H, Araki E, et al. Intensive insulin therapy prevents the progression of diabetic microvascular complications in Japanese patients with non-insulin-dependent diabetes mellitus: a randomized prospective 6-year study. Diabetes Res Clin Pract 1995;28(2):103–117.

14. Jorneskog G, Brismar K, Fagrell B. Skin capillary circulation severely impaired in toes of patients with IDDM, with and without late diabetic complications. Diabetologia 1995;38:474–480.
15. Goldenberg SG, Alex M, Joshi RA, Blumenthal HT. Nonatheromatous peripheral vascular disease of the lower extremity in diabetes mellitus. Diabetes 1959;8:261–273.
16. Barner HB, Kaiser GC, Willman VL. Blood flow in the diabetic leg. Circulation 1971;43:391–394.
17. Strandness DE Jr, Priest RE, Gibbons GE. Combined clinical and pathologic study of diabetic and nondiabetic peripheral arterial disease. Diabetes 1964;13:366–372.
18. LoGerfo FW, Coffman JD. Vascular and microvascular disease of the foot in diabetes. N Engl J Med 1984;311:1615–1619.
19. Nathan DM. Long-term complications of diabetes mellitus. N Engl J Med 1993;328:1676–1685.
20. Vanhoutte PM. The endothelium—modulator of vascular smooth-muscle tone. N Engl J Med 1988;319: 512–513.
21. Cohen RA. Dysfunction of vascular endothelium in diabetes mellitus. Circulation 1993;87:V67–V76.
22. Jaap AJ, Shore AC, Stockman AJ, Tooke JE. Skin capillary density in subjects with impaired glucose tolerance and patients with type 2 diabetes. Diabet Med 1996;13:160–164.
23. Rayman G, Malik RA, Sharma AK, Day JL. Microvascular response to tissue injury and capillary ultrastructure in the foot skin of type I diabetic patients. Clin Sci 1995;89:467– 474.
24. Malik RA, Metcalf I, Sharma AK, Day JL, Rayman G. Skin epidermal thickness and vascular density in type 1 diabetes. Diabet Med 1992;9:263–267.
25. Williamson JR, Kilo C. Basement membrane physiology and pathophysiology. In: Alberti KGMM, DeFronzo RA, Keen H, Zimmet P, (eds). International textbook of diabetes mellitus, second edition. John Wiley, Chichester, 1992, pp. 1245–1265.
26. Raskin P, Pietri A, Unger R, Shannon WA Jr. The effect of diabetic control on skeletal muscle capillary basement membrane width in patients with type 1 diabetes mellitus. New Engl J Med 1983;309:1546–1550.
27. Ajjam ZS, Barton S, Corbett M, et al. Quantitative evaluation of the dermal vasculature of diabetics. Q J Med 1985;215:229–239.
28. Tilton RG, Faller AM, Burkhardt JK, et al. Pericyte degeneration and acellular capillaries are increased in the feet of human diabetes. Diabetologia 1985;28:895–900.
29. Rayman G, Williams SA, Spencer PD, Smaje LH, Wise PH, Tooke JE. Impaired microvascular hyperaemic response to minor skin trauma in type 1 diabetes. Br Med J 1986;292:1295–1298.
30. Flynn MD, Tooke JE. Aetiology of diabetic foot ulceration: A role for the microcirculation? Diabet Med 1992;8:320–329.
31. Tooke JE. Microvascular function in human diabetes: A physiological perspective. Diabetes 1995;44: 721–726.
32. Parving HH, Viberti GC, Keen H, Christiansen JS, Lassen NA. Hemodynamic factors in the genesis of diabetic microangiopathy. Metabolism 1983;32:943–949.
33. Mullarkey CJ, Brownlee M. Biochemical basis of microvascular disease. In: Pickup JC, Williams G, (eds). Chronic complications of diabetes. Blackwell Scientific Publications, Oxford, 1994, pp. 20–29.
34. Schmidt AM, Hori O, Brett J, Yan SD, Wautier JL, Stern D. Cellular receptors for advanced glycation end products. Implications for induction of oxidant stress and cellular dysfunction in the pathogenesis of vascular lesions. Arteriosclerosis and Thrombosis 1994;14:1521–1528.
35. Makita Z, Radoff S, Rayfield EJ, et al. Advanced glycosylation end products in patients with diabetic nephropathy. N Engl J Med 1991;325:836–842.
36. Bucala R, Tracey KJ, Cerami A. Advanced glycosylation end products quench nitric oxide and mediate defective endothelium-dependent vasodilatation in experimental diabetes. J Clin Invest 1991; 87:432–438.
37. Sandeman DD, Shore AC, Tooke JE. Relation of skin capillary pressure in patients with insulin-dependent diabetes to complications and metabolic control. N Eng J Med 1992;327:760–764.
38. Shore AC, Price HJ, Sandeman DD, Green EM, Tripp JH, Tooke JE. Impaired microvascular hyperaemic response in children with diabetes mellitus. Diabet Med 1991;8:619–623.
39. Rendell M, Bergman T, O'Donnell G, Drobny E, Borgos J, Bonner RF. Microvascular blood flow, volume, and velocity measured by laser doppler techniques in IDDM. Diabetes 1989;38:819–824.
40. Tooke JE, Ostergren J, Fagrell B. Synchronous assessment of human skin microcirculation by laser doppler flowmetry and dynamic capillaroscopy. Int J Microcirc Clin Exp 1983;2:277–284.
41. Boulton AJM, Scarpello JHB, Ward JD. Venous oxygenation in the diabetic neuropathic foot: evidence of arteriovenous shunting? Diabetologia 1982;22:6–8.

42. Murray HJ, Boulton A. The pathophysiology of diabetic foot ulceration. Clin Podiatr Med Surg 1995; 12(1):1–17.

43. Conrad MC. Functional anatomy of the circulation to the lower extremities. Year Book Medical Publishers Inc., Chicago, IL, 1971.

44. Watkins PJ, Edmonds ME. Sympathetic nerve failure in diabetes. Diabetologia 1983;25:75–77.

45. Malik RA, Newrick PG, Sharma AK, et al. Microangiopathy in human diabetic neuropathy: relationship between capillary abnormalities and the severity of neuropathy. Diabetologia 1989;32:92–102.

46. Flynn MD, Tooke JE. Diabetic neuropathy and the microcirculation. Diabet Med 1995;12:298–301.

47. Edmonds ME, Roberts VC, Watkins PJ Blood flow in the diabetic neuropathic foot. Diabetologia 1982; 22:141–147.

48. Williams SB, Cusco JA, Roddy M, Johnstone MY, Creager MA. Impaired nitric oxide-mediated vasodilation in patients with non-insulin-dependent diabetes mellitus. J Am Coll Cardiol 1996;27:567–574.

49. Stehouwer CDA, Fischer HRA, Van Kuijk AWR, Polak BCP, Donker AJM Endothelial dysfunction precedes development of microalbuminuria in IDD. Diabetes 1995;44:561–564.

50. Caballero AE, Arora S, Saouaf R, et al. Microvascular and macrovascular reactivity is reduced in subjects at risk for type 2 diabetes. Diabetes 1999;48(9):1856–1862.

51. Veves A, Akbari CA, Primavera J, et al. Endothelial dysfunction and the expression of endothelial nitric oxide synthetase in diabetic neuropathy, vascular disease, and foot ulceration. Diabetes 1998;47:457–463.

52. Parkhouse N, LeQueen PM. Impaired neurogenic vascular response in patients with diabetes and neuropathic foot lesions. N Engl J Med 1988;318:1306–1309.

53. Walmsley D, Wiles PG Early loss of neurogenic inflammation in the human diabetic foot. Clin Sci 1991; 80:605–610.

54. Arora S, Smakowski P, Frykberg RG, et al. Differences in foot and forearm skin microcirculation in diabetic patients with and without neuropathy. Diabetes Care 1998;21(8):1339–1344.

55. Stansberry KB, Peppard HR, Babyak LM, Popp G, McNitt PM, Vinik AI. Primary nociceptive afferents mediate the blood flow dysfunction in non-glabrous (hairy) skin of type 2 diabetes. Diabetes Care 1999; 22(9):1549–1554.

56. Caselli A, Rich J, Hanane T, Uccioli L, Veves A. Role of C-nociceptive fibers in the nerve axon reflex-related vasodilation in diabetes. Neurology 2003;60:297–300.

57. Hamdy O, Abou-Elenin K, Smakowski P, et al. The contribution of nerve axon reflex-related vasodilation to the total skin vasodilation in diabetic patients with and without neuropathy. Diabetes Care 2001; 24(2):344–349.

58. Veves A, Uccioli L, Manes C, et al. Comparisons of risk factors for foot problems in diabetic patients attending teaching hospitals outpatient clinics in four different European states. Diabet Med 1994;11: 709–713.

59. Ward JD. Upright posture and the microvasculature in human diabetic neuropathy: a hypothesis. Diabetes 1997;46 (Suppl 2):S94–S97,61.

60. Jude EB, Boulton AJ, Ferguson MW, Appleton I. The role of nitric oxide synthase isoforms and arginase in the pathogenesis of diabetic foot ulcers: possible modulatory effects by transforming growth factor beta 1. Diabetologia 1999;42:748–757.

61. Szabo C, Zanchi A, Komjati K, et al. Poly(ADP-Ribose) Polymerase is activated in subjects at risk of developing type 2 diabetes and is associated with impaired vascular reactivity. Circulation 2002:2680–2686.

62. Frykberg RG, Kozak GP. The diabetic Charcot foot. In: Kozak GP, Campbell DR, Frykberg RG, Habershaw GM, (eds). Management of Diabetic Foot Problems, 2nd Ed. , SaundersPhiladelphia, PA, 1995, pp. 88–97.

II CLINICAL

C. Cardiovascular System: Peripheral Vascular System

20 Epidemiology of Peripheral Vascular Disease

Stephanie G. Wheeler, MD, MPH,
Nicholas L. Smith, PhD, MPH,
and Edward J. Boyko, MD, MPH

CONTENTS

INTRODUCTION

The epidemiology of several atherosclerotic arterial diseases and their association with diabetes will be covered in this chapter. This chapter will focus on peripheral vascular disease (PVD), arterial disease affecting the extremities, and will include more general epidemiological aspects of PVD, including associated conditions and mortality. Additionally, the epidemiology of cerebrovascular disease (CBD) and coronary artery disease (CAD) will also be discussed, primarily as they relate to diabetes.

EPIDEMIOLOGICAL PRINCIPLES RELEVANT TO THE STUDY OF ARTERIAL DISEASES

Measurement of disease prevalence and incidence is best conducted in a population-based sample of study subjects. Typically, such samples are obtained from defined populations, such as all residents of a certain geographic area, or using some other characteristic

From: *Contemporary Cardiology: Diabetes and Cardiovascular Disease, Second Edition*
Edited by: M. T. Johnstone and A. Veves © Humana Press Inc., Totowa, NJ

to define the population, such as enrollees of a health plan. Populations obtained from clinic-based or other medical care settings are likely to overestimate prevalence and incidence of arterial diseases because associated conditions that put such persons at higher risk of arterial diseases are likely to be present in higher proportion in these subjects who seek care rather than a random population-based sample.

In addition to measurements of disease incidence and prevalence, several methods are used by epidemiologists to assess whether an exposure (e.g., smoking, diabetes) is related to a change in risk of disease. Further methods are employed to determine if such an association may be causal, or instead as a result of confounding, selection, or measurement bias. Cross-sectional study designs provide weak information regarding causality. Retrospective study designs tend to be less compelling in establishing whether an exposure is related to a change in disease risk, because the passage of time between the onset of the exposure and disease development may result in inaccurate exposure classification, or a different mortality rate related to exposure and disease that may induce bias in the estimates of association. Prospective research is less likely to be biased by differences in probability of subject selection based on arterial disease and risk-factor presence. Prospective research is a stronger study design regarding inferring the possibility of causation, because the presence of risk factors may be determined prior to arterial disease onset. Many prospective studies exist on the epidemiology of CAD, but fewer have covered the topics of PVD and CBD.

The problem of measurement error in the assessment of the presence or absence of vascular disease is well recognized. Even coronary angiography for the diagnosis of CAD is likely to result in some degree of misclassification, for reasons described previously (1). A similar situation holds for the diagnosis of PVD. For example, it is likely that in some instances claudication will occur even with a normal or high ankle-arm index (AAI), if noncompressible, calcified vessels result in falsely high readings of the ankle systolic blood pressure (SBP) (2). This misclassification issue is even more problematic when a test result is used to formulate a clinical plan for an individual patient, as compared to epidemiological analysis in which population statistics are the result of interest. When misclassification of PVD status occurs nondifferentially regarding exposure (randomly), the net result is bias of any observed difference toward the null value (3). The same holds true for exposures that are nondifferentially misclassified regarding PVD. Therefore observed differences found in an epidemiological analysis of risk factors for PVD validly reflect potential causative factors for this complication, but probably underestimate the magnitude of the risk increase. Epidemiological studies may therefore draw valid conclusions regarding risk factors for PVD, CBD, and CAD even if the techniques used to measure either vascular disease or the potential risk factor are prone to nondifferential misclassification.

The American Diabetes Association produced a consensus statement in which they recommended using AAI to screen for PVD in patients with diabetes over the age of 50 (4). The issues of screening and misclassification and the limitations of the AAI were acknowledged. However, the problems were not felt to detract from the clinical usefulness of the AAI to screen for and diagnose PVD in patients with diabetes.

PERIPHERAL VASCULAR DISEASE INCIDENCE AND PREVALENCE

PVD affects a high proportion of older persons in general populations located in developed countries. Meijer and associates presented age- and gender-adjusted results of the prevalence of low AAI using different definitions (<0.75 to <0.94) for nine population-based surveys that ranged from 5.5% to 26.7% *(5)*. In very elderly (85–93 years) Japanese-American men living in Hawaii, prevalence of PVD was somewhat higher at 27.4% *(6)*. In a population of patients chosen because they were over age 70 or over age 50 but with a history of tobacco use or diabetes, the prevalence of PVD was 27% *(7)*.

Claudication is an insensitive measure of peripheral vascular disease, with symptomless diminished arterial flow estimated to occur at least two to five times as frequently as claudication *(8)*. The Rose questionnaire has been used by investigators to assess claudication prevalence, but it has been shown to have only moderate sensitivity (60%–68%) in capturing persons with this clinical diagnosis *(9)*. In the Edinburgh Artery Study, the prevalence of claudication in men increased from 2.2% in the 50- to 59-year age category to 7.7% in the 70- to 74-year age category *(10)*. Meijer and associates reviewed 13 population-based screening surveys for presence of claudication, and reported age- and gender-adjusted estimates ranging from 0.6% to 7.4%, with one additional study finding a prevalence as high as 14.4% *(5,11)*. Although it has been written that men are affected with symptomatic PVD between two to five times as frequently as women *(10)*, in the review of Meijer a twofold or higher prevalence of claudication was seen in only one of the 13 studies *(5)*.

Among patients who have type 1 diabetes, PVD is more common than for the general population. In the Pittsburgh Epidemiology of Diabetes Complications Study of childhood onset type 1 diabetes, women who had type 1 diabetes for 30 years were found to have a prevalence of PVD greater than 30% compared to only 11% for men when determined by AAI less than 0.8 at rest or after exercise *(12)*. The Epidemiology of Diabetes and Complications (EDIC) study, the long-term follow-up of the Diabetes Control and Complications Trial (DCCT), identified those patients with AAI less than 0.9. The EDIC study found that intensively treated participants, with an average duration of type 1 diabetes of about 14 years, had a prevalence of PVD of 8.8% among women and 4.6% among men *(13)*.

Patients with type 2 diabetes in the United Kingdom Prospective Diabetes Study (UKPDS) had a prevalence of PVD of 1.2% (95% confidence interval [CI], 0.9%–1.5%) at the time of diagnosis of their diabetes *(14)*. PVD in the UKPDS was defined as the presence of any two of the following: (a) AAI less than 0.8, (b) absence of both dorsalis pedis and posterior tibial pulses to palpation in at least one leg, and (c) claudication. At 6 years of follow-up in the UKPDS, 2.7% of participants (95% CI, 2.2%–3.2%) had PVD according to these criteria that was not present at diagnosis and 10.6% had at least one of these three abnormal measures. The prevalence of PVD increased to 12.5% in the smaller subgroup or participants followed for 18 years (95% CI 3.8%–21.1%). The Framingham Offspring Study examined 1554 males and 1759 females for PVD. In this population-based study, the odds ratio for PVD was 2.3 (95% CI, 1.5–3.6) among diabetic vs nondiabetic participants *(15)*. This odds ratio associated with diabetes for developing PVD, in addition to the odds ratios associated with hypertension, current smoking, and each additional 10 years of age, are shown in Fig. 1.

Vascular disease in people with diabetes is both morphologically and physiologically distinguished from nondiabetic atherosclerosis *(16)*. The femoropopliteal segments are most often affected, as in nondiabetic patients, but smaller vessels below the knee, such as the tibial and peroneal arteries are more severely affected in diabetic than in nondiabetic patients *(17,18)*. In practical terms, diabetes is associated with a high prevalence of

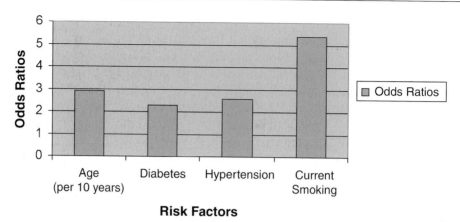

Fig. 1. Odds ratios for risk factors for peripheral vascular disease. Peripheral vascular disease (PVD) was defined as an ankle-brachial index less than 0.9. Data taken from the Framingham Offspring Study, a population-based study of PVD and its risk factors.

distal arterial disease, a propensity to earlier calcification, increased thrombogenicity, and generally poorer prognosis.

Racial differences in the prevalence of diabetes mellitus (DM) in the United States are well documented. The Atherosclerosis Risk in Communities (ARIC) Study included 4264 black and 11,479 white randomly selected men and women. This study found 19% of the black women were diabetic compared with 7% of white women and that 16% of black men were diabetic compared with 8% of white men (19). The National Health and Nutrition Examination Survey Epidemiologic Follow-up Study 1971–1992 (NHEFS) followed 14,407 subjects prospectively and found 10.6% of black subjects had diabetes at baseline compared to 6.8% of white subjects (20).

Similarly, there are racial differences in the complications of diabetes, including PVD. The NHEFS found that among subjects with incident DM during the study follow-up period, 3.4% of blacks had lower extremity amputations compared to 1.4% of whites. The authors of the study speculated that a combination of social and environmental factors may account for the apparent ethnic difference. To examine the question of whether the observed differences in complication rates were the result of disparate access to health care, a study of an ethnically diverse population with uniform health care coverage was undertaken by the Kaiser Permanente Medical Care Program in northern California. The study observed 63,432 diabetic patients, which included 12% Asians, 14% blacks, 10% Latinos, and 64% whites, for 4 years and measured nontraumatic lower extremity amputation and end-stage renal disease (ESRD) among other outcomes. Age- and sex-adjusted incidence rates of lower extremity amputation did not differ significantly between whites and blacks or Latinos, whereas Asians had a rate 64% lower than that of whites (21). On the other hand, age- and sex-adjusted incidence rates of ESRD were significantly higher for blacks, Asians, and Latinos relative to whites (112%, 44%, and 41% higher, respectively).

RISK FACTORS FOR PERIPHERAL VASCULAR DISEASE

The Framingham Heart Study found a strong relationship between the number of cigarettes smoked and the incidence of intermittent claudication and a multivariate analysis identified smoking as the strongest single risk factor for development of symptomatic obstructive arterial disease, regardless of gender *(22)*. The occurrence of intermittent claudication is twice as frequent in smokers as nonsmokers. In the Edinburgh Artery Study, peripheral arterial disease prevalence was strongly and positively related to life-time cigarette smoking *(23)*. Smoking was related to a higher relative prevalence of peripheral arterial disease (range of odds ratios [OR], 1.8–5.6) than heart disease (range of ORs, 1.1–1.6). A prospective analysis of this cohort over 5 years revealed an incidence of new claudication of 2.6% among nonsmokers, 4.5% in moderate smokers (<25 pack-years) and 9.8% in heavy smokers (>25 pack-years) *(24)*.

Hyperglycemia was found to be associated with an increased risk of incident PVD, independent of other risk factors including age, elevated SBP, low high-density lipopro-tein (HDL), smoking, prior cardiovascular disease (CVD), peripheral sensory neuropa-thy and retinopathy. Each 1% increase in hemoglobin (Hb)A1c was associated with a 28% increased risk of PVD (95% CI, 12–46) *(14)*.

Many conditions associated with DM may help explain the higher prevalence of PVD seen in persons with this condition, such as other PVD risk factors that comprise features of the metabolic syndrome (hypertension, dyslipidemia) *(25)*. Increased levels of hemo-static factors such as fibrinogen, von Willebrand factor, tissue plasminogen activator, fibrin D-dimer, and plasma viscosity explained in part the higher prevalence of PVD in subjects with diabetes or impaired glucose tolerance in the Edinburgh Artery Study *(26)*.

Hypertensive patients show a threefold increased risk of intermittent claudication at a 16-year follow-up *(27)*. Limb arterial obstructive disease occurs twice as frequently as CAD among hypertensive individuals and hypertension has been reported in 29% to 39% of patients with symptomatic PVD *(28)*. The Cardiovascular Health Study reported about a 50% higher prevalence of an AAI less than 0.9 associated with hypertension in a multivariate analysis adjusted for age, smoking, diabetes, and dyslipidemia *(29)*. Obser-vational data analysis among 3642 patients in the UKPDS showed that the aggregate endpoint of amputation or death from PVD was associated with a 16% decrease per 10 mmHg reduction in SBP, adjusted for age at diagnosis of diabetes, ethnic group, smoking status, presence of albuminuria, HbA1c, high-density lipoprotein (HDL) and low-density lipoprotein (LDL) cholesterol, and triglyceride *(30)*.

The association of hypercholesterolemia with atherosclerosis of the lower extremities has been known for 60 years *(31)*. The prevalence of claudication in patients with serum cholesterol levels over 260 mg/dL is on average over twice as high as in those with a concentration below this level. The prevalence of hyperlipidemia in patients with clinical manifestations of lower extremity arterial occlusive disease ranges in various studies from 31% to 57%. The Edinburgh Artery Study reported a higher prevalence of PVD in association with higher serum cholesterol and lower HDL cholesterol in multiple logistic regression analysis *(23)*. The Cardiovascular Health Study reached similar conclusions among its sample of 5084 subjects aged 65 years or older, with PVD defined as an AAI less than 0.9 *(29)*.

Other risk factors have been shown to be associated with a higher prevalence of PVD. Higher circulating levels of homocysteine have been demonstrated in this condition *(32)*, as have parallel low levels of folate in red blood cells and circulating vitamin B$_6$, which raises the possibility that supplementation with these vitamins may reduce the incidence of peripheral arterial disease *(33)*. One small, randomized, placebo-controlled study of secondary prevention has shown that oral therapy with folic acid, vitamin B$_{12}$, and vita-min B$_6$ decreased the need for revascularization in patients receiving percutaneous coronary intervention *(34)*. Higher levels of various hemostatic factors have been demonstrated in persons with lower AAI, suggesting that a hypercoagulable state predisposes to the development of PVD *(35,36)*. Infectious agents such as chlamydia pneumoniae have been implicated in the development of atherosclerosis in several vascular beds *(37,38)*. The prevalence of low AAI (<1.05) was highest among persons with a birth weight less than 6.6 pounds, a demonstration of the "thrifty phenotype" hypothesis that postulates fetal growth retardation as a cause of metabolic disorders and vascular disease in adult life *(39,40)*.

CONDITIONS ASSOCIATED WITH PERIPHERAL VASCULAR DISEASE

Atherosclerosis, the underlying cause of PVD, is a multifactorial, progressive condition that begins in childhood and involves multiple biological processes and foci. Therefore, it is not surprising that patients with PVD often have extensive CAD and CBD. The prevalence of CAD among persons with claudication in the general population is between two and four times higher than in nonclaudicants *(10)*. Around 50% of claudicants also suffer from angina, whereas patients with angina are six times more likely to have claudication *(41)*. When 200 consecutive patients admitted to a vascular surgery service in an academic teaching hospital were evaluated for concomitant diseases, CAD was present in 46%, 22% had symptomatic CAD, 37% had impaired cardiac function, and 32% had carotid artery disease *(12)*. Both claudication and asymptomatic PVD (AAI <0.9) in the Edinburgh Artery Study population were significantly associated with greater intima-media thickness (IMT) of the carotid arteries as assessed by ultrasound *(42)*.

MORTALITY ASSOCIATED WITH PERIPHERAL VASCULAR DISEASE

Although peripheral arterial disease rarely causes death, diminished long-term survival in these patients is well established. The causes of death associated with this condition are primarily cardiovascular. In the Framingham study 14% of men and 18% of women died within 6 years of the onset of intermittent claudication *(43)*. Mortality rates appear to be related to the severity of the obstructive process. Szilagyi and associates found the cumulative 6-year mortality rate was 62% in patients with symptoms sufficiently severe to require femoropopliteal bypass *(44)*. In the study of DeWeese and Rob, 48% of patients with claudication, 80% of those with ischemic rest pain and 95% of those with gangrene were dead within 10 years of undergoing femoropopliteal bypass grafting *(45)*.

Patients with severe or symptomatic PVD have four to seven times the risk of mortality from all causes and a 15-fold higher risk of mortality from CVD than persons who do not have PVD *(46)*. Simonsick and associates demonstrated that intermittent claudication was an important predictor of mortality and cardiovascular morbidity in ambulatory older adults independent of associated coronary ischemia and CVD risk factors *(47)*. Howell and associates found that independent of age or the presence or absence of diabetes, a low AAI was strongly associated with increased mortality *(48)*. Although the presence of arterial obstructive disease of the legs is a hallmark of generalized atherosclerosis and therefore would be expected to confer an increased risk of cardiovascular or cerebrovascular death, extremely severe PVD appears to carry a particularly ominous prognosis. These researchers noted that patients with an AAI less than 0.30 had a very high 6-year cumulative mortality rate (64%) *(48)*.

THE EPIDEMIOLOGY OF CAROTID AND VERTEBRAL ARTERIAL DISEASE

Atherosclerosis of the carotid and vertebral arteries is related to a higher risk of stroke *(49)*. Not all strokes, however, are as a result of atherosclerosis of the carotid or vertebral circulation. Some arise from embolic events or result from intracerebral vascular disease. The recent development of techniques to directly visualize the carotid artery has led to a recent surge in publications on risk factors for IMT of the carotid arterial wall and presence of plaques measured using B-mode ultrasonography. These methods permit detection of subclinical atherosclerosis. It has been shown that carotid wall thickness is predictive of incident clinical stroke *(50)*. Although visualization of the vertebral system is also possible using this same imaging technology, little epidemiological information is available to indicate the prevalence of this condition or associated risk factors.

A strong association exists between greater intima-media carotid arterial thickness and diabetes in a regression model adjusted for other CAD risk factors, as demonstrated by the Insulin Resistance Atherosclerosis Study, which was conducted among 1625 persons with different categories of glucose tolerance *(51)*. Subjects with normal and impaired glucose tolerance had similar IMT, suggesting that higher levels of hyperglycemia are required to promote carotid atherosclerotic lesions *(51)*. Low insulin sensitivity as measured using the minimal model technique was found to be related to greater IMT of the internal carotid artery among Caucasian and Hispanic participants in the IRAS study *(52)*. Several other CAD risk factors have been studied in relation to carotid wall thickness. The ARIC study found that low LDL cholesterol, high SBP, and smoking predicted greater carotid wall thickness among its 12,193 participants aged 45 to 64 years *(53)*. Carotid plaques demonstrated by ultrasound were very common in British men (57%) and women (58%) between the ages of 56 and 77 years *(54)*. Risk factors for presence of plaque differed depending on location but in general were associated with greater age, smoking, and higher SBP *(54)*. Greater carotid wall thickness has also been demonstrated among persons with lower birth weights and serological evidence of past infection to Chlamydia pneumoniae *(37,39)*. In general, the risk factors for PVD and CVD appear similar.

Intensive treatment of type 1 diabetes is associated with a decrease in IMT, although this effect was not evident after 1 year of follow-up of the DCCT cohort *(55)*. In the EDIC, the long-term follow-up of the DCCT, intensive insulin therapy, compared to conventional therapy, during the DCCT resulted in decreased progression of IMT 6 years after the end of the trial *(56)*. Progression of carotid IMT was associated with the traditional risk factors mentioned above, including age, SBP, smoking, the ratio of LDL to HDL cholesterol, urinary albumin excretion rate and with the mean glycosylated hemoglobin value during the mean duration of the DCCT. The glycosylated hemoglobin value during the DCCT explained 96% of the differences between groups in IMT of the common carotid artery at year 6 of follow-up.

THE EPIDEMIOLOGY OF CORONARY ARTERY DISEASE

The coronary arteries have received a far greater amount of clinical, public health, and research interest and resources than the arteries of other vascular beds. This focus can be attributed to the extraordinarily negative health impact CAD has had in the past century on most populations in Western societies. In the United States, CAD has been the leading cause of death for the past 80 years and, although the burden of disease is lessening in all major subpopulations, *(57)* it was still the primary cause of death in 2000, accounting for 35% of all mortality *(58)*. The hallmark of CAD is acute myocardial infarction (MI), but outcomes also include angina pectoris, acute coronary syndrome, sudden cardiac arrest, and heart failure. Although other coronary outcomes have decreased in prevalence in the United States, the prevalence of heart failure has increased *(59,60)*.

Adults with disorders of glucose metabolism are at higher risk of CAD than adults without such disturbances. Data from the Third National Health and Nutrition Examination Survey found that elevated blood pressure, increased body mass index, decreased HDL cholesterol, and increased triglycerides and LDL cholesterol were more prevalent in adults with glucose disorders (fasting glucose >110 mg/dL) than in those with normal fasting glucose (<110 mg/dL) *(61)*. Among those with glucose disorders, the prevalence of each CAD risk factor was generally greater in those with diabetes (fasting glucose >126 mg/dL) than in those with impaired fasting glucose (fasting glucose 110–125 mg/ dL). Inflammation measures such as fibrinogen and C-reactive protein were also markedly elevated in those with disturbances in glucose metabolism compared to those without. In a meta-analysis of data from 20 prospective studies that followed nearly 100,000 adults—primarily men—for an average of 12.4 years, fasting glucose and 2-hour postchallenge glucose were associated with an increased risk of incident CVD, which included MI, stroke, sudden cardiac arrest, and cardiovascular mortality. There was a 33% increase in cardiovascular risk (relative risk [RR], 1.3; 95% CI, 1.1–1.7) when a fasting glucose level of 110 mg/dL was compared to a level of 75 mg/dL and there was a 58% increase in risk (RR: 1.6; 95% CI, 1.3–2.1) when a 2-hour glucose level of 140 mg/ dL was compared to a 75 mg/dL level *(62)*. Among adults 65 years of age and older, 2-hour postchallenge glucose was a better predictors of cardiovascular events, primarily MI and coronary death, than fasting glucose in a biracial elderly population *(63)*. This observation has been supported by data in a younger population as well *(64)*. Other manifestations of impaired glucose metabolism such as insulin resistance—a component of the metabolic syndrome—has been associated with an increased risk of incident MI and cardiovascular morbidity and mortality in large, population-based studies *(65,66)*.

Several prospective community-based studies have demonstrated that adults with frank DM have a multifold increase in risk of incident CAD when compared to adults without diabetes. In middle-aged northern Europeans, the relative risk of incident MI in men was 2.9 (95% CI, 2.6–3.4) and in women it was 5.0 (95% CI, 3.9–6.3) when event rates of those with diabetes were compared to those without diabetes *(67)*. Risks of similar magnitude were seen for men and women with diabetes in a population of southern Europeans when compared to those without diabetes *(68)*. In older adults, when compared to those without diabetes, the relative risk of incident CAD (MI or angina) was 2.5 (95% CI, 1.9–3.4) for those with diabetes and subclinical CVD and was 1.3 (95% CI, 0.8–2.0) in those with diabetes and without subclinical CVD *(69)*. Data addressing the association of diabetes with the risk of coronary and cardiovascular mortality are similar to the coronary morbidity setting in which adults with diabetes—primarily Caucasian males—had a nearly fourfold increase in mortality risk compared to adults without diabetes (RR, 3.8; 95% CI, 3.1–4.7) *(70)*. In a different cohort of male Caucasians, the risk of all-cause and coronary mortality was two- to threefold higher in those with diabetes and without established CAD and was 4- to 10-fold higher in those with diabetes and established CAD when compared to those free of both *(71)*. Coronary mortality risk associated with diabetes was higher in those less than 60 years of age (RR = 6.2; 95% CI, 3.4–11.3) than in those 70 years of age or older (RR= 2.7; 95% CI, 2.0–3.6). In a cohort of middle-aged women, diabetes was associated with a sixfold (RR = 5.7; 95% CI, 4.8–6.6) increase in fatal coronary disease risk in those without a history of coronary disease and an 11-fold (RR = 10.7; 95% CI, 9.0–12.6) increase in risk in those with a history when compared to those without diabetes and without a coronary disease history *(72)*. The relative risk of incident CAD and all-cause mortality in adults with diabetes compared to those without appears to be similar in African-American and Euro-American women *(73)*. For men, however, risks may be lower in African-American and Afro-Caribbean men than in Caucasians *(74,75)*.

Risk factors for CAD in adults with diabetes are similar to those for coronary disease in populations without diabetes. Increased age, LDL cholesterol, and SBP and decreased HDL and smoking are all associated in a dose–response relationship with increase coronary disease risk *(76)*. Of the various risk factors, lipids by far have received the most research attention *(77-80)*. The difficulty in measuring the association between many of these factors and CAD risk in adults with diabetes is that risk factors often co-occur in individuals and causality is not easily inferred.

The underlying pathophysiology of impaired glucose metabolism that leads to an increased risk of CAD and atherosclerotic diseases of the other vascular beds is an expansive area of biological research that includes genetic and molecular investigations. The roles of endothelial cell and smooth muscle dysfunction and platelet and coagulation abnormalities appear to be key in atherosclerotic disease progression *(81)*. Many of these topics are covered in other chapters of this book.

CONCLUSIONS

Vascular disease of the peripheral, carotid, and coronary beds probably reflects a process of generalized atherosclerosis in most cases, because co-occurrence of stenoses at multiple sites is often seen, risk factors for disease at one site usually are related to higher risk at other sites, and peripheral disease confers a higher risk of death as a result of CAD. There are important differences to note. The effects of smoking and diabetes mellitus on PVD are associated with higher relative risks than the carotid and coronary arteries. It is not yet clear whether higher circulating homocysteine will be related to greater risk of CAD or CBD. Since many of these risk factors are reversible or treatable to some extent, there is hope that primary or secondary preventive interventions may yield further benefits in reducing the impacts of these diseases on mortality, morbidity, and health status/quality of life.

REFERENCES

1. Boyko EJ, Alderman BW, Baron AE. Reference test errors bias the evaluation of diagnostic tests for ischemic heart disease. J Gen Intern Med 1988;3:476–481.
2. Young MJ, Anderson GF, Boulton AJ, Cavanaugh PR. Medial arterial calcification in the feet of diabetic patients and matched non-diabetic control subjects. Diabetolgia 1993;36:615–621.
3. Rothman KJ. Modern Epidemiology. Philadelphia: Lippincott-Raven, 1998.
4. American Diabetes Association. Peripheral arterial disease in people with diabetes. Diabetes Care 2003;26:3333–3341.
5. Meijer WT, Hoes AW, Rutgers D, Bots ML, Hofman A, Grobbee DE. Peripheral arterial disease in the elderly: The Rotterdam Study. Arterioscler Thromb Vasc Biol 1998;18:185–192.
6. Curb JD, Kamal M, Rodriguez BL, et al. Peripheral artery disease and cardiovascular risk factors in the elderly. The Honolulu Heart Program. Arterioscler Thromb Vasc Biol 1996;16(12):1495–1500.

7. Hirsch A, Treat-Jacobson D, Regensteiner J, et al. Peripheral arterial disease detection, awareness, and treatment in primary care. JAMA 2001;286:1317–1324.
8. Criqui MH, Denenberg JO, Langer RD, Fronek A. The epidemiology of peripheral arterial disease: importance of identifying the population at risk. Vasc Med 1997;2(3):221–226.
9. Leng GC, Fowkes FG. The Edinburgh Claudication Questionnaire: an improved version of the WHO/Rose Questionnaire for use in epidemiological surveys. J Clin Epidemiol 1992;45:1101–1109.
10. Fowkes FG. Epidemiology of peripheral vascular disease. Atherosclerosis 1997;131(Suppl):S29–S31.
11. Hale WE, Marks RG, May FE, Moore MT, Stewart RB. Epidemiology of intermittent claudication: evaluation of risk factors. Age Ageing 1988;17:57–60.
12. Orchard TJ, Maser RE, Becker DJ, et al. Prevalence of complications in IDDM by sex and duration. Pittsburgh Epidemiology of Diabetes Complications Study II. Diabetes 1990;39(9):1116–1124.
13. Nathan DM, Lachin J, Cleary P, et al. Intensive diabetes therapy and carotid intima-media thickness in type 1 diabetes mellitus. N Engl J Med 2003;348(23):2294–2303.
14. Adler AI, Neil A, Stratton IM, Boulton AJM, Holman RR, for the UK Prospective Diabetes Study Group. UKPDS 59: hyperglycemia and other potentially modifiable risk factors for peripheral vascular disease in type 2 diabetes. Diabetes Care 2002;25:894–899.
15. Murabito JM, Nieto K, Larson MG, Levy D, Wilson PWF. Prevalence and clinical correlates of peripheral arterial disease in the Framingham Offspring Study. Am Heart J 2002;143:961–965.
16. Halperin JL. Arterial obstructive diseases of the extremities. In: Loscalzo CM, Dzau VJ, (eds). Vascular Medicine. Boston: Little Brown, 1992, pp. 835–865.
17. LoGerfo FW, Coffman JD. Current Concepts. Vascular and microvascular disease of the foot in diabetes. Implications in foot care. N Engl J Med 1984;311:1615–1619.
18. Jude EB, Oyibo SO, Chalmers N, Boulton AJ. Peripheral arterial disease in diabetic and nondiabetic patients: a comparison of severity and outcome. Diabetes Care 2001;24(8):1433–1437.
19. Hutchinson RG, Davis CE, Barnes R, et al. Racial differences in risk factors for atherosclerosis. Angiology 1997;48(4):279–290.
20. Resnick HE, Valsania P, Phillips CL. Diabetes mellitus and nontraumatic lower extremity amputation in black and white Americans: the National Health and Nutrition Examination Survey Epidemiologic Follow-up Study, 1971–1992. Arch Intern Med 1999;159:2470–2475.
21. Karter AJ, Liu JY, Moffet HH, Ackerson LM, Selby JV. Ethnic disparities in diabetic complications in an insured population. JAMA 2002;287(19):2519–2527.
22. Kannel WB, McGee D, Gordon T. A general cardiovascular risk profile: the Framingham Study. Am J Cardiol 1976;38(1):46–51.
23. Fowkes FG, Housley E, Riemersma RA, et al. Smoking, lipids, glucose tolerance, and blood pressure as risk factors for peripheral atherosclerosis compared with ischemic heart disease in the Edinburgh Artery Study. Am J Epidemiol 1992;135(4):331–340.
24. Price JF, Mowbray PI, Lee AJ, Rumley A, Lowe GD, Fowkes FG. Relationship between smoking and cardiovascular risk factors in the development of peripheral arterial disease and coronary artery disease: Edinburgh Artery Study. Eur Heart J 1999;20(5):344–353.
25. Liese AD, Mayer-Davis EJ, Haffner SM. Development of the multiple metabolic syndrome: an epidemiologic perspective. Epidemiol Rev 1998;20:157–172.
26. Lee AJ, MacGregor AS, Hau CM, et al. The role of haematological factors in diabetic peripheral arterial disease: the Edinburgh artery study. Br J Haematol 1999;105(3):648–654.
27. Kannel WB, McGee DL. Update on some epdemiologic features of intermittant claudication: the Framingham Study. J Am Geriatr Soc 1985;33(1):13–18.
28. Ogren M, Hedblad B, Isacsson SO, Janzon L, Jungquist G, Lindell SE. Non-invasively detected carotid stenosis and ischaemic heart disease in men with leg arteriosclerosis. Lancet 1993;342(8880):1138–1141.
29. Newman AB, Siscovick DS, Monolio TA, et al. Ankle-arm index as a marker of atherosclerosis in the Cardiovascular Health Study. Cardiovascular Heart Study (CHS) Collaborative Researac Group. Circulation 1993;88:837–845.
30. Adler AI, Stratton IM, Neil HA, et al., on behalf of the the UK Prospective Diabetes Study Group. Association of systolic blood pressure with macrovascular and microvascular complications of type 2 diabetes (UKPDS 36): prospective observational study. BMJ 2000;321:412–419.
31. Aschoff L. Observations concerning the relationship between cholesterol metabolism and vascular disease. BMJ 1932;2:1121.
32. Malinow MR, Kang SS, Taylor LM, et al. Prevalence of hyperhomo-cyst(e)inemia in patients with peripheral occlusive disease. Circulation 1989;79:1180–1188.

33. Robinson K, Arheart K, Refsum H, et al. Low circulating folate and vitamin B6 concentrations: risk factors for stroke, peripheral vascular disease, and coronary artery disease. European COMAC Group [see comments]. Circulation 1998;97(5):437–443.

34. Schnyder G, Roffi M, Flammer Y, Pin R, Hess OM. Effect of homocysteine-lowering therapy with folic acid, vitamin B12, vitamin B6 on clinical outcome after percutaneous coronary intervention. JAMA 2002;288(8):973–979.

35. Lowe GD, Dawes J, Donnan PT, Lennie SE, Housley SE. Blood viscosity, fibrinogen, and activation of coagulation and leukocytes in peripheral arterial disease and the normal population in the Edinburgh Artery Study. Circulation 1993;87:1915–1920.

36. Lee AJ, Fowkes FG, Lowe GD, Rumley A. Fibrin D-dimer, haemostatic factors and peripheral arterial disease. Thromb Haemost 1995;74:828–832.

37. Cook PJ, Lip GY. Lip, Infectious agents and atherosclerotic vascular disease. QJM 1996;89(10):727–735.

38. Gibbs RG, Carey N, Davies AH. Chlamydia pneumoniae and vascular disease. Br J Surg 1998;85(9): 1191–1197.

39. Martyn CN, Gale CR, Jespersen S, Sherriff SB. Impaired fetal growth and atherosclerosis of carotid and peripheral arteries. Lancet 1998;352(9123):173–178.

40. Hales CN, Desai M, Ozanne SE. The Thrifty Phenotype hypothesis: how does it look after 5 years? Diabet Med 1997;14(3):189–195.

41. Bainton D, Sweetman P, Baker I, Elwood P. Peripheral vascular disease: consequence for survival and association with risk factors in the Speedwell prospective heart disease study. Br Heart J 1994;72(2):128–132.

42. Allan PL, Mowbray PI, Lee AJ, Fowkes GR. Relationship between carotid intima-media thickness and symptomatic and asymptomatic peripheral arterial disease. The Edinburgh Artery Study. Stroke 1997;28(2):348–353.

43. Peabody CN, Karrnel WB, McNamara PM. Intermittant claudication. Surgical significance. Arch Surg 1974;109(5): 693–697.

44. Szilagyi DE, Smith RF, Elliott JP, Brown F, Dietz P. Autogenous vein grafting in femorpopliteal atherosclerosis: the limits of its effectiveness. Surgery 1979;86:836–851.

45. DeWeese JA, Rob CG. Autogenous venous grafts ten years later. Surgery 1977;82(6):755–784.

46. Criqui MH, Langer RD, Fronek A, et al. Mortality over a period of 10 years in patients with peripheral arterial disease. N Engl J Med 1992;326(6):381–386.

47. Simonsick EM, Guralnik JM, Hennekens CH, Wallace RB, Ostfeld AM. Intermittent claudication and subsequent cardiovascular disease in the elderly. J Gerontol A Biol Sci Med Sci 1995;50A:M17–M22.

48. Howell MA, Colgan MP, Seeger RW, Ramsey DE, Sumner DS. Relationship of severity of lower limb peripheral vascular disease to mortality and morbidity: a six-year follow-up study. J Vasc Surg 1989;9(5):691–696.

49. Hankey G. Stroke: how large a public health problem, and how can the neurologist help? Arch Neurol 1999;56:748–754.

50. Chambless LE, Folsom AR, Clegg LX, et al. Carotid wall thickness is predictive of incident clinical stroke: the Atherosclerosis Risk in Communities (ARIC) study. Am J Epidemiol 2000;151(5):478–487.

51. Wagenknecht LE Jr, D'Agostino RB, Haffner SM, Savage PJ, Rewers M. Impaired glucose tolerance, type 2 diabetes, and carotid wall thickness: the Insulin Resistance Atherosclerosis Study. Diabetes Care 1998;21(11):1812–1818.

52. Howard G, Zaccaro D, Haffner S, et al. Insulin sensitivity and atherosclerosis. The Insulin Resistance Atherosclerosis Study (IRAS) Investigators. Circulation 1996;93:1809–1817.

53. Sharrett AR, Sorlie PD, Chambless LE, et al. Relative importance of various risk factors for asymptomatic carotid atherosclerosis versus coronary heart disease incidence: the Atherosclerosis Risk in Communities Study. Am J Epidemiol 1999;149(9):843–852.

54. Ebrahim S, Papacosta O, Whincup P, et al. Carotid plaque, intima media thickness, cardiovascular risk factors, and prevalent cardiovascular disease in med and women: the British Regional Heart Study. Stroke 1999;30(4):841–850.

55. Anonymous. Effect of intensive diabetes treatment on carotid artery wall thickness in the epidemiology of diabetes interventions and complications. Epidemiology of Diabetes Interventions and Complications (EDIC) Research Group. Diabetes 1999;48(2):383–390.

56. Anonymous. Intensive blood-glucose control with sulphonylureas or insulin compared with conventional treatment and risk of complications in patients with type 2 diabetes (UKPDS 33). UK Prospective Diabetes Study Group. Lancet 1998;352(9131):837–853.

57. Decline in deaths from heart disease and stroke—United States 1900–1999. MMWR Morb Mortal Wkly Rep 1999;48(30):649–656.

58. Minino AM, Smith BL. Deaths: preliminary data for 2000. Natl Vital Stat Rep 2001;49(12):1–40.
59. Changes in mortality from heart failure—United States 1980–1995. MMWR Morb Mortal Wkly Rep 1998;47(30):633–637.
60. Croft JB, Giles WH, Pollard RA, Casper ML, Anda RF, Livengood JR. National trends in the initial hospitalization for heart failure. J Am Geriatr Soc 1997;45(3):270–275.
61. Alexander CM, Landsman PB, Teutsch SM. Diabetes mellitus, impaired fasting glucose, atherosclerotic risk factors, and prevalence of coronary heart disease. Am J Cardiol 2000;86(9):897–902.
62. Coutinho M, Gerstein HC, Wang Y, Yusuf S. The relationship between glucose and incident cardiovascular events. A metaregression analysis of published data from 20 studies of 95,783 individuals followed for 12.4 years. Diabetes Care 1999;22(2):233–240.
63. Smith NL, Barzilay JI, Shaffer D, et al. Fasting and 2-hour postchallenge serum glucose measures and risk of incident cardiovascular events in the elderly: the Cardiovascular Health Study. Arch Intern Med 2002;162(2):209–216.
64. Qiao Q, Pyorala K, Pyorala M, et al. Two-hour glucose is a better risk predictor for incident coronary heart disease and cardiovascular mortality than fasting glucose. Eur Heart J 2002;23(16): p 1267–75.
65. Isomaa B, Almgren P, Tuomi T, et al. Cardiovascular morbidity and mortality associated with the metabolic syndrome. Diabetes Care 2001;24(4):683–689.
66. Hedblad B, Nilsson P, Engstrom G, Berglund G, Janzon L. Insulin resistance in non-diabetic subjects is associated with increased incidence of myocardial infarction and death. Diabet Med 2002;19(6):470–475.
67. Lundberg V, Stegmayr B, Asplund K, Eliasson M, Huhtasaari F. Diabetes as a risk factor for myocardial infarction: population and gender perspectives. J Intern Med 1997;241(6):485–492.
68. Tavani A, Bertuzzi M, Gallus S, Negri E, La Vecchia C. Diabetes mellitus as a contributor to the risk of acute myocardial infarction. J Clin Epidemiol 2002;55(11):1082–1087.
69. Kuller LH, Velentgas P, Barzilay J, Beauchamp NJ, O'Leary DH, Savage PJ. Diabetes mellitus: subclinical cardiovascular disease and risk of incident cardiovascular disease and all-cause mortality. Arterioscler Thromb Vasc Biol 2000;20(3):823–829.
70. Cho E, Rimm EB, Stampfer MJ, Willett WC, Huf B. The impact of diabetes mellitus and prior myocardial infarction on mortality from all causes and from coronary heart disease in men. J Am Coll Cardiol 2002;40(5):954–960.
71. Lotufo PA, Gaziano JM, Chae CV, et al. Diabetes and all-cause and coronary heart disease mortality among US male physicians. Arch Intern Med 2001;161(2):242–247.
72. Hu FB, Stampfer MJ, Solomon GG, et al. The impact of diabetes mellitus on mortality from all causes and coronary heart disease in women: 20 years of follow-up. Arch Intern Med 2001;161(14):1717–1723.
73. Gillum RF, Mussolino ME, Madans JH. Diabetes mellitus, coronary heart disease incidence, and death from all causes in African American and European American women: The NHANES I epidemiologic follow-up study. J Clin Epidemiol 2000;53(5):511–518.
74. Gillum RF, Mussolino ME, Madans JH. Coronary heart disease incidence and survival in African-American women and men. The NHANES I Epidemiologic Follow-up Study. Ann Intern Med 1997;127(2):111–118.
75. Ethnicity and cardiovascular disease. The incidence of myocardial infarction in white, South Asian, and Afro-Caribbean patients with type 2 diabetes (U.K. Prospective Diabetes Study 32). Diabetes Care 1998;21(8):1271–1277.
76. Turner RC, Millns H, Neil HA, et al. Risk factors for coronary artery disease in non-insulin dependent diabetes mellitus: United Kingdom Prospective Diabetes Study (UKPDS: 23). BMJ 1998;316(7134):823–828.
77. Haffner SM. Lipoprotein disorders associated with type 2 diabetes mellitus and insulin resistance. Am J Cardiol 2002;90(8A):55i–61i.
78. Solfrizzi V, Panza F, Colacicco AM, et al. Relation of lipoprotein(a) as coronary risk factor to type 2 diabetes mellitus and low-density lipoprotein cholesterol in patients > or = 65 years of age (The Italian Longitudinal Study on Aging). Am J Cardiol 2002;89(7):825–829.
79. Laakso M, Lehtos, Penttlia I, Pyorala K. Lipids and lipoproteins predicting coronary heart disease mortality and morbidity in patients with non-insulin-dependent diabetes. Circulation 1993;88(4 Pt 1):1421–1430.
80. Barrett-Connor ET, Philippi, Khaw KT. Lipoproteins as predictors of ischemic heart disease in non-insulin-dependent diabetic men. Am J Prev Med 1987;3(4):206–210.
81. Beckman JA, Creager MA, Libby P. Diabetes and atherosclerosis: epidemiology, pathophysiology, and management. JAMA 2002;287(19):2570–2581.

21 Noninvasive Methods to Assess Vascular Function and Pathophysiology

Peter G. Danias, MD, PhD and Rola Saouaf, MD

CONTENTS

INTRODUCTION

Cardiovascular disease (CVD) carries significant morbidity and is the leading cause of death in the Western world (1). Direct visualization of the vascular system and assessment of its properties has been proposed as a reliable method to evaluate patients for the presence of atherosclerotic disease and to follow-up the effect of medical interventions and therapies. Moreover, evaluation of the vessels and their properties can enhance our understanding of the pathophysiological processes underlying CVD and enable taking knowledgeable steps toward health maintenance and prevention. This chapter will summarize the main noninvasive methods currently used to assess the macrovascular system and its pathophysiology.

The vascular system is a complex and dynamic organ composed of arteries, capillaries, and veins. The arteries are in turn structured in three layers: the intima, media, and adventitia, which are separated by the internal and external elastic laminae. The intima is composed of the endothelium, a monolayer of epithelial cells covering the entire vascular tree. The relative thickness of the media and adventitia, and the content of the vascular wall in collagen and elastin varies considerably depending on the diameter of the vessel. Accordingly, large vessels (aorta, carotids, iliofemorals) are characterized by relatively thick advetitia with abundant collagen and elastin content, although medium and small size arteries (brachial, radial, coronary, renal, and mesenteric arteries) have a more prominent muscular layer and lesser collagen/elastin content. The arterial wall

From: *Contemporary Cardiology: Diabetes and Cardiovascular Disease, Second Edition*
Edited by: M. T. Johnstone and A. Veves © Humana Press Inc., Totowa, NJ

components interplay with each other and so determine the function of the vascular system. In particular, the endothelium carries a most important regulatory function, especially for the small and medium size arteries in both normality and disease (2).

Assessment of the macrovascular system can be broadly categorized into anatomic imaging and functional evaluation of vascular reactivity. An anatomic approach is to evaluate the intima-media thickness, which is feasible noninvasively for arteries that are close to the body surface. One way to evaluate vascular reactivity is by assessing the endothelium-dependent function primarily at the small and medium size arteries. This can be accomplished by inducing and measuring flow-dependent vasodilation or venous occlusive plethysmography. An alternative approach to examine vascular reactivity is to assess the elastic properties, mainly of the medium and large size arteries, under physiological conditions. This can be accomplished with either ultrasonography or magnetic resonance imaging, both of which can quantify parameters such as arterial compliance, stiffness index, pressure-strain and Young's elastic modulus, and pulse wave velocity.

ANATOMIC IMAGING OF THE VESSELS

Intimal-Medial Thickness

An early morphological change in atherosclerosis is the increase of the IMT, which can be detected noninvasively with high-resolution ultrasound B-mode imaging. In early stages of the atherosclerotic process the vessel wall thickens, although the lumen maintains its internal diameter resulting in outward expansion of the vessel, a process termed positive remodeling (3). The lumen gets compromised late in the atherosclerotic process, with the development of diffuse or focal stenoses.

Pignoli and colleagues (4) studied in vitro specimens of human aortic and common carotid arteries to determine the anatomic structures involved in ultrasound energy reflection in the arterial wall and the feasibility of measurement of arterial wall thickness with B-mode real-time imaging. In addition to the in vitro studies, these investigators also evaluated the common carotid arteries of 10 young healthy volunteers in vivo using the same methodology. Imaging was performed with high-resolution real-time scanners equipped with 7–8 MHz probes. The vessels were grouped into macroscopically normal or with fatty streaks (class A), or vessels with atherosclerotic lesions (class B). The ultrasound pattern of class A group was characterized by two parallel echogenic lines separated by a hypoechoic or anechoic space. This scan pattern is defined as the "double line pattern." The inner (luminal) line was generally more regular, smooth, and thin than the outer one. Correlating these findings with gross specimens, it was postulated that the inner line represents the intima, the hypoechoic line the media and the outer echogenic line the adventitia. Therefore, measuring the distance from the inner echogenic line to the interface between the hypoechoic line and the second echogenic line represents the IMT of the vascular wall (Fig. 1). The B-mode measurements of IMT showed a significant correlation with values obtained by gross pathology and histology in both class A and class B specimens. Class A aortic IMT measured 1.22 ± 0.37 mm vs 1.13 ± 0.26 mm by gross pathology; and class B aortic IMT measured 2.06 ± 1.02 mm vs 1.93 ± 0.84 mm by gross pathology.

In early studies assessing the reproducibility of the technique, suboptimal performance was reported (5), with low intraobserver correlation coefficients (0.72–0.77) and poor interobserver agreement (0.48–0.65). However, in the study by O'Leary and colleagues (5), many technologists form different centers obtained images using various

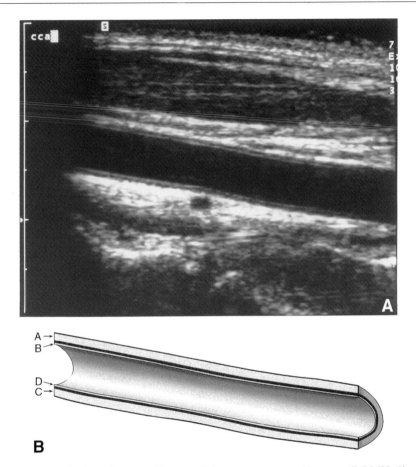

Fig. 1. (A) High-resolution ultrasound image of the common carotid artery (7.5 MHz linear array transducer). **(B)** Simplified diagram of the arterial wall boundaries indicating the adventitia-media (A) of the near wall, intima-blood boundaries (B) for the near wall and adventitia-media (C) and intima-blood boundaries (D) for the far wall.

equipment, and the images were analyzed off line from videotape, largely accounting for the high variability observed.

More recent studies demonstrated the good reproducibility of IMT measurements (6–8). Salonen and colleagues (6) reported an interobserver coefficient of variation of 10.5%, and an intraobserver coefficient of variation of 5.4% to 5.8%. The intraobserver variation accounted for only 4% of the total variability, whereas the remaining 96% was attributable to interobserver variation. Espeland and colleagues (7) also examined the reliability of longitudinal measurement of IMT from measurements obtained in the Asymptomatic Carotid Artery Progression Study. These investigators concurred that serial IMT data were highly reliable, demonstrating that multicenter studies using B-mode measurements are feasible and valid.

A more recent evaluation of the reproducibility of the technique for assessment of carotid IMT (9) examined different anatomic locations along the carotid artery, to identify which segment offers more robust measurements. It was concluded that evaluation of the common carotid artery is more reproducible than the bulbus and the internal carotid artery, likely as a result of better visualization. Based on these results, it may be prudent to serially measure the common carotid IMT in longitudinal studies assessing vascular pathology.

Application

Using B-mode ultrasound imaging, Howard and colleagues *(10)* examined the incidence of carotid atherosclerosis in the general population. The median wall thickness ranged from 0.5 to 1 mm at all ages, with more than 5% of the cohort having carotid wall thickness more than 2mm. Cross-sectional analysis suggested that age-related increases in wall thickness averaged approx 0.015 mm per year in women and 0.018 mm per year in men at the carotid bifurcation, 0.010 mm per year in women and 0.014 mm per year in men at the internal carotid artery, and 0.010 mm per year in both genders at the common carotid artery.

The association of IMT with conventional risk factors for atherosclerosis, including diabetes, hyperglycemia and fasting insulin, but also body mass index, waist-to-hip circumference ratio, and physical inactivity has been reported *(11)*. Abdominal adiposity, physical inactivity, and abnormal glucose metabolism are associated positively with carotid IMT, in line with their believed contribution to atherogenesis. Similarly, the Atherosclerosis Risk in Communities study showed that wall thickness is strongly associated with atherogenic lipids, tobacco smoking, and hypertension *(12)*, suggesting that the atherosclerotic process is reflected in the IMT measurements.

The prognostic value of IMT has been prospectively evaluated, and in multiple studies, increased IMT has been shown to be associated with increased cardiovascular morbidity (incidence of stroke and myocardial infarction [MI]) *(13–17)*. In a study involving more han 4400 subjects from the Cardiovascular Health Study with age over 65 years and no known CVD, IMT was a predictor of new stroke or heart attack, even after adjusting for traditional cardiovascular risk factors *(17)*.

ASSESSMENT OF VASCULAR REACTIVITY/ENDOTHELIAL FUNCTION

Flow-Mediated Vasodilation

The endothelium is an active paracrine organ. Among other functions, the endothelium maintains vasodilation and inhibits platelet aggregation and smooth muscle cell proliferation, through the release of the endothelium-derived relaxing factor (EDRF) *(18)*, now known as nitric oxide (NO) *(19)*. Endothelial cells also secrete vasoconstrictor factors, such as endothelin-1, and factors that affect the differentiation and growth of vascular smooth muscle cells *(20,21)*. Endothelial dysfunction occurs from the very early stages of the atherosclerotic process *(22)*, and may actually precede the development of structural changes of the arterial wall *(23)*.

Furchgott and Zawadski *(24)* first described that in the presence of intact endothelium, acetycholine produced dose-dependent relaxation of isolated arterial segments through the release of EDRF. Subsequently, it was shown that EDRF is NO, which is synthesized from L-arginine by NO synthase *(19,25)*. Various substances, including acetylcholine, bradykinin, adenosine triphosphate, adenosine diphosphate, thrombin, serotonin, histamine, and substance P are capable of releasing NO from endothelial cells. Shear stress or other physiological stimuli that increase blood flow, also act by releasing NO *(26–28)*, resulting in flow-mediated vasodilation (FMD) *(29)*.

With endothelial dysfunction, the ability to release NO becomes impaired *(24)*. Using invasive coronary angiography, Ludmer and colleagues *(30)* showed that acetylcholine caused dose-dependent vasodilation in patients with angiographically normal coronary arteries, and vasoconstriction occurred in those with atherosclerosis. Subsequent studies provided evidence that acetylcholine-induced coronary vasodilation in humans is mediated by NO *(31–33)*. In contrast, nitroglycerin is a vasodilator that acts directly on vascular smooth muscle and, therefore, its vasodilatory effect is endothelium-independent *(28)*. Atherosclerosis does not inhibit the vasodilatory effect of nitrates *(30,34)*.

For accurate FMD measurements, overnight fasting and withholding of all vasoactive medications for four half lives is recommended. Typically, the brachial artery is used for measurements, although the use of the superficial femoral, the carotid and the brachial artery has also been described. The diameter of the target artery is measured from two-dimensional ultrasound images with a no less than 7.0 MHz linear array transducer. Two-dimensional gray scale scans are taken at four time points: (a) baseline at rest, (b) during reactive hyperemia, (c) at rest following hyperemia (second baseline), and (d) after nitroglycerin administration at rest. The arterial flow velocity is measured at rest (first scan) by pulsed Doppler interrogation of the vessel at a 70° angle. Distal blood flow is then obstructed with a pneumatic cuff, which is inflated to a pressure of 300 mmHg for 4 to 5 minutes. The release of the cuff induces an increase in peripheral blood flow. The second scan is obtained during the period 30 seconds before to 2 minutes after cuff deflation, including a repeat flow velocity recording for the first 15 seconds after cuff release. Fifteen minutes are allowed for vessel recovery, and a second baseline (third scan) is obtained at rest. Sublingual nitroglycerin spray (400 μg) is then administered, and 3 to 4 minutes later, the final scan is obtained (fourth scan). The electrocardiogram (ECG) is monitored continuously, and used to define end-diastole (R wave of the ECG), at which the vessel diameter is measured (Fig. 2). A detailed description of the technique along with guidelines regarding the performance of FMD were recently published by the International Brachial Artery Reactivity Task Force *(35)*.

FMD measurements have been shown to be reproducible, with low interobserver difference (percent FMD of 1.7% [0%–7%]), and low coefficient of variation (1.4%) *(36)*. Good repeatability has also been demonstrated in normal subjects, in whom FMD can be consistently demonstrated, although the extent of dilation varies. Subjects with abnormal FMD response had reproducible failure to dilate. The measurement error (1%–3%) was significantly less than the difference between normal and abnormal FMD responses (7%–10%).

Subsequent studies have corroborated previous reports regarding the high reproducibility of this technique. Corretti and colleagues *(37)* reported a low intraobserver coefficient of variation (1.9%) for baseline arterial diameter. Another group showed similar directional response to reactive hyperemia and nitroglycerin in seven subjects, but reported higher estimated coefficient of variation (3.4%) between two visits *(38)*.

The brachial artery vasodilatory response has been examined by several investigators *(37,39)*. Using upper arm cuff occlusion proximally to the brachial artery under investigation, Corretti and colleagues *(37)* demonstrated significant vasodilation after 5 minutes of occlusion, whereas 1 and 3 minutes was not associated with statistically significant vasodilatatory response. Leeson and colleagues *(39)* used forearm cuff occlusion distally to the brachial artery under investigation, and demonstrated a linear relationship between length of cuff occlusion and FMD, up to a maximum occlusion time of 4.5 minutes. There

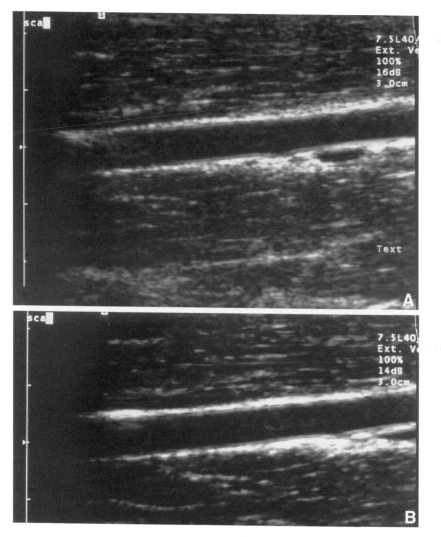

Fig. 2. (A) Brachial artery at rest. The diameter of the brachial artery measured 5.8 mm (7.5 MHz linear array transducer). **(B)** Brachial artery during reactive hyperemia. The brachial artery diameter has increased to 6.5 mm for flow-mediated vasodilation (FMD)% of 10.2%.

was no significant increase in vasodilatation with longer occlusion times. The increase in flow occurred immediately on release of occlusion and the maximal diameter change occurred at 1 minute. Vasodilation persisted for up to 20 minutes.

Saouaf and colleagues *(40)* compared the reactive hyperemic responses in the brachial artery between upper arm and forearm cuff occlusion. This study demonstrated no difference in the vasodilation achieved in response to 5 minutes of ischemia. There was however, a significant difference in the mean and peak systolic velocities that may be reflection of the extent of induced ischemia and increased flow response in conjunction with maximal FMD. Corretti and colleagues *(37)* also demonstrated no significant difference in vasodilatory response or flow when comparing upper arm and forearm cuff occlusion.

Application

Celermajer and colleagues *(36)* first addressed the clinical utility of FMD and demonstrated endothelial dysfunction in children and adults with risk factors for atherosclerosis, before there was any macroscopic evidence of plaque formation in the arteries studied. Children with familial hypercholesterolemia and adults who smoked or had known coronary artery disease (CAD) had significantly reduced or absent brachial artery FMD, when compared with appropriate controls. Nitroglycerin-induced dilatation was present in all groups. FMD has also been used to study endothelial function in relation to CAD risk factors, including essential hypertension *(38)*, insulin-dependent diabetes mellitus (IDDM) *(41)*, and familial predisposition to CAD *(42)*.

The brachial artery rarely develops structural changes typical of coronary atherosclerosis. Anderson and colleagues *(43)* assessed the relationship between endothelium-dependent vasodilator function in the brachial and coronary arteries in the same subjects. Patients who were undergoing conventional coronary angiograms also underwent acetylcholine and nitroglycerine challenge to assess coronary endothelial function. The paradoxical response of the coronary arteries to acetylcholine indicated endothelial dysfunction *(30,44)*, although all coronary arteries showed a normal vasodilatory response to nitroglycerine. Patients with coronary artery endothelial dysfunction or significant coronary stenoses manifested as vasoconstriction in response to acetylcholine had significantly impaired brachial artery FMD, compared with those without epicardial stenoses or with normal coronary endothelial function. Thus, there is a close relationship between coronary artery endothelium-dependent vasomotor response to acetylcholine and FMD in the brachial artery. These data suggest that endothelial dysfunction is a generalized process, and is not confined to vascular beds with clinically overt atherosclerosis. Enderle and colleagues *(45)* also assessed the relationship between impaired FMD and atherosclerotic coronary disease. A decreased FMD (<4.5%) of the brachial artery was shown to predict CAD with sensitivity of 71%, specificity of 81%, and positive predictive value of 95%. Enderle's cut off point of 4.5% dilatation or more was higher, but not too dissimilar to Anderson and colleagues *(43)*.

High-resolution ultrasound evaluation of vessel diameter for the evaluation of endothelial dysfunction has significant potential for assessing usefulness of various interventions. Plotnick and colleagues *(46)* evaluated the effect of antioxidant vitamins on endothelial function. They noted that a single high-fat meal transiently reduces endothelial function in healthy adults and this decrease is blocked by pretreatment with antioxidant vitamins C and E.

The acute response of the endothelial function to several drugs, including estrogen and progesterone *(47,48)*, statins *(48–50)*, angiotensin-converting enzyme (ACE) inhibitors and angiotensin II receptor blockers (ARBs) *(51,52)* and novel thromboxane A receptor inhibitor *(53)* has also been reported.

VENOUS PLETHYSMOGRAPHY

Venous plethysmography or venous occlusive plethysmography is a technique to measure forearm blood flow (FBF) and was first described by Hokanson and colleagues *(54)*. For this method, the patient sits comfortably with the forearm resting at or slightly above the level of the heart. A mercury in-silastic strain gauge coupled to a calibrated plethysmograph is placed at the upper third of the forearm (at maximum circumference). A wrist cuff is used by some laboratories and inflated to suprasystolic pressures to exclude hand circulation. Forearm venous occlusion is achieved by an arm blood pressure cuff inflated to 40 mmHg by a rapid cuff inflator (average venous occlusion pressure is 22 ± 1 mmHg). FBF measured during each experimental period composed at least five separate measurements performed at 10- to 15-second intervals. The experimental arm typically undergoes infusion of various agents in the brachial artery to assess vascular response. Typically, methacholine-induced endothelium-dependent dilatation and sodium nitroprusside-induced endothelium-independent dilatation are assessed similar to what has been previously described regarding FMD. The contralateral arm is used as a control. FBF is typically expressed in mL per minute per 100 mL of tissue, and forearm vascular resistance is calculated as the ratio of mean blood pressure (BP) to FBF. BP is measured via an arterial catheter that is attached to a pressure transducer. Heart rate is determined from simultaneous ECG recording.

Lind and colleagues (55) evaluated the short- and long-term reproducibility of this method to evaluate endothelial function. Ten subjects were studied on the same day 2 hours apart, and again after 3 weeks. The resting FBF obtained 2 hours apart were highly reproducible ($r = 0.91$). The same was found for FBF during metacholine and nitroprusside infusions ($r = 0.97$ and $r = 0.93$, respectively). Comparing the first and second measurements of resting FBF (3 weeks later), the reproducibility was poor ($r = 0.34$), but the values obtained during metacholine and nitroprusside infusions were still highly reproducible ($r = 0.92$ and $r = 0.90$, respectively). These results suggested that the vasodilatory response to metacholine or nitroprusside are not related to resting FBF and are highly reproducible. These investigators evaluated the use of the wrist cuff to exclude hand circulation and reported that it did not significantly influence the evaluation of endothelial function.

Lind and colleagues (55) evaluated the maximal blood flow during reactive hyperemia and concluded that FBF was not related to endothelial function. In that study however, arterial blood flow was occluded for only 3 minutes. To obtain maximal effect arterial occlusion should be maintained for 5 minutes (37,39) and therefore, Lind may have underestimated the vasodilatory effect.

Application

Assessment of endothelial function using venous occlusive plethysmography has been widely used (56–61). The effect of hypertension on FBF has been assessed by several investigators. Most studies (56,57) have reported decreased function of the forearm resistive vessels in response to muscarinic agonists. However, other investigators (62) have reported that selective impairment of the responsiveness of the forearm vasculature to muscarinic agonists is not universal in patients with essential hypertension. The effect of antihypertensive medications on endothelial function has also been investigated using venous occlusive plethysmography. Creager and colleagues (61) and Hirooka and colleagues (63) demonstrated improved endothelial function with chronic and acute administration of ACE inhibitors, respectively. Other agents such as calcium channel blockers, NO antagonists (64), and antioxidants (55,65) have also been used and shown to improve endothelial function and FBF. More recently, the effect of novel thromboxane A receptor inhibitors (53) and intra-arterial leptin infusion (66) on endothelial function (measured by venous plethysmography) has been reported.

Johnstone and colleagues (67) and Smits and colleagues (68) assessed the endothelial function in patients with IDDM and reported that the basal FBF was similar in patients with diabetes and control subjects. However, the forearm vasodilative response to vari-

Table 1
Indices Used to Characterize Arterial Elasticity With the Corresponding Units

Parameter	Definition	Units
Arterial distensibility	Relative diameter (or area) change for a pressure increment	mmHg −1
Arterial compliance	Absolute diameter (or area) change for a given pressure step at fixed vessel length	cm/mmHg or cm^2/mmHg
Volume elastic modulus	Pressure step required for a (theoretical) 100% increase in volume in which there is no change in length	mmHg
Elastic modulus	The pressure step required for a (theoretical) 100% stretch from resting diameter at fixed vessel length	mmHg
Young's modulus	Elastic modulus per unit area, i.e., the pressure step per cm^2 required for a (theoretical) 100% stretch from resting length	mmHg/cm
Pulse wave velocity	Speed of travel of the pulse along an arterial segment	cm per second
Pressure augmentation	Increase in aortic or carotid pressure after the peak of blood flow in the vessel	mmHg or as % of pulse pressure
Characteristic impedance	Relationship between pressure change and flow velocity in the absence of wave reflections	(mmHg/cm) per secons
Stiffness index	Ratio of logarithm (systolic/diastolic pressures) to (relative change in diameter)	Nondimensional
Artery elasticity index	Relationship between pressure fall and volume fall in the arterial tree during the exponential component of diastolic pressure decay	cm^3/mmHg
Small artery elasticity index	Relationship between oscillating pressure change and oscillating volume change around the exponential pressure decay during diastole	cm^3/mmHg

ous stimuli was lesser in the diabetics. These data suggest that there may be an association between the impaired endothelium-dependent vasodilatory response and high incidence of vascular disease in patients with diabetes.

ASSESSMENT OF VASCULAR REACTIVITY/ELASTICITY

Vascular Elastic Properties

The arteries behave as elastic tubes. Many models have been applied to explain the elastic properties of the large and medium size arteries. The oldest one is the Windkessel, a model that has been gradually abandoned as it is unrealistic (the elastic properties are not confined to one site of the arterial tree) and is seriously limited in many circumstances, although it still applies reasonably well for the very elderly and the very hypertensive (69). Under normal circumstances, during each cardiac cycle a bolus of blood is propulsed into the arterial system during ventricular ejection. Flow waves are thus created, which travel distally at a velocity that is largely determined by the elastic properties of the arterial wall and the distal conduit resistances, which induce reflectance waves. Many parameters have been used to describe vascular elasticity (69) and are summarized in Table 1.

To quantify the arterial elastic properties, one needs to obtain accurate measurements of the arterial diameter during the cardiac cycle and an accurate representation of the pulse wave at the site of measurement. Typically, for medium size arteries that are close to the body surface ultrasonography is used (M-Mode, B-mode and phase-locked echo-tracking, two-dimensional [gray scale] and color kinesis). For large size arteries the use of magnetic resonance imaging (MRI) has also been described (including spin-echo, gradient echo cine, and phase-contrast [flow encoded] approaches).

The reproducibility of noninvasive techniques for assessment of arterial elastic properties has been well documented. The ultrasonic echo-tracking system has been shown to have a coefficient of variation of 3.9% to 6% *(70)*. Similarly, the interobserver variability for measurement of the diameter throughout the cardiac cycle was reported to be approx 10% for the common carotid artery, and higher (~15% for the abdominal aorta and femoral artery) *(71)*. The interobserver variability for the pressure-strain elastic modulus and stiffness index (β) has been reported to be higher, in the range of 15%–25% *(71,72)*. Cine MRI has been reported to have better interobserver variability for area measurement. In a study assessing aortic distensibility in patients with Marfan syndrome using phase-contrast MRI, Groenink and colleagues *(73)* reported a variability of only 5%.

Using a conventional spin echo MRI method and a low field scanner, Mohiaddin and colleagues *(74)* demonstrated that in volunteers, mean regional compliance was greatest in the ascending aorta, lower in the arch and lowest in the descending aorta. Aortic compliance decreased with age, although in athletes it was significantly higher than in age-matched controls. Patients with CAD had significantly lower compliance compared with those without significant CAD. Total arterial compliance also decreased with age in those with CAD, although there was more variation in the pattern. This technique was also used to evaluate pulmonary arterial compliance *(75)*, aortic compliance of patients with coarctation following surgical repair *(76)*, and patients with ischemic heart disease *(77)*.

More recently, functional cine images are used to quantify the dimensions of the aorta throughout the cardiac cycle with high spatial and temporal resolution *(73,78–81)* (Fig. 3). Measurement of the peripheral pressure is used to calculate indices of vascular elasticity, including the aortic compliance, stiffness index, pressure-strain elastic modulus, and Young's elastic modulus. One of the main advantages of aortic elasticity measurement by MRI is that it is entirely noninvasive, and can be easily combined with other assessment of the cardiac structure and function, such as quantitation of left ventricular volumes, mass, and ejection fraction.

Application

Lehmann and colleagues *(82)* studied the vascular elasticity of type 1 and type 2 diabetic subjects. Adult type 2 diabetics had less distensible arteries than their normal counterparts. However, the type 1 diabetic subjects who were studied within 1 year of diagnosis had more distensible aortas than the age- and sex-matched nondiabetic controls. Salomaa and colleagues *(83)* concurred that subjects with noninsulin-dependent diabetes or borderline glucose intolerance had decreased aortic elasticity. More recent data on patients with type 2 diabetes and impaired glucose metabolism have corroborated the initial findings in this population. In a population-based cohort including 278 subjects with normal glucose metabolism, 168 with impaired glucose metabolism, and 301 patients with type 2 diabetes, arterial stiffness was ultrasonically estimated by distensibility and compliance of the carotid, femoral, and brachial arteries and by the

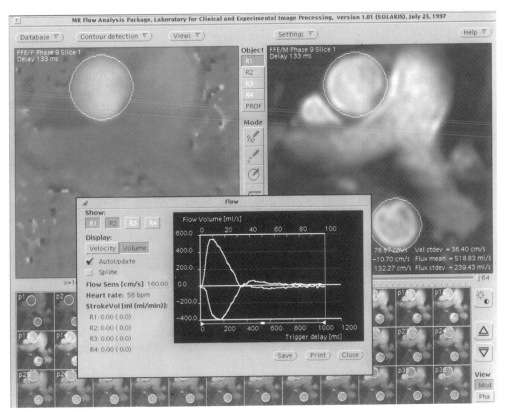

Fig. 3. Magnetic resonance imaging measurement of aortic elasticity. Contours of the ascending (upper circle) and descending (lower circle) aorta are drawn on the right-sided (modulus) image, encompassing the velocity-encoded area on the left-sided (phase) image. Mean velocity and flow can be calculated. (From ref. *73*.)

carotid elastic modulus. After adjustment for age, sex, and mean arterial pressure, type 2 diabetes was associated with increased carotid, femoral, and brachial stiffness, whereas impaired glucose metabolism was associated only with increased femoral and brachial stiffness. These data confirmed that impaired glucose metabolism and type 2 diabetes are associated with increased arterial stiffness, an important part of which appears to occur before the onset of clinical diabetes. This increase in arterial stiffness could not be explained neither by conventional cardiovascular risk factors nor by hyperglycemia or hyperinsulinemia *(84)*.

Lehmann and colleagues *(85)* have shown that young hypercholesterolemic patients have abnormal aortic compliance. It was suggested that the measurement of aortic compliance in this population may be a clinically useful noninvasive tool for assessing susceptibility to atherosclerosis.

Arterial stiffness has been shown to be impaired in young patients with end-stage renal disease (ESRD) *(86,87)*. Hypertension is a main determinant and might be a target for treatment of these potentially lethal arterial wall changes *(86)*. Abnormal aortic elasticity has been shown with a variety of approaches in patients with Marfan syndrome *(88–93)*. Therapy with β-blockers has been shown to improve aortic elasticity in these individuals

(94,95). Abnormal elastic properties have also been reported in patients with Takayashu disease *(96)*.

Further application of this methodology was to investigate systemic arteries in patients with MI *(97)* and chronic heart failure *(98)*. Both studies demonstrated that healthy subjects had more distensible vessels than patients with MI or congestive heart failure.

Danias and colleagues *(81)* has used cardiovascular MRI to examine the elastic properties of young otherwise healthy obese men and lean controls. Obese subjects had greater absolute maximal cross-sectional area of the ascending thoracic aorta (984 ± 252 vs 786 ± 109 mm^2, $p < 0.01$) and of the abdominal aorta (415 ± 71 vs 374 ± 51 mm^2, $p < 0.05$). The obese subjects also had decreased abdominal aortic elasticity, characterized by 24% lower compliance, 22% higher stiffness index (β), and 41% greater pressure-strain elastic modulus. At the ascending thoracic aorta, only the pressure-strain elastic modulus was 31% higher in the obese, but arterial compliance and stiffness index were not significantly different between groups. The differences in aortic elasticity could not be explained by small but significant blood pressure differences between the obese and lean subjects *(81)*.

PULSE WAVE VELOCITY

Another approach to assess the arterial elastic properties in vivo is by measuring the speed of forward propagation of the pulse wave (i.e., the pulse wave velocity [PWV]). PWV is dependent on the biophysical properties of the arterial conduit, and is increased in stiff arteries and decreased in more distensible vessels. The science of pulse wave recording is not new. In ancient China, the importance of pulse palpation in establishing a diagnosis was first recognized. Ars Sphygmica, the science of the pulse, was also established in the Western world from 200 BC, with Galen's texts (18 books on the topic preserved), and then in the Medieaval period by Struthius, who performed the first graphic pulse representation in 1540. The current technique, relative advantages and limitations of the technique are summarized in a recent review *(99)*.

Gosling and colleagues *(100)* used two Doppler probes simultaneously, proximal and distal to the vessel pathway, and the signals were displayed and read out simultaneously. Three parameters were measured from the two simultaneously displayed sonograms waveforms: pulsatility index (PI) = (peak to peak height of sonogram waveform)/(mean height over one cardiac cycle), damping factor (Δ) = (PI proximal)/(PI distal), and transit time (T) = (foot to foot distance between displayed waveforms)/(time base calibration of display).

The technique was further refined by Lehmann and colleagues *(101)* who described a structured and highly reproducible method to measure PWV. A Doppler ultrasound probe (8 Mhz) was placed in the left supraclavicular fossa to interrogate the left subclavian artery close to its origin from the aortic arch. Another probe (4 Mhz) was used to interrogate the abdominal aorta just proximal to the aorto-iliac bifurcation. Doppler-shifted signals from these transducers were processed for directionality and spectrally analyzed in real-time using the dual-channel audio-frequency analyzer. Thus, the "foot-to-foot" time delay between the sonograms was measured with an error of plus or minus 5 ms (Fig. 4). The aortic length was measured by locating the sternal notch and the position of the transducer tip on the abdomen.

Using this technique, the coefficient of variation for repeatability is 2.5% to 11.7% with a mean of 6.3%. The intraobserver coefficient of variation for the aortic compliance

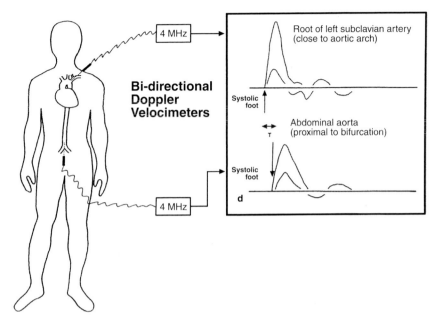

Fig. 4. Pulse wave velocity (PWV) measurements are obtained at the proximal left subclavian artery and the abdominal aorta. Doppler sonogram signals for the same heart beat. PWV equals to the distance between the proximal and distal measurement sites divided by the transit time.

values was 8% and the corresponding interobserver value was 9.4% *(102)*. Wright and colleagues *(103)* reported a similar reproducibility for this technique with a coefficient of variation ranging from 13.7 to 14.4% and a correlation coefficient for two separate measurements of 0.92 to 0.93.

The reproducibility of the Doppler assessment of PWV in various arterial segments was recently evaluated in 15 patients with coronary disease *(104)*. The authors concluded that pulsed wave Doppler analysis is a reproducible method to determine regional arterial stiffness quantified by PWV. There was a gradual increase in PWV from the proximal aorta to the femoral artery. The variation coefficients were low for all segments (4.6%–7.5% for intraobserver and 4.7%–8.6% for interobserver variability), maximum at the ascending aorta and minimal at the iliac segments.

Besides using Doppler ultrasound, MRI phase-contrast analysis can be used to quantify flow velocities at different levels of the same vessel (usually aorta) and the distance between these levels can be accurately measured *(105)*. BP is measured in a peripheral artery, which accounts for most of the errors of measurement with this approach. However, measurements obtained are very similar to the bibliography reported values *(105)*.

A more elaborate approach of measuring PWV in a single heartbeat has recently been described using MRI *(106)*. The method sinusoidally tags a column of blood within the vessel, and rapidly acquires a series single-dimensional projections of the tags as they move (in practice, 64 projections at 4-ms intervals). From these projections, the relative motion of blood at different positions along the vessel is measured. The PWV is then obtained by fitting a mathematical model of blood flow to the tag trajectories. This method was applied to four normal volunteers, in whom velocities of 3.6 to 5.3 m per second were measured *(106)*.

Application

The aging process and the changes in arterial elasticity have been investigated in diabetic and nondiabetic patients *(107)*. There are significant differences in the rate of age-related decline in vascular stiffness in elastic arteries of nondiabetic compared with diabetic arteries. The PWV in diabetic patients increased at an accelerated rate with aging and then reached a functional plateau.

Dietary ingredients can directly affect PWV. For example isoflavones *(108)* have been shown to improve vascular elasticity (decrease PWV), although caffeine worsens aortic elasticity (increases PWV) *(109)*. Folic acid has been shown to improve endothelium-dependent vasoreactivity in smokers and decrease BP, but did not significantly affect PWV *(110)*. Finally, acute vs chronic alcohol ingestion has been reported to have disparate effects on aortic PWV *(111)*.

The effect of antihypertensive medications on PWV has also been reported *(112)*. Patients with mild to moderate essential arterial hypertension were randomized to treatment with 10 mg per day of amlodipine (group 1), 20 mg per day of quinapril (group 2), or 2 × 50 mg per day of losartan (group 3) for a 6-month treatment period. Of the three drugs with comparableBP-lowering efficacy, only quinapril significantly decreased PWV, plasma aldosterone, and the plasma collagen I metabolite carboxy propeptide. Other investigators have reported that ACE-I and ARBs have comparable effect on aortic PWV *(113)*. Non-antihypertensive medications, such as statins *(114)*, have also been shown to have favorable effects on PWV

In patients with ESRD, abnormal PWV has been shown to be a poor prognostic marker *(115,116)*. PWV has also been shown to be a strong predictor of cardiovascular events in hypertensive patients without renal dysfunction. In a longitudinal study, 1715 essential hypertensive patients with no overt CVD or symptoms who had PWV measured at entry were followed up for a mean 7.9 years *(117)*. PWV significantly predicted the occurrence of stroke death in the whole population. There was a relative risk increase of 1.72 (95% CI, 1.48–1.96; $p < 0.0001$) for each standard deviation increase in PWV (4 m per second). The predictive value of PWV remained significant (RR = 1.39 [95% CI, 1.08–1.72]; p = 0.02) after full adjustment for classic cardiovascular risk factors, including age, cholesterol, diabetes, smoking, meanBP, and pulse pressure. Similar results were reported by Boutouyrie and colleagues *(118)*, who in 1045 patients with hypertension, using a multivariate analysis, found that PWV remained significantly associated with the occurrence of a coronary event after adjustment either of Framingham score (for 3.5 m per second: RR, 1.34; 95% CI, 1.01–1.79; p = 0.039) or classic risk factors (for 3.5 m per second: RR, 1.39; 95% CI, 1.08–1.79; p = 0.01). Parallel results were observed for all cardiovascular events.

In diabetics or patients with impaired glucose tolerance, age, sex, and systolic blood pressure (SBP) predicted mortality; the addition of PWV independently predicted all-cause and cardiovascular mortality (hazard ratio 1.08, 95% CI 1.03 to 1.14 for each 1 m per second increase) but displaced SBP as a predictor of outcome *(119)*.

CONCLUSIONS

Several methods are available to evaluate the macrovasculature both anatomically and functionally. Abnormal vascular properties can be identified in patients with CVD and those with predisposing conditions, even before atherosclerosis becomes clinically evident. Furthermore, indices of vascular structure and function have been shown to have prognostic value in patients with or at high risk for atherosclerosis. Various medical interventions with proven benefit for these patients have been demonstrated to improve vascular properties. Further research is needed to expand our understanding of the pathophysiological changes associated with atherogenesis and to validate how measurements related to the macrovascular system can be used on an individual patient level, to guide optimal therapy and follow-up for assessment of progression or regression of vascular disease.

REFERENCES

1. American Heart Association. 2002 Heart and Stroke Statistical Update. Dallas, TX, 2002.
2. Haller H. Endothelial function. General considerations. Drugs 1997;53(Suppl 1):1–10.
3. Glagov S, Weisenberg E, Zarins CK, Stankunavicius R, Kolettis GJ. Compensatory enlargement of human atherosclerotic coronary arteries. N Engl J Med 1987;316:1371–1375.
4. Pignoli P, Tremoli E, Poli A, Oreste P, Paoletti R. Intimal plus medial thickness of the arterial wall: a direct measurement with ultrasound imaging. Circulation 1986;74:1399–1406.
5. O'Leary DH, Bryan FA, Goodison MW, et al. Measurement variability of carotid atherosclerosis: real-time (B-mode) ultrasonography and angiography. Stroke 1987;18:1011–1017.
6. Salonen R, Haapanen A, Salonen JT. Measurement of intima-media thickness of common carotid arteries with high-resolution B-mode ultrasonography: inter- and intra-observer variability. Ultrasound Med Biol 1991;17:225–230.
7. Espeland MA, Craven TE, Riley WA, Corson J, Romont A, Furberg CD. Reliability of longitudinal ultrasonographic measurements of carotid intimal-medial thicknesses. Asymptomatic Carotid Artery Progression Study Research Group. Stroke 1996;27:480–485.
8. Riley WA, Barnes RW, Applegate WB, et al. Reproducibility of noninvasive ultrasonic measurement of carotid atherosclerosis. The Asymptomatic Carotid Artery Plaque Study. Stroke 1992;23:1062–1068.
9. Montauban van Swijndregt AD, De Lange EE, De Groot E, Ackerstaff RG. An in vivo evaluation of the reproducibility of intima-media thickness measurements of the carotid artery segments using B-mode ultrasound. Ultrasound Med Biol 1999;25:323–330.
10. Howard G, Sharrett AR, Heiss G, et al. Carotid artery intimal-medial thickness distribution in general populations as evaluated by B-mode ultrasound. ARIC Investigators. Stroke 1993;24:1297–1304.
11. Folsom AR, Eckfeldt JH, Weitzman S, et al. Relation of carotid artery wall thickness to diabetes mellitus, fasting glucose and insulin, body size, and physical activity. Atherosclerosis Risk in Communities (ARIC) Study Investigators. Stroke 1994;25:66–73.
12. Heiss G, Sharrett AR, Barnes R, Chambless LE, Szklo M, Alzola C. Carotid atherosclerosis measured by B-mode ultrasound in populations: associations with cardiovascular risk factors in the ARIC study. Am J Epidemiol 1991;134:250–256.
13. Salonen JT, Salonen R. Ultrasonographically assessed carotid morphology and the risk of coronary heart disease. Arterioscler Thromb 1991;11:1245–1249.
14. Chambless LE, Heiss G, Folsom AR, et al. Association of coronary heart disease incidence with carotid arterial wall thickness and major risk factors: the Atherosclerosis Risk in Communities (ARIC) Study, 1987–1993. Am J Epidemiol 1997;146:483–494.
15. Bots ML, Hoes AW, Koudstaal PJ, Hofman A, Grobbee DE. Common carotid intima-media thickness and risk of stroke and myocardial infarction: the Rotterdam Study. Circulation 1997;96:1432–1437.
16. Hodis HN, Mack WJ, LaBree L, et al. The role of carotid arterial intima-media thickness in predicting clinical coronary events. Ann Intern Med 1998;128:262–269.
17. O'Leary DH, Polak JF, Kronmal RA, Manolio TA, Burke GL, Wolfson SK, Jr. Carotid-artery intima and media thickness as a risk factor for myocardial infarction and stroke in older adults. Cardiovascular Health Study Collaborative Research Group. N Engl J Med 1999;340:14–22.
18. Moncada S, Higgs A. The L-arginine-nitric oxide pathway. N Engl J Med 1993;329:2002–2012.
19. Ignarro LJ, Byrns RE, Buga GM, Wood KS. Endothelium-derived relaxing factor from pulmonary artery and vein possesses pharmacologic and chemical properties identical to those of nitric oxide radical. Circ Res 1987;61:866–879.
20. Luscher TF, Barton M. Biology of the endothelium. Clin Cardiol 1997;20:II-3–II-10.
21. Brutsaert DL. Cardiac endothelial-myocardial signaling: its role in cardiac growth, contractile performance, and rhythmicity. Physiol Rev 2003;83:59–115.

22. Healy B. Endothelial cell dysfunction: an emerging endocrinopathy linked to coronary disease. J Am Coll Cardiol 1990;16:357–358.

23. Ross R. The pathogenesis of atherosclerosis: a perspective for the 1990s. Nature 1993;362:801–809.

24. Furchgott RF, Zawadzki JV. The obligatory role of endothelial cells in the relaxation of arterial smooth muscle by acetylcholine. Nature 1980;288:373–376.

25. Palmer RM, Ashton DS, Moncada S. Vascular endothelial cells synthesize nitric oxide from l-arginine. Nature 1988;333:664–666.

26. Rubanyi GM, Romero JC, Vanhoutte PM. Flow-induced release of endothelium-derived relaxing factor. Am J Physiol 1986;250:H1145–H1149.

27. Pohl U, Holtz J, Busse R, Bassenge E. Crucial role of endothelium in the vasodilator response to increased flow in vivo. Hypertension 1986;8:37–44.

28. Inoue T, Tomoike H, Hisano K, Nakamura M. Endothelium determines flow-dependent dilation of the epicardial coronary artery in dogs. J Am Coll Cardiol 1988;11:187–191.

29. Laurent S, Lacolley P, Brunel P, Laloux B, Pannier B, Safar M. Flow-dependent vasodilation of brachial artery in essential hypertension. Am J Physiol 1990;258:H1004–H1011.

30. Ludmer PL, Selwyn AP, Shook TL, et al. Paradoxical vasoconstriction induced by acetylcholine in atherosclerotic coronary arteries. N Engl J Med 1986;315:1046–1051.

31. Hodgson JM, Marshall JJ. Direct vasoconstriction and endothelium-dependent vasodilation. Mechanisms of acetylcholine effects on coronary flow and arterial diameter in patients with nonstenotic coronary arteries. Circulation 1989;79:1043–1051.

32. Collins P, Burman J, Chung HI, Fox K. Hemoglobin inhibits endothelium-dependent relaxation to acetylcholine in human coronary arteries in vivo. Circulation 1993;87:80–85.

33. Lefroy DC, Crake T, Uren NG, Davies GJ, Maseri A. Effect of inhibition of nitric oxide synthesis on epicardial coronary artery caliber and coronary blood flow in humans. Circulation 1993;88:43–54.

34. Nabel EG, Selwyn AP, Ganz P. Large coronary arteries in humans are responsive to changing blood flow: an endothelium-dependent mechanism that fails in patients with atherosclerosis. J Am Coll Cardiol 1990;16:349–356.

35. Corretti MC, Anderson TJ, Benjamin EJ, et al. Guidelines for the ultrasound assessment of endothelial-dependent flow-mediated vasodilation of the brachial artery: a report of the International Brachial Artery Reactivity Task Force. J Am Coll Cardiol 2002;39:257–265.

36. Celermajer DS, Sorensen KE, Gooch VM, et al. Non-invasive detection of endothelial dysfunction in children and adults at risk of atherosclerosis. Lancet 1992;340:1111–1115.

37. Corretti MC, Plotnick GD, Vogel RA. Technical aspects of evaluating brachial artery vasodilatation using high-frequency ultrasound. Am J Physiol 1995;268:H1397–H1404.

38. Li J, Zhao SP, Li XP, Zhuo QC, Gao M, Lu SK. Non-invasive detection of endothelial dysfunction in patients with essential hypertension. Int J Cardiol 1997;61:165–169.

39. Leeson P, Thorne S, Donald A, Mullen M, Clarkson P, Deanfield J. Non-invasive measurement of endothelial function: effect on brachial artery dilatation of graded endothelial dependent and independent stimuli. Heart 1997;78:22–27.

40. Saouaf R, Arora S, Smakowski P, Caballero AE, Veves A. Reactive hyperemic response of the brachial artery: comparison of proximal and distal occlusion. Acad Radiol 1998;5:556–560.

41. Veves A, Saouaf R, Donaghue VM, et al. Aerobic exercise capacity remains normal despite impaired endothelial function in the micro- and macrocirculation of physically active IDDM patients. Diabetes 1997;46:1846–1852.

42. Clarkson P, Celermajer DS, Powe AJ, Donald AE, Henry RM, Deanfield JE. Endothelium-dependent dilatation is impaired in young healthy subjects with a family history of premature coronary disease. Circulation 1997;96:3378–3383.

43. Anderson TJ, Uehata A, Gerhard MD, et al. Close relation of endothelial function in the human coronary and peripheral circulations. J Am Coll Cardiol 1995;26:1235–1241.

44. Yasue H, Matsuyama K, Okumura K, Morikami Y, Ogawa H. Responses of angiographically normal human coronary arteries to intracoronary injection of acetylcholine by age and segment. Possible role of early coronary atherosclerosis. Circulation 1990;81:482–490.

45. Enderle MD, Schroeder S, Ossen R, et al. Comparison of peripheral endothelial dysfunction and intimal media thickness in patients with suspected coronary artery disease. Heart 1998;80:349–354.

46. Plotnick GD, Corretti MC, Vogel RA. Effect of antioxidant vitamins on the transient impairment of endothelium-dependent brachial artery vasoactivity following a single high-fat meal. Jama 1997;278:1682–1686.

47. Gerhard M, Walsh BW, Tawakol A, et al. Estradiol therapy combined with progesterone and endothelium-dependent vasodilation in postmenopausal women. Circulation 1998;98:1158–1163.

48. Koh KK, Cardillo C, Bui MN, et al. Vascular effects of estrogen and cholesterol-lowering therapies in hypercholesterolemic postmenopausal women. Circulation 1999;99:354–360.

49. Kosch M, Barenbrock M, Suwelack B, Schaefer RM, Rahn KH, Hausberg M. Effect of a 3-year therapy with the 3-hydroxy-3-methylglutaryl coenzyme a reductase-inhibitor fluvastatin on endothelial function and distensibility of large arteries in hypercholesterolemic renal transplant recipient. Am J Kidney Dis 2003;41:1088–1096.

50. Jarvisalo MJ, Toikka JO, Vasankari T, et al. HMG CoA reductase inhibitors are related to improved systemic endothelial function in coronary artery disease. Atherosclerosis 1999;147:237–242.

51. Wilmink HW, Banga JD, Hijmering M, Erkelens WD, Stroes ES, Rabelink TJ. Effect of angiotensin-converting enzyme inhibition and angiotensin II type 1 receptor antagonism on postprandial endothelial function. J Am Coll Cardiol 1999;34:140–145.

52. Anderson TJ, Elstein E, Haber H, Charbonneau F. Comparative study of ACE-inhibition, angiotensin II antagonism, and calcium channel blockade on flow-mediated vasodilation in patients with coronary disease (BANFF study). J Am Coll Cardiol 2000;35:60–66.

53. Belhassen L, Pelle G, Dubois-Rande JL, Adnot S. Improved endothelial function by the thromboxane A2 receptor antagonist S 18886 in patients with coronary artery disease treated with aspirin. J Am Coll Cardiol 2003;41:1198–1204.

54. Hokanson DE, Sumner DS, Strandness DE, Jr. An electrically calibrated plethysmograph for direct measurement of limb blood flow. IEEE Trans Biomed Eng 1975;22:25–29.

55. Lind L, Sarabi M, Millgard J. Methodological aspects of the evaluation of endothelium-dependent vasodilatation in the human forearm. Clin Physiol 1998;18:81–78.

56. Linder L, Kiowski W, Buhler FR, Luscher TF. Indirect evidence for release of endothelium-derived relaxing factor in human forearm circulation in vivo. Blunted response in essential hypertension. Circulation 1990;81:1762–1767.

57. Panza JA, Quyyumi AA, Brush JE, Jr, Epstein SE. Abnormal endothelium-dependent vascular relaxation in patients with essential hypertension. N Engl J Med 1990;323:22–27.

58. Creager MA, Gallagher SJ, Girerd XJ, Coleman SM, Dzau VJ, Cooke JP. L-arginine improves endothelium-dependent vasodilation in hypercholesterolemic humans. J Clin Invest 1992;90:1248–1253.

59. McVeigh GE, Brennan GM, Johnston GD, et al. Impaired endothelium-dependent and independent vasodilation in patients with type 2 (non-insulin-dependent) diabetes mellitus. Diabetologia 1992;35:771–776.

60. Elliott TG, Cockcroft JR, Groop PH, Viberti GC, Ritter JM. Inhibition of nitric oxide synthesis in forearm vasculature of insulin-dependent diabetic patients: blunted vasoconstriction in patients with microalbuminuria. Clin Sci (Lond) 1993;85:687–693.

61. Creager MA, Roddy MA. Effect of captopril and enalapril on endothelial function in hypertensive patients. Hypertension 1994;24:499–505.

62. Cockcroft JR, Chowienczyk PJ, Benjamin N, Ritter JM. Preserved endothelium-dependent vasodilatation in patients with essential hypertension. N Engl J Med 1994;330:1036–1040.

63. Hirooka Y, Imaizumi T, Masaki H, et al. Captopril improves impaired endothelium-dependent vasodilation in hypertensive patients. Hypertension 1992;20:175–180.

64. Rees DD, Palmer RM, Schulz R, Hodson HF, Moncada S. Characterization of three inhibitors of endothelial nitric oxide synthase in vitro and in vivo. Br J Pharmacol 1990;101:746–752.

65. Ting HH, Timimi FK, Boles KS, Creager SJ, Ganz P, Creager MA. Vitamin C improves endothelium-dependent vasodilation in patients with non-insulin-dependent diabetes mellitus. J Clin Invest 1996;97:22–28.

66. Nakagawa K, Higashi Y, Sasaki S, Oshima T, Matsuura H, Chayama K. Leptin causes vasodilation in humans. Hypertens Res 2002;25:161–165.

67. Johnstone MT, Creager SJ, Scales KM, Cusco JA, Lee BK, Creager MA. Impaired endothelium-dependent vasodilation in patients with insulin-dependent diabetes mellitus. Circulation 1993;88:2510–2516.

68. Smits P, Kapma JA, Jacobs MC, Lutterman J, Thien T. Endothelium-dependent vascular relaxation in patients with type I diabetes. Diabetes 1993;42:148–153.

69. O'Rourke MF, Staessen JA, Vlachopoulos C, Duprez D, Plante GE. Clinical applications of arterial stiffness; definitions and reference values. Am J Hypertens 2002;15:426–444.

70. Imura T, Yamamoto K, Kanamori K, Mikami T, Yasuda H. Non-invasive ultrasonic measurement of the elastic properties of the human abdominal aorta. Cardiovasc Res 1986;20:208–214.

71. Hansen F, Bergqvist D, Mangell P, Ryden A, Sonesson B, Lanne T. Non-invasive measurement of pulsatile vessel diameter change and elastic properties in human arteries: a methodological study. Clin Physiol 1993; 13:631–643.

72. Gamble G, Zorn J, Sanders G, MacMahon S, Sharpe N. Estimation of arterial stiffness, compliance, and distensibility from M-mode ultrasound measurements of the common carotid artery. Stroke 1994;25: 11–16.

73. Groenink M, de Roos A, Mulder BJ, Spaan JA, van der Wall EE. Changes in aortic distensibility and pulse wave velocity assessed with magnetic resonance imaging following beta-blocker therapy in the Marfan syndrome. Am J Cardiol 1998;82:203–208.

74. Mohiaddin RH, Underwood SR, Bogren HG, et al. Regional aortic compliance studied by magnetic resonance imaging: the effects of age, training, and coronary artery disease. Br Heart J 1989;62:90–96.

75. Bogren HG, Klipstein RH, Mohiaddin RH, et al. Pulmonary artery distensibility and blood flow patterns: a magnetic resonance study of normal subjects and of patients with pulmonary arterial hypertension. Am Heart J 1989;118:990–999.

76. Rees S, Somerville J, Ward C, et al. Coarctation of the aorta: MR imaging in late postoperative assessment. Radiology 1989;173:499–502.

77. Bogren HG, Mohiaddin RH, Klipstein RK, et al. The function of the aorta in ischemic heart disease: a magnetic resonance and angiographic study of aortic compliance and blood flow patterns. Am Heart J 1989;118:234–247.

78. Matsumoto Y, Honda T, Hamada M, Matsuoka H, Hiwada K. Evaluation of aortic distensibility in patients with coronary artery disease by use of cine magnetic resonance. Angiology 1996;47:149–155.

79. Resnick LM, Militianu D, Cunnings AJ, Pipe JG, Evelhoch JL, Soulen RL. Direct magnetic resonance determination of aortic distensibility in essential hypertension: relation to age, abdominal visceral fat, and in situ intracellular free magnesium. Hypertension 1997;30:654–659.

80. Vulliemoz S, Stergiopulos N, Meuli R. Estimation of local aortic elastic properties with MRI. Magn Reson Med 2002;47:649–654.

81. Danias PG, Tritos NA, Stuber M, Botnar RM, Kissinger KV, Manning WJ. Comparison of aortic elasticity determined by cardiovascular magnetic resonance imaging in obese versus lean adults. Am J Cardiol 2003; 91:195–199.

82. Lehmann ED, Gosling RG, Sonksen PH. Arterial wall compliance in diabetes. Diabet Med 1992;9: 114–119.

83. Salomaa V, Riley W, Kark JD, Nardo C, Folsom AR. Non-insulin-dependent diabetes mellitus and fasting glucose and insulin concentrations are associated with arterial stiffness indexes. The ARIC Study. Athero-sclerosis Risk in Communities Study. Circulation 1995;91:1432–1443.

84. Henry RM, Kostense PJ, Spijkerman AM, et al. Arterial stiffness increases with deteriorating glucose tolerance status: the Hoorn Study. Circulation 2003;107:2089–2095.

85. Lehmann ED, Watts GF, Fatemi-Langroudi B, Gosling RG. Aortic compliance in young patients with heterozygous familial hypercholesterolaemia. Clin Sci (Lond) 1992;83:717–721.

86. Barenbrock M, Spieker C, Laske V, et al. Studies of the vessel wall properties in hemodialysis patients. Kidney Int 1994;45:1397–1400.

87. Groothoff JW, Gruppen MP, Offringa M, et al. Increased arterial stiffness in young adults with end-stage renal disease since childhood. J Am Soc Nephrol 2002;13:2953–2961.

88. Hirata K, Triposkiadis F, Sparks E, Bowen J, Wooley CF, Boudoulas H. The Marfan syndrome: abnormal aortic elastic properties. J Am Coll Cardiol 1991;18:57–63.

89. Adams JN, Brooks M, Redpath TW, et al. Aortic distensibility and stiffness index measured by magnetic resonance imaging in patients with Marfan's syndrome. Br Heart J 1995;73:265–269.

90. Lehmann ED, Hopkins KD, Gosling RG. Aortic distensibility measured by magnetic resonance imaging in patients with Marfan's syndrome. Heart 1996;75:214.

91. Franke A, Muhler EG, Klues HG, et al. Detection of abnormal aortic elastic properties in asymptomatic patients with Marfan syndrome by combined transoesophageal echocardiography and acoustic quantifi-cation. Heart 1996;75:307–311.

92. Fattori R, Bacchi Reggiani L, Pepe G, et al. Magnetic resonance imaging evaluation of aortic elastic properties as early expression of Marfan syndrome. J Cardiovasc Magn Reson 2000;2:251–256.

93. Sonesson B, Hansen F, Lanne T. Abnormal mechanical properties of the aorta in Marfan's syndrome. Eur J Vasc Surg 1994;8:595–601.

94. Groenink M, de Roos A, Mulder BJ, et al. Biophysical properties of the normal-sized aorta in patients with Marfan syndrome: evaluation with MR flow mapping. Radiology 2001;219:535–540.

95. Reed CM, Fox ME, Alpert BS. Aortic biomechanical properties in pediatric patients with the Marfan syndrome, and the effects of atenolol. Am J Cardiol 1993;71:606–608.

96. Raninen RO, Kupari MM, Hekali PE. Carotid and femoral artery stiffness in Takayasu's arteritis. An ultrasound study. Scand J Rheumatol 2002;31:85–88.

97. Hirai T, Sasayama S, Kawasaki T, Yagi S. Stiffness of systemic arteries in patients with myocardial infarction. A noninvasive method to predict severity of coronary atherosclerosis. Circulation 1989;80:78–86.

98. Ramsey MW, Goodfellow J, Jones CJ, Luddington LA, Lewis MJ, Henderson AH. Endothelial control of arterial distensibility is impaired in chronic heart failure. Circulation 1995;92:3212–3219.

99. Davies JI, Struthers AD. Pulse wave analysis and pulse wave velocity: a critical review of their strengths and weaknesses. J Hypertens 2003;21:463–472.

100. Gosling RG, King DH. Arterial assessment by Doppler-shift ultrasound. Proc R Soc Med 1974;67:447–449.

101. Lehmann ED, Gosling RG, Fatemi-Langroudi B, Taylor MG. Non-invasive Doppler ultrasound technique for the in vivo assessment of aortic compliance. J Biomed Eng 1992;14:250–256.

102. Lehmann ED, Hopkins KD, Gosling RG. Aortic compliance measurements using Doppler ultrasound: in vivo biochemical correlates. Ultrasound Med Biol 1993;19:683–710.

103. Wright JS, Cruickshank JK, Kontis S, Dore C, Gosling RG. Aortic compliance measured by non-invasive Doppler ultrasound: description of a method and its reproducibility. Clin Sci (Lond) 1990;78:463–468.

104. Baguet JP, Kingwell BA, Dart AL, Shaw J, Ferrier KE, Jennings GL. Analysis of the regional pulse wave velocity by Doppler: methodology and reproducibility. J Hum Hypertens 2003;17:407–412.

105. Boese JM, Bock M, Schoenberg SO, Schad LR. Estimation of aortic compliance using magnetic resonance pulse wave velocity measurement. Phys Med Biol 2000;45:1703–1713.

106. Macgowan CK, Henkelman RM, Wood ML. Pulse-wave velocity measured in one heartbeat using MR tagging. Magn Reson Med 2002;48:115–121.

107. Cameron JD, Bulpitt CJ, Pinto ES, Rajkumar C. The aging of elastic and muscular arteries: a comparison of diabetic and nondiabetic subjects. Diabetes Care 2003;26:2133–2138.

108. Teede HJ, McGrath BP, DeSilva L, Cehun M, Fassoulakis A, Nestel PJ. Isoflavones reduce arterial stiffness: a placebo-controlled study in men and postmenopausal women. Arterioscler Thromb Vasc Biol 2003;23:1066–1071.

109. Vlachopoulos C, Hirata K, O'Rourke MF. Effect of caffeine on aortic elastic properties and wave reflection. J Hypertens 2003;21:563–570.

110. Mangoni AA, Sherwood RA, Swift CG, Jackson SH. Folic acid enhances endothelial function and reduces blood pressure in smokers: a randomized controlled trial. J Intern Med 2002;252:497–503.

111. Mahmud A, Feely J. Divergent effect of acute and chronic alcohol on arterial stiffness. Am J Hypertens 2002;15:240–243.

112. Rajzer M, Klocek M, Kawecka-Jaszcz K. Effect of amlodipine, quinapril, andlosartan on pulse wave velocity andplasma collagen markers in patients withmild-to-moderate arterial hypertension. Am J Hypertens 2003;16:439–444.

113. Mahmud A, Feely J. Reduction in arterial stiffness with angiotensin II antagonist is comparable with and additive to ACE inhibition. Am J Hypertens 2002;15:321–325.

114. Raison J, Rudnichi A, Safar ME. Effects of atorvastatin on aortic pulse wave velocity in patients with hypertension and hypercholesterolaemia: a preliminary study. J Hum Hypertens 2002;16:705–710.

115. Guerin AP, Blacher J, Pannier B, Marchais SJ, Safar ME, London GM. Impact of aortic stiffness attenuation on survival of patients in end-stage renal failure. Circulation 2001;103:987–992.

116. London GM, Blacher J, Pannier B, Guerin AP, Marchais SJ, Safar ME. Arterial wave reflections and survival in end-stage renal failure. Hypertension 2001;38:434–438.

117. Laurent S, Katsahian S, Fassot C, et al. Aortic stiffness is an independent predictor of fatal stroke in essential hypertension. Stroke 2003;34:1203–1206.

118. Boutouyrie P, Tropeano AI, Asmar R, et al. Aortic stiffness is an independent predictor of primary coronary events in hypertensive patients: a longitudinal study. Hypertension 2002;39:10–15.

119. Cruickshank K, Riste L, Anderson SG, Wright JS, Dunn G, Gosling RG. Aortic pulse-wave velocity and its relationship to mortality in diabetes and glucose intolerance: an integrated index of vascular function? Circulation 2002;106:2085–2090.

22 Peripheral Vascular Disease in Patients With Diabetes Mellitus

Bernadette Aulivola, MD, Allen D. Hamdan, MD, and Frank W. LoGerfo, MD

CONTENTS

INTRODUCTION

The concomitant occurrence of atherosclerotic peripheral vascular disease in patients with diabetes mellitus is a major factor in the progression of diabetic foot pathology. The rate of lower extremity amputation in the diabetic population is 15 times that seen in the nondiabetic population *(1)*. This increased rate is a result of a number of factors present in the diabetic population that leads to foot pathology in a synergistic fashion. These factors include peripheral neuropathy, which leads to structural and sensory changes within the foot; microvascular changes, nonocclusive changes in the microcirculation leading to the impairment of normal cellular exchange; infection, often aggressive and polymicrobial and macrovascular disease, atherosclerosis of the peripheral arteries. Although the underlying pathogenesis of atherosclerotic disease in diabetics is similar to that noted in nondiabetics, there are several significant differences. Of note, the diabetic foot is more susceptible to moderate changes in perfusion than the nondiabetic foot, which results in a greater sensitivity to atherosclerotic occlusive disease. Compounding this scenario is the fact that diabetics have a fourfold increase in the prevalence of atherosclerosis, and a propensity for an accelerated form of atherosclerosis. This chapter reviews the pathobiology and anatomic distribution of diabetic peripheral arterial occlu-

From: *Contemporary Cardiology: Diabetes and Cardiovascular Disease, Second Edition*
Edited by: M. T. Johnstone and A. Veves © Humana Press Inc., Totowa, NJ

451

sive disease, its clinical presentation and the various diagnostic modalities of use in its evaluation. It concludes with a diagnostic and treatment protocol that can be used in patients presenting with this multifactorial disease process.

PATHOGENESIS

The understanding of the basic pathology of atherosclerosis in diabetics has evolved considerably over the past two decades. The commonly held belief that diabetics are prone to "small vessel disease" has been refuted by a number of investigators. This popular misconception, in which the arterioles of the ankle and foot are thought to be preferentially affected by atherosclerotic occlusive disease, originated from a publication by Goldenberg and associates (2). In this retrospective review of amputation specimens from diabetics and nondiabetics, a periodic acid-Schiff staining technique was used to examine the histology of the peripheral vasculature. The diabetic specimens were unique in that that they contained deposits that stained positive in the arterioles of the ankle and foot. These deposits were considered to be atherosclerotic lesions and were felt to be the principle cause of the worsened prognosis in diabetic patients. This assumption partly led to the prevailing idea that because the small vessels, or arterioles, were preferentially involved in the occlusive process, diabetics were not ideal candidates for distal revascularization procedures. In the past, this label of unreconstructable disease has led to unnecessary amputations in the diabetic population.

A number of research studies have attempted to determine whether a diffuse and unique type of atherosclerosis exists in diabetics. In a prospective analysis, Strandness and co-workers (3) performed a blinded histological review of amputation specimens prepared with periodic acid-Schiff staining and demonstrated no difference between diabetic and nondiabetic specimens. Both groups had similar patterns of atherosclerosis, namely a paucity of occlusive disease at the arteriolar level. In another prospective study by Conrad (4), a sophisticated casting technique was used to evaluate the peripheral vasculature. This study confirmed the similar characteristics of arteriolar atherosclerosis in both diabetic and nondiabetic patients. Barner and associates (5) aimed to dispel the theory that the peripheral vascular bed in diabetics was less reactive by measuring the flow rate in femoropopliteal bypass grafts in the two groups of patients. Differences in vessel reactivity after infusion of papaverine into the vascular outflow bed were assessed. Again, no difference was noted between diabetics and nondiabetics. These studies have reinforced the newer theory that a unique "small vessel disease" does not exist in diabetic patients.

Some aspects of atherosclerotic peripheral vascular disease in diabetics are, in fact, different from those in the nondiabetic population. As previously mentioned, diabetics have a fourfold higher prevalence of atherosclerosis, which progresses at a more rapid rate to occlusion. It is also noteworthy that diabetic patients present with the sequelae of atherosclerotic disease at a significantly younger age than their nondiabetic counterparts. Additionally, diabetics often have a unique distribution of atherosclerosis at the arterial level. Occlusive disease in these patients has the propensity to occur in the infrageniculate arteries in the calf. The typically affected arteries are the anterior tibial, posterior tibial and peroneal. These vessels often present with occlusion in diabetics. The more proximal arteries, including the popliteal, are often spared of disease in this population of patients (Fig. 1). Equally important is the observation that the arteries of the foot, specifically the dorsalis pedis, are often spared of occlusive disease (Fig. 2). This provides an excellent

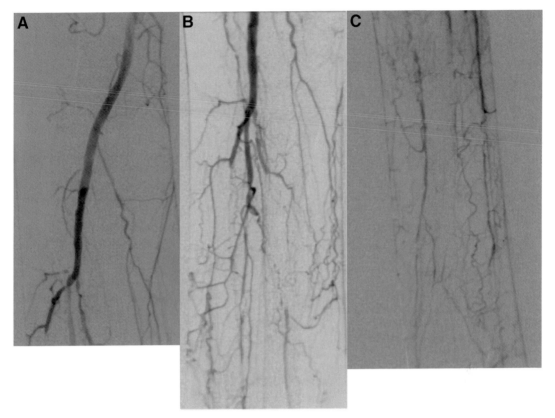

Fig. 1. Intra-arterial digital subtraction arteriogram of the right leg of a diabetic patient with a nonhealing right foot ulcer. Proximal vessels are not shown because they were all widely patent. (**A**) Knee view: The popliteal artery is patent, the anterior tibial artery occludes proximally and the tibioperoneal trunk is markedly narrowed. (**B**) Proximal calf view: The anterior tibial artery and tibioperoneal trunk are occluded proximally. Multiple small collateral vessels are seen. (**C**) Distal calf view: Collateral vessels reconstitute multiple focal segments of the calf vessels along their lengths.

option for a distal revascularization target. This pattern of occlusive disease is a generalization and by no means applies to all patients with diabetes, as some present with disease similar to that found more commonly in nondiabetic patients.

These observations have had a crucial impact on the manner in which peripheral vascular disease (PVD) is approached in the diabetic population. In the past, based on the false presumption of small vessel disease, diabetics were not treated as aggressively with revascularization as is now standard. Because diabetics were thought to have disease at the arteriolar level, bypass to the vessels of the foot was falsely considered futile. As our understanding of the disease process has been clarified, our treatment protocol has evolved. Through our current understanding that the calf vessels are typically more severely affected by atherosclerosis while the pedal vessels are spared, we have been able to modify our approach to the evaluation and treatment of the diabetic patient. A more aggressive attempt is made to identify pedal arteries suitable as distal bypass targets. This, in addition to more aggressive measures to control local infection, has radically altered the prognosis of PVD in the diabetic extremity.

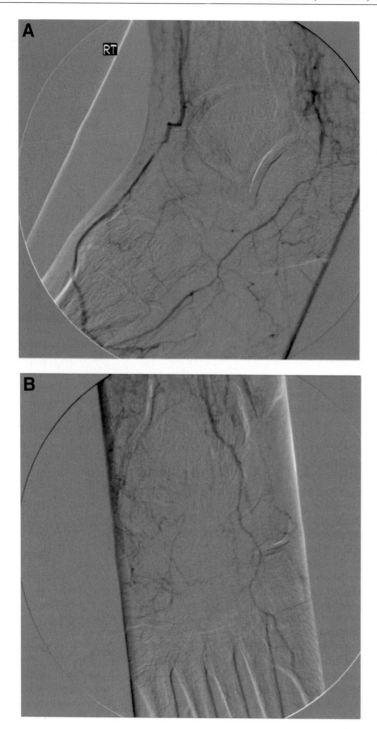

Fig. 2. Intra-arterial digital subtraction arteriography of the foot of the same patient as in Fig. 1. (**A**) Lateral foot view: The dorsalis pedis artery is patent, with runoff into patent tarsal branches. The plantar artery fills through the patent pedal arch. (**B**) Anteroposterior foot view: The presence of a patent dorsalis pedis artery is again seen.

CLINICAL PRESENTATION

It is important to understand the presentation of PVD in the nondiabetic patient to fully appreciate the differences in its presentation in the diabetic population. Atherosclerotic disease is manifest by a continuum of signs and symptoms that can be divided into three categories, in order of increasing severity: claudication, rest pain, and tissue loss. These categories represent the normal evolution of symptoms in the nondiabetic population with PVD. However, as a result of the effects of diabetic peripheral neuropathy, this sequence of progression of symptoms may differ in diabetics.

Claudication is defined as ischemic muscle pain that occurs as the result of inadequate blood flow. This poor tissue perfusion is as a result of proximal arterial occlusive disease, which results in diminished blood flow to the large muscle groups. Claudication of the thighs and buttocks can occur and is a result of occlusive disease of the aortoiliac system. More commonly, calf claudication is the initial presenting symptom. The pain is characteristic and is described as intermittent and cramping in nature. It is often aggravated by exercise and may be relieved after several minutes of rest. The patient's ability to quantify the distance he or she can walk before the onset of symptoms, termed initial claudication distance, is useful in tracking the progression of disease. This assessment is extremely valuable in clinical practice for the follow-up of patients with PVD. Claudication is an important early sign of PVD that should always be elicited in a patient's history. Careful follow-up and monitoring of claudication symptoms can identify patients with worsening occlusive disease before the progression to more severe pathology. Approximately 75% of patients with claudication will not have progression of their symptoms over time.

Rest pain is another symptom of PVD and usually indicates more severe occlusive disease. It is characterized as a burning pain involving either the forefoot or the region of the metatarsal heads. Unlike claudication, rest pain is constant, occurs most commonly at night and is relieved by dependent positioning of the extremity. Patients will often dangle the affected extremity off the side of the bed at night to gain symptomatic relief. Diabetic patients may not develop rest pain or it may be confused with the pain of peripheral neuropathy. The absence of this hallmark clinical sign may delay the diagnosis of severe foot ischemia in diabetics.

Tissue loss is the most severe presentation of PVD. Tissue loss may present in two distinct forms: foot ulceration and gangrene. Diabetic patients with tissue loss most commonly present with foot ulceration. Multiple synergistic factors contribute to the increased incidence of foot ulceration in these patients, including the increased propensity for unrecognized foot trauma in the presence of peripheral neuropathy. It is important to realize that ulceration in diabetics is rarely caused by ischemia alone, a fact that may guide treatment and preventative strategies. All diabetic patients presenting with foot ulceration should be promptly evaluated for PVD. Gangrene seen in diabetics and nondiabetics is quite similar. The gangrenous extremity is a hallmark of severe vascular occlusive disease. The diagnosis of gangrene is easily established on physical examination. The affected extremity appears black and shriveled, is insensate and has no motor function. Without the presence of coexisting infection, gangrene is of little systemic consequence. This is not the case when gangrenous tissue becomes secondarily infected, so-called wet gangrene. This separate clinical entity is characterized by the presence of gangrene in association with signs and symptoms of invasive infection including fever, chills, leukocytosis, erythema, cellulitis, purulent drainage, abscess, and osteomyelitis. Wet gangrene, in contrast to its uninfected counterpart, constitutes a surgical emergency.

Any discussion regarding the presentation of PVD would be incomplete without the mention of infection as a presenting condition. Infection is more often a presenting sign in diabetic rather than nondiabetic patients and may accompany foot ulceration or gangrene. These infections are often aggressive and polymicrobial in nature. They may cause significant tissue destruction and are the most common cause of amputation in the diabetic patient. It is crucial to realize that the signs of diabetic foot infection may be quite subtle. Because the normal immune response to infection is dampened in diabetics, patients with massive invasive infection may not have associated fever, chills, leukocytosis, or erythema. In fact, many diabetic patients with foot infection may present merely with hyperglycemia or an increased insulin requirement. Given these factors, the index of suspicion for foot infection in diabetics should always be high.

PRINCIPLES OF THERAPY

The pathobiology of the diabetic foot can be quite complex. However, successful results can be achieved by adhering to some basic principles of the care of these patients.

Drainage and Debridement

The management of the diabetic patient with foot ischemia should be approached in a premeditated and stepwise fashion. Aggressive evaluation for abscesses involving the foot is key, because, as previously mentioned, the standard signs of infection seen in nondiabetics may be blunted in the diabetic patient. Debridement of dry eschars without evidence of associated underlying infection is not necessary. The initial priority is the prompt and thorough drainage of any infected or necrotic tissue. This can be accomplished either by simple incision and drainage of an abscess or by more extensive debridement procedures, depending on what is warranted by the clinical situation. The goal of these procedures, whether extensive soft tissue debridement or amputation, is the complete eradication of an ongoing focus of sepsis. This may require daily operative debridements to ensure adequate results. Again, one must keep in mind that the signs of continued infection in diabetics are often blunted and accurate diagnosis requires a high level of suspicion. Due to the peripheral neuropathy that accompanies diabetes, some or all of the debridements may be performed without the need for local anesthesia.

Evaluation for Ischemia

The next step in the treatment of the diabetic foot is evaluation of the severity and level of ischemia. This step should not be delayed and may be pursued even in the presence of active infection. The diabetic patient who presents with a foot infection should always be evaluated for ischemia. Additionally, the presence of foot ulceration, even the so-called "neuropathic" ulcer located beneath the metatarsal head, should trigger an ischemic work-up. The absence of palpable dorsalis pedis or posterior tibial foot pulses is an indication of advanced occlusive disease and is a good predictor of the need for angiography, especially in the setting of tissue loss, poor healing and gangrene. In a small percentage of patients, significant ischemic disease can be present even in the face of a palpable foot pulse. In the absence of a palpable foot pulse, bedside Doppler evaluation should be performed and may elucidate the location of the vessels. Beyond the physical examination, various noninvasive and invasive diagnostic modalities are available to the clinician. Noninvasive modalities are preferred for screening and initial work-up. These include ankle-brachial indexes (ABI), pulse volume recordings (PVR), segmental pressures, toe pressures, and transcutaneous oxygen measurements. There are many conflicting arguments regarding the efficacy and reproducibility of these measurements, particularly in the diabetic patient. The continued controversy regarding these tests, in addition to their inapplicability in the diabetic population, has hampered their usefulness in clinical practice. The only invasive diagnostic test utilized in the evaluation of peripheral vascular disease is digital subtraction angiography (DSA). DSA remains the gold standard in the assessment of peripheral arterial occlusive disease. Magnetic resonance angiography (MRA) and computed tomography angiography (CTA) are less invasive alternatives and may be used in patients in whom DSA is contraindicated. This includes patients with severe renal insufficiency or contrast allergy. MRA and CTA have significant limitations and have not yet gained widespread acceptance as replacements for conventional angiography.

Noninvasive Studies

Noninvasive measurements can often yield a significant amount of information regarding the location and severity of arterial occlusive lesions. The ABI compares the systolic pressure of the upper extremity to that of the lower extremity. Using a Doppler probe and a blood pressure (BP) cuff, the systolic pressure in the dorsalis pedis and anterior tibial arteries is measured. The higher of these two measurements is compared with a similarly measured brachial artery systolic pressure. Again, the higher of the two measured brachial artery pressures (right and left) is used in this calculation. An ankle-brachial ratio of less than 1 is considered an indicator of impaired blood flow to the lower extremity. The ABI is of limited usefulness in the diabetic population as a result of the presence of arterial wall medial calcification. This calcification causes the affected arteries to be less compressible than other arteries, such as the brachial, at the same pressure. As a result, the ABI measurement is often falsely elevated and therefore may be unreliable. In some diabetics, the arterial wall calcification is so severe that the cuff pressure cannot occlude the arteries, deeming them noncompressible. For this reason, ABI measurements have limited clinical applicability in diabetic patients, although the thorough work-up for PVD should always include the ABI.

The technique of measuring segmental pressures from the high thigh down to the foot is a popular method of assessing the location of occlusive lesions. This test is performed by placing a series of pressure cuffs at various levels along the affected extremity. The systolic pressure measurements are indicators of the amount of tissue perfusion at the corresponding level. A drop in pressure from one level to the next is predictive of the presence of an occlusive lesion within the arterial system between those two levels. Unfortunately, this measurement is also affected by the arterial wall calcification found in diabetics and therefore may be unreliable in this patient population.

PVR assess the flow characteristics within the arterial system. A series of air plethysmography cuffs is placed along the extremity in question. The cuffs detect the small change in circumference of the leg between systole and diastole and record these findings as a waveform (Fig. 3). A progression from a triphasic to a monophasic or dampened waveform is indicative of occlusive disease. The advantage of this method is the fact that it is not hampered by arterial wall calcification. Although this technique does provide some information, it is mostly a qualitative, rather than quantitative, examination and is difficult to use as an absolute determinant of disease severity.

A

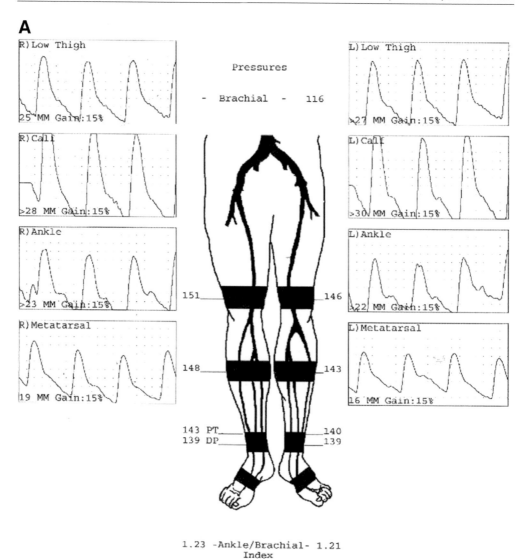

Fig. 3. Pulse volume recording. (**A**) Normal bilateral tracing with triphasic waveform and ABIs more than 1.0. (**B**) Tracing typical of tibial vessel disease with loss of triphasic waveform, drop in pressure measurements from thigh to foot and decreased ABIs.

Transcutaneous oxygen measurements have also been used to evaluate the amount of tissue perfusion in patients with vascular disease. This method has been used to predict the healing potential of the diseased extremity in cases of an existing wound or a potential wound, such as one created by performing a surgical procedure. This test is performed by placing a probe over the metatarsal region of the affected foot. After equilibrating to a specific temperature, the oxygen level is determined. Enthusiasm for this test has been hampered by the large degree of variability noted in the measurements. Many factors, including the site of measurement and the ambient temperature are thought to affect the oxygen reading. However, on review of multiple factors, no one factor was noted to

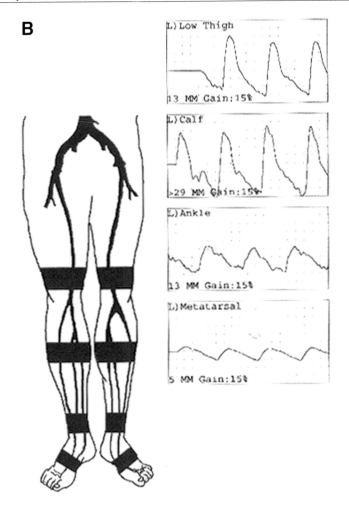

account for the variability in measurement *(6)*. Another review noted that the transcutaneous oxygen measurements were lower in diabetics than in nondiabetics when comparing groups with similar disease severity *(7)*. Although there exists some literature supporting the use of transcutaneous oxygen measurements in the evaluation of the diabetic foot *(8)*, results are difficult to interpret. This has lead to a gray zone of measurements without significant predictive value. The continued evaluation of this modality may lead to a better understanding of its role in the evaluation of the ischemic extremity.

As it became increasingly evident that the vessels of the foot were spared the atherosclerotic changes noted in the more proximal vessels, measurement of digital toe pressures was initiated. Subsequent study has confirmed that toe pressures are not hampered by the coexistence of diabetes. In fact, Vincent and associates *(9)* demonstrated that toe pressure is an accurate hemodynamic indicator of peripheral arterial occlusive disease in diabetics. Although this methodology can be a useful adjunct in the evaluation of vascular disease in the diabetic foot, its use is often obviated by the presence of ulceration, gangrene or previous toe amputation. Additionally, the lack of familiarity with this test at some hospitals also impedes its use.

To summarize, although noninvasive diagnostic tests are quite useful in the initial evaluation of nondiabetic patients with peripheral vascular disease, these tests are easy to misinterpret in the diabetic population. The combination of diabetic peripheral neuropathy and medial arterial wall calcification limits the ability to diagnose and accurately predict the location and severity of occlusive disease. Because the traditional approach to the work-up of peripheral vascular disease is not adequate in the diabetic patient, a separate algorithm in the management of these patients is often required.

Digital Subtraction Angiography

The gold standard in the evaluation of diabetic patients with peripheral vascular disease remains DSA. Intra-arterial DSA is a simple and effective methodology (10). The images of conventional angiography have been greatly enhanced with the advent of this technique, which utilizes subtraction of the bone and soft tissue components to provide better visualization of the contrast column (Figs. 1 and 2). The radiographer can follow the contrast bolus over a greater period of time and select the optimal images, which has resulted in improved visualization of the distal vasculature. In imaging diabetics, the most important point for a radiographer to understand is that, especially in the presence of tibial vessel occlusion, priority must be given to visualizing the pedal anatomy. Angiogram studies are often terminated prematurely in these situations with the misconception that tibial occlusion represents unreconstructable disease. Both anteroposterior and lateral views of the foot should be obtained. Care should be taken to avoid excessive plantar flexion of the foot during the exam, as this may impede flow to the dorsalis pedis artery. The prevailing concern in performing angiography is the risk of nephrotoxicity from contrast agents, especially in patients with pre-existing renal insufficiency. Careful consideration should be given to the type of contrast media used, with options including carbon dioxide gas, ionic and non-ionic agents. Recent data suggests decreased nephrotoxicity with the iso-osmolar dimeric non-ionic contrast agent iodixanol, when compared to a low-osmolar non-ionic agent in patients with renal insufficiency (11). Another important factor in the prevention of renal failure in these patients is the use of intravenous hydration prior to and following angiography (12). In conjunction with hydration, prophylactic oral administration of the antioxidant acetylcysteine has been shown to prevent the reduction in renal function induced by contrast agents in patients with underlying renal insufficiency (13). When renal failure does occur, it is almost always reversible (14), but it may delay the arterial reconstructive surgery for several days while the creatinine returns to baseline.

Alternative Imaging Modalities

MRA and spiral CTA have been investigated as alternatives to angiography in the evaluation of vascular occlusive disease. MRA with two-dimensional time of flight was used to assess the lower extremity vasculature in diabetics in comparison with digital subtraction angiography (15). Although MRA was shown to have acceptable sensitivity and specificity in the evaluation of the tibial vessels, it was not sufficiently capable of identifying patent pedal vessels. Three areas prone to error by MRA were the bifurcation of the peroneal artery at the ankle, the plantar arch and retrograde flow into the lateral plantar artery. These shortcomings are especially significant in the diabetic population, in whom the pedal vessels are often a target for revascularization. The role of CTA in the evaluation of peripheral vascular disease has also been investigated. Some reviews have reported an accuracy of 95% *(16)*. Interpretation of CTA is inaccurate in instances of overlapping leg veins and in the setting of vessel wall calcification. It is also limited by the amount of contrast required to image the vasculature from the distal aorta to the foot. For this reason, studies evaluating CTA have not included the pedal vessels in their evaluation and to do so would likely require prohibitively high-contrast doses. The combination of inaccuracy with calcification and the inability to visualize the pedal vessels makes CTA an ineffective means of evaluating vascular disease in the diabetic population.

Arterial Reconstruction

Once angiography is complete, planning for revascularization is undertaken. It cannot be emphasized enough that, especially in the face of tibial and peroneal occlusion, the pedal vessels should be thoroughly assessed for patency. The fundamental goal of any revascularization effort in the diabetic patient should be restoration of pulsatile blood flow to the foot.

Patient Selection

Once a patient has been evaluated through the aforementioned protocol and a patent dorsalis pedis or tibial vessel identified, consideration should be given to surgical revascularization. It is, of course, important that the site of the planned anastamosis is free of necrosis or active infection. However, patients with necrosis of the forefoot, plantar aspect of the foot or heel may all be suitable candidates for revascularization. Calcifications seen on plain film, specifically those involving the dorsalis pedis artery, should not be regarded as a contraindication to attempt at arterial reconstruction, as calcification does not imply occlusion. Details of the arteriogram are important in verifying the presence of a patent vessel in this setting.

Technical Considerations for Bypass

In the treatment of limb-threatening ischemia, bypass surgery should preferentially target those vessels with direct runoff into the foot, specifically via the anterior and posterior tibial arteries. However, results of bypass to the peroneal artery are also excellent. Given equal caliber and quality peroneal and dorsalis pedis arteries, the dorsalis pedis artery is used preferentially.

In our practice, which is comprised mainly (90%) of diabetic patients, bypass to the dorsalis pedis artery has become the most frequently performed lower extremity revascularization procedure, comprising nearly 30% of all such reconstructions. It should be reiterated that bypass to the dorsalis pedis artery should be avoided in cases of severe dorsal foot infection. All dorsalis pedis artery bypasses in our practice are performed for failing previous bypass grafts or limb-threatening ischemia. Our general approach to vein bypass grafting utilizes distal inflow sites with short, translocated saphenous vein grafts *(17)*. Our experience has indicated that the outcome of bypass is not influenced by the use of *in situ (18)*, reversed, translocated *(19)* or nonreversed saphenous vein grafts. The most appropriate conduit is saphenous vein from the ipsilateral leg, however, other options include contralateral saphenous vein, arm vein *(20),* or a composite of these. Whenever possible, the use of prosthetic graft is avoided. Preoperative duplex ultrasound vein mapping of potential arm and leg vein conduit plays an important role in revascularization planning.

Postoperative monitoring of dorsalis pedis bypass grafts is facilitated by the superficial location of the distal anastamosis. Patients are instructed to monitor the graft pulse by direct palpation over the dorsum of the foot. Routine graft surveillance with graft palpation and duplex ultrasound is performed every 3 months for the first year, every 6 months for the second year, and every year thereafter. Once revascularization has been accomplished, attention should be focused on the meticulous care of the initial foot lesion. Secondary revisions or closure may be required and can be carried out as a separate procedure.

RESULTS OF REVASCULARIZATION

In our series of more than 1000 dorsalis pedis bypasses performed over the past decade *(21),* almost 80% of patients had preoperative nonhealing foot ulcers, of which 30% were infected. Comparable healing rates for both forefoot and heel ulcers have been noted in patients having undergone dorsalis pedis artery bypass procedures (90.5% vs 86.5%) *(22).* Graft failure rate within 30 days of dorsalis pedis artery bypass was 4.2% in our series. Five-year secondary patency and limb-salvage rates were 62.7% and 78.2%, respectively. Of interest, we found that diabetic patients had improved patency rates at 5 years as compared to nondiabetics (65.9% vs 56.3%). In our experience, saphenous vein use was associated with improved 5-year patency rates when compared to all other conduit (67.6% vs 46.3%). Patient 30-day mortality associated with dorsalis pedis bypass was 1%, although the incidence of symptomatic myocardial infarction or acute congestive heart failure was 3%. Our increased use of this revascularization option has correlated almost precisely with a decline in the incidence of all levels of amputations in our practice *(23).* Dorsalis pedis artery bypass can therefore be performed with a high rate of success and low mortality, certainly equivalent to that achieved with other lower extremity grafts.

SECONDARY REVISIONS

Secondary revisions or closure of the open foot lesion may be required following revascularization and is usually performed as a separate procedure. This may involve further debridement, toe amputations, occasional transmetatarsal amputation, local flaps and, rarely, free flaps. In the revascularized foot, even in the presence of diabetes, all of these treatment options become available. The clinician caring for these patients must understand that the bypass operation is only one component of the overall surgical care necessary to obtain limb salvage. If the revascularization procedure is approached as a technical exercise without proper attention to the role of infection and neuropathy, results may be compromised.

SUMMARY

Without a doubt, the care and management of the diabetic patient presenting with the sequelae of peripheral vascular disease is a complex undertaking. A thorough knowledge of the pathobiology associated with the disease is essential. All aspects of the care of these patients, from initial evaluation to diagnosis to treatment must be approached in a manner unique to this population. As our understanding of this disease process has evolved, so has our ability to affect improvement in functional outcome.

Improvements in both angiography technique and results of distal arterial reconstruction have established extreme distal autogenous vein reconstruction to the foot vessels as a safe and effective treatment for limb-threatening ischemia. Accordingly, patients presenting with diabetic foot complications exacerbated by atherosclerotic occlusive disease are now treated very aggressively. Dorsalis pedis artery bypass has become a crucial component of the surgical armamentarium involved in the care diabetic patients, given their predilection for atherosclerotic lesions of the tibial vessels with relative sparing of the dorsalis pedis artery. This approach has led to improved results and a more optimistic prognosis in the diabetic population. A carefully planned approach, including prompt infection control, complete arteriography and arterial reconstruction to maximize foot perfusion, affords a likelihood of successful limb salvage in diabetics that should equal or exceed that in nondiabetics.

REFERENCES

1. Armstrong DG, Lavery LA. Diabetic foot ulcers: prevention, diagnosis and classification. Am Fam Physician 1998;57:1325–1332.
2. Goldenberg SG, Alex M, Joshi RA, et al. Nonatheromatous peripheral vascular disease of the lower extremity in diabetes mellitus. Diabetes 1959;8:261–273.
3. Strandness DE, Priest RE, Gibbons GE. Combined clinical and pathologic study of diabetic and nondiabetic peripheral arterial disease. Diabetes 1964;13:366–372.
4. Conrad MC. Large and small artery occlusion in diabetics and nondiabetics with severe vascular disease. Circulation 1967;36:83–91.
5. Barner HB, Kaiser GC, Willman VL. Blood flow in the diabetic leg. Circulation 1971;43:391–394.
6. Boyko EJ, Afroni JF. Predictors of transcutaneous oxygen tension in the lower limbs of diabetic subjects. Diabet Med 1996;13:549–554.
7. Rooke TW, Osmundson PJ. The influence of age, sex, smoking, and diabetes on lower limb transcutaneous oxygen tension in patients with arterial occlusive disease. Arch Intern Med. 1990;150:129–132.
8. Ballard JL, Ede CC, Bunt TJ, et al. A prospective evaluation of transcutaneous oxygen measurements in the management of diabetic foot problems. J Vasc Surg 1995;22:485–490.
9. Vincent DG, Salles-Cunha SX, Bernhard VM, et al. Noninvasive assessment of toe systolic pressures with special reference to diabetes mellitus. J Cardiovasc Surg 1983;24:22–28.
10. Blakeman BM, Littooy FM, Baker WH. Intra-arterial digital subtraction angiography as a method to study peripheral vascular diseases. J Vasc Surg 1986;4:168–173.
11. Aspelin P, Aubry P, Fransson SG, et al. Nephrotoxicity in high-risk patients: Study of iso-osmolar and low-osmolar non-ionic contrast media. N Engl J Med 2003;348:551–553.
12. Solomon R, Werner C, Mann D, et al. Effects of saline, mannitol, and furosemide on acute decreases in renal function by radiocontrast agents. N Engl J Med 1994;331:1416–1420.
13. Tepel M, Van der Giel M, Schwarzfeld C, et al. Prevention of radiographic-contrast-agent-induced reductions in renal function by acetylcysteine. N Engl J Med 2000;343:210–212.
14. Parfrey PS, Griffiths SM, Barret BJ, et al. Contrast material-induced renal failure in patients with diabetes mellitus, renal insufficiency, or both: a prospective controlled study. N Engl J Med 1989;320:143.
15. McDermott VG, Meakem TJ, Carpenter JP, et al. Magnetic resonance angiography of the distal lower extremity. Clin Radiol 1995;50:741–746.
16. Lawrence JA, Kim D, Kent KC, et al. Lower extremity spiral CT angiography versus catheter angiography. Radiology 1995;194:903–908.
17. Pomposelli FB, Jr., Jepsen SJ, Gibbons GW, et al. A flexible approach to infrapopliteal vein grafts in patients with diabetes mellitus. Arch Surg 1991;126:724–727.
18. Leather RP, Powers SR, Karmody AM. A reappraisal of the in situ saphenous vein arterial bypass: its use in limb salvage. Surgery 1979;86:453–461.

19. Thompson RW, Mannick JA, Whittemore AD. Arterial reconstruction at divers sites using nonreversed autogenous vein. Ann Surg 1987;205:747–751.
20. Faries PL, Arora S, Pomposelli FB, Jr., et al. The use of arm vein in lower extremity revascularization: Results of 520 procedures performed in eight years. J Vasc Surg 2000;31:50–59.
21. Pomposelli, FB, Jr., Kansal N, Hamdan AD, et al. A decade of experience with dorsalis pedis artery bypass: Analysis of outcome in more than 1000 cases. J Vasc Surg 2003;37:307–315.
22. Berceli SA, Chan AK, Pomposelli FB, Jr., et al. Efficacy of dorsal pedal artery bypass in limb salvage for ischemic heel ulcers. J Vasc Surg 1999;30:499–508.
23. LoGerfo FW, Gibbons GW, Pomposelli FB, Jr, et al. Trends in the care of the diabetic foot: expanded role of arterial reconstruction. Arch Surg 1992;127:617–621.

23 Therapeutic Interventions to Improve Endothelial Function in Diabetes

Lalita Khaodhiar, MD
and Aristidis Veves, MD, DSC

CONTENTS

INTRODUCTION

Endothelial dysfunction often marks an early stage in the development atherosclerosis and can be observed in coronary and peripheral arterial beds *(1,2)*. Endothelial dysfunction has been documented in patients with type 2 diabetes *(3–5)* and also type 1 diabetes particularly those who have microalbuminuria *(6)*. Recent data also showed its existence in individuals at high risk for developing diabetes *(7)* (e.g., impaired glucose tolerance [IGT], first-degree relatives of patients with type 2 diabetes and metabolic syndrome) and in women with pervious gestational diabetes *(8)*.

Several therapeutic interventions have been tested both in vitro and/or in vivo aim to improve endothelial function in patients with diabetes mellitus (DM). This includes insulin sensitizers, angiotensin-converting enzyme (ACE) inhibitor, lipid-lowering medications, and antioxidants. Estrogen therapy has also been studied in postmenopausal women. Finally, exercise and weight loss improve insulin resistance and potentially improve endothelial function.

From: *Contemporary Cardiology: Diabetes and Cardiovascular Disease, Second Edition*
Edited by: M. T. Johnstone and A. Veves © Humana Press Inc., Totowa, NJ

INSULIN SENSITIZERS

Abundant evidence has shown the association between insulin resistance and endothelial dysfunction. Prolonged hyperinsulinemia induced by a euglycemic insulin clamp has been shown to impair endothelial-dependent vasodilation *(9)*. Obese individuals without diabetes but with insulin resistance are found to have blunted endothelium-dependent, but normal endothelium-independent vasodilation *(10)*. Thus, treatments that can improve insulin sensitivity have been investigated.

Thiozolidenediones (TZDs), belong to a class of drugs known as peroxisome proliferator activating receptor (PPAR)γ agonists, enhance insulin sensitivity of peripheral tissues (fat and muscle). They are known as insulin sensitizers and are used for the treatment of type 2 diabetes. Recent evidence indicates that TZDs can improve some of the cardiovascular risk factors associated with insulin resistance syndrome, and they also have a direct effect in the vasculature *(11,12)*. Although PPARγ is predominantly expressed in adipose tissue, it is also expressed in endothelial cells and monocytes/macrophages and it is suggested to be involved in atherosclerosis *(13)*.

A study in endothelial-cell cultures using troglitazone, a PPARγ activator, has found that the drug inhibited expression of vascular cell adhesion molecule (VCAM)-1 and intercellular cell adhesion molecule (ICAM)-1. Additionally, it also reduced monocyte/macrophage homing to atherosclerotic plaques *(14)*. In other studies using umbilical vein endothelial cells, troglitazone was found to reduce, in a dose-dependent manner, the expression of VCAM-1, ICAM-1, E-selectin, and plasminogen activator inhibitor (PAI)-1 induced by different amounts of oxidized low-density lipoprotein (LDL) cholesterol and/or tumor necrosis factor (TNF)-α *(15,16)*.

Studies of TDZs on endothelial function have yielded conflicting results. Most of these studies, however, were short term and had small numbers of patients. Avena et al studied patients with peripheral vascular disease (PVD) and IGT and age- and sex-matched control *(17)*. The brachial artery blood flow was measured before and after 5 minutes of arterial occlusion (flow-mediated endothelium-dependent vasodilation [FMD]) during fasting and at 30 minutes, 1 hour, and 2 hours after oral glucose tolerance test (OGTT). At the beginning of the study, patients with PVD and IGT had an abnormal response to hyperemia. After 2 months of troglitazone therapy (400 mg/day), FMD results improved after oral glucose intake during the OGTT but not during fasting. By 4 months, FMD results normalized both while fasting and after oral glucose intake. Similarly, Watanabe and associates examined seven male subjects with abnormal OGTT and six male controls *(18)*. Insulin-resistant males had an impairment of FMD at baseline. After 2 months of troglitazone treatment, an improvement in both vascular response and insulin resistance were observed. Murakami and associates studied 10 diabetes patients with spontaneous or provoked coronary vasospasm and residual angina pectoris *(19)*. Administration of troglitazone for 4 months was associated with a significant reduction in the frequency and duration of anginal episodes and FMD of the brachial artery.

In one randomized, placebo-controlled, parallel-group study of 29 patients with type 2 DM, troglitazone (200 mg per day) increased the resistance of LDL to oxidation and decreased the adhesion molecule E-selectin *(20)*. Another study using rosiglitazone yielded similar results *(21)*. This data suggests that TDZs may have beneficial effects on the vascular wall and may slow down the development of atherosclerosis by modifying LDL-related atherogenic events.

TDZs have also been tested in obese, insulin-resistant subjects. One small study using troglitazone was conducted in an 8-week randomized, double-blind, cross-over fashion

(22). Fifteen obese subjects were included in the study, although only 13 of those had vascular evaluation. At baseline, insulin-induced vasodilation was blunted in obese subjects, but in contrast to other studies, endothelial vascular function (measured by forearm vasodilator responses [plethysmography] to intra-arterial administered acetylcholine (Ach) and sodium nitroprusside (SNP), and vasoconstrictor responses to NC-monomethyl-L-arginine [L-NMMA] during hyperinsulinemia) was normal and did not differ to their lean healthy controls. Not surprisingly, troglitazone had no effects on endothelium-dependent and -independent vascular responses in this study, although it improved insulin sensitivity.

A recent placebo-controlled study examined the effects of troglitazone on the endothelial function in early and late type 2 diabetes *(23)*. Twenty-seven patients who were recently diagnosed diabetes (<3 years) and no clinically evident macrovascular disease, 29 patients with long-term diabetes but no macrovascular complication and 31 patients with documented macrovascular disease were enrolled in the study. The result showed that 12 weeks of troglitazone treatment improved the FMD and fasting insulin only in a group of patients with recently diagnosed type 2 diabetes and no macrovascular complications (Fig. 1). The improvement of fasting insulin levels was strongly correlated to the increase in FMD (Fig. 2). Troglitazone resulted in no changes in nitroglycerin-induced dilation, microcirculation activity, or biochemical markers of endothelial dysfunction (e.g., von Willebrand factor [vWF], ICAM, VCAM) in all three groups.

The effect of rosiglitazone, another TDZ, on endothelial function was tested in insulin-resistant fatty Zucker rats, which displayed hypertension and abnormal endothelial cell function *(24)*. Treatment with rosiglitazone prevented the development of hypertension, improved fasting hyperinsulinemia, and partially protected against impaired endothelial functions in these animals. In humans, a recent 16-week, randomized, double-blind, placebo-controlled crossover to open-label, single-blind study in patients with type 2 DM showed that rosiglitazone significantly increased skin nitric oxide (NO) production and blood flow in the foot *(25)*.

In summary, evidence suggests a beneficial effect of insulin sensitizers on vascular endothelial function, at least for the short term (3–4 months). This effect may not be uniform and may be present in only certain group of populations (i.e., early diagnosed diabetes without clinically evidence macrovascular disease). Currently, there is no long-term data on drugs and cardiovascular endpoint. However, based on available data, further investigation on the role of insulin sensitizers in the prevention and the delay of atherosclerosis in patients with insulin resistance or type 2 diabetes may be warranted.

ANGIOTENSIN-CONVERTING ENZYME INHIBITORS AND ANGIOTENSIN II-RECEPTOR BLOCKERS

ACE plays an important role in the renin–angiotensin–aldosterone system (RAAS) and the kinin–kellekrien system. The RAAS is depicted in Fig. 3. The kidney releases renin into the systemic circulation in response to renal hypoperfusion, produced by hypotension or volume depletion, and increased sympathetic activity *(26)*. Renin converts angiotensinogen, made in the liver (and other organs including the kidney), to angiotensin I, which is inactive. Angiotensin I is then converted to angiotensin II (Ang II). The reaction is catalyzed by an ACE, which presents in the pulmonary circulation, and also in the endothelial cells. Ang II is a potent vasoconstrictor and promotes renal sodium and water reabsorption *(27)*. It also increases the production of aldosterone from the adrenal cortex, which also enhances sodium transport in the kidney. Furthermore, Ang II is a growth factor and potentiates thrombosis.

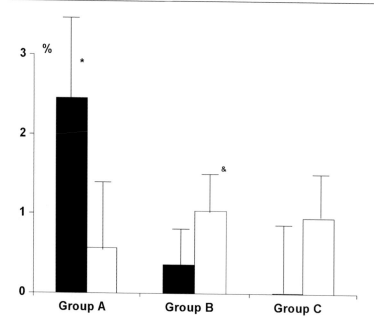

Fig. 1. The increase (difference between exit and baseline visits) in the flow-mediated endothe-lium-dependent vasodilation (FMD) in troglitazone (solid bar) and placebo-treated patients (hatched bar). The FMD was significantly increased in the troglitazone-treated patients with early type 2 diabetes (group A, $p = 0.038$). Additionally, a small, but significant increase was noticed in the placebo-treated patients with long-duration type 2 diabetes without macrovascular disease (group B, $p = 0.046$). No changes were found in the diabetic patients with macrovascular disease (group C). (Reproduced with permission from ref. *23*.)

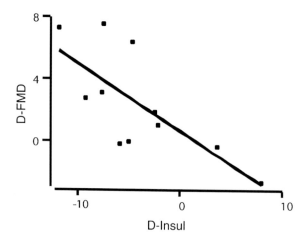

Fig. 2. The increase in flow-mediated endothelium-dependent vasodilation (FMD) was signifi-cantly correlated ($r = 0.73, p < 0.01$) with the reduction of fasting insulin levels in the troglitazone-treated patients with early diabetes (group A). (Reproduced with permission from ref. *23*.)

In the kinin–kallekrein system, bradykinin, a vasodilator, is produced in the kidney from an inactive precursor, kininogen. In the circulation, bradykinin is metabolized by kininases, one of which is ACE *(28)*. ACE inhibitors, therefore increase bradykinin levels

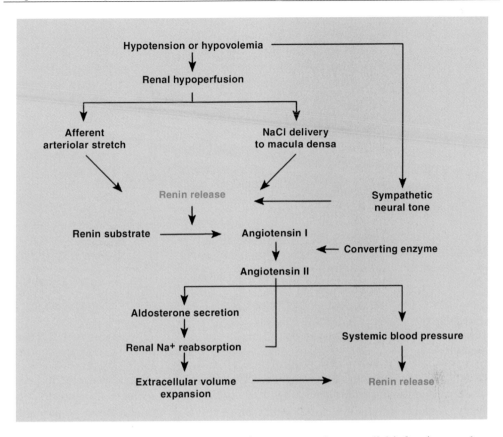

Fig. 3. Kaplan–Meier estimates of the composite outcome of myocardial infarction, stroke, or death from cardiovascular causes in the ramipril group and the placebo group. The relative risk of the composite outcome in the ramipril group as compared to the placebo group was 0.78 (95% CI, 0.7–0.86). (Reproduced with permission from ref. *30*. Copyright 2000 Massachusets Medical Society. All rights reserved.)

and results in vasodilation, mediated in part by release of NO at vascular endothelial cells and in part of the stimulation of endothelial production of prostacyclin *(29)*.

ACE inhibitors have been shown to improve micro- and macrovascular outcomes in patients with diabetes *(30–32)*. The Heart Outcomes Prevention Evaluation (HOPE) study *(32,33)* was a large randomized, clinical trial of 9541 adults at high risk for cardiac events. Subjects were at least 55 years old and had history of coronary artery disease (CAD), stroke, PVD, or diabetes plus at least one other cardiovascular risk factor (3577 had diabetes). They were randomly assigned to ramipril (10 mg per day) or placebo, and to vitamin E or placebo, according to a 2×2 factorial design. The study was terminated 6 months early (after 4.5 years) because of a consistent benefit of ramipril compared with placebo. Ramipril treatment in diabetes lowered the risk of myocardial infarction (MI) by 22%, stroke by 33%, cardiovascular death by 37%, and total mortality by 24% (Fig. 4). There were also significant reductions in cardiac revascularization, heart failure and complications related to diabetes (overt nephropathy). Additionally, treatment with ramipril was associated with a 34% decrease in the development of diabetes in the study population.

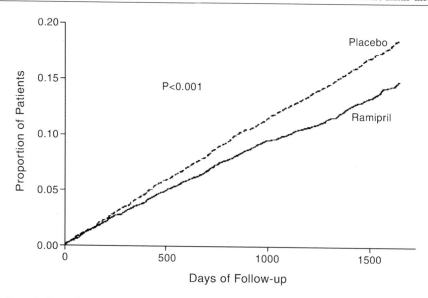

Fig. 4. Regulation of renin release: the renin–angiotensin–aldosterone system and the maintenance of sodium and volume balance.

In contrast, the Quinapril Ischemic Event Trial (QUIET) *(34,35)* failed to demonstrate a similar reduction in cardiac events. QUIET investigated the effects of quinapril 20 mg per day on ischemic events (cardiac death, cardiac arrest, nonfatal MI, coronary artery bypass grafting, coronary angioplasty, or hospitalization for angina pectoris) and the progression of CAD in patients without systolic left ventricular dysfunction. A total of 1750 patients who had undergone successful angioplasty or atherectomy were randomized to 20 mg of quinapril per day or placebo. After the mean follow-up of 27 months, there were no significant differences in the incidence of ischemic events, the incidence of patients having angiographic progression of CAD, or the rate of development of new coronary lesions in both groups. The quinapril group, however, reduced the incidence of angioplasty for previously unintervened vessels. It should be noted that subjects in this study already had advanced CAD and the study itself had several limitation including the inadequate sample size, the low dose of medication, and the short-treatment duration.

Although the mechanisms by which ACE inhibitors reduce cardiovascular risk are not well understood, available data suggest that these drugs exert a cardiovascular protection beyond lowering arterial blood pressure (BP) and suppression of Ang II *(36)*. Experimental and clinical trials show that ACE inhibitors possess pleiotropic properties by having secondary benefits on smooth muscle cell (SMC) proliferation and migration, atheroinflammatory changes, oxidative stress, and NO formation *(37)*. The pharmacological mechanisms appear to be different for various members within this class of agents and this may be a result of differences in binding affinity for plasma and tissue ACE. ACE inhibitors that have high affinity for tissue ACE, such as ramipril, quinapril, trandolapril, perindopril, and benazepril may have more direct effects on vascular reactivity and may directly inhibit atherosclerosis *(38)*.

Several studies have shown that treatment with ACE inhibitors improve the endothelial function in patients with hypertension and coronary heart disease. The Trial on

Reversing ENdothelial Dysfunction *(39)* examined the effect of quinapril in endothelial function in normotensive patients with CAD and no heart failure, cardiomyopathy, or major lipid abnormalities. The outcome was assessed by coronary artery diameter in response to incremental concentrations of Ach using quantitative coronary angiography. After 6 months of treatment, the quinapril group when compared to the placebo group, showed a significant improvement in vascular reactivity. The authors proposed that the benefits of ACE inhibition were likely the result of attenuation of the vasoconstrictive effects and superoxide-generating effects of Ang II and to the enhancement of NO release from endothelial cells secondary to reduced breakdown of bradykinin. Another study (BANFF study) *(40)* of 80 patients with CAD, only quinapril, but not enalapril, losartan or amlodipine treatment for 8 weeks was associated with significant improvement in FMD.

In contrast, current data on ACE inhibitors and endothelial function in patients with diabetes are still conflicting. One study included nine patients with type 1 diabetes and no evidence of micro- or macrovascular disease and eight healthy subjects *(41)*. At baseline, diabetes patients had an impairment of endothelium-dependent vasodilation (Ach infusion). Acute ACE inhibition with intra-arterial enalaprilat enhanced Ach responses in the diabetic patients. After 1 month of oral therapy with enalapril, Ach responses were normalized. ACE inhibition did not affect endothelial-independent vasodilation (SNP infusion). In another study, both enalapril and captopril were shown to restore the endothelial function in normotensive microalbuminuric type 1 diabetic patients *(42)*. In this study, captopril also improved endothelium-independent vasodilation. In contrary, one randomized double-blind study showed that enalapril therapy for 6 months resulted in no improvement in either FMD or glyceryl trinitrate (GTN) induced dilation in young adults with type 1 diabetes *(43)*. Similarly, in a randomized cross-over trial in 20 type 1 diabetes with known endothelial dysfunction, treatment with perindopril for 12 weeks had no effect on endothelial function *(44)*. One study reported a decreased in E-selectin with short-term (5-week) quinaril treatment in normotensive type 1 diabetic patients with normoalbuminuria or microalbuminuria, however, the medication did not affect FMD.

The effects of ACE inhibitors on endothelial function in type 2 diabetes are also not clear, although most of the studies suggest beneficial effects. O'Driscoll and associates studied the effects of enalapril on endothelium-dependent and -independent vasodilator function in 10 subjects with type 2 diabetes and no evidence of vascular disease. Enalapril treatment for 4 weeks increased the response to the endothelium-dependent vasodilator, Ach , and the vasoconstrictor response to the NO synthase inhibitor, L-NMMA45. Similarly, perindopril use for 12-week normalized the decreased vasodilating response to L-arginine, the natural precursor of NO, in patients with type 2 diabetes and mild hypertension *(46)*. In contrast, the data on long-term treatment (6 months) with perindopril did not show a positive effect on endothelial function in patients with type 2 diabetes and hypertension *(47)*. In our unit, we studied the effect of quinaril in 60 type 2 diabetes subjects without long-term complications. The result showed that the medication improved their endothelial function of the macrocirculation independent of any BP-lowering effect (unpublished data).

Angiotensin II type-1 receptor blockers (ARBs) have the theoretical potential to be efficient regarding the vascular endothelial function. ARBs can provide a sustained inhibition of the binding of Ang II to the angiotensin-1 (AT1) receptor, although during chronic ACE inhibitor therapy, AngII levels may return to normal over time. Also ARBs do not affect the angiotensin-2 (AT2) receptor function that includes vasodilatory and antiproliferative ability. However, the absence of augmentation of bradykinin through inhibition of the kininase pathway may lead to differences between the effects of ARBs and ACE inhibitors (48). Numerous studies in animal models have indicated that Ang II-receptor antagonists can have a beneficial effect on the endothelial function. A study in rats using experimental postischemic (coronary artery ligation) heart failure model, long-term but not short-term AT1-receptor blockade, prevented endothelial function degradation, improved coronary blood flow, prevented pericoronary fibrosis development, and improved systemic hemodynamics (49). In hypertensive female rats, irbesartan increased basal NO availability and enhanced the responsiveness of aortic rings to Ach and SNP, regardless of their estrogen status (50).

Presently, very limited information is available in humans. One study was conducted in 34 patients with mild to moderate essential hypertension (diastolic blood pressure 90–120 mmHg). They were randomized to receive either once daily 150 to 300 mg of irbesartan or 50 to 100 mg of atenolol for 3 months. Both medications resulted in the improvement in endothelial-dependent vasodilation (51). In contrary, another study using losartan in patients with coronary heart disease (CHD) did not find an improvement in FMD after 8 weeks (40). A randomized control study examining the effects of ARBs on endothelial function in patients with diabetes is now underway.

LIPID-LOWERING MEDICATIONS

The hydroxymethylglutaryl coenzyme A reductase inhibitors, or statins have been shown to significantly lower the serum lipid levels and reduce cardiovascular morbidity and mortality in patients with and without CHD (52). Because hypercholesterolemia and increased levels of oxidized LDL also impair endothelial function, it was initially thought that the beneficial effects of statins on cardiovascular disease (CVD) was solely related to their lipid lowering capacity. Over the last few years, however, it has been recognized that statins may act through mechanisms that are independent of LDL lowering (53). Recent evidence show that statins directly upregulate endothelial nitric oxide synthase, and enhance NO production; these effects of statins are seen in normocholesterolemic cells (54–56). By increasing NO production, statins may interfere with atherosclerotic lesion development, stabilize plaque, inhibit platelet aggregation, improve blood flow, exert anti-inflammatory actions, and protect against ischemia (57–58). Thus, it is currently accepted that statins have pleiotropic properties that contribute to the observed reduction in the CVD.

There are limited data regarding the effects of statins on human endothelial function as most information is derived either from nonrandomized, placebo-controlled trials or small studies with limited number of subjects and/or limited treatment period. The main conclusions from previously published trials are that treatment with statins improve the endothelial function of the brachial artery or the coronary arteries or regress the coronary intima-media thickness (IMT) in patients with CAD, hypercholesterolemia, and postmenopausal women with normal cholesterol levels (59–62).

Regarding diabetes, the previous nonrandomized studies have suggested no effect of treatment with statins on endothelial function. A small study of poorly controlled type 2 diabetes patients (mean HbA1c 9.3) who also had hypercholerolemia (LDL cholesterol >3.4 mmol/L) reported no improvement in endothelial function in the microcirculation with 3 months of simvastatin treatment (63). The authors concluded that LDL lowering does not appear to improve endothelial function without adequate glycemic control. Another small study in Taiwanese adults with type 2 diabetes and hypercholesterolemia, showed that simvastatin treatment for 6 months did not improve endothelial-dependent or -independent brachial artery vasoactivity despite cholesterol lowering *(64)*. This group of investigators also performed another study using simvastatin in 12 patients with type 2 diabetes and normal cholesterol (LDL cholesterol <80 mg/dL) *(65)*. In contrast to previous study, 12 weeks of medication significantly improved endothelial function in this group of patients. The authors suggested that more aggressive lowering of LDL cholesterol may be needed to improve endothelial function in patients with type 2 diabetes.

Recently, two randomized controlled trials examined effects of statins on endothelial markers and/or endothelial function in type 2 diabetic patients have been published. Both studies reported a beneficial outcome. The first study evaluated the effect of atorvastatin on indexes of leukocytes adhesion *(66)*. Twenty-five type 2 diabetic patients who had no microvascular complications and had LDL cholesterol less than 180 mg/dL were randomized to receive either atorvastatin or placebo for 12 months. The group that received atorvastatin significantly reduced E-selectin, VCAM-1, total- and LDL cholesterol. Another study used atorvastatin (10 mg per day) treatment for 6 months in patients with mean HbA1c 7.9 and mean LDL cholesterol 4.37 mmol/L *(67)*. Atorvastatin decreased plasma C-reactive protein (CRP) and improved endothelium-dependent vasodilation. This change in endothelium-dependent vasodilation correlated with the change in CRP, but not with changes in plasma lipids. Therefore, the authors suggested that the improvement in endothelial function might be partly related to the anti-inflammatory effects of the medication.

For type 1 diabetes, the effect of oral L-arginine and atorvastatin (40 mg per day) on vascular function were investigated in 84 type 1 diabetic adults *(68)*. All participants had normal cholesterol at baseline. Six-weeks of Atorvastatin treatment resulted in a 48 ± 10% decrease in serum LDL cholesterol levels and a significant increased in FMD. In contrast, L-arginine had no significant impact on endothelial function.

A recent study in our unit showed beneficial effect of atorvastatin in endothelial function in people at high risk for developing type 2 diabetes and patients with type 1 and type 2 diabetes. A 12-week treatment of atorvastatin significantly improved FMD, reduced CRP and TNF in high-risk subjects (Table 1). Similarly, there was a trend in improvement of FMD, and a significant reduction in PAI-1 and endothelin in diabetic subjects *(69)*.

In summary, available data suggest that statins improve endothelial function in patients with type 1 and type 2 diabetes, independent of their lipid-lowering capacity. However, other factors such as good glycemic control may also be needed to achieve the beneficial result from statins drug.

ESTROGENS

The risk of MI in diabetic patients without previous MI is equivalent to that in nondiabetic patients with a previous event *(70)*. Additionally, early mortality rate is substantially higher. CVD in patients with diabetes is multifactorial and includes a complex interaction between hyperglycemia, hyperinsulinemia, hyperlipidemia, oxidative stress, and alterations in coagulation and fibrinolysis *(71)*. Although CHD is less common in premenopausal women than in men, this difference begins to disappear after the onset of menopause, suggesting that estrogen and/or progesterone may be protective against

Table 1
Changes in Endothelial Function in the Two Groups That Completed a 3-Month Treatment
With Atorvastatin or Placebo

		At risk of T2DM		Diabetic patients	
		Active $n = 15$	Placebo $n = 15$	Active $n = 19$	Placebo $n = 18$
Brachial	Baseline	3.6 ± 0.9	3.1 ± 0.6	3.7 ± 0.8	3.5 ± 0.7
Artery	Exit	3.6 ± 0.9	3.1 ± 0.5	3.6 ± 0.8	3.3 ± 0.6
Diameter (mm)	p	NS	NS	NS	NS
FMD	Baseline	6. 6 (2.9–9.5)	7.1 (4.4–9.8)	4.2 (3.2–7.2)	5.8 (3.3–7.6)
	Exit	7.2 (2.9–9.6)	7.0 (4.2–9.1)	5.6 (3.9–7.9)	6.2 (3.6–8.8)
	p	< 0.05	NS	0.07	NS NID
	Baseline	14.1 (10.8–21.0)	15.2 (14.0–24.5)	12.5 (10.3–16.2)	16.3 (10.0–17.4)
	Exit	13.7 (11.6–19.3)	15.5 (12.1–23.2)	11.9 (10.7–15.8)	13.7 (10.6–17.5)
	p	NS	NS	NS	NS
Baseline	Baseline	0.94 ± 0.28	1.00 ± 0.25	1.00 ± 0.35	0.88 ± 0.23
Laser flux	Exit	1.00 ± 0.30	0.99 ± 0.21	1.01 ± 0.42	1.00 ± 0.26
(Volts)	p	NS	NS	NS	NS
Ach	Baseline	133 ± 55	159 ± 67	146 ± 86	163 ± 67
	Exit	121 ± 60	152 ± 75	157 ± 84	130 ± 78
	p	NS	NS	NS	NS
SNP	Baseline	67 ± 28	96 ± 54	94 ± 49	86 ± 41
	Exit	78 ± 52	97 ± 61	109 ± 75	90 ± 39
	p	NS	NS	NS	NS

T2DM, type 2 diabetes mellitus; NS, not significant; FMD, flow-mediated endothelium-dependent vasodilation; NID, nitroglycerin-induced dilation; Ach, acetylcholine; SNP, sodium nitroprusside. (From ref. 69.)

hypertension and CHD. Diabetes, however, appears to preclude the protective effects of female sex hormones (72).

Several epidemiological studies, which include predominantly nondiabetic women suggests that postmenopausal hormone replacement therapy (HRT), may reduce risk for coronary events in women without previous heart disease (73–75). The cardiovascular protective action of estrogen may be mediated indirectly by its effect on lipoprotein metabolism, insulin sensitivity. and prothrombotic factors, and by a direct effect on the vessel wall (76). Estrogen receptors are present in both endothelial cells and vascular smooth muscle. Estrogen administration results in vasodilation, in part by stimulating prostacyclin and NO synthesis.

Cross-sectional studies have shown that estrogen replacement might enhance endothelial-dependent and -independent vasodilation in nondiabetic women (77,78). Data from the Cardiovascular Health Study (78) showed that among women with established CVD, the brachial flow-mediated vasodilator responses was comparable between estrogen users and nonusers. However, among women without clinical or subclinical CVD or its risk factors, hormone users had a response that was 40% better than that of nonhormone users.

In contrast to observational studies, the recently published Women's Health Initiative, a large randomized, controlled primary prevention trial reported a significant health risk associated with combination hormone use *(79)*. Women were randomly assigned to either 0.625 mg of conjugated equine estrogens per day, plus 2.5 mg of medroxyprogesterone acetate per day in one tablet ($n = 8506$) or placebo ($n = 8102$). The study stopped early after a mean follow-up of 5.2 years because of excess health risks with hormone treatment. Women receiving estrogen plus progestin were at 29% higher risk for CHD, 41% higher risk for strokes, 2.1 times higher risk for venous thromboembolism, and 26% higher risk for invasive breast cancers as compared with women taking placebo. Additionally, HRT was associated with significant elevated CRP levels *(80)*. Thus, data suggested that overall health risks exceeded benefits from use of combined estrogen plus progestin among healthy postmenopausal women.

To date, there is little information on the effects of HRT on endothelial function in patients with diabetes. One small study examined the effects of short-term treatment (1 week) with conjugated estrogen in postmenopausal women with and without diabetes *(81)*. The basal endothelial-dependent vascular reactivity was decreased in patients with diabetes compared with nondiabetic postmenopausal women. Estrogen supplementation improved endothelial function not only in women with diabetes but also in postmenopausal women without diabetes. Lim and associates *(82)* studied six groups of women; pre- and postmenopausal healthy women, pre- and postmenopausal women with type 2 diabetes, postmenopausal healthy women on HRT and postmenopausal women with diabetes on HRT. Laser Doppler flowmetry was used to measure forearm cutaneous vasodilatation in response to iontophoresis of 1% Ach (endothelium-dependent) and 1% SNP (endothelium-independent). Both endothelium-dependent and -independent responses were significantly higher in premenopausal healthy women compared with premenopausal diabetic women. They were also higher in postmenopausal healthy women on HRT compared with postmenopausal healthy women without HRT, and postmenopausal diabetic women regardless of HRT treatment (Fig. 5). Furthermore, the levels of sICAM were lower in premenopausal women with diabetes and postmenopausal women with diabetes on HRT compared with the postmenopausal diabetic women without HRT. The data suggested that HRT substantially improved microvascular reactivity in postmenopausal healthy women, although the benefit was less apparent in postmenopausal diabetic patients. Similarly, a recent randomized, double-blinded, placebo-controlled, crossover trial reported no beneficial effects of HRT in postmenopausal women with type 2 diabetes. Women were randomized to 0.625 mg of conjugated equine estrogen per day or placebo for 8 weeks. Despite a significant decrease in LDL cholesterol ($15 \pm 23\%$), an increase in HDL cholesterol ($8 \pm 16\%$), and improvement in glycemic control (glycosylated hemoglobin lowered by $3 \pm 13\%$), estrogen did not significantly improve the percent flow-mediated dilatory response to hyperemia. Additionally, estrogen did not significantly change E-selectin, ICAM-1, VCAM-1, monocyte chemoattractant protein-1, or matrix metalloproteinase-9 levels *(83)*.

The effects of combined HRT preparations on plasma lipids, coagulation, endothelial markers in postmenopausal women with type 2 diabetes were recently reported *(84)*. Women were randomized to either to continuous transdermal estradiol (80-µg patches) in combination with oral norethisterone (1 mg daily) or to placebo. Those receiving HRT decreased total cholesterol and triglyceride concentrations by 8% and 22%, respectively. Factor VII activity decreased by 16%, and vWF antigen decreased by 7% with active treatment. Levels of fibrinogen, tissue plasminogen activator (t-PA), fibrin D-dimer, very low-density lipoprotein, LDL cholesterol, lipoprotein (a), and leptin were not sig-

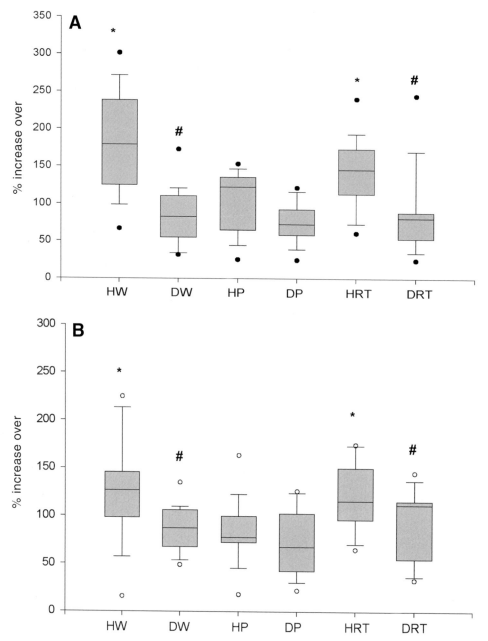

Fig. 5. The result of iontophoresis of acetylcholine **(A)** and sodium nitroprusside **(B)** on the forearm skin in healthy and diabetic women. The responses were higher in the premenopausal women (HW) and postmenopausal healthy women on hormone replacement therapy (HRT) when compared with the premenopausal diabetic women (DW) and postmenopausal diabetic women on HRT (DRT), respectively ($p < 0.001$). Premenopausal healthy women and postmenopausal healthy women on HRT had better responses compared with postmenopausal healthy women without HRT (HP) ($p < 0.001$). The responses between premenopausal diabetic women, postmenopausal diabetic women (DP), and postmenopausal diabetic women on HRT were not significantly different. (Reproduced with permission from ref. *82*.)

nificantly altered. Overall, lipid and coagulation changes were considered slightly beneficial with respect to CHD risk.

In summary, at present there is not enough information to recommend the use of HRT for the treatment of endothelial dysfunction in postmenopausal women with diabetes. Although estrogen has been shown to improve endothelial function in nondiabetic patients, the current evidence does not support hormone use for the purpose of preventing CVD. Furthermore, long- term use of estrogen plus progestin may increase risk of other diseases such as breast cancer, stroke, and thromboembolism.

EXERCISE

The association between type 2 DM with a cluster of disorders that includes obesity, hypertension, dyslipidemia, and atherosclerotic heart disease has long been recognized *(85)*, but until recently, there were no clinically relevant or widely accepted diagnostic criteria for this metabolic syndrome. The Third Report of the National Cholesterol Education Program Expert Panel on Detection, Evaluation, and Treatment of High Blood Cholesterol in Adults (Adult Treatment Panel III [ATP III]) *(86)*, released in 2001, changed this situation by emphasizing the importance of the metabolic syndrome, and providing a working definition of it (i.e., three or more of these criteria: abdominal obesity, hypertriglyceridemia, high high-density lipoprotein cholesterol, high BP, and high fasting glucose). According to ATP III criteria, metabolic syndrome affects an estimated 24% of US adults, or 47 million people *(87)*.

Therapeutic lifestyle changes (TLC), which include dietary changes, increased physical activity, and weight loss are mainstays for treating overweight persons with metabolic syndrome. Weight loss as low as 5% to 10% can improve insulin sensitivity and reduces blood glucose levels in both obese diabetic and nondiabetic individuals *(88)*. Additionally, recent studies have shown that modest weight reduction is also effective in preventing type 2 diabetes. In the Finnish Diabetes Prevention Study *(89)*, a diet and exercise program produced a 58% reduction in diabetes compared with control. The US Diabetes Prevention Program (DPP) *(90)*, a randomized clinical trial of more than 3200 overweight subjects at high risk for diabetes (i.e., IGT) also showed a 58% reduction in diabetes from 11% per year in the control group to 4.8% per year in the lifestyle-modification group, which lost 5% to 7% of initial body weight.

Although the positive impacts of weight loss and physical activity on insulin resistance have been well established, few data are available on the effects of these interventions on vascular reactivity and endothelial function. One group of investigators studied 56 healthy premenopausal obese women (mean body mass index [BMI] 37.2 kg/m^2) and 40 age-matched normal weight women *(91)*. At baseline, obese women had higher fasting glucose and insulin concentrations when compared with nonobese women. They also had higher levels of TNF-α, interleukin-6, P-selectin, ICAM-1, and VCAM-1, and impairment of vascular responses to L-arginine (3 g intravenously), the natural precursor of NO. After 1 year of a multidisciplinary program of weight reduction (diet, exercise, behavioral counseling), all obese women lost at least 10% of their original weight. Compared with baseline, weight loss was associated with improvement in insulin sensitivity, reduction of cytokine and adhesin concentrations, and improvement of vascular responses to L-arginine. The effect of weight loss, with or without exercise, on vessel wall properties of the brachial and common carotid artery has also been studied in healthy obese men *(92)*. After 3 months of energy-restricted diet, the mean BMI decreased from 32.3kg/ m^2

and to 27.6 kg/ m[2] and the mean BP decreased by 6%. Weight loss was accompanied by an increase in carotid artery distensibility, however, the addition of exercise to the regimen did not result in an additional effect.

Finally, a recent publication from our unit has shown positive impact of weight loss on endothelial function *(93)*. Twenty-four obese subjects (mean age 49 years, mean BMI 36.7 kg/ m[2]) with metabolic syndrome were studied at baseline and after 6 months of weight reduction as part of the DPP. All subjects had insulin resistance at the beginning of the study. The intervention resulted in 6.6% weight reduction and significant improvement in insulin sensitivity. FMD significantly improved but responses to GTN and microvascular reactivity did not change. ICAM-1 and PAI-1 significantly decreased, but there were no changes in the plasma concentration of vWF, VCAM, and t-PA. The improvement in endothelial-dependent vasodilation was strongly associated with the percentage of weight reduction.

In conclusion, the TLC and other weight-loss programs are not only useful for the treatment and prevention of diabetes, but they can also improve endothelial function and may ultimately decrease the risk of atherosclerosis and CVD in overweight or obese subjects with metabolic syndrome.

ANTIOXIDANTS

Growing evidence suggests that oxidation of LDL plays an important role in the development of atherosclerosis. Oxidized LDL is taken up more readily than native LDL by macrophages, which contributes directly to foam cell formation *(94,95)*. Oxidized LDL is a chemotactic for circulating monocytes *(96)*, and it also inhibits tissue macrophage motility *(97)*. Additionally, it may be cytotoxic to endothelial cells and may induce arterial vasoconstriction. Thus, the inhibition of the oxidation of LDL is a potential approach to reducing atherogenesis.

Vitamin E (α-tocopherol) is the most prevalent natural occurring antioxidants. In addition to its inhibitory effects on the oxidation of LDL particle, vitamin E also reduces the cytotoxic effects of oxidized LDL, inhibits SMC proliferation and improves endothelial function. The vitamin E derivative, tocopheral succinate, has been shown to prevent the adherence of monocytes to activated endothelium, which is one of the earliest events in the development of atherosclerosis *(98)*. Furthermore, vitamin E decreases enzyme protein kinase C (PKC) activation. The activation of PKC by physical stress, growth factors, inflammatory agents, or hyperglycemia results in superoxide anions production, the impairment of endothelial function, and the association with diabetes microvascular complications *(99)*.

Large epidemiological studies have shown an association between a high intake of vitamin E and a lower risk of CHD *(100,101)* or coronary artery lesion progression *(102)*. Animal models of atherosclerosis are mainly consistent with the concept that antioxidant vitamins reduce the progression of atherosclerosis *(103)*. However, results from randomized, clinical trials are conflicting. Data from the Cambridge Heart Antioxidant Study, a large double-blind, placebo-controlled trial of 2002 patients with angiographically proven coronary atherosclerosis reported that high doses of vitamin E (400–800 IU daily) reduced the rates of cardiovascular death and nonfatal MI by almost 50% after the mean follow-up of 510 days *(104)*. Another study (the Secondary Prevention with Antioxidants of Cardiovascular Disease in Endstage Renal Disease [SPACE] study) using high-dose vitamin E supplementation (800 IU per day) *(105)* also showed vitamin E reduced rates of CVD (MI, stroke, PVD, and unstable angina) in hemodialysis patients with pre-existing CVD. In contrast, the Gruppo Italiano per lo Studio della Sopravvivenza nell'Infarto Miocardio (GISSI)-Prevenzione Trial, an open-label, randomized, controlled trial in more than 11,000 MI survivors showed low-dose fish oil, but not vitamin E, significantly reduced the rates of all cause mortality, nonfatal MI, and nonfatal stroke *(106)*. In the MRC/BHF Heart Protection Study *(107)*, 20,536 patients with coronary disease, other occlusive arterial disease, or diabetes were randomly assigned to receive antioxidant vitamin supplementation (600 mg vitamin E, 250 mg vitamin C, and 20-mg β-carotene daily) or placebo. After 5 years, there were no significant differences between the two treatment groups in all-cause mortality, death as a result of vascular or nonvascular causes, nonfatal or fatal MI, nonfatal or fatal stroke, or coronary revascularization.

The data regarding vitamin E and CHD or endothelial function in diabetes are limited. The α-tocopheral levels in diabetic patients have been reported to be either reduced or normal *(108,109)*. Although several studies have suggested that vitamin E supplementation in diabetes may reduce the LDL susceptibility to oxidation, not all randomized placebo-controlled studies do support the positive results of vitamin E in CVD. The data from the HOPE trial showed no effects of the daily administration of 400 IU vitamin E for an average of 4.5 years on cardiovascular outcomes (MI, stroke, cardiovascular death) or nephropathy in middle-aged and elderly people with diabetes or CVD and at least one additional cardiac risk factor *(110)*. No effects of vitamin E were also found on the carotid IMT *(111)*. Similarly, one study examined 48 subjects with type 2 diabetes their endothelial function using venous occlusion plethysmography with endothelial independent (GTN), endothelial-dependent (Ach and bradykinin) vasodilators before and after daily supplementation of 1600 IU vitamin E or placebo for 8 weeks *(112)*. Results showed that vitamin E did not affect vasodilation to any of the three vasodilators tested. In contrast, a study used raxofelast, a new water-soluble vitamin E-like compound with antioxidant properties in men with type 2 diabetes showed a promising result *(113)*. Administration of raxofelast for 1 week was accompanied by a decrease oxidative stress and an increased in forearm blood-flow responses to Ach infusion. Likewise, the result from a randomized controlled trial using 1,000 IU vitamin E for 3 months in patients with type 1 diabetes showed that patients who received vitamin E had an improvement in FMD and blood-flow response to Ach *(114)*. The change in FMD was related to the change in vitamin E content in LDL particle and the oxidative capacity of LDL. Finally, a recent study from our unit reported that treatment of type 1 and 2 with 1800 IU daily for a 12-month period failed to offer any benefits and had a detrimental effect on the vascular reactivity of the micro- and macrocirculation when compared to placebo treatment. Therefore, the use of vitamin E, at least in large doses, cannot be recommended at present *(115)*.

Vitamin C is a low-molecular-weight antioxidant that scavenges free radicals. Evidence from observational studies or clinical trials do not always support cardiovascular benefits from vitamin C and data in diabetes are scant. In a short-term study, both vitamin C and E administration have been shown to prevent a transient decrease of FMD after acute oral glucose load in healthy subjects without diabetes *(116)*. Intracellular levels of vitamin C have been found to be reduced in patients with type 1 diabetes, especially in those with poor control *(117)*.

Endothelial function and oxidative stress in 20 type 2 diabetes patients (mean HbA1c 8.4%) have been assessed at baseline and following 6 weeks of insulin lispro and 1 g vitamin C daily or insulin lispro alone *(118)*. At the end of the study, insulin lispro improved fasting and postprandial endothelial function (FMD) and reduced oxidative stress. Simultaneous vitamin C therapy produced an additional improvement in endothelial function and oxidative stress. The authors suggested that potential benefits of insulin therapy on cardiovascular outcome in type 2 diabetes might be enhanced by vitamin C supplementation, although further studies will be required. Acute effects of vitamin C on endothelial function was also demonstrated in the study of 10 subjects with type 2 diabetic and 10 age-matched, nondiabetic controls *(119)*. Forearm blood flow was determined by venous occlusion plethysmography. Endothelium-dependent vasodilation was assessed by intra-arterial infusion of methacholine before and after intra-arterial administration of vitamin C (24 mg per minute). In diabetic subjects, endothelium-dependent vasodilation to methacholine was augmented by simultaneous infusion of vitamin C; in contrast, vitamin C administration did not alter endothelium-dependent vasodilation in healthy subjects. Similar results from the same group of investigators was also reported in patients with type 1 diabetes *(120)*. In contrast, short-term (3 weeks) treatment with oral vitamin C (1.5 g daily) was reported to have no impact on oxidative stress, BP, or endothelial function in patients with type 2 diabetes *(121)*. To date, there are no long-term data of vitamin C supplementation in patients with diabetes.

SUMMARY AND CONCLUSIONS

Endothelial dysfunction has been demonstrated in patients with type 1 and type 2 diabetes and obese individuals with insulin resistance. Data suggest that vascular endothelial dysfunction may contribute to the pathophysiology of clinical ischemia, especially angina pectoris, MI, and sudden cardiac death, as it emerges as one of the initial stages in the development of atherosclerosis. Endothelial dysfunction comprises of abnormalities in vascular tone, balance in thrombosis and fibrinolysis, control of inflammatory response, and the growth of smooth muscle. Over the past few years, several cardiovascular therapeutic interventions have been explored, although the results are still not clear. The interventions that are undoubtedly effective in endothelial function are diet therapy and weight loss. The role of insulin sensitizers, lipid-lowering drugs, ACE inhibitors, HRT, and antioxidant remains to be further explored.

REFERENCES

1. Furchgott RF, Zawadzki JV. The obligatory role of endothelial cells in the relaxation of arterial smooth muscle by acetylcholine. Nature 1980;288:373–476.
2. Quyyumi AA. Prognostic value of endothelial function. Am J Cardiol 2003;91:19H–24H.
3. McVeigh GE, Brennan GM, Johnston GD, et al. Impaired endothelium-dependent and independent vasodilation in patients with type 2 (non-insulin-dependent) diabetes mellitus. Diabetologia 1992;35:771–776.
4. Vallance P, Calver A, Collier J. The vascular endothelium in diabetes and hypertension. J Hypertens Suppl 1992;10:S25–S29.
5. Williams SB, Cusco JA, Roddy MA, Johnstone MT, Creager MA. Impaired nitric oxide-mediated vasodilation in patients with non-insulin-dependent diabetes mellitus. J Am Coll Cardiol 1996;27:567–574.
6. Johnstone MT, Creager SJ, Scales KM, Cusco JA, Lee BK, Creager MA. Impaired endothelium-dependent vasodilation in patients with insulin-dependent diabetes mellitus. Circulation 1993;88:2510–2516.
7. Caballero AE, Arora S, Saouaf R, et al. Microvascular and macrovascular reactivity is reduced in subjects at risk for type 2 diabetes. Diabetes 1999;48:1856–1862.
8. Anastasiou E, Lekakis JP, Alevizaki M, et al. Impaired endothelium-dependent vasodilatation in women with previous gestational diabetes. Diabetes Care 1998;21:2111–2115.

9. Arcaro G, Cretti A, Balzano S, et al. Insulin causes endothelial dysfunction in humans: sites and mechanisms. Circulation 2002;105:576–582.
10. Steinberg HO, Chaker H, Leaming R, Johnson A, Brechtel G, Baron AD. Obesity/insulin resistance is associated with endothelial dysfunction. Implications for the syndrome of insulin resistance. J Clin Invest 1996;97:2601–2610.
11. Fujiwara T, Horikoshi H. Troglitazone and related compounds: therapeutic potential beyond diabetes. Life Sci 2000;67:2405–2416.
12. Horikoshi H, Hashimoto T, Fujiwara T. Troglitazone and emerging glitazones: new avenues for potential therapeutic benefits beyond glycemic control. Prog Drug Res 2000;54:191–212.
13. Marx N, Bourcier T, Sukhova GK, Libby P, Plutzky J. PPARgamma activation in human endothelial cells increases plasminogen activator inhibitor type-1 expression: PPARgamma as a potential mediator in vascular disease. Arterioscler Thromb Vasc Biol 1999;19:546–551.
14. Pasceri V, Wu HD, Willerson JT, Yeh ET. Modulation of vascular inflammation in vitro and in vivo by peroxisome proliferator-activated receptor-gamma activators. Circulation 2000;101:235–238.
15. Cominacini L, Garbin U, Pasini AF, et al. The expression of adhesion molecules on endothelial cells is inhibited by troglitazone through its antioxidant activity. Cell Adhes Commun 1999;7:223–231.
16. Kato K, Satoh H, Endo Y, et al. Thiazolidinediones down-regulate plasminogen activator inhibitor type 1 expression in human vascular endothelial cells: A possible role for PPARgamma in endothelial function. Biochem Biophys Res Commun 1999;258:431–435.
17. Avena R, Mitchell ME, Nylen ES, Curry KM, Sidawy AN. Insulin action enhancement normalizes brachial artery vasoactivity in patients with peripheral vascular disease and occult diabetes. J Vasc Surg 1998;28:1024–1031; discussion 1031–1032.
18. Watanabe Y, Sunayama S, Shimada K, et al. Troglitazone improves endothelial dysfunction in patients with insulin resistance. J Atheroscler Thromb 2000;7:159–163.
19. Murakami T, Mizuno S, Ohsato K, et al. Effects of troglitazone on frequency of coronary vasospastic-induced angina pectoris in patients with diabetes mellitus. Am J Cardiol 1999;84:92–94, A8.
20. Cominacini L, Garbin U, Fratta Pasini A, et al. Troglitazone reduces LDL oxidation and lowers plasma E-selectin concentration in NIDDM patients. Diabetes 1998;47:130–133.
21. Martin-Nizard F, Furman C, Delerive P, et al. Peroxisome proliferator-activated receptor activators inhibit oxidized low-density lipoprotein-induced endothelin-1 secretion in endothelial cells. J Cardiovasc Pharmacol 2002;40:822–831.
22. Tack CJ, Ong MK, Lutterman JA, Smits P. Insulin-induced vasodilatation and endothelial function in obesity/insulin resistance. Effects of troglitazone. Diabetologia 1998;41:569–576.
23. Caballero AE, Saouaf R, Lim SC, et al. The effects of troglitazone, an insulin-sensitizing agent, on the endothelial function in early and late type 2 diabetes: a placebo-controlled randomized clinical trial. Metabolism 2003;52:173–180.
24. Walker AB, Chattington PD, Buckingham RE, Williams G. The thiazolidinedione rosiglitazone (BRL-49653) lowers blood pressure and protects against impairment of endothelial function in Zucker fatty rats. Diabetes 1999;48:1448–1453.
25. Vinik AI, Stansberry KB, Barlow PM. Rosiglitazone treatment increases nitric oxide production in human peripheral skin: a controlled clinical trial in patients with type 2 diabetes mellitus. J Diabetes Complications 2003;17:279–285.
26. Wagner C, Kurtz A. Regulation of renal renin release. Curr Opin Nephrol Hypertens 1998;7:437–441.
27. Ichikawi I, Harris RC. Angiotensin actions in the kidney: renewed insight into the old hormone. Kidney Int 1991;40:583–596.
28. Carretero OA, Scicli AG. The renal kallikrein-kinin system. Am J Physiol 1980;238:F247–F255.
29. Parmley WW. Evolution of angiotensin-converting enzyme inhibition in hypertension, heart failure, and vascular protection. Am J Med 1998;105:27S–31S.
30. Yusuf S, Sleight P, Pogue J, Bosch J, Davies R, Dagenais G. Effects of an angiotensin-converting-enzyme inhibitor, ramipril, on cardiovascular events in high-risk patients. The Heart Outcomes Prevention Evaluation Study Investigators. N Engl J Med 2000;342:145–153.
31. Effects of ramipril on cardiovascular and microvascular outcomes in people with diabetes mellitus: results of the HOPE study and MICRO-HOPE substudy. Heart Outcomes Prevention Evaluation Study Investigators. Lancet 2000;355:253–259.
32. Gerstein HC. Reduction of cardiovascular events and microvascular complications in diabetes with ACE inhibitor treatment: HOPE and MICRO-HOPE. Diabetes Metab Res Rev 2002;18 Suppl 3:S82–S85.

33. Gerstein HC. Diabetes and the HOPE study: implications for macrovascular and microvascular disease. Int J Clin Pract Suppl 2001:8–12.
34. Pitt B, O'Neill B, Feldman R, et al. The QUinapril Ischemic Event Trial (QUIET): evaluation of chronic ACE inhibitor therapy in patients with ischemic heart disease and preserved left ventricular function. Am J Cardiol 2001;87:1058–1063.
35. Cashin-Hemphill L, Holmvang G, Chan RC, Pitt B, Dinsmore RE, Lees RS. Angiotensin-converting enzyme inhibition as antiatherosclerotic therapy: no answer yet. QUIET Investigators. QUinapril Ischemic Event Trial. Am J Cardiol 1999;83:43–47.
36. Gryglewski RJ, Uracz W, Swies J, et al. Comparison of endothelial pleiotropic actions of angiotensin converting enzyme inhibitors and statins. Ann N Y Acad Sci 2001;947:229–245; discussion 245–246.
37. Garber AJ. Attenuating CV risk factors in patients with diabetes: clinical evidence to clinical practice. Diabetes Obes Metab 2002;4 Suppl 1:S5–S12.
38. Dzau VJ, Re R. Tissue angiotensin system in cardiovascular medicine. A paradigm shift? Circulation 1994;89:493–498.
39. Mancini GB, Henry GC, Macaya C, et al. Angiotensin-converting enzyme inhibition with quinapril improves endothelial vasomotor dysfunction in patients with coronary artery disease. The TREND (Trial on Reversing ENdothelial Dysfunction) Study. Circulation 1996;94:258–265.
40. Anderson TJ, Elstein E, Haber H, Charbonneau F. Comparative study of ACE-inhibition, angiotensin II antagonism, and calcium channel blockade on flow-mediated vasodilation in patients with coronary disease (BANFF study). J Am Coll Cardiol 2000;35:60–66.
41. O'Driscoll G, Green D, Rankin J, Stanton K, Taylor R. Improvement in endothelial function by angiotensin converting enzyme inhibition in insulin-dependent diabetes mellitus. J Clin Invest 1997;100:678–684.
42. Arcaro G, Zenere BM, Saggiani F, et al. ACE inhibitors improve endothelial function in type 1 diabetic patients with normal arterial pressure and microalbuminuria. Diabetes Care 1999;22:1536–542.
43. Mullen MJ, Clarkson P, Donald AE, et al. Effect of enalapril on endothelial function in young insulin-dependent diabetic patients: a randomized, double-blind study. J Am Coll Cardiol 1998;31:1330–1335.
44. McFarlane R, McCredie RJ, Bonney MA, et al. Angiotensin converting enzyme inhibition and arterial endothelial function in adults with Type 1 diabetes mellitus. Diabet Med 1999;16:62–66.
45. O'Driscoll G, Green D, Maiorana A, Stanton K, Colreavy F, Taylor R. Improvement in endothelial function by angiotensin-converting enzyme inhibition in non-insulin-dependent diabetes mellitus. J Am Coll Cardiol 1999;33:1506–1511.
46. Giugliano D, Marfella R, Acampora R, Giunta R, Coppola L, D'Onofrio F. Effects of perindopril and carvedilol on endothelium-dependent vascular functions in patients with diabetes and hypertension. Diabetes Care 1998;21:631–636.
47. Bijlstra PJ, Smits P, Lutterman JA, Thien T. Effect of long-term angiotensin-converting enzyme inhibition on endothelial function in patients with the insulin-resistance syndrome. J Cardiovasc Pharmacol 1995;25:658–664.
48. Mancini GB. Emerging role of angiotensin II type 1 receptor blockers for the treatment of endothelial dysfunction and vascular inflammation. Can J Cardiol 2002;18:1309–1316.
49. Gervais M, Fornes P, Richer C, Nisato D, Giudicelli JF. Effects of angiotensin II AT1-receptor blockade on coronary dynamics, function, and structure in postischemic heart failure in rats. J Cardiovasc Pharmacol 2000;36:329–337.
50. Riveiro A, Mosquera A, Alonso M, Calvo C. Angiotensin II type 1 receptor blocker irbesartan ameliorates vascular function in spontaneously hypertensive rats regardless of oestrogen status. J Hypertens 2002;20:1365–1372.
51. von zur Muhlen B, Kahan T, Hagg A, Millgard J, Lind L. Treatment with irbesartan or atenolol improves endothelial function in essential hypertension. J Hypertens 2001;19:1813–1818.
52. Randomised trial of cholesterol lowering in 4444 patients with coronary heart disease: the Scandinavian Simvastatin Survival Study (4S). Lancet 1994;344:1383–1389.
53. Maron DJ, Fazio S, Linton MF. Current perspectives on statins. Circulation 2000;101:207–213.
54. Laufs U. Beyond lipid-lowering: effects of statins on endothelial nitric oxide. Eur J Clin Pharmacol 2003;58:719–731.
55. Laufs U, Fata VL, Liao JK. Inhibition of 3-hydroxy-3-methylglutaryl (HMG)-CoA reductase blocks hypoxia-mediated down-regulation of endothelial nitric oxide synthase. J Biol Chem 1997;272:31725–31729.
56. Laufs U, Liao JK. Post-transcriptional regulation of endothelial nitric oxide synthase mRNA stability by Rho GTPase. J Biol Chem 1998;273:24266–24271.

57. Lefer AM, Scalia R, Lefer DJ. Vascular effects of HMG CoA-reductase inhibitors (statins) unrelated to cholesterol lowering: new concepts for cardiovascular disease. Cardiovasc Res 2001;49:281–287.

58. Lefer DJ. Statins as potent antiinflammatory drugs. Circulation 2002;106:2041–2042.

59. Simaitis A, Laucevicius A. [Effect of high doses of atorvastatin on the endothelial function of the coronary arteries]. Medicina (Kaunas) 2003;39:21–29.

60. Marchesi S, Lupattelli G, Siepi D, et al. Short-term atorvastatin treatment improves endothelial function in hypercholesterolemic women. J Cardiovasc Pharmacol 2000;36:617–621.

61. Taylor AJ, Kent SM, Flaherty PJ, Coyle LC, Markwood TT, Vernalis MN. ARBITER: Arterial Biology for the Investigation of the Treatment Effects of Reducing Cholesterol: a randomized trial comparing the effects of atorvastatin and pravastatin on carotid intima medial thickness. Circulation 2002;106:2055–2060.

62. Mercuro G, Zoncu S, Saiu F, Sarais C, Rosano GM. Effect of atorvastatin on endothelium-dependent vasodilation in postmenopausal women with average serum cholesterol levels. Am J Cardiol 2002;90:747–750.

63. Mansourati J, Newman LG, Roman SH, Travis A, Rafey M, Phillips RA. Lipid lowering does not improve endothelial function in subjects with poorly controlled diabetes. Diabetes Care 2001;24:2152–2153.

64. Sheu WH, Juang BL, Chen YT, Lee WJ. Endothelial dysfunction is not reversed by simvastatin treatment in type 2 diabetic patients with hypercholesterolemia. Diabetes Care 1999;22:1224–1225.

65. Sheu WH, Chen YT, Lee WJ. Improvement in endothelial dysfunction with LDL cholesterol level < 80 mg/dl in type 2 diabetic patients. Diabetes Care 2001;24:1499–1501.

66. Dalla Nora E, Passaro A, Zamboni PF, Calzoni F, Fellin R, Solini A. Atorvastatin improves metabolic control and endothelial function in type 2 diabetic patients: a placebo-controlled study. J Endocrinol Invest 2003;26:73–78.

67. Tan KC, Chow WS, Tam SC, Ai VH, Lam CH, Lam KS. Atorvastatin lowers C-reactive protein and improves endothelium-dependent vasodilation in type 2 diabetes mellitus. J Clin Endocrinol Metab 2002;87:563–568.

68. Mullen MJ, Wright D, Donald AE, Thorne S, Thomson H, Deanfield JE. Atorvastatin but not L-arginine improves endothelial function in type I diabetes mellitus: a double-blind study. J Am Coll Cardiol 2000;36:410–416.

69. Economides PA, Caselli A, Khaodhiar L, Horton ES, Veves A. The effects of atorvastatin on the endothelial function in diabetic patients and subjects at risk for type 2 diabetes. J Clin Endocrinol Metab. 2004;89(2):740–747.

70. Haffner SM, Lehto S, Ronnemaa T, Pyorala K, Laakso M. Mortality from coronary heart disease in subjects with type 2 diabetes and in nondiabetic subjects with and without prior myocardial infarction. N Engl J Med 1998;339:229–234.

71. Calles-Escandon J, Cipolla M. Diabetes and endothelial dysfunction: a clinical perspective. Endocr Rev 2001;22:36–52.

72. Sowers JR. Diabetes mellitus and cardiovascular disease in women. Arch Intern Med 1998;158:617–621.

73. Grodstein F, Manson JE, Colditz GA, Willett WC, Speizer FE, Stampfer MJ. A prospective, observational study of postmenopausal hormone therapy and primary prevention of cardiovascular disease. Ann Intern Med 2000;133:933–941.

74. Grodstein F, Stampfer MJ, Manson JE, et al. Postmenopausal estrogen and progestin use and the risk of cardiovascular disease. N Engl J Med 1996;335:453–461.

75. Hu FB, Grodstein F. Postmenopausal hormone therapy and the risk of cardiovascular disease: the epidemiologic evidence. Am J Cardiol 2002;90:26F–29F.

76. Farhat MY, Lavigne MC, Ramwell PW. The vascular protective effects of estrogen. Faseb J 1996;10:615–624.

77. Arora S, Veves A, Caballaro AE, Smakowski P, LoGerfo FW. Estrogen improves endothelial function. J Vasc Surg 1998;27:1141–1146; discussion 1147.

78. Herrington DM, Espeland MA, Crouse JR, 3rd, et al. Estrogen replacement and brachial artery flow-mediated vasodilation in older women. Arterioscler Thromb Vasc Biol 2001;21:1955–1961.

79. Rossouw JE, Anderson GL, Prentice RL, et al. Risks and benefits of estrogen plus progestin in healthy postmenopausal women: principal results From the Women's Health Initiative randomized controlled trial. JAMA 2002;288:321–333.

80. Pradhan AD, Manson JE, Rossouw JE, et al. Inflammatory biomarkers, hormone replacement therapy, and incident coronary heart disease: prospective analysis from the Women's Health Initiative observational study. Jama 2002;288:980–987.

81. Lee SJ, Lee DW, Kim KS, Lee IK. Effect of estrogen on endothelial dysfunction in postmenopausal women with diabetes. Diabetes Res Clin Pract 2001;54 Suppl 2:S81–S92.
82. Lim SC, Caballero AE, Arora S, et al. The effect of hormonal replacement therapy on the vascular reactivity and endothelial function of healthy individuals and individuals with type 2 diabetes. J Clin Endocrinol Metab 1999;84:4159–4164.
83. Koh KK, Kang MH, Jin DK, et al. Vascular effects of estrogen in type II diabetic postmenopausal women. J Am Coll Cardiol 2001;38:1409–1415.
84. Perera M, Sattar N, Petrie JR, et al. The effects of transdermal estradiol in combination with oral norethisterone on lipoproteins, coagulation, and endothelial markers in postmenopausal women with type 2 diabetes: a randomized, placebo-controlled study. J Clin Endocrinol Metab 2001;86:1140–1143.
85. Karam JH. Type II diabetes and syndrome X. Pathogenesis and glycemic management. Endocrinol Metab Clin North Am 1992;21:329–350.
86. National Heart, Lung, and Blood Institute. Third Report of the Expert Panel on Detection, Evaluation, and Treatment of High Blood Cholesterol In Adults (Adult Treatment Panel III). Bethesda, Md: National Cholesterol Education Program (NCEP), National Institutes of Health, 2001. Available at: http://www.nhlbi.nih.gov/ guidelines/cholesterol/ atp3_rpt.htm. Accessed August 15, 2002.
87. Ford ES, Giles WH, Dietz WH. Prevalence of the metabolic syndrome among US adults: findings from the third National Health and Nutrition Examination Survey. JAMA 2002;287:356–359.
88. Watts NB, Spanheimer RG, DiGirolamo M, et al. Prediction of glucose response to weight loss in patients with non-insulin-dependent diabetes mellitus. Arch Intern Med 1990;150:803–806.
89. Tuomilehto J, Lindstrom J, Eriksson JG, et al. Prevention of type 2 diabetes mellitus by changes in lifestyle among subjects with impaired glucose tolerance. N Engl J Med 2001;344:1343–1350.
90. Knowler WC, Barrett-Connor E, Fowler SE, et al. Reduction in the incidence of type 2 diabetes with lifestyle intervention or metformin. N Engl J Med 2002;346:393–403.
91. Ziccardi P, Nappo F, Giugliano G, et al. Reduction of inflammatory cytokine concentrations and improvement of endothelial functions in obese women after weight loss over one year. Circulation 2002;105:804–809.
92. Balkestein EJ, van Aggel-Leijssen DP, van Baak MA, Struijker-Boudier HA, Van Bortel LM. The effect of weight loss with or without exercise training on large artery compliance in healthy obese men. J Hypertens 1999;17:1831–1835.
93. Hamdy O, Ledbury S, Mullooly C, et al. Lifestyle modification improves endothelial function in obese subjects with the insulin resistance syndrome. Diabetes Care 2003;26:2119–2125.
94. Parthasarathy S, Steinberg D, Witztum JL. The role of oxidized low-density lipoproteins in the pathogenesis of atherosclerosis. Annu Rev Med 1992;43:219–225.
95. Parthasarathy S, Wieland E, Steinberg D. A role for endothelial cell lipoxygenase in the oxidative modification of low density lipoprotein. Proc Natl Acad Sci U S A 1989;86:1046–1050.
96. Quinn MT, Parthasarathy S, Fong LG, Steinberg D. Oxidatively modified low density lipoproteins: a potential role in recruitment and retention of monocyte/macrophages during atherogenesis. Proc Natl Acad Sci U S A 1987;84:2995–2998.
97. Quinn MT, Parthasarathy S, Steinberg D. Endothelial cell-derived chemotactic activity for mouse peritoneal macrophages and the effects of modified forms of low density lipoprotein. Proc Natl Acad Sci U S A 1985;82:5949–5953.
98. Erl W, Weber C, Wardemann C, Weber PC. alpha-Tocopheryl succinate inhibits monocytic cell adhesion to endothelial cells by suppressing NF-kappa B mobilization. Am J Physiol 1997;273:H634–H640.
99. Yuan SY, Ustinova EE, Wu MH, et al. Protein kinase C activation contributes to microvascular barrier dysfunction in the heart at early stages of diabetes. Circ Res 2000;87:412–417.
100. Rimm EB, Stampfer MJ, Ascherio A, Giovannucci E, Colditz GA, Willett WC. Vitamin E consumption and the risk of coronary heart disease in men. N Engl J Med 1993;328:1450–1456.
101. Stampfer MJ, Hennekens CH, Manson JE, Colditz GA, Rosner B, Willett WC. Vitamin E consumption and the risk of coronary disease in women. N Engl J Med 1993;328:1444–1449.
102. Hodis HN, Mack WJ, LaBree L, et al. Serial coronary angiographic evidence that antioxidant vitamin intake reduces progression of coronary artery atherosclerosis. Jama 1995;273:1849–1854.
103. Meagher E, Rader DJ. Antioxidant therapy and atherosclerosis: animal and human studies. Trends Cardiovasc Med 2001;11:162–165.

104. Stephens NG, Parsons A, Schofield PM, Kelly F, Cheeseman K, Mitchinson MJ. Randomised controlled trial of vitamin E in patients with coronary disease: Cambridge Heart Antioxidant Study (CHAOS). Lancet 1996;347:781–786.

105. Boaz M, Smetana S, Weinstein T, et al. Secondary prevention with antioxidants of cardiovascular disease in endstage renal disease (SPACE): randomised placebo-controlled trial. Lancet 2000;356: 1213–1218.

106. Stone NJ. The Gruppo Italiano per lo Studio della Sopravvivenza nell'Infarto Miocardio (GISSI)-Prevenzione Trial on fish oil and vitamin E supplementation in myocardial infarction survivors. Curr Cardiol Rep 2000;2:445–451.

107. MRC/BHF Heart Protection Study of antioxidant vitamin supplementation in 20,536 high-risk individuals: a randomised placebo-controlled trial. Lancet 2002;360:23–33.

108. Nourooz-Zadeh J, Rahimi A, Tajaddini-Sarmadi J, et al. Relationships between plasma measures of oxidative stress and metabolic control in NIDDM. Diabetologia 1997;40:647–653.

109. Granado F, Olmedilla B, Gil-Martinez E, Blanco I, Millan I, Rojas-Hidalgo E. Carotenoids, retinol and tocopherols in patients with insulin-dependent diabetes mellitus and their immediate relatives. Clin Sci (Lond) 1998;94:189–195.

110. Lonn E, Yusuf S, Hoogwerf B, et al. Effects of vitamin E on cardiovascular and microvascular outcomes in high-risk patients with diabetes: results of the HOPE study and MICRO-HOPE substudy. Diabetes Care 2002;25:1919–1927.

111. Lonn E, Yusuf S, Dzavik V, et al. Effects of ramipril and vitamin E on atherosclerosis: the study to evaluate carotid ultrasound changes in patients treated with ramipril and vitamin E (SECURE). Circulation 2001;103:919–925.

112. Gazis A, White DJ, Page SR, Cockcroft JR. Effect of oral vitamin E (alpha-tocopherol) supplementation on vascular endothelial function in Type 2 diabetes mellitus. Diabet Med 1999;16:304–311.

113. Chowienczyk PJ, Brett SE, Gopaul NK, et al. Oral treatment with an antioxidant (raxofelast) reduces oxidative stress and improves endothelial function in men with type II diabetes. Diabetologia 2000;43:974–977.

114. Skyrme-Jones RA, O'Brien RC, Berry KL, Meredith IT. Vitamin E supplementation improves endothelial function in type I diabetes mellitus: a randomized, placebo-controlled study. J Am Coll Cardiol 2000;36:94–102.

115. Economides PA, Khaodhiar L, Caselli A, et al. The effect of vitamin E on the endothelial function of the micro- and macrocirculation and the left ventricular function of type 1 and 2 diabetic patients. Diabetes 2005;54:204–211.

116. Title LM, Cummings PM, Giddens K, Nassar BA. Oral glucose loading acutely attenuates endothelium-dependent vasodilation in healthy adults without diabetes: an effect prevented by vitamins C and E. J Am Coll Cardiol 2000;36:2185–2191.

117. Cunningham JJ, Ellis SL, McVeigh KL, Levine RE, Calles-Escandon J. Reduced mononuclear leukocyte ascorbic acid content in adults with insulin-dependent diabetes mellitus consuming adequate dietary vitamin C. Metabolism 1991;40:146–149.

118. Evans M, Anderson RA, Smith JC, et al. Effects of insulin lispro and chronic vitamin C therapy on postprandial lipaemia, oxidative stress and endothelial function in patients with type 2 diabetes mellitus. Eur J Clin Invest 2003;33:231–238.

119. Ting HH, Timimi FK, Boles KS, Creager SJ, Ganz P, Creager MA. Vitamin C improves endothelium-dependent vasodilation in patients with non-insulin-dependent diabetes mellitus. J Clin Invest 1996;97:22–28.

120. Timimi FK, Ting HH, Haley EA, Roddy MA, Ganz P, Creager MA. Vitamin C improves endothelium-dependent vasodilation in patients with insulin-dependent diabetes mellitus. J Am Coll Cardiol 1998;31:552–557.

121. Darko D, Dornhorst A, Kelly FJ, Ritter JM, Chowienczyk PJ. Lack of effect of oral vitamin C on blood pressure, oxidative stress and endothelial function in Type II diabetes. Clinical Science. 2002;103:339–344.

122. Rose B, Post T. Clinical Physiology of Acid-Base and Electrolyte Disorders. New York: McGraw-Hill, 2001.

II

CLINICAL

D. Cardiovascular System: Cardiac

24   Preoperative Assessment and Perioperative Management of the Surgical Patient With Diabetes Mellitus

Alanna Coolong, MD
and Mylan C. Cohen, MD, MPH

CONTENTS

From: *Contemporary Cardiology: Diabetes and Cardiovascular Disease, Second Edition*
Edited by: M. T. Johnstone and A. Veves © Humana Press Inc., Totowa, NJ

INTRODUCTION

Patients with diabetes mellitus (DM) are more likely than patients without diabetes to undergo surgery and may be at higher than average risk to suffer perioperative complications, usually because of frequent concomitant cardiovascular disease (CVD). The manifestations of CVD in patients with diabetes are often atypical, making identification and management more difficult (1,2). The role of the physician asked to provide preoperative consultation is to work with the surgical team in assessing and reducing the risk of complications in the perioperative period, and to identify opportunities to make a favorable impact on long-term health. In caring for the patient with diabetes perioperatively, heightened awareness of the higher incidence of coronary artery disease (CAD), silent ischemia, and increased predisposition to postoperative complications of infection, hyperglycemia, and hypoglycemia is necessary to permit the best outcomes to occur.

EPIDEMIOLOGY

Perioperative Cardiac Morbidity

Each year in the United States approx 34.1 million patients undergo noncardiac operations (3,4), more than 1 million individuals have noncardiac surgery complicated by perioperative cardiac morbidity and mortality (5). The risk of perioperative cardiac complications is substantially higher in patients with CAD, advanced congestive heart failure (CHF), major valvular abnormalities, or significant arrhythmias (3,6,7). The risk of cardiac complications is also institution- and procedure-specific. A higher incidence of complications is associated with intrathoracic, intraperitoneal, and vascular procedures and procedures performed in an emergency (8–10).

Cardiac outcomes have improved over the past decades, and the risk of a perioperative myocardial infarction (MI) is relatively low in the overall surgical population (<2%) (8,11,12). The risk for MI and other complications is higher in patients with a prior MI. Reports from the 1970s placed the operative risk of reinfarction or cardiac death within 3 months of the previous MI as high as 30%, within 3 and 6 months at 15%, and after 6 months at about 5% (9,10). More recent estimates show an improvement: a 6% risk if within 3 months from the infarct and 2% if between 3 and 6 months (13,14). In a study evaluating the morbidity associated with vascular surgeries between 1955 and 1981, the operative mortality decreased from 8% in the 1950s to 2.9% in 1981(15). The incidence of perioperative MI in elective vascular surgeries has been estimated at 2.8% to 7.3% (16,17). More recent estimates differentiate between those patients with ischemic heart disease and those without such history. A retrospective study of 6948 patients from the Cleveland Clinic undergoing vascular surgery from January 1989 to June 1997 found the incidence of perioperative MI to be 1.54% (18). Two recent prospective studies found the incidence of perioperative MI after noncardiac surgery in patients with a history of ischemic heart disease to be 4.1–5.6% (19,20).

It is recognized, however, that when a perioperative infarction occurs it carries an extremely high risk of recurrent cardiac complications, including death, postoperatively (9,10,18,20–22) and in the long-term (23,24). Mortality for perioperative MI has been estimated to be from 17% to 41% (18,20,25).

SURGERY IN THE DIABETIC PATIENT

Seventeen million Americans have diabetes and the incidence of the disease is on the rise. The diagnosis of diabetes in US adults increased 61% from 1991 and is projected to more than double by 2050 *(26)*. It has been estimated that a patient with DM has a 50% lifetime chance of having a surgical procedure *(27)*, and is more likely to undergo particular types of surgeries, related to complications of diabetes. In 1980, 11.3% of operations in diabetic patients were on the cardiovascular system, as compared to 4.3% in nondiabetic patients *(28)*; nearly 12% of all patients undergoing coronary artery bypass surgery have diabetes *(29,30)*. Other surgical procedures performed more frequently in diabetic patients include cataract extraction and vitrectomy, renal transplantation, ulcer debridement, and penile prosthesis implantation *(31)*.

For many reasons, the surgical patient with diabetes has long been regarded as being at high risk for both cardiovascular and noncardiovascular complications. In the early 20th century, diabetic patients were denied all but the most necessary surgery. Over time, the use of insulin and antibiotics, improvements in surgical and anesthetic techniques, intravenous fluid management, and transfusion therapy have all served to improve postsurgical survival. With these advances, postoperative sepsis and ketoacidosis have become less common, and cardiovascular complications have become the primary cause of perioperative morbidity and mortality among patients with DM. Data from the 1960s suggest that surgery in the diabetic patient was associated with 4% to 13% mortality, mainly as a result of cardiovascular causes, making surgery a major cause of death in diabetics *(32)*. Although improved anesthetic and surgical techniques and better cardiovascular treatment have helped decrease the risks, the gains have been partially offset by the increasing age of the diabetic population and the greater complexity of procedures now undertaken in these patients.

However, whether DM is definitely an independent risk factor for adverse perioperative outcomes, cardiac or noncardiac, is debatable. Studies of diabetes as a risk factor are predominantly retrospective, and much of the data is derived from subanalyses of studies looking at a broader surgical population (Table 1).

A modest number of studies show a statistically significant association between diabetes and adverse operative outcomes (Table 1). In developing their risk index, Eagle and associates found that in 200 patients undergoing major vascular surgery, diabetes was an independent risk factor and predictive of postoperative events or deaths ($p = 0.03$), sensitivity of 33% (confidence interval [CI], 18–53) and specificity of 96% (CI, 25–100) *(33)*. Other investigators have subsequently reported that DM is a risk factor for adverse cardiac events in patients undergoing noncardiac surgery *(34–37)*. An association was suggested in two other reports *(12,38)*, but failed to reach statistical significance. More recently, L'Italien and colleagues *(39)* assessed a Bayesian model for perioperative cardiac risk in a cohort of vascular surgical patients, and in the validation of their model they found diabetes to be an independent predictor of adverse outcomes with an odds ratio (OR) of 2.0 ($p = 0.048$; CI, 1.0–4.1).

Conversely, several studies have shown that outcomes in diabetics and nondiabetics are not significantly different (Table 1). Two prospective studies by Goldman and associates *(21)* and Pedersen associates *(40)*, failed to show that DM is associated with a significantly increased risk for perioperative complications. Another prospective study

Table 1
Perioperative Outcomes in Patients With Diabetes Mellitus

Author (reference)	Surgery dates	Patients	Surgery	Overall outcomes	Diabetic outcomes	Statistical significance
Mauney 1970 (48)	1968–1969	365 patients with abnormal ECGs	Major Noncardiac	Postoperative ECG changes and MIs	No significant increase in ECG Changes or MIs	NS
Steen 1978 (9)	1974–1975	587 patients with prior MIs (121 diabetics)	Noncardiac	6.1% had reinfarctions	7.4% diabetics had reinfarctions 5.9% nondiabetics had reinfarctions	NS
Goldman 1978 (21)	1975–1976	1001 patients >40 years old	Noncardiac	1.8% had MIs prospective	Diabetes was not a significant factor	NS
Crawford 1981 (15)	1955–1981	949 patients (113 diabetics)	Aortoiliac	3.8% mortality	Diabetes was not a significant factor (decreased long-term [at 5 and 10 years] survival in diabetics)	NS
Von Knorring 1981 (22)	1975–1977	214 patients with evidence of CAD	Major Noncardiac	17.7% had MIs	23% diabetics had MIs 17% nondiabetics had MIs	NS
Walsh 1982 (49)	1975–1979	175 patients (80 diabetics)	Gallbladder (acute and chronic)	1.1% had MIs 5.2% mortality	1.3% diabetics had MIs 1% nondiabetics had MIs 5% diabetic mortality 5.3% nondiabetic mortality	NS NS
Hertzer 1982 (50)		951 patients (284 diabetics)	Vascular	8.8% mortality	Diabetes was not a significant factor	NS
Hjortrup 1985 (47)	1975–1983	224 diabetics 224 nondiabetics	Major noncardiac matched	20.5% had general complications	20.5% diabetics had complications 20.5% nondiabetics had complications 30% of complications were cardiac in diabetics 43% of complications were cardiac in nondiabetics	NS NS
Foster 1986 (36)	1978–1981	1600 patients CASS patients (12% diabetics)	Noncardiac	Mortality and cardiac morbidity	Diabetics had more events	p = 0.004
Larsen 1987 (12)	1981–1983	2609 patients >40 years old (176 diabetics)	Major Noncardiac	2.6% had cardiac complications 0.8% had cardiac mortality	7.3% diabetics had complications 2.3% nondiabetics had complications 1.7% diabetics had cardiac mortality 0.8% nondiabetics had cardiac mort.	Regr coefficient Cardiac event p = 1.06
Leppo 1987 (38)	1984–1985	80 patients for dip. thallium	Vascular	16.8% had cardiac events	47% patients with events had diabetes 24% patients without events had diabetes	NS

Study	Years	Patients	Surgery	Outcome	Results	p-value
Eagle 1989 (33)	1984–1987	200 patients for dip. thallium (30% diabetics)	Vascular	15% had ischemic events	33% patients with events had diabetes / 12% patients without events had diabetes	$p = 0.03$
Younis 1990 (51)	1984–1989	111 patients for dip thallium (30% diabetics)	Vascular	7.2% had MIs	30% patients with MIs had diabetes / 29% patients without MIs had diabetes	NS
Pedersen 1990 (40)	1986–1987	7306 patients (141 diabetics)	Noncardiac Nonvascular	9.4% had complications / 6.3% had cardiac events	9.2% diabetics had cardiac events	NS
Lette 1992 (37)		355 patients for dip thallium	Major Noncardiac	8.5% had cardiac event	47% patients with events had diabetes / 19% patients without events had diabetes	$p = 0.0004$
Hollenberg 1992 (34)	1987–1989	474 male VA patients (105 diabetics)	Noncardiac	Postoperative ischemia	Diabetes was a significant risk factor	$p = 0.01$
Ashton 1993 (7)	1987–1989	835 male VA patients (194 diabetics)	Noncardiac	1.8% had MIs	Diabetes was not a significant factor	NS
Brown 1993 (35)	1988–1990	231 patients	Noncardiac	8.2% had cardiac events	53% patients with events had diabetes / 20% patients without events had diabetes	$p < 0.005$
L'Italien 1996 (39)	1984–1991	567 patients in "training" set / 514 patients in "validation" set	Vascular	8.1% had cardiac events / 7.6% had cardiac events	37% patients with events had diabetes / 20% patients without events had diabetes / 69% patients with events had diabetes / 53% patients without events had diabetes	$p = 0.008$ / $p = 0.048$
Treiman 1994 (41)	1964–1988	153 patients DM / 970 patients non-DM	Abdominal aortic		5.2% patients with DM had PMI / 2.1% patients without DM had PMI	$p = 0.0434$
Melliere 1999 (42)	1992–1996	169 patients DM / 834 patients non-DM	Vascular		8.9% mortality in patients with DM / 0.8% mortality in patients without DM	$p < 0.001$
Dardik 1999 (43)	1990–1995	2335 patients (168 diabetics)	Abdominal aortic	3.5% mortality	Diabetes was not a significant factor	NS
Berry 2001 (44)	1986–1996	856 patients (106 diabetics)	Abdominal aortic	1.3% mortality	Diabetes was not a significant factor	NS
Ballotta 2001 (45)	1992–1999	199 patients DM / 348 pts nonDM	CEA	Overall mortality 0.5%	Diabetes was not a significant factor	NS
Rayan 2002 (46)	1990–1999	421 patients (52 diabetics)	Abdominal aortic	1.7% mortality	3.8% mortality in patients with DM / 1.4% mortality in patients without DM	$p = 0.19$

ECG, electrocardiograph; NS, not significant; MI, myocardial infarction; CASS, Coronary Artery Surgery Study dip thallium, dipyridamole thallium; DM, diabetes mellitus; CEA, carotid endarterectomy.

by Ballotta and associates *(45)*, looking at the perioperative outcome of carotid endart-erectomy in diabetic patients vs nondiabetic patients found no significant difference between the two groups with respect to cardiac morbidity and mortality. Recently, several studies have compared outcomes between diabetic and nondiabetic patients undergoing abdominal aortic aneurysm repair and have found no differences in mortality *(43,44,46)*. Other studies have also shown similar rates of postoperative complications, including perioperative MI, in diabetics and nondiabetics undergoing both vascular and nonvascular surgical procedures *(7,9,15,22,47–51)*.

PATHOPHYSIOLOGY

Pathophysiology of Perioperative Cardiovascular Complications

Anesthesia and surgery have profound effects on overall metabolism and on the cardiovascular system, and several mechanisms have been implicated in the pathophysiology of perioperative cardiac complications. In the perioperative period there can be remarkable changes in the loading conditions of the heart, as a result of either volume loss or volume overload. There is stimulation of the sympathetic autonomic system resulting from hemodynamic changes and from other stressors such as pain and anxiety. Catecholamine-mediated tachycardia and hypertension may cause significant myocardial ischemia as a result of a mismatch in oxygen supply and demand, in the setting of fixed CAD or catecholamine-induced coronary spasm *(52–54)*. A hypercoagulable state exists postoperatively, associated with decreased fibrinolytic and increased prothrombotic activity *(55–58)*. Such a milieu may predispose to plaque rupture and coronary thrombosis in patients undergoing surgery *(59,60)*. In the setting of these disturbances, the presence of underlying CVD raises the likelihood for complications.

Perioperative Pathophysiology Related to Diabetes Mellitus

The diabetic patient is more likely than the nondiabetic patient to have CAD *(61)*, and cardiovascular causes are responsible for the majority of deaths in diabetic individuals. In fact, the risk of heart disease mortality is two to four times higher in diabetic patients than in nondiabetics *(62)*. The diabetic patient is more likely to have diffuse CAD with involvement of smaller caliber vessels *(63,64)*. In the event of MI, the incidence of heart failure is higher and the overall in-hospital mortality is higher for diabetic patients than for nondiabetics, especially in women *(65)*. It has been repeatedly demonstrated that a large proportion of the diabetic population has CAD that is manifested atypically *(66–69)*, making diagnosis more difficult.

DM appears to increase the likelihood of developing CHF from any cause. And aside from identifiable causes, the existence of a cardiomyopathy related specifically to DM has been described, particularly in women, associated with increased cardiovascular mortality *(63)*.

Autonomic dysfunction is estimated to be present in 20% to 40% of patients with diabetes, and 82% of patients with peripheral neuropathy have evidence for autonomic dysfunction *(70)*. Autonomic dysfunction is characterized by the loss of appropriate heart rate and blood pressure (BP) modulation, and may cause significant cardiovascular instability. The diabetic patient with autonomic dysfunction is more likely to have depressed ventricular function *(71,72)*, to suffer an MI or sudden death, and the MI is more likely to be have been clinically unrecognized *(73–76)*. Autonomic dysfunction may impair cardiovascular reflexes and prevent the appropriate response to the hemodynamic effects of anesthetic induction and other surgical stresses, and may be related to an increased mortality seen in some diabetic surgical patients.

Insulin normally serves as an anabolic hormone, affecting the metabolism of carbohydrates, proteins, and fats. In general, the stress response to surgery produces neurohormonal changes, which disturb the normal role of insulin, and promote intense catabolism. In the postoperative period, insulin secretion is normally decreased relative to the degree of hyperglycemia (although absolute levels may be normal or high). Perioperative fasting will tend to induce further catabolism. In the diabetic patient, in the setting of pre-existing insulin deficiency or resistance, the catabolic consequences of surgery are pronounced and severe hyperglycemia and ketosis can develop, along with attendant acidosis, fluid depletion, and electrolyte disturbances (77). To minimize the effects of these metabolic events, attention to glycemic metabolic control is necessary.

Finally, postoperative wound-healing is impaired in the diabetic patient. In vitro and animal models have shown a correlation between impaired deep wound-healing and hyperglycemia, which may cause deficiencies in granulation tissue and collagen, and decreased capillary ingrowth (78,79). Reversible in vitro neutrophil dysfunction is also associated with hyperglycemia (80,81). Neuropathy and occlusive vascular disease are factors likely affecting wound-healing, and experts suggest that surgical success and adequate healing may be related to the presence or absence of these factors, rather than humoral factors or specific levels of blood glucose in the postoperative period (82).

The impact of DM on numerous organ systems can make perioperative management challenging. Years of hyperglycemia may be manifested in abnormalities of the renal, immune, neurological, autonomic, endocrine, and cardiovascular systems, and will have implications for the perioperative course and outcome. The stressful effects of the perioperative period will be pronounced when superimposed on the pre-existing disturbances related to diabetes and its associated co-morbidities.

RISK ASSESSMENT

The clinician performing the preoperative assessment should evaluate the patient's current medical status and provide a clinical risk profile that the patient, primary physician, anesthesiologist, and surgeon can use in making treatment decisions. The evaluation is intended to identify the patient who is at increased risk for a complication as a result of the proposed procedure, and to identify any patient-related or surgery-specific variables that can be modified to lower the risk. An important part of the evaluation is the decision regarding further testing to identify and characterize the severity and stability of underlying CVD.

CLINICAL EVALUATION

Clinical Risk Indices

Various schemata have been developed to risk stratify surgical patients based on clinical characteristics and comorbidities (Table 2). The vast majority of cardiovascular complications occur in patients with known cardiac disease, and predominantly in patients who have or are at risk for CAD (3). Therefore, much of the focus of perioperative cardiac risk assessment, and the research in the field, is on the identification and management of coronary disease. The development of the above models has been based mainly

Table2
Two Commonly Used Indexes of Perioperative Cardiac Risk

Factor	Original[a] Definition	No. of points	Detsky et al.[a] Definition	No. of points
Ischemic heart disease	MI within 6 months	10	MI within 6 months	10
			MI more than 6 months earlier	5
			CCS class III angina	10
			CCS class IV angina	20
			Unstable angina within 6 months	10
Congestive heart failure	S$_3$ gallop or jugular venous distention	11	Pulmonary edema within 1 week any time in the past	10 / 5
Cardiac rhythm	Rhythm other than sinus or PACs on last preoperative ECG >5 PVCs/minute at any time preop.	7	Rhythm other than sinus or PACs on last preoperative ECG 7	5
Valvular heart disease	Important aortic stenosis	3	Suspected critical aortic stenosis	20
General medical status	PO2 <60 mmHg, PCO2 >50 mmHg, potassium <3 mmol/L, bicarbonate <20 mmol/L, BUN >50 mg/dL, creat. >3 mg/dL, abnormal AST, signs of chronic liver disease, patient bedridden for noncardiac causes	3	Same as for original index	
Age	>70 years	5	>70 years	5
Type of surgery	Intraperitoneal, intrathoracic, or aortic operation	3	Emergency operation	10
	Emergency operation	4		

MI, myocardial infarction; CCS, Canadian Cardiovascular Society classification of angina; PAC, premature atrial contraction; ECG, electrocardiogram;PVC, premature ventricular contraction; PO$_2$, partial pressure of oxygen; PCO$_2$, partial pressure of carbon dioxide; BUN, blood urea nitrogen; AST, aspartate aminotransferase.
[a]Adapted with permission from refs. *8,11,213*.

on observational or retrospective studies, and little data is available from prospective or randomized studies.

The original Cardiac Risk Index developed by Goldman and colleagues was the first validated multivariate model developed to predict cardiac complications in a general surgical population *(8)*. A modified index by Detsky and associates added "significant angina" and included the type of planned surgery *(11)*. High scores assessed by these indices, reflecting the presence of multiple risk factors, have proved helpful in risk-stratifying unselected, consecutive patients undergoing general surgery. In patients undergoing vascular surgery, which is generally considered to be relatively high-risk surgery, Eagle and colleagues were able to identify patients who were at low risk for complications by the absence of advanced age, angina, history of ventricular ectopic activity, Q waves on electrocardiogram (ECG), and DM *(33)*. The American College of Cardiology (ACC) and the American Heart Association (AHA) jointly published guidelines for the perioperative management of noncardiac surgical patients in 1996, which were recently updated (Fig. 1) *(83,84)*.

There is no unified approach to how the diagnosis of DM should be factored into the process of preoperative risk stratification. In the report of the original risk index Goldman noted that the "conspicuously insignificant variables in our analysis includes diabetes," and DM was not included as one of the nine risk factors *(8)*. Similarly, diabetes is not included as a risk factor in the index by Detsky *(11)*, and Detsky's recent position paper on preoperative risk assessment for the American College of Physicians does not address diabetes *(85)*. Eagle's schema, on the other hand, uses DM as a significant risk factor *(33)*. Expert opinions can be conflicting, and recent reviews have drawn opposite conclusions *(3,82)*. The ACC/AHA guidelines on perioperative management include DM among the "intermediate predictors" for perioperative cardiovascular risk, which were defined as "well-validated markers of enhanced risk of perioperative cardiac complications which justify careful assessment of the patient's current status" *(83)*.

Clearly, not all diabetic surgical patients are at high perioperative risk. There is a need to define clinical risk factors that might aid the physician in identifying the individual diabetic patient who is at an increased risk. A significant deficiency of the available epidemiological data is the lack of information on the risk associated with particular subgroups of the diabetic population.

Subgroups of Patients With Diabetes Mellitus

As with surgical patients in general, diabetic patients with manifestations of CVD are at a higher risk in the perioperative period. MacKenzie and associates showed that serious morbidity and mortality in diabetic patients were predicted by the presence of pre-existing cardiac disease. They identified diabetic patients with heart failure and significant valvular disease as being at increased risk, and suggested that diabetics without these two conditions were not likely to have cardiac or noncardiac complication *(86)*. In a study by Zarich and associates *(68)*, all adverse events occurred in patients with clinical markers for coronary disease (history of angina or CHF, pathological Q waves on ECG). No adverse events occurred in the patients without clinical markers of coronary disease, despite the 58% prevalence of abnormal dipyridamole thallium scans, in the setting of similar vascular procedures, anesthetic techniques, and perioperative use of nitroglycerin and hemodynamic monitoring.

Farrow and associates have suggested that DM may be more associated with cardiac events in certain types of surgery *(87)*. These investigators found that diabetes figured prominently as a risk factor in orthopedic procedures, operations of the larynx and trachea, and of the upper gastrointestinal tract; it was not a significant factor in laparotomies, esophageal and colorectal surgery, and amputations. Conspicuously absent was major vascular surgery. On the other hand, Hjortrup and colleagues found no difference in the incidence of postoperative complications amongst diabetic patients in three groups of surgical procedures—major abdominal surgery, major vascular surgery, and orthopedic surgery *(47)*.

For diabetics and nondiabetics alike, vascular surgery is undertaken at a higher risk for cardiac events than many other surgical procedures. The increased risk may be partly related to the risks inherent to the procedure itself and partly because of the high prevalence of concomitant coronary disease in these patients *(69,88,89)*. Patients undergoing infrainguinal vascular bypass, compared to those having aortic procedures, tend to have

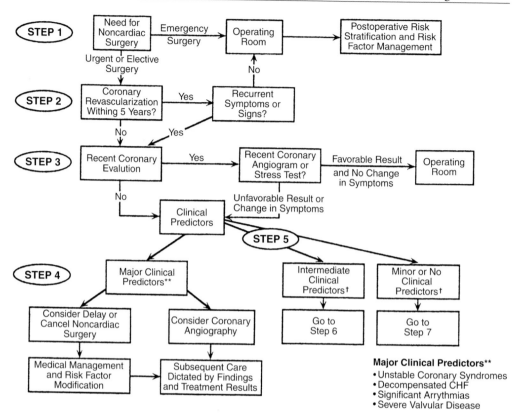

Fig. 1. Stepwise approach to preoperative cardiac assessment. *Subsequent care may include cancellation or delay of surgery, coronary revascularization, or intensified care. (Reprinted with permission from ref. *83*.)

a higher prevalence of CAD *(90,91)*. The increased cardiac morbidity, early and late, observed in patients undergoing peripheral vascular procedures is likely related to the increased prevalence of concomitant CAD.

Institutional factors will influence postoperative outcomes. The experience and expertise of the surgical team and the medical consultants in the management of diabetes are likely to favorably affect outcomes. On the other hand, an institution specializing in the management of diabetes may undertake procedures that are more complex and risky, and may attract referrals of high-risk patients.

As discussed previously, patients with autonomic dysfunction are a group of diabetics particularly prone to CVD, associated with increased atypical or silent ischemia, ventricular dysfunction, and hemodynamic instability. Diabetic patients who manifest autonomic dysfunction are at an increased risk for perioperative hemodynamic instability, cardiorespiratory arrest, and death *(92–94)*. Therefore, the patient with autonomic dysfunction should be considered to be at a high risk for perioperative complications. Such a patient may warrant particularly close cardiovascular evaluation, hemodynamic monitoring, and surveillance for cardiovascular events.

The incidence of postoperative complications is not necessarily related to the duration of diabetes *(67,68,86)*, and previously has not been felt to be related to the form of treatment of the diabetes (i.e., insulin vs oral agents) *(47,67,68,86)*. But a recent retro-

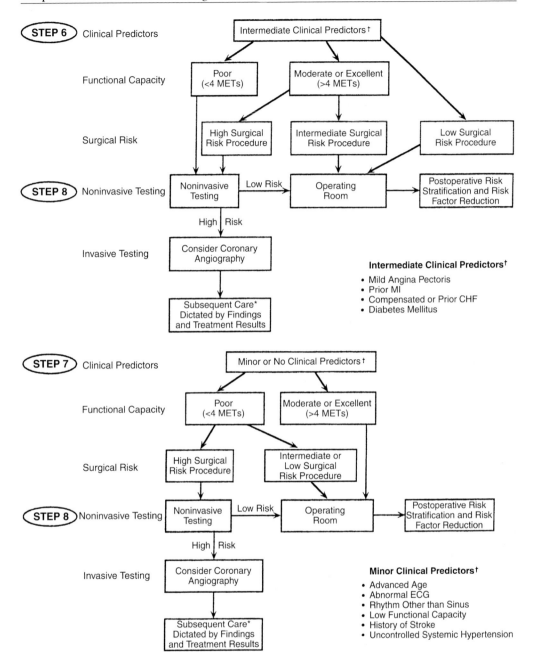

STEP 6 — Clinical Predictors — Intermediate Clinical Predictors[†]

Functional Capacity: Poor (<4 METs) / Moderate or Excellent (>4 METs)

Surgical Risk: High Surgical Risk Procedure / Intermediate Surgical Risk Procedure / Low Surgical Risk Procedure

STEP 8 — Noninvasive Testing — Noninvasive Testing — Low Risk — Operating Room — Postoperative Risk Stratification and Risk Factor Reduction

High | Risk

Invasive Testing — Consider Coronary Angiography

Subsequent Care* Dictated by Findings and Treatment Results

Intermediate Clinical Predictors[†]
- Mild Angina Pectoris
- Prior MI
- Compensated or Prior CHF
- Diabetes Mellitus

STEP 7 — Clinical Predictors — Minor or No Clinical Predictors[†]

Functional Capacity: Poor (<4 METs) / Moderate or Excellent (>4 METs)

Surgical Risk: High Surgical Risk Procedure / Intermediate or Low Surgical Risk Procedure

STEP 8 — Noninvasive Testing — Noninvasive Testing — Low Risk — Operating Room — Postoperative Risk Stratification and Risk Factor Reduction

High | Risk

Invasive Testing — Consider Coronary Angiography

Subsequent Care* Dictated by Findings and Treatment Results

Minor Clinical Predictors[†]
- Advanced Age
- Abnormal ECG
- Rhythm Other than Sinus
- Low Functional Capacity
- History of Stroke
- Uncontrolled Systemic Hypertension

spective VA study by Axelrod et al. examining the impact of DM on perioperative outcomes in patients who underwent major vascular surgery found that patients treated with insulin were at increased risk for cardiovascular complications (OR 1.48; 95% CI, 1.15–1.91) but not death *(95)*. In their derivation and prospective validation of a simple index for prediction of cardiac risk in major noncardiac surgery, Lee and associates also found preoperative treatment with insulin to be an independent predictor of cardiac complications (96). Thus, it would appear that patients with diabetes are not uniformly at risk for adverse outcomes and those patients treated with insulin may represent a subgroup of diabetics at higher risk.

CLINICAL EVALUATION OF THE PATIENT WITH DIABETES MELLITUS

A limitation to the clinical evaluation of the patient with DM is the concern for atypical manifestations of CVD (73,74,97,98). Uncertainty in defining ischemia and MI has important consequences for the reliability of the preoperative assessment and the reliability of the perioperative surveillance for cardiac events. Physicians, therefore, may not feel as confident in basing their assessment on the clinical evaluation of a diabetic patient, as compared with a nondiabetic patient.

Despite the atypical nature of presentation, careful evaluation can often yield a history of symptoms ascribable to an ischemic event. A number of studies have shown that it is a minority of patients who are asymptomatic at the time of their acute MI and that in most cases symptoms can be determined, albeit atypical in nature in up to 42% of cases (99,100). Atypical symptoms are more common in elderly diabetic patients, as in nondiabetic patients (101). Autonomic dysfunction increases the likelihood for atypical ischemic symptoms and for silent ischemia (73–75). In patients with peripheral vascular disease (PVD), limitations in activity imposed by claudication may make evaluating symptoms of CAD particularly difficult. Therefore, careful attention is required for atypical manifestations in elderly patients, in patients with autonomic dysfunction, and in patients with PVD.

The presence of anginal symptoms in a patient with DM is prognostically important. There is evidence that diabetics have a higher threshold for feeling angina and, therefore, the presence of symptoms may be indicative of more severe ischemia. Zarich and associates (68) and Lane and associates (67) found that a history of angina in a patient with DM was associated with a higher incidence of cardiac complications.

With a heightened vigilance the physician can identify historical clues and physical findings which are associated with increased perioperative risk. Additionally, surgery- and institution-specific factors should be considered.

NONINVASIVE TESTING

Preoperative noninvasive testing is intended to evaluate the severity of CAD, whether suspected or already diagnosed. It is also intended to assess the functional capacity of the patient in whom clinical evaluation alone cannot provide that information.

EXERCISE-TOLERANCE TESTING

Exercise-tolerance testing to evaluate exercise capacity and electrocardiocraphic response has been used to risk-stratify patients awaiting general noncardiac (102) and vascular surgery (103,104). The efficacy of the exercise-tolerance test relies greatly on defining functional capacity, and the predictive value depends on an adequate stress level (85% maximal predicted heart rate) during the test. Significant confounders of exercise testing are any physical condition that will limit the patient's ability to exercise, such as claudication resulting from severe PVD, or medications such as β-blockers that might blunt the heart rate response to exercise. Peripheral neuropathy and autonomic neuropathy in diabetics impair the ability of the patient to exercise adequately, and may alter the hemodynamic response to exercise *(70)*.

NONINVASIVE IMAGING

The addition of imaging, such as thallium scintigraphy, significantly improves the sensitivity of exercise testing, even if suboptimal levels of stress are achieved *(105)*. In patients who are unable to exercise adequately, pharmacological testing with dipyridamole and dobutamine in conjunction with imaging modalities are useful. Dipyridamole-thallium scintigraphy has been studied extensively in the preoperative setting.

The utility of thallium defects in predicting perioperative risk has been shown repeatedly, particularly in vascular patients *(33,35,37,89,106–108)*. The sensitivity for coronary disease has been as high as 100%, and the positive predictive value for cardiac complications ranges from 10% to 30% in the larger studies. The extent of abnormality has been found to be significant, and the nature of the defects (i.e., reversible vs fixed). The probability of long-term event-free survival can also be assessed with these preoperative results *(51,109,110)*. Perfusion imaging with scintigraphy may have greater functional and a prognostic utility than angiography, because perfusion imaging provides information on the extent of myocardium that may be in jeopardy in association with a coronary stenosis.

Although the presence of a transient thallium defect is associated with an increase in the relative risk among patients referred for testing, the association weakens as the test is applied to unselected patients. This applies even in patients with PVD *(111,112)*, considered to be at higher risk to begin with. The importance of combining clinical with scintigraphic data was demonstrated by Eagle and associates *(33)* (Fig. 2), and subsequently confirmed in a multicenter study by L'Italien and associates *(39)*.

The data on dobutamine echocardiography to assess perioperative risk are few relative to those available for nuclear perfusion imaging. The positive predictive value ranges from 7% to 23% for deaths or MIs, and the negative predictive value ranges from 93% to 100% *(113,114)*. The extent of wall motion abnormalities and ischemia manifested by new wall motion abnormalities at low dobutamine doses appear to be significant. Although the results seem comparable to perfusion modalities, the published experience is still limited. Stress echocardiography may be potentially useful in evaluating patients with valvular disease.

Resting left ventricular function as determined by echocardiography or radionuclide angiography is of limited utility in risk stratifying patients. Although patients with a left ventricular ejection fraction of less than 35% may be at risk for developing perioperative CHF, resting left ventricular function is not a reliable predictor of ischemic events *(115–117)*.

USE OF NONINVASIVE IMAGING IN PATIENTS WITH DIABETES MELLITUS

Preoperative nuclear imaging is used extensively in patients with diabetes. Because CVD is likely to be atypical in patients with diabetes, there has been a tendency to rely on further testing, particularly thallium scintigraphy, to identify patients with significant disease. Numerous investigators have shown that in the absence of a history of angina,

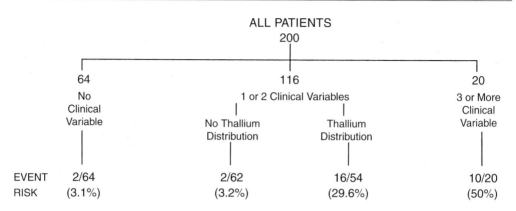

Fig. 2. Results of using clinical variables and results of dipyridamole thallium imaging to stratify cardiac risk as applied to a group of 200 patients. (Reprinted with permission from ref. *35.*)

CHF, or infarct up to 59% of diabetic patients being evaluated for vascular surgery have abnormal thallium scans (fixed or reversible) *(66–69)*. In comparison, only 17% of asymptomatic nondiabetic patients with PVD have reversible defects *(118)*.

Patients with diabetes who have additional coronary risk factors are more likely to have significant thallium abnormalities. Nesto and co-workers studied 165 patients with diabetes and PVD *(69)*, 30 of whom did not have clinical evidence of coronary disease. Of these 30 patients, 87% of the smokers, 71% of the hypertensives, and all with both of these risk factors had abnormal scans, although the 6 patients without either risk factor had normal scans. Diabetes alone, therefore, is not a strong predictor for the high prevalence of thallium-perfusion defects observed in diabetic patients, even in the population with PVD. The presence of additional risk factors is more predictive of significant thallium abnormalities.

Lane and co-workers studied 101 diabetic patients undergoing dipyridamole thallium scintigraphy prior to vascular surgery *(67)*. An abnormal thallium scan alone was not significantly predictive of cardiovascular risk. However, the specificity and positive predictive value improved with an increasing number of reversible defects. The positive predictive value of the presence of angina was similar to that of two reversible defects. This was confirmed by Brown and associates *(35)*, who determined that the probability of perioperative cardiac deaths or nonfatal MI increased relative to the number of thallium-perfusion defects, a relationship more pronounced in patients with DM when compared with nondiabetics. These results suggest that the risk of vascular surgery in patients with diabetes can be assessed by quantitating the extent of myocardial ischemia by dipyridamole thallium screening. To assess the utility of dipyridamole thallium in patients with and without clinical evidence of cardiac disease, Zarich and colleagues prospectively performed dipyridamole thallium scintigraphy in 133 patients with diabetes undergoing peripheral vascular surgery (more than 90% for limb-threatening ischemia) *(68)*. Clinical evidence of CAD was found in 57 patients, 36 patients were without clinical evidence of CAD, and 40 patients were excluded for reasons not related to the thallium results. All adverse events occurred in patients with clinical markers for CAD (history of angina or CHF, pathological Q waves on ECG) despite similar vascular procedures, anesthetic techniques, and perioperative use of nitroglycerin and hemodynamic monitoring. No adverse events occurred in the patients without clinical markers of CAD, despite the 58% prevalence of abnormal dipyridamole thallium scans. Among those with clinical markers of CAD, the number of thallium defects was an independent risk factor for postoperative events. In patients who do not have clinical markers for coronary disease, an abnormal thallium scan may not be predictive of cardiac events perioperatively.

The long-term prognostic value of dipyridamole thallium imaging in diabetics undergoing peripheral vascular surgery was evaluated in a prospective study by Cohen and associates (119). The presence of more than two reversible thallium defects was associated with a median survival of only 1.8 years. The thallium findings also further risk-stratified clinically high- and low-risk patients; whereas high-risk patients with normal scans had a median survival similar to low-risk patients (8.6 years), the presence of any thallium abnormality markedly reduced median survival to 3.7 years ($p < 0.001$). Conversely, low-risk patients with more than two reversible defects had a median survival of 4 years. Thus, dipyridamole thallium imaging in diabetic patients would seem to identify a subset of patients requiring more aggressive medical or surgical intervention.

Thus, thallium scintigraphy is a powerful tool in the risk assessment of the surgical candidate. Thallium scanning has impressive sensitivity in detecting the presence and severity of CAD. In diabetics and nondiabetics alike, the overuse of the test will lower its predictive value and therefore its clinical utility. Although patients with DM are more likely to have abnormal scans, this does not necessarily translate into an increased perioperative risk. Thallium scanning in diabetics without clinical evidence for CVD has little prognostic utility in the perioperative period. And in patients with clinical evidence for CVD, little is added to the overall assessment by a nuclear scan unless there are multiple defects suggestive of extensive ischemia. As with any diagnostic test, a Bayesian approach should be applied. Further testing should depend on the likely influence of the test on the overall assessment and how that in turn will affect further management decisions.

ANGIOGRAPHY

The patient who is determined to be at high risk by virtue of the preoperative evaluation should be referred for angiography to define the coronary anatomy. This is done with the expectation that coronary revascularization will be performed if feasible.

Patients with unstable angina or a recent MI warrant evaluation by coronary angiography prior to urgent surgery, foregoing preliminary noninvasive testing. Other patients who are at increased risk for adverse cardiac events and might benefit from angiography will be identified by clinical factors and noninvasive tests, as outlined above. Guidelines issued by the ACC and the AHA have outlined generally accepted indications for angiography in the nonoperative setting (120,121). In general, the indications for preoperative coronary angiography should parallel those for the nonoperative setting, and the recent ACC/AHA guidelines for perioperative cardiac risk assessment incorporated the above guidelines for angiography (83,84). Recently, Cohen and Eagle compiled the opinions of 30 experts regarding indications for angiography based on specific results of preoperative noninvasive tests (122). There is general agreement that a noninvasive result that indicates large zones of myocardial ischemia warrants further evaluation. The decision to pursue angiography should take into account the risk of this procedure itself and subsequent revascularization.

SPECIAL SITUATIONS: RENAL TRANSPLANTATION

The prevalence of CAD among diabetic patients with end-stage renal disease (ESRD) is as high as 55% *(105,122–126)*. The duration or type of diabetes may not have an effect on the severity of the coronary disease *(123,126)*, but hemodialysis may accelerate atherosclerosis *(127)*. There is a striking impact of coronary disease on survival in these patients. Two-year survival ranges from 22% to 45% in diabetics with ESRD *(123,126)*. Approximately 50% of deaths before *(105,126,129,130)* and after *(131–133)* transplantation resultfrom cardiac causes, with an average cardiac mortality rate of 7.8% per year. And in the perioperative period there is an increased incidence of cardiac complications with renal and pancreatic transplants *(134,135)*.

Evaluation of the diabetic renal transplant candidate is fraught with difficulties unique to ESRD. These patients will often have multiple risk factors for coronary disease and will frequently have numerous atypical cardiac and noncardiac complaints, often leading to many false-positive and false-negative clinical assessments.

The experience with noninvasive testing for CAD in patients with ESRD has yielded disappointing results. These patients are frequently unable to achieve adequate stress levels on exercise stress testing *(105)*. In one series, only 7% of the patients achieved target heart rates *(136)*. Various limiting factors include anemia *(137)*, debilitation, PVD, neuropathy *(70)*, and peritoneal dialysis *(138)*.

Although thallium has been shown to increase the sensitivity of exercise testing in these patients *(105)* and has been found to be useful when combined with dipyridamole in some studies *(129,130)*, the overall predictive value of thallium has been poor. In a series of 45 patients being evaluated for transplantation (only 1 patient with DM included), Marwick and colleagues *(139)* found that the sensitivity of dipyridamole thallium for CAD compared with angiography was only 37% (much lower than in patients without ESRD) and the specificity 73%. Of prognostic importance is that in this cohort, five of the six cardiac deaths occurred in patients who had normal scans and who all had significant CAD by catheterization. Other studies have confirmed the poor utility of this testing in this particular patient population *(128,130,140)*.

Dipyridamole can have a blunted hemodynamic effect in patients with ESRD as a result of high levels of endogenous adenosine in this population. This may account for a higher false-negative rate of dipyridamole thallium imaging in these patients *(141)*.

Given the grave perioperative and long-term implications of CAD in patients with diabetes and ESRD, and the poor efficacy of noninvasive testing, many experts recommend routine angiography prior to transplantation *(105,123,126,142–144)*. If noninvasive assessment is utilized the clinician should have a very high index of suspicion for CAD and a low threshold for referral to coronary angiography.

There is some limited evidence that coronary revascularization improves survival in diabetic patients being considered for renal transplantation. One study showed that in 26 patients randomly assigned to medical treatment or revascularization (angioplasty or coronary bypass surgery) *(145)* the frequency of cardiac events was lower in patients who underwent revascularization among the insulin-dependent diabetic patients with chronic renal failure.

RISK REDUCTION

After determining the magnitude of perioperative risk, the consultant's next task is to make recommendations aimed at lowering the risk. Risk lowering may be achieved by medical management, preoperative revascularization, and perioperative surveillance. In some instances, changing or canceling the procedure may be necessary. Data for specific recommendations is generally limited, and particularly so for patients with DM.

MEDICAL INTERVENTIONS

β-Blockers

Outside of the perioperative period, β-blockers have repeatedly been shown to improve survival in the setting of chronic coronary insufficiency and acute coronary syndromes. Data is limited regarding use of β-blockade perioperatively. In randomized and nonrandomized studies, β- blockers have been shown to decrease ischemic events, acute MIs, and death in the perioperative period *(146–149,150,151)*. There are no data regarding diabetics specifically, however, some clinicians have been reluctant to use β-blockers in patients with DM as a result of the potential effect on an already abnormal chronotropic response, and because of the theoretical concern for predisposing diabetic patients to hypoglycemia and altering the symptoms associated with hypoglycemia *(152)*. On the contrary, β-blockers are well tolerated clinically *(153,154)*. They are clearly beneficial in diabetic patients with CAD *(155,156)* and the reduction of postinfarction mortality and reinfarction rates associated with β-blockers appears to be especially pronounced in diabetic patients *(157–160)*.

In summary, the benefits of β-blockers in reducing perioperative mortality and MI warrant at least a perioperative course of treatment, although the optimal duration of therapy needing to be better established by clinical trials.

NITRATES

Intravenous nitroglycerin has been used to reverse ischemia in various clinical settings, including intraoperatively. However, its prophylactic intraoperative use in two small studies was not associated with improved outcomes *(161,162)*, and may actually lead to cardiovascular decompensation by decreasing preload. Additionally, the vasodilatory effects may be accentuated by the action of various anesthetic agents and by impaired autonomic function. Therefore, nitroglycerin administration should be reserved for the high-risk patient who has required nitrates prior to surgery for the control of angina and for the patient who develops signs of active ischemia.

ANESTHETIC AGENTS

There are many potential approaches to the anesthetic care of the patient with CVD. Most often the decisions regarding the anesthetic regimen are deferred to the anesthesiology team responsible for the patient. Patient co-morbidities and the surgical procedure itself usually outweigh any effects the anesthetic technique may have on outcome *(163)*.

All anesthetic techniques are associated with cardiovascular side effects. Spinal and epidural techniques can cause neural blockade, particularly sympathetic blockade, and can bring about profound afterload and preload changes. The intravenous agents used for induction of anesthesia typically lower the systemic BP by up to 30% in healthy patients, and often by even more in the hypertensive patient. This lowering is followed shortly thereafter by a predictable rise in BP during laryngoscopy and intubation. Inhalational agents may cause myocardial depression and afterload reduction. There are no significant differences among the commonly used inhalational agents (i.e., isoflurane, halothane, enflurane) *(164)*. Epidural anesthesia, spinal blocks, and splanchnic nerve blocks have been shown to ameliorate the endocrine, hematological and metabolic response to surgery *(165–167)*. Overall, however, studies have failed to show a myocardial benefit of any one regimen *(58,167,168)*.

The consequences of inadequate anesthesia should not be underestimated. Bode reported that the highest complication rate was in patients who failed regional anesthesia and were switched over to general anesthesia in the same setting *(169)*. Because of that finding it was recommended that patients who fail regional anesthesia should be brought back on another day.

The use of anesthesia in the diabetic patient involves some special considerations. Hypoglycemia has occasionally been documented after epidural anesthesia and after infiltration of large amounts of lidocaine *(170,171)*. Ether was associated with hyperglycemia and ketosis in the past, but the newer inhalational agents such as halothane and enflurane can be used safely *(172)*. The presence of impaired cardiovascular reflexes may prevent the appropriate response to the hemodynamic effects of anesthesia and surgery, and may be related in part to the increased mortality seen in diabetic surgical patients *(92,93)*. Therefore, particular caution should be used when administering anesthesia to patients with autonomic dysfunction.

REVASCULARIZATION

Retrospective and observational data have suggested that preoperative revascularization may confer some protection in patients who are determined to be at high risk for adverse cardiac outcomes. It should be noted, although, that no randomized, controlled trials have assessed the benefit of coronary artery bypass grafting (CABG) or percutaneous coronary intervention (PCI) before noncardiac surgery *(173)*.

Preoperative coronary artery bypass grafting lowers the operative mortality compared to medical therapy in patients undergoing noncardiac surgery. Among 1600 patients enrolled in the Coronary Artery Surgery Study (CASS) registry, Foster and associates *(36)* found that the operative mortality for noncardiac surgery was similar in patients without significant angiographic disease (0.5%) and in patients who had undergone CABG (0.9%), whereas it was significantly higher (2.4%) in patients with CAD treated medically. There was no significant difference in the incidence of perioperative MI, heart failure, or arrhythmias in the three groups. In a series of 1001 Cleveland Clinic patients undergoing elective vascular surgery *(174)*, the postoperative mortality rate was 1.4% in patients with no CAD, 3.6% in patients with advanced but compensated CAD (well collateralized territory, or already infarcted in area of involved vessel), 1.5% in patients who had preoperative coronary bypass, and 14% in patients with severe but inoperable coronary disease.

The potential benefit of preoperative revascularization must be weighed against the surgical risks of the coronary bypass itself and the delay to the proposed noncardiac surgery. The operative mortality of coronary artery bypass usually exceeds the risks inherent to the proposed noncardiac procedure, 5.3% in the Cleveland Clinic series *(174)* and 2.3% in the CASS registry *(36)*.

There is data to suggest that patients who have both CAD and PVD are at increased long-term cardiac risk, and long-term survival seems to be improved in patients undergoing CABG *(174,175)*. This is an effect on the chronic coronary disease rather than an immediate perioperative benefit. But the decision on whether to pursue revascularization before noncardiac surgery is controversial. In the short term, the perioperative mortality from elective vascular surgery is lower than prophylactic CABG surgery *(176)*. However, the major cause of long-term mortality in this patient population is cardiac; prompting some physicians to adopt a more aggressive stance on revascularization.

Patients with diabetes have increased morbidity and mortality after coronary revascularization compared with nondiabetic patients *(177,178)*. The randomized Bypass Angioplasty Revascularization Investigation (BARI) trial, although it did not specifically study patients undergoing noncardiac surgery, demonstrated that patients with treated diabetes (with insulin or oral agents) and multivessel disease had a significantly decreased 5.4-year cardiac mortality if assigned to an initial strategy of coronary bypass (5.8%), compared with percutaneous transluminal coronary angioplasty (20.6%) *(179)*. This survival benefit was pronounced in patients with internal mammary artery grafts, as compared to patients who received only venous conduits. In the diabetic patient with multivessel disease, the decision between angioplasty and bypass surgery should be guided by the results of this trial. In patients with single-vessel coronary disease, percutaneous revascularization is probably an acceptable, less-invasive alternative. Treatment options for patients with DM will be better defined with the completion of the BARI II trial. The study group in BARI II consists of 2600 patients with type 2 DM and stable CAD who are suitable for elective revascularization. Importantly, this trial should provide greater insight regarding the practice of single or multivessel stenting as it compares to CABG *(180)*.

Several small series have shown a protective benefit from preoperative percutaneous coronary balloon angioplasty, with a lower complication rate than with bypass surgery *(181–184)*. Recently, two studies have looked at postoperative outcomes in patients who have undergone coronary stenting before noncardiac surgery *(185,186)*. Kaluza and associates examined the outcomes of a group of patients who had undergone noncardiac surgery within 6 weeks of stenting. Of 40 patients, there were 7 MIs, 11 major bleeding episodes, and 8 deaths. All deaths and MIs, and 8 of 11 bleeds, occurred in patients undergoing surgery less than 14 days after stent placement. Most deaths were accounted for by stent thrombosis. Wilson and associates, in attempting to determine the optimal delay following stent placement prior to noncardiac surgery, reviewed the clinical course of 207 patients who underwent noncardiac surgery in the 2 months following stent placement. Eight patients (4%) died or suffered an MI or stent thrombosis. All 8 patients underwent noncardiac surgery within 6 weeks of stent placement. From these studies, it would seem advisable to wait 6 weeks poststent placement before proceeding with noncardiac surgery when possible.

In summary, the indications for preoperative revascularization should parallel those in the nonsurgical population. Patients with diabetes awaiting elective noncardiac surgery who are found to have high-risk coronary anatomy, and in whom short- or long-term outcome would likely be improved by revascularization, should generally undergo CABG before elective high-risk noncardiac surgery. In patients who have undergone PCI with stent placement, elective noncardiac surgery should be performed at least 6 weeks after stent placement.

PERIOPERATIVE MONITORING

The detection of a cardiovascular event perioperatively ideally would lead to prompt and appropriate treatment. In the perioperative period, multiple confounders may not allow for the detection of cardiovascular problems. An altered sensorium as a result of analgesics and sedatives may prevent the patient from appropriately recognizing or expressing symptoms. A focus on the surgical site and related issues may cause the patient and caretakers to mistake cardiovascular symptoms for problems associated with the surgery itself. Atypical symptoms may be further distorted in this context and particularly difficult to characterize; an issue especially relevant in some diabetic patients.

It would seem reasonable, then, to consider the perioperative use of a pulmonary artery catheter in selected patients undergoing procedures deemed high risk. But current evidence from randomized trials evaluating the use of pulmonary artery catheters in abdominal aortic surgery and vascular surgery have shown no difference in perioperative MI or mortality (187–189,173,151). The American Society of Anesthesiologists has published guidelines for the intraoperative use of pulmonary artery catheters according to patient disease, surgical procedure, and practice setting (190). The ACC/AHA guidelines are in accordance with these recommendations. And although there is no class I indication for the intraoperative use of pulmonary artery catheters, their use may benefit high-risk patients undergoing procedures in which large intraoperative and postoperative fluid shifts are anticipated (83).

The optimal method for documenting perioperative MI has not been determined. Various protocols have been examined, although serial electrocardiography and serial cardiac enzymes have been used most commonly. The efficacy of these methods has varied considerably in different studies, depending on the diagnostic criteria used. Rettke and associates found that higher creatinine kinase (CK)-MB levels after abdominal aortic surgery correlated with worse outcomes (191). Charlson and associates demonstrated that electrocardiography immediately after noncardiac surgery and subsequently on the first and second postoperative days had a higher sensitivity than enzyme analysis (192).

Given the fact that CK-MB is released from noncardiac tissue, troponin T and I potentially provide better specificity perioperatively (193–199). Adams and associates prospectively evaluated 108 patients undergoing noncardiac surgery with baseline echocardiograms, serial ECGs, and serial CK-MB and troponin I. On the third postoperative day, a repeat echocardiogram was obtained. Eight patients developed new segmental wall motion abnormalities; all eight patients had elevations of troponin I, and six patients had elevations of CK-MB. Of the 100 patients without perioperative MI by echocardiography, 19 had elevations of CK-MB, with only 1 with a slight elevation of troponin I (193). In another study evaluating the prognostic significance of troponin T elevation after noncardiac surgery, patients with elevated troponin T had a relative risk for cardiac events of 5.4, whereas CK-MB was not correlated with postdischarge cardiac events (194).

Real-time ST-segment monitoring has been used to detect perioperative ischemia. Postoperative ischemic changes in the ST segment, especially of prolonged duration in high-risk patients, have been shown to be predictive of perioperative cardiac events (54,200,201) and predictive of worse long-term survival in patients (23). Computerized ST-segment analysis and trending is superior to visual interpretation and will greatly improve the sensitivity of this monitoring modality. Although ST-segment monitoring may detect ischemia, the clinical significance of transient ST-segment changes and their impact on outcome has not been established (202).

Per ACC/AHA guidelines regarding the optimal strategy for surveillance and detection of perioperative MI in patients with high or intermediate clinical risk undergoing high- or intermediate-risk surgery, it is recommended that ECGs be obtained at baseline, immediately postoperatively, and on postoperative days 1 and 2 with troponin measurements 24 hours postoperatively and on day 4 or hospital discharge *(83)*.

METABOLIC MANAGEMENT

As discussed previously, the catabolic consequences of surgery are pronounced in the diabetic patient, and severe hyperglycemia and ketosis can develop along with acidosis, fluid depletion, and electrolyte disturbances. To minimize the effects of these metabolic events, close attention to glycemic control is necessary. Insulin administration inhibits lipolysis, ketogenesis, and protein catabolism. Glucose administration also helps to inhibit these. All insulin-dependent patients should be treated with insulin, glucose, and fluids during the perioperative period. Noninsulin-dependent patients may also require insulin.

There is little evidence regarding the ideal level of glycemic control. Hypoglycemia may be associated with neurological effects, and a sympathetic surge and a potentially deleterious cardiovascular response. Therefore, blood glucose levels should be maintained above 120 mg/dL. To avoid osmotic diuresis and the effects of relative hypoinsulinemia discussed above, blood glucose levels should ideally be maintained below 180 mg/dL *(77,82)*. Hjortrup et al. observed that the mean blood glucose levels preoperatively and during the first postoperative day were significantly lower in the diabetic patient with complications, as compared to the patients without complications *(47)*. More recently, however, studies of patients with DM undergoing cardiac surgery have shown an association between perioperative hyperglycemia and wound infections *(203,204,205)*. These patients have less infectious complications when glycemic control is obtained with a continous insulin infusion and blood glucose was maintained below 200 mg/dL. For elective procedures it is generally felt that good glucose control should be achieved before surgery, and this may mean initiating insulin therapy or changing current dosing *(82)*. This can take several days or even weeks. In this era of cost containment, most patients are admitted on the day of surgery regardless of co-morbidities or fragility of glucose control, thereby complicating metabolic management. Patients with well-controlled noninsulin-dependent diabetes should have oral agents held on the day of surgery until the first postoperative meal. If blood glucose is above 200 mg/dL during the perioperative period, insulin and glucose should be instituted, either in addition to or in place of the oral agent.

Insulin requirements depend on patient and surgical characteristics, and on the postoperative course. The highest insulin requirements occur in patients undergoing cardiopulmonary bypass surgery. Obesity, liver disease, steroid therapy, and sepsis will cause higher insulin requirements. However, because of impaired gluconeogenesis patients with hepatic disease are also prone to hypoglycemia during insulin administration *(206)*.

Several regimens exist for perioperative glycemic management. Only a few prospective randomized studies in small numbers of patients have compared the subcutaneous and intravenous administration of insulin. Although intravenous regimens yield tighter control of glucose levels, subcutaneous administration is effective in achieving adequate control *(207–209)*. Theoretically, the absorption of subcutaneous insulin may be affected by postoperative interstitial edema and by alterations in cutaneous flow (e.g., during hypotension, shock, use of vasopressors) *(77)*. Intravenous insulin is recommended for patients with ketoacidosis who require emergency surgery, for "brittle" diabetics, and for patients in whom insulin requirements are extremely high. The choice of regimen for glycemic control will depend greatly on the treating physician's familiarity with the various protocols and the insulin requirements of the patient.

The use of subcutaneous insulin is common, and is currently recommended by the Joslin Clinic in Boston (82) for the majority of insulin-requiring patients. One-half or two-thirds of the usual daily dose of protamine or lente insulin is given on the morning of the surgery. Glucose must be infused, usually as a 5% solution. Glucose levels should be measured at 4-hour intervals. Administration of additional subcutaneous regular insulin prevents high glucose levels.

A variable rate insulin infusion is an effective alternative for achieving glycemic control. Regular insulin is infused at an initial rate of 0.5 to 1.0 U per hour, along with a glucose infusion at a rate of 5 to 10 g per hour the insulin rate is adjusted according to blood glucose levels. Glucose measurements at one or two hour intervals are required. This technique has been shown to achieve smooth and rapid glycemic control (208).

A fixed-rate insulin infusion can also be used, as one adjusts the rate of the glucose infusion. However, in patients with high insulin requirements, the administered glucose might not be sufficient to suppress catabolism if the initial insulin dose is low (209). This approach has not yet been evaluated in a large series.

An alternative strategy is the glucose–insulin–potassium method. The three components are mixed in a single solution. The insulin concentration is adjusted if the blood glucose levels are outside the targeted goals. Any such change requires a new solution to be mixed. However, once the desired proportions are determined for a particular patient it becomes simple to manage (210), assuming stable insulin requirements.

Attention to fluids and electrolytes is extremely important. Potassium levels should be checked regularly. Dextrose is usually administered at a rate of 5 to 10 g per hour, although the optimal glucose required to prevent protein and fat metabolism has not been determined (77). If fluid restriction is necessary, the more concentrated dextrose solutions can be used. Lactate supplementation in intravenous fluids may increase glucose levels, as a substrate of gluconeogenesis (77).

ROLE OF THE CONSULTANT

Preoperative risk assessment and perioperative management of the surgical patient is a frequent cause for consultation for family practitioners, internists, cardiologists, and other medical specialists. A critical role of the consultant is to communicate the severity and stability of the patient's cardiovascular condition and to determine whether the patient is in a reasonable medical condition in the context of the surgical illness. The consultant may recommend changes in medications and suggest preoperative tests or procedures.

A crucial aspect of the consultative process is the exchange of information between the consultant and the physician who has requested the consultation. The consultant's assessment and recommendations must be communicated with brevity and clarity. As well as writing a complete note in the chart or sending a letter, there is no substitute for direct personal contact with the primary physician (211).

Follow-up increases compliance with recommendations (212) and allows for modifications in the original management plan as the clinical context changes. Many medical conditions require long-term follow-up, and the involvement of the consultant in the perioperative care of a patient offers the physician the opportunity to make recommendations that will also affect the long-term management of the patient.

With regard to CVD, even if frank manifestations are not found in the initial assessment, the preoperative encounter affords the opportunity to pursue primary and secondary preventative measures, particularly in the patient with DM who is at an increased risk for CVD. Every effort should be made to urge the patient and the primary care provider to focus on any modifiable risk factors identified during the preoperative assessment. The cardiologist may be asked to participate in subsequent surveillance for manifestations of CVD in the patient at increased risk.

REFERENCES

1. Alpert JS, Chipkin SR, Aronin N. Diabetes mellitus and silent myocardial ischemia. Adv Cardiol 1990;37:279–303.
2. Titus BG, Sherman CT. Asymptomatic myocardial ischemia during percutaneous transluminal coronary angioplasty and importance of prior Q-wave infarction and diabetes mellitus. Am J Cardiol 1991;68:735–739.
3. Mangano DT. Perioperative cardiac morbidity. Anesthesiology 1990;72(1):153–184.
4. National Center for Health Statistics. Available from http://www.cdc.gov/nchs/fastats/insurg.htm. Accessed July 17, 2003.
5. Massie BM, Mangano DT. Risk stratification for noncardiac surgery. How (and why)? [editorial; comment] [see comments]. Circulation 1993;87(5):1752–1755.
6. Rose SD, Corman LC, Mason DT. Cardiac risk factors in patients undergoing noncardiac surgery. Med Clin North Am 1979;63(6):1271–1288.
7. Ashton CM, Petersen NJ, Wray NP, et al. The incidence of perioperative myocardial infarction in men undergoing noncardiac surgery [see comments]. Ann Intern Med 1993;118(7):504–510.
8. Goldman L, Caldera DL, Nussbaum SR, et al. Multifactorial index of cardiac risk in noncardiac surgical procedures. N Engl J Med 1977;297(16):845–850.
9. Steen PA, Tinker JH, Tarhan S. Myocardial reinfarction after anesthesia and surgery. JAMA 1978;239(24):2566–2570.
10. Tarhan S, Moffitt EA, Taylor WF, Giuliani ER. Myocardial infarction after general anesthesia. JAMA 1972;220(11):1451–1454.
11. Detsky AS, Abrams HB, McLaughlin JR, et al. Predicting cardiac complications in patients undergoing non-cardiac surgery. J Gen Intern Med 1986;1(4):211–219.
12. Larsen SF, Olesen KH, Jacobsen E, et al. Prediction of cardiac risk in non-cardiac surgery. Eur Heart J 1987;8(2):179–185.
13. Rao TL, Jacobs KH, El Etr AA. Reinfarction following anesthesia in patients with myocardial infarction. Anesthesiology 1983;59(6):499–505.
14. Shah KB, Kleinman BS, Sami H, Patel J, Rao TL. Reevaluation of perioperative myocardial infarction in patients with prior myocardial infarction undergoing noncardiac operations. Anesth Analg 1990;71(3):231–235.
15. Crawford ES, Bomberger RA, Glaeser DH, Saleh SA, Russell WL. Aortoiliac occlusive disease: factors influencing survival and function following reconstructive operation over a twenty-five year period. Surgery 1981;90(6):1055–1067.
16. Taylor Jr. LM, Yeager RA, Moneta GL, McConnell DB, Porter JM. The incidence of perioperative myocardial infarction in general vascular surgery. J Vasc Surg 1991;15:52–61.
17. Mamode N, Scott RN, McLaughlin SC, McLelland A, Pollock JG: Perioperative myocardial infarction in peripheral vascular surgery. Br Med J 1996;312(7043):1396–1397.
18. Sprung J, Abdelmakak B, Gottlieb A, Mayhew C, Hammel J, Levy PJ, O'Hara P, Hertzer NR: Analysis of risk factors for myocardial infarction and cardiac mortality after major vascular surgery. Anesthesiology 2000;93:129–140.
19. Ashton CM, Petersen NJ, Wray NP, et al. The incidence of perioperative myocardial infarction in men undergoing noncardiac surgery. Ann Intern Med 1993;118:504–510.
20. Badner NH, Knill RL, Brown JE, Novick TV, Gelb AW: Myocardial infarction after noncardiac surgery. Anesthesiology 1998;88:572–578.

21. Goldman L, Caldera DL, Southwick FS, et al. Cardiac risk factors and complications in non-cardiac surgery. Medicine (Baltimore) 1978;57(4):357–370.
22. von Knorring J. Postoperative myocardial infarction: a prospective study in a risk group of surgical patients. Surgery 1981;90(1):55–60.
23. Mangano DT, Browner WS, Hollenberg M, Li J, Tateo IM. Long-term cardiac prognosis following noncardiac surgery. The Study of Perioperative Ischemia Research Group [see comments]. JAMA 1992;268(2):233–239.
24. Yeager RA, Moneta GL, Edwards JM, Taylor LM, Jr., McConnell DB, Porter JM. Late survival after perioperative myocardial infarction complicating vascular surgery. J Vasc Surg 1994;20(4):598–604.
25. Gedebou TM, Barr ST, Hunter G, Sinha R, Rappaport W, VillaReal K. Risk factors in patients undergoing major nonvascular abdominal operations that predict perioperative myocardial infarction. Am J Surg; 1997;174(6):755–758.
26. Centers for Disease Control and Prevention. Diabetes: Disabling, Deadly, and on the Rise 2003. Available from http://www.cdc.gov/nccdphp/aag/pdf/aag_ddt2003.pdf. Accessed
27. Root HF. Preoperative medical care of the diabetic patient. Postgrad Med 1966;40(4):439–444.
28. Sinnock P. Hospital utilization for diabetes. In: Harrison M, Hamman R, editors. Diabetes in America (National Diabetes Data Group), NIH Publication 85–1468. Washington, DC: US Department of Health and Human Services, 1985, pp. XXVI-1–XXVI-11.
29. Salomon NW, Page US, Okies JE, Stephens J, Krause AH, Bigelow JC. Diabetes mellitus and coronary artery bypass. Short-term risk and long-term prognosis. J Thorac Cardiovasc Surg 1983;85(2):264–271.
30. Johnson WD, Pedraza PM, Kayser KL. Coronary artery surgery in diabetics: 261 consecutive patients followed four to seven years. Am Heart J 1982;104(4 Pt 1):823–827.
31. Hirsch IB, McGill JB, Cryer PE, White PF. Perioperative management of surgical patients with diabetes mellitus [see comments]. Anesthesiology 1991; 74(2):346–359.
32. Alberti K, Marshall S. In: Alberti KGM, Krall L, editors. The Diabetes Annual/4. Amsterdam: Elsevier, 1988, pp. 248–271.
33. Eagle KA, Coley CM, Newell JB, et al. Combining clinical and thallium data optimizes preoperative assessment of cardiac risk before major vascular surgery. Ann Intern Med 1989;110(11):859–866.
34. Hollenberg M, Mangano DT, Browner WS, London MJ, Tubau JF, Tateo IM. Predictors of postoperative myocardial ischemia in patients undergoing noncardiac surgery. The Study of Perioperative Ischemia Research Group [see comments]. JAMA 1992;268(2):205–209.
35. Brown KA, Rowen M. Extent of jeopardized viable myocardium determined by myocardial perfusion imaging best predicts perioperative cardiac events in patients undergoing noncardiac surgery. J Am Coll Cardiol 1993;21(2):325–330.
36. Foster ED, Davis KB, Carpenter JA, Abele S, Fray D. Risk of noncardiac operation in patients with defined coronary disease: The Coronary Artery Surgery Study (CASS) registry experience. Ann Thorac Surg 1986;41(1):42–50.
37. Lette J, Waters D, Cerino M, Picard M, Champagne P, Lapointe J. Preoperative coronary artery disease risk stratification based on dipyridamole imaging and a simple three-step, three-segment model for patients undergoing noncardiac vascular surgery or major general surgery. Am J Cardiol 1992;69(19):1553–1558.
38. Leppo J, Plaja J, Gionet M, Tumolo J, Paraskos JA, Cutler BS. Noninvasive evaluation of cardiac risk before elective vascular surgery. J Am Coll Cardiol 1987;9(2):269–276.
39. L'Italien GJ, Paul SD, Hendel RC, et al. Development and validation of a Bayesian model for perioperative cardiac risk assessment in a cohort of 1,081 vascular surgical candidates [see comments]. J Am Coll Cardiol 1996;27(4):779–786.
40. Pedersen T, Eliasen K, Henriksen E. A prospective study of risk factors and cardiopulmonary complications associated with anaesthesia and surgery: risk indicators of cardiopulmonary morbidity. Acta Anaesthesiol Scand 1990;34(2):144–155.
41. Treiman GS, Treiman RL, Foran RF, Cossman DV, Cohen JL, Levin PM, Wagner WH, Davidson MB: The influence of diabetes mellitus on the risk of abdominal aortic surgery. The Am Surgeon; 1994;60:436–440.
42. Melliere D, Berrahal D, Desgranges EA, Becquemin JP, Perlemuter L, Simon D. Influence of diabetes on revascularization procedures of the aorta and lower limb arteries: early results. Eur J Vasc Endovasc Surg;1999;17:438–441.
43. Dardik A, Lin JW, Gordon TA, Williams GM, Perler BA. Results of elective abdominal aortic aneurysm repair in the 1990s: a population-based analysis of 2335 cases. J Vasc Surg; 1999; 30:985–95.

44. Berry AJ, Smith III RB, Weintraub WS, et al. Age versus comorbidities as risk factors for complications after elective abdominal aortic reconstructive surgery. J Vasc Surg; 2001;33:345–52.

45. Ballotta E, Giuseppe DG, Renon L. Is diabetes mellitus a risk factor for carotid endarterectomy? A prospective study. Surgery; 2001;129:146–152.

46. Rayan SS, Hamdan AD, Campbell DR, et al. Is diabetes a risk factor for patients undergoing open abdominal aortic aneurysm repair? Vasc Endovasc Surg;2002;36:33–40.

47. Hjortrup A, Sorensen C, Dyremose E, Hjortso NC, Kehlet H. Influence of diabetes mellitus on operative risk. Br J Surg 1985;72(10):783–785.

48. Mauney FM, Jr., Ebert PA, Sabiston DC, Jr. Postoperative myocardial infarction: a study of predisposing factors, diagnosis and mortality in a high risk group of surgical patients. Ann Surg 1970;172(3):497–503.

49. Walsh DB, Eckhauser FE, Ramsburgh SR, Burney RB. Risk associated with diabetes mellitus in patients undergoing gallbladder surgery. Surgery 1982;91(3):254–257.

50. Hertzer NR. Fatal myocardial infarction following peripheral vascular operations. A study of 951 patients followed 6 to 11 years postoperatively. Cleve Clin Q 1982;49(1):1–11.

51. Younis LT, Aguirre F, Byers S, et al. Perioperative and long-term prognostic value of intravenous dipyridamole thallium scintigraphy in patients with peripheral vascular disease. Am Heart J 1990;119(6):1287–1292.

52. Ellis SG, Hertzer NR, Young JR, Brener S. Angiographic correlates of cardiac death and myocardial infarction complicating major nonthoracic vascular surgery. Am J Cardiol 1996;77(12):1126–1128.

53. Ouyang P, Gerstenblith G, Furman WR, Golueke PJ, Gottlieb SO. Frequency and significance of early postoperative silent myocardial ischemia in patients having peripheral vascular surgery. Am J Cardiol 1989;64(18):1113–1116.

54. Fleisher LA, Nelson AH, Rosenbaum SH. Postoperative myocardial ischemia: etiology of cardiac morbidity or manifestation of underlying disease? J Clin Anesth 1995;7(2):97–102.

55. Knight MT, Dawson R, Melrose DG. Fibrinolytic response to surgery. Labile and stable patterns and their relevance to post-operative deep venous thrombosis. Lancet 1977;2(8034):370–373.

56. Sautter RD, Myers WO, Ray JF, III, Wenzel FJ. Relationship of fibrinolytic system to postoperative thrombotic phenomena. Arch Surg 1973;107(2):292–296.

57. Paramo JA, Alfaro MJ, Rocha E. Postoperative changes in the plasmatic levels of tissue-type plasminogen activator and its fast-acting inhibitor—relationship to deep vein thrombosis and influence of prophylaxis. Thromb Haemost 1985;54(3):713–716.

58. Tuman KJ, McCarthy RJ, March RJ, DeLaria GA, Patel RV, Ivankovich AD. Effects of epidural anesthesia and analgesia on coagulation and outcome after major vascular surgery [see comments]. Anesth Analg 1991;73(6):696–704.

59. Dawood MM, Gutpa DK, Southern J, Walia A, Atkinson JB, Eagle KA. Pathology of fatal perioperative myocardial infarction: implications regarding pathophysiology and prevention. Int J Cardiol 1996;57(1):37–44.

60. Cohen M, Aretz TSM. Fatal postoperative myocardial infarction is often caused by coronary plaque rupture. J Am Coll Cardiol 1997;29:53A. Abstr.

61. Garcia MJ, McNamara PM, Gordon T, Kannel WB. Morbidity and mortality in diabetics in the Framingham population. Sixteen year follow-up study. Diabetes 1974;23(2):105–111.

62. National Institutes of Health, National Institute of Diabetes and Digestive and Kidney Diseases. Diabetes in America. 2nd Ed. NIH publication no. 95–1468, 1995, p. 4.

63. Fein FS, Sonnenblick EH. Diabetic cardiomyopathy. Prog Cardiovasc Dis 1985;27(4):255–270.

64. Robertson WB, Strong JP. Atherosclerosis in persons with hypertension and diabetes mellitus. Lab Invest 1968;18(5):538–551.

65. Savage MP, Krolewski AS, Kenien GG, Lebeis MP, Christlieb AR, Lewis SM. Acute myocardial infarction in diabetes mellitus and significance of congestive heart failure as a prognostic factor. Am J Cardiol 1988;62(10 Pt 1):665–669.

66. Rubler S, Gerber D, Reitano J, Chokshi V, Fisher VJ. Predictive value of clinical and exercise variables for detection of coronary artery disease in men with diabetes mellitus. Am J Cardiol 1987;59(15):1310–1313.

67. Lane SE, Lewis SM, Pippin JJ, et al. Predictive value of quantitative dipyridamole-thallium scintigraphy in assessing cardiovascular risk after vascular surgery in diabetes mellitus. Am J Cardiol 1989;64(19):1275–1279.

68. Zarich SW, Cohen MC, Lane SE, et al. Routine perioperative dipyridamole 201Tl imaging in diabetic patients undergoing vascular surgery. Diabetes Care 1996;19(4):355–360.

69. Nesto RW, Watson FS, Kowalchuk GJ, et al. Silent myocardial ischemia and infarction in diabetics with peripheral vascular disease: assessment by dipyridamole thallium-201 scintigraphy. Am Heart J 1990;120(5):1073–1077.
70. Roy TM, Peterson HR, Snider HL, et al. Autonomic influence on cardiovascular performance in diabetic subjects. Am J Med 1989;87(4):382–388.
71. Kahn JK, Zola B, Juni JE, Vinik AI. Radionuclide assessment of left ventricular diastolic filling in diabetes mellitus with and without cardiac autonomic neuropathy. J Am Coll Cardiol 1986;7(6):1303–1309.
72. Zola B, Kahn JK, Juni JE, Vinik AI. Abnormal cardiac function in diabetic patients with autonomic neuropathy in the absence of ischemic heart disease. J Clin Endocrinol Metab 1986;63(1):208–214.
73. Niakan E, Harati Y, Rolak LA, Comstock JP, Rokey R. Silent myocardial infarction and diabetic cardiovascular autonomic neuropathy. Arch Intern Med 1986;146(11):2229–2230.
74. Murray DP, O'Brien T, Mulrooney R, O'Sullivan DJ. Autonomic dysfunction and silent myocardial ischaemia on exercise testing in diabetes mellitus. Diabet Med 1990;7(7):580–584.
75. Ambepityia G, Kopelman PG, Ingram D, Swash M, Mills PG, Timmis AD. Exertional myocardial ischemia in diabetes: a quantitative analysis of anginal perceptual threshold and the influence of autonomic function. J Am Coll Cardiol 1990;15(1):72–77.
76. Ewing DJ, Campbell IW, Clarke BF. The natural history of diabetic autonomic neuropathy. Q J Med 1980;49(193):95–108.
77. Peters A, Kerner W. Perioperative management of the diabetic patient. Exp Clin Endocrinol Diabetes 1995;103(4):213–218.
78. Yue DK, McLennan S, Marsh M, et al. Effects of experimental diabetes, uremia, and malnutrition on wound healing. Diabetes 1987;36(3):295–299.
79. Gottrup F, Andreassen TT. Healing of incisional wounds in stomach and duodenum: the influence of experimental diabetes. J Surg Res 1981;31(1):61–68.
80. Robertson HD, Polk HC, Jr. The mechanism of infection in patients with diabetes mellitus: a review of leukocyte malfunction. Surgery 1974;75(1):123–128.
81. Bagdade JD, Stewart M, Walters E. Impaired granulocyte adherence. A reversible defect in host defense in patients with poorly controlled diabetes. Diabetes 1978;27(6):677–681.
82. Palmisano J. Surgery and Diabetes. In: Kahn C, Weir G, (eds). Joslin's Diabetes Mellitus. Lea & Febiger, Philadelphia, 1994, pp. 955–961.
83. Eagle KA, Berger PB, Calkins H, et al. ACC/AHA guideline update for perioperative cardiovascular evaluation for noncardiac surgery: a report of the American College of Cardiology/American Heart Association Task Force on Practice Guidelines (Committee to Update the 1996 Guidelines on Perioperative Cardiovascular Evaluation for Noncardiac Surgery), 2002.
84. Eagle KA, Brundage BH, Chaitman BR, et al. Guidelines for perioperative cardiovascular evaluation for noncardiac surgery. Report of the American College of Cardiology/American Heart Association Task Force on Practice Guidelines (Committee on Perioperative Cardiovascular Evaluation for Noncardiac Surgery). J Am Coll Cardiol 1996;27(4):910–948.
85. Palda VA, Detsky AS. Perioperative assessment and management of risk from coronary artery disease. Ann Intern Med 1997;127(4):313–328.
86. MacKenzie CR, Charlson ME. Assessment of perioperative risk in the patient with diabetes mellitus. Surg Gynecol Obstet 1988;167(4):293–299.
87. Farrow SC, Fowkes FG, Lunn JN, Robertson IB, Sweetnam P. Epidemiology in anaesthesia: a method for predicting hospital mortality. Eur J Anaesthesiol 1984;1(1):77–84.
88. Hertzer NR, Beven EG, Young JR, et al. Coronary artery disease in peripheral vascular patients. A classification of 1000 coronary angiograms and results of surgical management. Ann Surg 1984;199(2):223–233.
89. Boucher CA, Brewster DC, Darling RC, Okada RD, Strauss HW, Pohost GM. Determination of cardiac risk by dipyridamole-thallium imaging before peripheral vascular surgery. N Engl J Med 1985;312(7):389–394.
90. L'Italien GJ, Cambria RP, Cutler BS, et al. Comparative early and late cardiac morbidity among patients requiring different vascular surgery procedures. J Vasc Surg 1995;21(6):935–944.
91. Krupski WC, Layug EL, Reilly LM, Rapp JH, Mangano DT. Comparison of cardiac morbidity rates between aortic and infrainguinal operations: two-year follow-up. Study of Perioperative Ischemia Research Group. J Vasc Surg 1993;18(4):609–615.
92. Burgos LG, Ebert TJ, Asiddao C, Turner LA, Pattison CZ, Wang-Cheng R et al. Increased intraoperative cardiovascular morbidity in diabetics with autonomic neuropathy. Anesthesiology 1989; 70(4):591–597.

93. Vohra A, Kumar S, Charlton AJ, Olukoga AO, Boulton AJ, McLeod D. Effect of diabetes mellitus on the cardiovascular responses to induction of anaesthesia and tracheal intubation. Br J Anaesth 1993;71(2):258–261.

94. Charlson ME, MacKenzie CR, Gold JP. Preoperative autonomic function abnormalities in patients with diabetes mellitus and patients with hypertension. J Am Coll Surg 1994;179(1):1–10.

95. Axelrod DA, Upchurch GR Jr, DeMonner S, et al. Perioperative cardiovascular risk stratification of patients with diabetes who undergo elective major vascular surgery. J Vasc Surg; 2002;35:894–901.

96. Lee TH, Marcantonio ER, Mangione CM, et al. Derivation and prospective validation of a simple index for prediction of cardiac risk of major noncardiac surgery. Circulation; 1999;100:1043–1049.

97. Nesto RW, Phillips RT. Asymptomatic myocardial ischemia in diabetic patients. Am J Med 1986;80(4C):40–47.

98. Nesto RW, Phillips RT, Kett KG, et al. Angina and exertional myocardial ischemia in diabetic and nondiabetic patients: assessment by exercise thallium scintigraphy [published erratum appears in Ann Intern Med 1988;108(4):646]. Ann Intern Med 1988;108(2):170–175.

99. Kannel WB, Abbott RD. Incidence and prognosis of unrecognized myocardial infarction. An update on the Framingham study. N Engl J Med 1984; 311(18):1144–1147.

100. Soler NG, Bennett MA, Pentecost BL, Fitzgerald MG, Malins JM. Myocardial infarction in diabetics. Q J Med 1975;44(173):125–132.

101. Uretsky BF, Farquhar DS, Berezin AF, Hood WB, Jr. Symptomatic myocardial infarction without chest pain: prevalence and clinical course. Am J Cardiol 1977; 40(4):498–503.

102. Carliner NH, Fisher ML, Plotnick GD, et al. Routine preoperative exercise testing in patients undergoing major noncardiac surgery. Am J Cardiol 1985;56(1):51–58.

103. Cutler BS, Wheeler HB, Paraskos JA, Cardullo PA. Applicability and interpretation of electrocardiographic stress testing in patients with peripheral vascular disease. Am J Surg 1981;141(4):501–506.

104. McPhail N, Calvin JE, Shariatmadar A, Barber GG, Scobie TK. The use of preoperative exercise testing to predict cardiac complications after arterial reconstruction. J Vasc Surg 1988;7(1):60–68.

105. Philipson JD, Carpenter BJ, Itzkoff J, et al. Evaluation of cardiovascular risk for renal transplantation in diabetic patients. Am J Med 1986;81(4):630–634.

106. Cutler BS, Leppo JA. Dipyridamole thallium 201 scintigraphy to detect coronary artery disease before abdominal aortic surgery. J Vasc Surg 1987;5(1):91–100.

107. Sachs RN, Tellier P, Larmignat P, et al. Assessment by dipyridamole-thallium-201 myocardial scintigraphy of coronary risk before peripheral vascular surgery. Surgery 1988;103(5):584–587.

108. Bry JD, Belkin M, O'Donnell TF, Jr., et al. An assessment of the positive predictive value and cost-effectiveness of dipyridamole myocardial scintigraphy in patients undergoing vascular surgery. J Vasc Surg 1994;19(1):112–121.

109. Cutler BS, Hendel RC, Leppo JA. Dipyridamole-thallium scintigraphy predicts perioperative and long-term survival after major vascular surgery. J Vasc Surg 1992;15(6):972–979.

110. Hendel RC, Layden JJ, Leppo JA. Prognostic value of dipyridamole thallium scintigraphy for evaluation of ischemic heart disease [see comments]. J Am Coll Cardiol 1990;15(1):109–116.

111. Baron JF, Mundler O, Bertrand M, et al. Dipyridamole-thallium scintigraphy and gated radionuclide angiography to assess cardiac risk before abdominal aortic surgery [see comments]. N Engl J Med 1994;330(10):663–669.

112. Mangano DT, London MJ, Tubau JF, et al. Dipyridamole thallium-201 scintigraphy as a preoperative screening test. A reexamination of its predictive potential. Study of Perioperative Ischemia Research Group [see comments]. Circulation 1991;84(2):493–502.

113. Poldermans D, Fioretti PM, Forster T, et al. Dobutamine stress echocardiography for assessment of perioperative cardiac risk in patients undergoing major vascular surgery [see comments]. Circulation 1993;87(5):1506–1512.

114. Eichelberger JP, Schwarz KQ, Black ER, Green RM, Ouriel K. Predictive value of dobutamine echocardiography just before noncardiac vascular surgery. Am J Cardiol 1993;72(7):602–607.

115. Pedersen T, Kelbaek H, Munck O. Cardiopulmonary complications in high-risk surgical patients: the value of preoperative radionuclide cardiography. Acta Anaesthesiol Scand 1990;34(3):183–189.

116. Pasternack PF, Imparato AM, Riles TS, Baumann FG, Bear G, Lamparello PJ et al. The value of the radionuclide angiogram in the prediction of perioperative myocardial infarction in patients undergoing lower extremity revascularization procedures. Circulation 1985;72(3 Pt 2):II13–II17.

117. Mosley JG, Clarke JM, Ell PJ, Marston A. Assessment of myocardial function before aortic surgery by radionuclide angiocardiography. Br J Surg 1985;72(11):886–887.

118. Eagle KA, Singer DE, Brewster DC, Darling RC, Mulley AG, Boucher CA. Dipyridamole-thallium scanning in patients undergoing vascular surgery. Optimizing preoperative evaluation of cardiac risk. JAMA 1987;257(16):2185–2189.

119. Cohen MC, Curran PJ, L'Italien GJ, Mittleman MA, Zarich SW: Long-term prognostic value of preoperative dipyridamole thallium imaging and clinical indexes in patients with diabetes mellitus undergoing peripheral vascular surgery. Am J Cardiol; 1999;83:1038–1042.

120. Guidelines for coronary angiography. A report of the American College of Cardiology/American Heart Association Task Force on Assessment of diagnostic and therapeutic cardiovascular procedures (subcommittee on coronary angiography). J Am Coll Cardiol 1987;10(4):935–950.

121. Scanlon PJ, Faxon DP, Audet AM, et al. ACC/AHA guidelines for coronary angiography: executive summary and recommendations: a report of the American College of Cardiology/American Heart Association Task Force on Practice Guidelines (Committee on Coronary Angiography). Circulation 1999;99:2345–2357.

122. Cohen MC, Eagle KA. Expert opinion regarding indications for coronary angiography before noncardiac surgery. Am Heart J 1997;134(2 Pt 1):321–329.

123. Braun WE, Phillips DF, Vidt DG, et al. Coronary artery disease in 100 diabetics with end-stage renal failure. Transplant Proc 1984;16(3):603–607.

124. Bennett WM, Kloster F, Rosch J, Barry J, Porter GA. Natural history of asymptomatic coronary arteriographic lesions in diabetic patients with end-stage renal disease. Am J Med 1978;65(5):779–784.

125. Braun WE, Phillips D, Vidt DG, et al. Coronary arteriography and coronary artery disease in 99 diabetic and nondiabetic patients on chronic hemodialysis or renal transplantation programs. Transplant Proc 1981;13(1 Pt 1):128–135.

126. Weinrauch L, D'Elia JA, Healy RW, Gleason RE, Christlieb AR, Leland OS Jr. Asymptomatic coronary artery disease: angiographic assessment of diabetics evaluated for renal transplantation. Circulation 1978;58(6):1184–1190.

127. Lindner A, Charra B, Sherrard DJ, Scribner BH. Accelerated atherosclerosis in prolonged maintenance hemodialysis. N Engl J Med 1974;290(13):697–701.

128. Khauli RB, Steinmuller DR, Novick AC, et al. A critical look at survival of diabetics with end-stage renal disease. Transplantation versus dialysis therapy. Transplantation 1986;41(5):598–602.

129. Brown KA, Rimmer J, Haisch C. Noninvasive cardiac risk stratification of diabetic and nondiabetic uremic renal allograft candidates using dipyridamole-thallium-201 imaging and radionuclide ventriculography. Am J Cardiol 1989;64(16):1017–1021.

130. Camp AD, Garvin PJ, Hoff J, Marsh J, Byers SL, Chaitman BR. Prognostic value of intravenous dipyridamole thallium imaging in patients with diabetes mellitus considered for renal transplantation. Am J Cardiol 1990;65(22):1459–1463.

131. Ibels LS, Stewart JH, Mahony JF, Sheil AG. Deaths from occlusive arterial disease in renal allograft recipients. Br Med J 1974;3(5930):552–554.

132. Washer GF, Schroter GP, Starzl TE, Weil R, III. Causes of death after kidney transplantation. JAMA 1983;250(1):49–54.

133. Rao KV, Andersen RC. The impact of diabetes on vascular complications following cadaver renal transplantation. Transplantation 1987;43(2):193–197.

134. Sutherland DE, Goetz C, Najarian JS. Pancreas transplantation at the University of Minnesota: donor and recipient selection, operative and postoperative management, and outcome. Transplant Proc 1987;19(4 Suppl 4):63–74.

135. Manske CL, Wang Y, Thomas W. Mortality of cadaveric kidney transplantation versus combined kidney- pancreas transplantation in diabetic patients [see comments]. Lancet 1995;346(8991–8992):1658–1662.

136. Morrow CE, Schwartz JS, Sutherland DE, et al. Predictive value of thallium stress testing for coronary and cardiovascular events in uremic diabetic patients before renal transplantation. Am J Surg 1983;146(3):331–335.

137. Mayer G, Thum J, Cada EM, Stummvoll HK, Graf H. Working capacity is increased following recombinant human erythropoietin treatment. Kidney Int 1988;34(4):525–528.

138. Ohmura N, Ohta M, Tamura H, Kawaguchi Y, Miyahara T. The influence of dialysis solution on the exercise capacity in patients on CAPD. In: Khanna R, Nolph K, Prowant B, Twardowski Z, Oreopoulos D, (eds). Advances in peritoneal dialysis. University of Toronto Press, Toronto, Canada, 1989, pp. 46–48.

139. Marwick TH, Steinmuller DR, Underwood DA, et al. Ineffectiveness of dipyridamole SPECT thallium imaging as a screening technique for coronary artery disease in patients with end-stage renal failure. Transplantation 1990;49(1):100–103.

140. Holley JL, Fenton RA, Arthur RS. Thallium stress testing does not predict cardiovascular risk in diabetic patients with end-stage renal disease undergoing cadaveric renal transplantation. Am J Med 1991;90(5):563–570.

141. Melissinos K, Delidou A, Grammenou S, Markopoulos P. Study of the activity of lymphocyte adenosine deaminase in chronic renal failure. Clin Chim Acta 1983;135(1):9–12.

142. Lorber MI, Van Buren CT, Flechner SM, et al. Pretransplant coronary arteriography for diabetic renal transplant recipients. Transplant Proc 1987;19(1 Pt 2):1539–1541.

143. Lemmers MJ, Barry JM. Major role for arterial disease in morbidity and mortality after kidney transplantation in diabetic recipients. Diabetes Care 1991;14(4):295–301.

144. Friedman E. Management of diabetes and diabetic complications in patients with diabetic renal disease. In: Jacobson H, Striker G, Klahr S, (eds). Principles and practice of nephrology. BC Decker Inc., Philadelphia, 1991, pp. 483–491.

145. Manske CL, Wang Y, Rector T, Wilson RF, White CW. Coronary revascularisation in insulin-dependent diabetic patients with chronic renal failure. Lancet 1992;340(8826):998–1002.

146. Stone JG, Foex P, Sear JW, Johnson LL, Khambatta HJ, Triner L. Myocardial ischemia in untreated hypertensive patients: effect of a single small oral dose of a beta-adrenergic blocking agent. Anesthesiology 1988;68(4):495–500.

147. Pasternack PF, Imparato AM, Baumann FG, et al. The hemodynamics of beta-blockade in patients undergoing abdominal aortic aneurysm repair. Circulation 1987;76(3 Pt 2):III1–III7.

148. Pasternack PF, Grossi EA, Baumann FG, et al. Beta blockade to decrease silent myocardial ischemia during peripheral vascular surgery. Am J Surg 1989;158(2):113–116.

149. Mangano DT, Layug EL, Wallace A, Tateo I. Effect of atenolol on mortality and cardiovascular morbidity after noncardiac surgery. Multicenter Study of Perioperative Ischemia Research Group [see comments] [published erratum appears in N Engl J Med 1997;336(14):1039]. N Engl J Med 1996;335(23):1713–1720.

150. Poldermans D, Boersma E, Bax JJ, et al. The effect of bisoprolol on preoperative mortality and myocardial infarction in high-risk patients undergoing vascular surgery. N Engl J Med 1999;341:1789–1794.

151. Boersma E, Poldermans D, Bax JJ, et al. Predictors of cardiac events after major vascular surgery: role of clinical characteristics, dobutamine echocardiography, and [beta]-blocker therapy. JAMA 2001;285(14):1865–1873.

152. Christlieb A. Hypertension in the diabetic patient. In: Kahn C, Weir G, (eds). Joslin's Diabetes Mellitus. Lea & Febiger, Philadelphia, 1985:538–599.

153. Shorr RI, Ray WA, Daugherty JR, Griffin MR. Antihypertensives and the risk of serious hypoglycemia in older persons using insulin or sulfonylureas [see comments]. JAMA 1997;278(1):40–43.

154. Efficacy of atenolol and captopril in reducing risk of macrovascular and microvascular complications in type 2 diabetes: UKPDS 39. UK Prospective Diabetes Study Group [see comments]. BMJ 1998;317(7160):713–720.

155. Tight blood pressure control and risk of macrovascular and microvascular complications in type 2 diabetes: UKPDS 38. UK Prospective Diabetes Study Group [see comments] [published erratum appears in BMJ 1999;318(7175):29]. BMJ 1998;317(7160):703–713.

156. Jonas M, Reicher-Reiss H, Boyko V, et al. Usefulness of beta-blocker therapy in patients with non-insulin- dependent diabetes mellitus and coronary artery disease. Bezafibrate Infarction Prevention (BIP) Study Group. Am J Cardiol 1996;77(15):1273–1277.

157. Kjekshus J, Gilpin E, Cali G, Blackey AR, Henning H, Ross J Jr. Diabetic patients and beta-blockers after acute myocardial infarction. Eur Heart J 1990;11(1):43–50.

158. Malmberg K, Herlitz J, Hjalmarson A, Ryden L. Effects of metoprolol on mortality and late infarction in diabetics with suspected acute myocardial infarction. Retrospective data from two large studies. Eur Heart J 1989;10(5):423–428.

159. Rodda BE. The Timolol Myocardial Infarction Study: an evaluation of selected variables. Circulation 1983;67(6 Pt 2):I101–I106.

160. Furberg CD, Byington RP. What do subgroup analyses reveal about differential response to beta-blocker therapy? The Beta-Blocker Heart Attack Trial experience. Circulation 1983; 67(6 Pt 2):I98–I101.

161. Coriat P, Daloz M, Bousseau D, Fusciardi J, Echter E, Viars P. Prevention of intraoperative myocardial ischemia during noncardiac surgery with intravenous nitroglycerin. Anesthesiology 1984; 61(2):193–196.

162. Dodds TM, Stone JG, Coromilas J, Weinberger M, Levy DG. Prophylactic nitroglycerin infusion during noncardiac surgery does not reduce perioperative ischemia [see comments]. Anesth Analg 1993;76(4):705–713.

163. Cohen MM, Duncan PG, Tate RB. Does anesthesia contribute to operative mortality? [see comments]. JAMA 1988;260(19):2859–2863.

164. Slogoff S, Keats AS. Randomized trial of primary anesthetic agents on outcome of coronary artery bypass operations. Anesthesiology 1989; 70(2):179–188.

165. Kehlet H. Epidural analgesia and the endocrine-metabolic response to surgery. Update and perspectives. Acta Anaesthesiol Scand 1984;28(2):125–127.

166. Shirasaka C, Tsuji H, Asoh T, Takeuchi Y. Role of the splanchnic nerves in endocrine and metabolic response to abdominal surgery. Br J Surg 1986;73(2):142–145.

167. Christopherson R, Beattie C, Frank SM, et al. Perioperative morbidity in patients randomized to epidural or general anesthesia for lower extremity vascular surgery. Perioperative Ischemia Randomized Anesthesia Trial Study Group [see comments]. Anesthesiology 1993;79(3):422–434.

168. Baron JF, Bertrand M, Barre E, et al. Combined epidural and general anesthesia versus general anesthesia for abdominal aortic surgery. Anesthesiology 1991;75(4):611–618.

169. Bode RH, Jr., Lewis KP, Zarich SW, et al. Cardiac outcome after peripheral vascular surgery. Comparison of general and regional anesthesia [see comments]. Anesthesiology 1996;84(1):3–13.

170. Janda A, Salem C. [Hypoglycemia caused by lidocaine overdosage]. Reg Anaesth 1986;9(3):88–90.

171. Romano E, Gullo A. Hypoglycaemic coma following epidural analgesia. Anaesthesia 1980;35(11): 1084–1086.

172. Pierce E. Anesthesia in the diabetic. In: Kozak G, (ed). Clinical diabetes mellitus. WB Saunders, Philadelphia, 1982, pp. 246–251.

173. Grayburn PA, Hillis DL. Cardiac events in patients undergoing noncardiac surgery: shifting the paradigm from noninvasive risk stratification to therapy. Ann Intern Med 2003;138:506–511.

174. Hertzer NR, Young JR, Beven EG, et al. Late results of coronary bypass in patients with peripheral vascular disease. I. Five-year survival according to age and clinical cardiac status. Cleve Clin Q 1986;53(2):133–143.

175. Long-term results of prospective randomised study of coronary artery bypass surgery in stable angina pectoris. European Coronary Surgery Study Group. Lancet 1982;2(8309):1173–1180.

176. McFalls EO, Ward HB, Santilli S, Scheftel M, Chesler E, Doliszny K. The influence of perioperative myocardial infarction on long-term prognosis following elective vascular surgery. Chest 1998;113(3): 681–686.

177. Stein B, Weintraub WS, Gebhart SP, et al. Influence of diabetes mellitus on early and late outcome after percutaneous transluminal coronary angioplasty. Circulation 1995;91(4):979–989.

178. Brandrup-Wognsen G, Haglid M, Karlsson T, Berggren H, Herlitz BJ. Preoperative risk indicators of death at an early and late stage after coronary artery bypass grafting. Thorac Cardiovasc Surg 1995;43(2):77–82.

179. Influence of diabetes on 5-year mortality and morbidity in a randomized trial comparing CABG and PTCA in patients with multivessel disease: the Bypass Angioplasty Revascularization Investigation (BARI) [see comments]. Circulation 1997;96(6):1761–1769.

180. Kelsey SF. Patients with diabetes did better with coronary bypass graft surgery than with percutaneous transluminal coronary angioplasty: was this BARI finding real? Am Heart J 1999;138:S387–S393.

181. Elmore JR, Hallett JW Jr, et al. Myocardial revascularization before abdominal aortic aneurysmorrhaphy: effect of coronary angioplasty [see comments]. Mayo Clin Proc 1993;68(7): 637–641.

182. Huber KC, Evans MA, Bresnahan JF, Gibbons RJ, Holmes DR Jr. Outcome of noncardiac operations in patients with severe coronary artery disease successfully treated preoperatively with coronary angioplasty [see comments]. Mayo Clin Proc 1992;67(1):15–21.

183. Jones SE, Raymond RE, Simpfendorfer CC, Whitlow PL. Cardiac outcome of major noncardiac surgery in patients undergoing preoperative coronary angioplasty. J Invasive Cardiol 1993;5(6):212–218.

184. Allen JR, Helling TS, Hartzler GO. Operative procedures not involving the heart after percutaneous transluminal coronary angioplasty. Surg Gynecol Obstet 1991;173(4):285–288.

185. Kaluza GL, Joseph J, Lee JR, Raizner ME, Raizner AE. Catastrophic outcomes of noncardiac surgery soon after coronary stenting. J Am Coll Cardiol 2000;35:1288–1294.

186. Wilson SH, Fasseas P, Orford JL, et al. Clinical outcomes of patients undergoing non-cardiac surgery in the two months following coronary stenting. J Am Coll Cardiol 2003;42:234–240.

187. Joyce WP, Provan JL, Ameli FM, McEwan MM, Jelenich S, Jones DP. The role of central haemodynamic monitoring in abdominal aortic surgery. A prospective randomised study. Eur J Vasc Surg 1990;4(6):633–636.

188. Isaacson IJ, Lowdon JD, Berry AJ, Smith RB, III, Knos GB, Weitz FI et al. The value of pulmonary artery and central venous monitoring in patients undergoing abdominal aortic reconstructive surgery: a comparative study of two selected, randomized groups. J Vasc Surg 1990;12(6):754–760.

189. Berlauk JF, Abrams JH, Gilmour IJ, O'Connor SR, Knighton DR, Cerra FB. Preoperative optimization of cardiovascular hemodynamics improves outcome in peripheral vascular surgery. A prospective, randomized clinical trial [see comments]. Ann Surg 1991;214(3):289–297.

190. Practice guidelines for pulmonary artery catheterization. A report by the American Society of Anesthesiologists Task Force on Pulmonary Artery Catheterization [see comments]. Anesthesiology 1993;78(2):380–394.

191. Rettke SR, Shub C, Naessens JM, Marsh HM, O'Brien JF. Significance of mildly elevated creatine kinase (myocardial band) activity after elective abdominal aortic aneurysmectomy. J Cardiothorac Vasc Anesth 1991;5(5):425–430.

192. Charlson ME, MacKenzie CR, Ales K, Gold JP, Fairclough G Jr, Shires GT. Surveillance for postoperative myocardial infarction after noncardiac operations. Surg Gynecol Obstet 1988;167(5):407–414.

193. Adams JE, Sicard GA, Allen BT, et al. Diagnosis of perioperative myocardial infarction with measurement of cardiac troponin I. N Engl J Med 1994;330:670–674.

194. Lopez-Jimenez F, Goldman L, Sacks DB, Thomas EJ, Johnson PA, Cook EF, Lee TH. Prognostic value of cardiac troponin T after noncardiac surgery: 6-month follow-up data. J Am Coll Cardiol 1997;29:1241–1245.

195. Metzler H, Gries M, Rehak P, Lang TH, Fruhwald S, Toller W. Perioperative myocardial cell injury: the role of troponins. Br J Anaesth 1997;78:386–390.

196. Lee TH, Thomas EJ, Ludwig LE, et al. Troponin T as a marker for myocardial ischemia in patients undergoing major noncardiac surgery. Am J Cardiol 1996;77:1031–1036.

197. Badner NH, Knill RL, Brown JE, Novick TV, Gelb AW. Myocardial infarction after noncardiac surgery. Anesthesiology 1998;88:572–578.

198. Godet G, Ayed SB, Bernard M, et al. Cardiac troponin I cutoff values to predict postoperative cardiac complications after circulatory arrest and profound hypothermia. J Cardiothorac Vasc Anesth 1999;13:272–275.

199. Benoit MO, Paris M, Silleran J, Fiemeyer A, Moatti N. Cardiac troponin I: its contribution to the diagnosis of preoperative myocardial infarction and various complications of cardiac surgery. Crit Care Med 2001;29(10):1880–1886.

200. Mangano DT, Browner WS, Hollenberg M, London MJ, Tubau JF, Tateo IM. Association of perioperative myocardial ischemia with cardiac morbidity and mortality in men undergoing noncardiac surgery. The Study of Perioperative Ischemia Research Group [see comments]. N Engl J Med 1990;323(26):1781–1788.

201. Landesberg G, Luria MH, Cotev S, et al. Importance of long-duration postoperative ST-segment depression in cardiac morbidity after vascular surgery [see comments]. Lancet 1993;341(8847):715–719.

202. Fleisher LA, Zielski MM, Schulman SP. Perioperative ST-segment depression is rare and may not indicate myocardial ischemia in moderate-risk patients undergoing noncardiac surgery. J Cardiothorac Vasc Anesth 1997;11(2):155–159.

203. Golden SH, Peart-Vigilance C, Kao WHL, Brancati FL. Perioperative glycemic control and the risk of infectious complications in a cohort of adults with diabetes. Diabetes Care 1999;22:1408–1414.

204. Furnary AP, Zerr KJ, Grunkemeier GL, Starr A. Continuous intravenous insulin infusion reduces the incidence of deep sternal wound infection in diabetic patients after cardiac surgical procedures. Ann Thorac Surg 1999;67:352–362.

205. Rassias AJ, Marrin CAS, Arruda J, Whalen PK, Beach M, Yeager MP. Insulin infusion improves neutrophil function in diabetic cardiac surgery patients. Anesth Analg. 1999;88:1011–1016.

206. Gill GV, Sherif IH, Alberti KG. Management of diabetes during open heart surgery. Br J Surg 1981;68(3):171–172.

207. Taitelman U, Reece EA, Bessman AN. Insulin in the management of the diabetic surgical patient: continuous intravenous infusion vs subcutaneous administration. JAMA 1977;237(7):658–660.

208. Pezzarossa A, Taddei F, Cimicchi MC, Rossini E, Contini S, Bonora E et al. Perioperative management of diabetic subjects. Subcutaneous versus intravenous insulin administration during glucose-potassium infusion. Diabetes Care 1988;11(1):52–58.

209. Goldberg NJ, Wingert TD, Levin SR, Wilson SE, Viljoen JF. Insulin therapy in the diabetic surgical patient: metabolic and hormone response to low dose insulin infusion. Diabetes Care 1981;4(2):279–284.

210. Alberti KG, Gill GV, Elliott MJ. Insulin delivery during surgery in the diabetic patient. Diabetes Care 1982;(5 Suppl 1):65–77.

211. Goldman L, Lee T, Rudd P. Ten commandments for effective consultations. Arch Intern Med 1983;143(9):1753–1755.
212. Horwitz RI, Henes CG, Horwitz SM. Developing strategies for improving the diagnostic and management efficacy of medical consultations. J Chronic Dis 1983; 36(2):213–218.
213. Mangano DT, Goldman L. Preoperative assessment of patients with known or suspected coronary disease. N Engl J Med 1995;333(26):1750–1756.

25 Diabetes and Percutaneous Interventional Therapy

David P. Lorenz, MD, Joseph P. Carrozza, MD, and Lawrence Garcia, MD

CONTENTS

IMPORTANCE OF THE PROBLEM
PRECATHETERIZATION CONSIDERATIONS
HYDRATION
NONIONIC CONTRAST AGENTS
N-ACETYLCYSTEINE
ACCESS
OTHER ISSUES
CORONARY INTERVENTION
EMERGENT CORONARY INTERVENTIONS
CONCURRENT ANTIPLATELET THERAPY
CORONARY ARTERY BYPASS GRAFTING
PERCUTANEOUS CORONARY INTERVENTION VS CORONARY ARTERY
    BYPASS GRAFTING
PERIPHERAL ARTERIAL INTERVENTIONS
INFRAPOPLITEAL INTERVENTIONS
RENAL INTERVENTIONS
CAROTID INTERVENTIONS
CONCLUSION
REFERENCES

IMPORTANCE OF THE PROBLEM

With the aging of the US population and increasing prevalence of both diabetes and coronary artery disease (CAD), the number of interventional coronary and peripheral arterial procedures has markedly increased in an attempt to prevent morbid and mortal events. Unfortunately, the cardiovascular mortality of the diabetic patient remains high; the risk of a myocardial infarction (MI) at 7 years is equivalent for the diabetic without CAD and the nondiabetic who has already suffered an MI *(1)*. It has been estimated that

From: *Contemporary Cardiology: Diabetes and Cardiovascular Disease, Second Edition*
Edited by: M. T. Johnstone and A. Veves © Humana Press Inc., Totowa, NJ

the spontaneous risk of MI in diabetics with three-vessel disease is 10% to 15% per year *(2)*. Total mortality after this MI is higher than in the nondiabetic population. Over the last two decades, the number of diabetics undergoing percutaneous coronary intervention (PCI) has doubled, and the age, lesion complexity, and proportion of unstable patients has increased *(3)*.

The diabetic patient who undergoes elective or urgent PCI has an increased risk of early death compared with the nondiabetic. A retrospective review of more than 20,000 patients undergoing PCI from 1980 to 1999 demonstrated almost a doubling of diabetic in-hospital mortality in both the elective (0.8% vs 1.4%; $p < 0.001$) and emergent (6.9% vs 12.7%; $p < 0.001$) setting *(4)*. Fortunately, by 1995, the mortality rate in the elective PCI had become equivalent to that of nondiabetics, *(4)* likely secondary to technological advances.

Cardiologists are increasingly being asked to become caretakers of the entire vascular bed. This evolved as multiple studies demonstrated that disease in one area of the vascular tree frequently predicted asymptomatic disease in another. Symptomatic cerebrovascular disease has been associated with approximately a 20% to 40% rate of silent cardiac disease in several series *(5)*. The increased prevalence of lower extremity arterial disease in the diabetic patient is also well documented, and has significant effects on morbidity and mortality. In the Bypass Angioplasty Revascularization Investigation (BARI) trial, the patients with peripheral arterial disease (PAD) had a 4.9 times increased risk of death ($p < 0.01$) at 5 years (14%) *(6)*, results that were also seen in the original Coronary Artery Surgery Study (CASS) Trial *(7)*.

Diabetes is the leading cause of atraumatic amputation in the United States, and the relative risks of claudication, occlusive infra-popliteal disease, and need for lower extremity amputation range from 4 to 12 times that of the general population *(8,9)*. Diabetics have a two- to fourfold increase in the risk of PAD, and the severity of the disease directly correlates with its duration *(10,11)*. Lower extremity intervention has increasingly been used to prevent, replace, or work synergistically with surgical revascularization, and advancing technology continues to allow for the success of more complex interventions. Renal and carotid stenting are newer procedures whose indications and outcomes will be better defined in the early part of this century.

PRECATHETERIZATION CONSIDERATIONS

The vast majority of patients are referred for cardiac catheterization on an elective or semi-urgent basis. There are a number of modifiable risks that can and should be addressed prior to the patient entering the catheterization laboratory.

Renal Protection

Of the potentially avoidable complications of cardiac catheterization, acute renal failure related to contrast-induced nephrotoxicity remains one associated with significant morbidity and mortality. Transient mild impairment in renal function defined by elevation of the serum creatinine is frequently seen even in patients with normal renal function *(12)*. Currently identified risk factors include pre-existing baseline renal insufficiency, diabetes, poor forward flow states (congestive heart failure [CHF]), and the volume of contrast used *(13–15)*. The incidence of acute renal failure, although low, has a significant bearing on outcomes. In a recent retrospective analysis of 7586 patients at Mayo Clinic, 3.3% developed acute renal failure, defined as an increase over baseline of 0.5 mg/

dL *(14)*. Those who developed acute renal failure during the initial hospitalization had a mortality rate of 22% vs 1.4% for those without renal failure. Diabetic patients with a serum creatinine under 2.0 mg/dL were at higher risk than nondiabetic patients with the same creatinine, whereas all patients became high risk once the creatinine rose over 2.0 mg/dL. A number of strategies exist to prevent this morbid complication.

HYDRATION

Hydration with normal saline or one-half normal saline is routinely used to decrease the incidence of contrast nephropathy. Whether one regimen is superior to another is unclear, but a recently published randomized trial of 1620 patients comparing the two demonstrated a 2% incidence of contrast nephropathy with one-half normal saline vs 0.7% with normal saline *(16)*. Diabetics, women, and patients receiving more than 250 cc of contrast were subgroups that were noted to have greater benefit with isotonic saline. Conflicting results exist regarding whether oral hydration the night before as an outpatient is equivalent to 12 hours of intravenous hydration as an inpatient *(17,18)*. Our practice is to admit patients with renal insufficiency as documented by a creatinine greater than 1.7 mg/dL the night prior to catheterization for intravenous hydration.

NONIONIC CONTRAST AGENTS

The benefits of non-ionic contrast agents in the diabetic population for the prevention of contrast nephropathy have been reported but not fully established. In one study of 1196 patients, diabetics were noted to have a 15% absolute risk reduction in the development on renal failure with the use of the non-ionic agent iohexil *(19)* compared with nondiabetics. This benefit has been noted in other studies and appears to be greatest in diabetics with pre-existing renal disease *(20,21)*. Recent interest has focused on the use of iso-osmolar contrast agents to further decrease the risk of nephropathy. A recent study of an iso-osmolar agent iodixanol vs the non-ionic agent iohexol in diabetic patients with serum creatinine between 1.5 and 3.5 mg/dL demonstrated a statistically significant 23% risk reduction in an increase of creatinine of more than 0.5 mg/dL *(22)* (Fig. 1).

N-ACETYLCYSTEINE

The antioxidant acetylcysteine in combination with low-ionic contrast and hydration has been shown in certain studies to attenuate the degree of contrast nephropathy in those with pre-existing renal dysfunction *(23,24)*. Current data is conflicting and most studies have enrolled small numbers of patients, which makes interpretation of its effects on the diabetic subgroups difficult. Given the benign nature of the drug and potential benefit, we currently give 600 mg twice a day on the day of and prior to an elective catheterization in diabetic patients with a serum creatinine greater than 2.0 mg/dL.

ACCESS

Approximately 95% of interventional cardiac catheterization procedures are performed by access of the femoral artery *(25)*. This is technically straightforward, allows for patient and operator comfort, and the delivery of the relatively bulkier interventional equipment with less difficulty and arterial trauma. Given the high prevalence of peripheral vascular disease in the diabetic patient, however, greater consideration must be given to the pos-

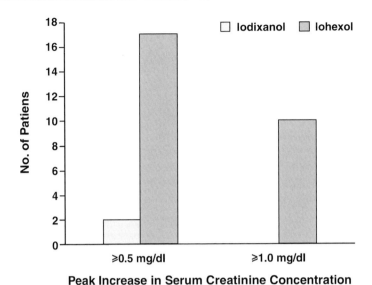

Peak Increase in Serum Creatinine Concentration

Fig. 1. From ref. *22* with permission.

sibility of aortic aneurysm, femoral/iliac occlusion, and the presence of femoral arterial grafts. Although access may be obtained via the brachial or radial arteries, this may make delivery of interventional equipment or rapid placement of an intra-aortic balloon pump (IABP) in an unstable patient challenging.

OTHER ISSUES

Allergic reactions to intra-arterial contrast dye occur roughly 1% of the time *(25,26)*. This may be avoided by the prophylactic use of low-ionic contrast media and premedication with corticosteroids. The oral biguanide Metformin should be discontinued prior to catheterization, as it may cause a severe type B lactic acidosis in patients with a serum creatinine over 1.5 mg/dL or CHF.

Consideration must also be given to the diabetic patient's tolerance of an anticoagulation regimen. Severe retinopathy is a relative contraindication to antiplatelet therapy. Clearance of the small molecule IIB/IIIA inhibitors is affected by renal clearance and appropriate adjustments must be made in the dosing or use of abciximab should be considered. Although abciximab may be dialyzed in an emergency or reversed with platelet transfusions, the effectiveness of this approach has not been documented with the small molecule IIB/IIIA inhibitors *(186)*.

CORONARY INTERVENTION

Elective

Diabetics currently comprise approximately one-quarter of patients referred for PCI *(27–29)*. When matched for other patient characteristics, they have more extensive and diffuse CAD *(29)*. Data from large populations of diabetics in the National Heart, Lung, and Blood Institute (NHLBI) Dynamic Registry demonstrate that despite comparable

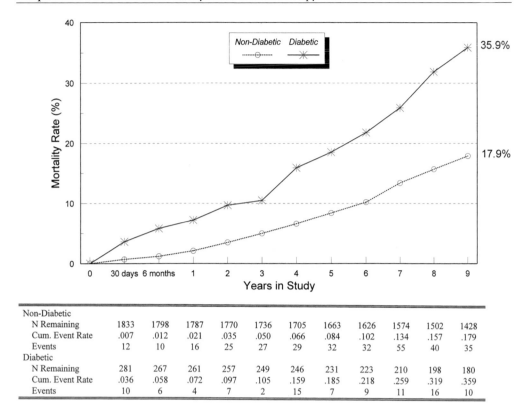

Non-Diabetic											
N Remaining	1833	1798	1787	1770	1736	1705	1663	1626	1574	1502	1428
Cum. Event Rate	.007	.012	.021	.035	.050	.066	.084	.102	.134	.157	.179
Events	12	10	16	25	27	29	32	32	55	40	35
Diabetic											
N Remaining	281	267	261	257	249	246	231	223	210	198	180
Cum. Event Rate	.036	.058	.072	.097	.105	.159	.185	.218	.259	.319	.359
Events	10	6	4	7	2	15	7	9	11	16	10

Fig. 2. From ref. *29* with permission.

acute procedural results to nondiabetics, diabetics have decreased long-term survival, freedom from MI, and increased target lesion revascularization *(29,30)*. Kip and colleagues *(29)* in the NHLBI Registry documented a doubling of diabetic mortality at 9 years (35.9% vs 17.9%), with more than 50% of the diabetic patients with three-vessel disease dying in this time frame (51.3% vs 25.1%) (Fig. 2). This marked increase in mortality rates persists in the modern era, despite the availability of superior medical therapy and coronary stents *(31)*.

One of the primary reasons for the poorer outcomes of the diabetic patient is the impact of aggressive restenosis. The cause of restenosis is multifactorial; aggressive smooth muscle hyperplasia, accelerated fibrosis, enhanced endogenous thrombogenicity, and increased recoil have all been implicated *(32–34)*. Owing to this proliferative restenotic response, diabetics are almost twice as likely to present with complete vessel occlusion *(35)*. This appears to be a key determinant for long-term survival. A recent study demonstrated that 10-year mortality for diabetic patients with no restenosis, nonocclusive restenosis, and occlusive restenosis was 24%, 35%, and 59%, respectively *(36)*.

Initial treatment with balloon angioplasty provides similar procedural success and relief of angina for patients with diabetes *(31)*. However, the initial report from the NHLBI Angioplasty Registry indicated that the angiographic restenosis rate in the diabetic patients was 47%, compared with 32% in the nondiabetic patients *(37)*. Subsequent studies confirmed this, with reported restenosis rates of 49%-71% among diabetic patients *(38–40)*.

The use of intracoronary stents provide for greater acute luminal gain, attenuating some of the effects of the exaggerated intimal hyperplasia and also preventing acute vessel recoil after percutaneous transluminal coronary angioplasty (PTCA). Multiple studies have demonstrated the efficacy of stents in decreasing restenosis relative to PTCA in patients with diabetes; however, the reported rates remain in the 24% to 55% range (33,35,41). Interpretation of these numbers must be taken in context, as higher restenosis rates were reported for stents placed in saphenous vein grafts, smaller vessels, and longer lesions. Recently, Van Belle and colleagues reported less in-stent restenosis compared with balloon angioplasty in 314 diabetic patients (27% vs 62%; $p < 0.0001$) for uncomplicated native coronary artery stenting of average vessel sizes of 3.06 mm and lesion lengths of 9 mm (27). There was an associated decrease in 4-year cardiac mortality and nonfatal MI (14.8% vs 26%; $p = 0.02$) and target lesion revascularization (35.4 vs 52.1%; $p = 0.001$) (27) (Fig. 3). The lower rate of restenosis correlated with lower rates of vessel occlusion (4% vs 13%; $p < 0.005$) and a statistically significant higher ejection fraction. Comparable in-stent restenosis rates (24% at 6 months) were reported in the recently published STRESS Trial, a randomized trial including 92 diabetics, but survival data is not yet available (41).

Attempts to treat this restenotic process have been difficult. In addition to stenting a previously unstented area, the only proven effective modality for treatment of restenosis is brachytherapy. Stenting results in greater maximum luminal diameter but also a greater intimal hyperplastic response, so a significant number of patients still present with restenosis. Intra-coronary brachytherapy, which significantly inhibits smooth muscle cell division, has been shown in multiple trials to reduce the recurrence of treated in-stent restenosis. A recent study of brachytherapy vs placebo in 303 diabetics demonstrated a reduction in restenosis (63.8% vs 15.7%, $p < 0.0001$), target lesion revascularization (66.7% vs 17.6%, $p < 0.0001$) and target vessel revascularization (TVR) (70.6% vs 22.9%, $p < 0.0001$) at 6 months (42). Additionally, compared with the 371 nondiabetics, the diabetics treated with brachytherapy had similar restenosis (15.6% vs 10.7% $p = 0.33$) and TVR rates (22.9% vs 28.2% $p = 0.41$) (42) (Fig. 4).

The introduction of drug-coated stents has demonstrated great promise in early results from clinical trials. Multiple agents aimed at reducing the antiproliferative response and promoting vascular healing are currently under investigation, but the two most well studied at this point are sirolimus and paclitaxel. These drugs are generally bound to the stent via a polymer that allows for delayed and prolonged release into the area of injured endothelium.

Two large clinical trials, Randomized Study with the Sirolimus-Coated Bx Velocity Balloon-Expandable Stent in the Treatment of Patients with de Novo Native Coronary Artery Lesions (RAVEL) and Sirolimus-Coated BX Velocity Balloon-Expandable Stent in the Treatment of Patients with De Novo Coronary Artery Lesions (SIRIUS), have demonstrated the efficacy of sirolimus in preventing restenosis and major adverse cardiac events. RAVEL randomized 238 patients (42 diabetics) with *de novo* coronary lesions to drug-eluting vs bare-metal stents. The authors reported 0% vs 26% restenosis at 6-month and 1-year major adverse cardiac events of 5.8% vs 28%; $p < 0.001$ (43). The larger SIRIUS study enrolled 1058 patients (279 diabetics) and demonstrated a reduction in target segment restenosis of 36.3% to 8.9% at 6 months. Although the diabetic subgroup in the sirolimus arm had a higher rate of restenosis (17.6% vs 8.9%), their relative risk reduction was preserved, as the diabetics in the bare-metal stenting arm had a

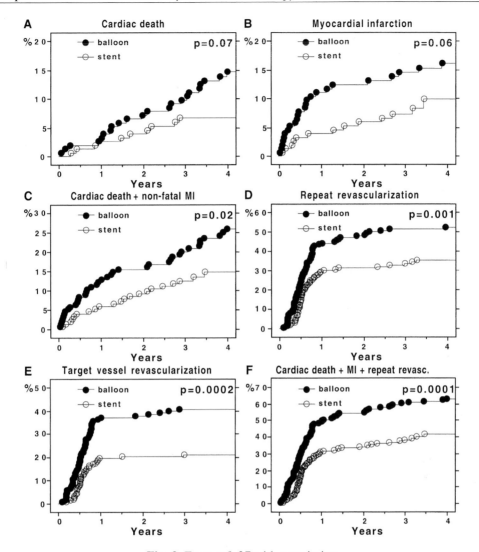

Fig. 3. From ref. *27* with permission.

restenosis rate of 50.5% *(43a)*. Similar results were recently reported for paclitaxel in the TAXUS IV trial. The TVR for all patients was 12% vs 4.7% ($p < 0.0001$) with binary restenosis of 24.4% vs. 5.5% ($p < 0.0001$). The incidence of binary restenosis at 9 months in the diabetic patients strongly favored the drug-eluting stent (42.9% vs 7.7% $p < 0.007$) *(43b)*. A trial enrolling only diabetics is currently underway to evaluate sirolimus, and future trials will compare the two agents for superiority.

EMERGENT CORONARY INTERVENTIONS

In the setting of an acute coronary syndrome, the vascular bed is a thrombogenic milieu of damaged endothelium, activated platelets and fresh clot. Pharmacological and mechanical revascularization of this area is frequently undertaken with balloon angioplasty and/or stenting with or without rheolytic thrombectomy and distal protection in an attempt to restore arterial patency, stabilize the active lesion, and prevent further infarction.

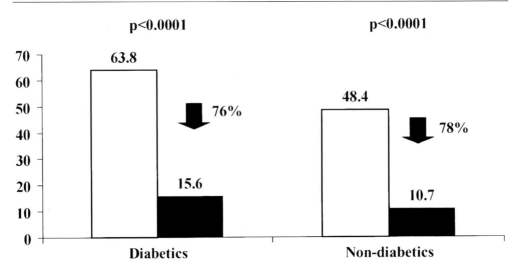

Fig. 4. Reprinted from ref. *42* with permission.

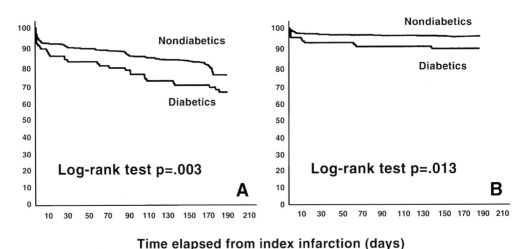

Time elapsed from index infarction (days)

Fig. 5. Reprinted from ref. *46* with permission from Excerpta Medica, Inc.

Diabetic patients have higher early and late mortality than nondiabetics in part because of older age, later presentation, and a greater prevalence of multivessel CAD *(44–46)* (Fig. 5). It has also been recognized that no-reflow, a phenomenon resulting from obstruction and spasm of the microvasculature causing increased infarct size and poorer clinical outcomes, is associated with hyperglycemia, and may contribute to this increased mortality *(47)*.

In the acute ST elevation setting, emergent balloon angioplasty has been proven highly effective in restoring infarct vessel patency, and in multiple studies has been shown to be superior to thrombolytic therapy *(48–51)*. Although there are no randomized trials comparing the outcome of diabetics as a prespecified group, analysis of Global Use of Strategies to Open Occluded Arteries in Acute Coronary Syndromes demonstrated decreased re-infarction and recurrent ischemia for angioplasty over fibrinolysis, and similar 12-month mortality of the diabetics and nondiabetics within the angioplasty arm *(52)*. A subsequent nonrandomized, retrospective analysis of 202 diabetic patients involving the use of both coronary stents (94.2% of patients) and IIB/IIIA inhibitors (63.1% of patients) demonstrated lower in-hospital recurrent ischemia for primary revascularization (5.8% vs 17.2%, $p = 0.011$) and target lesion revascularization at 1 year (19.4% vs 36.4%, $p = 0.007$) *(53)*. Death or re-infarction at 1 year was also reduced among those treated with angioplasty/stenting (17.5% vs 31.3%, $p = 0.02$) *(53)*.

In the urgent setting, percutaneous revascularization has also been demonstrated to be beneficial. In the TACTICS-TIMI 18 Study, which evaluated the efficacy of a conservative approach to NSTEMI vs an aggressive interventional strategy in 2220 patients, diabetics comprised 28% of the population. The diabetic cohort had a 27% risk reduction of death, MI, re-hospitalization at 6 months (27.7% vs 20.1%, $p < 0.05$) *(54)* with the more aggressive strategy to include angiography and PCI.

CONCURRENT ANTIPLATELET THERAPY

The use of intravenous glycoprotein IIB/IIIA inhibitors followed by an outpatient oral thienopyridine has become standard for the prevention of acute and chronic complications of percutaneous revascularization. The IIB/IIA inhibitors abciximab, eptifibatide and tirofiban have been the most studied in the early interventional period. For the diabetic patient, there is no apparent differential effect of the diabetes itself on the drugs ability to maintain platelet inhibition *(55)*. Indeed, much excitement has been generated by demonstration that the use of a IIB/IIA inhibitor at the time of percutaneous revascularization decreased death and MI rates to levels approaching or comparable to those of nondiabetics.

In the Enhanced Suppression of the Platelet IIb/IIIa Receptor With Integrilin Therapy trial, use of eptifibatide in the diabetic patient undergoing stent implantation resulted in similar degrees of reduction of death, MI, and TVR as compared to the nondiabetic *(56)* (Fig. 6). One-year mortality was reduced from 3.5% to 1.3% with eptifibatide, comparable to 1.4% in nondiabetic group *(56)*. A similar benefit was seen for abciximab in the Evaluation of Platelet IIb/IIIa Inhibitor for Stenting study with a reduced risk of death, MI, and urgent 30-day revascularization from 12.1% to 5.6% in stented diabetics, comparable to the nondiabetics (5.2%) *(57)*. There was a 65% decrease in the 1-year risk of death and MI (13.9% to 10.4%) *(57)*.

Direct head-to-head comparisons are rare with the IIb/IIIa agents. No apparent benefit of abciximab over tirofiban was for diabetic patients seen in the Do Tirofiban and ReoPro Give Similar Efficacy Outcomes Trial for the composite of death, MI, and TVR *(58)*. As with all agents, there appears to be no effect of the IIB/IIA inhibitor on restenosis, as patients with diabetes had a higher incidence of TVR at 6 months as compared with nondiabetics (10.3% vs 7.8%; $p = 0.008$) *(58)*.

The oral thienopyridine agents clopidogrel and ticlopidine are generally continued anywhere from one to twelve months post procedure, depending on the presence of drug-eluting stents, the use of intracoronary brachytherapy, and severity of coronary disease. Ticlopidine has generally been supplanted by clopidogrel as a result of its risk of hematological toxicity. The drugs serve primarily to prevent stent thrombosis during endothelialization of the device, but more recent data suggests that they may protect

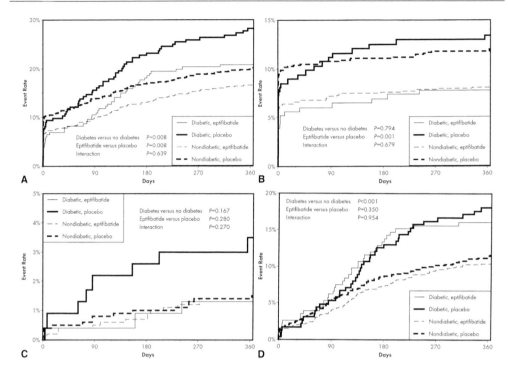

Fig. 6. From ref. *56* with permission.

against future events. In the Effects of Pretreatment with Clopidogrel and Aspirin Followed by Long-Term Therapy in Patients Undergoing Percutaneous Coronary Intervention study, cardiovascular death or MI at 1 year decreased from 16.5% to 12.9% in the diabetic population *(59)*. Whether or not aggressive preprocedure loading of clopidogrel can provide equivalent clinical benefit to IIB/IIA inhibition is currently under investigation.

CORONARY ARTERY BYPASS GRAFTING

Coronary artery bypass grafting (CABG) is a highly effective procedure in the diabetic population for both relief of angina and myocardial revascularization. Although perioperative mortality and relief of anginal symptoms are equivalent to those of the nondiabetic population *(60)*, diabetics suffer from higher infection rates and longer hospital stays *(61,62)*. Although the rate of chest wound infection remains consistently higher in the diabetic population, there is conflicting data regarding whether the use of unilateral or even bilateral mammary grafting increases this risk *(63–65)*. This is an important issue, as the presence of an internal mammary artery (IMA) graft confers much of the benefit of the operation *(66)*.

With regard to long-term outcomes, the survival of the diabetic remains consistently lower than that of the nondiabetic *(66,67)*. In one large retrospective analysis of 9,920 nondiabetics and 2278 diabetic patients undergoing CABG between 1978 and 1993, the 5-year (78% vs 88%, $p < 0.05$) and 10-year (50% vs 71%, $p < 0.05$) survival was lower for the diabetics *(68)*. This has been attributed to increased rates of saphenous vein graft failure as a result of aggressive intimal hyperplasia in the few years following CABG. However, a recent study addressing the effect of long-term effect of diabetic bypass grafts status did not support this hypothesis. Despite the fact that patients with diabetes were more likely to have smaller distally grafted vessels (<1.5mm) and vessels of poor quality (9% vs 6%), there was no statistical difference in likelihood of having either a left internal mammarian artery or saphenous vein graft (SVG) stenosis at a mean of 4 years follow-up *(69)*.

PERCUTANEOUS CORONARY INTERVENTION VS CORONARY ARTERY BYPASS GRAFTING

CABG was accepted as the preferred form of revascularization for multi-vessel disease over angioplasty throughout the early days of percutaneous intervention. However, increasing interest in multivessel PCI led to many large trials of CABG vs angioplasty in the early 1990s. Too few diabetics were enrolled in most of the trials of multivessel angioplasty (EAST, RITA, ERACI, and GABI) vs CABG to make a meaningful assessment of its impact on survival. However, the BARI Trial raised concerning questions regarding the appropriateness of multivessel PCI in the diabetic patient.

In BARI, 1829 patients randomized to either multivessel PCI or CABG demonstrated no significant difference in 5-year mortality (10.7% CABG vs 13.7% PTCA, $p = 0.19$), however, additional revascularization was required with increased frequency in the PTCA arm (8% vs 54%, $p < 0.001$). The diabetic population ($n = 353$) showed a significantly lower 5-year CABG mortality (19.4% vs 34.5%; $p < 0.003$) *(70)* and 7-year mortality (23.6% vs 44%; $p = 0.001$) *(71)* (Fig. 7). These results raised concern about selection of revascularization procedures in diabetic patients with multivessel CAD, and prompted a NHLBI clinical alert stating that CABG should be the preferred initial revascularization in medically treated diabetics with multivessel CAD *(72)*.

A subsequent report from the BARI investigators indicated that the survival benefit of CABG is limited to diabetics receiving IMA grafts, a finding that has been verified in other trials (63,66,73). Cardiac mortality after 5.4 years was 2.9% when IMA was used and 18.2% when only SVG conduits were used. The latter rate was similar to that in patients receiving PTCA (20.6%) *(72)*. The mortality benefit afforded by IMA was most apparent in those experiencing a Q-wave MI during follow-up, an effect also seen in nondiabetic patients *(74)*. This greater protective effect (90% mortality reduction) of the IMA bypass was likely related to either reduction of hypoperfusion during coronary occlusion, distal vessel protection from proximal disease progression, or the more complete revascularization offered by CABG over PTCA allowing for greater collateral recruitment during periods of active ischemia. In BARI, 3.1 grafts were placed per patient undergoing CABG *(75)*, whereas the mean number of successfully treated lesions in the PTCA group was 2 *(28)*. Recently, a study of the diabetic BARI population at 1-year re-look angiogram indicated a greater amount of jeopardized myocardium present in those who underwent PTCA than CABG (42% vs 24%, $p = 0.05$) *(76)*. Many previous CABG studies have emphasized that it is this ability to obtain complete revascularization that is responsible for CABG's survival benefit over PTCA.

The current guidelines for revascularization of the diabetic with multivessel CAD favor CABG, reflecting the outcomes seen in the BARI trial *(77)*. However, support for these guidelines is not universal for multiple reasons. Interestingly, in the BARI registry of nonrandomized diabetic patients, there was no significant difference in long-term survival between the two strategies *(2)* (Fig. 8). This difference has been partially attributed to increased education and activity levels and decreased smoking rates in the registry

A **Survival-All Patients**

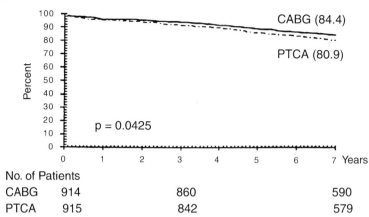

No. of Patients
CABG   914   860   590
PTCA   915   842   579

B **Survival-Patients with Treated Diabetes**

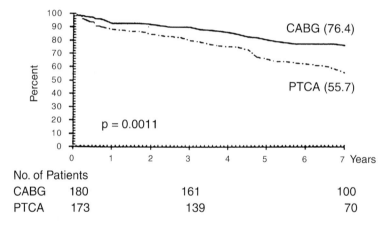

No. of Patients
CABG   180   161   100
PTCA   173   139   70

C **Survival-Patients without Treated Diabetes**

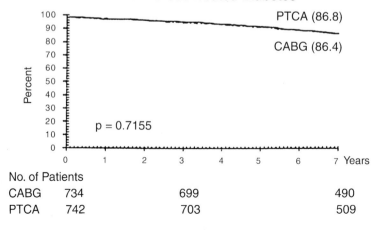

No. of Patients
CABG   734   699   490
PTCA   742   703   509

Fig. 7. Reprinted from ref. *71* with permission from the American College of Cardiology.

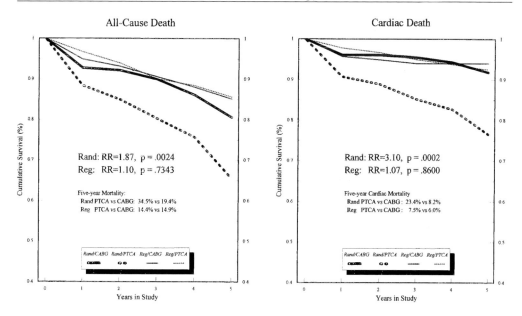

All-Cause Death

Cardiac Death

Rand: RR=1.87, p = .0024
Reg: RR=1.10, p = .7343

Five-year Mortality:
 Rand PTCA vs CABG: 34.5% vs 19.4%
 Reg PTCA vs CABG: 14.4% vs 14.9%

Rand: RR=3.10, p = .0002
Reg: RR=1.07, p = .8600

Five-year Cardiac Mortality
 Rand PTCA vs CABG : 23.4% vs 8.2%
 Reg PTCA vs CABG :   7.5% vs 6.0%

Rand/CABG Rand/PTCA Reg/CABG Reg/PTCA

Years in Study

Rand/CABG Rand/PTCA Reg/CABG Reg/PTCA

Years in Study

Fig. 8. From ref. *2* with permission.

diabetics. A recent analysis of the registry patients revealed that they had more frequent single vessel PCI (76% vs 33%, $p < 0.001$), greater use of stents (76% vs 1%, $p < 0.001$), and greater use of IIB/IIIA inhibitors (24% vs 0%, $p < 0.001$) *(78)*. Because BARI patients did not receive the current PCI standard of care, involving the use of stents and glycoprotein IIB/IIIA antagonists, many argue that the results may not be applicable to current practice.

Three recent trials have incorporated the use of intracoronary stents. In the Arterial Revascularization Therapies Study Group (ARTS) trial, multivessel stenting vs CABG was compared in 1205 patients, with approx 100 diabetics in each arm *(79)*. The diabetics in the stenting arm had the lowest 1-year event-free survival (63.4%) vs CABG (84%; $p < 0.001$), almost entirely as a result of TVR. The need for repeat procedures in the PCI arm of 25% was notably decreased compared to prior trials. Diabetics and nondiabetics treated with CABG had comparable 1-year event free rates of 84.4% and 88.4% *(80)*. Five-year mortality numbers in the diabetic population will be necessary to fully assess the significance of this trial, however, the authors point out that future use of newer off-pump procedures in the CABG arm and use of IIB/IIIA inhibitors in the PCI arm may further lower the mortality rates.

In the Stents or Surgery trial, which that enrolled 988 patients, the incidence of death or Q-wave MI was similar in both groups (PCI 9%, CABG 10%; $p = 0.80$) at 2 years *(81)*. The need for TVR was higher in the PCI group 21% vs 6% CABG group; $p < 0.0001$). Data on the 150 diabetic patients enrolled is not yet available. Similar to ARTS, the use of an IIB/IIIA (8%) was not widely employed.

The Angina With Extremely Serious Operative Mortality Evaluation (AWESOME) trial evaluated a sicker patient population. AWESOME was a veterans study from 1995 to 2000 of 454 (144 diabetics) patients for PCI vs CABG with one of five high-risk features to include prior CABG, MI within 7 days, ejection fraction less than 35%, age greater than 70 years, or IABP for hemodynamic stabilization. Additionally, a separate analysis of 1650 (525 diabetics) nonrandomizable physician-directed registry patients and 327 (89 diabetics) self-directed registry patients was performed. CABG and PCI mortality for diabetics at 3 years was 72% and 81% for randomized patients (p = ns), 85% and 89% for patient choice (p = ns) and 73% and 71% for physician choice (p = ns) *(82)*. Coronary stents were used in 54% of patients and IIB/IIIA inhibitors in 11%.

Although the current standard of care remains CABG for most diabetic patients with multivessel coronary disease, the paradigm may begin to shift in the next decade. Although further follow-up from the initial stent vs CABG studies will offer insight, the field has already begun to move beyond these trials. Trials such as FREEDOM, ARTS-II, CARDia are all looking at the use of coated stents vs CABG for multivessel disease. Additionally, greater and more sustained use of both intravenous and oral platelet inhibitors and the use of hybrid operative and PCI procedures will also change practice patterns. Finally, given the dramatic advances in medical therapy in the last decade, the question had been raised regarding whether revascularization remains a superior treatment to best medical care. The medical care in the BARI patient cohort has been criticized because there was no change in the average low-density lipoprotein of approx 140 mg/dL over the 5-year trial period *(70)*. The BARI 2D trial will randomize 2600 diabetic patients with stable coronary disease to medical therapy vs PCI/CABG, and is currently enrolling patients *(83)*.

PERIPHERAL ARTERIAL INTERVENTIONS

General

Among Americans, there is up to a 10% prevalence rate of peripheral arterial occlusive disease. Fortunately, the vast majority of patients are asymptomatic, given the ability of the vascular bed to recruit robust collaterals. However, in patients with CAD the rate is closer to 50%, and in patients with diabetes the rate may approach 80%.

Lower Extremity

Approximately half of all lower extremity amputations in the United States are performed on patients with diabetes. Peripheral arterial interventions are increasingly being used in the treatment of symptomatic lower extremity peripheral disease after traditional exercise and smoking cessation programs have failed. Although rest pain, nonhealing ulcers, and critical limb ischemia have traditionally been treated through surgical revascularization, the less-invasive nature of peripheral intervention has lowered the threshold for percutaneous revascularization. Owing to the fact that diabetics tend to present with peripheral arterial disease that is both more diffuse, multilevel, and severe, these procedures are frequently used for correction of significant iliac disease in conjunction with surgery. This allows for distal surgery without the risks associated with cross-clamping the aorta. Although diabetes persists as a significant risk factor for decreased long-term patency after lower extremity PCI *(84)*, amputation rates continue to decrease.

Aorto-Iliac Intervention

Diabetics present more frequently with limb ischemia than claudication, the etiology of which is usually as a result of multilevel disease. Although lesions in the lower extremity vascular tree occur in tandem, the significance of the cumulative pressure drop may be alleviated by PCI on the proximal (inflow) lesion, and may delay or obviate the need for surgery. Early studies such as the Veterans Administration Cooperative Study, that included 29% diabetics, demonstrated similar rates of death and amputation at 4 years follow-up for balloon angioplasty vs surgery, albeit at a greater need for repeat target limb revascularization in the angioplasty arm *(85)*. A study by Spence and colleagues evaluating the efficacy of percutaneous intervention vs aorto-iliac bypass grafting in the setting of the diabetic limb-threatening ischemia (rest pain, nonhealing ulcers, gangrene) also demonstrated comparable salvage rates of 85% at 4 years *(86)*.

Primary vs provisional stenting remains an area of investigation. The Dutch Iliac Stent Trial demonstrated no significant differences in long-term outcome for primary stenting (compared to percutaneous transluminal angioplasty (PTA) alone or bailout stenting), despite greater periprocedural success *(87)*. A meta-analysis of primary stenting for aorto-iliac disease, however, demonstrated better acute and long-term outcomes with primary stenting *(88)*. The authors separated the results based on both the indication for the procedure, claudication or critical ischemia, and for the initial angiographic findings of stenosis or occlusion. They found higher patency rates for stenosis over occlusions (77% vs 61%; 67% vs 53%; $p < 0.05$) after stent placement to treat claudication and critical ischemia respectively.

With acute procedural success rates in excess of 95%, the initial Food and Drug Administration (FDA) recommendation in 1993 was that decision to stent be based on the presence of extensive dissection, residual stenosis greater than 30%, or residual mean gradient over 5 mmHg *(89)*. Mean gradient pressure measurements are an integral part of PCI assessment as an adjunct to visual estimate. The presence of tandem stenoses, long segments of diffuse disease, and need for significant inflow with ambulation all make lesion significance difficult to gage, and the presence of a mean gradient over 10 mmHg is considered significant. Despite the recommendations for provisional stenting, many interventionalists have a lower threshold toward proceeding with a primary stenting technique.

Key principles derived from early trials include the following. Angiographic criteria of total occlusion, poor distal run-off, and the clinical setting of critical limb ischemia have all been demonstrated to be negative predictors of long-term patency. This is important, as diabetics are more likely than nondiabetics to have vessel occlusion, and the presence of multilevel vascular disease is seen in half the population *(90)*. For iliac disease alone, however, the presence of diabetes does not clearly prognosticate a worse long-term result *(86,91)* than the nondiabetic.

Serious complications are uncommon. Risks of emergent surgery for arterial perforation (0.1%) and acute vessel closure are rare because of the increased use of stents *(92)*. The risk of stent thrombosis is increased by the presence of long lesions, total occlusions, and poor outflow, but appears to be attenuated by the use of clopidogrel in conjunction with aspirin *(93,94)*. Vascular access issues (hematoma, pseudoaneursym, arteriovenous fistula) remain the most prevalent complications (~5%), but are generally readily recognized and managed in both diabetic and nondiabetic patients *(94,95)*.

Femoral-Popliteal Intervention

The track record of interventional arterial therapy below the common femoral artery is less impressive than with aorto-iliac disease. The common femoral itself is considered the territory of the surgeon, as it is the only supply to the leg outside of the abdomen, and the surgical durability of the femoral-popliteal graft at 5 years approaches 80%. Up to this point, the Achilles heel of the superficial femoral and popliteal intervention has been long-term primary patency rates that approach only 70% and a lack of clear benefit of stenting. Standard interventional principles predict outcome; longer lesion lengths, higher complexity lesions, poor run-off, and the presence of total occlusion of the vessel all impact negatively on outcome. Balloon angioplasty for lesion lengths of greater than 10 cm have been associated with patency rates as low as 20% at 1 year (84).

Advances in technology have improved the outcomes following intervention. Stenting provides acute success rates of over 95% and a greater reduction in transluminal gradient than with balloon angioplasty alone (96). A recent trial evaluating stenting vs angioplasty for short lesions (<5cm) demonstrated higher acute success rates (99% vs 84%; p (< 0.009) but no difference in 1- or 2-year primary patency rates (73% vs 74%) (97). In one single center study, stenting also led to higher technical success and greater 6-month patency (87% vs 25%; p (< 0.02) at 2 years with corresponding improvement in ankle-brachial indexes (98). At this point, however, the benefit to primary stenting below the inguinal ligament is debatable.

Complication rates are similar to those discussed for iliac intervention. Owing the increased instance of restenotic disease, there has been significant interest in intravascular radiation therapy recurrent disease. Small studies have demonstrated efficacy with restenosis rates of about 30%, however, there is a significant risk (up to 27%) of late thrombotic occlusion after discontinuing clopidogrel in patients with stents (100–103a). (Given the relatively high secondary patency rate with a second procedure, many operators choose to primarily stent, as occlusive restenosis in a stent is easier to deal with technically than native restenotic occlusion.

INFRAPOPLITEAL INTERVENTIONS

The clinical outcomes of critical limb ischemia resulting from infrapopliteal arterial disease is dismal, with 1-year mortality rates approaching 30% and amputation rates close to 20% (103). Angioplasty is of questionable sustainable benefit; published literature is generally retrospective as procedures are performed in a last attempt at limb salvage. Generally, surgery remains the standard of care for these patients, although it is associated with lower patency rates than more proximal procedures. Recently, Dorros and colleagues published a nonrandomized series of 529 tibeoperoneal lesions and reported a 5-year limb-salvage rate of 91% and survival of 56% (104). These results will need to be duplicated, but provide some hope for improving the bleak outcomes associated with this arterial disease at this level.

RENAL INTERVENTIONS

Diabetic renal disease and hypertension are the leading indications for initiation of hemodialysis in the United States. Estimates of the prevalence of renovascular disease as the underlying etiology for chronic renal failure range from 6% to 20% (105). The risk of progression of underlying renovascular disease is doubled by the presence of diabetes (106). Increasingly, percutaneous revascularization of the renal arteries is undertaken for renal preservation, hypertension control, and prevention of recurrent pulmonary edema, although the indications are in evolution and the subject of intense debate.

The evaluation of response to renal intervention remains problematic. Serum creatinine and glomerular filtration rate (GFR) are inadequate screening tests for renal dysfunction, as stenosis and hypoperfusion of one kidney secondary to stenosis may result in hyperfusion and damage to the contralateral kidney with little change in either marker. A recent study of consecutive patients with unilateral stenosis demonstrated normalization by nuclear scintigraphy of split renal function and GFR in both kidneys after PTA of renal stenosis *(107)*.

The measurement by ultrasound of renal resistive indices has also been used to predict the response to renal revascularization. Radermacher and colleagues demonstrated that among 96 patients (17% diabetics) with resistive indices less than 80, demonstrating the absence of chronic renal parenchymal injury, 94% of patients had a greater than 10% blood pressure response ($p < 0.001$) to PTA for stenoses greater than 50% ($p < 0.001$) *(107a)*.

Results of three randomized controlled trials for PTA for unilateral or bilateral renal artery stenosis demonstrated equivocal results with respect to renal preservation and hypertension control *(108–110)*. Small numbers and limited enrollment make interpretation of these results difficult. However, these trials demonstrated a high rate of angiographic recoil, particularly with ostial lesions, and led to increasing stent use *(111)*.

In one of the largest series available, Dorros and associates looked at 1058 patients (283 diabetics) who underwent stenting of 1443 atherosclerotic renal arteries (64% unilateral and 36% bilateral) for poorly controlled hypertension (85%), preservation of renal function (59%), and CHF (15%) *(112)*. Renal function after unilateral or bilateral stent revascularization demonstrated stabilization or lowering of the serum creatinine (bilateral: 1.7 ± 1.2 to 0.8 ± 0.6; unilateral: 1.7 ± 1.1 to 1.4 ± 0.8; $p < 0.05$) for all groups *(112)*. However, long-term follow-up at 4 years demonstrated worse renal function and overall survival (62% vs 78%) in the diabetic patients *(112)*. Future direction will include more randomized trials, distal embolic protection, and less-toxic contrast agents.

CAROTID INTERVENTIONS

Diabetes is a potent risk factor for a cerebrovascular accident. Even for the well-controlled diabetic, the stroke risk is up to three times greater than a nondiabetic *(113)*. Although diabetics suffer strokes at the same age as their nondiabetic counterparts, these strokes are associated with more significant limb weakness, dysarthria, and a poorer functional recovery *(114)*.

Atherosclerotic disease of the carotid artery commonly occurs at the bifurcation of the external and internal carotid. Up until recently, the standard of care for patients with symptomatic or asymptomatic high-grade carotid lesions was repair by a vascular surgeon *(115,116)*. However, over the last decade, published series of carotid angioplasty and stenting in patients with high-surgical risk heightened interest in head-to-head comparisons of surgical endarterectomy vs stenting. The Carotid and Vertebral Artery Transluminal Angioplasty Study *(117)*, published in 2001, randomized 504 patients (67 diabetics, 13%) with symptomatic high-grade carotid lesions to endarterectomy vs PTCA with bailout stenting. The outcome of disabling stroke or death was similar at 30 days in both groups (6.4% vs 5.9%; $p = $ ns), however, the high rates of complication compared to prior surgical trials led to questioning of the trial's applicability.

Given the inherent risk of plaque liberalization and distal embolization associated with carotid intervention, the current standard of care for percutaneous intervention has incorporated distal embolic protection devices of either balloon occlusive or filter designed systems. The recently reported Stenting and Angioplasty with Protection in Patients at High Risk for Endarterectomy study (*117a*) randomized patients with symptomatic or asymptomatic greater than 80% carotid lesions with at least one of the following high-risk features: age greater than 80 years, the presence of congestive heart failure, severe chronic obstructive pulmonary disease, previous endarterectomy with restenosis, previous radiation therapy or radical neck surgery, or lesions distal or proximal to the usual cervical location. Stenting with distal embolic protection was associated with a decreased rate of death, stroke, or MI at 30 days (5.8% vs 12.6%; $p = 0.047$), with trends toward significance of all components of the major end points and the greatest benefit from lack of MI. At 1 year, the data have continued with benefit from the stenting group compared with the surgical group with MI 2.5% vs 7.9% stent vs. surgical group ($p < 0.05$) and with major ipsilateral stroke at 0% vs 3.3% stenting vs surgery ($p < 0.05$). Data on the diabetic patients enrolled in the trial is not yet available.

Similar benefit was recently reported by Wholey and colleagues for 30-day results of the Acculink for Revascularization of Carotids in High-Risk Patients trial. In a single-arm study, the authors enrolled 437 patients with asymptomatic high-grade or more than 50% symptomatic carotid lesions and one high-risk characteristic, including uncontrolled diabetes mellitus, to carotid stenting with distal embolic protection. Event rates were not been reported for the diabetics as a subgroup, but rates of overall ipsilateral major stroke (1.4%), stoke-related death (0.7%), and Q wave MI (0.7%) were quite low (*117b*).

The Carotid Revascularization vs Stenting Trial is currently randomizing 2500 symptomatic patients with more than 50% stenosis to stenting with distal protection or endarterectomy, and will offer further insight into the management of this disease.

CONCLUSION

The diffuse and aggressive nature of diabetic vascular disease will continue to provide a significant challenge to the interventional cardiologist in the next century.

Diabetes has been best managed at our institution with a team approach involving multiple physician specialties, nurses, and dieticians, and making the patient responsible for his/her own care. Advances in medical technology will continue to provide innovative and satisfying temporizing therapies, but ultimate progress will come in the form of education and prevention.

REFERENCES

1. Haffner SM, et al. Mortality from coronary heart disease in subjects with type 2 diabetes and in nondiabetic subjects with and without prior myocardial infarction. N Engl J Med 1998;339(4):229–234.
2. Detre KM, et al. Coronary revascularization in diabetic patients: a comparison of the randomized and observational components of the Aypass Angioplasty Revascularization Investigation (BARI). Circulation 1999;99(5):633–640.
3. Williams DO, et al. Percutaneous coronary intervention in the current era compared with 1985–1986: the National Heart, Lung, and Blood Institute Registries. Circulation 2000;102(24):2945–2951.
4. Marso SP, et al. Diabetes mellitus is associated with a shift in the temporal risk profile of inhospital death after percutaneous coronary intervention: an analysis of 25,223 patients over 20 years. Am Heart J 2003;145(2):270–277.
5. Adams RJ, et al. Coronary risk evaluation in patients with transient ischemic attack and ischemic stroke: a scientific statement for healthcare professionals from the Stroke Council and the Council on Clinical Cardiology of the American Heart Association/American Stroke Association. Circulation 2003;108(10):1278–1290.

6. Burek KA, et al. Prognostic importance of lower extremity arterial disease in patients undergoing coronary revascularization in the Bypass Angioplasty Revascularization Investigation (BARI). J Am Coll Cardiol 1999;34(3):716–721.
7. Barzilay JI, et al. Coronary artery disease in diabetic patients with lower-extremity arterial disease: disease characteristics and survival. A report from the Coronary Artery Surgery Study (CASS) registry. Diabetes Care 1997;20(9):1381–1387.
8. Uusitupa MI, et al. 5-year incidence of atherosclerotic vascular disease in relation to general risk factors, insulin level, and abnormalities in lipoprotein composition in non-insulin-dependent diabetic and non-diabetic subjects. Circulation 1990;82(1):27–36.
9. Diabetes-related amputations of lower extremities in the Medicare population—Minnesota 1993–1995. MMWR Morb Mortal Wkly Rep 1998;47(31):649–652.
10. Jude EB, et al. Peripheral arterial disease in diabetic and nondiabetic patients: a comparison of severity and outcome. Diabetes Care 2001;24(8):1433–1437.
11. Newman AB, et al. Ankle-arm index as a predictor of cardiovascular disease and mortality in the Cardiovascular Health Study. The Cardiovascular Health Study Group. Arterioscler Thromb Vasc Biol 1999;19(3):538–545.
12. Davidson CJ, et al. Cardiovascular and renal toxicity of a nonionic radiographic contrast agent after cardiac catheterization. A prospective trial. Ann Intern Med 1989;110(2):119–24.
13. Parfrey PS, et al. Contrast material-induced renal failure in patients with diabetes mellitus, renal insufficiency, or both. A prospective controlled study. N Engl J Med 1989;320(3):143–149.
14. Rihal CS, et al. Incidence and prognostic importance of acute renal failure after percutaneous coronary intervention. Circulation 2002;105(19):2259–2264.
15. Cigarroa RG, et al. Dosing of contrast material to prevent contrast nephropathy in patients with renal disease. Am J Med 1989;86(6 Pt 1):649–652.
16. Mueller C, et al. Prevention of contrast media-associated nephropathy: randomized comparison of 2 hydration regimens in 1620 patients undergoing coronary angioplasty. Arch Intern Med 2002;162(3): 329–336.
17. Taylor AJ, et al. PREPARED: Preparation for Angiography in Renal Dysfunction: a randomized trial of inpatient vs outpatient hydration protocols for cardiac catheterization in mild-to-moderate renal dysfunction. Chest 1998;114(6):1570–1574.
18. Trivedi HS, et al. A randomized prospective trial to assess the role of saline hydration on the development of contrast nephrotoxicity. Nephron Clin Pract 2003;93(1):C29–C34.
19. Rudnick MR, et al. Nephrotoxicity of ionic and nonionic contrast media in 1196 patients: a randomized trial. The Iohexol Cooperative Study. Kidney Int 1995;47(1):254–261.
20. Barrett BJ, et al. Contrast nephropathy in patients with impaired renal function: high versus low osmolar media. Kidney Int 1992;41(5):1274–1279.
21. Barrett BJ, Carlisle EJ. Metaanalysis of the relative nephrotoxicity of high- and low-osmolality iodinated contrast media. Radiology 1993;188(1):171–178.
22. Aspelin P, et al. Nephrotoxic effects in high-risk patients undergoing angiography. N Engl J Med 2003;348(6):491–499.
23. Tepel M, et al. Prevention of radiographic-contrast-agent-induced reductions in renal function by acetylcysteine. N Engl J Med 2000;343(3):180–184.
24. Shyu KG, Cheng JJ, Kuan P. Acetylcysteine protects against acute renal damage in patients with abnormal renal function undergoing a coronary procedure. J Am Coll Cardiol 2002;40(8):1383–1388.
25. Noto TJ Jr, et al. Cardiac catheterization 1990: a report of the Registry of the Society for Cardiac Angiography and Interventions (SCA&I). Cathet Cardiovasc Diagn 1991;24(2):75–83.
26. Wyman RM et al. Current complications of diagnostic and therapeutic cardiac catheterization. J Am Coll Cardiol 1988;12(6):1400–1406.
27. Van Belle E et al. Effects of coronary stenting on vessel patency and long-term clinical outcome after percutaneous coronary revascularization in diabetic patients. J Am Coll Cardiol 2002;40(3):410–417.
28. Influence of diabetes on 5-year mortality and morbidity in a randomized trial comparing CABG and PTCA in patients with multivessel disease: the Bypass Angioplasty Revascularization Investigation (BARI). Circulation 1997;96(6):1761–1769.
29. Kip KE, et al. Coronary angioplasty in diabetic patients. The National Heart, Lung, and Blood Institute Percutaneous Transluminal Coronary Angioplasty Registry. Circulation 1996;94(8):1804–1806.
30. Laskey WK, et al. Comparison of in-hospital and one-year outcomes in patients with and without diabetes mellitus undergoing percutaneous catheter intervention (from the National Heart, Lung, and Blood Institute Dynamic Registry). Am J Cardiol 2002;90(10): 1062–1067.

31. Stein B, et al. Influence of diabetes mellitus on early and late outcome after percutaneous transluminal coronary angioplasty. Circulation 1995;91(4):979–989.
32. Moreno PR, et al. Tissue characteristics of restenosis after percutaneous transluminal coronary angioplasty in diabetic patients. J Am Coll Cardiol 1999;34(4):1045–1049.
33. Carrozza JP Jr, et al. Restenosis after arterial injury caused by coronary stenting in patients with diabetes mellitus. Ann Intern Med 1993;118(5):344–349.
34. Kornowski R, et al. Increased restenosis in diabetes mellitus after coronary interventions is due to exaggerated intimal hyperplasia. A serial intravascular ultrasound study. Circulation 1997;95(6):1366–1369.
35. Elezi S, et al. Diabetes mellitus and the clinical and angiographic outcome after coronary stent placement. J Am Coll Cardiol 1998;32(7):1866–1873.
36. Van Belle E, et al. Patency of percutaneous transluminal coronary angioplasty sites at 6- month angiographic follow-up: A key determinant of survival in diabetics after coronary balloon angioplasty. Circulation 2001;103(9):1218–1224.
37. Holmes DR Jr, et al. Restenosis after percutaneous transluminal coronary angioplasty (PTCA): a report from the PTCA Registry of the National Heart, Lung, and Blood Institute. Am J Cardiol 1984;53(12): 77C–81C.
38. Weintraub WS, et al. Can restenosis after coronary angioplasty be predicted from clinical variables? J Am Coll Cardiol 1993;21(1):6–14.
39. Vandormael MG, et al. Multilesion coronary angioplasty: clinical and angiographic follow-up. J Am Coll Cardiol 1987;10(2):246–252.
40. Quigley PJ, et al. Repeat percutaneous transluminal coronary angioplasty and predictors of recurrent restenosis. Am J Cardiol 1989;63(7):409–413.
41. Savage MP, et al. Coronary intervention in the diabetic patient: improved outcome following stent implantation compared with balloon angioplasty. Clin Cardiol 2002;25(5):213–217.
42. Gruberg L, et al. The effect of intracoronary radiation for the treatment of recurrent in-stent restenosis in patients with diabetes mellitus. J Am Coll Cardiol 2002;39(12):1930–1936.
43. Morice MC, et al. A randomized comparison of a sirolimus-eluting stent with a standard stent for coronary revascularization. N Engl J Med 2002;346(23):1773–1780.
43a. Leon M. The SIRIUS trial. Presented at the Transcatheter Therapeutics meeting, September 24, 2002, Washington, DC.
43b. Stone G. TAXUS-IV. The pivotal, prospective, randomized trial of the slow-rate release polymer-based paclitaxel-eluting TAXUS stent. Clinical overview and subset analysis. Presented at the Transcatheter Therapeutics Meeting, September 16, 2003, Washington, DC.
44. Mak KH, et al. Influence of diabetes mellitus on clinical outcome in the thrombolytic era of acute myocardial infarction. GUSTO-I Investigators. Global Utilization of Streptokinase and Tissue Plasminogen Activator for Occluded Coronary Arteries. J Am Coll Cardiol 1997;30(1):171–179.
45. Harjai KJ, et al. Comparison of outcomes of diabetic and nondiabetic patients undergoing primary angioplasty for acute myocardial infarction. Am J Cardiol 2003;91(9):1041–1045.
46. Bolognese L, et al. Angiographic findings, time course of regional and global left ventricular function, and clinical outcome in diabetic patients with acute myocardial infarction treated with primary percutaneous transluminal coronary angioplasty. Am J Cardiol 2003;91(5):544–549.
47. Iwakura K, et al. Association between hyperglycemia and the no-reflow phenomenon in patients with acute myocardial infarction. J Am Coll Cardiol 2003;41(1):1–7.
48. Grines CL, et al. A comparison of immediate angioplasty with thrombolytic therapy for acute myocardial infarction. The Primary Angioplasty in Myocardial Infarction Study Group. N Engl J Med 1993;328(10): 673–679.
49. Nunn CM, et al. Long-term outcome after primary angioplasty: report from the primary angioplasty in myocardial infarction (PAMI-I) trial. J Am Coll Cardiol 1999;33(3):640–646.
50. Zijlstra F, et al. A comparison of immediate coronary angioplasty with intravenous streptokinase in acute myocardial infarction. N Engl J Med 1993;328(10):680–684.
51. Zijlstra F, et al. Long-term benefit of primary angioplasty as compared with thrombolytic therapy for acute myocardial infarction. N Engl J Med 1999;341(19):1413–1419.
52. Hasdai D, et al. Diabetes mellitus and outcome after primary coronary angioplasty for acute myocardial infarction: lessons from the GUSTO-IIb Angioplasty Substudy. Global Use of Strategies to Open Occluded Arteries in Acute Coronary Syndromes. J Am Coll Cardiol 2000;35(6):1502–1512.
53. Hsu LF, et al. Clinical outcomes of patients with diabetes mellitus and acute myocardial infarction treated with primary angioplasty or fibrinolysis. Heart 2002;88(3):260–265.

54. Cannon CP, et al. Comparison of early invasive and conservative strategies in patients with unstable coronary syndromes treated with the glycoprotein IIb/IIIa inhibitor tirofiban. N Engl J Med 2001;344(25):1879–1887.

55. Steinhubl SR, et al. Attainment and maintenance of platelet inhibition through standard dosing of abciximab in diabetic and nondiabetic patients undergoing percutaneous coronary intervention. Circulation 1999;100(19):1977–1982.

56. Labinaz M, et al. Comparison of one-year outcomes following coronary artery stenting in diabetic versus nondiabetic patients (from the Enhanced Suppression of the Platelet IIb/IIIa Receptor With Integrilin Therapy [ESPRIT] Trial). Am J Cardiol 2002;90(6):585–590.

57. Topol EJ, et al. Outcomes at 1 year and economic implications of platelet glycoprotein IIb/IIIa blockade in patients undergoing coronary stenting: results from a multicentre randomised trial. EPISTENT Investigators. Evaluation of Platelet IIb/IIIa Inhibitor for Stenting. Lancet 1999;354(9195):2019–2024.

58. Roffi M, et al. Impact of different platelet glycoprotein IIb/IIIa receptor inhibitors among diabetic patients undergoing percutaneous coronary intervention: do Tirofiban and ReoPro Give Similar Efficacy Outcomes Trial (TARGET) 1-year follow-up. Circulation 2002;105(23):2730–2736.

59. Mehta SR, et al. Effects of pretreatment with clopidogrel and aspirin followed by long- term therapy in patients undergoing percutaneous coronary intervention: the PCI-CURE study. Lancet 2001;358(9281): 527–533.

60. Barzilay JI, et al. Coronary artery disease and coronary artery bypass grafting in diabetic patients aged > or = 65 years (report from the Coronary Artery Surgery Study [CASS] Registry). Am J Cardiol 1994;74(4):334–339.

61. Fietsam R Jr, Bassett J, Glover JL. Complications of coronary artery surgery in diabetic patients. Am Surg 1991;57(9):551–557.

62. Slaughter MS, et al. A fifteen-year wound surveillance study after coronary artery bypass. Ann Thorac Surg 1993;56(5):1063–1068.

63. Hirotani T, et al. Effects of coronary artery bypass grafting using internal mammary arteries for diabetic patients. J Am Coll Cardiol 1999;34(2):532–538.

64. Gummert JF, et al. Mediastinitis and cardiac surgery—an updated risk factor analysis in 10,373 consecutive adult patients. Thorac Cardiovasc Surg 2002;50(2):87–91.

65. Gansera B, et al. End of the millenium—end of the single thoracic artery graft? Two thoracic arteries— standard for the next millenium? Early clinical results and analysis of risk factors in 1,487 patients with bilateral internal thoracic artery grafts. Thorac Cardiovasc Surg 2001;49(1):10–15.

66. Morris JJ, et al. Influence of diabetes and mammary artery grafting on survival after coronary bypass. Circulation 1991;84(5 Suppl):III275–III284.

67. Herlitz J, Bang A, Karlson BW. Mortality, place and mode of death and reinfarction during a period of 5 years after acute myocardial infarction in diabetic and non-diabetic patients. Cardiology 1996;87(5): 423–428.

68. Thourani VH, et al. Influence of diabetes mellitus on early and late outcome after coronary artery bypass grafting. Ann Thorac Surg 1999;67(4):1045–1052.

69. Schwartz L, et al. Coronary bypass graft patency in patients with diabetes in the Bypass Angioplasty Revascularization Investigation (BARI). Circulation 2002;106(21):2652–2658.

70. Comparison of coronary bypass surgery with angioplasty in patients with multivessel disease. The Bypass Angioplasty Revascularization Investigation (BARI) Investigators. N Engl J Med 1996;335(4): 217–225.

71. BARI Investigators. Seven-year outcome in the Bypass Angioplasty Revascularization Investigation (BARI) by treatment and diabetic status. J Am Coll Cardiol 2000;35(5):1122–1129.

72. Ferguson JJ. NHLI BARI clinical alert on diabetics treated with angioplasty. Circulation 1995;92(12): 3371.

73. Farinas JM, et al. Comparison of long-term clinical results of double versus single internal mammary artery bypass grafting. Ann Thorac Surg 1999;67(2):466–470.

74. Detre KM, et al. The effect of previous coronary-artery bypass surgery on the prognosis of patients with diabetes who have acute myocardial infarction. Bypass Angioplasty Revascularization Investigation Investigators. N Engl J Med 2000;342(14):989–997.

75. Schaff HV, et al. Clinical and operative characteristics of patients randomized to coronary artery bypass surgery in the Bypass Angioplasty Revascularization Investigation (BARI). Am J Cardiol 1995;75(9): 18C–26C.

76. Kip KE, et al. Differential influence of diabetes mellitus on increased jeopardized myocardium after initial angioplasty or bypass surgery: bypass angioplasty revascularization investigation. Circulation 2002;105(16):1914–1920.

77. Braunwald E, et al. ACC/AHA guidelines for the management of patients with unstable angina and non-ST-segment elevation myocardial infarction. A report of the American College of Cardiology/American Heart Association Task Force on Practice Guidelines (Committee on the Management of Patients With Unstable Angina). J Am Coll Cardiol 2000;36(3):970–1062.
78. Srinivas VS, et al. Contemporary percutaneous coronary intervention versus balloon angioplasty for multivessel coronary artery disease: a comparison of the National Heart, Lung and Blood Institute Dynamic Registry and the Bypass Angioplasty Revascularization Investigation (BARI) study. Circulation 2002;106(13):1627–1633.
79. Serruys PW, et al. Comparison of coronary-artery bypass surgery and stenting for the treatment of multivessel disease. N Engl J Med 2001;344(15):1117–1124.
80. Abizaid A, et al. Clinical and economic impact of diabetes mellitus on percutaneous and surgical treatment of multivessel coronary disease patients: insights from the Arterial Revascularization Therapy Study (ARTS) trial. Circulation 2001;104(5):533–538.
81. Coronary artery bypass surgery versus percutaneous coronary intervention with stent implantation in patients with multivessel coronary artery disease (the Stent or Surgery trial): a randomised controlled trial. Lancet 2002;360(9338):965–970.
82. Sedlis SP, et al. Percutaneous coronary intervention versus coronary bypass graft surgery for diabetic patients with unstable angina and risk factors for adverse outcomes with bypass: outcome of diabetic patients in the AWESOME randomized trial and registry. J Am Coll Cardiol 2002;40(9):1555–1566.
83. Sobel BE, Frye R, Detre KM. Burgeoning dilemmas in the management of diabetes and cardiovascular disease: rationale for the Bypass Angioplasty Revascularization Investigation 2 Diabetes (BARI 2D) Trial. Circulation 2003;107(4):636–642.
84. Capek, P, McLean GK, Berkowitz HD. Femoropopliteal angioplasty. Factors influencing long-term success. Circulation 1991;83(2 Suppl):I70–I80.
85. Wolf GL, et al. Surgery or balloon angioplasty for peripheral vascular disease: a randomized clinical trial. Principal investigators and their Associates of Veterans Administration Cooperative Study Number 199. J Vasc Interv Radiol 1993;4(5):639–648.
86. Spence LD, et al. Diabetic versus nondiabetic limb-threatening ischemia: outcome of percutaneous iliac intervention. AJR Am J Roentgenol 1999;172(5):1335–1341.
87. Tetteroo E, et al. Randomised comparison of primary stent placement versus primary angioplasty followed by selective stent placement in patients with iliac-artery occlusive disease. Dutch Iliac Stent Trial Study Group. Lancet 1998;351(9110):1153–1159.
88. Bosch JL, Hunink MG. Meta-analysis of the results of percutaneous transluminal angioplasty and stent placement for aortoiliac occlusive disease. Radiology 1997;204(1):87–96.
89. Palmaz JC, et al. Placement of balloon-expandable intraluminal stents in iliac arteries: first 171 procedures. Radiology 1990;174(3 Pt 2):969–975.
90. Laborde JC, et al. Influence of anatomic distribution of atherosclerosis on the outcome of revascularization with iliac stent placement. J Vasc Interv Radiol 1995;6(4):513–521.
91. Cambria RP, et al. Percutaneous angioplasty for peripheral arterial occlusive disease. Correlates of clinical success. Arch Surg 1987;122(3):283–287.
92. Belli AM, et al. The complication rate of percutaneous peripheral balloon angioplasty. Clin Radiol 1990;41(6):380–383.
93. Strecker EP, Boos IB, Gottmann D, Vetter S. Clopidogrel plus long-term aspirin after femoro-popliteal stenting. The CLAFS project: 1- and 2-year results. Eur Radiol 2004;14(2):302–308.
94. Flexible tantalum stents for the treatment of iliac artery lesions: long-term patency, complications, and risk factors. Eur Radiol 2003;10(3):10.
95. Strecker EP, Boos IB, Hagen B. Flexible tantalum stents for the treatment of iliac artery lesions: long-term patency, complications, and risk factors. Radiology 1996;199(3):641–647.
96. Ballard JL, et al. Complications of iliac artery stent deployment. J Vasc Surg 1996;24(4):545–553; discussion 553–555.
97. Cho L, et al. Superficial femoral artery occlusion: nitinol stents achieve better flow and reduce the need for medications than balloon angioplasty alone. J Invasive Cardiol 2003;15(4):198–200.
98. Cejna M, et al. PTA versus Palmaz stent placement in femoropopliteal artery obstructions: a multicenter prospective randomized study. J Vasc Interv Radiol 2001;12(1):23–31.
99. Saxon RR, et al. Long-term Results of ePTFE Stent-Graft versus Angioplasty in the Femoropopliteal Artery: Single Center Experience from a Prospective, Randomized Trial. J Vasc Interv Radiol 2003;14(3):303–311.

100. Bonvini R, et al. Late acute thrombotic occlusion after endovascular brachytherapy and stenting of femoropopliteal arteries. J Am Coll Cardiol 2003;41(3):409–412.

101. Wolfram RM, et al. Endovascular brachytherapy for prophylaxis against restenosis after long-segment femoropopliteal placement of stents: initial results. Radiology 2001;220(3):724–729.

102. Minar E, et al. Endovascular brachytherapy in peripheral arteries. Vasa 2003;32(1):3–9.

103. Krueger K, et al. Endovascular gamma irradiation of femoropopliteal de novo stenoses immediately after PTA: interim results of prospective randomized controlled trial. Radiology 2002;224(2):519–528.

103a. Pokrajac B, Wolfram r, Lileg B, Minar E. Endovascular brachytherapy in peripheral arteries: solution f or restenosis or false hopes? Curr Treat Options Cardiovasc Med 2003;5(2):121–126.

104. Holdsworth RJ, McCollum PT. Results and resource implications of treating end-stage limb ischaemia. Eur J Vasc Endovasc Surg 1997;13(2):164–173.

105. Dorros G, et al. Tibioperoneal (outflow lesion) angioplasty can be used as primary treatment in 235 patients with critical limb ischemia: five-year follow-up. Circulation 2001;104(17):2057–2062.

106. Stansby G, Hamilton G, Scoble J. Atherosclerotic renal artery stenosis. Br J Hosp Med 1993;49(6): 388–395,398.

107. Caps MT, et al. Prospective study of atherosclerotic disease progression in the renal artery. Circulation 1998;98(25):2866–2872.

107a. Radermacher J, Chavan A, Bleck J, et al. Use of Doppler ultrasonography to predict the outcome of therapy for renal-artery stenosis. N Engl J Med 2001:344(6):410–417.

108. La Batide-Alanore A, et al. Split renal function outcome after renal angioplasty in patients with unilateral renal artery stenosis. J Am Soc Nephrol 2001;12(6):1235–1241.

109. van Jaarsveld BC, et al. The effect of balloon angioplasty on hypertension in atherosclerotic renal-artery stenosis. Dutch Renal Artery Stenosis Intervention Cooperative Study Group. N Engl J Med 2000;342(14):1007–1014.

110. Webster J, et al. Randomised comparison of percutaneous angioplasty vs continued medical therapy for hypertensive patients with atheromatous renal artery stenosis. Scottish and Newcastle Renal Artery Stenosis Collaborative Group. J Hum Hypertens 1998;12(5):329–335.

111. Plouin PF, et al. Blood pressure outcome of angioplasty in atherosclerotic renal artery stenosis: a randomized trial. Essai Multicentrique Medicaments vs Angioplastie (EMMA) Study Group. Hypertension 1998;31(3):823–829.

112. Blum U, et al. Treatment of ostial renal-artery stenoses with vascular endoprostheses after unsuccessful balloon angioplasty. N Engl J Med 1997;336(7):459–465.

113. Dorros G, et al. Multicenter Palmaz stent renal artery stenosis revascularization registry report: four-year follow-up of 1,058 successful patients. Catheter Cardiovasc Interv 2002;55(2):182–188.

114. Himmelmann A, et al. Predictors of stroke in the elderly. Acta Med Scand 1988;224(5):439–443.

115. Megherbi SE, et al. Association between diabetes and stroke subtype on survival and functional outcome 3 months after stroke: data from the European BIOMED Stroke Project. Stroke 2003;34(3): 688–694.

116. Hobson RW 2nd, et al. Efficacy of carotid endarterectomy for asymptomatic carotid stenosis. The Veterans Affairs Cooperative Study Group. N Engl J Med 1993;328(4):221–227.

117. Beneficial effect of carotid endarterectomy in symptomatic patients with high-grade carotid stenosis. North American Symptomatic Carotid Endarterectomy Trial Collaborators. N Engl J Med 1991;325(7): 445–453.

117a. Yadav J. Stenting and angioplasty with protection in patients at high risk for enderterectomy (the SAPPHIRE study). Presented at the American Heart Association November 19, 2002, Chicago, IL.

117b. Wholey MH. The ARCHeR trial: prospective clinical trial for carotid stenting in high surgical risk patients, preliminary thirty-day results. Presented at the American College of Cardiology Meeting, March 30, 2003, Chicago, IL.

118. Endovascular versus surgical treatment in patients with carotid stenosis in the Carotid and Vertebral Artery Transluminal Angioplasty Study (CAVATAS): a randomised trial. Lancet 2001;357(9270): 1729–1737.

26 Cardiac Surgery and Diabetes Mellitus

Tanveer A. Khan, MD, Pierre Voisine, MD, and Frank W. Sellke, MD

CONTENTS

INTRODUCTION

Diabetes mellitus (DM) is an established risk factor for the development and progression of cardiovascular disease (CVD). The prevalence of coronary artery disease (CAD) has been estimated as high as 55% in the diabetic population. It has been shown that diabetes is a major independent risk factor for CVD after adjustment for risk factors such as age, hypertension, hypercholesterolemia, and tobacco abuse *(1)*. Patients with diabetes appear to develop more severe CAD with a greater tendancy toward adverse events. The relative risk of myocardial infarction (MI) is 50% greater in diabetic men and 150% greater in diabetic women *(2)*. Approximately 20% of patients who have undergone coronary artery bypass grafting (CABG) have DM *(3)*. Thus, diabetic patients undergoing surgical coronary revascularization represent a large and complex patient population. In the past decade, advancements in both percutaneous coronary intervention (PCI), primarily the use of stents, and surgical techniques, such as off-pump CABG and the use of arterial grafts, have continued to improve methods of coronary revascularization. Although there is evidence to suggest these new techniques have improved outcomes in diabetic patients, the optimal treatment for multivessel CAD continues to evolve for the diabetic patient population, which despite improvements in revascularization still suffers from significantly worse outcomes when compared to the general population.

From: *Contemporary Cardiology: Diabetes and Cardiovascular Disease, Second Edition*
Edited by: M. T. Johnstone and A. Veves © Humana Press Inc., Totowa, NJ

Table 1

Risks Associated With Diabetes Mellitus and Cardiac Surgery

Increased morbidity
    Stroke
    Low cardiac output syndrome
    Renal failure
    Wound infection
Increased mortality

OPERATIVE RISKS OF CARDIAC SURGERY IN DIABETIC PATIENTS

Operative Morbidity and Mortality

In diabetic patients, CAD is more prevalent compared with nondiabetic patients, but also is more extensive, involves multiple vessels, and rapidly progressive. Such patients with diabetes represent a significant proportion of the patient population requiring myocardial revascularization, and a surgical challenge as a result of the diffuse nature of their coronary disease. In this diabetic population with more severe CAD, CABG is associated with increased rates of perioperative complications and mortality as compared with nondiabetic patients (Table 1). Diabetes has been well established as an independent risk factor for increased early and late mortality in patients treated with CABG (4–6). A review of 9920 patients with diabetes and 2278 patients without diabetes from a single center over 15 years revealed lower survival rates in diabetics vs nondiabetics at 5-year (78% vs 88%) and 10-year (50% vs 71%) of follow-up (6). In addition to decreased survival, patients with diabetes have been shown to have increased rates of sternal wound infection (7–9). Diabetes appears to increase the risk of both superficial sternal wound infections and mediastinitis (10) and saphenous vein harvest-site infections (11). Diabetes also has been associated with increased rates of neurological and renal complications and prolonged, postoperative intensive care unit stays (12). Stroke has an incidence of approx 2% to 5% during heart operations, with diabetes reported as an independent predictor of stroke in several studies (13–15). The relative risk of renal dysfunction in diabetic patients is fivefold compared with nondiabetics during cardiac surgery (12). Diabetes increases the risk of stroke and renal failure with CABG and valve surgery (16,17). Postoperative myocardial dysfunction appears to be exacerbated by diabetes as it is an independent predictor of postoperative low cardiac output syndrome (18). Finally, once patients with diabetes have been discharged from the hospital, evidence suggests that this group of patients is at high-risk for re-admission (19). Thus, diabetics present a challenging patient population for cardiac surgeons. In these patients, severe, multivessel coronary disease often necessitates surgical revascularization, which in this diabetic population is associated with increased morbidity and mortality.

CORONARY ARTERY BYPASS GRAFTING IN DIABETIC PATIENTS

Coronary Artery Bypass Grafting vs Percutaneous Transluminal Coronary Angioplasty

Several large, published clinical studies have demonstrated that patients with diabetes suffering from multivessel CAD have an increased survival benefit when treated with surgically with CABG as compared to percutaneous transluminal coronary angioplasty

(PTCA). The Bypass Angioplasty Revascularization Investigation (BARI) study was initiated by the National Heart, Lung, and Blood Institute in 1987 to test the hypothesis that in patients with multivessel CAD, initial revascularization by PTCA does not result in a poorer outcome than CABG during a follow-up period of 5 months. The study was a multicenter, randomized trial that assigned patients with multivessel CAD to an initial treatment strategy of either CABG ($n = 914$) or PTCA ($n = 915$). Average follow-up was 5.4 years. The 5-year survival rate was 89.3% for patients assigned to CABG and 86.3% for those assigned to PTCA. Five-year survival rates free from Q-wave MI were 80.4% for CABG and 78.7% for PTCA. By 5 years of follow-up, 8% of the patients assigned to CABG had undergone additional revascularization procedures, although 54% of patients assigned to PTCA required further revascularization. Among diabetic patients treated with either oral hypoglycemic agents or insulin, 5-year survival was greater in the CABG group at 80.6% compared to 65.5% in the PTCA group *(20)*.

Several follow-up studies to the BARI trial provided more information. A study that examined the finding of increased survival in diabetic patients who had CABG vs PTCA determined that the improved survival was as a result of reduced cardiac mortality. Furthermore, the reduced cardiac mortality was confined to those who received at least one internal mammary artery (IMA) graft, suggesting that long-term patency of the IMA graft contributed to the reduction in cardiac mortality *(21)*. In another follow-up study of MI after CABG or PTCA, diabetic patients that had undergone CABG had a greatly reduced risk of death from Q-wave MI compared to those who were treated with PTCA. Patients with diabetes were 10 times more likely to die of their MI if treated with PTCA as compared to CABG *(22)*. A study of 7-year outcome found that diabetic patients in the CABG group had an even greater survival advantage over those in the PTCA group *(23)*. Overall, CABG was shown to be the treatment of choice for diabetic patients with multivessel CAD based on these results that showed improved long-term survival when compared to PTCA.

Coronary Artery Bypass Grafting vs Percutaneous Coronary Intervention

Since the BARI study compared CABG with PTCA and demonstrated a survival advantage for diabetic patients treated surgically, the use of stents and glycoprotein IIb/IIIa inhibitors have become central to the treatment of coronary disease by PCI with demonstrated clinical benefits over PTCA *(24)*. Furthermore, the more common use of arterial conduits for CABG has improved surgical outcomes as well. The Arterial Revascularization Therapies Study (ARTS) randomly assigned 1205 patients with multivessel CAD to either stent placement or CABG. The primary clinical end points were freedom from cardiac or cerebrovascular events at 1 year. There was no significant difference between groups in terms of rates of death, stroke, or MI. However, 16.8% of patients in the stent group required a second revascularization compared to only 3.5% in the surgery group *(25)*. A study of the outcomes of diabetic patients in the ARTS trial showed that diabetics treated with stenting had a 1-year event-free survival of 63.4% compared with nondiabetics at 76.2%. In contrast, patients with diabetes and without diabetes treated by CABG had similar 1-year event-free survival at 84.8% and 88.4%, thus revealing significantly greater event-free survival when compared to the stenting group. Thus, event-free survival of diabetic patients was lower in the stenting group at 1 year compared to the CABG group as a result of a higher incidence of repeat revascularization in the stenting group *(26)*. A follow-up study examined the 2-year outcomes of the patients enrolled in the ARTS trial. Again, at 2 years, freedom from death, stroke, and MI was equivalent in the stent and CABG groups. Similarly, event-free survival was greater in the CABG group (84.8%) than in the stent group (69.5%). In diabetic subgroup, the difference was more pronounced with event-free survival of 82.3% in the surgery group and 56.3% in the stent group. The follow-up study concluded that the greater need for revascularization in the stent group seen at 1 year remained essentially unchanged at 2 years, particularly in the diabetic group, suggesting that surgery is the preferable form of treatment for these patients (27).

Although a number of studies have provided evidence that diabetic patients have better outcomes with surgery than PCI primarily from decreased need for revascularization, the Angina With Extremely Serious Operative Mortality Evaluation trial focused on the benefit of PCI vs CABG in diabetic patients medically refractory myocardial ischemia and high-risk for surgery, defined as those with previous CABG, MI within 7 days, left ventricular ejection fraction less than 35%, age greater than 70 years, or intraortic ballon pump requirement for stabilization. This prospective, randomized trial showed that for patients randomized to CABG or PCI, 36-month survival rates were similar at 85% and 89%, respectively. Although there was no survival advantage to CABG, diabetic patients treated surgically has less recurrent angina and a decreased need for revascularization (28). Thus, CABG appears to provide for decreased recurrent angina and a lower rate of revascularization as compared to PCI in patients with diabetes.

Surgical Outcomes in Diabetic Patients

Another follow-up study of the BARI trial examined the group of patients who underwent CABG and evaluated CABG patency in patients with and without treated DM. The results of this study showed that diabetic patients were more likely to have grafts to small (<1.5 mm) distal vessels and coronary arteries of poor distal quality. Angiographic evaluation at a mean follow-up of 3.9 years showed that graft patency was equivalent for diabetic and nondiabetic patients for both IMA grafts (89% vs 85%, respectively; $p = 0.23$) and vein grafts (71% and 75%, respectively, $p = 0.40$). The authors concluded that despite having smaller distal target vessels of poorer quality, patients with treated DM do not have adverse effects on graft patency at an average of nearly 4 years follow-up and therefore graft patency does not explain differences in survival that as been observed in diabetic and nondiabetic patients following CABG (29). Although the findings of this study are important, a difference in mortality rate between the diabetic and nondiabetic populations may have introduced a bias that would affect the patients that were studied by angiography, that is those that survived for follow-up.

SURGICAL TREATMENT OPTIONS IN DIABETIC PATIENTS

CABG

The effect of CABG without cardiopulmonary bypass generally has been favorable in terms of morbidity and mortality, although some conflicting data has been reported (30–33). Although it is unclear whether patients with diabetes benefit from survival advantage with off-pump CABG, diabetics appear to have fewer postoperative complications including lower rates of atrial fibrillation, renal failure, and respiratory failure (34). Another technique that has been suggested to improve outcome of CABG is the use of arterial bypass grafts (35). In diabetics, the use of arterial grafts has been suggested to improve outcomes of survival *(3)*. CABG with at least one IMA graft should be standard practice in diabetic patients. Bilateral IMA grafts appear to be safe in patients with diabetes and may have a survival advantage *(36,37)*. Finally, diabetes has been shown to be a risk factor for wound infection of the saphenous vein graft harvest site. The newer technique of endoscopic vein harvesting has been suggested to decrease wound infections of the lower extremity after vein harvest in high-risk patients such as those with diabetes *(11)*. In our institution, endoscopic saphenous vein harvest had become the procedure of choice for elective CABG, particularly in diabetic patients.

Postoperative Care

Hyperglycemia has been associated with adverse outcomes in patients with CVD. In patients with MI, glucose values in excess of 110 to 144 mg/dL were associated with a threefold increase in mortality and a greater risk of heart failure *(38)*. Diabetic patients with ischemic stroke have a threefold increase in mortality with glucose levels above 108 to 144 mg/dL *(39)*. An aggressive approach to the treatment of hyperglycemia with continuous insulin infusion therapy has been shown to reduce morbidity and mortality in critically ill patients. A study of intensive care patients treated with intensive insulin therapy to maintain blood glucose at or below 110 mg/dL demonstrated a reduced mortality of 8% compared to 4.6% with conventional therapy that treated glucose levels above 215 mg/dL by insulin infusion. Among these patients in the study, more than 60% had undergone cardiac surgery *(40)*. Continuous insulin infusion therapy also has been shown to reduce deep sternal wound infection in cardiac surgical patients with diabetes *(41)*. In our institution, a larger portion of our patient population is diabetic at nearly 50% of patients that undergo cardiac surgery. We currently use a fairly aggressive approach to that management of hyperglycemia that starts continuous insulin infusion therapy for blood glucose levels above 150 mg/dL. Since initiating this protocol, our deep sternal wound infection rate has decreased from approx 1.8% to 0.8% in recent months. Overall, hyperglycemia has been demonstrated to increase the risk of adverse outcomes in critically ill patients with CVD, and evidence suggests that the early use of continuous insulin infusions in the treatment of hyperglycemia improves the morbidity and mortality associated with elevated blood glucose levels after cardiac surgery.

FUTURE DIRECTIONS

Early Coronary Revascularization in Diabetes

As a follow-up to the BARI trial, the BARI 2D trial seeks to improve our understanding of why the favorable decline in cardiovascular mortality over the past two decades has not been seen in the diabetic population. The prospective clinical trial presents two important questions: (a) will treatment targeted to reduce insulin resistance favorably alter the course of CAD compared to therapy that augments endogenous insulin resistance, regardless of coronary revascularization, and (b) does early coronary intervention improve the clinical course of patients without severe symptoms or signs of CAD refractory to medical management? A key aspect of the trial will be that PCI in the BARI 2D trial will include traditional and coated stents and glycoprotein IIb/IIIa inhibitors, none of which were evaluated in the BARI trial *(42)*. Thus, this follow-up trial may determine whether early CABG offers a survival advantage to diabetic patients compared to PCI with its contemporary armamentarium.

Molecular Mechanisms in Diabetes During Cardiac Surgery

ENDOTHELIN-1 AND OXIDATIVE STRESS

A multitude of molecular mechanisms likely contribute to the clinical manifestations of diabetes in cardiac surgery. Recently, there has been evidence to suggest that endothelin-1 (ET-1) and nitric oxide (NO) play important roles in the pathophysiology of diabetics undergoing cardiac surgery. The response of the myocardium in diabetics to cardiac surgery and the associated reperfusion injury is characterized by alterations in neutrophil adhesion, endothelial function, myocyte contractility, and oxidative stress. ET-1 is a potent, endogenous vasoconstrictor that has been associated with endothelial dysfunction and vasospasm. In a study of 25 patients (13 diabetic and 12 nondiabetic) who underwent cardiopulmonary bypass with cardioplegic arrest, levels of ET-1 in the coronary sinus effluent of diabetic patients was greater than that from nondiabetics. Furthermore, coronary microvessels from the diabetic patients showed increased vasocontriction to ET-1 and diminished NO-mediated vasodilation. These responses were blocked by endothelin antagonism *(43)*. These results suggest that ET-1 may contribute to reperfusion injury in diabetic patients as seen in dysfunction of the coronary microcirculation, which is a major determinant of myocardial perfusion. Furthermore, there has been evidence to suggest that endothelin receptors mediate reperfusion injury of cardiomyocytes under conditions of hyperglycemia *(44)*.

Oxidative stress has been shown to play a significant role in the response to cardiopulmonary bypass and reperfusion injury. In a study of patients with diabetes ($n = 20$) and without diabetes ($n = 20$) who underwent cardiac surgery, the response to cardiopulmonary bypass and cardioplegic arrest was measured in terms of oxidative stress. Cardiopulmonary bypass with cardioplegic arrest induced a greater oxidative stress in patients with diabetes compared with nondiabetics as measured by plasma lipid hydroperoxides and protein carbonyls. These results suggest that oxidative stress in response to cardiac surgery is increased in diabetic patients *(45)*. Considering that oxidative stress is associated with reperfusion injury, alterations in the coronary microcirculation, and myocardial contractile dysfunction, further investigation of the role of increased oxidative stress in the pathophysiological responses of diabetics to cardiac surgery may be warranted. Decreased oxidative stress in off-pump CABG compared to CABG with cardiopulmonary bypass may represent a mechanism by which diabetics benefit from the off-pump technique *(46)*.

GENE EXPRESSION PROFILES OF DIABETIC PATIENTS AFTER CARDIAC SURGERY WITH CARDIOPULMONARY BYPASS AND CARDIOPLEGIA

As diabetes is an independent risk factor for postoperative complications and mortality after CABG, we sought to examine and compare myocardial gene expression responses to cardiopulmonary bypass and cardioplegic arrest in patients with and without diabetes by the use of cDNA array analysis. Ten atrial myocardial samples were harvested from five insulin-treated diabetic and five matched nondiabetic patients undergoing CABG, before and after cardiopulmonary bypass and cardioplegia.

Each gene whose expression was uniformly modified by a median ratio of fourfold or greater magnitude was the object of a literature search and reported, along with its GenBank number, according to the current nomenclature of Online Mendelian Inheritance in Man. Of 12,625 genes examined, 851 were upregulated in the diabetic group and 480 in the control group ($p < 0.001$). Less genes were downregulated in diabetic (443)

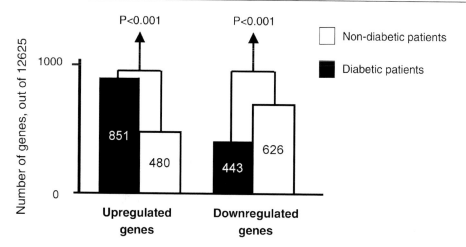

Fig. 1. Differential gene expression after cardiopulmonary bypass and cardioplegic arrest in myocardial tissue of diabetic and nondiabetic patients.

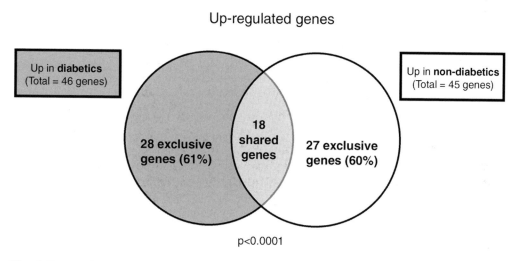

Fig. 2. Expression profile for fourfold (or greater) up-regulated genes in diabetic vs nondiabetic patients after cardiopulmonary bypass and cardioplegic arrest.

compared with nondiabetic (626) patients ($p < 0.001$; Fig. 1). Thirty-nine genes showed greater than fourfold upregulation in the diabetic group, as did 35 genes in the nondiabetic group. Of these, 17 were upregulated in both groups, whereas 22 and 18 were respectively upregulated exclusively in the diabetic and nondiabetic patients, respectively, a highly significant different expression profile (Fig. 2 and Table 2). We concluded that the gene expression profile after cardiopulmonary bypass and cardioplegic arrest is quantitatively and qualitatively different in patients with diabetes. These results have important implications for the design of tailored myocardial protection and operative strategies for diabetic patients undergoing cardiac surgery.

Table 2

Select Genes Exhibiting an Increase in Expression in Myocardial Samples From Diabetic Patients After Cardiopulmonary Bypass and Cardioplegic Arrest

Gene name	Symbol	Fold increase	Function
Amphiregulin	AREG	16:1	Autocrine growth factor
Interleukin (IL)-1β	IL-1B	9:1	Inflammatory cytokine
Nuclear receptor subfamily 4, group A, member 3	NR4A3	8:1	Transcription factor
Regulator of G protein signaling 1	RGS1	8:1	Immediate-early response gene
Activating transcription factor 3	ATF3	8:1	Transcription factor
Insulin receptor substrate 1	IRS1	7:1	Substrate of the insulin receptor tyrosine kinase
V-maf musculoaponeurotic fibrosarcoma oncogene	MAFF	7:1	Transcription regulator
Ras homolog gene family, Member B (Rho B)	ARHB	6:1	Growth factor-responsive early gene
Complement component 1, q Subcom, R1	C1QR1	6:1	Regulation of phagocytic activity
Nuclear antigen SP100	SP100	6:1	Role in autoimmunity, infections, tumorigenesis
Chemokine (CC motif) ligand4	CCL4	6:1	Chemotactic factor for monocytes
Interleukin 8	IL8	5:1	Mediates neutrophils chemotaxis and migration
Interleukin 1 receptor	IL1RN	5:1	Inhibits Interleukin 1-alpha and –beta antagonist
Oncogene MYC	MYC	5:1	Transcription factor
Vascular Endothelial Growth Factor	VEGF	5:1	Growth factor, mitogen primarily for vascular endothelial cells
Chemokine (C-X-C motif), ligand 3	CXCL3	5:1	Chemotactic factor for monocytes

CONCLUSIONS

DM is a well-established risk factor for increased morbidity and mortality associated with cardiac surgery. Patients with diabetes have been shown to have worse outcomes than nondiabetics from both surgical and percutaneous catheter-based techniques of revascularization. Clinical trials have demonstrated increased event-free survival for diabetic patients treated surgically, likely in part as a result of the completeness of revascularization considering that freedom from repeat revascularization procedures has been the most consistent benefit shown from CABG when compared to current PCI including stenting. The best method of selection of revascularization should be based on the severity and extent of coronary disease and the potential for complete revascularization. Currently, surgical revascularization rather than PCI for diabetic patients with multivessel CAD is appropriate, particularly for those patients with extensive coronary disease and myocardial dysfunction. However, this treatment recommendation may change in the future as improving technologies and therapies such as coated stents, antiplatelet agents, and insulin-providing agents as opposed to insulin-sensitizing agents may alter the course of coronary disease and restenosis. Surgical treatment options that potentially decrease morbidity associated with diabetes include off-pump CABG, arterial grafting, endoscopic saphenous vein harvest, and aggressive management of hyperglycemia with continuous insulin infusions. A research technique that may provide important information on the molecular mechanisms, specifically gene expression profile, involved in the diabetic response to cardiac surgery is cDNA microarray analysis. We found significant differences in the gene expression response to cardiopulmonary bypass with cardioplegic arrest between diabetic and nondiabetic patients. These results will enable further investigation of identified molecular pathways by this technique that may contribute to the pathophysiology of diabetes related to cardiac surgery.

REFERENCES

1. Kannel WB,McGee DL. Diabetes and cardiovascular risk factors: the Framingham study. Circulation 1979;59:8–13.
2. Waller BF, Palumbo PJ, Lie JT, Roberts WC. Status of the coronary arteries at necropsy in diabetes mellitus with onset after age 30 years. Analysis of 229 diabetic patients with and without clinical evidence of coronary heart disease and comparison to 183 control subjects. Am J Med 1980;69:498–506.
3. Morris JJ, Smith LR, Jones RH, et al. Influence of diabetes and mammary artery grafting on survival after coronary bypass. Circulation 1991;84:III275–III284.
4. Smith LR, Harrell FE Jr, Rankin JS, et al. Determinants of early versus late cardiac death in patients undergoing coronary artery bypass graft surgery. Circulation 1991;84:III245–II253.
5. Calafiore AM, Di Mauro M, Di Giammarco G, et al. Effect of diabetes on early and late survival after isolated first coronary bypass surgery in multivessel disease. J Thorac Cardiovasc Surg 2003;125:144–54.
6. Thourani VH, Weintraub WS, Stein B, et al. Influence of diabetes mellitus on early and late outcome after coronary artery bypass grafting. Ann Thorac Surg 1999;67:1045–1052.
7. Fietsam R Jr, Bassett J, Glover JL. Complications of coronary artery surgery in diabetic patients. Am Surg 1991;57:551–557.
8. Carson JL, Scholz PM, Chen AY, Peterson ED, Gold J, Schneider SH. Diabetes mellitus increases short-term mortality and morbidity in patients undergoing coronary artery bypass graft surgery. J Am Coll Cardiol 2002;40:418–423.
9. Szabo Z, Hakanson E,Svedjeholm R. Early postoperative outcome and medium-term survival in 540 diabetic and 2239 nondiabetic patients undergoing coronary artery bypass grafting. Ann Thorac Surg 2002;74:712–719.
10. Zacharias A, Habib RH. Factors predisposing to median sternotomy complications. Deep vs superficial infection. Chest 1996;110:1173–1178.

11. Carpino PA, Khabbaz KR, Bojar RM, et al. Clinical benefits of endoscopic vein harvesting in patients with risk factors for saphenectomy wound infections undergoing coronary artery bypass grafting. J Thorac Cardiovasc Surg 2000;119:69–75.

12. Morricone L, Ranucci M, Denti S, et al. Diabetes and complications after cardiac surgery: comparison with a non-diabetic population. Acta Diabetol 1999;36:77–84.

13. Bucerius J, Gummert JF, Borger MA, et al. Stroke after cardiac surgery: a risk factor analysis of 16,184 consecutive adult patients. Ann Thorac Surg 2003;75:472–478.

14. Hogue CW Jr, Murphy SF, Schechtman KB, Davila-Roman VG. Risk factors for early or delayed stroke after cardiac surgery. Circulation 1999;100:642–647.

15. Newman MF, Wolman R, Kanchuger M, et al. Multicenter preoperative stroke risk index for patients undergoing coronary artery bypass graft surgery. Multicenter Study of Perioperative Ischemia (McSPI) Research Group. Circulation 1996;94:II74–II80.

16. Grayson AD, Khater M, Jackson M, Fox MA. Valvular heart operation is an independent risk factor for acute renal failure. Ann Thorac Surg 2003;75:1829–1835.

17. Sharony R, Grossi EA, Saunders PC, et al. Aortic valve replacement in patients with impaired ventricular function. Ann Thorac Surg 2003;75:1808–1814.

18. Rao V, Ivanov J, Weisel RD, Ikonomidis JS, Christakis GT, David TE. Predictors of low cardiac output syndrome after coronary artery bypass. J Thorac Cardiovasc Surg 1996;112:38–51.

19. Ferraris VA, Ferraris SP, Harmon RC, Evans BD. Risk factors for early hospital readmission after cardiac operations. J Thorac Cardiovasc Surg 2001;122:278–286.

20. Comparison of coronary bypass surgery with angioplasty in patients with multivessel disease. The Bypass Angioplasty Revascularization Investigation (BARI) Investigators. N Engl J Med 1996;335:217–225.

21. Influence of diabetes on 5-year mortality and morbidity in a randomized trial comparing CABG and PTCA in patients with multivessel disease: the Bypass Angioplasty Revascularization Investigation (BARI). Circulation 1997;96:1761–1769.

22. Detre KM, Lombardero MS, Brooks MM, et al. The effect of previous coronary-artery bypass surgery on the prognosis of patients with diabetes who have acute myocardial infarction. Bypass Angioplasty Revascularization Investigation Investigators. N Engl J Med 2000;342:989–997.

23. Seven-year outcome in the Bypass Angioplasty Revascularization Investigation (BARI) by treatment and diabetic status. J Am Coll Cardiol 2000;35:1122–1129.

24. Srinivas VS, Brooks MM, Detre KM, et al. Contemporary percutaneous coronary intervention versus balloon angioplasty for multivessel coronary artery disease: a comparison of the National Heart, Lung and Blood Institute Dynamic Registry and the Bypass Angioplasty Revascularization Investigation (BARI) study. Circulation 2002;106:1627–1633.

25. Serruys PW, Unger F, Sousa JE, et al. Comparison of coronary-artery bypass surgery and stenting for the treatment of multivessel disease. N Engl J Med 2001;344:1117–1124.

26. Abizaid A, Costa MA, Centemero M, et al. Clinical and economic impact of diabetes mellitus on percutaneous and surgical treatment of multivessel coronary disease patients: insights from the Arterial Revascularization Therapy Study (ARTS) trial. Circulation 2001;104:533–538.

27. Unger F, Serruys PW, Yacoub MH, et al. Revascularization in multivessel disease: comparison between two-year outcomes of coronary bypass surgery and stenting. J Thorac Cardiovasc Surg 2003;125:809–820.

28. Sedlis SP, Morrison DA, Lorin JD, et al. Percutaneous coronary intervention versus coronary bypass graft surgery for diabetic patients with unstable angina and risk factors for adverse outcomes with bypass: outcome of diabetic patients in the AWESOME randomized trial and registry. J Am Coll Cardiol 2002;40:1555–1566.

29. Schwartz L, Kip KE, Frye RL, Alderman EL, Schaff HV, Detre KM. Coronary bypass graft patency in patients with diabetes in the Bypass Angioplasty Revascularization Investigation (BARI). Circulation 2002;106:2652–2658.

30. Arom KV, Flavin TF, Emery RW, Kshettry VR, Janey PA, Petersen RJ. Safety and efficacy of off-pump coronary artery bypass grafting. Ann Thorac Surg 2000;69:704–710.

31. Taggart DP. Respiratory dysfunction after cardiac surgery: effects of avoiding cardiopulmonary bypass and the use of bilateral internal mammary arteries. Eur J Cardiothorac Surg 2000;18:31–37.

32. Taggart DP, Browne SM, Halligan PW, Wade DT. Is cardiopulmonary bypass still the cause of cognitive dysfunction after cardiac operations? J Thorac Cardiovasc Surg 1999;118:414–420; discussion 420–421.

33. Buffolo E, de Andrade CS, Branco JN, Teles CA, Aguiar LF, Gomes WJ. Coronary artery bypass grafting without cardiopulmonary bypass. Ann Thorac Surg 1996;61:63–66.

34. Magee MJ, Dewey TM, Acuff T, et al. Influence of diabetes on mortality and morbidity: off-pump coronary artery bypass grafting versus coronary artery bypass grafting with cardiopulmonary bypass. Ann Thorac Surg 2001;72:776–780; discussion 780–781.

35. Farinas JM, Carrier M, Hebert Y, et al. Comparison of long-term clinical results of double versus single internal mammary artery bypass grafting. Ann Thorac Surg 1999;67:466–470.

36. Endo M, Tomizawa Y, Nishida H. Bilateral versus unilateral internal mammary revascularization in patients with diabetes. Circulation 2003;108:1343–1349.

37. Taggart DP, D'Amico R, Altman DG. Effect of arterial revascularisation on survival: a systematic review of studies comparing bilateral and single internal mammary arteries. Lancet 2001;358:870–875.

38. Capes SE, Hunt D, Malmberg K, Gerstein HC. Stress hyperglycaemia and increased risk of death after myocardial infarction in patients with and without diabetes: a systematic overview. Lancet 2000;355:773–778.

39. Capes SE, Hunt D, Malmberg K, Pathak P, Gerstein HC. Stress hyperglycemia and prognosis of stroke in nondiabetic and diabetic patients: a systematic overview. Stroke 2001;32:2426–2432.

40. van den Berghe G, Wouters P, Weekers F, et al. Intensive insulin therapy in the critically ill patients. N Engl J Med 2001;345:1359–1367.

41. Furnary AP, Zerr KJ, Grunkemeier GL, Starr A. Continuous intravenous insulin infusion reduces the incidence of deep sternal wound infection in diabetic patients after cardiac surgical procedures. Ann Thorac Surg 1999;67:352–360; discussion 360–362.

42. Sobel BE, Frye R, Detre KM. Burgeoning dilemmas in the management of diabetes and cardiovascular disease: rationale for the Bypass Angioplasty Revascularization Investigation 2 Diabetes (BARI 2D) Trial. Circulation 2003;107:636–642.

43. Verma S, Maitland A, Weisel RD, et al. Increased endothelin-1 production in diabetic patients after cardioplegic arrest and reperfusion impairs coronary vascular reactivity: reversal by means of endothelin antagonism. J Thorac Cardiovasc Surg 2002;123:1114–1119.

44. Verma S, Maitland A, Weisel RD, et al. Hyperglycemia exaggerates ischemia-reperfusion-induced cardiomyocyte injury: reversal with endothelin antagonism. J Thorac Cardiovasc Surg 2002;123:1120–1124.

45. Matata BM, Galinanes M. Cardiopulmonary bypass exacerbates oxidative stress but does not increase proinflammatory cytokine release in patients with diabetes compared with patients without diabetes: regulatory effects of exogenous nitric oxide. J Thorac Cardiovasc Surg 2000;120:1–11.

46. Matata BM, Sosnowski AW, Galinanes M. Off-pump bypass graft operation significantly reduces oxidative stress and inflammation. Ann Thorac Surg 2000;69:785–791.

27 Heart Failure and Cardiac Dysfunction in Diabetes

Lawrence H. Young, MD,
Raymond R. Russell, III, MD, PhD,
and Deborah Chyun, RN, PhD

CLINICAL EPIDEMIOLOGY

Heart failure is a well-recognized clinical problem in patients with diabetes. The Framingham Heart Study demonstrated that patients with diabetes have an increased incidence of heart failure, which contributes significantly to their high cardiovascular morbidity and mortality *(1,2)*. The age-adjusted risk of developing heart failure was 2.4 times higher in diabetic than in nondiabetic men. In women, the impact of diabetes was even more striking, with the risk of heart failure being 5.1 times greater in the presence of diabetes. The incidence of heart failure in older patients was substantial: 22–27 per

From: *Contemporary Cardiology: Diabetes and Cardiovascular Disease, Second Edition*
Edited by: M. T. Johnstone and A. Veves © Humana Press Inc., Totowa, NJ

1000 patient years over 18 years. Although Framingham and many other studies did not distinguish between patients with type 1 and type 2 diabetes, the majority of their patients had type 2 diabetes. However, in the era before treatment with combined oral hypoglycemic agents, many patients with type 2 diabetes were treated with insulin and such patients had a four- to fivefold increased risk of heart failure compared to nondiabetic patients.

Despite more contemporary therapy, heart failure still remains a common problem in patients with diabetes. In the Kaiser Permanent study, middle-aged individuals with type 2 diabetes had an 11.8% prevalence of heart failure as compared to 4.5% in those without diabetes *(3)*. In elderly Medicare patients with diabetes, 22% had a diagnosis of heart failure and the prevalence increased with age *(4)*. Additionally, new diagnoses of heart failure were two- to threefold more common in Medicare patients with diabetes. Similarly, in a prospective study of very elderly patients in a long-term health care facility, heart failure developed in 39% of those with diabetes and 23% of those without diabetes over 43 months *(5)*. Thus, heart failure remains extremely common in patients with diabetes and this risk is highest in the very elderly.

What accounts for the increase in heart failure in patients with diabetes? In many cases the presence of coronary artery disease (CAD) or hypertension plays an important role because type 2 diabetes is often associated with hypertension, CAD, and obesity *(6)*. The co-existence of hypertension, obesity, glucose intolerance, dyslipidemia, and insulin resistance is now widely recognized and has been codified as the metabolic syndrome *(7,8)*. In many epidemiological studies, it is difficult to discern whether diabetes truly increases the risk of heart failure in such patients independent of these other factors. For instance, in the Framingham study, the diabetes-associated risk of heart failure persisted after adjustment for age, hypertension, hypercholesterolemia, and obesity, and clinically evident CAD *(2)*. However, many of these patients had CAD, hypertension, or rheumatic heart disease, although other patients likely had unrecognized CAD, which is extremely common in type 2 diabetes even in the absence of angina or ischemic electrocardiographic findings *(9)*. Although the prevalence of CAD was similar in heart failure patients with and without diabetes, the extent of CAD was not specifically evaluated and more extensive CAD in diabetic patients may well have contributed to their higher incidence of heart failure. Nonetheless, the high risk for heart failure has been consistently observed in diabetes. Follow-up analysis of Framingham patients and their offspring also indicated that diabetes is an independent and important predictor of heart failure, along with hypertension, left ventricular hypertrophy (LVH), and CAD *(10)*. These results are also supported by recent cohort studies that have also implicated diabetes as an important risk for heart failure *(11,12)*, although CAD was excluded simply on the basis of clinical history or discharge diagnosis.

A number of clinical factors have been associated with heart failure in patients with diabetes. In the Kaiser Permanent report, existing heart failure was associated with older age, female sex, longer diabetes duration, insulin use, higher serum creatinine, and the presence of CAD or hypertension *(3)*. The new development of heart failure was associated with older age, longer diabetes duration, insulin or oral agent use, CAD at baseline, and the development of new ischemic heart disease *(3)*. In the Medicare population, older age, lower socioeconomic status, CAD and the presence of diabetes-related co-morbidities, particularly nephropathy, were associated with both prevalent and incident heart failure *(4)*. In more general populations such as the First National Health and Nutrition

Examination Survey study, in addition to diabetes, development of heart failure was associated with male sex, lower level of education, low physical activity, cigarette smoking, overweight, hypertension, valvular heart disease, and CAD *(13)*. Thus, not unexpectedly, heart failure is most common in older patients with CAD, hypertension, or other diabetes-related co-morbidity.

Heart failure is frequently encountered in patients with diabetes in many areas of clinical practice, including the primary-care setting, diabetes clinic, and cardiology care units. Additonally, as many as 15% to 30% of patients enrolled in randomized heart failure clinical trials have diabetes *(14,15)*, much greater than the 5% to 8% of the population with diabetes. With the prevalence of heart failure in the United States estimated to be 5 million people, more than 1 million diabetic patients have heart failure. Indeed, this is a conservative estimate given the growing number of patients with type 2 diabetes *(16,17)*, and is likely a result of aging, increasing obesity and the more inclusive criteria for the diagnosis of diabetes *(18)*.

CORONARY ARTERY DISEASE, DIABETES, AND HEART FAILURE

Just as CAD is the most common cause of heart failure in the overall US population *(10)*, underlying CAD is often the reason for the development of symptomatic heart failure in patients with diabetes *(2)*. Myocardial ischemia may cause heart failure through impairment in either systolic or diastolic left ventricular function. In some cases, previous myocardial infarction (MI) leads to adverse remodeling, progressive left ventricular systolic dysfunction, and symptomatic heart failure *(19)*. In other patients with diabetes, diffuse CAD causes patchy necrosis and fibrosis, even in the absence of clinically recognized MI, leading to progressive deterioration in ventricular systolic function. Coronary hypoperfusion may also lead to stunned or hibernating myocardium with significant left ventricular dysfunction in patients with diabetes even in the absence of myocardial necrosis.

Diastolic dysfunction is also an important cause of heart failure in patients with CAD *(20–22)*. Diastolic dysfunction further compromises cardiac performance in the presence of systolic dysfunction, but also sometimes causes clinical heart failure in the absence of overt systolic dysfunction. Impaired left ventricular relaxation and compliance culminate in elevated diastolic filling pressures *(23)*. Decreased left ventricular compliance may also result from myocardial fibrosis associated with previous MI. Additionally, as discussed here, diabetes *per se* may cause diastolic dysfunction.

HYPERTENSION, DIABETES, AND HEART FAILURE

Hypertension is extremely common in type 2 diabetes, occurring in 40% to 60% of patients *(24)*. Hypertension is the most common cause of heart failure in patients without CAD, accounting for 24% of cases of heart failure in the overall population *(25)*. The combination of diabetes and hypertension is especially problematic. For reasons that are not well understood, this is particularly the case in women: diabetes increases the risk of developing heart failure 3.7-fold in hypertensive women as compared to 1.8-fold in hypertensive men *(26)*. Patients with hypertension and diabetes often develop heart failure despite normal systolic function, sometimes referred to as diastolic heart failure *(27,28)*. From a physiological viewpoint, diastolic dysfunction is a result of impaired left ventricular relaxation, and increased stiffness or decreased compliance of the left ventricular chamber *(21,22)*. From a structural viewpoint, diastolic dysfunction is often seen in hypertensive patients with a small or wound-sized left ventricular chamber and increased wall thickness. Although cardiac hypertrophy increases the risk of heart failure dramatically, patients with diabetes may also have diastolic dysfunction even in the absence of LVH *(28)*. In patients with poorly controlled hypertension, systolic dysfunction sometimes develops with impaired contractility and remodeling leading to left ventricular dilation *(29)*.

DIABETIC CARDIOMYOPATHY

The diagnosis of diabetic cardiomyopathy is sometimes invoked when a patient with diabetes has heart failure in the absence of an identifiable etiology. This term was initially suggested almost 30 years ago, based on the pathological findings in a small series of patients with diabetic nephropathy who had unexplained heart failure *(30)*. These patients had myofibrillar hypertrophy and diffuse interstitial fibrosis in the absence of significant CAD. Although the contribution of renal insufficiency and undiagnosed hypertension to these findings was not accounted for, interstitial accumulation of periodic acid-Schiff-positive material and collagen have been reported in other pathological studies *(31–33)*. However, none of these findings are specific to diabetes, which makes it difficult to confirm the diagnosis of diabetic cardiomyopathy based on biopsy or pathological findings. Nonetheless, it seems likely that changes in the extracellular matrix (ECM) may contribute to the decreased left ventricular compliance and impaired diastolic function observed in patients with diabetes.

Another mechanism potentially contributing to cardiac dysfunction in patients with diabetes is impaired coronary blood flow. Even in the absence of CAD, minor structural abnormalities in the coronary microvasculature have been reported in hearts from patients with diabetes, including perivascular fibrosis and thickening of myocardial capillary basement membranes *(34–37)*. Perhaps more importantly, abnormal coronary flow reserve occurs in both type 1 *(38)* and type 2 *(39)* diabetes patients without clinically evident CAD. Abnormal coronary flow reserve appears to be related to poor glycemic control, suggesting that elevated glucose concentrations have detrimental effects on endothelial function *(40)*. In type 2 diabetes, vascular inflammation and dyslipidemia also are important contributors to impaired nitric oxide signaling and endothelial dysfunction. Additionally, older patients with diabetes have impaired nonendothelium-dependent vasodilation, presumably reflecting changes in vascular smooth muscle function. Interestingly, diastolic dysfunction has been associated with abnormal flow reserve in patients with type 2 diabetes and normal coronary arteries *(41)*.

In some populations, diabetes has been associated with an increase in left ventricular mass in the absence of clinical hypertension, particularly in women *(42,43)*. This may result from insulin resistance and the effects of resulting hyperinsulinemia on heart muscle growth. In type 2 diabetes, both hyperinsulinemia and insulin resistance have been correlated with left ventricular mass *(44)*. Proteins in the left ventricle continuously undergo breakdown and re-synthesis *(45)*, and high insulin concentrations decrease the rates of heart protein breakdown *(46)*, which would tend to promote increased muscle mass and hypertrophy.

PROGNOSIS OF PATIENTS WITH DIABETES AND HEART FAILURE

Diabetes increases the morbidity and mortality in patients with heart failure. In the Framingham study, diabetes was an independent predictor of death in women with heart failure, increasing their mortality 1.8-fold *(2)*. The Studies of Left Ventricular Dysfunction demonstrated that diabetes increased the risk of heart failure, and all-cause morbidity and mortality in patients with low left ventricular ejection fractions (LVEF). This risk was independent of age, LVEF, and the etiology of heart failure, but increased with diabetes duration and was particularly apparent in women *(47)*. Further analysis revealed that the higher mortality risk was confined to those with ischemic cardiomyopathy, although diabetes was not associated with an increased risk in those with nonischemic cardiomyopathy *(48)*. Similar findings have been demonstrated in the Beta-Blocker Evaluation of Survival Trial *(49)*.

After MI or coronary revascularization, patients with diabetes also have a high morbidity and mortality that results from the development of heart failure *(50–52)*. In elderly Medicare patients in the year following MI, 11% of patients without diabetes, 17% of patients with diabetes on oral agents, and 25% of those treated with insulin were admitted for heart failure *(53)*. Older age, insulin treatment, previous coronary artery bypass graft surgery, renal insufficiency, low LVEF, or clinical heart failure were all associated with an increased risk of subsequent heart failure admission. In the Cholesterol and Recurrent Events trial, diabetes along with age, low LVEF, hypertension, previous MI, and baseline heart rate were also associated with an increased risk of developing heart failure after MI *(54)*. Additionally, women with diabetes have a particularly high risk of death following hospitalization for heart failure *(55)*.

HEART FAILURE TREATMENT

In patients with diabetes, the management of heart failure follows standard American College of Cardiology/American Heart Association Task Force recommendations, including intensive treatment of co-existent hypertension, CAD, renal disease, and hyperglycemia. Guidelines for the overall management of these patients, based on the four stages of heart failure are shown in Table 1 *(56)*. Heart failure is extremely common in elderly patients with diabetes *(28)* in whom co-morbidities, such as chronic renal insufficiency, may complicate treatment *(57)*. These patients are very susceptible to fluid retention, which not only causes exertional intolerance but can also precipitate pulmonary edema. Interesting recent evidence also suggests that pulmonary dysfunction may be present in heart failure patients with diabetes and may contribute to their exercise intolerance *(58–60)*. Optimal treatment of hypertension is critical to both the prevention and treatment of heart failure in patients with diabetes. The United Kingdom Prospective Diabetes Study of patients with newly diagnosed type 2 diabetes, demonstrated that more intensive blood pressure (BP) control decreased the incidence of heart failure by 40% *(61)*. Although the level at which medication should be started is still debated *(62,63)*, there is little question that an attempt should be made to lower the BP to below 130/80.

Angiotensin-converting enzyme (ACE) inhibitors are the cornerstone of prevention and treatment of heart failure in diabetic patients. In the Heart Outcomes Prevention Evaluation (HOPE) study, ACE inhibitors prevented cardiac events in high-risk patients without heart failure or known low LVEF *(64)*. HOPE included but was not limited to patients with type 2 diabetes. ACE inhibitors also improve clinical outcome in diabetic patients with known heart failure, decreasing subsequent hospitalization and death *(47)*. Additionally, their renal protective benefit may have long-term benefit to prevent the development or worsening of heart failure in patients with diabetes *(65,66)*. Angiotensin-receptor blockers (ARBs) are also used widely for the prevention and treatment of heart failure, particularly when patients are unable to use ACE inhibitors as a result of the

Table 1
Recommendations for Treatment of Heart Failure

High risk of developing (stage A)	LV dysfunction without symptoms (stage B)	LV dysfunction with current or prior symptoms (stage C)	Refractory end-stage (stage D)
Blood pressure control Lipid control Avoid smoking, alcohol, and illicit drugs			
ACE inhibitors with DM	ACE inhibitors and β-blockers with prior MI	ACE inhibitors and β-blockers in all unless contraindicated	
Control of ventricular rate Treatment of thyroid disorders			
Periodic evaluation for signs and symptoms of heart failure	Regular evaluation for signs and symptoms of heart failure Valve replacement or repair for hemodynam- ically significant stenoses regurgitation		
		Diuretics if evidence of fluid retention Digitalis unless contraindicated Withdrawal of drugs known to adversely affect clinical status	
			Meticulous identifica- tion and control of fluid retention Referral for cardiac transplantation and heart failure program
	Other as in stage A	Other as in stages A and B	Other as in stages A, B, and C

LV, left ventricular; ACE, angiotensin-converitng enzyme; DM, diabetes mellitus; MI, myocardial infarction. (From ref. 56.)

development of cough. In the Reduction of Endpoints in noninsulin-dependent diabetics (NIDDM) with the Angiotensin II Antagonist Losartan study, the incidence of heart failure in patients with nephropathy was reduced by 32% over 4 years of follow-up (67). In the Losartan Intervention for Endpoint reduction in hypertension study, which in-cluded hypertensive patients with LVH, ARBs reduced the combined endpoint of cardio-vascular death, MI, or stroke, and hospitalizations for heart failure (68). In patients with diabetes in the Valsartan in Acute Myocardial Infarction study, ARB treatment was comparable to ACE inhibition in preventing the combined endpoint of cardiovascular death, MI, and heart failure in the diabetic subgroup after MI (69).

There is sometimes reluctance to use β-blockers in treating patients with diabetes with symptomatic heart failure, as a result of concerns for worsening insulin resistance, masking hypoglycemia, or aggravating orthostatic hypotension. However, these concerns need to be carefully considered within the context of the clear benefit of these agents in patients with diabetes with heart failure. A recent meta-analysis of six major clinical trials studying β-blocker therapy indicated that they significantly decreased mortality in diabetic patients with heart failure (70). β-Blockers improve ventricular function and survival in patients with chronic heart failure and depressed left ventricular function (49,71,72). They also reduce the incidence of MI, heart failure hospitalization, and mortality in diabetic patients with advanced heart failure (49). Finally, β-blockers have an established benefit after MI in high-risk patients (73), and are instrumental in the treatment of angina and hypertension. Thus, their benefits are substantial and every attempt should be made to include these agents in treating heart failure in patients with diabetes.

Diuretics have a well-recognized role in the treatment of symptomatic heart failure, particularly in diabetic patients who tend to be volume sensitive because of diastolic dysfunction and have a tendency to retain fluid because of renal impairment. Loop diuretics are the mainstay of treatment, but recent evidence indicates that aldosterone antagonists (74,75) may have an important role in the treatment of advanced symptomatic heart failure. These agents may slow the progression of myocardial fibrosis and have the added benefit that they prevent hypokalemia resulting from loop diuretics. However, serum potassium concentrations should be carefully monitored in patients with diabetes, particularly those taking ACE inhibitors or ARBs and when renal insufficiency is present, because of the potential for hyperkalemia (74).

In younger patients with diabetes who are unresponsive to medical therapy, their candidacy for cardiac transplantation is carefully considered. A recent analysis of the Columbia Presbyterian experience showed no significant reduction in survival in patients with diabetes, and overall 70% were still alive 5 years later after transplantation (76). Diabetes has been reported as a risk factor for significant rejection (77), but this is a relatively infrequent occurrence with current immunosuppressive therapy. Renal insufficiency is relatively common after heart transplantation and the presence of pre-existing nephropathy increases this risk and therefore is often a contraindication to heart transplantation. Insulin-requiring diabetes was also once considered to be a contraindication, but the survival of insulin-requiring patients without end-organ disease is quite good and selected individuals are considered for transplantation. Patients with diabetes typically require high doses of insulin or oral hypoglycemic agents after transplantation as a result of the use of corticosteroids for immunosuppression. Patients with advanced heart failure who are awaiting transplantation sometimes require left ventricular assist device support. Although the risk of infection is somewhat increased in patients with diabetes, these devices are in many cases are life saving.

The treatment of diabetic patients with heart failure in the absence of significant systolic dysfunction is challenging and requires special comment. Symptomatic heart failure as a result of diastolic dysfunction occurs in diabetic patients with hypertension, particularly in the presence of LVH. Poorly controlled hypertension, tachycardia, atrial fibrillation, active myocardial ischemia, and volume overload can all potentially exacerbate heart failure in these patients (21,22,28). There are no specific therapies with proven benefit in diastolic dysfunction, but aggressive BP control (<130/80), sodium restriction, and diuretics remain the mainstays of therapy for symptomatic patients (28).

Although the benefit of ACE inhibitors is clear in the treatment of systolic dysfunction, their effectiveness for diastolic dysfunction has not been proven (72). However, they are often used with the rationale that inhibition of the renin–angiotensin–aldosterone system prevents adverse neurohormonal activation, reduces left ventricular mass and may prove useful in reversing diastolic dysfunction (78).

Recent evidence has suggested that insulin resistance is common in heart failure patients (79), and sometimes contributes to the development of diabetes (80). The role of intensive metabolic control has not been studied in patients with diabetes and heart failure, but optimizing blood glucose may prove to be important. In type 2 diabetes, cardiac insulin resistance and excessive fatty acid metabolism may also play a role in heart failure patients. Highly innovative therapies that inhibit heart fatty acid oxidation and promote glucose utilization have been used in small studies in Europe (81). Metabolic therapy appears to improve left ventricular function and symptoms in patients with type 2 diabetes and heart failure, although also improving peripheral insulin sensitivity, blood glucose, and reducing endothelin-1 (81). These agents may offer a novel approach to heart failure treatment in the future, but are not yet approved for use in the United States and require further study to determine their efficacy in large clinical trials.

DIABETES TREATMENTS AND HEART FAILURE

Heart failure complicates the treatment of patients with type 2 diabetes, because the oral hypoglycemic agents metformin and thiazolidinediones (TZDs) are not recommended in patients with moderate to severe heart failure. Decreased clearance of metformin in patients with heart failure and renal insufficiency can lead to potentially dangerous lactic acidosis. TZDs are commonly associated with weight gain, and a small number of patients (2%–5%) also develop fluid retention and pedal edema, particularly those on insulin. Actual heart failure is a very infrequent occurrence with TZD treatment, but may occur with higher doses, concomitant insulin treatment, or active heart failure (82). The Cleveland Clinic experience with class I–III heart failure patients suggested that fluid retention and edema were much more usual occurrences with TZDs than worsening heart failure (83). Nonetheless, these agents are not recommended for patients with class III–IV heart failure. A recent consensus statement regarding the use of TZDs recommends clinical assessment prior to initiation of therapy and careful ongoing monitoring for heart failure (82). Low starting doses with gradual dose escalation should be used in the presence of known structural heart disease or a prior history of heart failure.

In current clinical practice, both metformin and TZDs are used in patients with type 2 diabetes and heart failure (84). The long-term effects of these agents in patients with type 2 diabetes are uncertain. Both medications are effective in improving glycemic control and whether they can be used judiciously to the benefit of patients with well-compensated heart failure remains to be determined. TZDs have a number of biological effects that may be beneficial to the myocardium in the long-term and also lower systemic vascular resistance (82). However, alternative strategies including insulin and insulin secretagogues are often required in heart failure patients. Although insulin treatment has been associated with poor outcomes in patients with heart failure, this largely reflects patient selection and the presence of more advanced microvascular and macrovascular disease. Interestingly, in the Diabetes Insulin-Glucose in Acute Myocardial Infarction study, tighter control of blood glucose during MI and after discharge from the hospital significantly reduced the subsequent rate of heart failure (85–87).

ABNORMALITIES IN CARDIAC FUNCTION IN PATIENTS WITH DIABETES

Even in the absence of symptomatic heart failure, patients with either type 1 or type 2 diabetes have been shown to have abnormalities in cardiac function. Cardiac abnormalities are found in young, otherwise healthy patients with type 1 diabetes in the absence of confounding hypertension or clinically evident CAD *(88)*. These observations support the idea that diabetes alone can cause cardiac abnormalities. Additionally, many studies in patients with type 2 diabetes have also excluded the presence of occult CAD with exercise testing. Abnormalities in left ventricular function have included both diastolic parameters and systolic function, and have been detected using a number of techniques.

Left ventricular diastolic dysfunction has been reported in as many as 60% of subjects with well-controlled type 2 diabetes who were carefully screened for CAD with exercise stress testing and myocardial perfusion imaging *(89)*. Diastolic abnormalities have been widely documented in patients with diabetes. Echocardiographic studies have demonstrated prolonged isovolumic relaxation time *(90–92)*, delayed opening of the mitral valve and a decreased rate of left ventricular diastolic filling *(93–95)* and abnormal transmitral flow velocities *(95–99)*. Radionuclide ventriculography studies have demonstrated abnormalities in both left ventricular peak filling rate and the time to peak filling in type 1 and 2 diabetes *(98,100–102)*. Diastolic abnormalities may be present earlier than systolic abnormalities in patients with diabetes *(103)*. Such studies have been criticized because many of the indices used to assess diastolic function are highly influenced by preload and heart rate *(21,22)*. However, more recent tissue Doppler studies that assess myocardial diastolic velocity, provide confirmatory evidence that diastolic function is altered in patients with diabetes *(104)*. Several molecular abnormalities may contribute to diastolic dysfunction in diabetes. Additionally, ventricular relaxation is an active energy-dependent process and recent studies have found that impaired diastolic function is associated with changes in myocardial energy stores in patient with type 2 diabetes *(105)*.

Mild abnormalities in left ventricular systolic function have also been reported in diabetic subjects, including prolonged pre-ejection interval and shortened systolic ejection time *(93,106–108)*, diminished LVEF *(107,109–111)*, increased systolic dimension and mass *(112,113)*, and decreased left ventricular strain *(114)*. Although mean values in the diabetic and nondiabetic subjects have differed significantly in these studies, typically the absolute values have been within the range of normal for the laboratory. Additionally, some laboratories have reported results indicating that fractional shortening may be increased in diabetic patients *(115)*, particularly in those with microalbuminuria *(116)*.

Abnormal contractile responses to exercise have also been documented in diabetic patients. Impaired augmentation of LVEF during exercise occurs in up to 40% of diabetic patients, including those with type 1 and type 2 diabetes *(100,117–121)*. Impaired LVEF response has been somewhat variably defined as a decrease, no change, or a subnormal increase (<3–5%) in LVEF with exercise. Blunted systolic reserve might be interpreted to reflect intrinsic abnormalities in the diabetic heart. However, in one such study, dobutamine-stimulated LVEF was normal in young diabetic patients despite abnormal exercise LVEF *(122)*, suggesting the alternate possibility that exercise abnormalities may reflect the influence of either altered loading conditions or autonomic activation, rather than cardiac muscle dysfunction *per se*. Similarly, recent studies also indicate that the response to dobutamine is preserved in type 2 diabetes *(114)*.

RELATIONSHIP BETWEEN CONTRACTILE ABNORMALITIES AND DIABETES COMPLICATIONS

Diastolic dysfunction has been associated with poor glycemic control in both type 1 and type 2 diabetes (88,123,124). Abnormalities of ventricular function sometimes improve after intensive treatment which improves glycemic control (108,110). Abnormal cardiac indices also have been associated with microangiopathy (91,92,107). Cardiac dysfunction in type 2 diabetes has also been associated with microalbuminuria (125), which in turn is often associated with endothelial dysfunction. Recent attention has focused on the relationship between autonomic neuropathy and cardiac function. Abnormal cardiac autonomic dysfunction is present in up to 40% of type 1 diabetics at the time of diagnosis (126–128). In one study, more than 90% of diabetic patients with exercise-induced systolic dysfunction had cardiac autonomic dysfunction, and more than half of diabetic patients with cardiac autonomic neuropathy had systolic dysfunction (120). Diastolic dysfunction has also been associated with cardiac autonomic dysfunction in type 1 diabetes (129). Most studies have examined indices of heart rate variation that reflect both parasympathetic and sympathetic innervation, but abnormal contractile reserve in type 1 diabetics has been associated with cardiac sympathetic denervation, demonstrated by metaiodobenzylguanidine scintigraphy (130). Diastolic dysfunction has been associated with autonomic dysfunction in type 2 diabetes. Autonomic neuropathy is a predictor of overall mortality in patients with diabetes (131), and improved methods of assessing cardiac autonomic function may further our understanding of cardiac function in diabetes.

We have recently demonstrated frequent abnormalities of cardiac function in patients with diabetes complicated by peripheral neuropathy, who did not have CAD or significant hypertension (117). Abnormal left ventricular systolic contractile reserve and low peak diastolic filling rates were identified in 18% and 47% of these patients, respectively. After 1 year, patients on placebo experienced decreases in left ventricular stroke volume and cardiac output during exercise, but patients treated with an aldose reductase inhibitor, which blocks glucose flux into the polyol pathway (see later), increased their exercise LVEF. These results support the hypothesis that patients with diabetes and neuropathy have a tendency to progressive cardiac dysfunction that may be preventable with treatment.

CELLULAR AND MOLECULAR ABNORMALITIES IN THE DIABETIC HEART

A variety of animal models have been used to study the cellular and molecular complications of diabetes, including surgical pancreatectomy, chemically induced, diet, spontaneous genetic models, and recombinant genetic models. Because of the simplicity of the model, most of the work on the cardiac effects of diabetes has been performed in animals with chemically induced diabetes, using streptozotocin or alloxan, which cause destruction of the ß-cells of the pancreas. The induction of diabetes with these agents leads to depressed cardiac function in rats (132). However, this agent can cause hypothyroidism, anorexia, weight loss, and has other potentially toxic effects, which may also compromise cardiac function. More recently, with recombinant gene technology, diabetic animals have been developed, either by overexpressing genes or by deleting genes for experimental studies.

Insulin causes peripheral vasodilation and has a mild positive inotropic effect in animals (133,134) and humans (135), the latter related to sympathetic activation (136). In insulin-deficient models, the lack of insulin may have hemodynamic consequences. However, there are also a number of fundamental cardiac cellular and molecular abnormalities in diabetic animal models that affect the normal contraction and relaxation of myofibrillar proteins. Physiological function of the heart depends on the integrity of cellular and molecular mechanisms involved in regulating calcium flux, contractile protein function, and substrate and energy metabolism in the heart. Abnormalities in each of these essential pathways have been described in experimental models of diabetes *(137–139)*, although they remain less well understood in humans.

Systolic contraction depends on calcium release from the sarcoplasmic reticulum, which modulates the interaction between actin and myosin filaments. Diastolic relaxation of the heart is an active process involving the pumping of calcium from the cytosol back into the sarcoplasmic reticulum. Several alterations in calcium homeostasis have been described in experimental models of diabetes, including abnormal sarcolemmal calcium binding *(140)*, calcium pump activity *(141)*, sodium–calcium exchange *(141)*, and decreased sarcoplasmic reticulum calcium pump activity *(142,143)*. Recent studies have shown a prolonged increase in intracellular calcium concentration in isolated cardiac myocytes from diabetic rats *(144)*. Interestingly, overexpression of the sarcoplasmic reticulum Ca^{2+}- adenosine triphosphate (ATP)ase in the hearts of diabetic mice improved contractile performance (145). Additionally, abnormalities in mitochondrial calcium homeostasis in the diabetic heart have been shown to decrease the activity of calcium-dependent mitochondrial enzymes, thereby decreasing mitochondrial ATP synthesis *(146)*. Hyperglycemia also activates protein kinase C, which may have a role in cardiac dysfunction in view of findings that mice with transgenic over-expression of the β2-isoform of this protein develop cardiomyopathy *(147)*. Thus, alterations in calcium flux and calcium signaling are likely to be important in so much as impaired calcium handling may impair diastolic relaxation in patients with diabetes.

Abnormalities in myofibrillar proteins may also contribute to impaired cardiac contractile function in diabetes. These include depressed calcium-ATPase activity of actin-myosin and a shift to the lower activity isoform of the myosin heavy chain *(148,149)*. Additonally, altered phosphorylation of troponin I and the myosin light-chain proteins, which regulate contractile activity may also interfere with function in the diabetic heart *(150,151)*. Abnormal collagen crosslinking as a result of glycosylation of ECM proteins may contribute to the decreased compliance and diastolic dysfunction *(152)*. Recent studies have shown that increased plasma concentrations of advanced glycosylation endproducts are associated with diastolic dysfunction in patients with diabetes *(153,154)*. Additional mechanisms such as increased reactive oxygen species (ROS) may also contribute to cardiac dysfunction in the diabetic heart. Many of the molecular abnormalities in experimental models of insulin-deficient diabetes are reversed with insulin therapy *(154)*, suggesting that they are a result of insulin deficiency, hyperglycemia, or other metabolic perturbations. In this regard, high extracellular glucose and low insulin concentrations directly impair relaxation and electromechanical coupling in cultured rat myocytes *(155,156)*. Thus, overall experimental data provide a potential rationale for intensive treatment of diabetes to improve cardiac function in patients with diabetes.

METABOLIC ABNORMALITIES IN THE DIABETIC HEART

To meet the energetic demands of contractile function, maintenance of ionic homeostasis and protein synthesis, the heart utilizes a variety of substrates including glucose, fatty acids, lactate, ketone bodies, and amino acids. The relative contribution of these substrates varies depending on the hormonal milieu, the concentrations of available substrates (including oxygen), the workload imposed on the heart, and blood flow. In both type 1 and type 2 diabetes, significant alterations in the arterial concentrations of substrates also contribute to changes in metabolism and metabolic gene expression.

Glucose Transport

Although glucose contributes approximately only 10% to 15% of the energy required by the heart under normal conditions, glucose metabolism increases during insulin stimulation, exercise, and ischemia (157). Heart glucose uptake is mediated by the facilitative transporter glucose transporter (GLUT)4 and to a lesser extent GLUT1 (158). Stimulation of heart glucose transport involves the translocation of GLUT proteins from intracellular storage membranes to the cell surface in which they facilitate glucose entry into the cell. Both insulin and myocardial ischemia cause GLUT4 translocation in the heart and the two stimuli have additive effects on GLUT4 translocation (158,159). GLUT1 is responsible for basal glucose uptake in the heart, but also is present in intracellular storage membranes and is recruited to a modest degree by insulin and ischemia (158,159). The amount of heart GLUT1 and GLUT4 is reduced in rats (160–163) and pigs (164,165) with chemically induced diabetes, and in Zucker obese diabetic rats (166,167).

The ability of the diabetic heart to take up glucose has been studied both in animal models and in patients. Both basal and insulin-stimulated myocardial glucose uptake is blunted in diabetic animals (168). Heart glucose uptake is also reduced in diabetic rats (160). On the other hand, glucose uptake increases normally during dobutamine infusion in diabetic pigs (165). When glucose uptake is imaged with the glucose analog fluorodeoxyglucose (FDG) using positron emission tomography, moderate reductions in insulin-stimulated myocardial FDG uptake are found in patients with type 2 diabetes and CAD (169,170). Other reports indicate that FDG uptake is preserved in the absence of CAD (171) and in regions of myocardium with normal flow in type 2 patients with CAD (172). In patients with type 1 diabetes, fasting heart glucose uptake is decreased (173), but insulin-stimulated FDG uptake appears to be normal (174). Atrial pacing increases myocardial glucose uptake in patients with type 1 diabetes, suggesting that they have normal glucose transporter recruitment with increased workload. This is in keeping with the recent finding that the activity of adenosine monophosphate-activated protein kinase, the stress kinase that is responsible for ischemia- and workload-mediated increases in myocardial glucose uptake and GLUT4 translocation (175,176), is similar in diabetic and nondiabetic hearts (177). Thus, the heart glucose appears to altered in some, although not all, settings, and may contribute to the abnormalities seen in the diabetic heart.

Glucose Metabolism

Once transported into the heart, glucose primarily undergoes glycolysis to pyruvate and is oxidized, or is stored as glycogen. In diabetes, glycolytic flux is impaired because of decreased hexokinase activity (178) and diminished flux through phosphofructokinase (PFK), because of increases in the citrate derived from increased fatty acid utilization (179), and as a result of decreases in the PFK activator fructose 2,6-bisphosphate (178). Despite a decrease in glycogen synthase activity in the diabetic heart (180,181), there is a paradoxical increase in the glycogen content, resulting from the increased utilization of fatty acids and ketone bodies that shunt glucose into glycogen (182,183).

A minor fate of glucose in the heart is the polyol pathway, which may be responsible for diabetes complications such as neuropathy. Glucose is reduced to sorbitol by aldose reductase and then oxidized to fructose by sorbitol dehydrogenase. The first reaction consumes nicotinamide adenine dinucleotide phosphate (NADPH), which is needed to reduce glutathione and increased flux through aldose reductase leads to increased oxidative stress. The second reaction generates nicotinamide adenine dinucleotide phosphate (NADH), which may alter the redox state and cause "pseudo-hypoxia" with adverse effects on cellular function (184). Treatment of diabetic rats with aldose reductase inhibitors increases glycolytic flux (185) and may have beneficial effects during myocardial ischemia (186,187). Additionally, uncoupling of myocardial glycolytic flux from glucose oxidation because of inhibition of pyruvate dehydrogenase (PDH) in the diabetic heart may increase flux through the pentose phosphate and hexosamine biosynthetic pathways. Recent work has highlighted the importance of alterations in the diabetic heart that induce the expression of glucose regulated transcriptional factors (USF 1/2 and Sp1) and alter metabolic gene expression (188). Combined with the increased production of ROS that occurs with hyperglycemia (189), glucose toxicity may contribute to alterations in cardiac function in diabetes.

Furthermore, the oxidation of carbohydrate is impaired in the diabetic heart. Patients with type 1 diabetes without evidence of CAD have abnormal lactate utilization by the heart (173), as do animals with streptozotocin (STZ)-induced diabetes (165). Lactate is taken up by cells via the monocarboxylic acid transporter, which does not appear to be significantly affected by diabetes (190,191), but is then oxidized to pyruvate, which is transported into the mitochondria in which it undergoes oxidative decarboxylation by PDH to form acetyl-coenzyme A (CoA). In STZ-diabetic rats, myocardial PDH activity is decreased basally because of a decrease in total PDH activity (192). Pyruvate dehydrogenase kinase-4, which is upregulated in the diabetic heart, also inactivates PDH (193). Thus, PDH activity does not increase normally in response to either insulin stimulation or increased workload (194,195). Additionally, there is increased feedback inhibition of PDH by higher acetyl-CoA/CoA and NADH/NAD ratios (196), which result from increased metabolism of free fatty acids and ketone bodies. The net effect of these changes is that oxidative metabolism of carbohydrates is impaired.

Fatty Acid Metabolism

Circulating fatty acid concentrations are often elevated in diabetes, resulting in increased uptake and oxidation of free fatty acids (FFAs) in hearts from spontaneously diabetic (type 1) rats and diabetic db/db mice (197–200). In contrast, decreased myocardial fatty acid oxidation has been reported in insulin-resistant Zucker obese rats (201), and hearts from rats with STZ-induced diabetes also have decreased rates of fatty acid oxidation (202). Clinical studies have reported normal rates of myocardial FFA oxidation in diabetic patients, based on myocardial kinetics of ^{125}I-heptadecanoic acid uptake using single-photon emission tomography (203). Although the use of FFA for energy production may be normal or increased, the concentration of triglycerides is significantly elevated in the diabetic heart (201,204), suggesting that uptake exceeds the rate of oxidation. Excessive FFA uptake and oxidation may play a role in the decreased cardiac function seen in the diabetic rat, and several pharmacological interventions directed at decreasing fatty acid utilization and increasing glucose oxidation have been proposed (205). Inhibition of carnitine palmitoyltransferase-1, a key enzyme responsible for FFA oxidation, improves function in diabetic rats. Increasing PDH activity and glucose oxidation by treatment with dichloroacetate also improves function in the working diabetic rat heart *(206)*. It has been found that overexpression of GLUT4 in diabetic db/db mice normalizes glucose and fatty acid metabolism and restores normal contractile function *(200,207)*, emphasizing the important link between altered metabolic activity and impaired contractile function in the diabetic heart.

Excess FFA uptake results in increased concentrations of long chain acyl-CoA fatty acid intermediates, which may be toxic to the cell. Treatment of diabetic animals with L-carnitine decreases the concentration of these intermediates and improves function in the diabetic heart *(208)*. Thus, metabolic manipulations aimed at increasing glucose oxidation and decreasing FFA utilization appear to have some beneficial effect on cardiac function, at least in the animal model. On the other hand, it is important to recognize that glucose alone is not adequate substrate for the heart, and particularly not for the diabetic heart. Specifically, the function of the diabetic heart improves significantly with the addition of FFA to the perfusate compared to glucose alone perfusion *(209)*.

An important regulator of myocardial fatty acid metabolism, peroxisome proliferator-activated receptor (PPAR)α, deserves particular attention with respect to the diabetic heart. PPARα is activated by FFAs, fibrates, and novel drugs that are under development for the treatment of diabetes, which are combined PPARγ/PPARα agonists. PPARα-activated genes are responsible for fatty acid transport, esterification and β-oxidation, all of which are upregulated in the setting of diabetes *(210)*. Mice over-expressing PPARα in the heart demonstrate a decrease in fractional shortening that is worsened if the animals are made diabetic or fed a high fat diet *(210)* and is associated with triglyceride accumulation in the cardiac myocytes. In contrast, knocking out PPARα protects against the development of left ventricular dysfunction in diabetic animals *(210)*. However, knocking out PPARα in the normal mouse heart can also cause lipid accumulation and early death in male mice, that is reversed by treatment with estradiol *(211)*. Interestingly, treatment of diabetic mice (with intact PPARα) with a PPARα activator can correct abnormalities in fatty acid and glucose metabolism but does not improve depressed left ventricular contractile function *(212)*. Thus, the biology is complex and further work is necessary to determine the exact role of PPARα in regulating fatty acid metabolism in the diabetic heart and its role in the development of diabetic cardiomyopathy in humans.

KETONE BODY METABOLISM

Ketoacidosis may occur in the setting of uncontrolled diabetes and the heart readily oxidizes ketones bodies *(213)*. The ketones, acetoacetate and β-hydroxybutyrate, are transesterified to acetoacetyl-CoA and converted to two molecules of acetyl-CoA. As a result, the intracellular content of free, nonesterified CoA decreases, which may inhibit citric acid cycle flux *(214,215)*. This inhibition of the citric acid cycle by ketone oxidation is associated with decreases in contractile function in vitro *(214,216)*. Increasing the myocardial content of CoA, by providing the CoA precursor, pantothenic acid, prevents both the inhibition of citric acid cycle flux and the resulting contractile dysfunction in isolated hearts oxidizing ketone bodies *(215)*. Thus, it is possible that ketone bodies may contribute to reversible cardiac dysfunction during metabolic decompensation in the setting of ketoacidosis. Interestingly, studies in isolated cardiac myocytes from diabetic rats have demonstrated that the presence of ketones inhibits fatty acid oxidation and increases the accumulation of intracellular triglycerides and fatty acids, augmenting the potential detrimental effects of fatty acids in the diabetic heart *(217)*.

HIGH-ENERGY PHOSPHATES

Mitochondrial oxidative phosphorylation is responsible for the majority of ATP synthesis in the heart. The generation of ATP involves the production of reducing equivalents by the citric acid cycle, which are used to generate an electrochemical gradient of protons across in the inner mitochondrial membrane. This proton gradient drives the F0F1-ATPase (ATP synthase) that converts intramitochondrial adenosine diphosphate (ADP) to ATP although depleting the proton gradient. The newly synthesized ATP is transported out of the mitochondria by the adenine nucleotide translocase in exchange for ADP. The mitochondrial proton gradient can also be dissipated by the uncoupling proteins, UCP-2 and UCP-3, which do not generate ATP, and therefore "uncouple" citric acid cycle flux from mitochondrial ATP synthesis. Recent studies have demonstrated that UCP-3 is upregulated in the diabetic heart *(162,218,219)*, but that F0F1-ATPase expression is unchanged *(220)*. Thus, it is possible that increased expression of UCPs in the diabetic heart may alter mitochondrial ATP synthesis, rendering the diabetic heart less energy efficient.

Cytosolic ATP concentrations are maintained through equilibration between ADP and creatine phosphate, which is mediated by the enzyme creatine kinase. Initial studies suggested that abnormalities in the creatine kinase system might contribute to the impairment in ventricular function in diabetes *(221)*, but more recent studies demonstrated that at high workloads, creatine kinase does not limit the availability of ATP in diabetic rats *(222)*. Nuclear magnetic resonance studies in diabetic patients without evidence of CAD revealed a lower creatine phosphate–ATP ratio, suggesting that ATP concentrations are being maintained at the expense of creatine phosphate depletion *(223,224)*. However, whether such energetic changes in the diabetic heart contribute to diastolic dysfunction or predispose to heart failure in the ischemic setting remains uncertain, but is an important question.

CHANGES IN METABOLIC GENE EXPRESSION IN THE DIABETIC HEART

In addition to affecting the regulation of metabolic, contractile, and ionic channel genes, diabetes can affect the regulation of basic cellular function. Specifically, all cells, including cardiac myocytes, have intrinsic circadian clocks that regulate the expression of metabolic genes that are upregulated in anticipation of changes in nutritional status *(225)*. In the diabetic heart, this circadian rhythm is phase shifted so that the heart is no longer normally synchronized with the environment *(226)*. However, it remains to be determined whether this change in the cyclic pattern of metabolic enzyme expression is associated with the development of cardiac dysfunction.

SUMMARY

Thus, clinical and epidemiological evidence strongly indicate that diabetes increases the incidence of heart failure, particularly in older patients with type 2 diabetes in the presence of CAD or hypertension. Numerous cellular and molecular abnormalities in heart function are present in animal models of diabetes, which potentially may have relevance to patients. Additional alterations in the autonomic innervation of the heart and the integrity of its microvasculature may also compromise the diabetic heart. These abnormalities together impair the ability of the diabetic heart to compensate in the presence of other cardiac insults. Intensive measures to prevent and treat heart failure in patients with diabetes are warranted and therapies targeted at metabolic abnormalities may provide novel approaches to treating patients with diabetes in the future.

REFERENCES

1. Garcia MJ, McNamara PM, Gordon T, Kannell WB. Morbidity and mortality in diabetics in the Framingham population. Diabetes 1973;23:105–111.
2. Kannel WB, Hjortland M, Castelli WP. Role of diabetes in congestive heart failure: The Framingham Study. Am J Cardiol 1974;34:29–34.
3. Nichols GA, Erbey JR, Hillier TA, Brown JB. Congestive heart failure in type 2 diabetes. Diabetes Care 2001;24:1614–1619.
4. Bertoni AG, Bonds DE, Hundley WG, et al. Heart failure prevalence, incidence, and mortality in the elderly with diabetes. Diabetes Care 2004;27:699–703.
5. Aronow WS, Ahn C. Incidence of heart failure in 2,737 older persons with and without diabetes mellitus. Chest. 1999;115:867–868.
6. Stamler J, Vaccaro O, Neaton JD, et al. Diabetes, other risk factors, and 12-year cardiovascular mortality for men screened in the Multiple Risk Factor Intervention Trial. Diabetes Care 1993;16:434–444.
7. Executive Summary of the Third Report of The National Cholesterol Education Program (NCEP) Expert Panel on Detection Evaluation, and Treatment of High Blood Cholesterol in Adults (Adult Treatment Panel III. JAMA 2001;285:2486–2497.
8. Alberti K, Zimmet P. Definition, diagnosis and classification of diabetes mellitus and its complications; Part 1: diagnosis and classification of diabetes mellitus provisional report of a WHO consultation. Diabetic Med 1998;15:539–553.
9. Wackers FJT, Young LH, Inzucchi SE, et al. Detection of silent myocarial ischemia in asymptomatic patients with type 2 diabetes—The DIAD Study. Diabetes Care 2004;27:1954–1961.
10. Ho KK, Pinsky JL, Kannel WB, Levy D. The epidemiology of heart failure: the Framingham Study. J Am Coll Cardiol 1993;22:6A–13A.
11. Chen YT, Vaccarino V, Williams CS, et al. Risk factors for heart failure in the elderly: a prospective community-based study. Am J Med 1999;106:605–612.
12. Chae CU, Pfeffer MA, Glynn RJ, et al. Increased pulse pressure and risk of heart failure in the elderly. JAMA 1999;281:634–639.
13. He J, Ogden LG, Bazzano LA, et al. Risk factors for congestive heart failure in US men and women: NHANES I epidemiologic follow-up study. Archives of Internal Medicine. 2001;161:996–1002.
14. Massie BM, Cleland JG, Armstrong PW, et al. Regional differences in the characteristics and treatment of patients participating in an international heart failure trial. The Assessment of Treatment with Lisinopril and Survival (ATLAS) Trial Investigators. J Card Fail 1998;4:3–8.
15. Pitt B, Segal R, Martinez FA, et al. Randomised trial of losartan versus captopril in patients over 65 with heart failure (Evaluation of Losartan in the Elderly Study, ELITE). Lancet 1997;349:747–752.
16. Harris MI, Flegal KM, Cowie CC, et al. Prevalence of diabetes, impaired fasting glucose tolerance in US adults: The Third National Health and Nutrition Examination Survey, 1988–1994. Diabetes Care 1998;21:518–524.
17. Mokdad AH, Engelgau MM, Ford ES, et al. Diabetes trends in the US: 1900–1998. Diabetes Care 2000;23:1278–1283.
18. Expert Committee on the Diagnosis and Classification of Diabetes Mellitus. Follow-up report on the diagnosis of diabetes mellitus. Diabetes Care 2003;26:3160–3167.
19. Dash H, Johnson RA, Dinsmore RE, et al. Cardiomyopathic syndrome due to coronary artery disease. Br Heart J 1977;39:740–747.
20. Litwin SE, Grossman W. Diastolic dysfunction as a cause of heart failure. J Am Coll Cardiol 1993;22:49A–55A.
21. Zile MR, Brutsaert DL. New concepts in diastolic dysfunction and diastolic heart failure: Part II: causal mechanisms and treatment. Circulation 2002;105:1503–1508.
22. Zile MR, Brutsaert DL. New concepts in diastolic dysfunction and diastolic heart failure: Part I: diagnosis, prognosis, and measurements of diastolic function. Circulation 2002;105:1387–1393.
23. Zile MR, Baicu CF, Gaasch WH. Diastolic heart failure—abnormalities in active relaxation and passive stiffness of the left ventricle. N Engl J Med 2004;350:1953–1959.

24. Hypertension in Diabetes Study Group. HDS 1: Prevalence of hypertension in newly presenting type 2 diabetic patients and the association with risk factors or cardiovascular disease. J Hypertension 1993;11:309–317.
25. Ho KKL, Anderson KM, Kannel WB, et al. Survival after the onset of congestive heart failure in Framingham Heart Study subjects. Circulation 1993;88:107–115.
26. Levy D, Larson MG, Vasan RS, et al. The progression from hypertension to congestive heart failure. JAMA 1996;275:1557–1562.
27. Vasan RS, Levy D. Defining diastolic heart failure: a call for standardized diagnostic criteria. Circulation 2000;101:2118–2121.
28. Piccini JP, Klein L, Gheorghiade M, Bonow RO. New insights into diastolic heart failure: role of diabetes mellitus. Am J Med 2004;116(Suppl 5A):64S–75S.
29. Grossman E, Messerli FH. Diabetic and hypertensive heart disease. Ann Intern Med 1996;125:304–310.
30. Rubler S, Dlugash J, Yuceoglu YZet al. New type of cardiomyopathy associated with diabetes glomerulosclerosis. Am J Cardiol 1972;30:595–602.
31. Factor SM, Minase T, Sonnenblick EH. Clinical and morphological features of human hypertensive-diabetic cardiomyopathy. Am Heart J 1980;99:446–458.
32. van Hoeven KH, Factor SM. A comparison of the pathological spectrum of hypertensive, diabetic, and hypertensive-diabetic heart disease. Circulation 1990;82:848–855.
33. Regan TJ, Lyons MM, Ahemd SS, et al. Evidence for cardiomyopathy in familial diabetes mellitus. J Clin Invest 1977;60:885–899.
34. Blumenthal HT, Alex M, Goldenberg S. A study of lesions of the intramural coronary artery branches in diabetes mellitus. Arch Pathol 1960;70:27–42.
35. Ledet T. Histological and histochemical changes in the coronary arteries of old diabetic patients. Diabetologia 1968;4:268–272.
36. Zoneraich S, Silverman G, Zoneraich O. Primary myocardial disease, diabetes mellitus, and small vessel disease. Am Heart J 1980;100:754–755.
37. Factor SM, Okun EM, Minase T. Capillary microaneurysms in the human diabetic heart. N Engl J Med 1980;302:384–388.
38. Johnstone M, Creager S, Scales K, et al. Impaired endothelium-dependent vasodilation in patients with insulin-dependent diabetes mellitus. Circulation 1993;88:2510–2516.
39. Yokoyama I, Momomura S, Ohtake T, et al. Reduced myocardial flow reserve in non-insulin-dependent diabetes mellitus. J Am Coll Cardiol 1997;30:1472–1477.
40. Yokoyama I, Ohtake T, Momomura S, et al. Hyperglycemia rather than insulin resistance is related to reduced coronary flow reserve in NIDDM. Diabetes 1998;47:119–124.
41. Strauer BE, Motz W, Vogt M, Schwartzkopff B. Evidence for reduced coronary flow reserve in patients with insulin-dependent diabetes. A possible cause for diabetic heart disease in man. Exp Clin Endocrinol Diabetes 1997;105:15–20.
42. Galderisi M, Anderson KM, Wilson PW, Levy D. Echocardiographic evidence for the existence of a distinct diabetic cardiomyopathy (the Framingham Heart Study). Am J Cardiol 1991;68:85–91.
43. Howard BV, Cowan LD, Go O, Welty TK, Robbins DC, Lee ET. Adverse effects of diabetes on multiple cardiovascular risk factors in women. Diabetes Care 1998;14:1258–1265.
44. Ohya Y, Abe I, Fujii K, et al. Hyperinsulinemia and left ventricular geometry in a work-site population in Japan. Hypertension 1996;27:729–734.
45. Young LH, McNulty PH, Morgan C, et al. Myocardial protein turnover in patients with coronary artery disease. Effect of branched chain amino acid infusion. Journal of Clinical Investigation 1991;87: 554–560.
46. McNulty P, Louard R, Deckelbaum L, et al. Hyperinsulinemia inhibits myocardial protein degradation in patients with cardiovascular disease and insulin resistance. Circ 1995;92:2151–2156.
47. Shindler DM, Kostis JB, Yusuf S, et al. Diabetes mellitus, a predictor of morbidity and moratlity in the Studies of Left Ventricular Dysfunction (SOLVD) Trials and Registry. Am J Cardiol 1996;77:1017–1020.
48. Dries DL, Sweitzer NK, Drazner MH, et al. Prognostic impact of diabetes mellitus in patients with heart failure according to the etiology of left ventricular systolic dysfunction. Journal of the American College of Cardiology. 2001;38:421–428.
49. Domanski M, Krause-Steinrauf H, Deedwania P, et al. The effect of diabetes on outcomes of patients with advanced heart failure in the BEST trial. Journal of the American College of Cardiology. 2003;42:914–922.

50. Hildebrandt P, Kaiser-Nielsen P, Seibæk M, Køber L. Myocardial infarction in diabetic patients: Presentation, residual systolic function and heart failure. Circulation 1996;94.

51. Stone PH, Muller JE, Hartwell T, et al. The effect of diabetes mellitus on prognosis and serial left ventricular function after acute myocardial infarction: Contribution of both coronary disease and diastolic left ventricular dysfunction to adverse prognosis. Journal of the American College of Cardiology 1989;14:49–57.

52. Jaffe AS, Spadaro JJ, Schechtman K, et al. Increased congestive heart failure after myocardial infarction of modest extent in patients with diabetes mellitus. American Heart Journal 1984;108:31–37.

53. Chyun D, Vaccarino V, Murillo J, et al. Cardiac outcomes after myocardial infarction in elderly patients with diabetes mellitus. American Journal of Critical Care 2002;11:504–519.

54. Lewis EF, Moye LA, Rouleau JL, et al. Predictors of late development of heart failure in stable survivors of myocardial infarction: the CARE study. Journal of the American College of Cardiology. 2003;42:1446–1453.

55. Gustafsson I, Brendorp B, Seibaek M, et al. Influence of diabetes and diabetes-gender interaction on the risk of death in patients hospitalized with congestive heart failure. J Am Coll Cardiol 2004;43:771–777.

56. American College of Cardiology/American Heart Association Task Force on Practice Guidelines. ACC/AHA Guidelines for the evaluation and management of chronic heart failure in the adult: Executive summary. Circulation 2001;104:2996.

57. Havranek EP, Masoudi FA, Westfall KA, et al. Spectrum of heart failure in older patients: results from the National Heart Failure project. American Heart Journal. 2002;143:412–417.

58. Guazzi M, Brambilla R, Pontone G, et al. Effect of non-insulin-dependent diabetes mellitus on pulmonary function and exercise tolerance in chronic congestive heart failure. American Journal of Cardiology. 2002;89:191–197.

59. Guazzi M, Brambilla R, De Vita S, Guazzi MD. Diabetes worsens pulmonary diffusion in heart failure, and insulin counteracts this effect.[see comment]. American Journal of Respiratory & Critical Care Medicine. 2002;166:978–982.

60. Guazzi M, Tumminello G, Matturri M, Guazzi MD. Insulin ameliorates exercise ventilatory efficiency and oxygen uptake in patients with heart failure-type 2 diabetes comorbidity.[see comment]. Journal of the American College of Cardiology. 2003;42:1044–1050.

61. UK Prospective Diabetes Study Group. Tight blood pressure control and risk of macrovascular and microvascular complications in type 2 diabetes: UKPDS 38. Br Med J 1998;317:703–713.

62. Chobanian AV, Bakris GL, Black HR, et al. The seventh report of the Joint National Committee on Prevention, Detection, Evaluation and Treatment of High Blood Pressure. JAMA 2003;289:1560–1572.

63. American Diabetes Association. Treatment of hypertension in diabetes. Diabetes Care 2003;26:S80–S82.

64. Investigators THOPES. Effects of an angiotensin-converting enzyme inhibitor, ramipril, on cardiovascular events in high-risk patients. N Engl J Med 2000;342:145–153.

65. Lewis EJ, Hunsicker LG, Bain RP, Rohde RD. The effect of angiotensin-converting-enzyme inhibition on diabetic nephropathy. The Collaborative Study Group [see comments] [published erratum appears in N Engl J Med 1993;330(2):152]. N Engl J Med 1993;329:1456–1462.

66. Maschio G, Alberti D, Janin G, et al. Effect of the angiotensin-converting-enzyme inhibitor benazepril on the progression of chronic renal insufficiency. The Angiotensin-Converting-Enzyme Inhibition in Progressive Renal Insufficiency Study Group [see comments]. N Engl J Med 1996;334:939–945.

67. Brenner BM, Cooper ME, de Zeeuw D, et al. Effects of losartan on renal and cardiovascular outcomes in patients with type 2 diabetes and nephropathy. N Engl J Med 2001;345:861–869.

68. Lindholm LH, Ibsen H, Borch-Johnsen K, et al. Risk of new-onset diabetes in the Losartan Intervention For Endpoint reduction in hypertension study. J Hypertens 2002;20:1879–1886.

69. Pfeffer MA, McMurray JJV, Velazquez EJ, et al. Valsartan, Captopril, or both in myocardial infarction complicated by heart failure, left ventricular dysfunction, or both. N Engl J Med 2003;349:1893–1906.

70. Haas SJ, Vos T, Gilbert RE, Krum H. Are beta-blockers as efficacious in patients with diabetes mellitus as in patients without diabetes mellitus who have chronic heart failure? A meta-analysis of large-scale clinical trials. Am Heart J 2003;146:848–853.

71. Bristow MR, Gilbert EM, Abraham WT, et al. Carvedilol produces dose-related improvements in left ventricular function and survival in subjects with chronic heart failure. MOCHA Investigators [comment] [see comments]. Circulation 1996;94:2807–2816.

72. Shekelle PG, Rich MW, Morton SC, et al. Efficacy of angiotensin-converting enzyme inhibitors and beta-blockers in the management of left ventricular systolic dysfunction according to race, gender, and diabetic status: a meta-analysis of major clinical trials. Journal of the American College of Cardiology 2003;41:1529–1538.

73. Viscoli CM, Horwitz RI, Singer BH. Beta-blockers after myocardial infarction: influence of first-year clinical course on long-term effectiveness. Ann Intern Med 1993;118:99–105.
74. Pitt B, Zannad F, Remme WJ, et al. The effect of spironolactone on morbidity and mortality in patients with severe heart failure. Randomized Aldactone Evaluation Study Investigators [see comments]. New England Journal of Medicine 1999;341:709–717.
75. Pitt B ,Perez A. Spironolactone in patients with heart failure. NEJ.M. 2000;342:132.
76. Morgan JA, John R, Weinberg AD, et al. Heart transplantation in diabetic recipients: A decade review of 161 patients at Columbia Presbyterian. J Thorac Cardiovasc Surg 2004;127:1486–1492.
77. Mills RM, Naftel DC, Kirklin JK, et al. Heart transplant rejection with hemodynamic compromise: a multiinstitutional study of the role of endomyocardial cellular infiltrate. Cardiac Transplant Research Database. J Heart Lung Transplant 1997;16:813–821.
78. Wachtell K, Bella JN, Rokkedal J, et al. Change in diastolic left ventricular filling after one year of antihypertensive treatment: The Losartan Intervention For Endpoint Reduction in Hypertension (LIFE) Study. Circulation 2002;105:1071–1076.
79. Grundy SM. Higher incidence of new-onset diabetes in patients with heart failure.[comment]. American Journal of Medicine. 2003;114:331–332.
80. Tenenbaum A, Motro M, Fisman EZ, et al. Functional class in patients with heart failure is associated with the development of diabetes.[see comment]. American Journal of Medicine. 2003;114:271–275.
81. Fragasso G, Piatti Md PM, Monti L, et al. Short- and long-term beneficial effects of trimetazidine in patients with diabetes and ischemic cardiomyopathy. Am Heart J 2003;146:E18.
82. Nesto RW, LeWinter M, Bell D, et al. Thiazolidinedione use, fluid retention, and congestive heart failure. Diabetes Care 2004;27:256–263.
83. Tang WH, Francis GS, Hoogwerf BJ, Young JB. Fluid retention after initiation of thiazolidinedione therapy in diabetic patients with established chronic heart failure. J Am Coll Cardiol 2003;41:1394–1398.
84. Masoudi FA, Wang Y, Inzucchi SE, et al. Metformin and thiazolidinedione use in Medicare patients with heart failure. JAMA 2003;290:81–85.
85. Malmberg K, Ryden L, Suad E, et al. Randomized trial of insulin-glucose infusion followed by subcutaneous insulin treatment in diabetic patients with acute myocardial infarction (DIGAMI Study): Effects on mortality at 1 year. Journal of the American College of Cardiology 1995;26:57–65.
86. Malmberg K, Ryden L, Hamsten A, et al. Effects of insulin treatment on cause-specific one-year mortality and morbidity in diabetic patients with acute myocardial infarction. European Heart Journal 1996;17:1337–1344.
87. Malmberg K. Prospective randomised study of intensive insulin treatment on long term survival after acute myocardial infarction in patients with diabetes mellitus. DIGAMI (Diabetes Mellitus, Insulin Glucose Infusion in Acute Myocardial Infarction) Study Group [see comments]. British Medical Journal 1997;314:1512–1515.
88. Shishehbor MH, Hoogwerf BJ, Schoenhagen P, et al. Relation of hemoglobin A1c to left ventricular relaxation in patients with type 1 diabetes mellitus and without overt heart disease. Am J Cardiol 2003;91:1514–1517, A9.
89. Poirier P, Marois L, Bogaty P, et al. Diastolic dysfunction in normotensive men with well-controlled type 2 diabetes. Diabetes Care 2001;24:5–10.
90. Rynkiewicz A, Semetkowska-Jurkiewicz E, Wyrzykowski B. Systolic and diastolic time intervals in young diabetics. Br Heart J 1980;44:280–283.
91. Shapiro LM, Howat AP, Calter MM. Left ventricular function in diabetes mellitus I: Methodology, and prevalence and spectrum of abnormalities. British Heart Journal 1981;45:122–128.
92. Shapiro LM, Leatherdale BA, MacKinnon J, Fletcher RF. Left ventricular function in diabetes mellitus II: Relation between clinical features and ventricular function. British Heart Journal 1981;45:129–132.
93. Sanderson JE, Brown DJ, Rivellese A, Kohner E. Diabetic cardiomyopathy? An echocardiographic study of young diabetics. Br Med J 1978;1:404–407.
94. Hausdorf G, Rieger U, Koepp P. Cardiomyopathy in childhood diabetes mellitus: incidence, time of onset, and relation to metabolic control. Internat J Cardiol 1988;19:225–236.
95. Danielsen R. Factors contributing to left ventricular diastolic dysfunction in long-term type 1 diabetic subjects. Acta Med Scand 1988;224:249–256.
96. Zarich SW, Arbuckle BE, Cohen LR, et al. Diastolic abnormalities in young asymptomatic diabetic patients assessed by pulsed Doppler echocardiography. J Am Coll Cardiol 1988;12:114–120.
97. Takenaka K, Sakamoto T, Amano K, et al. Left ventricular filling determined by doppler echocardiography in diabetes mellitus. Am J Cardiol 1988;61:1140–1143.

 98. Bouchard A, Sanz N, Botvinick EH, et al. Noninvasive assessment of cardiomyopathy in normotensive diabetic patients between 20 and 50 years old. Am J Med 1989;87:160–166.

 99. Paillole C, Dahan M, Paycha F, et al. Prevalence and significance of left ventricular filling abnormalities determined by doppler echocardiography in type I (insulin-dependent) diabetic patients. Am J Cardiol 1989;64:1010–1016.

100. Mustonen JN, Uusitupa MIJ, Tahvanainen K, et al. Impaired left ventricular systolic function during exercise in middle-aged insulin-dependent and noninsulin-dependent diabetic subjects without clinically evident cardiovascular disease. Am J Cardiol 1988;62:1273–1279.

101. Kahn JK, Zola B, Juni JE, Vinik AI. Decreased exercise heart rate and blood pressue response in diabetic subjects with cardiac autonomic neuropathy. Diabetes Care 1986;9:389–394.

102. Ruddy TD, Shumak SL, Liu PP, et al. The relationship of cardiac diastolic dysfunction to concurrent hormonal and metabolic status in type I diabetes mellitus. J Clin Endocrin Met 1988;66:113–118.

103. Raev DC. Which left ventricular function is impaired earlier in the evolution of diabetic cardiomyopathy? Diabetes Care 1994;17:633–639.

104. Boyer JK, Thanigaraj S, Schechtman KB, Perez JE. Prevalence of ventricular diastolic dysfunction in asymptomatic, normotensive patients with diabetes mellitus. Am J Cardiol 2004;93:870–875.

105. Diamant M, Lamb HJ, Groeneveld Y, et al. Diastolic dysfunction is associated with altered myocardial metabolism in asymptomatic normotensive patients with well-controlled type 2 diabetes mellitus. J Am Coll Cardiol 2003;42:328–335.

106. Ahmed SS, Jaferi GA, Narang RM, Regan TJ. Preclinical abnormality of left ventricular function in diabetes melitus. Am Heart J 1975;89:153–158.

107. Seneviratne BIB. Diabetic cardiomyopathy: The preclinical phase. Br Med J 1977;1:1444–1446.

108. Sykes CA, Wright AD, Malins JM, Pentecost BL. Changes in systolic time intervals during treatment of diabetes mellitus. Br Heart J 1977;39:255–259.

109. Zoneraich S, Zoneraich O, Rhee JJ. Left ventricular performance in diabetic patients without clinical heart disease. Chest 1977;72:748–751.

110. Shapiro LM, Leatherdale BA, Coyne ME, et al. Prospective study of heart disease in untreated maturity onset diabetics. Br Heart J 1980;44:342–348.

111. Uusitupa M, Siitonen O, Pyorala K, Lansimies E. Left ventricular function in newly diagnosed non-insulin-dependent (type 2) diabetics evaluated by systolic time intervals and echocardiography. Acta Med Scand 1985;217:379–388.

112. Friedman NE, Levitsky LL, Edidin DV, et al. Echocardiographic evidence of impaired performance in children with type I diabetes mellitus. Am J Med 1982;73:846–850.

113. Lababidi ZA ,Goldstein DE. High prevalence of echocardiographic abnormalities in diabetic youths. Diabetes Care 1983;6:18–22.

114. Fang ZY, Yuda S, Anderson V, et al. Echocardiographic detection of early diabetic myocardial disease. J Am Coll Cardiol 2003;41:611–617.

115. Thuesen L, Christiansen JS, Falstie-Jensen N, et al. Increased myocardial contractility in short-term type 1 diabetic patients: an echocardiographic study. Diabetologia 1985;28:822–826.

116. Thuesen L, Christiansen JS, Mogensen CE, Henningsen P. Cardiac hyperfunction in insulin-dependent diabetic patients developing microvascular complications. Diabetes 1988;37:851–856.

117. Johnson BF, Nesto RW, Pfeifer MA, et al. Cardiac abnormalities in diabetic patients with neuropathy: Effects of aldose reductase inhibitor administration. Diabetes Care 2004;27:448–454.

118. Mildenberger RR, Bar-Shlomo B, Druck MN. Clinically unrecognized ventricular dysfunction in young diabetic patients. J Am Coll Cardiol 1984;4:234–238.

119. Vered Z, Battler A, Sega P, et al. Exercise-induced left ventricular dysfunction in young men with asymptomatic diabetes mellitus (diabetic cardiomyopathy). American Journal of Cardiology 1984;54:633–637.

120. Zola B, Kahn JK, Juni JE, Vinik AI. Abnormal cardiac function in diabetic patients with autonomic neuropathy in the absence of ischemic heart disease. J Clin Endocrinol Metab 1986;63:208–214.

121. Arvan S, Singal B, Knapp R, Vagnucci A. Subclinical left ventricular abnormalities in young diabetics. Chest 1988;93:1031–1034.

122. Borow KM, Jaspan JB, Williams KA, et al. Myocardial mechanics in young adult patients with diabetes mellitus: effects of altered load, inotropic state and dynamic exercise. J Am Coll Cardiol 1990;15:1508–1517.

123. Fraser GE, Luke R, Thompson S, et al. Comparison of echocardiographic variables between type I diabetics and normal controls. Am J Cardiol 1995;75:141–145.

124. Vinereanu D, Nicolaides E, Tweddel AC, et al. Subclinical left ventricular dysfunction in asymptomatic patients with Type II diabetes mellitus, related to serum lipids and glycated haemoglobin. Clin Sci (Lond) 2003;105:591–599.
125. Liu JE, Robbins DC, Palmieri V, et al. Association of albuminuria with systolic and diastolic left ventricular dysfunction in type 2 diabetes: the Strong Heart Study. J Am Coll Cardiol 2003;41:2022–2028.
126. Hilsted J ,Jeensen SB. A simple test for autonomic neuropathy in juvenile diabetics. Acta Med Scand 1979:385–387.
127. Fava S, Azzopardi J, Muscatt HA, Fenech FF. Factors that influence outcomes in diabetic subjects with myocardial infarction. Diabetes Care 1993:1615–1618.
128. Page MM, Watkins PJ. The heart in diabetes: automomic neuropathy and cardiomyopathy. Clin Endocrinol Metab 1977:377–388.
129. Didangelos TP, Arsos GA, Karamitsos DT, et al. Left ventricular systolic and diastolic function in normotensive type 1 diabetic patients with or without autonomic neuropathy: a radionuclide ventriculography study. Diabetes Care 2003;26:1955–1960.
130. Scognamiglio R, Avogaro A, Casara D, et al. Myocardial dysfunction and adrenergic cardiac innervation in patients with insulin-dependent diabetes mellitus. J Am Coll Cardiol 1998;31:404–412.
131. Vinik AI, Maser RE, Mitchell BD, Freeman R. Diabetic autonomic neuropathy. Diabetes Care 2003;26:1553–1579.
132. Fein FS, Kornstein LB, Strobeck JE, et al. Altered myocardial mechanics in diabetic rats. Circ Res 1980;47:922–933.
133. Lucchesi B, Medina M, Kniffen F. The positive inotropic action of insulin in the canine heart. Eur J Pharmacol 1972;18:107–115.
134. Farah A ,Alousi A. The actions of insulin on cardiac contractility. Life Sciences 1981;29:975–1000.
135. Russell RR, III, Chyun D, Song S, et al. Cardiac responses to insulin-induced hypoglycemia in non-diabetic and intensively treated type 1 diabetic patients. Am J Physiol Endocrinol Metab 2001;281: E1029–E1036.
136. Scherrer U ,Sartori C. Insulin as a vascular and sympathoexcitatory hormone: Implications for blood pressure regulation, insulin sensitivity, and cardiovascular morbidity. Circulation 1997;96:4104–4113.
137. Schaffer SW, Mozaffari MS, Artman M, Wilson GL. Basis for myocardial mechanical defects associated with non-insulin-dependent diabetes. Am J Physiol 1989;19: E25–E30.
138. Schaffer SW. Cardiomyopathy associated with noninsulin-dependent diabetes. [Review]. Mol Cell Biochem 1991;107:1–20.
139. Rodrigues B ,McNeill JH. The diabetic heart: metabolic causes for the development of a cardiomyopathy. Cardiovascular Research 1992;26:913–922.
140. Pierce GN, Dhalla NS. Sarcolemmal Na+-K+ ATPase activity in diabetic rat heart. American Journal of Physiology 1983;245:241–247.
141. Heyliger CE, Prakash A, McNeill JH. Alterations in cardiac sarcolemmal Ca2+ pump activity during diabetes mellitus. Am J Physiol 1987;252:540–544.
142. Lopaschuk GD, Tahiliani A, Vadlamudi RVSV, et al. Cardiac sarcoplasmic reticulum function in insulin or carnitine-treated diabetic rats. Am J Physiol 1983;245:969–976.
143. Penpargkul S, Fein FS, Sonnenblick EH, Scheuer J. Depressed cardiac sarcoplasmic reticular function from diabetic rats. J Mol Cell Cardiol 1981;13:303–309.
144. Lagadic-Gossmann D, Buckler KJ, Le Prigent K, Feuvray D. Altered Ca2+ handling in ventricular myocytes isolated from diabetic rats. Am J Physiol 1996;270:H1529–H1537.
145. Trost SU, Belke DD, Bluhm WF, et al. Overexpression of the sarcoplasmic reticulum Ca2+-ATPase improves myocardial contractility in diabetic cardiomyopathy. Diabetes 2002;51:1166–1171.
146. Flarsheim CE, Grupp IL, Matlib MA. Mitochondrial dysfunction accompanies diastolic dysfunction in diabetic rat heart. Am J Physiol 1996;271:H192–H202.
147. Wakasaki H, Koya D, Schoen FJ, et al. Targeted overexpression of protein kinase C beta2 isoform in myocardium causes cardiomyopathy. Proc Natl Acad Sci U S A 1997;94:9320–9325.
148. Dillmann WH. Diabetes mellitus induces changes in cardiac myosin of the rat. Diabetes 1980;29: 579–582.
149. Malhotra A, Penpargkul S, Fein FS, et al. The effect of streptozotocin-induced diabetes in rats on cardiac contractile proteins. Circ Res 1981;49:1243–12450.
150. Liu X, Takeda N, Dhalla NS. Troponin I phosphorylation in heart homogenate from diabetic rat. Biochem Biophys Acta 1996;1316:78–84.

151. Liu X, Takeda N, Dhalla NS. Myosin light-chain phosphorylation in diabetic cardiomyopathy in rats. Metabolism 1997;46:71–75.

152. Norton GR, Candy G, Woodiwiss AJ. Aminoguanidine prevents the decreased myocardial compliance produced by streptozotocin-induced diabetes mellitus in rats. Circulation 1996;93:1905–1912.

153. Berg TJ, Snorgaard O, Faber J, et al. Serum levels of advanced glycation end products are associated with left ventricular diastolic function in patients with type 1 diabetes. Diabetes Care 1999;22:1186–1190.

154. Watts GF, Marwick TH. Ventricular dysfunction in early diabetic heart disease: detection, mechanisms and significance. Clin Sci (Lond) 2003;105:537–540.

155. Davidoff AJ, Ren J. Low insulin and high glucose induce abnormal relaxation in cultured adult rat ventricular myocytes. Am J Physiol 1997;272: H159–H167.

156. Ren J, Gintant GA, Miller RE, Davidoff AJ. High extracellular glucose impairs cardiac E-C coupling in a glycosylation-dependent manner. Am J Physiol 1997;273:H2876–H2883.

157. Young LH, Russell RR, Yin R, et al. Regulation of myocardial glucose uptake and transport during ischemia and energetic stress. Am J Cardiol 1999;83:25H–30H.

158. Young LH, Renfu Y, Russell RR, et al. Low-flow ischemia leads to translocation of canine heart GLUT-4 and GLUT-1 glucose transporters to the sarcolemma in vivo. Circulation 1997;95:415–422.

159. Russell RR, Yin R, Caplan MJ, et al. Additive effects of hyperinsulinemia and ischemia on myocardial GLUT1 and GLUT4 translocation in vivo. Circulation 1998;98:2180–2186.

160. Kainulainen H, Breiner M, Schurmann A, et al. In vivo glucose uptake and glucose transporter proteins GLUT1 and GLUT4 in heart and various types of skeletal muscle from streptozotocin-diabetic rats. Biochim Biophys Acta 1994;1225:275–282.

161. Garvey WT, Hardin D, Juhaszova M, Dominguez JH. Effects of diabetes on myocardial glucose transport system in rats: implications for diabetic cardiomyopathy. American Journal of Physiology 1993;264:837–844.

162. Depre C, Taegtmeyer H. Metabolic aspects of programmed cell survival and cell death in the heart. Cardiovasc Res 2000;45:538–548.

163. Burcelin R, Printz RL, Kande J, et al. Regulation of glucose transporter and hexokinase II expression in tissues of diabetic rats. Am J Physiol 1993;265: E392–E401.

164. Hall J, Sexton W, Stanley W. Exercise training attenuates the reduction in myocardial GLUT-4 in diabetic rats. J Appl Physiol 1995;78:76–81.

165. Hall J, Stanley W, Lopaschuk G, et al. Impaired pyruvate oxidation but normal glucose uptake in diabetic pig heart during dobutamine-induced work. Am J Physiol 1996;271: H2320–H2329.

166. Slieker LJ, Sundell KL, Heath WF, et al. Glucose transporter levels in tissues of spontaneously diabetic Zucker fa/fa rat (ZDF/drt) and viable yellow mouse (Avy/a). Diabetes 1992;41:187–193.

167. Liu L, Azhar G, Gao W, et al. Bcl-2 and Bax expression in adult rat hearts after coronary occlusion: age-associated differences. American Journal of Physiology 1998;275: R315–R322.

168. Barrett EJ, Schwartz RG, Young LH, et al. Effect of chronic diabetes on myocardial fuel metabolism and insulin sensitivity. Diabetes 1988;37:943–948.

169. Voipio-Pulkki LM, Nuutila P, Knuuti MJ, et al. Heart and skeletal muscle glucose disposal in type 2 diabetic patients as determined by positron emission tomography. J Nucl Med 1993;34:2064–2067.

170. Ohtake T, Yokoyama I, Watanabe T, et al. Myocardial glucose metabolism in noninsulin-dependent diabetes mellitus patients evaluated by FDG-PET. J Nucl Med 1995;36:456–463.

171. Utriainen T, Takala T, Luotolahti M, et al. Insulin resistance characterizes glucose uptake in skeletal muscle but not in the heart in NIDDM. Diabetologia 1998;41:555–559.

172. Maki M, Nuutila P, Laine H, et al. Myocardial glucose uptake in patients with NIDDM and stable coronary artery disease. Diabetes 1997;46:1491–1496.

173. Avogaro A, Nosadini R, Doria A, et al. Myocardial metabolism in insulin-deficient diabetic humans without coronary artery disease. Am J Physiol 1990;258:E606–E618.

174. Nuutila P, Knuuti J, Ruotsalainen U, et al. Insulin resistance is localized to skeletal but not heart muscle in type 1 diabetes. Am J Physiol 1993;264:E756–E762.

175. Russell R, Bergeron R, Shulman G, Young L. Translocation of myocardial GLUT4 and increased glucose uptake through activation of AMP-activated protein kinase by AICAR. Am J Physiol 1999;277:H643–H649.

176. Coven DL, Hu X, Cong L, et al. Physiological role of AMP-activated protein kinase in the heart: graded activation during exercise. Am J Physiol 2003;285:E629–E636.

177. Atkinson LL, Kozak R, Kelly SE, et al. Potential mechanisms and consequences of cardiac triacylglycerol accumulation in insulin-resistant rats. Am J Physiol 2003;284:E923–E930.

178. Sochor M, Kunjara S, Ali M, McLean P. Vanadate treatment increases the activity of glycolytic enzymes and raises fructose 2,6-bisphosphate concentration in hearts from diabetic rats. Biochem Int 1992;28:525–531.

179. Randle P, Garland P, Hales C, Newsholme E. The glucose fatty-acid cycle. Its role in insulin sensitivity and the metabolic disturbances of diabetes mellitus. Lancet 1963;1:785–789.

180. Laughlin MR, Petit WA, Shulman RG, Barrett EJ. Measurement of myocardial glycogen synthesis in diabetic and fasted rats. Am J Physiol 1990;258:E184–E190.

181. Laughlin MR, Morgan C, Barrett EJ. Hypoxic stimulation of heart glycogen synthase and synthesis. Effects of insulin and diabetes mellitus. Diabetes 1991;40:385–390.

182. Laughlin M, Taylor J, Chesnick A, Balaban R. Nonglucose substrates increase glycogen synthesis in vivo in dog heart. Am J Physiol 1994;267:H217–H223.

183. Russell R, Cline G, Guthrie P, et al. Regulation of exogenous and endogenous glucose metabolism by insulin and acetoacetate in the isolated working rat heart: A three tracer study of glycolysis, glycogen metabolism and glucose oxidation. J Clin Invest 1997;100:2892–2899.

184. Williamson JR, Chang K, Frangos M, et al. Hyperglycemic pseudohypoxia and diabetic complications. Diabetes 1993;42:801–813.

185. Trueblood N, Ramasamy R. Aldose reductase inhibition improves altered glucose metabolism of isolated diabetic rat hearts. Am J Physiol 1998;275:H75–H83.

186. Ramasamy R, Oates PJ, Schaefer S. Aldose reductase inhibition protects diabetic and nondiabetic rat hearts from ischemic injury. Diabetes 1997;46:292–300.

187. Ramasamy R, Trueblood N, Schaefer S. Metabolic effects of aldose reductase inhibition during low-flow ischemia and reperfusion. Am J Physiol 1998;275:H195–H203.

188. Young ME, McNulty P, Taegtmeyer H. Adaptation and maladaptation of the heart in diabetes: Part II: potential mechanisms. Circulation. 2002;105:1861–1870.

189. Rosen SG, Linares OA, Sanfield JA, et al. Epinephrine kinetics in humans: radiotracer methodology. J Clin Endocrinol Metab 1989;69:753–761.

190. Py G, Lambert K, Milhavet O, et al. Effects of streptozotocin-induced diabetes on markers of skeletal muscle metabolism and monocarboxylate transporter 1 to monocarboxylate transporter 4 transporters. Metabolism 2002;51:807–813.

191. Enoki T, Yoshida Y, Hatta H, Bonen A. Exercise training alleviates MCT1 and MCT4 reductions in heart and skeletal muscles of STZ-induced diabetic rats. J Appl Physiol 2003;94:2433–2438.

192. Seymour AM, Chatham JC. The effects of hypertrophy and diabetes on cardiac pyruvate dehydrogenase activity. J Mol Cell Cardiol 1997;29:2771–2778.

193. Wu P, Sato J, Zhao Y, et al. Starvation and diabetes increase the amount of pyruvate dehydrogenase kinase isoenzyme 4 in rat heart. Biochem J 1998;329:197–201.

194. Kobayashi K, Neely J. Effects of increased cardiac work on pyruvate dehydrogenase activity in hearts from diabetic animals. J Mol Cell Cardiol 1983;15:347–357.

195. Chatham JC, Forder JR. A 13C-NMR study of glucose oxidation in the intact functioning rat heart following diabetes-induced cardiomyopathy. J Mol Cell Cardiol 1993;25:1203–1213.

196. Randle P, Priestman D, Mistry S, Halsall A. Mechanisms modifying glucose oxidation in diabetes mellitus. Diabetologia 1994;37:S155–S161.

197. Ballard FB, Danforth WH, Naegle S, Bing RJ. Myocardial metabolism of fatty acids. J Clin Invest 1960;39:717–723.

198. Garland P, Randle P. Regulation of glucose uptake by muscle. 10. Effects of alloxan-diabetes, starvation, hypophysectomy and andrenalectomy, and of fatty acids, ketone bodies and pyruvate on the glycerol ouput and concentrations of free fatty acids, long-chain fatty acyl-coenzyme A, glycerol phosphate and citrate-cycle intermediates in rat heart and diaphragm muscles. Biochem J 1964;93:678–687.

199. Lopaschuk G, Tsang H. Metabolism of palmitate in isolated working hearts from spontaneously diabetic 'BB' Wistar rats. Cir Res 1987;61:853–858.

200. Belke DD, Larsen TS, Gibbs EM, Severson DL. Altered metabolism causes cardiac dysfunction in perfused hearts from diabetic (db/db) mice. Am J Physiol 2000;279:E1104–E1113.

201. Young ME, Guthrie PH, Razeghi P, et al. Impaired long-chain fatty acid oxidation and contractile dysfunction in the obese Zucker rat heart. Diabetes 2002;51:2587–2595.

202. Chatham JC, Gao ZP, Forder JR. Impact of 1 wk of diabetes on the regulation of myocardial carbohydrate and fatty acid oxidation. Am J Physiol 1999;277:E342–E351.

203. Turpeinen AK, Kuikka JT, Vanninen E, Uusitupa MI. Abnormal myocardial kinetics of 123I-heptadecanoic acid in subjects with impaired glucose tolerance. Diabetologia 1997;40:541–549.
204. Denton RM, Randle PJ. Concentration of glycerides and phospholipids in rat heart and gastrocnemius muscles. Biochem J 1967;104:416–422.
205. Rodrigues B, Cam MC, McNeill JH. Metabolic disturbances in diabetic cardiomyopathy. Molecular Cellular Biochemistry 1998;180:53–57.
206. Nicholl T, Lopaschuk G, McNeill J. Effects of free fatty acids and dichloroacetate on isolated working diabetic rat heart. Am J Physiol 1991;261: H1053–H1059.
207. Semeniuk LM, Kryski AJ, Severson DL. Echocardiographic assessment of cardiac function in diabetic db/db and transgenic db/db-hGLUT4 mice. Am J Physiol 2002;283:H976–H982.
208. Rodrigues B, Xiang H, McNeill JH. Effect of L-carnitine treatment on lipid metabolism and cardiac performance in chronically diabetic rats. Diabetes 1988;37:1358–1364.
209. Chatham JC, Forder JR. Relationship between cardiac function and substrate oxidation in hearts of diabetic rats. Am J Physiol 1997;273:H52–H58.
210. Finck BN, Han X, Courtois M, Aimond F, et al. A critical role for PPARa-mediated lipotoxicity in the pathogenesis of diabetic cardiomyopathy: Modulation by dietary fat content. PNAS 2003;100: 1226–1231.
211. Djouadi F, Weinheimer CJ, Saffitz JE, et al. A gender-related defect in lipid metabolism and glucose homeostasis in peroxisome proliferator-activated receptor alpha-deficient mice. J Clin Invest 1998;102:1083–1091.
212. Aasum E, Belke DD, Severson DL, et al. Cardiac function and metabolism in type 2 diabetic mice after treatment with BM 17.0744, a novel PPAR-alpha activator. Am J Physiol 2002;283:H949–H957.
213. Williamson J, Krebs H. Acetoacetate as fuel of respiration in the perfused rat heart. Biochem J 1961;80:540–547.
214. Taegtmeyer H. On the inability of ketone bodies to serve as the only energy providing substrate for rat heart at physiological work load. Basic Res Cardiol 1983;78:435–450.
215. Russell R, Taegtmeyer H. Coenzyme A sequestration in rat hearts oxidizing ketone bodies. J Clin Invest 1992;89:968–973.
216. Zimmermann A, Meijler F, Hülsmann W. The inhibitory effect of acetoacetate on myocardial contraction. Lancet 1962;2:757–758.
217. Hasselbaink DM, Glatz JF, Luiken JJ, et al. Ketone bodies disturb fatty acid handling in isolated cardiomyocytes derived from control and diabetic rats. Biochem J 2003;371:753–760.
218. Young ME, Patil S, Ying J, et al. Uncoupling protein 3 transcription is regulated by peroxisome proliferator-activated receptor a in the adult rodent heart. FASEB J 2001;15:833–845.
219. Hidaka S, Kakuma T, Yoshimatsu H, et al. Streptozotocin treatment upregulates uncoupling protein 3 expression in the rat heart. Diabetes 1999;48:430–435.
220. Turko IV, Murad F. Quantitative protein profiling in heart mitochondria from diabetic rats. J Biol Chem 2003;278:35844–35849.
221. Matsumoto Y, Kaneko M, Kobayashi A, et al. Creatine kinase kinetics in diabetic cardiomyopathy. Am J Physiol 1995;268:E1070–E1076.
222. Spindler M, Saupe K, Tian R, et al. Altered creatine kinase enzyme kinetics in diabetic cardiomyopathy. A 31P NMR magentization transfer study of the intact beating rat heart. J Mol Cell Cardiol 1999;31:2175–2189.
223. Metzler B, Schocke MF, Steinboeck P, et al. Decreased high-energy phosphate ratios in the myocardium of men with diabetes mellitus type I. J Cardiovasc Magn Reson 2002;4:493–502.
224. Scheuermann-Freestone M, Madsen PL, Manners D, et al. Abnormal cardiac and skeletal muscle energy metabolism in patients with type 2 diabetes. Circulation 2003;107:3040–3046.
225. Young ME, Razeghi P, Taegtmeyer H. Clock genes in the heart: characterization and attenuation with hypertrophy. Circ Res 2001;88:1142–1150.
226. Young ME, Wilson CR, Razeghi P, et al. Alterations of the circadian clock in the heart by streptozotocin-induced diabetes. J Mol Cell Cardiol 2002;34:223–231.

28 Diabetes Mellitus and Heart Disease

Michael T. Johnstone, MD, CM, FRCP(C) and George P. Kinzfogl, MD

INTRODUCTION

Editor's Note: The aim of this chapter is to not only serve as a review of the topic of diabetes mellitus and coronary artery disease, but also to serve as a synopsis of the chapters that have covered diabetes, risk factors, and macrovascular disease (except for peripheral arterial disease.

Heart disease was thought to be associated with diabetes as early as 1883 when Vegley recommended testing the urine of patients with angina for glucose *(1)*. However, as more diabetic patients survived with the discovery of insulin and improved treatments for renal failure and infection, there was a marked relative increase in morbidity and mortality from cardiovascular disease (CVD). Diabetes is the seventh leading cause of death in the United States, with much of that mortality as a result of CVD *(2)*. However because these statistics are based on the underlying cause of death, they underestimate the true impact of diabetes on mortality.

From: *Contemporary Cardiology: Diabetes and Cardiovascular Disease, Second Edition*
Edited by: M. T. Johnstone and A. Veves © Humana Press Inc., Totowa, NJ

Ultimately, atherosclerosis accounts for 65–80% of all deaths among North American diabetic patients, compared with one-third of all deaths in the general North American population *(3–5)*. A two- to fourfold excess in coronary artery disease (CAD) mortality among diabetic individuals has been noted in a number of prospective studies encompassing a variety of ethnic and racial groups *(6)*. Diabetes also increases the likelihood of severe carotid atherosclerosis *(7,8)* and mortality from stroke is increased almost threefold in diabetic patients *(9)*. Both type 1 and type 2 diabetes mellitus (DM) are therefore powerful and independent risk factors for CAD, stroke, and peripheral arterial disease *(3,9,10)*. Furthermore, when patients with diabetes develop clinical events, they sustain a worse prognosis compared with nondiabetics *(11)*. Coupled with these macrovascular complications are such microvascular complications as retinopathy, neuropathy and nephropathy, all of which accounts for most of the morbidity and mortality associated with DM. Thus, although diabetes may be a problem of glucose metabolism, the American Heart Association (AHA) has recently stated that, "diabetes is a cardiovascular disease" *(3)*.

EPIDEMIOLOGY

More than 10 million Americans carry the diagnosis of DM and another 5 million are estimated to have undiagnosed diabetes *(3)*. The prevalence of type 2 diabetes, which accounts for 90% of all cases of diabetes, is increasing in the United States and around the world because of the advancing age of the population, improved screening and detection, and the increase in risk factors such as obesity and physical inactivity. A growing ethnic diversity in the United States, including ethnic groups that are particularly susceptible to type 2 diabetes, such as Hispanics, blacks, and South Asians also contribute to the increasing prevalence of diabetes *(3,12)*. The obesity epidemic will result in an increasing number of patients of DM. Obesity now affects 18% of the US population in 1998 *(13)*. The problem of obesity is anticipated to grow with the increasing weight of the US population. Between 1991 and 1998, the body weight of the American male has increased by 3%, whereas that of the American female has increased by 5%.

Diabetes and Cardiovascular Mortality

A meta-analysis of several studies estimated the risk of death from CAD in patients with diabetes is 2.58 in men and 1.85 in women *(14)*. These values are in contrast to the Rancho Bernado study *(15)*, which followed subjects ages 40 to 79 for 14 years and found that although death rates were also increased in diabetics, the risk factor-adjusted relative odds was 3.3 in women and 1.9 in men. Factors associated with an increase in mortality rates of diabetics include male gender, black race, longer duration of diabetes, and insulin use *(16)*. Overall, CVD, which includes CAD and cerebrovascular disease, accounts for 65% of all deaths among diabetics. Although much of this data is based on findings in patients with type 2 diabetes, patients with type 1 diabetes have similar causes of death including CAD and renal failure *(17,18)*.

As a result of diabetes, life expectancy is shortened, on average, 9.1 fewer years of life for diabetic men and 6.7 for diabetic women relative to their nondiabetic counterparts *(19)*. Haffner and colleagues examined the mortality in 1000 type 2 diabetic and 1300 nondiabetic Finnish subjects and found that the mortality of the diabetics was similar to the nondiabetics who had a myocardial infarction (MI) *(20)* (Fig. 1). This data suggests that caregivers should treat individuals with type 2 diabetes as if they had experienced a

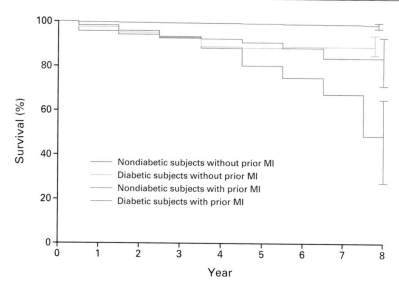

Fig. 1. Kaplan–Meier estimates of the probability of death from coronary heart disease in 1059 subjects with 2ype 2 diabetes and 1378 nondiabetic subjects with and without prior myocardial infarction. Error bars denote 95% confidence intervals. (Reproduced with permission from ref.*20*.)

MI. Mukamal *(21)* studied 1935 patients hospitalized with an acute MI and found that the mortality of the diabetic patients in the short-term period was similar to those of the nondiabetic patients who had a previous MI and twice those that of the nondiabetics who had suffered their first acute coronary event. Malmberg evaluated the findings of the Organization to Assess Strategies for Ischemic Syndromes (OASIS) registry and found that diabetic patients hospitalized for unstable angina or a non-Q wave MI had the same long-term morbidity and mortality as nondiabetic patients with established CVD *(22)*.

Over the past three decades, there has been a significant decrease in cardiovascular mortality in the United States. However, the effect on mortality in patients with diabetes has lagged well behind the general population *(23)*. The death rate of nondiabetic men with CAD decreased by 36.4% compared to 13.1% for diabetic men. The death rate for nondiabetic women decreased by 27% compared to a 23% increase for diabetic women *(23)*.

Prevalence and Risk Factors for Coronary Artery Disease in Insulin-Dependent Diabetes Mellitus

Long-term follow-up of patients with type 1 DM has demonstrated that the first cases of clinically manifest CAD occur late in the third decade or in the fourth decade of life regardless of whether diabetes developed early in childhood or in late adolescence. CAD risk increases rapidly after the age of 40, and by the age of 55 years, 35% of men and women with type 1 DM die of CAD *(18)* compared with 8% for nondiabetics. Women with type 1 DM lose most of their inherent protection from CAD observed in nondiabetic women is *(18,24,25)*. The occurrence of severe coronary atherosclerosis in a subset of type 1 DM patients before the age of 55 regardless of whether diabetes developed in childhood or adolescence, suggests that diabetes mainly accelerates the progression of early atherosclerotic lesions that commonly occur, even in the absence of diabetes, at a young age in the general population *(18)*.

Diabetic nephropathy, which develops in approx 30% to 40% of type 1 DM patients, dramatically increases the prevalence of CAD (18,26). Patients with persistent proteinuria followed in the Steno Memorial Hospital had a 37-fold increased mortality from CVD relative to the general population although patients without proteinuria had a cardiovascular mortality that was only 4.2 times higher (26). Type 1 DM patients followed from the onset of microalbuminuria, developed CAD eight times more frequently than in patients without microalbuminuria (27). Krolewski and associates reported that the risk of development of CAD in patients with persistent proteinuria was 15 times higher compared with those without proteinuria (17) Angiographic studies have shown that nearly all patients with diabetic nephropathy over the age of 45 have one or more clinically significant coronary stenoses (28). Microalbuminuria in type 1 DM is therefore, not only a marker for renal disease, but also a potent risk marker of CAD.

Several mechanisms contribute to the atherosclerotic process in the presence of diabetic nephropathy including hypertension, lipid abnormalities, fibrinolysis and coagulation alterations, all of which are detectable in the early stages of diabetic nephropathy when renal function is still normal (29). Hypertension is frequently present in patients with diabetic nephropathy even when the creatinine concentrations remain normal and can intensify CAD in type 1 DM patients. Diabetic nephropathy is associated with an atherogenic lipoprotein profile that includes elevated low-density lipoprotein (LDL) and very low-density lipoprotein (VLDL) levels, decreased high-density lipoprotein (HDL) levels, and elevated lipoprotein (a) levels (30–32). Furthermore, a hypercoagulable state, characterized by increased plasminogen activator inhibitor (PAI)-1, factor VII, and (plasma) fibrinogen levels, has been described in microalbuminuric type 1 DM patients (33). Finally, reduced renal function leads to the accumulation of advanced glycosylation end-products (AGE) in the circulation and tissue (34,35).

The risk for the development of diabetic nephropathy is only partially determined by glycemic control, and is highly influenced by genetic susceptibility (26,27). Several studies have established that a genetic susceptibility contributes to the high prevalence of CAD among type 1 patients with nephropathy. CAD is twice as common a cause of death among parents of diabetic patients with nephropathy then among parents of diabetic patients without nephropathy. Among diabetics with nephropathy, those who had a cardiovascular event are six times more likely to have a familial history of CVD then those who had no such event. A history of CVD in both parents or in the father of type I DM patient increases the risk of nephropathy in the offspring 10- and 3-fold respectively (36). Parents of diabetic offspring with nephropathy also have higher levels of blood pressure (BP) then do parents whose diabetic offspring do not have diabetic nephropathy (37).

Interestingly, recent studies have shown that an association between angiotensin-converting enzyme (ACE) inhibitors I/D polymorphism, potentially affecting the level of angiotensins and kinins in the kidney can affect the development of renal disease in type I DM patients (38). The same polymorphism has been linked to MI in nondiabetic subjects (39), and in type I (40,41) and type 2 (42) patients.

Prevalence and Risk Factors for Coronary Artery Disease
in Noninsulin-Dependent Diabetes Mellitus

Type 2 DM increases relative risk of CVD by two- to fourfold compared to the general population (43–46). The increased cardiovascular risk is particularly high in women. The protection that premenopausal women have against atherosclerosis is almost completely lost when diabetes is present (47,48).

Although traditional risk factors play an important role in the development of athero-sclerosis in diabetic subjects, the rate of cardiovascular mortality and morbidity in dia-betics exceeds that predicted by these risk factors by 50%. Several other risk factors may account for this discrepancy. Possible nontraditional risk factors include insulin resis-tance, insulin levels, and hyperglycemia.

Many of these type 2 diabetic patients have several of these risk factors for CAD. The term, "metabolic syndrome" was first used by Gerald Reaven in 1988 (49) to describe this clustering of risk factors including hypertension, dyslipidemia, hyperglycemia and insu-lin resistance. The National Cholesterol Education Panel (NCEP) Adult Treatment Panel III (ATPIII)guidelines for cholesterol management in 2001 recognized that the metabolic syndrome or atherogenic dyslipidemia as a collection of the risk factors mentioned above, and abdominal obesity.

PATHOPHYSIOLOGY OF DIABETIC CARDIOVASCULAR COMPLICATIONS

The increased risk of CVD in diabetics is partly explained by the clustering of risk factors including dyslipidemia, hypertension, hyperglycemia, hyperinsulinemia, and prothrombotic factors. Some of these risk factors will be described in detail in this chapter.

Insulin Levels, Insulin Resistance, and Hyperglycemia

Insulin resistance that is present many years or more before the clinical onset of overt diabetes resistance is associated with other atherogenic risk factors such as hypertension, lipid abnormalities, and a procoagulant state (50–56) (Table 1), that promotes atheroscle-rosis many years before overt hyperglycemia ensues (57,58). Indeed, several studies have shown an inverse correlation between insulin sensitivity and atherosclerosis (59–61). Investigators using the Bruneck Study database suggest (62) that these risk factors are present in 84% of patients with type 2 diabetes. Thus, an increased prevalence of CAD is apparent in patients with impaired glucose tolerance (44,46,63) and in newly diagnosed type 2 subjects (64,65). The duration of insulin resistance among hyperglycemic and diabetic individuals probably contributes to the development atherosclerosis. However, no obvious association between the extent or severity of macrovascular complications and the duration or severity of type 2 (24,66) has been found, which most likely stems from the fact the duration of insulin resistance is often unknown.

Another possibility is that the serum insulin level and not insulin resistance may have direct cardiovascular effects. Despres (67) and colleagues followed 2000 nondiabetic men without clinically overt CAD for 5 years and found that those subjects who had a cardiovascular event had 18% higher serum insulin levels than controls.

Serum glucose levels may be an important risk factor for CVD. Anderssen and col-leagues (68) demonstrated that the fasting serum glucose levels are independently related to all-cause and cardiovascular mortality. The San Antonio Heart Study (69) showed similar findings with subjects in the highest quartile of fasting glucose levels had a 4.7 times greater risk of CVD than the lowest two quartile levels combined.

The direct relationship between glucose levels and CVD is also seen in patients with type 1 diabetes. A 1% increase in glycosylated hemoglobin levels doubled the increase in CVD (70). Several studies have shown a direct relationship with the level of serum glucose on clinical events, including MI and strokes, with glucose levels ranging from abnormal glucose tolerance test to frank diabetes (71–73). This graded effect of serum

Table 1
Cardiovascular Risk Factors Associated With Insulin Resistance

Hypertension *(50,51)*
Abdominal obesity *(56,52)*
Dyslipidemia *(53–55,281)*
   Increased VLDL-triglyceride
   Decreased HDL
   Small dense atherogenic LDL particles
   Postprandial lipemia
Elevated PAI-1 activity *(57)*

Numbers in parenthesis represent reference citations. VLDL, very low-density lipoprotein; HDL, high-density lipoprotein; LDL,low-density lipoprotein; PAI-1, plasminogen activator inhibitor.

glucose on clinical events may in part be as a result of a direct effect on the vasculature as evidenced by a similar direct relationship of serum glucose levels to the intima-media thickness (IMT) of the carotid (as a marker for the presence and degree of atherosclerosis). The Atherosclerosis Risk in Communities study demonstrated that the effect of fasting glucose tolerance on carotid wall thickness in individuals free of symptomatic CVD *(8)*.

The level of chronic hyperglycemia, as determined by measurements of glycosylated hemoglobin, may also be an independent risk factor for coronary heart disease, particularly in women *(74,75)*. Recent prospective studies demonstrated that microalbuminuria in type 2 diabetic patients, is also an independent predictor of increased cardiovascular mortality *(76,77)*. In a substudy of the Heart Outcomes Prevention Evaluation Study (HOPE) trial, the MICRO-HOPE demonstrated that increasing levels of microalbuminuria correlated with an increased risk of major cardiovascular events (MI, stroke, cardiovascular death, and a secondary endpoint of hospitalization for heart failure) *(211)*. Insulin resistance may play an important role as a risk factor in the development of diabetic CVD. Hyperinsulinemia may be the mechanism by which the effect of hyperglycemia results in atherosclerosis. Insulin is elevated in patients with the metabolic syndrome. The possibility that insulin resistance could result in an increase in CVD was first demonstrated in population studies, which showed an association between fasting insulin levels and cardiovascular mortality *(59,78–80)*. In the Insulin Resistance Atherosclerosis Study, subjects were evenly divided between patients with normal serum glucose, hyperglycemia with normal glucose tolerance along with diabetes. The relationship of insulin levels and CVD is further strengthened by basic research studies which showed the effect of insulin on various possible mediators for the development of atherosclerosis, specifically the increase in PAI-1 and the mitogenic effect on smooth muscle cells (SMC) in vitro *(81)*.

Dyslipidemia

An important mechanism for the development of diabetic atherosclerosis is dyslipidemia (*see also* Chapter 15).

The central feature of diabetic dyslipidemia is increased levels of VLDLs, as a result of both increased production of VLDL, and decreased catabolism of triglyceride-rich lipoproteins, including chylomicrons. Increased hepatic production of VLDL is in response to increased fatty acid delivery from (a) decreased free fatty acid (FFA) uptake from the striated muscle and (b) increased delivery of the FFAs from the increased adipose tissue associated with central obesity.

The increase in triglyceride-rich lipoproteins not only accumulates because of increased VLDL production but also as a result of decreased catabolism of triglyceride lipoproteins. Lipoprotein lipase, which plays an important role in the metabolism of triglyceride-rich lipoproteins and in particular chylomicrons, is decreased in uncontrolled type 2 diabetes.

The increased triglyceride-rich lipoproteins provide an increased substrate for the cholesterol ester transfer protein. This promotes the flux of cholesterol from HDL particles, which result in decreased HDL levels, a common finding in type 2 DM. Yet other mechanisms must be involved because low HDL levels can occur in the absence of hypertriglyceridemia. The degree of HDL reduction is not related to the degree of control of diabetes or the mode of treatment in type 2 diabetes. One mechanism for the protective effect of HDL against atherosclerosis may be as a result of its ability to prevent oxidation of LDL. There may be qualitative differences in the HDL from patients of poorly controlled DM, which may make it a less effective antioxidant than HDL from normal individuals (82).

Although the dyslipidemia of DM is not characterized by marked elevations of LDL, there are differences in the LDL type found in type 2 diabetics. Specifically, the LDL is smaller and denser than typical LDL particles (83). These smaller denser LDL particles have a greater tendency to undergo oxidation, which accelerates the atherosclerotic process.

Increased Oxidative Stress in Diabetes Mellitus

There is recent evidence that increased oxidative stress in DM contributes to the development of diabetic complications (84). This increased stress may in part be as a result of the decreased availability of antioxidants such as ascorbic acid, vitamin E, uric acid, and glutathionine. Additionally, there may be increased lipid peroxidation products and superoxide anion products. The increase in these products along with the production of superoxide anion production observed in diabetic patients may lead to altered vascular function (84–86).

This increased in oxidative stress may be the result of several pathways including AGE production, small, dense LDL formation, altered polyol activity, or imbalance in the redox state (87). The activation of this polyol pathway is as a result of the conversion of glucose to sorbitol via aldolase reductase, which has been associated with microvascular complications (88,89).

The recent data from the HOPE trial have shown that the treatment with the antioxidant vitamin E at 400 IU per day for a mean of 4.5 years had no apparent effect on cardiovascular morbidity or mortality in both diabetics and nondiabetics (90). Dr. King's group (see Chapter 2) has demonstrated rather intriguing results demonstrating that high-dose vitamin E therapy (1800 IU per day) normalizes retinal hemodynamic abnormalities and improves renal function without improving glycemic control in type I diabetic patients of short duration (91). Whether this effect is via antioxidant-dependent or -independent pathways remains to be elucidated.

Oxidative stress also precedes the formation of some AGEs including pentosidine and N-(carboxymethyl) lysine (CML) and the activation of the diacylglycerol-protein kinase C pathway (DAG-PKC).

Advanced Glycation End-Products in Diabetes Mellitus

Those products, which occur as a result of the nonenzymatic glycation of both lipids and proteins, are termed AGEs (*see also* Chapter 11). Initially a labile covalent bond develops between the aldehyde of the glucose molecule and the amino acid side chain on both sugars and lipids. Specifically, glucose is covalently bound mainly to lysine residues in proteins, forming fructose-lysine residues. This reaction, results in the development of a Schiff base, which, in turn, undergoes another chemical reaction to form a ketoamine, termed an Amadori product. These products result in cumulative oxidative damage to proteins. These products include CML *(92)* and pentosidine *(93)*. The increased levels of pentosidine and CML correlate with the severity of diabetic complications including nephropathy, retinopathy, and vascular disease. One such Amadori product is glycated hemoglobin A1c, which is commonly used to monitor glycemic control in diabetic patients. Because both free radical oxidation and glycation are involved, these substances are also called glyoxidation products.

AGEs crosslink to the proteins composing the extracellular matrix (ECM) and vascular basement membrane, which result in reduced solubility and decreased enzymatic digestion *(94,95)*. AGE formation prevents proper assembly of basement proteins thereby altering its function. This in turn may alter the ability of cells to bind to their substrates.

AGEs are also derived from oxidation of lipids *(96,97)*. The side chains of unsaturated fatty acids chains undergo oxidation, which yield reactive carbonyl-containing fragments (MDA, glyoal, 4-HNE) and then react with amino groups, mainly lysine residues.

Enhanced glycation, oxidation and glyoxidation of lipoproteins have been postulated as a possible cause for the development of diabetic macrovascular disease. Certainly there are increased levels of AGE-modified LDL apoprotein and LDL lipid relative to nondiabetics *(98)*. This would suggest that even in the face of similar glycemic control and other cardiovascular risk factors, the development of diabetic vascular complications would depend on differences of oxidative stress and the tissue level of antioxidants.

The evidence for this possible role of these altered lipoproteins include the presence of oxidized lipoproteins in the vessel wall *(99,100)* and the demonstration of lesion regression with antioxidants *(101)*. One study *(102)* showed the susceptibility to oxidation of LDL correlated with the degree of atherosclerosis in 35 male survivors of a MI.

Vlassara *(103)* identified a specific receptor for AGEs on monocyte/macrophages, termed RAGE (receptor for AGEs). The subsequent interaction with the AGE and its receptor may induce the release of cytokines tumor necrosis factor and interleukin-1 *(104)*. Other cytokines that have been demonstrated include the synthesis and release of procoagulant activity and platelet-activating factor by endothelial cells *(105,106)* and the induction of platelet-derived growth factor-AA, which can be indirectly responsible for fibroblast and smooth muscle proliferation *(107)*. Furthermore increased RAGE interaction has been shown to result in the enhanced expression of the vascular cell adhesion molecule *(108–110)*, which in turn results in increased atherogenesis.

The important role of RAGE in the development of atherosclerosis was further strengthened by the demonstration that usually atherosclerotic apolipoprotein E-knockout mice had less atherosclerosis when they were administered an antibody-fragment, which neutralized RAGE *(111)*. This effect was seen without any effect on glycemic control or lipoprotein profile.

Thrombosis and Fibrinolysis in Diabetes Mellitus

Plaque disruption with overlying thrombosis is a major cause of acute coronary syndromes (ACS) including MI and sudden death and strokes (*see also* Chapter 6). Because patients with both type I and particularly type II DM have higher rates of both ACS than the nondiabetic population, heightened arterial prothrombotic reactivity may play a pivotal role in the development of these macrovascular complications.

There are three underlying mechanisms for this prothrombosis. This includes heightened platelet reactivity, increased procoagulant activity, and decreased antithrombotic and fibrinolytic activity. The principal components of a thrombus include platelets and fibrin. The coagulation is initiated by the exposure of tissue factor within the arterial plaque at time of plaque disruption. This results in the activation of factor VII/VIIa, which forms the tenase complex with factors X and V resulting in the activation of thrombin. Thrombin stimulates platelet reactivity and the conversion of fibrinogen to fibrin, producing a thrombus.

The platelets of diabetic individuals appear to have increased adherence to the vessel wall an increased circulating platelet mass (*112*). Platelet aggregometry studies which measures in vitro platelet reactivity have demonstrated increased aggregation of platelets in response to agonists adenosine diphosphate, collagen, and thrombin and even spontaneous aggregation of platelets without any agonist (*113–117*). Assessment of platelet reactivity in vivo by measurement of blood or urine metabolites released from activated platelets like thromboxane B2 are increased relative to normal healthy controls (*113,114*).

Patients with DM have increased concentrations of fibrinogen, von Willebrand factor and factor VII (*118–120*). Although the mechanisms of the increased concentrations of these factors have yet to be elucidated, the level of serum fibrinogen correlates with the level of proinsulin and insulin in the blood (*121*). However, the plasma level of fibrinogen level is not reduced with improved metabolic control nor is there a reduction of plasma prothrombin fragment 1 + 2, a cleavage product of prothrombin.

Several reports indicate that the activity of antithrombotic factors, including protein C and anti-thrombins, are decreased in diabetic subjects, which further potentiates the hypercoaguable state (*122–125*).

Fibrinolysis is also impaired in diabetic individuals, particularly type 2 diabetics (*126,127*). This impairment may be as a result of the increased activity of PAI-1 in the blood, which counteracts native tissue plasminogen activator (t-PA) or t-PA's action to induce fibrinolysis. PAI-1 is elevated not only in resting states but also in response to physiological stimuli. The serum level of PAI-1 may be elevated as a result of several factors including elevated serum insulin, serum lipids, and glucose levels (*128*). The impairment of the fibrinolysis system can potentially exacerbate the development and persistence of thrombi, resulting in an increased risk of vascular occlusion.

Endothelial Function and Diabetes Mellitus

Alterations in endothelial function may play an important role in the development of diabetic complications (*see also* Chapters 2 and 10). Decreased blood flow in many organs has been reported, including the kidney, retina, and peripheral retinal nerves. Recent diabetics have decreased retinal blood flow on the basis of increased vascular resistance. The mechanism of this increased vascular resistance is probably in part as a result of the increase in the intercellular signal transduction kinase, protein kinase C

(PKC) (129-132). This increase in PKC may result in an increase in endothelin-1. It has been documented that abnormalities in hemodynamic profiles precede diabetic nephropathy. This increase in glomerular filtration is probably as a result of the effect of hyperglycemia has on arteriolar resistance.

The vascular endothelium has been shown to be important in modulating blood cell–vessel wall interaction, regulating blood flow, angiogenesis, lipoprotein metabolism, and vasomotion. An important mediator in maintaining vascular homeostasis is endothelium-derived relaxing factor (EDRF) (133). EDRF has since been found to be nitric oxide (NO) (134). The release of NO activates soluble guanylate cyclase, resulting in the formation of cyclic guanosine monophosphate (cGMP), which, in turn, activates cGMP-dependent protein kinases resulting in vascular smooth muscle relaxation (135–138). Alterations in its elaboration or activity may play an important role in the initiation and progression of both micro- and macrovascular disease. Several studies have shown that endothelial-dependent vasodilator function is impaired in patients with type 1 DM without hypertension and dyslipidemia (139). This is in contradistinction to patients with type 2 DM, which have an impairment of both endothelial-dependent and endothelial-independent (smooth muscle) vasodilator function (140,141).

Although the mechanism for the impaired endothelial-dependent vasodilation is unknown, several possibilities are present. Acute hyperglycemia impairs endothelial-dependent vasodilation in both macro- and microvessels (142). Normally, insulin also may play a role. Insulin results in vasodilation in part as a result of NO production. However, glucose clamp experiments with insulin infusion in type 2 diabetic subjects have shown little improvement in endothelial-dependent vasodilation relative to nondiabetic subjects (142). As stated previously, there appears to be an increase in oxygen-derived free radicals in the diabetic state. Several studies have shown that high doses of vitamin C can improve endothelial-dependent vasodilation in both type 1 and type 2 diabetics (143,144). Intensive lipid lowering by statin therapy does not improve vasoreactivity in patients with type 2 diabetes, suggesting that mechanisms than dyslipidemia are responsible for endothelial dysfunction (145).

Another possible culprit for this impairment of endothelial function found in diabetic individuals may be the endogenous competitive inhibitor of NO synthase, asymmetric dimethylarginine (ADMA) (146). ADMA has been found to be elevated in diabetic subjects (147,148).

CLINICAL FEATURES OF CARDIOVASCULAR DISEASE IN DIABETES MELLITUS

Angiographic Features of CAD in Diabetic Patients

Autopsy, angiographic, and angioscopic studies have documented the severe and diffuse nature of the atherosclerotic coronary involvement in diabetic patients. Early autopsy data has shown that diabetic patients have a greater number of coronary vessels involved with more diffuse distribution of atherosclerotic lesions (149,150). Large angiographic studies comparing diabetics to matched controls in the setting of acute MI (151), elective angioplasty (152), or prior to coronary bypass surgery (153) have all shown that diabetes is associated with significantly more severe proximal and distal CAD (Table 2). An important finding regarding the pathogenesis of ACS is the autopsy (154) and angioscopic (155) evidence suggesting a significant increase in plaque ulceration and thrombosis in diabetic compared to nondiabetic patients.

Table 2
Angiographic Studies in Diabetic Patients[a]

Study (reference)	Patients (n)		% of patients with multivessel disease[b]		p Value
	Diabetics	Nondiabetic	Diabetic	Nondiabetic	
TAMI (151)	148	923	65[c]	46	0.0001
TIMI-II (382)	439[d]	2900	40.8	26.8	< 0.001
Orlander (180)	236	348	58.2	41.6	< 0.001
Stein et al. (152)	1133	9300	32.4[e]	28.2	< 0.004
BARI (228)	353	1476	46	40	< 0.05
NHLBI (247)	281	1833	27.7	17.7	< 0.01
CASS (153)	317	1843	85.8	77.7	< 0.001

[a]Because most patients undergoing initial angioplasty have single-vessel disease, they have milder coronary artery disease than patients with acute myocardial infarction who have an array of single-, double-, and triple-vessel disease, or patients undergoing coronary bypass grafting who usually have double- and triple-vessel disease.

[b]Multivessel disease is defined by the presence of two or more vessels with at least one stenosis >75%.

[c]For men. Corresponding values for women are 63% and 41%.

[d]Not all patients underwent angiography.

[e]Patients were selected for angioplasty and therefore this study includes a larger portion of patients with single-vessel disease.

TAMI, Thrombolysis and Angioplasty in Myocardial Infarction; TIMI, Thrombolysis in Myocardial Infarction; BARI, Bypass Angioplasty Revascularization Investigation; NHLBI, National Heart, Lung, and Blood Institute; CASS, Coronary Artery Surgery Study.

Silent Ischemia

The propensity of diabetic patients to present with either silent or unrecognized MI is well established (156,157). Atypical symptoms such as confusion, dyspnea, fatigue, or nausea and vomiting were the presenting complaint in 32% to 42% of diabetic patients with MI compared to 6% to 15% of nondiabetic patients (156,158). Several groups have reported that the detection of silent ischemia using various noninvasive techniques including treadmill exercise testing (159,160) ambulatory holter monitoring (161), or exercise thallium scintigraphy (162–165), is more common in diabetics than in nondiabetics. This finding, however, is not supported by all studies (166,167).

A plausible explanation for painless infarction and ischemia episodes in diabetics is autonomic neuropathy with involvement of the sensory supply to the heart is. In autopsies of diabetic patients who died of silent MIs, typical diabetic neuropathic changes were found in the intracardiac sympathetic and parasympathetic fibers (168), and several studies correlated abnormalities in autonomic function in patients with silent ischemia (159,161,163,169). The anginal perceptual threshold—the time from the onset of myocardial ischemia (assessed by ST-segment depression) to the onset of chest pain during exercise testing is prolonged in diabetic patients compared with nondiabetics. This delay in the perception of pain may be related to the impairment of autonomic nervous function (169). This association of silent ischemia with autonomic neuropathy was strengthened with the recent results of the Detection of Ischemia in Asymptomatic Diabetics (DIAB) study (170), which found that 22% of asymptomatic patients had abnormal stress perfusion tests. Abnormal results were not associated with traditional risk factors but rather a low heart rate response to Valsalva maneuvers, indicating this association with autonomic neuropathy.

ACUTE CORONARY SYNDROMES IN DIABETIC PATIENTS

Acute ischemic events represent a major cause of death in the diabetic population *(64)*. Diabetics who suffer MIs have a higher mortality than nondiabetics both in the acute phase and on long-term follow-up. Numerous studies have shown that in-hospital mortality rates from MIs in diabetic patients are 1.5- to twofold higher than in nondiabetic patients *(151,171–174)*. DM remains an independent predictor for a poor prognosis in the thrombolytic era. In the Thrombolysis and Angioplasty in Myocardial Infarction (TAMI) trials the in hospital mortality rate was nearly twice as high in patients with diabetes, with more congestive heart failure (CHF) and twice the rate of clinically recognized reinfarction *(151)*. In the Global Utilization of Streptokinase and Tissue Plasminogen Activator for Occluded Coronary Arteries (GUSTO)-I trial, mortality at 30 days was highest among diabetic patients treated with insulin (12.5%) compared with noninsulin-treated diabetic (9.7%) and nondiabetic (6.2%) patients ($p < 0.001$) *(175)*. Similar results have been reported from the other large studies *(176–178)*. Diabetes is also a risk factor for cardiogenic shock in the setting of acute ischemic syndromes *(179)*. Overall, despite the overall improvement in survival from an acute MI with thrombolysis, the in-hospital mortality rates in diabetics remain 1.5–2 times higher than in nondiabetics *(175,178)*.

Increased in-hospital mortality among diabetic patients with acute MI is predominantly as a result of a higher increased incidence of CHF *(172,174,180,181)*, although increased reinfarction, infarct extension, and recurrent ischemia have also been reported *(172–174,181,182)*.

Studies using serial determinations of total creatine kinase activity *(180,181)*, radionuclide ventriculography *(183)*, or echocardiography have shown no evidence that diabetic patients sustain more extensive infarctions than their nondiabetic counterparts *(184)*. Thus, CHF and cardiogenic shock are more common and more severe in diabetic subjects than would be expected from the size of the index infarction *(178,180,181,183,185,186)*. The observation that clinical manifestations of heart failure occur in diabetic patients despite a modest decrease in left ventricular ejection fraction (LVEF), led to the suggestion that pre-existing diastolic dysfunction is a major culprit of the congestive symptoms *(174)*. Indeed, subclinical diabetic cardiomyopathy, which is characterized by diastolic dysfunction *(187)*, is likely to be an important factor in this setting.

However, it should be emphasized that a reduction in both LVEF *(183,188)* and the regional ejection fraction (EF) of the noninfarcted myocardium *(151,183,187)* have been well-documented in diabetic patients following MI compared with nondiabetics. One such study examined early angiography in the TAMI cohort and found worse noninfarct zone ventricular function in diabetics *(151)* relative to the nondiabetic controls.

The performance of the left ventricle following MI is largely determined by extent of coronary disease *(189)* and the quality of collateral circulation. Thus, the diffuse nature of coronary atherosclerosis (Table 2) in diabetes may contribute to systolic dysfunction of the noninfarcted myocardium. Moreover, a recent study has shown that diabetic patients have a reduced ability to develop collateral blood vessels in the presence of CAD *(190)*, a finding that may also explain the more frequent occurrence of postinfarction angina and infarct extension *(173,174,182,184)* in diabetic subjects.

Diabetic patients surviving MI also suffer high late mortality rates compared with nondiabetics *(174,182,191–193)*. Late mortality is mainly related to both recurrent MI and the development of new congestive heart failure *(176,178,184,192–194)*.

MEDICAL THERAPY OF CORONARY ARTERY DISEASE IN DIABETIC PATIENTS

Diabetes exerts a deleterious effect on both short- and long-term course following MI through diverse mechanisms, some of which (e.g., cardiomyopathy) cannot be modified at the time of presentation. Because diabetic patients are at greater risk, application of effective preventive and treatment measures may result in a particularly large survival benefit.

Insulin

One possible mechanism for the increased mortality of diabetic patients with acute MI may be the altered metabolism of the myocardium. The diabetic state results in increased fatty acid metabolism, compromising glycolysis in both ischemic and nonischemic territories. FFAs and their intermediates may potentiate ischemic injury. One way to attenuate FFA oxidation is by the infusion of insulin-glucose. It was that rationale that led Malmberg and colleagues *(195)* to evaluate the effect of insulin-glucose infusion followed by multidose insulin treatment in diabetic patients (Diabetes Mellitus Insulin-Glucose Infusion in Acute Myocardial Infarction [DIGAMI] study) (Fig. 2). Diabetic patients with an acute MI within the previous 24 hours were randomized to two separate arms. Insulin-glucose infusion was given for the first 24 hours and until stable normoglycemia. in the experimental arm. Then subcutaneous multidose insulin was given to maintain normoglycemia for a 3-month period. Control patients received standard coronary care unit care and did not receive insulin unless clinically indicated.

The 3-month mortality was not significantly different between the control and experimental groups. However, the 1-year mortality was 18.6% in the experimental group and 26% in the control group, or a relative risk reduction of approx 30%. This improvement of mortality continued for 3.4 years, with an absolute reduction of mortality of 11% *(196)*.

A recent study investigating the benefit of glucose–insulin–potassium (GIK) infusion as adjunctive therapy to percutaneous transluminal coronary angioplasty (PTCA) in acute ST-elevation MI (Glucose-Insulin-Potassium Study) demonstrated a significant reduction in the 30-day mortality but only if those patients that had no signs or symptoms of heart failure *(195)*. There was a 3% absolute risk reduction (1.2% vs 4.2%) in the 30-day mortality seen in those patients presenting with Killip Class I and who received GIK.

Aspirin

Studies have shown an increased platelet adhesiveness and aggregability *(197)*, with a concomitant increased release of thromboxane A2 *(114)* in diabetic subjects. Based on these data, several authors stated that diabetics may require larger doses of aspirin to suppress thromboxane A2 synthesis *(114,198)*. Furthermore, in the International Study of Infarction Survival-2 there was no reduction in mortality in diabetics receiving 160 mg of aspirin daily *(199)*.

The Antiplatelet Trialist Collaboration meta-analysis quantified the benefit of aspirin in diabetic patients who have had a previous cardiovascular event *(200)*. The relative benefit on vascular events was 17% in the diabetic patients and 22% in those without diabetes. Although the number was lower for diabetic patients than for nondiabetic patients in terms of percentage benefit, the absolute number of events prevented was similar in the two groups (38 ± 12 per thousand compared with 36 ± 3 per thousand, respectively) probably because of the higher event rates in diabetic patients. Data from

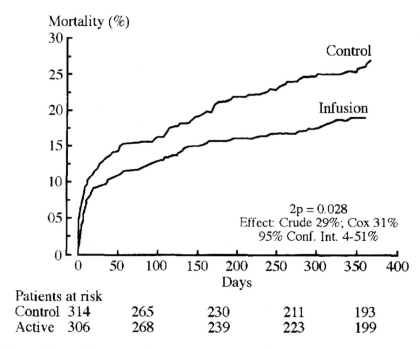

Fig. 2. Actuarial mortality curves in the patients receiving insulin-glucose infusion and in he control goup of the present Diabetes Mellitus Insulin-Glucose Infusion in Acute Myocardial Infarction study during 1 year of follow-up. Numbers below graph, number of patients at different times of observation. Active, patients receiving infusion; Con. Int., confidence interval. (Reproduced with permission from ref. *195*.)

the US Physicians' Health Study and the Early Treatment Diabetic Retinopathy Study (ETDRS) indicates that aspirin may also be efficacious as primary prevention in diabetic patients *(201)*.

A major risk of aspirin therapy is gastric mucosal injury and gastrointestinal hemorrhage. These effects are dose-related and are reduced to placebo levels when enteric-coated preparations of 75–325 mg per day are used once daily *(202)*. The ETDRS established that aspirin therapy is not associated with an increased risk of retinal or vitreous hemorrhage using serial retinal photography.

The American Diabetes Association recommends the use of aspirin therapy (81–325 mg per day) as secondary prevention in any patient with evidence of large vessel disease. Aspirin is also recommended as primary prevention in diabetic patients with the following: (a) family history of CAD, (b) cigarette smoking, (c) hypertension, (d) obesity, (e) albuminuria, (f) LDL greater than 130 mg/dL (g) HDL less than 40 mg/dL, (h) triglycerides over 250 mg/dL *(202)*.

β-*Blockers*

β-blockers are effective in reducing reinfarction and sudden death in diabetic patients, perhaps to a greater extent than in nondiabetics. Early treatment of MI with β-blockers resulted in a 37% mortality reduction in diabetics compared with a 13% mortality reduction in all patients, whereas long-term mortality reduction was 48% and 33% in diabetics and all patients, respectively *(203)*.

In a controlled study evaluating the use of atenolol in patients with, or at risk for CAD who had noncardiac surgery, diabetes was the strongest predictor of death after 2 years follow-up, with twice the mortality compared with nondiabetics *(204)*. Compared with nondiabetic patients, diabetic patients on atenolol had no increased risk of death, whereas those given placebo had a fourfold increase in risk *(204)*. It should be emphasized that the deterioration in glycemic control or blunted counterregulatory response to hypoglycemia are seldom a serious clinical problem, especially when cardioselective β1-blockers are used *(203,205)*.

Angiotensin-Converting Enzyme Inhibition

ACE inhibition is now unequivocally associated with a substantial mortality reduction in patients surviving MI with left ventricular dysfunction (EF <40%) *(206)*. The Italian Study Group for Streptokinase in Myocardial Infarction-3 investigators compared the effect of early administration (within 24 hours of admission) of lisinopril in patients with and without diabetes presenting with MI *(207)*. Compared to placebo, lisinopril dramatically reduced both 6 week (30% vs 5%) and 6-month (20% vs 0%) mortality in diabetics vs nondiabetics. These finding are corroborated by subgroup analysis of the Survival and Ventricular Enlargement Study (SAVE) study *(208)*. A retrospective analysis of data from the Trandolapril Cardiac Evaluation study, a randomized, double-blind, placebo-controlled trial evaluating trandolapril in patients after acute MI with an EF less than or equal to 35%, has shown a 36% reduction of death from any cause and a 62% reduction in the risk of progression to severe heart failure *(209)*. Recently, the HOPE study has shown that ramipril substantially lower the risk of death, MI, stroke, coronary revascularization, heart failure, and complications related to DM in a high-risk group of patients with pre-existing vascular disease *(210,211)* (Fig. 3). Interestingly, there was also a 33% relative risk reduction in the incidence of new cases of DM in the ramipril arm of the HOPE study.

ACE inhibitors have become the primary agents of choice for the treatment of hypertension associated with DM, because they do not adversely affect the glycemic control and lipid profile *(212,213)*. In fact, ACE inhibitors may actually enhance insulin sensitivity in noninsulin-dependent diabetes mellitus (NIDDM) patients, with or without hypertension *(214–216)*. ACE inhibitors are especially desirable in patients with evidence of diabetic nephropathy.

Serum potassium and creatinine should be monitored closely in the first few weeks of therapy. A rapid decline in renal function can occur in patients with bilateral renal artery stenosis, which is more common in diabetics. Hyporeninemic hypoaldosteronism (type IV renal tubular acidosis) is frequently associated with diabetes and predisposes the patients to clinically significant hyperkalemia when ACE inhibitors are initiated.

Glycoprotein IIb/IIIa Antagonists

These antiplatelet agents have become an important therapeutic modality in the treatment of unstable angina and non-Q wave MIs. In particular, these agents have been shown to be equal if not more beneficial in the diabetic population than its nondiabetic counterpart. The Platelet Receptor Inhibition in Ischemic Syndrome Management in Patients Limited by Unstable Signs and Symptoms (PRISM-PLUS) study *(217,218)* compared heparin to heparin and the glycoprotein (Gp)IIb/IIIa inhibitor tirofiban in 1208 patients, with 362 patients being diabetic. The cumulative end-point at 7 days of death, MI,

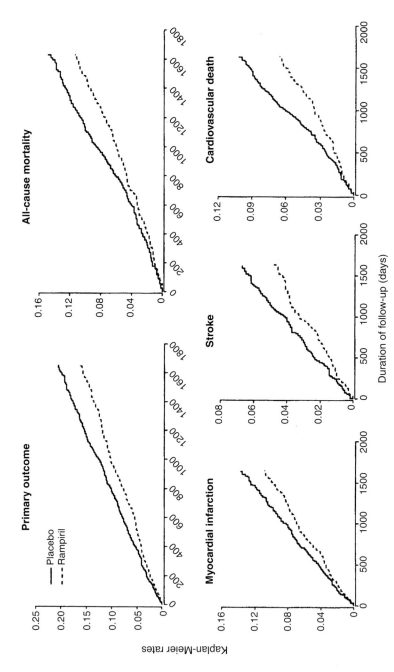

Fig. 3. Kaplan–Meier survival curves for study participants with diabetes in the HOPE Study comparing the use of ramipril (——) vs placebo (-). (Reproduced with permission from ref. *211*.)

refractory angina or re-hospitalizations for unstable angina was reduced from 21.4% on heparin alone and 14.8% on heparin plus tirofiban in the diabetic group and 16.7% on heparin alone to 12.4% with the addition of tirofiban in the nondiabetic group. There was no difference in the ability of the standard dose of tirofiban required to result in an over 80% inhibition of platelet aggregation after a 12-hour infusion in the diabetic and non-diabetic patients, despite the hyperaggregability of diabetic platelets.

The EPILOG study (219), which evaluated percutaneous coronary angioplasty plus the GpIIb/IIIa, abciximab to angioplasty alone, found no significant difference in acute events although the longer-term follow-up revealed a higher rate of subsequent revascularization involving the target vessel in diabetic subjects. The Evaluation of Platelet IIb/IIIa Inhibitor for Stenting Trial (EPISTENT) (220), which evaluated coronary stenting plus abciximab and heparin vs stenting plus heparin alone demonstrated a marked decrease of target vessel revascularization in diabetic patients. The rate of target vessel revascularization in diabetic patients randomized to stenting and heparin was 16.6% although those randomized to stenting and abciximab had a rate of 8.1%, a 50% decrease. One recent study (221) did not demonstrate a difference in efficacy between two GpIIb/IIIa receptor inhibitors, abciximab or tirofiban, when used in diabetic patients undergoing percutaneous coronary intervention (PCI).

Thrombolytic Therapy

Thrombolytic therapy is of substantial benefit in diabetic patients. In the GUSTO-I angiographic substudy, early infarct-related artery patency (TIMI flow grade 3) and reocclusion rates were similar among diabetics and nondiabetics (222). Diabetic patients treated with various fibrinolytic agents benefit by the same mortality reduction as non-diabetic patients (151,223) (Table 3). In an overview of fibrinolytic trials in patients with MI, the relative reduction in 35-day mortality was slightly, but not significantly, greater in diabetic patients than in nondiabetic patients (21.7% vs 14.3%) (223). In these trials, no increase in serious bleeding complications or stroke was observed in patients with diabetes. Retinal bleeding is an extremely uncommon complication of thrombolytic therapy in diabetic patients. In the GUSTO-I study, 300 of 6011 diabetic patients had proliferative retinopathy, but none developed intraocular hemorrhage (224). It is unlikely that thrombolytic therapy would increase vitreous hemorrhage, which is the result of vitreous detachment in patients with diabetic retinopathy. Thus, the concern that many clinicians have, regarding thrombolytic therapy in patients with diabetic retinopathy, is not supported by the results of large clinical trials. It is probably unjustified to deny these patients the proven life saving benefit of thrombolysis.

REVASCULARIZATION PROCEDURES IN DIABETIC PATIENTS

Because CAD is a major health problem in patients with diabetes, the need for revascularization procedure arises frequently (*see also* Chapters 25, 26). Therefore, many diabetic patients require some form of revascularization procedure. Significant and increasing proportion of patients undergoing angioplasty is diabetic. In the 1977 to 1981 National Heart, Lung, and Blood Institute (NHLBI) registry, 9% of patients undergoing angioplasty were diabetics (225). Recent large trials suggest that the prevalence of diabetes in patients undergoing angioplasty increased to approx 17% to 19% (226,227). The influence of diabetes on outcome after revascularization procedures received attention following the results of the Bypass Angioplasty Revascularization Investigation (BARI)

Table 3
Effect of Thrombolytic Therapy in Diabetic Patients

Study (reference)	Thrombolytic agent	Patients (n)		In-hospital/short term ortality (%)		
		Nondiabetics	Diabetics	Nondiabetics	Diabetics	p Value
ISIS-2 (199)	SK	15694	1287	8.9	11.8[b]	NR
FTT collaborative group (223)	SK, rt-PA, UK, APSAC	38814	4529	8.7	13.6[c]	NR
TAMI (151)	rt-PA, UK	923	148	6	11	< 0.02
International t‑PA/ SK (223)	rt-PA, SK	8055	833	7.5[d]	11.8	< 0.001[e]
Streptokinase mortality trial						
GISSI-2 (178)	rt-PA, SK	8069	1266	5.8[f]	8.7	NR
TIMI (382)	rt-PA	2900	439	4.1	10.2	
GUSTO (222)	rt-PA, SK	34705	6125	6.2	10.6	< 0.0001[h]

study, which suggested that diabetic patients with significant CAD involving the left anterior descending coronary artery had improved mortality if they underwent a coronary artery bypass grafting (CABG) *(228)*. The results of the Coronary Angioplasty vs Bypass Revascularization Investigation investigators *(229)* demonstrated that the mortality of diabetics is double that of nondiabetics, independent of the means of revascularization, be it CABG or PTCA. Among diabetics or nondiabetics there was no significant mortality difference between PTCA or CABG, although there was a trend favoring CABG, especially in the diabetic population *(229)*.

Percutaneous Coronary Interventions

PCI provides effective relief of angina in most patients and performed with similar success in diabetics as in nondiabetics *(152)*. However, increased restenosis rates in diabetic patients greatly limit long-term benefit from such interventions. The importance of diabetes as a clinical risk factor restenosis after PCI has been demonstrated in multiple studies. The initial report from the NHLBI Angioplasty Registry indicated that the angiographic restenosis rate in diabetic patients was 47%, as compared to 32% in nondiabetic patients *(230)*, and subsequent studies have reported restenosis rates of 49%-71% among diabetic patients *(231–236)*. New angioplasty devices also initially failed to make any major impact on the restenosis rate among diabetics. Diabetes is associated with a twofold increase in recurrent clinical events after directional coronary atherectomy *(237) (238,239)*, have with higher restenosis rates after excimer laser angioplasty *(240)*. Recently, intracoronary stents have been shown to decrease restenosis compared with PTCA *(241)*. Even with stents, several groups have reported that diabetic patients have higher restenosis rates compared to nondiabetic patients *(242–245)* although this finding is debated *(246)*.

The full impact of the higher PCI restenosis, on cardiovascular morbidity of diabetic patients is significant. Numerous studies have shown that diabetic patients experience a greater need for repeat revascularization (angioplasty or CABG), a high cardiac event rate, and lower overall survival rates, following coronary angioplasty compared with their nondiabetic counterparts *(152,237,239,247–250)*. Recent data from the EPISTENT and other studies *(251)* suggest that the combination of stenting with platelet GpIIb/IIIa blockade may decrease the incidence of death, MI, and target-vessel revascularization among diabetic patients *(252)*.

Although vessel recoil may also contribute to loss of luminal size, the increased restenosis rate seen in diabetics following stent placement underscores the role of enhanced SMC proliferation as the major mechanism for restenosis in these patients, because coronary artery stenting decreases elastic recoil and vascular spasm at the treated site *(244)*. In a study using intravascular ultrasound, exaggerated intimal proliferation was found in diabetic patients at the site of angioplasty-induced arterial injury, and this proliferative response was particularly striking in restenotic lesions *(253)*. Thus, the diabetic state promotes SMC proliferation and ECM deposition following arterial injury. Surprisingly, the possibility that strict glycemic control may reduce restenosis rates among diabetics *(254)* has not been addressed clinically or experimentally. There are studies ongoing, which are examining means to reduce the restenosis rate including β-radiation (ANTI-PrOliferative Effect of Beta-Radiation on Restenosis Prevention in Diabetic Patients after Coronary Stent Implantation).

In diabetic subjects with restenosis post-PCI, there is a reduced intimal hypercellular tissue in the restenotic lesion relative to nondiabetic patients *(255)*. Sobel's group has found an increase in the intramural synthesis of PAI-1 in the vessel walls of experimental rabbits that were subjected to experimental angioplasty *(256,257)*. PAI-1 synthesis is stimulated by insulin. In turn, PAI-1 may inhibit the remodeling and proteolysis that normally occurs post PCI, resulting in the accumulation of the ECM and lipid, with a relative decrease in the relative amount of SMC migration and proliferation. One recent development has suggested that haptoglobin phenotype may determine which diabetic patients may develop restenosis after coronary stent implantation *(258)*.

Coronary Artery Bypass Surgery

CABG is effective in relieving anginal symptoms in diabetic patients as in nondiabetic patients *(153)* *(see also* Chapter 26). Diabetes is not associated with increased perioperative mortality during bypass graft surgery, although wound infections and the average hospital stay are increased *(259,260)*. Several reports have noted decreased survival of vein grafts in diabetic patients *(261–263)*. Intimal proliferation that causes luminal loss in the first years following bypass surgery with venous conduit may be accelerated in diabetics *(264)*. In contrast, the benefit of internal mammary artery (IMA) conduits is well documented among diabetics *(263,265)*. Data from the Duke registry indicate that the long-term benefit of one IMA graft is at least as great in patients with diabetes as in those without *(265)*. Nonetheless, long-term survival rate after bypass surgery remains consistently lower in diabetic then in nondiabetic patients *(265–267)*.

Percutaneous Coronary Intervention vs Coronary Artery Bypass Surgery in Multivessel CAD

Coronary angioplasty with or without stenting has been widely accepted as the initial revascularization procedure for treatment of most single-vessel CAD, although CABG has been the standard form of revascularization for multivessel disease. However, in the last decade, angioplasty has been proposed and evaluated as an alternative to CABG in patients with multivessel disease.

The influence of diabetes on outcome after PCI for patients with multivessel disease received attention following the results of the Bypass Angioplasty Revascularization Investigation (BARI) study *(228)*. The BARI study enrolled 1829 patients (including 353 diabetics) with angiographycally documented multivessel CAD and either clinically severe angina or objective evidence of marked myocardial ischemia requiring revascularization. Cause of death was classified as cardiac if occurring less than one hour after onset of cardiac symptoms or within one hour to 30 days after a documented or probable MI, or occurring as a result of intractable CHF, cardiogenic shock, or other documented cardiac cause.

A review of 5-year all-cause mortality rates showed a near doubling of mortality among diabetics on insulin or oral therapy assigned to multivessel angioplasty compared with those assigned to surgery (35% vs 19%, $p = 0.003$). In contrast, the 5-year mortality in nondiabetics and diabetics not on drug treatment was 9% with both revascularization strategies. Cause-specific 5.4-year cardiac mortality rates were three-and-a-half times higher in the PTCA group (20.6 % vs 5.8%) *(228)*. These results raised concern about selection of revascularization procedures in diabetic patients with multivessel coronary artery disease, and prompted a NHLBI clinical alert stating that CABG should be the preferred initial revascularization choice in medically treated diabetics with multivessel CAD *(268)*.

A subsequent report from the BARI investigators indicated that the survival benefit of CABG is limited to diabetics receiving an IMA graft. Cardiac mortality after 5.4 years was 2.9% when IMA was used and 18.2% when only saphenous vein graft (SVG) conduits were used. The latter rate was similar to patient receiving PTCA (20.6%) *(269)*. The mortality benefit afforded by IMA was most apparent in those experiencing MI during follow-up (an effect seen also in nondiabetic patients). The cardiac death rate in those diabetics sustaining MI was 36% for diabetics who had a PTCA, 60% for those diabetics who underwent a CABG with only an SVG, and only 7.4% for diabetics who had a CABG with a LIMA. For diabetic patients not sustaining post-randomization MI, a less marked but nonetheless substantial decrease in cardiac mortality was associated with IMA use (5 year cardiac death rates without MI: diabetics who underwent PTCA, 16.8%; diabetics who had a CABG with SVG, 10.7%; TDM-IMA, 1.8%). As an IMA graft is less susceptible to atherosclerosis it may provide an alternative source of perfusion to maintain ventricular function in regions of hypoperfusion resulting from coronary occlusion.

Three recent studies examined the effect of revascularization strategies in diabetic patients. In a large prospective cohort of 3220 patients with multivessel disease, of whom 770 (24%) were diabetics, Barsness and associates evaluated the relationship between diabetes and survival after revascularization with either PTCA or CABG *(270)*. Although diabetes was strongly associated with a worse long-term prognosis, the 5-year survival for diabetics undergoing PTCA was 76%, whereas for nondiabetics the rate was 88%. Similarly, in the group of patients undergoing CABG, 5-year survival was 74% in diabetics and 86% in patients without diabetes. Unlike other studies, however, there was no significant differential effect of diabetes on outcome between patients treated with PTCA and those treated with CABG. In a similar study, Weintraub *(271)* and associates prospectively compared the outcome of PTCA (*n* = 834) and CABG (*n* = 1805) in diabetic patients with multivessel coronary disease using an observational database. Corrected for baseline differences, there was no difference in survival for the group as a whole. However, in the insulin-requiring subgroup, 5- and 10-year survival rates were 68% and 36% after PTCA and 75% and 47% after CABG, respectively.

Gum and associates performed a retrospective outcome analysis of 525 diabetic patients who underwent coronary revascularization. Overall actuarial survival curves showed a nonsignificant trend favoring the CABG group for survival at 6 years (30% vs 37%; *p* = 0.04) *(248)*.

A crucial question is why CABG may be superior to PTCA in diabetic patients in the setting of multivessel disease. The only difference between the diabetic groups in the BARI study is the revascularization procedure chosen. Hence, the prognosis difference is likely to be related to the relative efficacy of these revascularization procedures.

The major advantage of CABG over PTCA is the ability to achieve complete revascularization *(272,273)*. The superiority of CABG over angioplasty in providing complete revascularization is exemplified in the BARI study itself. In the BARI population, 3.1 grafts were placed per patient undergoing CABG *(274)*, whereas the mean number of successfully treated lesions in the PTCA group was 2 *(269)*. Similar numbers are reported by other studies comparing multivessel angioplasty and CABG *(248, 270,271)*.

Previous CABG studies have emphasized that complete revascularization is essential for obtaining survival benefit in patients with multivessel disease *(273)*. If complete revascularization (which is accomplished almost exclusively through CABG surgery) is essential for survival benefit, the successful application of multivessel angioplasty (which entails a selective high-priority lesion-targeting strategy) requires that a comparable proportion of myocardium supplied through high-priority lesions be revascularized by each of the two strategies. Because when multivessel angiograplasty is preformed, multiple treatment sites can result in restenosis independently *(243)*, it is likely that this goal is frequently not achieved in diabetic patients given their high restenosis rates (Table 2). Thus, the worse outcome of diabetic patients undergoing PCI may be mediated in part by the frequent occurrence of incomplete revascularization *(248)*. Van Belle and colleagues suggest that restenosis, especially in its occlusive form is a major determinant of long-term mortality in diabetic patients after coronary angioplasty. When these investigators studied 604 diabetic patients who underwent angioplasty, followed by a 6-month follow-up angiogram and long-term follow-up. They found the group, which had no restenosis, had a 10-year mortality of 24% compared to a 35% mortality in the group with nonocclusive restenosis and a 59% mortality in the group that had occlusive restenosis ($p < 0.0001$) *(256,275)*. The impact of incomplete revascularization may be more pronounced in view of the more diffuse and distal CAD *(153,247)* and worse coronary vasodilatory reserve in diabetic patients *(276)*. Thus PTCA, rather then leading to increased mortality, may fail to alter the aggressive natural course of CAD in diabetic patients *(269)*. The use of sirolimus-coated stents reduces restenosis post-PCI significantly, especially in diabetics, which may improve the long term outlook in diabetic patients undergoing multivessel PCI.

MANAGEMENT OF RISK FACTORS

It is important to identify the risk factors of an individual patient to develop a plan for risk reduction. The goals for risk reduction are summarized in Table 4, adapted from a review from an AHA Executive Summary *(277)*.

Cholesterol Reduction

The Scandinavian Simvastatin Survival Study (4S) has demonstrated the effectiveness of cholesterol-lowering therapy *(278,279)* for secondary prevention of death and morbidity in patients with angina or prior infarction (*see also* Chapter 15). Compared with the placebo group, the relative total mortality and cardiovascular mortality were 0.57 and 0.64, respectively.

Subjects in the 4S study had relatively high LDL cholesterol levels at baseline (~185 mg/dL). However, the majority of patients with coronary disease (including diabetics) have lower LDL cholesterol levels. The Cholesterol and Recurrent Events study (CARE), which included 586 diabetic patients, determined the effect of cholesterol-lowering therapy in patients with coronary disease with average cholesterol levels (mean 139 mg/dL). In the 586 diabetic subjects with CAD, 40 mg of pravastatin was associated with a 25% decrease in coronary events and revascularization procedures, similar to a 23% decrease observed in nondiabetic patients *(280)*.

These results strongly suggest that cholesterol lowering improves the prognosis of diabetic patients with CAD. The absolute clinical benefit achieved by cholesterol lowering may be greater in diabetic than in nondiabetic patients with CAD because diabetic

Table 4
Goals for Risk Factor Management in Patients With Diabetes

Risk factor	Goal of therapy	Recommending body
Cigarette smoking	Complete cessation	ADA
Blood pressure	<130/85 mmHg	JNC 6 (NHLBI)
	</80 mmHg	ADA
LDL cholesterol	<100 mg/dL (^{a}<70 mg/dL)	ATPIII (NHLBI), ADA
Triglycerides 200–499 mg/dL	Non-HDL cholesterol <130 mg/dL	ATPIII (NHLBI)
HDL cholesterol <40 mg/dL	Raise HDL (No set goal)	ATPIII (NHLBI)
Prothrombotic state	Low-dose aspirin therapy (patients with CHD and other high-risk patients)	ADA
Glucose	Hemoglobin A1c <7%	ADA
Overweight and obesity (BMI ≥ 25 kg/m^2)	Lose 10% of body weight in 1 year	OEI (NEHBI)
Physical inactivity	Exercise prescription dependent on patient status	ADA
Adverse nutrition	See text	ADA, AHA, and NHLBI's ATPIII, OEI, and JNC VI

^{a}Patients with diabetes mellitus (DM) and coronary aretery disease (CAD) or DM without CAD should clinical judgment warrant (383). ADA, American Diabetes Association; JNC 6, Sixth report of the Joint National Committee on Prevention, Evaluation, and Treatment of High Blood Pressure; NHLBI, National Heart, Lung, and Blood Institute; ATPIII, National Cholesterol Education Program Adult Treatment Panel III; HDL, high-density lipoprotein; and OEI, Obesity Education Initiative Expert Panel on Identification, Evaluation, and Treatment of Overweight and Obesity in Adults; BMI, body mass index. (Reproduced with permission from ref. 384.)

patients have a higher absolute risk of recurrent CAD, higher case fatality rates (184), or because LDL cholesterol in diabetic patients is more atherogenic (57,98,281,282). The Heart Protection Study (HPS) investigated the treatment of patients at high risk for CVD (known CAD, peripheral vascular disease (PVD), or DM) with simvastatin independent of cholesterol levels for 5 years follow-up. There was a significant 24% reduction in any major vascular event including cardiac death. The proportional reduction in the event rates were similar and statistically significant in all subcategories including diabetics and in those whose initial LDL cholesterol was less than 116 mg/dL. The risk reduction was not affected by the pretreatment cholesterol concentrations. A study conducted by the HPS study group in which 5963 individuals with diabetes (283) were randomized to simvastatin 40 mg by mouth daily reduced the first-event cardiovascular events (including MIs, strokes, revascularization) by 25%. In 2912 patients with diabetes and without CVD, simvastatin therapy reduced the risk of a cardiovascular event by one-third. Event rates for diabetic patients with an LDL less than 116 mg/dL were 27% lower on simvastatin therapy. There was a marginally greater (30%) reduction in cardiac events in diabetes without evidence of CVD (see Figs. 4 and 5). This study suggests that high-risk individuals (5-year event rates of 20%–30%) should be considered for statin therapy independent of their cholesterol levels.

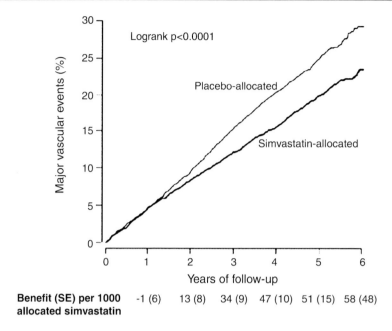

Fig. 4. Life-table plot of effects of simvastatin allocation on percentages of diabetic participants having major vascular events. (Reproduced with permission from ref. *283*.)

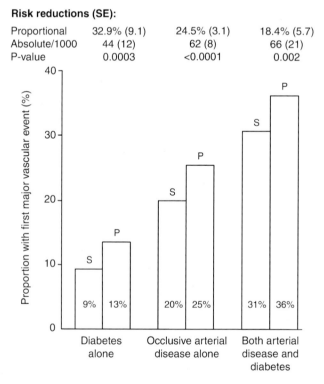

Fig. 5. Absolute effects of simvastatin allocation on 5-year rates of first major vascular event among participants with diabetes, occlusive arterial disease, or both. S, simvastatin treatment group. P, placebo group. (Reproduced with permission from ref. *283*.)

These findings were further strengthened by the recently completed Collaborative Atorvastatin Diabetes Study, which specifically examined the effect of lipid-lowering in type 2 diabetic patients without a history of CVD (284). The study was a multi-center trial conducted in the United Kingdom and Ireland and included 2838 patients with type 2 diabetes over the age of 40 who had a relatively low cholesterol (baseline LDL was 118 mg/dL) and at least one cardiovascular risk factors for CVD. Patients were randomized to atorvastatin 10 mg by mouth daily or placebo. The primary outcome was a composite of major cardiovascular events, revascularization, unstable angina, resuscitated cardiac arrest and stroke. The study was terminated 2 years early after a median 3.9 years follow-up and found a 37% relative risk reduction in the primary outcome with a 48% relative risk reduction in stroke. This benefit was independent of baseline LDL levels with a 38% reduction in events in primary outcomes with LDL greater than 120 mg/dL and 37% reduction with LDL levels less than 120 mg/dL. These investigators, like those of the HPS group, concluded that all diabetic patients should be on a statin independent of the LDL level.

The effect of LDL lowering in patients with acute CVD was specifically examined in the Pravastatin or Atorvastatin Evaluation and Infection-Thrombolysis in Myocardial Infarction (PROVE-IT) trial. The PROVE-IT trial (22) was designed to determine whether a more intensive LDL lowering will reduce major coronary events. In this study, there were 4162 patients who were hospitalized with ACS within preceding 10 days and randomized to two statins, 80 mg of atorvastatin compared to pravastatin 40 mg by mouth daily. The composite end-point for cardiovascular end-points after 2 years was reduced by 16% in favor of atorvarstatin although the difference was insignificant for MI and cardiovascular mortality.

This data has resulted in a modification of the NCEP-ATP III guidelines (285) suggesting that all patients with known CVD should have a LDL target level of 70 mg/dL. While the recommendations for diabetic patients without known vascular disease remains at least at 100 mg/dL or lower based on the clinical judgment of the treating physician, it is these authors' recommendation that all patients with diabetes have a target LDL level of 70 mg/dL. The rationale for this approach, which has been discussed above, stems from both the high event rates in diabetic patients without clinical evidence of CAD (presumably as a result of the very high rates of subclinical atherosclerosis) (20) and the worse prognosis in patients who have had a clinical event compared to nondiabetic subjects (184). Epidemiological studies and clinical trials demonstrate that in higher-risk populations these patients have a risk for CVD events approximately equal to that of nondiabetic patients with established CVD.

Tight glycemic control is the cornerstone of therapy for diabetic dyslipidemia. Hydroxymethylglutaryl-coenzyme-A (HMG-CoA) reductase inhibitors reduce coronary risk even when the LDL level lies within the average range in type II diabetic individuals (286,287). However, tight glycemic control does not completely reverse the lipid profile in patients with type 2 diabetes. Tan and colleagues (284) found that patients with excellent control of their glucose levels (average HbA1C levels <6.6%) continued to have a low HDL and a predominance of small dense LDL particles.

If the triglyceride level is more than 200mg/dL even in the face of an LDL less than 100 mg/dL, consideration should be made for fibrate therapy. The recent VA-HIT trial demonstrated that the fibrate gemfibrozil reduced both coronary events and strokes (288). Recent data suggests that when the LDL level is less than 125 mg/dL, the triglyceride and

HDL levels are significantly stronger predictors of recurrent cardiac events than those with LDL levels greater than 125 mg/dL *(289)*. This only strengthens the rationale for treating low HDL or elevated triglyceride levels.

Nicotinic acid can both lower triglyceride and raise HDL. However, its beneficial effect on lipids in the diabetic patient is offset by its tendency to worsen hyperglycemia, making it relatively contraindicated in such patients

Treatment of Hypertension

Hypertension occurs about twice as frequently in patients with diabetes as in the general population *(290,291)* (*see also* Chapter 14). Isolated systolic hypertension is considerably more common in diabetics. The combined presence of hypertension and diabetes considerably accelerates the development of both macrovascular and microvascular diabetic complications. However, the most significant manifestation of this combination of diseases is that they confer a greater risk of ischemic heart disease, stroke, and PVD in affected individuals. The high cardiovascular risk associated with the co-existence of hypertension and diabetes led the Joint National Committee on prevention, detection, evaluation, and treatment of high BP, to include hypertensive patients with diabetes in the same risk group as hypertensive patients who have clinically manifest CVD *(292)*. These patients should be considered for prompt pharmacological therapy even if they have high-normal BP.

Current evidence suggests that, for the prevention of cardiovascular events, ACE inhibitors *(293,294)* and low-dose diuretics *(295)* are the preferred first-line agents for hypertensive patients with diabetes. A controversy exists regarding the efficacy of calcium antagonists in preventing cardiovascular complications *(296)*. In the Appropriate Blood Pressure Control in Diabetes (ABCD) trial, patients in the nisoldipine group had a fivefold higher risk of fatal and nonfatal acute MI than did the enalapril group *(293)*. In the Fosinopril Versus Amlodipine Cardiovascular Events Randomized Trial (FACET) patients receiving fosinopril had half the risk of the combined outcome of acute MI, stroke, or hospitalized angina than those receiving amlodipine *(297)*. However, combination therapy resulted in a lower incidence of cardiovascular events than either treatment alone and could be interpreted as evidence that combination therapy is the preferred strategy *(297)*. Importantly, hypertension control is unlikely to be achieved by monotherapy in diabetic patients, as demonstrated in the ABCD trial *(293)*.

The Systolic Hypertension in Europe (Syst-Eur) compared outcomes of treatments with nitrendipine vs placebo in patients with isolated systolic hypertension. End-point reduction achieved by active treatment was significantly larger in the diabetic subgroup (–69% vs –26% cardiovascular events), indicating a remarkable benefit from first-line treatment with a calcium antagonist *(298)*. Similarly, the results of the Hypertension and Optimal Treatment (HOT) trial showed a reduction of MI event rates in diabetic patients (*N* = 1501, representing the largest calcium antagonist trial in diabetic patients) using the long-acting dihydropyridine calcium antagonist felodipine *(299)*.

The evidence for aggressive antihypertensive treatment in patients with insulin-dependent diabetes mellitus (IDDM), hypertension, and nephropathy is now overwhelming *(300,301)*. ACE inhibitors are particularly useful in this population with clear evidence that these agents reduced the progression of kidney dysfunction and the number of patients who will develop end-stage renal failure *(215,216)*.

The HOPE study (and the MICRO-HOPE substudy) (Fig. 3) demonstrated that ramipril significantly reduced the rates of MI, stroke and deaths in diabetic patients without overt CVD and one other risk factor *(211)*. The importance of blocking the renin–angiotensin system was further strengthened by the results of the Losartan Intervention for Endpoint Reduction in Hypertension (LIFE) study *(302)*. These results demonstrated that lorsartan reduced total and cardiovascular mortality more that atenolol did in diabetic patients with hypertension and left ventricular hypertrophy.

The sixth report of the Joint National Committee on prevention, Detection, Evaluation, and Treatment of High Blood Pressure (JNC 6) have incorporated these principals for the treatment of hypertension in the presence of diabetes and have included a more aggressive program of BP reduction, aiming for a target of less than 135/85 mmHg in both IDDM and NIDDM patients *(292)*. The American Diabetes Association (ADA) aims for the lower target BP of 130/80 *(291)*.

Additionally, the guidelines included a target of 125/75 mmHg in patients with greater than 1 g per day proteinuria. ACE inhibitors are often regarded as the initial antihypertensive drug of choice in diabetic patients *(292,300,301)*.

Glycemic Control

A central issue in the treatment of diabetic patients is whether tight glycemic control will reduce CAD morbidity and mortality. The Diabetes Control and Complications Trial (DCCT) conclusively showed that the greater the average blood glucose in patients with IDDM, (as assessed by HbA1C), the greater the risk of developing retinopathy, neuropathy and nephropathy *(303)*. Although the number of combined major macrovascular events was almost twice as high in the conventionally treated group as in the intensive-treatment group, the differences were not statistically significant ($p = 0.08$) because patients participating in this study were young and early in the course of their disease *(303,304)*. However, hyperglycemic animals develop fatty streaks resembling those of human type II atherosclerotic lesions in the absence of hyperinsulinemia *(305)*, and data from the Stockholm Diabetes Intervention Study indicate that tight control retards the development of atherosclerosis in IDDM patients as measured by the development of carotid IMT *(306)*. Thus, tight control is indicated in IDDM patients for prevention of both microvascular and macrovascular complications. It is noteworthy that the average total insulin dose in the intensive treatment group of the DCCT trial was less than 10% higher in the conventional treatment group. Thus, unless acceleration of atherosclerosis is exquisitely sensitive to small differences in exogenous insulin dose, it is unlikely that this form of therapy increases the risk for CVD.

The United Kingdom Prospective Diabetes Study (UKPDS) was a prospective, randomized, trial aiming to determine whether patients with NIDDM can obtain clinical benefit from intensive glycemic control. In the UKPDS, 3867 newly diagnosed patients with NIDDM were randomly assigned to an intensive treatment program or to a conventional treatment program. Compared to the conventional-treatment group, the intensive-treatment group demonstrated a 16% risk reduction ($p = 0.052$) for fatal and nonfatal MI, but all-cause mortality did not differ between the intensive and conventional groups *(307)*. In this study, intensive therapy resulted in a 0.9% difference in median HbA1C between the intensive (7%) and conventional (7.9%) groups over 10 years. The threshold above which hyperglycemia becomes atherogenic is unknown, but may be higher. Alternatively, as recent data from the DCCT indicates for all microvascular complications

(308), a continuous relative risk reduction relationship over the range of HbA1C may exist for CAD. Thus, an additional benefit may be obtained in many diabetic patients because HbA1C is generally only in the 9% to 10% in this population *(309)*.

The current recommendations of the ADA set the goal for glycemic control in NIDDM patients at a fasting (preprandial) glucose level of less than 120 mg/dL and a glycosylated hemoglobin of less than 7% (normal range 4%–6%) *(310)*. It is reasonable to believe that the mechanisms by which hyperglycemia promotes atherosclerosis and cardiovascular events are operative in all individuals with hyperglycemia. Because the major morbidity and mortality in NIDDM is a consequence of accelerated atherosclerosis, improved glycemic control is likely to result in a reduction of macrovascular events and probably in mortality.

Specific metabolic abnormalities induced by diabetes can adversely affect mechanical performance, or increase the myocardial vulnerability to ischemic insults. Thus, insulin administration and improved metabolic control during the acute phase of MI may reduce myocardial damage, improve contractility, and decrease mortality *(184)*. In one study insulin-glucose infusion in the immediate period after infarction resulted in a significant fall in mortality *(311)*. However, this approach has not been proven to be useful in the acute phase of MI in other studies *(195,196)*.

In one recent study, intensive glycemic control in diabetic patients with MI was associated with a 52% reduction in the 1-year mortality rate *(196)*, and the survival advantage was maintained for up to 5 years *(312,313)*. These findings demonstrate that glycemic control may be valuable even in diabetics with established CAD. More studies are needed to better delineate the importance of metabolic derangements in diabetic patients during myocardial ischemia.

The Metabolic Syndrome

The ATPIII guidelines present an opportunity for physicians to identify patients with the metabolic syndrome who are at increased risk for developing CAD. The Diabetes Prevention Program demonstrated that either a rigorous regimen of diet and exercise or metformin, can prevent or delay diabetes *(314)* *(see* Fig. 6). By diagnosing the metabolic syndrome in individuals would allow earlier treatment of these patients and thereby reduce the likelihood of developing CAD.

CONGESTIVE HEART FAILURE AND DIABETES

Paralleling the incidence of CAD in patients with diabetes, is the incidence of heart failure *(see also* Chapter 27). Heart failure is a frequent clinical manifestation of the end-stage of cardiovascular complications that afflicts diabetics. The Framingham Study was the first study that showed the risk of symptomatic heart failure was increased 2.4-fold in diabetic men and fivefold in diabetic women *(315)*. Population-based studies have revealed that 15% to 25% of heart failure patients are diabetic as are 25% to 30% of patients hospitalized for heart failure *(316–318)*.

However, these epidemiological studies do not reveal the frequency of diabetic cardiomyopathy. Whether diabetic cardiomyopathy exists as a separate entity, is controversial. The diagnosis of diabetic cardiomyopathy is defined as heart failure in the absence of an identifiable etiology. The presence of congestive heart failure in the diabetic, in the absence of CAD and hypertension is uncertain.

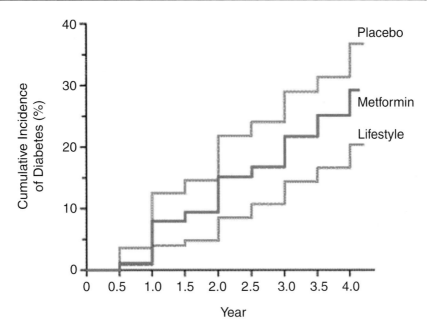

Fig. 6. Cumulative incidence of diabetes according to study group. The incidence of diabetes differed significantly among the three groups ($p < 0.001$ for each comparison). (Reproduced with permission from Diabetes Prevention Program Research Group N Engl J Med 2002;346:393–403).

In the Framingham study *(315)*, few of these patients with heart failure did not have CAD, hypertension, or rheumatic disease. The presence of CAD was diagnosed solely on the basis of clinical symptoms and electrocardiographic evidence, and not by noninvasive testing or coronary angiography. Therefore, CAD that did not manifest symptoms or typical electrocardiographic changes may have led to the development of heart failure. Diabetic patients are more prone to silent MIs accounting up to 30% of cases *(319)*. CAD is the most common cause of congestive heart in the overall United States *(320)* and also the diabetic *(315)* population. Diffuse CAD can lead to nontransmural infarction with patchy necrosis and myocardial fibrosis resulting in an impairment of systolic function. Myocardial ischemia may result in not only systolic dysfunction, but also diastolic dysfunction *(321,322)*. In the setting of a MI, diabetic patients are more likely to develop heart failure *(323)*, occurring in up to 50% of patients who suffer a MI *(324)*. The GUSTO-1 trial demonstrated that heart failure developed in 27% of the insulin-dependent diabetics compared to 20% of those diabetics not taking insulin and 15% of those in the nondiabetic group. This amounts to heart failure occurring almost twice as frequently in the diabetic population relative to the nondiabetic *(175)*. Diabetics are also almost twice as likely to develop heart failure as a result of an acute coronary syndrome (7.2 vs 3.8%) compared to nondiabetics.

Not surprisingly, the presence of heart failure in the diabetic population is associated with a poorer long-term prognosis. The GUSTO-1 study demonstrated that cardiac mortality at 30 days in the insulin-dependent diabetic was 12.5% compared to 9.7% in the noninsulin-dependent diabetic and 6.2% in the nondiabetic. This poorer outcome was not as a result of a larger MI. The MILIS database demonstrated that the prognosis of diabetics was worse relative to nondiabetic patients (4-year cardiac mortality rates of

25.9% in the diabetic and 14.5% in the nondiabetic) despite the presence of smaller infarcts (as measured by peak creatine phosphokinase [CPK] or area under the curve) and fewer Q-wave infarcts *(174)*. The GUSTO-1 study also found that vessel patency post-MI did not explain this worse prognosis either because there were similar degrees of infarct-related patency at 90 minutes in the diabetic and nondiabetic patient *(222)*. Compensatory hyperkinesis of the noninfarcted walls, which is frequently found in the non-diabetic subject immediately post-MI patient, is often blunted in the diabetic *(222)*.

As discussed earlier in this chapter, hypertension occurs in 40% to 60% of patients with type 2 diabetes *(325)*. Hypertension is the most common cause of heart failure in diabetic after CAD, accounting for 24% of the cases. Diabetes increases the likelihood of development of heart failure 1.8-fold in hypertensive men and 3.7-fold in hypertensive women *(325)*.

Substudy analysis of the BEST trial demonstrated that patients with diabetes and advanced heart failure have a significantly worse prognosis than those patients without diabetes *(322A)*. The prognostic effect of diabetes on mortality was limited to those patients with an ischemic etiology for their heart failure.

Diabetic Cardiomyopathy

The question whether diabetes itself, distinct from CAD and hypertension, results in a dilated cardiomyopathy, remains controversial. The term, diabetic cardiomyopathy was first coined by Rubler in 1972 *(326)*. In the 35- to 64-year-old Framingham cohort, diabetes increased the risk of CHF in men by fourfold and in women by eightfold, even after adjustment for BP, age, cholesterol, weight, and a history of CAD *(315)*. The more recent Washington DC Dilated Cardiomyopathy Study used case-controlled analyses determined that there was an association between diabetes and idiopathic cardiomyopathy *(327,328)*.

Diabetics, and especially women, have increased left ventricular mass and higher heart rates than their nondiabetic counterparts. Some studies report that diabetics may have an abnormal exercise response, with an attenuation of augmentation of LVEF relative to normals *(329–333)*. Furthermore, diastolic abnormalities have been reported by various groups using various parameters including prolonged isovolumic relaxation time *(334–336)*, decreased rates of left ventricular diastolic filling *(337–339)* and abnormal transmitral flow velocities *(187,339–342)*. Increased echodensity has also been reported despite normal wall thicknesses, which could suggest increased collagen deposition present in the myocardium *(343)*.

Pathologically, postmortem studies of patients with diabetic cardiomyopathy have revealed that they have features similar to other forms of nonischemic cardiomyopathy. This includes myocyte hypertrophy, interstitial fibrosis, and infiltration with periodic acid-Schiff-positive materials, with coronary arterioles that have thickened basement membranes and intramyocardial microangiopathy *(344–346)*.

Many theories abound regarding the possible mechanism(s) underlying diabetic cardiomyopathy. These include both cellular and molecular pertubations and metabolic abnormalities. Insulin may play a central role to the cellular and molecular mechanisms of diabetic cardiomyopathy. In studies with a line of transgenic mice in which the gene for the insulin-regulated glucose transporter GLUT4 has been deleted demonstrate hyperinsulinemia and cardiomyopathy *(347,348)*. Calcium homeostasis may be altered and have been reported in various animal models of diabetes, which suggests a diminished but prolonged increase in intracellular calcium concentration *(349)*. Further research with transgenic models have demonstrated that mice that overexpress the β2 isoform of PKC. Hyperglycemia increases calcium-activated signaling through PKC, which may, in turn, result in cardiac dysfunction. Abnormalities in myofibrillar proteins, including altered phosphorylation of troponin I and myosin light chains, may also play a role in diabetes-associated impairment of contractile function *(350,351)*. Advanced glycosylation results in abnormal collagen crosslinking, which may contribute to decreased compliance and, in turn, diastolic dysfunction *(352)*.

Several metabolic pertubations may contribute to the development of diabetic cardiomyopathy. Glucose contributes 10% to 15% of the energy of the heart under normal conditions. However during insulin stimulation, increased workload, and ischemia, glucose metabolism is increased. Studies using diabetic animal models have demonstrated that diabetic hearts have a blunted uptake of basal and insulin-stimulated myocardial glucose *(353)*. The glucose that is transported into the heart of a diabetic animal is often shunted to glycogen because of increased fatty acid utilization *(354,355)*. Increased fatty acid uptake and oxidation itself may decrease cardiac function. Ketoacidosis may occur in diabetes. The ketones produced are avidly taken up by the diabetic heart and reduce coenzyme A, which in turn, inhibits the citric acid cycle, thereby reducing the energy capability of the muscle and resulting in myocardial dysfunction *(356,357)*.

DIABETIC AUTONOMIC NEUROPATHY AND THE HEART

Autonomic neuropathy is a common complication of both type 1 and 2 DM. Common clinical manifestations of diabetic autonomic neuropathy include orthostatic hypotension, gastroparesis, and resting tachycardia *(358)*. Cardiovascular autonomic neuropathy (CAN) of DM confer both an increased risk for the development of CVD and a poorer prognosis for those individuals once they develop clinically apparent CAD *(359–362)*. The symptoms of CAN include postural hypotension and resting tachycardia described above and painless myocardial ischemia. Diabetic patients with CAN do not have the morning increase in MIs and acute CVD events ("circadian variation") as are found in the nondiabetic patients but rather, show a even distribution of such events throughout the day *(363–365)*. Parasympathetic nerve fibers are affected first, leading to a relative increase in sympathetic tone that results in a resting tachycardia and attenuation of the expected increase in heart rate and BP with exercise *(366,367)*. The decrease of parasympathetic tone may be responsible for the exaggerated coronary vasoconstriction, which may result in worsening ischemia *(368,369)*. Postural hypotension is a principal clinical manifestation of sympathetic dysfunction *(370)*.

The development of CAN parallels the occurrence of end-organ damage including retinopathy and nephropathy and generally occurs in those patients with diabetes of long duration with poorer glycemic control. However, subclinical CAN may occur relatively early in the disease. An important method for early detection is reduced heart-rate variability, which is measured over a 24-hour period *(371,372)*. Alternative methods for early detection of CAN include cardiac radionuclide imaging using the norepinephrine analogue metaiodobenzylguanidine (MIBG), which evaluates cardiac sympathetic activity. The activity is reduced in diabetic patients with CAN, suggesting reduced sympathetic activity *(373)*.

The estimates of the prevalence of CAN vary depending on the methods used to diagnose its presence and the population studied. In a series of newly diagnosed type 1 patients with IDDM individuals the incidence is 8% *(371)* although in a large series of both type 1 and 2 diabetic patients, there is a 50% incidence of reduced heart-rate variability (372). In one small series, 75% of patients with DM for 10 years and no significant CAD had evidence of adrenergic denervation as determined by MIBG imaging (373).

As stated above, the diagnosis of CAN is a harbinger for serious cardiovascular complications and increased mortality in diabetic individuals (360–362). The 5-year mortality in a cohort of individuals with type 1 DM and CAN was fivefold greater than type 1 diabetics without CAN (361). The presence of CAN in type 2 DM is not as well characterized as in type I diabetes. One study did show that those individuals with type 2 DM with CAN 5 years after being diagnosed with diabetes conferred an increased cardiovascular mortality in the subsequent 5 years than those type 2 diabetics free of CAN (359).

Numerous experimental and clinical studies have shown that the perturbations in autonomic activity may be important in the development of cardiac arrhythmias. Diabetic individuals, who demonstrate a restricted heart rate variability, have been shown to be associated with the development of both cardiac arrhythmias and sudden cardiac death, particularly in those patients post-MI with left ventricular dysfunction (374–376). The severity of autonomic dysfunction has been shown to be associated a higher incidence of arrhythmias. Because individuals with symptomatic clinical CAN usually have had diabetes for a longer period of time and have poorer glucose control, this may represent a subgroup with a more advanced disease and more cardiovascular complications including previous MIs.

The mechanisms for the increased morbidity and mortality associated with CAN include increased risk of ventricular arrhythmia, silent myocardial ischemia, impaired coronary vasomotor regulation, and increased resting heart rate. Sudden cardiac death has long been known to be associated with DM in the absence of CVD (360). Transient decreases in heart rate variability preceded the onset of ST segment shift and precipitated life-threatening arrhythmias in a group of diabetics with CAD who were survivors of sudden cardiac death (377). The Honolulu Heart Program also demonstrated that diabetes was independently associated with the risk of sudden cardiac death (378). Prolongation of the QT interval in diabetic individuals has been shown to correlate with the degree of autonomic neuropathy (379) and may be a method to screen for diabetics at risk for sudden cardiac death. One group used QT dispersion as a means to evaluate for the presence and degree of autonomic neuropathy. QT dispersion was defined as the difference between the longest corrected QT interval and the shortest corrected QT interval. These investigators found that the greater the QT dispersion, the greater the risk for ventricular arrythmias and this increased dispersion was more likely found in diabetic individuals with CAN (379).

It has long been recognized that diabetic patients frequently have less severe anginal pain or even no pain at all associated with myocardial ischemia (159,168,169,380). Diabetic patients may present with rather atypical symptoms including shortness of breath, diaphoresis gastrointestinal complaints or profound fatigue. Zarich and colleagues (364) showed that 90% of ischemic episodes were asymptomatic in a group of diabetic patients with documented CAD who underwent ambulatory electrocardiogram (ECG) monitoring. This blunted or altered pain response to myocardial ischemia in diabetic patients has been attributed to CAN. In the recent DIAB study (170), 22% of a cohort of asymptomatic diabetic patients had abnormal stress perfusion testing. The abnormal test results were not associated with traditional risk factors but to autonomic neuropathy.

The altered anginal response is further complicated by the resting tachycardia, which alters the threshold for myocardial ischemia. Myocardial oxygen-demand is largely determined by the heart rate-BP product. The resting tachycardia, as a result of parasympathetic denervation, increases myocardial oxygen demand. Therefore any activity puts the diabetic patient with CAD closer to his or hers ischemic threshold. Cardiac autonomic neuropathy can also affect coronary blood flow independent of the altered endothelial function (368). One study evaluated the cold pressor test in diabetic patients and found that the increase in flow in response to cold was lower in the diabetics with sympathetic nerve dysfunction compared to those without sympathetic nerve dysfunction (369).

The presence of autonomic neuropathy results in a two- to threefold increase in cardiac morbidity and mortality in diabetic patients undergoing noncardiac surgery. This increased risk of general anesthesia in this group of diabetic patients may, in part, be as a result of the relative hemodynamic instability that often occurs (381).

SCREENING FOR THE PRESENCE OF CORONARY ARTERY DISEASE

Little is known regarding the appropriate screening tests for CAD in patients with no clear evidence of CAD. The ADA /American College of Cardiology (ACC) (313) have developed a consensus regarding: which patients are at increased risk for cardiac events; which patients should be screened; and what is the appropriate follow-up to a positive test result. The potential benefit of diagnosing CAD in patients with DM allow for the initiation of both preventative measures and anti-ischemic therapy including medication or revascularization therapy. Although no evidence exists for risk intervention in diabetic patients and asymptomatic coronary artery disease, aggressive therapy has been shown to reduce cardiovascular mortality in diabetic individuals with known CAD (as discussed earlier in this chapter). Thus, the identification of CAD in asymptomatic patients is important to institute aggressive secondary preventative measures.

Although stress testing is clearly indicated with those diabetic individuals who have established CAD, it is not clear what test would be appropriate in patients who do not have known CAD. Table 5 lists those indications set by the ADA/ACC Consensus Panel (313). Stress testing is warranted if the patient has typical or atypical cardiac symptoms. Silent ischemia is a frequent occurrence in diabetic individuals. A resting ECG showing evidence of an infarction or ischemia warrants stress testing. The presence of peripheral or carotid occlusive arterial disease is strongly associated with CAD. Therefore, any diabetic individual with evidence of PVD should undergo stress testing. Multiple risk factors in the same patient increase the possibility of identifying significant CAD. The addition of two other risk factors to diabetes increases the cardiovascular death rate by threefold. Autonomic neuropathy has been strongly associated with cardiac morbidity and mortality however there is insufficient data regarding whether this is an independent risk factor. According to the Consensus Panel, the presence of autonomic neuropathy is enough to warrant stress testing. Microalbuminuria is also an important risk factor for cardiovascular mortality and therefore its presence should warrant stress testing.

Asymptomatic patients with diabetes and one or fewer risk factors and a normal ECG do not require cardiac testing. Those patients with carotid or peripheral vascular disease, beginning a vigorous exercise program, minor ST-T wave changes on ECG or two or more risk factors, should undergo an exercise stress test. If these patients have a baseline ECG making a proper assessment of an ECG stress test difficult, or those patients with

Table 5
Indications for Cardiac Testing in Diabetic Patients

1. Typical or atypical cardiac symptoms
2. Resting electrocardiographic suggestive of ischemia or infarction
3. Peripheral or carotid occlusive arterial disease
4. Sedentary lifestyle, age 35 years, and plans to begin a vigorous exercise program
5. Two or more of the risk factors listed below (a–e) in addition to diabetes:
   a. Total cholesterol 240 mg/dL, LDL cholesterol 160 mg/dL, or HDL cholesterol <35 mg/dL
   b. Blood pressure >140/90 mmHg
   c. Smoking
   d. Family history of premature CAD
   e. Positive micro/macroalbumininuria test

LDL, low-density lipoprotein; HDL, high-density lipoprotein; CAD, coronary artery disease. (Reproduced with permission from ref. *313*.)

clear evidence of an MI or have ischemia on their ECG, should undergo stress perfusion imaging or a stress echo.

If these patients are limited by an inability to exercise they should undergo they should undergo pharmacological testing (dobutamine echo or persantine thallium).

A negative test at a high workload, defined as completing 9 minutes or stage 3 of a Bruce treadmill protocol should provide some reassurance that have a favorable prognosis with regards to CVD. However, these patients must be routinely followed and should their symptoms change, undergo a repeat stress test. Those individuals who have mildly positive tests (defined as 1–1.5 mm ST depression at a moderate to high exercise level [Bruce stage 3]) are also in a low-risk group. These patients may require perfusion imaging or a stress echo to determine if this is a false-positive result, especially because many of these patients underwent stress testing prior to beginning a vigorous exercise program. If either of these tests is negative, these patients can have regular clinical evaluations and have a repeat stress-testing every 2 years or when they develop new symptoms. A moderately positive test in an asymptomatic diabetic should warrant a stress echo or cardiac nuclear test because a large perfusion defect indicates a significant risk for cardiac events in the next 1 to 2 years. If the defect is moderate or large as determined by echo or perfusion testing, there should be a low threshold to have the patient undergo a cardiac catheterization. A markedly positive stress test is defined as hypotension with exercise, a positive test at a heart rate of less than 120 beats per minute, an exercise capacity of less than 6 minutes, and greater than 2 mm ST depression. The asymptomatic diabetic patient who has such a test should undergo a cardiac catheterization.

Emerging technologies such as cardiac magnetic resonance imaging (MRI) and cardiac computed tomography (CT), including coronary calcium scoring, have an as yet unknown role in the screening of diabetic patients for "occult" CAD. Coronary calcium may be a marker for subclinical atherosclerosis that can be detected by electron beam CT scanning. Asymptomatic diabetics patients have increased amounts of coronary calcium when compared to age-matched nondiabetics *(383,384)*. However, although coronary calcium scores have some predictive value for future cardiovascular events in nondiabetics this has been shown not to be the case in the asymptomatic diabetic population *(385,386)*.

MRI is comparable to transesophageal echocardiography for the visualiztion of aortic atherosclerosis *(387)*. MRI can be used to perform noninvasive coronary angiography. Coronary MR angiography has a high sensitivity, negative predictive value, and overall accuracy for detecting CAD, especially in subjects with left main CAD or three-vessel disease *(388)*. MRI coronary angiography is currently limited by low specificity, and inability to visualize well the mid and distal vessel walls. Coronary wall-imaging which assesses coronary wall thickness and atherosclerosis burden is also under investigation for the evaluation of preclinical CAD *(389,390)*.

EVALUATION OF RISK FACTORS

Table 5 (adapted from the AHA) *(277)*, reviews the evaluation of the risk factors in such diabetic patients. In summary, it is important to identify the risk factors of an individual patient to develop a plan for risk reduction. To evaluate for risk factors in diabetic patients, it is important that the patient have a careful medical history and physical examination along with certain laboratory tests. Such tests include a lipoprotein analysis to evaluate not only the LDL but also the level of HDL and triglycerides. Predisposing risk factors need to be assessed including family history, and degree of obesity and level of physical activity. This assessment should also include an evaluation of the renal status including the determination for the presence of micro- or macroalbuminuria. The presence of microalbuminuria in the type 2 diabetic signifies an increased risk for CVD. Patients with greater than 1 g per day proteinuria may require more aggressive goals for BP control to less than 125/75 mmHg. ACE inhibitors are often regarded as the initial antihypertensive drug of choice in diabetic patients *(292,300,301)*.

The medical management of patients with clinical CVD includes risk reduction and can be defined as secondary prevention. However, there is a significant portion of the diabetic population that has no overt evidence of CVD. Such evidence would make it necessary to institute less aggressive cardiovascular risk factor management for primary prevention.

In patients with type 2 diabetes, the years of insulin resistance can result in atherogenesis long before the onset of hyperglycemia. Clinical evidence of insulin resistance includes abdominal obesity, high-normal BP, high-normal triglycerides (150–250 mg/dL), reduced HDL (<40 mg/dL in men; <50 mg/dL in women), borderline high-risk LDL (130–159 mg/dL) and, in some patients, with impaired fasting glucose (110–126 mg/dL). The detection of IFG is a strong risk factor for Type 2 DM. Therefore, it becomes important to follow the guidelines in Table 4 to not only reduce the risk of CVD, but delay the onset of type 2 DM.

Recent evidence would suggest that either lifestyle intervention or treatment with metformin can also reduce the development of diabetes in persons who are at high risk (Fig. 6) *(314)*. It is presumed that, measures that reduce the development of DM, will also reduce the incidence of diabetes most important sequelae, CVD.

REFERENCES

1. Vergely P. De l'angine de poitrine dans ses rapports avec le diabete. Gaz Hebd Med Chir (Paris) (Series 2) 1883;20:364–368.
2. Control CfD. Trends in diabetes mortality. MMWR Morb Mortal Wkly Rep 1988;38:285–288.
3. Grundy SM, et al. Diabetes and cardiovascular disease: a statement for healthcare professionals from the American Heart Association. Circulation 1999;100(10):1134–1146.

4. Barrett-Connor E, Orchard T. Diabetes and heart disease, in National Diabetes Data Group, Diabetes Data Compiled 1984,1985, U.S. Dept. of Health and Human Services: Washington, DC, 1985, pp. XVI-1–XVI-41.

5. American Diabetes Association. Consensus Statement: role of cardiovascular risk factors in prevention and treatment of macrovascular disease in diabetes. Diabetes Care 1993;16:72–78.

6. Pyorala K, Laakso M, Uusitupa M. Diabetes and atherosclerosis: an epidemiologic view. Diabetes Metab Rev 1987;3:463–524.

7. O'Leary D, et al. Distribution and correlates of sonographically detected carotid artery disease in the Cardiovascular Health Study. The CHS Collaborative Research Group. Stroke 1992;23(12):1752–1760.

8. Folsom AR, et al. Relation of carotid artery wall thickness to diabetes mellitus, fasting glucose and insulin, body size, and physical activity. Atherosclerosis Risk in Communities (ARIC) Study Investigators. Stroke 1994;25(1):66–73.

9. Stamler J, et al. Diabetes, other risk factors, and 12-yr cardiovascular mortality for men screened in the Multiple Risk Factor Intervention Trial. Diabetes Care 1993;16(2):434–444.

10. Schwartz CJ, et al. Pathogenesis of the atherosclerotic lesion. Implications for diabetes mellitus. Diabetes Care 1992;15(9):1156–1167.

11. Aronson D. Pharmacologic modulation of autonomic tone: implications for the diabetic patient. Diabetologia 1997;40(4):476–481.

12. Carter JS, Pugh JA, Monterrosa A. Non-insulin-dependent diabetes mellitus in minorities in the United States [see comments]. Ann Intern Med 1996;125(3):221–232.

13. Mokdad AH, et al. The spread of the obesity epidemic in the United States 1991–1998. Jama 1999;282(16):1519–1522.

14. Lee WL, et al. Impact of diabetes on coronary artery disease in women and men: a meta- analysis of prospective studies. Diabetes Care 2000;23(7):962–968.

15. Barrett-Connor EL, et al. Why is diabetes mellitus a stronger risk factor for fatal ischemic heart disease in women than in men? The Rancho Bernardo Study [published erratum appears in JAMA 1991;265(24): 3249]. JAMA 1991;265(5):627–631.

16. Gu, K, Cowie CC, Harris MI. Mortality in adults with and without diabetes in a national cohort of the U.S. population, 1971–1993. Diabetes Care 1998;21(7):1138–1145.

17. Krolewski AS, et al. Magnitude and determinants of coronary artery disease in juvenile- onset, insulin-dependent diabetes mellitus. Am J Cardiol 1987;59(8):750–755.

18. Krolewski AS, et al. Epidemiologic approach to the etiology of type I diabetes mellitus and its complications. N Engl J Med 1987;317(22):1390–1398.

19. Bale GS, Entmacher PS. Estimated life expectancy of diabetics. Diabetes 1977;26(5):434–438.

20. Haffner SM, et al. Mortality from coronary heart disease in subjects with type 2 diabetes and in nondiabetic subjects with and without prior myocardial infarction. N Engl J Med 1998;339(4):229–234.

21. Mukamal KJ, et al. Impact of diabetes on long-term survival after acute myocardial infarction: comparability of risk with prior myocardial infarction. Diabetes Care 2001;24(8):1422–1427.

22. Malmberg K, et al. Impact of diabetes on long-term prognosis in patients with unstable angina and non-Q-wave myocardial infarction: results of the OASIS (Organization to Assess Strategies for Ischemic Syndromes) Registry. Circulation 2000;102(9):1014–1019.

23. Gu, K, Cowie CC, Harris MI. Diabetes and decline in heart disease mortality in US adults. JAMA 1999;281(14):1291–1297.

24. Donahue RP, Orchard TJ. Diabetes mellitus and macrovascular complications. An epidemiological perspective. Diabetes Care 1992;15(9):1141–1155.

25. Maser RE, et al. Cardiovascular disease and arterial calcification in insulin-dependent diabetes mellitus: interrelations and risk factor profiles. Pittsburgh Epidemiology of Diabetes Complications Study-V. Arterioscler Thromb 1991;11(4):958–965.

26. Borch-Johnsen K, et al. Is diabetic nephropathy an inherited complication? Kidney Int 1992;41(4):719–722.

27. Jensen T, et al. Coronary heart disease in young type 1 (insulin-dependent) diabetic patients with and without diabetic nephropathy: incidence and risk factors. Diabetologia 1987;30(3):144–148.

28. Manske CL, et al. Coronary revascularisation in insulin-dependent diabetic patients with chronic renal failure. Lancet 1992;340(8826):98–1002.

29. Deckert T, et al. Microalbuminuria. Implications for micro- and macrovascular disease. Diabetes Care 1992;15(9):1181–1191.

30. Jensen T, Stender S, Deckert T. Abnormalities in plasmas concentrations of lipoproteins and fibrinogen in type 1 (insulin-dependent) diabetic patients with increased urinary albumin excretion. Diabetologia 1988;31(3):142–145.

31. Jones SL, et al. Plasma lipid and coagulation factor concentrations in insulin dependent diabetics with microalbuminuria. Bmj 1989;298(6672):487–490.

32. Winocour PH, et al. Influence of early diabetic nephropathy on very low density lipoprotein (VLDL), intermediate density lipoprotein (IDL), and low density lipoprotein (LDL) composition. Atherosclerosis 1991;89(1):49–57.

33. Gruden G, et al. PAI-1 and factor VII activity are higher in IDDM patients with microalbuminuria. Diabetes 1994;43(3):426–429.

34. Makita Z, et al. Advanced glycosylation end products in patients with diabetic nephropathy [see comments]. N Engl J Med 1991;325(12):836–842.

35. Makita Z, et al. Reactive glycosylation endproducts in diabetic uraemia and treatment of renal failure. Lancet 1994;343(8912):1519–1522.

36. Earle K, et al. Familial clustering of cardiovascular disease in patients with insulin- dependent diabetes and nephropathy. N Engl J Med 1992;326(10):673–677.

37. Krolewski AS, et al. Predisposition to hypertension and susceptibility to renal disease in insulin-dependent diabetes mellitus. N Engl J Med 1988;318(3):140–145.

38. Marre M, et al. Contribution of genetic polymorphism in the renin-angiotensin system to the development of renal complications in insulin-dependent diabetes: Genetique de la Nephropathie Diabetique (GENEDIAB) study group. J Clin Invest 1997;99(7):1585–1595.

39. Cambien F, et al. Deletion polymorphism in the gene for angiotensin-converting enzyme is a potent risk factor for myocardial infarction [see comments]. Nature 1992;359(6396):641–644.

40. Tarnow L, et al. Insertion/deletion polymorphism in the angiotensin-I-converting enzyme gene is associated with coronary heart disease in IDDM patients with diabetic nephropathy [see comments]. Diabetologia 1995;38(7):798–803.

41. Ruiz J, et al. Insertion/deletion polymorphism of the angiotensin-converting enzyme gene is strongly associated with coronary heart disease in non-insulin- dependent diabetes mellitus. Proc Natl Acad Sci U S A 1994;91(9):3662–3665.

42. Keavney BD, et al. UK prospective diabetes study (UKPDS) 14: association of angiotensin- converting enzyme insertion/deletion polymorphism with myocardial infraction in NIDDM. Diabetologia 1995;38(8):948–952.

43. Kannel WB, McGee DL. Diabetes and cardiovascular disease. The Framingham study. JAMA 1979;241(19):2035–2038.

44. Jarrett RJ, McCartney P, Keen H. The Bedford survey: ten year mortality rates in newly diagnosed diabetics, borderline diabetics and normoglycaemic controls and risk indices for coronary heart disease in borderline diabetics. Diabetologia 1982;22(2):79–84.

45. Jarrett RJ, Shipley MJ. Type 2 (non-insulin-dependent) diabetes mellitus and cardiovascular disease—putative association via common antecedents; further evidence from the Whitehall Study. Diabetologia 1988;31(10):737–740.

46. Fontbonne A, et al. Hypertriglyceridaemia as a risk factor of coronary heart disease mortality in subjects with impaired glucose tolerance or diabetes. Results from the 11-year follow-up of the Paris Prospective Study. Diabetologia 1989;32(5):300–304.

47. Nathan DM. Long-term complications of diabetes mellitus. N Engl J Med 1993;328(23):1676–1685.

48. Barrett-Connor E, Wingard DL. Sex differential in ischemic heart disease mortality in diabetics: a prospective population-based study. Am J Epidemiol 1983;118(4):489–496.

49. Reaven G. Syndrome X: 10 years after. Drugs 1999;58(Suppl 1):19–20; discussion 75–82.

50. Ferrannini E, et al. Insulin resistance in essential hypertension. N Engl J Med 1987;317(6):350–357.

51. Zavaroni I, et al. Risk factors for coronary artery disease in healthy persons with hyperinsulinemia and normal glucose tolerance [see comments]. N Engl J Med 1989;320(11):702–706.

52. Larsson B, et al. Abdominal adipose tissue distribution, obesity, and risk of cardiovascular disease and death: 13 year follow up of participants in the study of men born in 1913. Br Med J (Clin Res Ed) 1984;288(6428):1401–1404.

53. Laakso M, Barrett-Connor E. Asymptomatic hyperglycemia is associated with lipid and lipoprotein changes favoring atherosclerosis. Arteriosclerosis 1989;9(5):665–672.

54. Laws A, et al. Relation of fasting plasma insulin concentration to high density lipoprotein cholesterol and triglyceride concentrations in men. Arterioscler Thromb 1991;11(6):1636–1642.

55. Modan M, et al. Hyperinsulinemia is characterized by jointly disturbed plasma VLDL, LDL, and HDL levels. A population-based study. Arteriosclerosis 1988;8(3):227–236.

56. Peiris AN, et al. Adiposity, fat distribution, and cardiovascular risk. Ann Intern Med 1989;110(11):867–872.

57. Reaven GM. Role of insulin resistance in human disease (syndrome X): an expanded definition. Annu Rev Med 1993;44:121–131.

58. Reaven GM, Laws A. Insulin resistance, compensatory hyperinsulinaemia, and coronary heart disease. Diabetologia 1994;37(9):948–952.

59. Howard G, et al. Insulin sensitivity and atherosclerosis. The Insulin Resistance Atherosclerosis Study (IRAS) Investigators [see comments]. Circulation 1996;93(10):1809–1817.

60. Laakso M, et al. Asymptomatic atherosclerosis and insulin resistance. Arterioscler Thromb 1991;11(4):1068–1076.

61. Agewall S, et al. Urinary albumin excretion is associated with the intima-media thickness of the carotid artery in hypertensive males with non-insulin-dependent diabetes mellitus. J Hypertens 1995;13(4):463–469.

62. Bonora E, et al, Prevalence of insulin resistance in metabolic disorders: the Bruneck Study. Diabetes 1998;47(10):1643–1649.

63. Fuller JH, et al. Coronary-heart-disease risk and impaired glucose tolerance. The Whitehall study. Lancet 1980;1(8183):1373–1376.

64. Morrish NJ, et al. Aprospective study of mortality among middle-aged diabetic patients (the London Cohort of the WHO Multinational Study of Vascular Disease in Diabetics) II: Associated risk factors [published erratum appears in Diabetologia 1991 Apr;34(4):287]. Diabetologia 1990;33(9):542–548.

65. Uusitupa M, et al. The relationship of cardiovascular risk factors to the prevalence of coronary heart disease in newly diagnosed type 2 (non-insulin- dependent) diabetes. Diabetologia 1985;28(9):653–659.

66. Head J, Fuller JH. International variations in mortality among diabetic patients: the WHO Multinational Study of Vascular Disease in Diabetics. Diabetologia 1990;33(8):477–481.

67. Despres JP, et al. Hyperinsulinemia as an independent risk factor for ischemic heart disease. N Engl J Med 1996;334(15):952–957.

68. Andersson DK, Svardsudd K. Long-term glycemic control relates to mortality in type II diabetes. Diabetes Care 1995;18(12):1534–1543.

69. Wei M, et al. Effects of diabetes and level of glycemia on all-cause and cardiovascular mortality. The San Antonio Heart Study. Diabetes Care 1998;21(7):1167–1172.

70. Klein, R, Klein BE, Moss SE. The Wisconsin Epidemiologic Study of Diabetic Retinopathy. XVI. The relationship of C-peptide to the incidence and progression of diabetic retinopathy. Diabetes 1995;44(7):796–801.

71. Wingard DL, et al. Prevalence of cardiovascular and renal complications in older adults with normal or impaired glucose tolerance or NIDDM. A population-based study. Diabetes Care 1993;16(7):1022–1025.

72. Kuusisto J, et al. Non-insulin-dependent diabetes and its metabolic control are important predictors of stroke in elderly subjects. Stroke 1994;25(6):1157–1164.

73. Rodriguez BL, et al. Glucose intolerance and 23-year risk of coronary heart disease and total mortality: the Honolulu Heart Program. Diabetes Care 1999;22(8):1262–1265.

74. Singer DE, et al. Association of HbA1c with prevalent cardiovascular disease in the original cohort of the Framingham Heart Study. Diabetes 1992;41(2):202–208.

75. Kuusisto J, et al. NIDDM and its metabolic control predict coronary heart disease in elderly subjects. Diabetes 1994;43(8):960–967.

76. Mattock MB, et al. Prospective study of microalbuminuria as predictor of mortality in NIDDM. Diabetes 1992;41(6):736–741.

77. Neil A, et al. Aprospective population-based study of microalbuminuria as a predictor of mortality in NIDDM. Diabetes Care 1993;16(7):996–1003.

78. Ducimetiere P, et al. Relationship of plasma insulin levels to the incidence of myocardial infarction and coronary heart disease mortality in a middle-aged population. Diabetologia 1980;19(3):205–210.

79. Pyorala K. Relationship of glucose tolerance and plasma insulin to the incidence of coronary heart disease: results from two population studies in Finland. Diabetes Care 1979;2(2):131–141.

80. Welborn TA, Wearne K. Coronary heart disease incidence and cardiovascular mortality in Busselton with reference to glucose and insulin concentrations. Diabetes Care 1979;2(2):154–160.

81. Stout RW. Insulin and atheroma 20-yr perspective. Diabetes Care 1990;13(6):631–654.

82. Gowri MS, et al. Decreased protection by HDL from poorly controlled type 2 diabetic subjects against LDL oxidation may be due to the abnormal composition of HDL. Arterioscler Thromb Vasc Biol 1999;19(9):2226–2233.

83. Tsai EC, et al. Reduced plasma peroxyl radical trapping capacity and increased susceptibility of LDL to oxidation in poorly controlled IDDM. Diabetes 1994;43(8):1010–1014.

84. Baynes JW, Thorpe SR. Role of oxidative stress in diabetic complications: a new perspective on an old paradigm. Diabetes 1999;48(1):1–9.

85. Ceriello A, et al. Evidence for a possible role of oxygen free radicals in the abnormal functional arterial vasomotion in insulin dependent diabetes. Diabete Metab 1990;16(4):318–322.
86. Kilhovd BK, et al. Serum levels of advanced glycation end products are increased in patients with type 2 diabetes and coronary heart disease. Diabetes Care 1999;22(9):1543–1548.
87. Baynes JW. Role of oxidative stress in development of complications in diabetes. Diabetes 1991;40(4):405–412.
88. King GL, et al. Cellular and molecular abnormalities in the vascular endothelium of diabetes mellitus. Annu Rev Med 1994;45:179–188.
89. Gabbay KH. The sorbitol pathway and the complications of diabetes. N Engl J Med 1973;288(16):831–836.
90. Yusuf S, et al. Vitamin E supplementation and cardiovascular events in high-risk patients. The Heart Outcomes Prevention Evaluation Study Investigators. N Engl J Med 2000;342(3):154–160.
91. Bursell SE, et al. High-dose vitamin E supplementation normalizes retinal blood flow and creatinine clearance in patients with type 1 diabetes. Diabetes Care 1999;22(8):1245–1251.
92. Ahmed MU, Thorpe SR, Baynes JW. Identification of N epsilon-carboxymethyllysine as a degradation product of fructoselysine in glycated protein. J Biol Chem 1986;261(11):4889–4894.
93. Sell DR, Monnier VM. Structure elucidation of a senescence cross-link from human extracellular matrix. Implication of pentoses in the aging process. J Biol Chem 1989;264(36):21,597–21,602.
94. Baron AD. Insulin and the vasculature—old actors, new roles. J Investig Med 1996;44(8):406–412.
95. Moncada S. Eighth Gaddum Memorial Lecture. University of London Institute of Education, December 1980. Biological importance of prostacyclin. Br J Pharmacol 1982;76(1):3–31.
96. Fu MX, et al. The advanced glycation end product, Nepsilon-(carboxymethyl)lysine, is a product of both lipid peroxidation and glycoxidation reactions. J Biol Chem 1996;271(17):9982–9986.
97. Requena JR, et al. Quantification of malondialdehyde and 4-hydroxynonenal adducts to lysine residues in native and oxidized human low-density lipoprotein. Biochem J 1997;322(Pt 1):317–325.
98. Bucala R, et al. Lipid advanced glycosylation: pathway for lipid oxidation in vivo. Proc Natl Acad Sci U S A 1993;90(14):6434–6438.
99. Haberland ME, Fong D, Cheng L. Malondialdehyde-altered protein occurs in atheroma of Watanabe heritable hyperlipidemic rabbits. Science 1988;241(4862):215–218.
100. Rosenfeld ME, et al. Distribution of oxidation specific lipid-protein adducts and apolipoprotein B in atherosclerotic lesions of varying severity from WHHL rabbits. Arteriosclerosis 1990;10(3):336–349.
101. Carew TE, Schwenke DC, Steinberg D. Antiatherogenic effect of probucol unrelated to its hypocholesterolemic effect: evidence that antioxidants in vivo can selectively inhibit low density lipoprotein degradation in macrophage-rich fatty streaks and slow the progression of atherosclerosis in the Watanabe heritable hyperlipidemic rabbit. Proc Natl Acad Sci U S A 1987;84(21):7725–7729.
102. Regnstrom J, et al. Susceptibility to low-density lipoprotein oxidation and coronary atherosclerosis in man. Lancet 1992;339(8803):1183–1186.
103. Vlassara H, Brownlee M, Cerami A. Novel macrophage receptor for glucose-modified proteins is distinct from previously described scavenger receptors. J Exp Med 1986;164(4):1301–1309.
104. Vlassara H, et al. Cachectin/TNF and IL-1 induced by glucose-modified proteins: role in normal tissue remodeling. Science 1988;240(4858):1546–1548.
105. Bevilacqua MP, et al. Interleukin 1 (IL-1) induces biosynthesis and cell surface expression of procoagulant activity in human vascular endothelial cells. J Exp Med 1984;160(2):618–623.
106. Breviario F, et al. IL-1-induced adhesion of polymorphonuclear leukocytes to cultured human endothelial cells. Role of platelet-activating factor. J Immunol 1988;141(10):3391–3397.
107. Raines EW, Dower SK, Ross R. Interleukin-1 mitogenic activity for fibroblasts and smooth muscle cells is due to PDGF-AA. Science 1989;243(4889):393–396.
108. O'Brien KD, et al. Vascular cell adhesion molecule-1 is expressed in human coronary atherosclerotic plaques. Implications for the mode of progression of advanced coronary atherosclerosis. J Clin Invest 1993;92(2):945–951.
109. Beekhuizen H, van Furth R. Monocyte adherence to human vascular endothelium. J Leukoc Biol 1993;54(4):363–378.
110. Pohlman TH, et al. An endothelial cell surface factor(s) induced in vitro by lipopolysaccharide, interleukin 1, and tumor necrosis factor-alpha increases neutrophil adherence by a CDw18-dependent mechanism. J Immunol 1986;136(12):4548–4553.
111. Park L, et al. Suppression of accelerated diabetic atherosclerosis by the soluble receptor for advanced glycation endproducts. Nat Med 1998;4(9):1025–1031.
112. Brown AS, et al. Megakaryocyte ploidy and platelet changes in human diabetes and atherosclerosis. Arterioscler Thromb Vasc Biol 1997;17(4):802–807.

113. Winocour PD, Watala C, Kinglough-Rathbone RL. Membrane fluidity is related to the extent of glycation of proteins, but not to alterations in the cholesterol to phospholipid molar ratio in isolated platelet membranes from diabetic and control subjects. Thromb Haemost 1992;67(5):567–571.

114. Davi G, et al. Thromboxane biosynthesis and platelet function in type II diabetes mellitus. N Engl J Med 1990;322(25):1769–1774.

115. Ishii H, Umeda F, Nawata H. Platelet function in diabetes mellitus. Diabetes Metab Rev 1992;8(1):53–66.

116. Hendra T, Betteridge DJ. Platelet function, platelet prostanoids and vascular prostacyclin in diabetes mellitus. Prostaglandins Leukot Essent Fatty Acids 1989;35(4):197–212.

117. Menys VC, et al. Spontaneous platelet aggregation in whole blood is increased in non- insulin-dependent diabetes mellitus and in female but not male patients with primary dyslipidemia. Atherosclerosis 1995;112(1):115–122.

118. Kannel WB, et al. Diabetes, fibrinogen, and risk of cardiovascular disease: the Framingham experience. Am Heart J 1990;120(3):672–676.

119. Lufkin EG, et al. Increased von Willebrand factor in diabetes mellitus. Metabolism 1979;28(1):63–66.

120. Kannel WB, et al. Fibrinogen and risk of cardiovascular disease. The Framingham Study. Jama 1987;258(9):1183–1186.

121. Eliasson M, et al. Proinsulin, intact insulin, and fibrinolytic variables and fibrinogen in healthy subjects. A population study. Diabetes Care 1997;20(8):1252–1255.

122. Ceriello A, et al. Decreased antithrombin III activity in diabetes may be due to non- enzymatic glycosylation—a preliminary report. Thromb Haemost 1983;50(3):633–634.

123. Brownlee M, Vlassara H, Cerami A. Inhibition of heparin-catalyzed human antithrombin III activity by nonenzymatic glycosylation. Possible role in fibrin deposition in diabetes. Diabetes 1984;33(6):532–535.

124. Ceriello A, et al. Daily rapid blood glucose variations may condition antithrombin III biologic activity but not its plasma concentration in insulin-dependent diabetes. A possible role for labile non-enzymatic glycation. Diabete Metab 1987;13(1):16–19.

125. Ceriello A, et al. Protein C deficiency in insulin-dependent diabetes: a hyperglycemia- related phenomenon. Thromb Haemost 1990;64(1):104–107.

126. Auwerx J, et al. Tissue-type plasminogen activator antigen and plasminogen activator inhibitor in diabetes mellitus. Arteriosclerosis 1988;8(1):68–72.

127. McGill JB, et al. Factors responsible for impaired fibrinolysis in obese subjects and NIDDM patients. Diabetes 1994;43(1):104–109.

128. Nordt TK, Schneider DJ, Sobel BE. Augmentation of the synthesis of plasminogen activator inhibitor type-1 by precursors of insulin. A potential risk factor for vascular disease. Circulation 1994;89(1):321–330.

129. Small KW, Stefansson E, Hatchell DL. Retinal blood flow in normal and diabetic dogs. Invest Ophthalmol Vis Sci 1987;28(4):672–675.

130. Clermont AC, et al. Normalization of retinal blood flow in diabetic rats with primary intervention using insulin pumps. Invest Ophthalmol Vis Sci 1994;35(3):981–990.

131. Bursell SE, et al. Retinal blood flow changes in patients with insulin-dependent diabetes mellitus and no diabetic retinopathy. Invest Ophthalmol Vis Sci 1996;37(5):886–897.

132. Miyamoto K, et al. Evaluation of retinal microcirculatory alterations in the Goto-Kakizaki rat. A spontaneous model of non-insulin-dependent diabetes. Invest Ophthalmol Vis Sci 1996;37(5):898–905.

133. Furchgott RF, Zawadzki JV. The obligatory role of endothelial cells in the relaxation of arterial smooth muscle by acetylcholine. Nature 1980;288(5789):373–376.

134. Palmer RM, Ferrige AG, Moncada S. Nitric oxide release accounts for the biological activity of endothelium-derived relaxing factor. Nature 1987;327(6122):524–526.

135. Ignarro LJ, et al. Endothelium-derived relaxing factor produced and released from artery and vein is nitric oxide. Proc Natl Acad Sci U S A 1987;84(24):9265–9269.

136. Dinerman JL, Lowenstein CJ, Snyder SH. Molecular mechanisms of nitric oxide regulation. Potential relevance to cardiovascular disease. Circ Res 1993;73(2):217–222.

137. Lincoln TM, Cornwell RL, Taylor AE. cGMP-dependent protein kinase mediates the reduction of Ca^{2+} by cAMP in vascular smooth muscle cells. Am J Physiol 1990;258(3 Pt 1):C399–C407.

138. Collins P, et al. Differences in basal endothelium-derived relaxing factor activity in different artery types. J Cardiovasc Pharmacol 1986;8(6):1158–1162.

139. Johnstone MT, et al. Impaired endothelium-dependent vasodilation in patients with insulin- dependent diabetes mellitus. Circulation 1993;88(6):2510–2516.

140. McVeigh GE, et al. Impaired endothelium-dependent and independent vasodilation in patients with type 2 (non-insulin-dependent) diabetes mellitus. Diabetologia 1992;35(8):771–776.

141. Williams SB, et al. Impaired nitric oxide-mediated vasodilation in patients with non- insulin-dependent diabetes mellitus. J Am Coll Cardiol 1996;27(3):567–574.

142. Steinberg HO, et al. Obesity/insulin resistance is associated with endothelial dysfunction. Implications for the syndrome of insulin resistance. J Clin Invest 1996;97(11):2601–2610.

143. Ting HH, et al. Vitamin C improves endothelium-dependent vasodilation in patients with non-insulin-dependent diabetes mellitus. J Clin Invest 1996;97(1):22–28.

144. Timimi FK, et al. Vitamin C improves endothelium-dependent vasodilation in patients with insulin-dependent diabetes mellitus. J Am Coll Cardiol 1998;31(3):552–557.

145. van Etten RW, et al. Intensive lipid lowering by statin therapy does not improve vasoreactivity in patients with type 2 diabetes. Arterioscler Thromb Vasc Biol 2002;22(5):799–804.

146. Cooke JP. Does ADMA cause endothelial dysfunction? Arterioscler Thromb Vasc Biol 2000;20(9):2 032–2037.

147. Fard A, Tuck C, Di Tullio MR, et al. Plasma assymetric dimethylarginine is elevated and endothelial function is impaired after a high fat meal in type 2 diabetics. Circulation 1999;100(Supplement II):3700(abstr).

148. Asagami T, Li W, Abbasi FA, Tsao, PS, Cooke JP, Reaven G. Metformin attenuates plasma asymetric dimethylarginine and monocyte adhesion in type 2 diabetes. Circulation 1999;102(Supplement II):1129(abstr).

149. Vigorita VJ, Moore GW, Hutchins GM. Absence of correlation between coronary arterial atherosclerosis and severity or duration of diabetes mellitus of adult onset. Am J Cardiol 1980;46(4):535–542.

150. Waller BF, et al. Status of the coronary arteries at necropsy in diabetes mellitus with onset after age 30 years. Analysis of 229 diabetic patients with and without clinical evidence of coronary heart disease and comparison to 183 control subjects. Am J Med 1980;69(4):498–506.

151. Granger CB, et al. Outcome of patients with diabetes mellitus and acute myocardial infarction treated with thrombolytic agents. The Thrombolysis and Angioplasty in Myocardial Infarction (TAMI) Study Group. J Am Coll Cardiol 1993;21(4):920–925.

152. Stein B, et al. Influence of diabetes mellitus on early and late outcome after percutaneous transluminal coronary angioplasty. Circulation 1995;91(4):979–989.

153. Barzilay JI, et al. Coronary artery disease and coronary artery bypass grafting in diabetic patients aged > or = 65 years (report from the Coronary Artery Surgery Study [CASS] Registry). Am J Cardiol 1994;74(4):334–339.

154. Davies MJ, et al. Factors influencing the presence or absence of acute coronary artery thrombi in sudden ischaemic death. Eur Heart J 1989;10(3):203–208.

155. Silva JA, et al. Unstable angina. A comparison of angioscopic findings between diabetic and nondiabetic patients. Circulation 1995;92(7):1731–1736.

156. Bradley RF, Schonfeld A. Diminished pain in diabetic patients with acute myocardial infarction. Geriatrics 1962;17:322–326.

157. Margolis JR, et al. Clinical features of unrecognized myocardial infarction-silent and asymptomatic. Eighteen year follow-up: the Framingham study. Am J Cardiol 1973;32:1–7.

158. Soler NG, et al. Myocardial infarction in diabetics. Q J Med 1975;44(173):125–232.

159. Marchant B, et al. Silent myocardial ischemia: role of subclinical neuropathy in patients with and without diabetes. J Am Coll Cardiol 1993;22(5):1433–1437.

160. Hume L, et al. Asymptomatic myocardial ischemia in diabetes and its relationship to diabetic neuropathy: an exercise electrocardiography study in middle- aged diabetic men. Diabetes Care 1986;9(4):384–388.

161. O'Sullivan J, et al. Silent ischaemia in diabetic men with autonomic neuropathy. Br Heart J 1991;66(4):313–315.

162. Nesto RW, et al. Angina and exertional myocardial ischemia in diabetic and nondiabetic patients: assessment by exercise thallium scintigraphy [published erratum appears in Ann Intern Med 1988 Apr;108(4):646]. Ann Intern Med 1988;108(2):170–175.

163. Abenavoli T, et al. Exercise testing with myocardial scintigraphy in asymptomatic diabetic males. Circulation 1981;63(1):54–64.

164. Langer A, et al. Detection of silent myocardial ischemia in diabetes mellitus [see comments]. Am J Cardiol 1991;67(13):1073–1078.

165. Milan Study on Atherosclerosis and Diabetes (MiSAD) Group, Prevalence of unrecognized silent myocardial ischemia and its association with atherosclerotic risk factors in noninsulin-dependent diabetes mellitus. Am J Cardiol 1997;79(2):134–139.

166. Callaham PR, et al. Exercise-induced silent ischemia: age, diabetes mellitus, previous myocardial infarction and prognosis. J Am Coll Cardiol 1989;14(5):1175–1180.
167. Caracciolo EA, et al. Diabetics with coronary disease have a prevalence of asymptomatic ischemia during exercise treadmill testing and ambulatory ischemia monitoring similar to that of nondiabetic patients. An ACIP database study. ACIP Investigators. Asymptomatic Cardiac Ischemia Pilot Investigators [see comments]. Circulation 1996;93(12):2097–2105.
168. Faerman I, et al. Autonomic neuropathy and painless myocardial infarction in diabetic patients. Histologic evidence of their relationship. Diabetes 1977;26(12):1147–1158.
169. Ambepityia G, et al. Exertional myocardial ischemia in diabetes: a quantitative analysis of anginal perceptual threshold and the influence of autonomic function. J Am Coll Cardiol 1990;15(1):72–77.
170. Wackers FJ, et al. Detection of silent myocardial ischemia in asymptomatic diabetic subjects: the DIAD study. Diabetes Care 2004;27(8):1954–1961.
171. Jaffe AS, et al. Increased congestive heart failure after myocardial infarction of modest extent in patients with diabetes mellitus. Am Heart J 1984;108(1):31–37.
172. Savage MP, et al. Acute myocardial infarction in diabetes mellitus and significance of congestive heart failure as a prognostic factor. Am J Cardiol 1988;62(10 Pt 1):665–669.
173. Malmberg K, Ryden L. Myocardial infarction in patients with diabetes mellitus. Eur Heart J 1988;9(3):259–264.
174. Stone PH, et al. The effect of diabetes mellitus on prognosis and serial left ventricular function after acute myocardial infarction: contribution of both coronary disease and diastolic left ventricular dysfunction to the adverse prognosis. The MILIS Study Group. J Am Coll Cardiol 1989;14(1):49–57.
175. Mak KH, et al. Influence of diabetes mellitus on clinical outcome in the thrombolytic era of acute myocardial infarction. GUSTO-I Investigators. Global Utilization of Streptokinase and Tissue Plasminogen Activator for Occluded Coronary Arteries. JAm.Coll.Cardiol 1997;30(1):171–179.
176. Barbash GI, et al. Significance of diabetes mellitus in patients with acute myocardial infarction receiving thrombolytic therapy. Investigators of the International Tissue Plasminogen Activator/Streptokinase Mortality Trial. J Am Coll Cardiol 1993;22(3):707–713.
177. Lee KL, et al. Predictors of 30-day mortality in the era of reperfusion for acute myocardial infarction. Results from an international trial of 41,021 patients. GUSTO-I Investigators [see comments]. Circulation 1995;91(6):1659–1668.
178. Zuanetti G, et al. Influence of diabetes on mortality in acute myocardial infarction: data from the GISSI-2 study. J Am Coll Cardiol 1993;22(7):1788–1794.
179. Holmes DR Jr, et al. Cardiogenic shock in patients with acute ischemic syndromes with and without ST-segment elevation. Circulation 1999;100(20):2067–2073.
180. Orlander PR, et al. The relation of diabetes to the severity of acute myocardial infarction and postmyocardial infarction survival in Mexican-Americans and non-Hispanic whites. The Corpus Christi Heart Project. Diabetes 1994;43(7):897–902.
181. Lehto S, et al. Myocardial infarct size and mortality in patients with non-insulin- dependent diabetes mellitus. J Intern Med 1994;236(3):291–297.
182. Ulvenstam G, et al. Long-term prognosis after myocardial infarction in men with diabetes. Diabetes 1985;34(8):787–792.
183. Iwasaka T, et al. Residual left ventricular pump function after acute myocardial infarction in NIDDM patients. Diabetes Care 1992;15(11):1522–1526.
184. Aronson D, Rayfield EJ, Chesebro JH. Mechanisms determining course and outcome of diabetic patients who have had acute myocardial infarction. Ann Intern Med 1997;126(4):296–306.
185. Fava S, et al. Factors that influence outcome in diabetic subjects with myocardial infarction. Diabetes Care 1993;16(12):1615–168.
186. Gwilt DJ, et al. Myocardial infarct size and mortality in diabetic patients. Br Heart J 1985;54(5):466–472.
187. Zarich SW, et al. Diastolic abnormalities in young asymptomatic diabetic patients assessed by pulsed Doppler echocardiography. J Am Coll Cardiol 1988;12(1):114–120.
188. Takahashi N, et al. Left ventricular regional function after acute anterior myocardial infarction in diabetic patients. Diabetes Care 1989;12(9):630–635.
189. The GUSTO Angiographic Investigators, The effects of tissue plasminogen activator, streptokinase, or both on coronary-artery patency, ventricular function, and survival after acute myocardial infarction. N Engl J Med 1993;329(22):1615–1622.
190. Abaci A, et al. Effect of diabetes mellitus on formation of coronary collateral vessels. Circulation 1999;99(17):2239–2242.

191. Herlitz J, et al. Mortality and morbidity during a five-year follow-up of diabetics with myocardial infarction. Acta Med Scand 1988;224(1):31–38.
192. Capone RJ, et al. Events in the cardiac arrhythmia suppression trial: baseline predictors of mortality in placebo-treated patients. J Am Coll Cardiol 1991;18(6):1434–1438.
193. Gilpin E, et al. Factors associated with recurrent myocardial infarction within one year after acute myocardial infarction. Am Heart J 1991;121(2 Pt 1):457–465.
194. Taylor GJ, et al. Six-year survival after coronary thrombolysis and early revascularization for acute myocardial infarction. Am J Cardiol 1992;70(1):26–30.
195. Malmberg K, et al. Randomized trial of insulin-glucose infusion followed by subcutaneous insulin treatment in diabetic patients with acute myocardial infarction (DIGAMI study): effects on mortality at 1 year [see comments]. J Am Coll Cardiol 1995;26(1):57–65.
196. Malmberg K. Prospective randomised study of intensive insulin treatment on long term survival after acute myocardial infarction in patients with diabetes mellitus. DIGAMI (Diabetes Mellitus, Insulin Glucose Infusion in Acute Myocardial Infarction) Study Group [see comments]. BMJ 1997;314(7093):1512–1515.
197. Tschoepe D, et al. Platelets in diabetes: the role in the hemostatic regulation in atherosclerosis. Semin Thromb Hemost 1993;19(2):122–128.
198. DiMinno G, et al. Trial of repeated low-dose aspirin in diabetic angiopathy. Blood 1986;68(4):886–891.
199. Randomized trial of intravenous streptokinase, o.a, both, or neither among 17,187 cases of suspected acute myocardial infarction: ISIS-2. ISIS-2 (Second International Study of Infarct Survival) Collaborative Group,, Lancet 1988;2:349–360.
200. Antiplatelet Trialist' Collaboration, Collaborative overview of randomized trials of antiplatelet therapy. I. Prevention of death, myocardial infarction, and stroke by prolonged antiplatelet therapy in various categories of patients. BMJ 1994;308:81–106.
201. Colwell JA. Aspirin therapy in diabetes. Diabetes Care 1997;20(11):1767–1771.
202. Association AD. Aspirin therapy in diabetes. Diabetes Care 1997;20(11):1772–1773.
203. Kendall MJ, et al. Beta-blockers and sudden cardiac death [see comments]. Ann Intern Med 1995;123(5):358–367.
204. Mangano DT, et al. Effect of atenolol on mortality and cardiovascular morbidity after noncardiac surgery. Multicenter Study of Perioperative Ischemia Research Group [see comments] [published erratum appears in N Engl J Med 1997 Apr 3;336(14):1039]. N Engl J Med 1996;335(23):1713–1720.
205. Shorr RI, et al. Antihypertensives and the risk of serious hypoglycemia in older persons using insulin or sulfonylureas [see comments]. JAMA 1997;278(1):40–43.
206. Pfeffer MA. ACE inhibitors in acute myocardial infarction: patient selection and timing [editorial; comment]. Circulation 1998;97(22):2192–2194.
207. Zuanetti G, et al. Effect of the ACE inhibitor lisinopril on mortality in diabetic patients with acute myocardial infarction: data from the GISSI-3 study [see comments]. Circulation 1997;96(12):4239–4245.
208. Moye LA, et al. Uniformity of captopril benefit in the SAVE Study: subgroup analysis. Survival and Ventricular Enlargement Study. Eur Heart J 1994;15 (Suppl B):2–8; discussion 26–30.
209. Gustafsson I, et al. Effect of the angiotensin-converting enzyme inhibitor trandolapril on mortality and morbidity in diabetic patients with left ventricular dysfunction after acute myocardial infarction. Trace Study Group. J Am Coll Cardiol 1999;34(1):83–89.
210. Yusuf S, et al. Effects of an angiotensin-converting-enzyme inhibitor, ramipril, on cardiovascular events in high-risk patients. The Heart Outcomes Prevention Evaluation Study Investigators. N Engl J Med 2000;342(3):145–153.
211. Effects of ramipril on cardiovascular and microvascular outcomes in people with diabetes mellitus: results of the HOPE study and MICRO-HOPE substudy. Heart Outcomes Prevention Evaluation Study Investigators. Lancet 2000;355(9200):253–259.
212. Torlone E, et al. ACE-inhibition increases hepatic and extrahepatic sensitivity to insulin in patients with type 2 (non-insulin-dependent) diabetes mellitus and arterial hypertension. Diabetologia 1991;34(2):119–125.
213. Pollare T, Lithell H, Berne C. A comparison of the effects of hydrochlorothiazide and captopril on glucose and lipid metabolism in patients with hypertension [see comments]. N Engl J Med 1989;321(13):868–873.
214. Bak JF, et al. Effects of perindopril on insulin sensitivity and plasma lipid profile in hypertensive non-insulin-dependent diabetic patients. Am J Med 1992;92(4B):69S–72S.

215. Lewis EJ, et al. The effect of angiotensin-converting-enzyme inhibition on diabetic nephropathy. The Collaborative Study Group [see comments] [published erratum appears in N Engl J Med 1993;330(2): 152]. N Engl J Med 1993;329(20):1456–1462.

216. Ravid M, et al., Long-term stabilizing effect of angiotensin-converting enzyme inhibition on plasma creatinine and on proteinuria in normotensive type II diabetic patients [see comments]. Ann Intern Med 1993;118(8):577–581.

217. Inhibition of the platelet glycoprotein IIb/IIIa receptor with tirofiban in unstable angina and non-Q-wave myocardial infarction. Platelet Receptor Inhibition in Ischemic Syndrome Management in Patients Limited by Unstable Signs and Symptoms (PRISM-PLUS) Study Investigators. N Engl J Med 1998;338(21):1488–14897.

218. Steinhubl SR, et al. Attainment and maintenance of platelet inhibition through standard dosing of abciximab in diabetic and nondiabetic patients undergoing percutaneous coronary intervention. Circulation 1999;100(19):1977–1982.

219. Platelet glycoprotein IIb/IIIa receptor blockade and low-dose heparin during percutaneous coronary revascularization. The EPILOG Investigators. N Engl J Med 1997;336(24):1689–1696.

220. Randomised placebo-controlled and balloon-angioplasty-controlled trial to assess safety of coronary stenting with use of platelet glycoprotein- IIb/IIIa blockade. The EPISTENT Investigators. Evaluation of Platelet IIb/IIIa Inhibitor for Stenting. Lancet 1998;352(9122):87–92.

221. Roffi M, et al. Impact of different platelet glycoprotein IIb/IIIa receptor inhibitors among diabetic patients undergoing percutaneous coronary intervention: : Do Tirofiban and ReoPro Give Similar Efficacy Outcomes Trial (TARGET) 1-year follow-up. Circulation 2002;105(23):2730–2736.

222. Woodfield SL, et al. Angiographic findings and outcome in diabetic patients treated with thrombolytic therapy for acute myocardial infarction: the GUSTO-I experience. J Am.Coll.Cardiol 1996;28(7):1661–1669.

223. Fibrinolytic Therapy Trialists' (FTT) Collaborative Group:, indications for fibrinolytic therapy in suspected acute myocardial infarction: collaborative overview of early mortality and major morbidity results from all randomized trials of more then 1000 patients. Lancet 1994;343:311–322.

224. Mahaffey KW, et al. Diabetic retinopathy should not be a contraindication to thrombolytic. J Am Coll Cardiol 1997;30(7):1606–1610.

225. Detre K, et al. Percutaneous transluminal coronary angioplasty in 1985–1986 and 1977–1981. The National Heart, Lung, and Blood Institute Registry. N Engl J Med 1988;318:265–270.

226. Adelman A, et al. A comparison of directional atherectomy with balloon angioplasty for lesions of the left anterior descending coronary artery [see comments]. N Engl J Med 1993;329:228–233.

227. Parisi A, Folland E, Hartigan P. A comparison of angioplasty with medical therapy in the treatment of single-vessel coronary artery disease. N Engl J Med 1993;326:10–16.

228. The Bypass Angioplasty Revascularization Investigation (BARI) Investigators, Comparison of coronary bypass surgery with angioplasty in patients with multivessel disease. N Engl J Med 1996;335(4):217–225.

229. Kurbaan AS, et al. Difference in the mortality of the CABRI diabetic and nondiabetic populations and its relation to coronary artery disease and the revascularization mode. Am J Cardiol 2001;87(8):947–950,A3.

230. Holmes DJ, et al. Restenosis after percutanous transluminal coronary angioplasty (PTCA): a report from the PTCA Registry of the National Heart, Lung, and Blood Institute. Am J Cardiol 1984;53:77C–81C.

231. Weintraub W, et al. Can restenosis after coronary angioplasty be predicted from clinical variables. J Am Coll Cardiol 1993;21:6–14.

232. Vandormael MG, et al. Multilesion coronary angioplasty: clinical and angiographic follow-up. J Am.Coll.Cardiol 1987;10(2):246–252.

233. Quigley PJ, et al. Repeat percutaneous transluminal coronary angioplasty and predictors of recurrent restenosis. Am J Cardiol 1989;63(7):409–413.

234. Rensing BJ, et al. Luminal narrowing after percutaneous transluminal coronary angioplasty. A study of clinical, procedural, and lesional factors related to long-term angiographic outcome. Coronary Artery Restenosis Prevention on Repeated Thromboxane Antagonism (CARPORT) Study Group. Circulation 1993;88(3):975–985.

235. Bach R, et al. Factors affecting the restenosis rate after percutaneous transluminal coronary angioplasty. Thromb Hemost 1994;74:(Suppl 1):S55–S77.

236. Lambert M, et al. Multiple coronary angioplasty: a model to discriminate systemic and procedural factors related to restenosis. J Am Coll Cardiol 1988;12(2):310–314.

237. Popma JJ, et al. Clinical and angiographic outcome after directional coronary atherectomy. A qualitative and quantitative analysis using coronary arteriography and intravascular ultrasound. Am.JCardiol 1993;72(13):55E–64E.

238. Warth D, et al. Rotational atherectomy multicenter registry: acute results, complications and 6-month angiographic follow-up in 709 patients. J Am Coll Cardiol 1994;24:641–648.

239. Levine GN, et al. Impact of diabetes mellitus on percutaneous revascularization (CAVEAT-I). CAVEAT-I Investigators. Coronary Angioplasty Versus Excisional Atherectomy Trial. Am J Cardiol 1997;79(6):748–755.

240. Rabbani L, et al. Relation of restenosis after excimer laser angioplasty to fasting insulin levels. Am J Cardiol 1994;73:323–327.

241. Fischman DL, et al. A randomized comparison of coronary-stent placement and balloon angioplasty in the treatment of coronary artery disease. Stent Restenosis Study Investigators [see comments]. N Engl J Med 1994;331(8):496–501.

242. Kastrati A, et al. Predictive factors of restenosis after coronary stent placement. J Am Coll Cardiol 1997;30:1428–1436.

243. Kastrati A, et al. Interlesion dependence of the risk for restenosis in patients with coronary stent placement in in multiple lesions. Circulation 1998;97(24):2396–2401.

244. Carrozza J, et al. Restenosis after arterial injury caused by coronary stenting in patients with diabetes mellitus. Ann Intern Med 1993;118:344–349.

245. Wang N, et al. Percutaneous transluminal coronary angioplasty failures in patients with multivessel disease. Is there an increased risk? J Thorac Cardiovasc Surg 1995;110(1):214–221; discussion 221–223.

246. Van Belle E, et al. Restenosis rates in diabetic patients: a comparison of coronary stenting and balloon angioplasty in native coronary vessels. Circulation 1997;96:1454–1460.

247. Kip KE, et al. Coronary angioplasty in diabetic patients. The National Heart, Lung, and Blood Institute Percutaneous Transluminal Coronary Angioplasty Registry [see comments]. Circulation 1996;94(8): 1818–1825.

248. Gum P, et al. Bypass surgery versus coronary angioplasty for revascularization of treated diabetic patients. Circulation 1997;96(9 Suppl):II–II710.

249. Ellis CJ, et al. Results of percutaneous coronary angioplasty in patients <40 years of age. Am J Cardiol 1998;82(2):135–139.

250. Dauerman HL, et al, Mechanical debulking versus balloon angioplasty for the treatment of diffuse in-stent restenosis. Am J Cardiol 1998;82(3):277–284.

251. Walton BL, et al, Diabetic patients treated with abciximab and intracoronary stenting. Catheter Cardiovasc Interv 2002;55(3):321–325.

252. Marso SP, et al. Optimizing the percutaneous interventional outcomes for patients with diabetes mellitus: results of the EPISTENT (Evaluation of platelet IIb/IIIa inhibitor for stenting trial) diabetic substudy [see comments]. Circulation 1999;100(25):2477–2484.

253. Kornowski R, et al. Increased restenosis in diabetes mellitus after coronary interventions is due to exaggerated intimal hyperplasia. A serial intravascular ultrasound study. Circulation 1997;95(6):1366–1369.

254. Aronson D, Bloomgarden Z, Rayfield EJ. Potential mechanisms promoting restenosis in diabetic patients. J Am Coll Cardiol 1996;27(3):528–535.

255. Moreno PR, et al. Coronary composition and macrophage infiltration in atherectomy specimens from patients with diabetes mellitus. Circulation 2000;102(18):2180–2184.

256. Sobel BE. Acceleration of restenosis by diabetes: pathogenetic implications. Circulation 2001;103(9): 1185–1187.

257. Sobel BE. Increased plasminogen activator inhibitor-1 and vasculopathy. A reconcilable paradox. Circulation 1999;99(19):2496–2498.

258. Roguin A, et al. Haptoglobin phenotype and the risk of restenosis after coronary artery stent implantation. Am J Cardiol 2002;89(7):806–810.

259. Fietsam R Jr, Bassett J, Glover JL. Complications of coronary artery surgery in diabetic patients. Am Surg 1991;57(9):551–557.

260. Slaughter MS, et al. A fifteen-year wound surveillance study after coronary artery bypass. Ann Thorac Surg 1993;56(5):1063–1068.

261. Palac RT, et al. Risk factors related to progressive narrowing in aortocoronary vein grafts studied 1 and 5 years after surgery. Circulation 1982;66(2 Pt 2):I40–I44.

262. Lytle BW, et al. Long-term (5 to 12 years) serial studies of internal mammary artery and saphenous vein coronary bypass grafts. J Thorac Cardiovasc Surg 1985;89(2):248–258.

263. Hirotani T, et al. Effects of coronary artery bypass grafting using internal mammary arteries for diabetic patients. J Am Coll Cardiol 1999;34(2):532–538.

264. Davies M, et al. Diabetes mellitus and experimental vein graft structure and function. J Vasc Surg 1994;19:1031–1043.

265. Morris JJ, et al. Influence of diabetes and mammary artery grafting on survival after coronary bypass. Circulation 1991;84(5 Suppl):III275–III284.

266. Herlitz J, et al. Mortality and morbidity during a period of 2 years after coronary artery bypass surgery in patients with and without a history of hypertension. J Hypertens 1996;14(3):309–314.

267. Lawrie GM, Morris GC Jr, Glaeser DH. Influence of diabetes mellitus on the results of coronary bypass surgery. Follow-up of 212 diabetic patients ten to 15 years after surgery. JAMA 1986;256(21):2967–2971.

268. Ferguson J. NHLBI BARI clinical alert on diabetics treated with angioplasty. Circulation 1995;92:3371.

269. The Bypass Angioplasty Revascularization Investigation (BARI), Influence of diabetes on 5-year mortality and morbidity in a randomized trial comparing CABG and PTCA in patients with multivessel disease [see comments]. Circulation 1997;96(6):1761–1769.

270. Barsness GW, et al. Relationship between diabetes mellitus and long-term survival after coronary bypass and angioplasty. Circulation 1997;96(8):2551–2556.

271. Weintraub W, et al. Outcome of coronary bypass surgery versus coronary angioplasty in diabetic patients with multivessel coronary artery disease. J Am Coll Cardiol 1998;31:10–19.

272. Zhao X, et al. Effectiveness of revascularization in the Emory angioplasty versus surgery trial. A randomized comparison of coronary angioplasty with bypass surgery. Circulation 1996;93:1954–1962.

273. Bell MR, et al. Effect of completeness of revascularization on long-term outcome of patients with three-vessel disease undergoing coronary artery bypass surgery. A report from the Coronary Artery Surgery Study (CASS) Registry. Circulation 1992;86(2):446–457.

274. Schaff HV, et al. Clinical and operative characteristics of patients randomized to coronary artery bypass surgery in the Bypass Angioplasty Revascularization Investigation (BARI). Am J Cardiol 1995;75(9):18C–26C.

275. Van Belle E, et al. Patency of percutaneous transluminal coronary angioplasty sites at 6- month angiographic follow-up: A key determinant of survival in diabetics after coronary balloon angioplasty. Circulation 2001;103(9):1218–1224.

276. Nashar P, et al. Maximal coronary flow reserve and metabolic coronary vasodilation in patients with diabetes mellitus. Circulation 1995;91:635–640.

277. Grundy SM, et al. Prevention Conference VI: Diabetes and Cardiovascular Disease: executive summary: conference proceeding for healthcare professionals from a special writing group of the American Heart Association. Circulation 2002;105(18):2231–2239.

278. Scandinavian Simvastatin Survival Study Group, Randomized trial of cholesterol lowering in 4444 patients with coronary heart disease: Scandinavian Simvastatin Survival Study (4S). Lancet 1994;334:1383–1389.

279. Pyorala K, et al. Cholesterol lowering with simvastatin improves prognosis of diabetic patients with coronary heart disease. A subgroup analysis of the Scandinavian Simvastatin Survival Study (4S) [see comments]. Diabetes Care 1997;20(4):614–620.

280. Sacks FM, et al. Relationship between plasma LDL concentrations during treatment with pravastatin and recurrent coronary events in the Cholesterol and Recurrent Events trial. Circulation 1998;97(15):1446–1452.

281. Selby JV, et al. LDL subclass phenotypes and the insulin resistance syndrome in women. Circulation 1993;88(2):381–387.

282. Lyons TJ. Glycation and oxidation: a role in the pathogenesis of atherosclerosis. Am J Cardiol 1993;71(6):26B–31B.

283. Collins R, et al. MRC/BHF Heart Protection Study of cholesterol-lowering with simvastatin in 5963 people with diabetes: a randomised placebo-controlled trial. Lancet 2003;361(9374):2005–2016.

284. Colhoun HM, et al. Primary prevention of cardiovascular disease with atorvastatin in type 2 diabetes in the Collaborative Atorvastatin Diabetes Study (CARDS): multicentre randomised placebo-controlled trial. Lancet 2004;364(9435):685–696.

285. Grundy SM, et al. Implications of recent clinical trials for the National Cholesterol Education Program Adult Treatment Panel III guidelines. Circulation 2004;110(2):227–239.

286. Goldberg RB, et al. Cardiovascular events and their reduction with pravastatin in diabetic and glucose-intolerant myocardial infarction survivors with average cholesterol levels: subgroup analyses in the

cholesterol and recurrent events (CARE) trial. The Care Investigators. Circulation 1998;98(23):2513–2519.

287. Haffner SM. Epidemiological studies on the effects of hyperglycemia and improvement of glycemic control on macrovascular events in type 2 diabetes. Diabetes Care 1999;22(Suppl 3):C54–C56.

288. Rubins HB, et al. Gemfibrozil for the secondary prevention of coronary heart disease in men with low levels of high-density lipoprotein cholesterol. Veterans Affairs High-Density Lipoprotein Cholesterol Intervention Trial Study Group. N Engl J Med 1999;341(6):410–418.

289. Sacks FM, et al. Coronary heart disease in patients with low LDL-cholesterol: benefit of pravastatin in diabetics and enhanced role for HDL-cholesterol and triglycerides as risk factors. Circulation 2002;105(12):1424–1428.

290. National High Blood Pressure Education Program Working group report on Hypertension and Diabetes, Hypertension 1994;23:145–158.

291. American diabetes association, Consensus statement on the treatment of hypertension in diabetes. Diabetes Care 1993;16:1394–1401.

292. The sixth report of the Joint National Committee on prevention, d, evaluation, and treatment of high blood pressure,, Arch Intern Med 1997;157(21):2413–2446.

293. Estacio RO, et al, The effect of nisoldipine as compared with enalapril on cardiovascular outcomes in patients with non-insulin-dependent diabetes and hypertension [see comments]. N Engl J Med 1998;338(10):645–652.

294. Tatti P, et al. Outcome results of the Fosinopril Versus Amlodipine Cardiovascular Events Randomized Trial (FACET) in patients with hypertension and NIDDM. Diabetes Care 1998;21(4):597–603.

295. Curb JD, et al. Effect of diuretic-based antihypertensive treatment on cardiovascular disease risk in older diabetic patients with isolated systolic hypertension. Systolic Hypertension in the Elderly Program Cooperative Research Group [published erratum appears in JAMA 1997;277(17):1356] [see comments]. JAMA 1996;276(23):1886–1892.

296. Pahor M, Psaty BM, Furberg CD. Treatment of hypertensive patients with diabetes [see comments]. Lancet 1998;351(9104):689–690.

297. Sowers JR. Comorbidity of hypertension and diabetes: the fosinopril versus amlodipine cardiovascular events trial (FACET). Am J Cardiol 1998;82(9B):15R–19R.

298. Tuomilehto J, et al. Effects of calcium-channel blockade in older patients with diabetes and systolic hypertension. Systolic Hypertension in Europe Trial Investigators [see comments]. N Engl J Med 1999;340(9):677–684.

299. Hansson L, et al. Effects of intensive blood-pressure lowering and low-dose aspirin in patients with hypertension: principal results of the Hypertension Optimal Treatment (HOT) randomised trial. HOT Study Group [see comments]. Lancet 1998;351(9118):1755–1762.

300. Cooper ME. Pathogenesis, prevention, and treatment of diabetic nephropathy. Lancet 1998;352(9123):213–219.

301. Parving HH. Renoprotection in diabetes: genetic and non-genetic risk factors and treatment. Diabetologia 1998;41(7):745–759.

302. Lindholm LH, et al. Cardiovascular morbidity and mortality in patients with diabetes in the Losartan Intervention For Endpoint reduction in hypertension study (LIFE): a randomised trial against atenolol. Lancet 2002;359(9311):1004–1010.

303. The effect of intensive treatment of diabetes on the development and progression of long-term complications in insulin-dependent diabetes mellitus. The Diabetes Control and Complications Trial Research Group. N Engl J Med 1993;329(14):977–986.

304. Effect of intensive diabetes management on macrovascular events and risk factors in the Diabetes Control and Complications Trial. Am J Cardiol 1995;75(14):894–903.

305. Kunjathoor VV, Wilson DL, LeBoeuf RC. Increased atherosclerosis in streptozotocin-induced diabetic mice. J Clin Invest 1996;97(7):1767–1773.

306. Jensen-Urstad KJ, et al. Early atherosclerosis is retarded by improved long-term blood glucose control in patients with IDDM. Diabetes 1996;45(9):1253–1258.

307. UK Prospective Diabetes Study (UKPDS) Group, Intensive blood-glucose control with sulphonylureas or insulin compared with conventional treatment and risk of complications in patients with type 2 diabetes (UKPDS 33). Lancet 1998;352(9131):837–853.

308. The absence of a glycemic threshold for the development of long-term complications: the perspective of the Diabetes Control and Complications Trial. Diabetes 1996;45(10):1289–1298.

309. Klein R, et al. Glycosylated hemoglobin in a population-based study of diabetes. Am J Epidemiol 1987;126(3):415–428.

310. Consensus statement, The pharmacological treatment of hyperglycemia in NIDDM. Diabetes Care 1995;18:1510–1518.
311. Clark RS, et al. Effect of intravenous infusion of insulin in diabetics with acute myocardial infarction. Br Med J (Clin Res Ed) 1985;291(6491):303–305.
312. Malmberg K, et al. Glycometabolic state at admission: important risk marker of mortality in conventionally treated patients with diabetes mellitus and acute myocardial infarction: long-term results from the Diabetes and Insulin- Glucose Infusion in Acute Myocardial Infarction (DIGAMI) study. Circulation 1999;99(20):2626–2632.
313. Consensus development conference on the diagnosis of coronary heart disease in people with diabetes: 10–11 February 1998, Miami, Florida. American Diabetes Association. Diabetes Care 1998;21(9): 1551–1559.
314. Knowler WC, et al. Reduction in the incidence of type 2 diabetes with lifestyle intervention or metformin. N Engl J Med 2002;346(6):393–403.
315. Kannel WB, Hjortland M, Castelli WP. Role of diabetes in congestive heart failure: the Framingham study. Am J Cardiol 1974;34(1):29–34.
316. Croft JB, et al. National trends in the initial hospitalization for heart failure. J Am Geriatr Soc 1997;45(3):270–275.
317. Polanczyk CA, et al. Ten-year trends in hospital care for congestive heart failure: improved outcomes and increased use of resources. Arch Intern Med 2000;160(3):325–332.
318. Reis SE, et al. Treatment of patients admitted to the hospital with congestive heart failure: specialty-related disparities in practice patterns and outcomes. J Am Coll Cardiol 1997;30(3):733–738.
319. Butler R, et al. The clinical implications of diabetic heart disease. Eur Heart J 1998;19(11):1617–1627.
320. Garcia MJ, et al. Morbidity and mortality in diabetics in the Framingham population. Sixteen year follow-up study. Diabetes 1974;23(2):105–111.
321. Hamby RI, Zoneraich S, Sherman L. Diabetic cardiomyopathy. Jama 1974;229(13):1749–1754.
322. Litwin SE, Grossman W. Diastolic dysfunction as a cause of heart failure. J Am Coll Cardiol 1993;22(4 Suppl A):49A–55A.
323. Melchior T, et al. The impact of heart failure on prognosis of diabetic and non-diabetic patients with myocardial infarction: a 15-year follow-up study. Eur J Heart Fail 2001;3(1):83–90.
324. Timmis AD. Diabetic heart disease: clinical considerations. Heart 2001;85(4):463–469.
325. Hypertension in Diabetes Study (HDS): II. Increased risk of cardiovascular complications in hypertensive type 2 diabetic patients. J Hypertens 1993;11(3):319–325.
326. Rubler S, et al. New type of cardiomyopathy associated with diabetic glomerulosclerosis. Am J Cardiol 1972;30(6):595–602.
327. Coughlin SS, et al. Diabetes mellitus and risk of idiopathic dilated cardiomyopathy. The Washington, DC Dilated Cardiomyopathy Study. Ann Epidemiol 1994;4(1):67–74.
328. Coughlin SS, Tefft MC. The epidemiology of idiopathic dilated cardiomyopathy in women: the Washington DC Dilated Cardiomyopathy Study. Epidemiology 1994;5(4):449–455.
329. Mildenberger RR, et al. Clinically unrecognized ventricular dysfunction in young diabetic patients. J Am Coll Cardiol 1984;4(2):234–238.
330. Vered A, et al. Exercise-induced left ventricular dysfunction in young men with asymptomatic diabetes mellitus (diabetic cardiomyopathy). Am J Cardiol 1984;54(6):633–637.
331. Zola B, et al. Abnormal cardiac function in diabetic patients with autonomic neuropathy in the absence of ischemic heart disease. J Clin Endocrinol Metab 1986;63(1):208–214.
332. Mustonen JN, et al. Impaired left ventricular systolic function during exercise in middle- aged insulin-dependent and noninsulin-dependent diabetic subjects without clinically evident cardiovascular disease. Am J Cardiol 1988;62(17):1273–1279.
333. Arvan S, et al. Subclinical left ventricular abnormalities in young diabetics. Chest 1988;93(5):1031–1034.
334. Rynkiewicz A, Semetkowska-Jurkiewicz E, Wyrzykowski B. Systolic and diastolic time intervals in young diabetics. Br Heart J 1980;44(3):280–283.
335. Shapiro LM, et al. Left ventricular function in diabetes mellitus. II: Relation between clinical features and left ventricular function. Br Heart J 1981;45(2):129–132.
336. Shapiro LM, Howat AP, Calter MM. Left ventricular function in diabetes mellitus. I: Methodology, and prevalence and spectrum of abnormalities. Br Heart J 1981;45(2):122–128.
337. Sanderson JE, et al. Diabetic cardiomyopathy? An echocardiographic study of young diabetics. Br Med J 1978;1(6110):404–407.
338. Hausdorf G, Rieger U, Koepp P. Cardiomyopathy in childhood diabetes mellitus: incidence, time of onset, and relation to metabolic control. Int J Cardiol 1988;19(2):225–236.

339. Danielsen R. Factors contributing to left ventricular diastolic dysfunction in long- term type I diabetic subjects. Acta Med Scand 1988;224(3):249–256.

340. Takenaka K, et al. Left ventricular filling determined by Doppler echocardiography in diabetes mellitus. Am J Cardiol 1988;61(13):1140–1143.

341. Bouchard A, et al. Noninvasive assessment of cardiomyopathy in normotensive diabetic patients between 20 and 50 years old. Am J Med 1989;87(2):160–166.

342. Paillole C, et al. Prevalence and significance of left ventricular filling abnormalities determined by Doppler echocardiography in young type I (insulin- dependent) diabetic patients. Am J Cardiol 1989;64(16):1010–1016.

343. Di Bello V, et al. Increased echodensity of myocardial wall in the diabetic heart: an ultrasound tissue characterization study. J Am Coll Cardiol 1995;25(6):1408–1415.

344. Factor SM, et al. Myocardial alterations in diabetes and hypertension. Diabetes Res Clin Pract 1996;31 (Suppl):S133–S142.

345. van Hoeven KH, Factor SM. A comparison of the pathological spectrum of hypertensive, diabetic, and hypertensive-diabetic heart disease. Circulation 1990;82(3):848–855.

346. Hardin NJ. The myocardial and vascular pathology of diabetic cardiomyopathy. Coron Artery Dis 1996;7(2):99–108.

347. Katz EB, et al. Cardiac and adipose tissue abnormalities but not diabetes in mice deficient in GLUT4. Nature 1995;377(6545):151–155.

348. Stenbit AE, et al. GLUT4 heterozygous knockout mice develop muscle insulin resistance and diabetes. Nat Med 1997;3(10):1096–1101.

349. Lagadic-Gossmann D, et al. Altered Ca2+ handling in ventricular myocytes isolated from diabetic rats. Am J Physiol 1996;270(5 Pt 2):H1529–H1537.

350. Liu X, Takeda N, Dhalla NS. Troponin I phosphorylation in heart homogenate from diabetic rat. Biochim Biophys Acta 1996;1316(2):78–84.

351. Liu X, Takeda N, Dhalla NS. Myosin light-chain phosphorylation in diabetic cardiomyopathy in rats. Metabolism 1997;46(1):71–75.

352. Norton GR, Candy G, Woodiwiss AJ. Aminoguanidine prevents the decreased myocardial compliance produced by streptozotocin-induced diabetes mellitus in rats. Circulation 1996;93(10):1905–1912.

353. Barrett EJ, et al. Effect of chronic diabetes on myocardial fuel metabolism and insulin sensitivity. Diabetes 1988;37(7):943–948.

354. Laughlin MR, et al. Nonglucose substrates increase glycogen synthesis in vivo in dog heart. Am J Physiol 1994;267(1 Pt 2):H219–H223.

355. Russell RR 3rd, et al. Regulation of exogenous and endogenous glucose metabolism by insulin and acetoacetate in the isolated working rat heart. A three tracer study of glycolysis, glycogen metabolism, and glucose oxidation. J Clin Invest 1997;100(11):2892–2899.

356. Taegtmeyer H. On the inability of ketone bodies to serve as the only energy providing substrate for rat heart at physiological work load. Basic Res Cardiol 1983;78(4):435–450.

357. Russell RR 3rd, Taegtmeyer H. Coenzyme A sequestration in rat hearts oxidizing ketone bodies. J Clin Invest 1992;89(3):968–973.

358. Spallone V, Menzinger G. Autonomic neuropathy: clinical and instrumental findings. Clin Neurosci 1997;4(6):346–358.

359. Toyry JP, et al. Occurrence, predictors, and clinical significance of autonomic neuropathy in NIDDM. Ten-year follow-up from the diagnosis. Diabetes 1996;45(3):308–315.

360. Sampson MJ, et al. Abnormal diastolic function in patients with type 1 diabetes and early nephropathy. Br Heart J 1990;64(4):266–271.

361. O'Brien IA, McFadden JP, Corrall RJ. The influence of autonomic neuropathy on mortality in insulin-dependent diabetes. Q J Med 1991;79(290):495–502.

362. Orchard TJ, et al. Why does diabetic autonomic neuropathy predict IDDM mortality? An analysis from the Pittsburgh Epidemiology of Diabetes Complications Study. Diabetes Res Clin Pract 1996;34 Suppl:S165–S171.

363. Muller JE, Tofler GH, Stone PH. Circadian variation and triggers of onset of acute cardiovascular disease. Circulation 1989;79(4):733–743.

364. Zarich S, et al, Effect of autonomic nervous system dysfunction on the circadian pattern of myocardial ischemia in diabetes mellitus. J Am Coll Cardiol 1994;24(4):956–962.

365. Bernardi L, et al. Impaired circadian modulation of sympathovagal activity in diabetes. A possible explanation for altered temporal onset of cardiovascular disease. Circulation 1992;86(5):1443–1452.

366. Kahn JK, et al. Decreased exercise heart rate and blood pressure response in diabetic subjects with cardiac autonomic neuropathy. Diabetes Care 1986;9(4):389–394.

367. Hilsted J, Galbo H, Christensen NJ. Impaired cardiovascular responses to graded exercise in diabetic autonomic neuropathy. Diabetes 1979;28(4):313–319.

368. Di Carli MF, et al. Effects of cardiac sympathetic innervation on coronary blood flow. N Engl J Med 1997;336(17):1208–1215.

369. Di Carli MF, et al. Effects of autonomic neuropathy on coronary blood flow in patients with diabetes mellitus. Circulation 1999;100(8):813–819.

370. Spallone V, Menzinger G. Diagnosis of cardiovascular autonomic neuropathy in diabetes. Diabetes 1997;46 (Suppl 2):S67–S76.

371. Ziegler D, et al. Prevalence of cardiovascular autonomic dysfunction assessed by spectral analysis and standard tests of heart-rate variation in newly diagnosed IDDM patients. Diabetes Care 1992; 15(7):908–911.

372. Ewing DJ, et al. Twenty four hour heart rate variability: effects of posture, sleep, and time of day in healthy controls and comparison with bedside tests of autonomic function in diabetic patients. Br Heart J 1991;65(5):239–244.

373. Kreiner G, et al. Myocardial m-[123I]iodobenzylguanidine scintigraphy for the assessment of adrenergic cardiac innervation in patients with IDDM. Comparison with cardiovascular reflex tests and relationship to left ventricular function. Diabetes 1995;44(5):543–549.

374. Kleiger RE, et al. Decreased heart rate variability and its association with increased mortality after acute myocardial infarction. Am J Cardiol 1987;59(4):256–262.

375. Farrell TG, et al. Risk stratification for arrhythmic events in postinfarction patients based on heart rate variability, ambulatory electrocardiographic variables and the signal-averaged electrocardiogram. J Am Coll Cardiol 1991;18(3):687–697.

376. Bigger JT Jr, et al. Frequency domain measures of heart period variability and mortality after myocardial infarction. Circulation 1992;85(1):164–171.

377. Pozzati A, et al. Transient sympathovagal imbalance triggers "ischemic" sudden death in patients undergoing electrocardiographic Holter monitoring. J Am Coll Cardiol 1996;27(4):847–852.

378. Curb JD, et al. Sudden death, impaired glucose tolerance, and diabetes in Japanese American men. Circulation 1995;91(10):2591–2595.

379. Kahn JK, Sisson JC, Vinik AI. QT interval prolongation and sudden cardiac death in diabetic autonomic neuropathy. J Clin Endocrinol Metab 1987;64(4):751–754.

380. Burgos LG, et al. Increased intraoperative cardiovascular morbidity in diabetics with autonomic neuropathy. Anesthesiology 1989;70(4):591–597.

381. Keyl C, et al. Cardiovascular autonomic dysfunction and hemodynamic response to anesthetic induction in patients with coronary artery disease and diabetes mellitus. Anesth Analg 1999;88(5):985–991.

382. Mueller HS, et al. Predictors of early morbidity and mortality after thrombolytic therapy of acute myocardial infarction. Analyses of patient subgroups in the Thrombolysis in Myocardial Infarction (TIMI) trial, phase II. Circulation 1992;85(4):1254–1264.

383. Wong ND, et al. The metabolic syndrome, diabetes, and subclinical atheroscleroisi assessed by coronary calcium. JACC 2003;41(9):1547–1553.

384. Hoff JA, et al. The prevalence of coronary calcium among diabetic individuals without known coronary artery disease. JACC 2003;41(6):1008–1012.

385. Qu W, et al. Value of coronary artery calcium scanning by computed tomography for predicting coronary heart disease in diabetic subjects. Diabetes Care 2003;26(3):905–910.

386. Arad Y, Spardaro LA, Goodman K, et al. Prediciton of coronary events with electron beam computed tomography. J Am Coll Cardiol 2000;36:1253.

387. Fayad AZ, et al. In vivo magnetic resonance evaluation of atherosclerotic plaques in the human thoracic aorta: a comparison with transesophageal echocardiography. Circulation 2000;101:2503–2509.

388. Kim WY, Danias PG, Stuber M, Flamm SD. Coronary magnetic resonance angiography for the detection of coronary stenoses. N Engl J Med 2001;345:1863.

389. Fayad ZA, Fuster V, Fallon J, et al. Noninvasive in vivo human coronary artery lumen and wall imaging using black-blood magnetic resonance imaging. Circulation 2000;102:506–510.

390. Botnar RM, et al. Noninvasive coronary vessel wall and plaque imaging with magnetic resonance imaging. Circulation 2000;102:2582–2587.

INDEX